Springer
Berlin
Heidelberg
New York
Barcelona
Budapest
Hong Kong
London
Milano
Paris
Tokyo

A. Gullo (Ed.)

Anaesthesia, Pain, Intensive Care and Emergency Medicine - A.P.I.C.E.

Proceedings of the
10th Postgraduate Course in Critical Care Medicine
Trieste, Italy - November 13-19, 1995

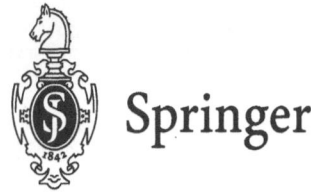 Springer

Prof. ANTONINO GULLO, M.D.
Head, Department of Anaesthesiology and Intensive Care
Trieste University School of Medicine
Trieste, Italy

ISBN-13: 978-3-540-75014-7   e-ISBN-13: 978-88-470-2203-4
DOI: 10.1007/978-88-470-2203-4

The use of general descriptive names, registered names, trademarks, etc. in this publication does not imply, even in the absence of a specific statement, that such names are exempt from the relevant protective laws and regulations and therefore free for general use.

Product liability: The publishers cannot guarantee the accuracy of any information about dosage and application contained in this book. In every individual case the user must check such information by consulting the relevant literature.

Table of Contents

CELLULAR AND HUMORAL ACTIVITY IN TRAUMA AND SEPSIS

CHEST IMAGING IN THE ICU

NEW MODES OF ARTIFICIAL VENTILATION

ARTIFICIAL VENTILATION AT THE BEDSIDE

ADVANCES IN RESPIRATORY MECHANICS

INVASIVE AND NONINVASIVE HAEMODYNAMIC MONITORING

TRAUMA OPERATIVE PROCEDURES (T.O.P.)

CEREBRAL AND SPINAL DYSFUNCTION

Authors Index

Bonivento B.
II Dept. of Anaesthesia and Intensive Care, Regional Hospital "S. Maria dei Battuti", Treviso (Italy)

Bonomo L.
Dept. of Radiodiagnostic, Radiological Sciences, SS. Annunziata Hospital, Chieti (Italy)

Borghi B.
I Unit of Anaesthesia and Intensive Care, IRCCS Rizzoli Orthopaedic Institutes, Bologna (Italy)

Bortolotto P.
Dept. of Radiology, Maggiore Hospital, Trieste (Italy)

Bosco E.
II Dept. of Anaesthesia and Intensive Care, Regional Hospital "S. Maria dei Battuti", Treviso (Italy)

Bozza P.
Dept. of Anaesthesiology and Intensive Care, Catholic University of Sacro Cuore, Policlinico A. Gemelli, Rome (Italy)

Brain A.I.J.
Royal Berkshire Hospital, Reading, Berks (U.K.) and Institute of Laryngology, University of London, London (UK)

Bramanti P.
Dept. of Neurology, University of Messina, Messina (Italy)

Brandolese R.
Dept. of Anaesthesia and Intensive Care, General Hospital, Padua (Italy)

Brimacombe J.R.
Dept. of Anaesthesia, Cairns Base Hospital, The Esplanade, Cairns (Australia)

Buzzi F.
I Dept. of Anaesthesia and Intensive Care, Hospital of Parma, Parma (Italy)

Calderini E.
Dept. of Intensive Care, S. Luigi Centre, "S. Raffaele" Hospital, Milan (Italy)

Carli P.
Department of Anaesthesia and Surgical Intensive Care, Necker Hospital, Paris (France)

Casali R.
Dept. of Anaesthesiology and Intensive Care, University of Florence, Policlinico Careggi, Florence (Italy)

Castagneto M.
Division of Organ Transplantation, Dept. of Surgery, University of Sacro Cuore, Rome (Italy)

Ceccarelli P.
I Dept. of Anaesthesia and Intensive Care, Hospital of Parma, Parma (Italy)

Cerisara M.
Dept. of Anaesthesia and Intensive Care, Maggiore Hospital, Milan (Italy)

Cestelli A.
Dept. of Cellular and Developmental Biology, University of Palermo, Palermo (Italy)

Chatignol D.
I.N.S.E.R.M., National Institute of Health and Medical Research, Unit 281, Lyon (France)

Classen B.
University Clinic of Anaesthesiology, ATV Section, University of Ulm, Ulm (Germany)

Clemente A.
Dept. of Anaesthesiology and Intensive Care, Catholic University of Sacro Cuore, Policlinico A. Gemelli, Rome (Italy)

Cole W.G.
Dept. of Medical Education, University of Washington, Seattle (USA)

Colò F.
Dept. of Anaesthesiology and Intensive Care, Udine University School of Medicine, Udine (Italy)

Colombo I.
Dept. of Anaesthesia and Intensive Care, S. Raffaele Hospital, Milan (Italy)

Coriat P.
Dept. of Anaesthesia and Intensive Care, Pitié-Salpétrière Hospital, Paris (France)

Cormio M.
I Dept. of Anaesthesia and Intensive Care, Hospital of Parma, Parma (Italy)

Cotev S.
Dept. of Anaesthesiology and Critical Care Medicine, Hadassah School of Medicine, Jerusalem (Israel)

Croci M.
Dept. of Anaesthesia and Intensive Care, Maggiore Hospital, Milan (Italy)

D'Uva R.
Dept. of Anaesthesiology and Intensive Care, University of Cagliari, S. Giovanni di Dio Hospital, Cagliari (Italy)

De Filippi G.L.
Dept. of Intensive Care "William Osler", Santa Corona Hospital, Garbagnate Milanese, Milan (Italy)

De Monte A.
II Dept. of Anaesthesia and Intensive Care, Santa Maria della Misericordia Hospital, Udine (Italy)

de Simone N.
I Unit of Anaesthesia and Intensive Care, IRCCS Rizzoli Orthopaedic Institutes, Bologna (Italy)

Dei Poli M.
Dept. of Intensive Care "William Osler", Santa Corona Hospital, Garbagnate Milanese, Milan (Italy)

Della Corte F.
Dept. of Anaesthesiology and Intensive Care, Catholic University of Sacro Cuore, Policlinico A. Gemelli, Rome (Italy)

Delooz H.H.
Dept. of Emergency Medicine, University Hospital Gasthuisberg, Leuven (Belgium)

Di Filippo A.
Dept. of Anaesthesiology and Intensive Care, University of Florence, Policlinico Careggi, Florence (Italy)

Di Liegro I.
Dept. of Cellular and Developmental Biology, University of Palermo, Palermo (Italy)

Doldi S.B.
Dept. of General Surgery and Surgical Oncology, University of Milan, Maggiore Hospital, Milan (Italy)

Eidelman L.A.
Dept. of Anaesthesiology and Critical Care Medicine, Hadassah School of Medicine, Jerusalem (Israel)

Facco E.
Dept. of Anaesthesiology and Intensive Care, University of Padua, Padua (Italy)

Falsini S.
Dept. of Anaesthesiology and Intensive Care, University of Florence, Policlinico Careggi, Florence (Italy)

Fantoni A.
Dept. of Anaesthesiology and Intensive Care, San Carlo Borromeo Hospital, Milan (Italy)

Fava C.
Dept. of Radiology, Le Molinette Hospital, Turin (Italy)

Favara A.
Dept. of General Surgery and Surgical Oncology, University of Milan, Maggiore Hospital, Milan (Italy)

Favaro M.
Dept. of Intensive Care "William Osler", Santa Corona Hospital, Garbagnate Milanese, Milan (Italy)

Feoli M.A.
I Unit of Anaesthesia and Intensive Care, IRCCS Rizzoli Orthopaedic Institutes, Bologna (Italy)

Ferrari G.
Dept. of Anaesthesia and Intensive Care, Maggiore Hospital, Milan (Italy)

Ferrario P.
Dept. of Intensive Care "William Osler", Santa Corona Hospital, Garbagnate Milanese, Milan (Italy)

Filley S.
Dept. of Anaesthesia, Cardiovascular and Pneumological Hospital "Louis Pradel", Lyon (France)

Fischer S.
Dept. of Anaesthesiology and Intensive Care, Westfälische Wilhelm University, Münster (Germany)

Fochi C.
Dept. of Anaesthesia and Intensive Care, Maggiore Hospital, Milan (Italy)

Foëx P.
Nuffield Dept. of Anaesthetics, The Radcliffe Infirmary, University of Oxford, Oxford (UK)

Friesdorf W.
University Clinic of Anaesthesiology, ATV Section, University of Ulm, Ulm (Germany)

Galli J.
Dept. of Radiology, Le Molinette Hospital, Turin (Italy)

Gandini E.
Dept. of Anaesthesiology and Intensive Care, University of Florence, Policlinico Careggi, Florence (Italy)

Gargioni G.
I Unit of Anaesthesia and Intensive Care, IRCCS Rizzoli Orthopaedic Institutes, Bologna (Italy)

Gasparetto A.
Dept. of Anaesthesiology and Intensive Care, University "La Sapienza", Policlinico Umberto I, Rome (Italy)

Gašparović V.
Dept. of Emergency Internal Medicine, Rebro University Hospital, Zagreb (Croatia)

George M.
Dept. of Anaesthesia, Cardiovascular and Pneumological Hospital "Louis Pradel", Lyon (France)

Gianotti L.
II Division of General Surgery, University of Milan, Milan (Italy)

Girard C.
Dept. of Anaesthesia, Cardiovascular and Pneumological Hospital "Louis Pradel", Lyon (France)

Giuliani G.
Dept. of Neurosurgery, M. Bufalini Hospital, Cesena (Italy)

Giuliani R.
Dept. of Anaesthesia and Intensive Care, University of Bari, Policlinico, Bari (Italy)

Gjurašin M.
Dept. of Emergency Internal Medicine, Rebro University Hospital, Zagreb (Croatia)

Gomes R.F.M.
Laboratory of Respiration Physiology, Institute of Biophysics "Carlos Chagas Filho", Federal University of Rio de Janeiro, Rio de Janeiro (Brasil)

Goodman L.R.
Section of Thoracic Radiology, Dept. of Radiology, Medical College of Wisconsin, Milwaukee, Wisconsin (USA)

Grasso S.
Dept. of Anaesthesia and Intensive Care, University of Bari, Policlinico, Bari (Italy)

Gregoretti C.
Dept. of Anaesthesia and Intensive Care, Orthopaedic Trauma Centre, Turin (Italy)

Grosso M.
Dept. of Radiology, Le Molinette Hospital, Turin (Italy)

Grop A.
Dept. of Anaesthesiology and Intensive Care, Trieste University School of Medicine, Trieste (Italy)

Gryglewski R.J.
Dept. of Pharmacology, Jagiellonian University Medical College, Cracow (Poland)

Gullo A.
Dept. of Anaesthesiology and Intensive Care, Trieste University School of Medicine, Trieste (Italy)

Gutierrez G.
Dept. of Pulmonary and Critical Care Medicine, University of Texas, Houston Health Science Center, Houston, Texas (USA)

Haglund U.
Dept. of Surgery, Uppsala University Hospital, Uppsala (Sweden)

Heusslein R.
Pall GmbH Biomedizin, Scientific and Laboratory Service, Dreieich-Sprendlingen (Germany)

Iamello R.
Dept. of Anaesthesia and Intensive Care, New Hospital S. Giovanni di Dio, Florence (Italy)

Ivanović D.
Dept. of Emergency Internal Medicine, Rebro University Hospital, Zagreb (Croatia)

Jossinet J.
I.N.S.E.R.M., National Institute of Health and Medical Research, Unit 281, Lyon (France)

Kakarigi D.
Dept. of Emergency Internal Medicine, Rebro University Hospital, Zagreb (Croatia)

Kellum J.A.
Dept. of Critical Care Medicine, University of Pittsburgh, Pittsburgh, Pennsylvania (USA)

Koller W.
University Clinic of Anaesthesia and General Intensive Care Medicine, University of Innsbruck, Innsbruck (Austria)

Kremžar B.
Intensive Care Unit, Institute of Anaesthesiology, University Medical Center, Ljubljana (Slovenia)

Kvarantan M.
Dept. of Emergency Internal Medicine, Rebro University Hospital, Zagreb (Croatia)

Lachmann B.
Dept. of Anaesthesiology, Erasmus University, Rotterdam (The Netherlands)

Latimer R.D.
Dept. of Anaesthesia, Papworth Hospital NHS Trust, Cambridge (UK)

Lavandier B.
I.N.S.E.R.M., National Institute of Health and Medical Research, Unit 281, Lyon (France)

Lehot J.J.
Dept. of Anaesthesia, Cardiovascular and Pneumological Hospital "Louis Pradel", Lyon (France)

Lissoni A.
Dept. of Anaesthesia and Resuscitation, Maggiore Hospital, Milan (Italy)

List W.F.
University Clinic of Anaesthesiology, University of Graz, Regional Hospital, Graz (Austria)

Little J.P.
Dept. of Anaesthesia, Papworth Hospital NHS Trust, Cambridge (UK)

Lucangelo U.
Dept. of Anaesthesiology and Intensive Care, Trieste University School of Medicine, Trieste (Italy)

Lunkenheimer P.P.
Dept. of Experimental Cardiac- and Thoracovascular Surgery, Westfälische Wilhelm University, Münster (Germany)

Maffessanti M.
Dept. of Radiology, Trieste University School of Medicine, Trieste (Italy)

Maglione B.
Dept. of Emergency Medicine, San Paolo Hospital, Naples (Italy)

Mangani V.
Dept. of Anaesthesia and Intensive Care, New Hospital S. Giovanni di Dio, Florence (Italy)

Manni C.
Dept. of Anaesthesiology and Intensive Care, Catholic University School of Medicine, Rome (Italy)

Marosi M.
Dept. of Neurology, University of Innsbruck, Innsbruck (Austria)

Martinelli G.
Dept. of Anaesthesiology and Intensive Care, Policlinico S. Orsola-Malpighi, Bologna (Italy)

Marzatico F.
Dept. of Pharmacology, University of Pavia, Pavia (Italy)

Mascia L.
Dept. of Anaesthesia and Intensive Care, University of Bari, Policlinico, Bari (Italy)

Melloni C.
Dept. of Anaesthesiology and Intensive Care, Policlinico S. Orsola-Malpighi, Bologna (Italy)

Merkler M.
Dept. of Emergency Internal Medicine, Rebro University Hospital, Zagreb (Croatia)

Merli M.
III Dept. of Anaesthesia and Intensive Care, Centre "A. De Gasperis" Niguarda Ca' Granda Hospital, Milan (Italy)

Messeri E.
Dept. of Anaesthesia and Intensive Care, New Hospital S. Giovanni di Dio, Florence (Italy)

Metnitz G.H.
Dept. of Cardiothoracic and Vasculosurgical Anaesthesia, University Clinic of Anaesthesia and General Intensive Care Medicine, University of Vienna, Vienna (Austria)

Meurer G.
Dept. of Experimental Cardiac- and Thoracovascular Surgery, Westfälische Wilhelm University, Münster (Germany)

Micheletto G.
Dept. of General Surgery and Surgical Oncology, University of Milan, Maggiore Hospital, Milan (Italy)

Miksch S.
Austrian Research Institute for Artificial Intelligence (ÖFAI), Vienna (Austria)

Milazzo F.
III Dept. of Anaesthesia and Intensive Care, Centre "A. De Gasperis" Niguarda Ca' Granda Hospital, Milan (Italy)

Milic-Emili J.
Respiratory Division, Meakins-Christie Laboratories, McGill University, Montreal (Canada)

Miller J.D.
Dept. of Clinical Neurosciences, Surgical Neurology, The University of Edinburgh, Western General Hospitals, Edinburgh (UK)

Milne E.N.C.
Dept. of Radiological Sciences, University of California, Irvine, Medical Center, Orange, California (USA)

Montebugnoli M.
I Unit of Anaesthesia and Intensive Care, IRCCS Rizzoli Orthopaedic Institutes, Bologna (Italy)

Muchada R.
Dept. of Anaesthesia and Intensive Care, Clinique Mutualiste "Eugène André", Lyon (France)

Müller E.
Center of Anaesthesiology, Heinrich Heine University, Düsseldorf (Germany)

Nanni G.
Dept. of Organ Transplantation, Dept. of Surgery, University of Sacro Cuore, Rome (Italy)

Nardi G.
II Dept. of Anaesthesia and Intensive Care, Santa Maria della Misericordia Hospital, Udine (Italy)

Nardin L.
II Dept. of Anaesthesia and Intensive Care, Regional Hospital "S. Maria dei Battuti", Treviso (Italy)

Nasi M.T.
Dept. of Neurosurgery, M. Bufalini Hospital, Cesena (Italy)

Novelli G.P.
Dept. of Anaesthesiology and Intensive Care, University of Florence, Policlinico Careggi, Florence (Italy)

Ogg T.W.
Day Surgery Unit, Addenbrooke's Hospital, Cambridge (UK)

Oggioni R.
Dept. of Anaesthesia and Intensive Care, New Hospital S. Giovanni di Dio, Florence (Italy)

Orsi P.
Dept. of Anaesthesiology and Intensive Care, University "La Sapienza", Policlinico Umberto I, Rome (Italy)

Paladino F.
Dept. of Emergency Medicine, San Paolo Hospital, Naples (Italy)

Panocchia N.
Dept. of Organ Transplantation, Dept. of Surgery, University of Sacro Cuore, Rome (Italy)

Paolin A.
II Dept. of Anaesthesia and Intensive Care, Regional Hospital "S. Maria dei Battuti", Treviso (Italy)

Pasetto A.
Dept. of Anaesthesiology and Intensive Care, Udine University School of Medicine, Udine (Italy)

Paver-Eržen V.
Institute of Anaesthesiology, University Medical Center, Ljubljana (Slovenia)

Pedoto A.
Dept. of Anaesthesia and Intensive Care, Maggiore Hospital, Milan (Italy)

Peduto V.A.
Dept. of Anaesthesiology and Intensive Care, University of Cagliari, S. Giovanni di Dio Hospital, Cagliari (Italy)

Pelosi P.
Dept. of Anaesthesia and Intensive Care, Maggiore Hospital, Milan (Italy)

Pennisi M.A.
Dept. of Anaesthesiology and Intensive Care, Catholic University of Sacro Cuore, Policlinico A. Gemelli, Rome (Italy)

Perel A.
Dept. of Anaesthesiology, Sheba Medical Center, Tel Hashomer (Israel)

Perilli V.
Dept. of Anaesthesiology and Intensive Care, Catholic University of Sacro Cuore, Policlinico A. Gemelli, Rome (Italy)

Petrini F.
Dept. of Anaesthesiology and Intensive Care, Policlinico S. Orsola-Malpighi, Bologna (Italy)

Philip B.K.
Day Surgery Unit, Dept. of Anaesthesia, Harvard Medical School, Brigham and Women's Hospital, Boston, Massachusetts (USA)

Piazza O.
Dept. of Anaesthesiology and Intensive Care, Catholic University of Sacro Cuore, Policlinico A. Gemelli, Rome (Italy)

Pieraccioli E.
Dept. of Anaesthesiology and Intensive Care, University of Florence, Policlinico Careggi, Florence (Italy)

Pinsky M.R.
Dept. of Critical Care Medicine, University of Pittsburgh, Pittsburgh, Pennsylvania (USA)

Pöhlau D.
Neurological Clinic of the Ruhr University, Bochum (Germany)

Proietti R.
Dept. of Anaesthesiology and Intensive Care, Catholic University School of Medicine, Rome (Italy)

Radonić R.
Dept. of Emergency Internal Medicine, Rebro University Hospital, Zagreb (Croatia)

Ranieri M.
Dept. of Anaesthesia and Intensive Care, University of Bari, Policlinico, Bari (Italy)

Ranieri R.
Dept. of Anaesthesiology and Intensive Care, Catholic University of Sacro Cuore, Policlinico A. Gemelli, Rome (Italy)

Räsänen J.
Dept. of Anaesthesiology, University Children's Hospital, Helsinki (Finland)

Redmann K.
Dept. of Experimental Cardiac- and Thoracovascular Surgery, Westfälische Wilhelm University, Münster (Germany)

Rehak L.
Dept. of General Pathology, University of Pavia, Pavia (Italy)

Reinhart K.
Clinic of Anaesthesiology and Intensive Care Medicine, "Friedrich Schiller" University of Jena, Jena (Germany)

Restelli A.
Dept. of General Surgery and Surgical Oncology, University of Milan, Maggiore Hospital, Milan (Italy)

Reu R.Chr.
University Clinic of Anaesthesiology, ATV Section, University of Ulm, Ulm (Germany)

Rixen D.
New Jersey Medical School, New Jersey (USA) and University of Cologne, Cologne (Germany)

Rossi S.
I Dept. of Anaesthesia and Intensive Care, Hospital of Parma, Parma (Italy)

Rother S.
Pall GmbH Biomedizin, Scientific and Laboratory Service, Dreieich-Sprendlingen (Germany)

Saltuari L.
Dept. of Neurology, University of Innsbruck, Innsbruck (Austria)

Salvo I.
Dept. of Anaesthesia and Intensive Care, S. Raffaele Hospital, Milan (Italy)

Sandroni C.
Dept. of Anaesthesiology and Intensive Care, Catholic University School of Medicine, Rome (Italy)

Savettieri G.
Dept. of Systematic Pathology, "Federico II" University, Naples (Italy)

Schiraldi F.
Dept. of Emergency Medicine, San Paolo Hospital, Naples (Italy)

Schmutzhard E.
Clinic of Neurology, University of Innsbruck, Innsbruck (Austria)

Servadei F.
Dept. of Neurosurgery, M. Bufalini Hospital, Cesena (Italy)

Sganga G.
Dept. of Surgery and C.N.R. Shock Centre, Catholic University, Rome (Italy)

Siegel J.H.
New Jersey Trauma Center, UMDNJ, New Jersey's University of the Health Sciences, Newark, New Jersey (USA)

Singer M.
Bloomsbury Institute of Intensive Care Medicine, UCL Medical School, London (UK)

Sjöstrand U.H.
Dept. of Anaesthesiology and Intensive Care Medicine, University Hospital, Uppsala (Sweden)

Soiat M.
Dept. of Anaesthesiology and Intensive Care, Trieste University School of Medicine, Trieste (Italy)

Sollazzi L.
Dept. of Anaesthesiology and Intensive Care, Catholic University of Sacro Cuore, Policlinico A. Gemelli, Rome (Italy)

Sostman H.D.
Dept. of Radiology, New York Hospital-Cornell Medical Center, New York, New York (USA)

Špec-Marn A.
Intensive Care Unit, Institute of Anaesthesiology, University Medical Center, Ljubljana (Slovenia)

Stella L.
Dept. of Intensive Care, S. Luigi Centre, "S. Raffaele" Hospital, Milan (Italy)

Stocchetti N.
I Dept. of Anaesthesia and Intensive Care, Hospital of Parma, Parma (Italy)

Tacchino R.
Dept. of Organ Transplantation, Dept. of Surgery, University of Sacro Cuore, Rome (Italy)

Takala J.
Dept. of Intensive Care, Kuopio University Hospital, Kuopio (Finland)

Tarenzi L.
Dept. of Anaesthesia and Intensive Care, Maggiore Hospital, Milan (Italy)

Tecklenburg A.
Medical Direction, Altona Hospital, Hamburg (Germany)

Tiengo M.
Dept. of Pain Therapy, University of Milan, Milan (Italy)

Torri C.
Dept. of Pharmacology, Pavia University School of Medicine, Pavia (Italy)

Trivellato A.
Dept. of Intensive Care "William Osler", Santa Corona Hospital, Garbagnate Milanese, Milan (Italy)

Trömel C.
Dept. of Zoology, University of Frankfurt, Frankfurt (Germany)

Tulli G.
Dept. of Anaesthesia and Intensive Care, New Hospital S. Giovanni di Dio, Florence (Italy)

Uracz W.
Dept. of Pharmacology, Jagiellonian University Medical College, Cracow (Poland)

Van der Linden P.
Dept. of Intensive Care, Erasme University Hospital, Bruxelles (Belgium)

Varutti A.M.
Dept. of Anaesthesiology and Intensive Care, Udine University School of Medicine, Udine (Italy)

Veltri A.
Dept. of Radiology, Le Molinette Hospital, Turin (Italy)

Veneziani A.
Dept. of Anaesthesia and Intensive Care, New Hospital S. Giovanni di Dio, Florence (Italy)

Vicardi P.
Dept. of Anaesthesia and Intensive Care, Maggiore Hospital, Milan (Italy)

Vincent J.-L.
Dept. of Intensive Care, Erasme University Hospital, Bruxelles (Belgium)

Visigalli M.M.
III Dept. of Anaesthesia and Intensive Care, Centre "A. De Gasperis" Niguarda Ca' Granda Hospital, Milan (Italy)

Viviani M.
Dept. of Anaesthesiology and Intensive Care, Trieste University School of Medicine, Trieste (Italy)

Voga G.
Dept. of Intensive Internal Medicine, General Hospital, Celje (Slovenia)

Volpini M.
Dept. of Anaesthesiology and Intensive Care, Policlinico S. Orsola-Malpighi, Bologna (Italy)

Weiskopf R.B.
Dept. of Anaesthesia, Physiology and Cardiovascular Research Institute, University of California, San Francisco, California (USA)

Weiss Y.G.
Dept. of Anaesthesiology and Critical Care Medicine, Hadassah School of Medicine, Jerusalem (Israel)

Wollinsky K.H.
Dept. of Anaesthesiology and Intensive Care, Rehabilitation Hospital, University of Ulm, Ulm (Germany)

Zhang H.
Dept. of Intensive Care, Erasme University Hospital, Bruxelles (Belgium)

Zin W.A.
Laboratory of Respiration Physiology, Institute of Biophysics "Carlos Chagas Filho", Federal University of Rio de Janeiro, Rio de Janeiro (Brasil)

Abbreviations

ABF, Aortic Blood Flow

ACE Ihn, Angiotensin Converting Enzyme Inhibitors

AD, Alzheimer's Disease

ADP, Adenosine Diphosphate

AEM, Ambulatory ECG Monitoring

AI, Artificial Intelligence

AIDS, Acquired Immunodeficiency Syndrome

AIS, Abbreviated Injury Scale

AISM, Australian Incident Monitoring Study

ALS, Advanced Life Support

ALS, Amyotrophic Lateral Sclerosis

AMC, American College of Surgeons

AMI, Acute Myocardial Infarction

ANS, Autonomic Nervous System

APACHE, Acute Physiology and Chronic Health Evaluation (system)

APRV, Airway Pressure Release Ventilation

APSAC, Anisolated Plasminogen Streptokinase Activator Complex

ARDEATH, APACHE II Derived Risk of Hospital Death

ARDS, Acute Respiratory Distress Syndrome

ARF, Acute Respiratory Failure

ARF, Acute Renal Failure

ASA, American Society of Anaesthesiologists

ASCOT, American Surgeons Committee on Trauma

ATLS, Advanced Trauma Life Support

ATM, Asynchronous Transfer Mode

ATP, Adenosin Triphosphate

AVDO$_2$, Arteriovenous Differences of Oxygen

BAL, Bronchoalveolar Lavage

BD, Brain Death

BGA, Blood Gas Analysis

BLS, Basic Life Support

BMI, Body Mass Index

BNI, Blind Nasal Intubation

CABG, Cardiopulmonary Arterial Bypass Graft

CAD, Coronary Arterial Disease

CAI, Computer Aided Instruction

CAO, Chronic Airway Obstruction

CASS, Coronary Artery Study

CAT, Catalase

CBF, Cerebral Blood Flow

CBPs, Cytokines-Binding Proteins

CCB, Calcium Channel Blocker

CCU, Coronary Care Unit

CDC, Centers for Disease Control

Cdyn, Dynamic Compliance

CFAV, Continuous Flow Apneic Ventilation

CHF, Congestive Heart Failure

CI, Cardiac Index

CIPU, Clinical Information Processing Unit

CJD, Creutzfeldt-Jacob Disease

CMRO$_2$, Cerebral Metabolic Rate of Oxygen

CNS, Central Nervous System

CNTF, Ciliary Neurotrophic Factor

CO, Cardiac Output

COPD, Chronic Obstructive Pulmonary Disease

COX-1, Cyclooxigenase 1

CPAP, Continuous Positive Airway Pressure

CPB, Cardiopulmonary Bypass

CPEO, Chronic Progressive External Ophtalmoplegia

CPP, Cerebral Perfusion Pressure

CPR, Cardiopulmonary Resuscitation

CPS, Central Pain Syndrome

Crs, Compliance of total respiratory system

CSF, Cerebral Spinal Fluid

CT, Computed Tomography

Cts,rs, respiratory static Compliance

CVP, Central Venous Pressure

CVVH, Continuous Veno-Venous Hemofiltration

CXR, Chest X-Ray

cyclic-AMP, cyclic Adenosine Monophosphate

DAP, Diastolic Arterial Pressure

DCA, Dichloro Acetate

DIC, Disseminated Intravascular Coagulation

DKA, Diabetic Ketoacidosis

DLT, Double Lung Transplantation

DO$_2$, Oxygen Delivery

DRGs, "Diagnosis-Related Groups" system

DVT, Deep Venous Thrombosis

ECCO$_2$-R, Extracorporeal CO_2 Removal

ECG, Electrocardiography

ECMO, Extracorporal Membrane Oxygenation

ecNOS, endothelial constitutive Nitric Oxide Synthase

EDPVR, End-Diastolic Pressure-Volume Relationship

EDRF, Endothelium-Derived Relaxing Factor

EEG, Electroencephalogram

EF, Ejection Fraction

EGFs, Epidermal Growth Factors

EIOM, End Inflation Occlusion Method

EM, Electron Microscopy

EMG, Electromyography

EMHS, Emergency Medical Helicopter Service

EMS, Emergency Medical Service

EOA, Esophageal Obturator Airway

EST, Exercise Stress Testing

Est,L, Lung Elastance

Est,rs, respiratory Elastance

Est,w, chest wall Elastance

ET 1-3, Endothelins

ETT, Endotracheal tube

ETT, Endotracheal intubation

EVLW, Extravascular Lung Water

FEV1, Forced Expiratory Volume in one second

FFB, Flexible Fibreoptic Bronchoscopy

FFI, Fatal Familial Insomnia

FGF, Fresh Gas Flow

FGFs, Fibroblast Growth Factors

FiO$_2$, Fractional inspiratory Oxygen

FMR1, Fragile X Mental Retardation 1

FRC, Functional Residual Capacity

GA, General Anaesthesia

GCS, Glasgow Coma Scale

GOS, Glasgow Outcome Score

GPI, Glycosylphosphatidyl Inositol

GSH-Px, Glutathione Peroxidase

GSS, Gerstmann-Straussler-Scheinker Disease

GUI, Graphical User Interfaces

HD, Huntington Disease

HeCa, Calcium Heparin

HFJV, High Frequency Jet Ventilation

HFPPV, High Frequency Positive Pressure Ventilation

HFV, High Frequency Ventilation

HIS, Hospital Information System

HIV, Human Immunodeficiency Virus

HNK-1, Human Natural Killer-1

HR, Heart Rate

HTLV III/LAV, Human T-Lymphotrophic Virus type III / Lymphadenopathy-Associated Virus

IABP, Intra-Aortic Balloon Pump

ICIS, Intensive Care Information Systems

ICP, Intracranial Pressure

IFN, Interferon

IGFs, Insuline-like Growth Factors

IL, Interleukin

INF-gamma, Interferon-gamma

iNOS, inducible Nitric Oxide Synthase

IPPV, Intermittent Positive Pressure Ventilation

ISS, Injury Severity Score

ITPV, Intratracheal Pulmonary Ventilation

IVRT, Isovolumic Relaxation Time

L-NAME, N^G-nitro-L-arginine methyl ester

L-NIO, N-iminoethyl-L-ornitine

L-NMMA, N^G-monomethyl-L-arginine

LAL, Limus Amoebocyte Lysate

LAN, Local Area Network

LI, Linear Interpolation

LIF, Lymphocyte Migration Inhibitory Factor

LM, Light Microscopy

LMA, Laryngeal Mask Airway

LMWH, Low-Molecular-Weight Heparin

LNS, Limb Norris Scale

LOI, Lactate Oxygen Index

LOOH, Lipid Hydroperoxides

LOS, Lower Oesophageal Sphincter

LO°, Lipid Alcoxides

LP, Lipid Peroxidation

LPS, Lipopolysaccharide

LVEDP, Left Ventricular End-Diastolic Pressure

LVEF, Left Ventricular Ejection Fraction

LVET, Left Ventricular Ejection Time

mAb, Monoclonal Antibody

MAC, Minimal Alveolar Concentration

MAO, Mono Amine Oxidase

MAP, Mean Arterial Pressure

MDA, Malondialdehyde

MDF, Myocardial Depressant Factor

MELAS, Myopathy, Encephalopathy, Lactic Acidosis and Stroke-like Episodes

MEPs, Multimodality Evoked Potentials

MERRF, Myoclonic Epilepsy with Ragged Red Fibres

MI, Myocardial Infarction
MIF, Macrophage Migration Inhibitory Factor
MIP, Maximal Inspiratory Airway Pressure
MISS, Modified Injury Severity Scale
MLA, Monophosphoryl Lipid A
MODFS, Multiple Organ Dysfunction Failure Syndrome
MODS, Multi-Organ Dysfunction Syndrome
MOF, Multi-Organ Failure
MR, Magnetic Resonance
mRNAs, messenger Ribonucleic Acids
MS, Multiple Sclerosis
MTC, Multimedial Telecommunication
MTOS, Major Trauma Outcome Study
MV, Mechanical Ventilation
MVO$_2$, Myocardial Oxygen Consumption
NAC, N-Acetyl-Cysteina
NANC, Non-Adrenergic Non-Cholinergic
ncNOS, neuronal constitutive Nitric Oxide Synthase
NFkB, Nuclear Factor kappa B
NGS, Nerve Growth Factor
NIRS, Near Infrared Spectroscopy
NMR, Nuclear Magnetic Resonance
NO, Nitric Oxide
NOS, Nitric Oxide Synthase
NSAID, Nonsteroidal Anti-Inflammatory Drug
NTs, Neurotrophins
O$_2$ER, Oxygen Extraction
ODM, Oesophageal Doppler Machine
OECD, Organization for Economic Cooperation and Development
OG, Osmonal Gap
OGTA, Oesophageal Gastric Tube Airway
ONOO⁻, Peroxinitrite Anion
OR°, Oxygen Radical
OSF, Organ System Failure
P(A-a)O$_2$, Alveolar-Arterial Oxygen tension difference
PAC, Pulmonary Artery Catheterization
PaCO$_2$, Partial Pressure of Arterial CO$_2$
PACS, Picture Archiving and Communication System
PAF, Platelet Activating Factor
PAFC, Pulmonary Artery Flotation Catheter
PAG, Periaqueductal Gray
PAI-1, Plasminogen Activator Inhibitor
PaO$_2$, Partial Pressure of Arterial Oxygen
PAP, Pulmonary Arterial Pressure

PAS, Systolic Artery Pressure
PAV, Proportional Assist Ventilation
PBV, Pulmonary Blood Volume
PC, Pressure Controlled
PCA, Patient Controlled Analgesia
PCEA, Patient Controlled Epidural Analgesia
PCP, Pneumocystis Carinii Pneumonia
PCP, Pulmonary Capillary Pressure
PCVAE, Perioperative Cardiovascular Adverse Events
PCWP, Pulmonary Capillary Wedge Pressure
PDGF-β, Platelet-Derived Growth Factor β
PDH, Pyruvate Dehydrogenase
PDMS, Patient Data Management Systems
PE, Pulmonary Embolism
PEEP, Positive End Expiratory Pressure
PEEPi, Positive End Expiratory Pressure Intrinsic PEEP
PEP, Pre-Ejection Period
PET, Peak Ejection Time
PetCO$_2$, End-Tidal CO$_2$ Pressure
PG, Prostaglandin
PGE1, Prostaglandin E1
PGE2, Prostaglandin E2
PGHS-1, Prostaglandin H Synthase-1
PGI2, Prostacyclin
PHi, Intragastric PH
PHT, Pulmonary Hypertension
PHv, Venous PH
Pimax, Maximum (Peak) Airway Pressure
PIP, Peak Inspiratory Pressure
PMN, Polymorphonuclear Neutrophil
PN, Parenteral Nutrition
pO$_2$, Partial Pressure of Oxygen
PONV, Postoperative Nausea and Vomiting
POSM, Plasmatic Osmolality
Pplat, plateau Pressure
PRQ, Pressure/heart Rate Quotient
PRVC, Pressure Regulated Volume Controlled Ventilation
PS, Phosphatidyl Serine
PSSC, Physiologic State Severity Classification
PSV, Pressure Support Ventilation
PSVfc, flow-cycled PSV
PSVtc, time-cycled PSV
PT, Prothrombin Time
PTI, Pressure Time Index
PTLA, Pharyngotracheal Lumen Airway

PVC, Premature Ventricular Contraction

PVC, Pressure-Volume-Controlled Ventilation

pvO$_2$, partial mixed venous Oxygen pressure

PVS, Persistent Vegetative State

QRS, Electrocardiographic Signal

Qs/Qt, Intrapulmonary Shunt Fraction

RAO, Rapid Airway Occlusion

RAP, Right Atrial Pressure

RES, Reticulo-Endothelial System

RI, Retrograde Intubation

RI, Respiratory Index

Rint,rs, Airway Resistance

Rmax,rs, Maximum Respiratory Resistance

Rmin,rs, Minimum Respiratory Resistance

RNA, Radionuclide Angiography

ROS, Oxygen Radical Species

RR(es-aw), difference between respiratory rate calculated on esophageal and airway pressure curve

Rrs, Total Respiratory System Resistance

RTS, Revised Trauma Score

RVEDP, Right Ventricular End-Diastolic Pressure

RVEF, Right Ventricular Ejection Fraction

RVI, Right Ventricular Infarction

SAH, Subarachnoid Haemorrage

SaO$_2$, Arterial Oxygen Saturation

SAP, Systolic Arterial Pressure

SAPS, Simplified Acute Physiology Score

SB, Spontaneous Breathing

SDD, Selective Digestive Decontamination

SDR,L, Specific Additional Lung Resistance

SID, Strong Ion Difference

SIDa, Apparent Strong Ion Difference

SIDe, Effective Strong Ion Difference

SIMV, Synchronized intermittent Mandatory Ventilation

SIRS, Systemic Inflammatory Response Syndrome

SjO$_2$, Jugular Venous Oxygen Saturation

SjvO$_2$, Arteriojugular Venous Oxygen Saturation

SLT, Single Lung Transplantation

SOD, Superoxide Dismutase

SPECT, Single Photon Emission Computed Tomography

SQL, Standard Query Language

ST, Surgical Tracheostomy

STI, Systolic Time Interval

STK, Streptokinase

SV, Stroke Volume

SvO$_2$, Mixed Venous Oxygen Saturation

SVR, Systemic Vascular Resistance

SW, Swan-Ganz

t-PA, Plasminogen Activator

TAL, Thick Ascendent Limb

TCD, Transcranial Doppler

TCDB, Traumatic Coma Data Bank

TD, Thermo Dilution

TDT, Thermal Dye Technique

TEA, Thoracic Epidural Anaesthesia

TEE, Transesophageal Echocardiography

TGFβ, Transforming Growth Factor β

TI/TTOT, Inspiratory Time/Total Time

TISS, Therapeutic Intervention Scoring System

TIVA, Total Intravenous Anaesthesia

TNFα, Tumour Necrosis Factor α

TOE, Transoesophageal Echocardiography

TOF, Time-Of-Flight

TPA, Plasminogen Activator

TPR, Total Peripheral Resistance

TRAM, Transfer Module

TRIO, Tracheal Insufflation of Oxygen

TRISS, Trauma Injury Severity Score

TRM, Thrombomodulin

TSVR, Total Systemic Vascular Resistance

TT, Tracheal Tube

TXA2, Thromboxane A2

UAG, Urinary Anion Gap

v-WF, von-Willebrandt Factor

V/Q, Ventilation Flow

VC, Volume Controlled

VCAM-1, Vascular Cell Adhesion Molecule-1

VD/VT, Dead Space Tidal Volume Ratio

VE, Minute Ventilation

VO$_2$, Oxygen Consumption

VPW, Vascular Pedicle Width

VT, Tidal Volume

Vt/Ti, Mean Inspiratory Flow

WAN, Wide Area Network

WHO, World Health Organization

WOB, Work Of Breathing

XD, Xanthine Hydroxydase

XO, Xanthine Oxidase

ΔPes, Δ Oesophageal Pressure

ΔRrs, additional Resistance of the respiratory system

BASICS OF CRITICAL CARE MEDICINE

ANAESTHESIA

Why Are Hypertensive Patients at Risk in the Perioperative Period?

J.J. Lehot, C. Girard, S. Filley, M. George, O. Bastien

Hypertension is defined as systolic arterial pressure greater than or equal to 160 mmHg and/or diastolic arterial pressure greater than 95 mmHg measured in the sitting position under quiet conditions at least on two occasions (WHO). If there is any doubt noninvasive ambulatory blood pressure (Holter) can be measured.

Hypertension is found in 8% of males and 10% of females and its frequency increases with age.

Perioperative risk is increased in hypertensive patients because of chronic visceral consequences of hypertension and acute consequences of hypertension occurring during the perioperative period.

Causes of hypertension

Essential hypertension is the most frequent cause of hypertension. Increased peripheral vascular resistance is its primary mechanism. However, other causes must be looked for (Table 1).

Consequences of hypertension

Chronic consequences

Hypertension increases the risk of stroke, nephroangiosclerosis (media hypertrophy), retinopathy and coronary artery disease (CAD). The risk of myocardial ischaemia is increased by compensatory thickening of the left ventricular (LV) wall. Essential hypertension is associated with increased systemic resistance in all organs and decreased venous capacitance. Hypovolaemia results from reduced venous capacitance and diuretic treatment. The baroreflex is reset toward higher arterial pressure (1, 2).

Table 1. Causes of hypertension

Measurement errors (size of cuff, migration of zero)	
Metabolic:	• Hypercapnia
	• Hypercalcaemia
	• Sodium overload
Circumstantial:	• Pain
	• Decreased anaesthesia level
	• Arterial surgical clamping
	• Stress
	• Anxiety
Endocrinopathy:	• Phaeochromocytoma
	• Cohn disease
	• Cushing syndrome
	• Adrenogenital syndrome
	• Acromegalia
Renal disease:	Renal artery stenosis, glomerulopathy, chronic renal failure
Aortic coarctation	
Cerebral:	Stroke, intracranial hypertension, preeclampsia
Toxic:	Narcotic dependence, cocaine, heavy metals (mercury, lead, thallium)
Medicines:	Decongestant sympathomimetics, antidepressive drugs (including selective MAO inhibitors), anorexigens, steroids

These circumstances require aetiologic treatments

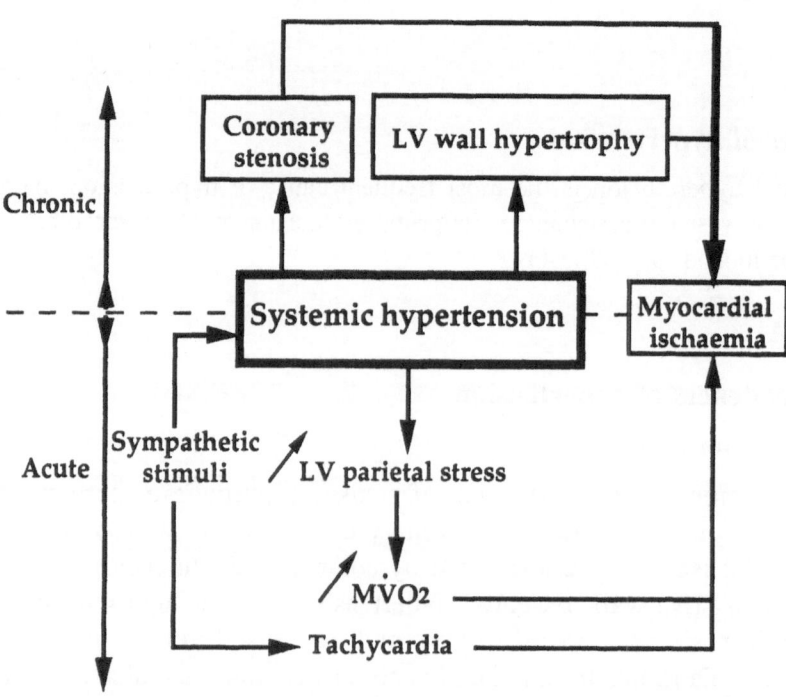

Fig. 1. Causes of myocardial ischaemia in hypertensive patients

Acute consequences

Hypertensive episodes result from acute arteriolar vasoconstriction due to sympathetic overreactivity (3) during nociceptive stimulations (tracheal intubation, surgery, awakening).

Increased vascular impedance decreases LV emptying, resulting in elevated LV telesystolic volume, reduced stroke volume and LV ejection fraction. Increased LV parietal stress elevates myocardial oxygen consumption.

Subendocardial ischaemia is majored by increased LV diastolic pressure caused by reduced LV compliance (Fig. 1).

Myocardial ischaemia itself reduces LV ejection fraction leading to LV failure. Moreover myocardial ischaemia favours arrhythmia and the occurrence of atrial fibrillation may drop cardiac output by more than 30% in patients with LV hypertrophy. Indeed, when arterial pressure is equal to or greater than 160/90 mmHg in spite of antihypertensive treatment pre- and postoperative myocardial ischaemia occurs in 74% (4).

The cerebral arteries only contain few precapillary sphincters; therefore they are directly submitted to blood pressure elevation, leading to increased capillary permeability and interstitial oedema. Haemorrhagic lesions are rare except after carotid endarterectomy (5).

Renal artery vasoconstriction leads to renal impairment and increased plasma renin concentration enhances systemic hypertension.

Moreover, hypertension may increase surgical bleeding.

The risks of perioperative *hypotension* are enhanced in hypertensive patients because of frequent hypovolaemia, decreased venous return to the heart, and decreased LV compliance leading to decreased cardiac output. Most anaesthetic agents decrease venous return (except ketamine, etomidate and nitrous oxide) and peripheral vascular resistance, leading to hypotension. Cerebral blood flow autoregulation is chronically altered in hypertensive patients. *Hypotension decreases perfusion pressure and regional output, particularly in the myocardium and the brain, leading to ischaemic episodes.*

Preoperative risk evaluation

According to arterial pressure value

Patients with persistent hypertension

Patients with diastolic arterial pressure greater than 100 mmHg are exposed to unstable perioperative blood pressure: hypotension at induction of anaesthesia and hypertension during surgical stimulations and awakening.

Patients with arterial pressure controlled by treatment are at standard risk except when hypertension is associated with CAD or when surgery itself is a risk.

Nonemergency operations in severe hypertensive patients should be delayed until normalization of arterial pressure.

According to operation

Patients undergoing vascular surgery (including carotid endarterectomy) and surgery with large liquid or blood losses are at major risks for haemodynamic instability.

According to associated visceral diseases

CAD increases the operative risk but ST monitoring cannot be reliably used in patients with hypertrophic LV. Thallium pyridamole scintigraphy may detect CAD.

Transthoracic echocardiography may diagnose LV hypertrophy and associated abnormalities such as aortic valve stenosis.

Preoperative treatment

Some treatments may prevent perioperative events whereas others must be stopped prior to elective surgery.

Beta-blockers

Beta-blocker therapy must be pursued also preoperatively in order to stabilize perioperative haemodynamics and reduce the occurrence of myocardial ischaemia and possibly myocardial infarction.

In previously nontreated moderately hypertensive patients undergoing non cardiac surgery, Stone et al. (6) administered one single tablet of beta-blocker preoperatively. Myocardial ischaemia during tracheal intubation and awakening occurred in only 2% of the beta-blocker patients versus 28% of the control group. Heart rate, arterial pressure, and arrhythmia were significantly reduced in the treated patients.

Calcium channel-blockers (CCB)

Though no randomized study has been performed these drugs are usually administered in treated patients until the induction of anaesthesia. They prevent perioperative hypertension (7-9) and possibly myocardial ischaemia.

Alpha-2-agonists

In patients administered clonidine chronically, the usual treatment must be administered preoperatively but the induction doses of anaesthetics must be decreased by 40% (10). However, enhancement of pressor response to i.v. phenylephrine following oral clonidine medication has been reported in awake and anaesthetized patients (11).

Conversely, the discontinuation of these three drug categories may lead to withdrawal syndrome with tachycardia, hypertension and angina pectoris.

Diuretics

Hypovolaemia may lead to intraoperative hypotension. Therefore withdrawal of this treatment 48 h prior to anaesthesia has been advocated (12).

Reserpine

Reserpine should be withdrawn 8 days prior to anaesthesia and replaced by another antihypertensive treatment, usually a dihydropyridine (13).

Angiotensin converting enzyme inhibitors (ACE Inh)

They may induce intraoperative hypotension and should be stopped when prescribed for *hypertension*. Captopril has a short half-life and may be stopped 18 h prior to induction. The others have a longer half-life and may be stopped more than 24 h prior to induction. They are usually replaced by a dihydropyridine up to the induction of anaesthesia.

If ACE Inh have been prescribed for chronic *cardiac failure*, their withdrawal may induce a relapse. Therefore it seems preferable to continue these drugs until the eve of anaesthesia and give anaesthesia with close monitoring of haemodynamic parameters.

Intraoperative management

Monitoring

Because hypertensive patients may present with hypovolaemia and many antihypertensive treatments increase venous capacitance or decrease baroreflex responsiveness, *avoiding hypovolaemia* is the main rule. Therefore monitoring of volaemia through pulmonary artery catheter, systolic pressure variations during mechanical ventilation or transoesophageal echocardiography may be helpful according to the surgical procedure.

Monitoring of arterial pressure is best performed by arterial catheter or, at least, automatic inflation cuff devices.

Monitoring of myocardiac ischaemia is usually performed by ST segment monitoring (CM5) and monitoring of arrhythmia by D2 lead.

Anaesthesia

The *induction* of anaesthesia may induce *hypotension*. Therefore, preinduction volume loading is mandatory. Drugs such as thiopental and methohexital are avoided because of their depressant effects on myocardium and vessel tone. Ketamine is avoided because of the risk of sympathetic stimulation and hypertension. Fentanyl (6-8 µg kg^{-1}) and midazolam (10-20 µg kg^{-1}) are well tolerated. Pancuronium (0.1 mg kg^{-1}) prevents the risk of bradycardia associated with beta-blocker, diltiazem, verapamil or clonidine administered prior to induction, and with high dose fentanyl administered at induction.

The *maintenance* of anaesthesia may be performed with reinjections of induction agents, propofol infusion and nitrous oxide. Halogenated anaesthetics are titrated according to arterial pressure. Leone et al. (14) showed that in dogs with a critical coronary constriction, an increase in halothane inspired concentration over 1% causes regional LV dysfunction. Interestingly this dysfunction could be prevented by i.v. oxprenolol.

Due to a similar mechanism of action, halogenated agents and CCB possess additive cardiovascular effects that can be easily controlled by modulating halogenated gas concentration. High concentrations (> 1.5 MAC) must be avoided in patients administered CCB preoperatively (Table 2).

Table 2. Relative effects of CCB and halogenated agents

CCB	Halogenated agent	Negative inotropic effect	Negative dromotropic effect	Arterial vasodilator
Verapamil	Enflurane	+++	+++	+
Diltiazem	Halothane	++	++	++
Dihidropyridine	Isoflurane			
	Desflurane	+	+	+++
	Sevoflurane			

Medullar anaesthesia is also possible provided hypovolaemia is absent; in this case, pressure variations due to medullar anaesthesia are similar in hypertensive and normal patients (15).

Treatment of haemodynamic disturbances

Acute hypertension

Prior to cardiovascular agent administration every effort must be made to eliminate hypercarbia and to suppress the effects of the exogenous stimulations by deepening the anaesthesia level, though Philbin et al. (16) showed a poor relationship between cardiovascular stability and narcotic dosages. Isoflurane, desflurane and sevoflurane decrease arterial pressure predominantly through depressing arterial tone, hence preserving the LV ejection fraction. Conversely halothane and enflurane decrease arterial pressure, predominantly by decreasing myocardial contractility, and are less desirable.

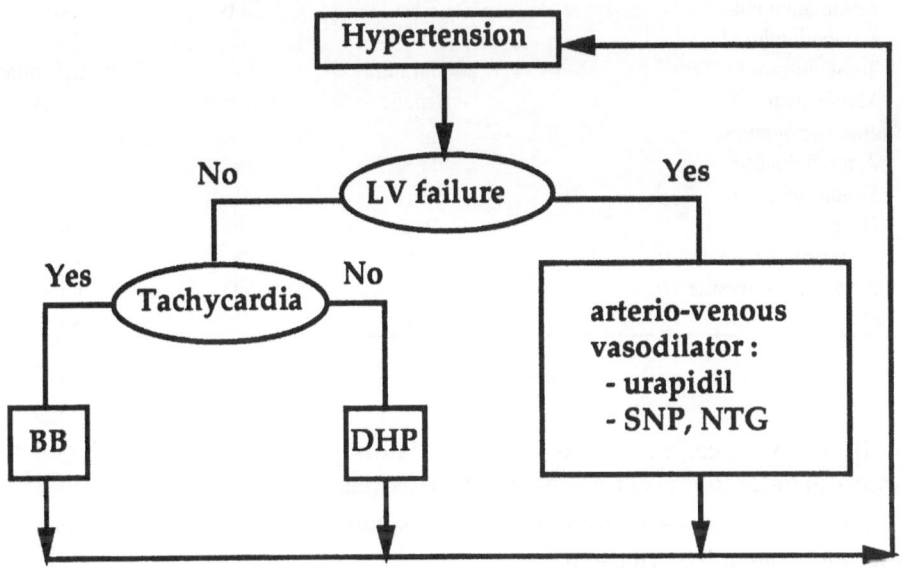

Fig. 2. Treatment of intraoperative hypertension. *LV*, left ventricular; *BB*, beta-blocker; *DHP*, dihydropyridine; *SNP*, sodium nitroprusside; *NTG*, nitroglycerine

When halogenated agents are ineffective, cardiovascular agents are administered i.v.:

- In the presence of tachycardia, beta-blocker (labetalol, acebutolol, esmolol) or diltiazem (starting with 0.15 mg kg⁻¹) increments are administered after correction of hypovolaemia in patients with satisfactory LV systolic function (preoperative LV ejection fraction > 50%).
- In other circumstances vasodilators are used:
  - If LV systolic function is satisfactory nicardipine is administered (1 mg every 3 min according to effects). However, on rare occasions, LV

failure occurred after nicardipine injection due to suppression of sympathetic activation during anaesthesia.
- Therefore if LV systolic function is poor, arteriovenous vasodilators such as urapidil, ketanserin, nitroglycerine or sodium nitroprusside are preferred (Fig. 2).

Table 3. New i.v. antihypertensive agents

	Urapidil	Nicardipine	Esmolol
Pharmacological class	Alpha-1 blocker	CCB	Beta-blocker
Pharmacokinetics			
• Distribution half-life	35 min	–	2 min
• Elimination half-life	3 hrs	4 hrs	9 min
• Protein binding (%)	80	98	55
• Total clearance	200 ml.min^{-1}	–	33 ml.kg^{-1}.min^{-1}
• Metabolism	Hepatic	Hepatic	Erythrocyte
Pharmacodynamics			
• Arterial dilation	++	++	0
• Venous dilation	++	0	0
• Heart rate	# 0	↗	↘
• Myocardial contractility	0	↘	↘↘
• Intracranial pressure	# 0	↗	# 0
Cost	++	0	++

In our practice, we administer vasodilators prior to stopping halogenated agents in order to prevent postoperative hypertension.

Alpha- and beta-adrenergic receptor blockers can be safely used in patients with intracranial hypertension (17).

Acute hypotension

While volume loading is administered, incremental doses of vasoconstrictors are injected i.v. to obtain more rapid elevation of arterial pressure. Ephedrine is selected when the heart rate is low and phenylephrine when heart rate is satisfactory. An overreactivity to sympathomimetics has been observed, with hypertension and arrhythmia, leading to *"Russian mountain syndrome"*.

Postoperative management

Patients at risk

Patients undergoing cardiac surgery, carotid endarterectomy and aortic surgery are particularly at risk of postoperative hypertension.

Monitoring

Continuous or frequent arterial pressure measurements are compulsory because of the high incidence of hypertensive episodes during this period. Myocardial ischaemia monitoring is also recommended but difficult to perform over several days in most institutions.

Reduction of global oxygen consumption during awakening

Hypertension may occur when cardiac output increases to meet the high O_2 demand. Therefore O_2 demand can be decreased by preventing pain, hypothermia and shivering.

Cardiovascular agents

Increased systemic resistance due to high sympathetic tone is the most frequent cause of postoperative hypertension. I.V. *droperidol* or *chlorpromazine* may be useful in ventilated patients.

In addition to agents used during anaesthesia i.v. *clonidine* decreases elevation of plasma noradrenaline concentration immediately after surgery (18) and can be administered intravenously. We prescribe 75 μg every 3 h if systolic arterial pressure is greater than 160 mmHg in the surgical ward. Its sedative effect is often appreciated. If not, we prescribe i.v. urapidil (25 to 50 mg) every 3 h under the same conditions.

Preoperative treatments must be resumed as soon as normal arterial pressure is established. They are started at lower doses after major operations and when low proteinaemia may increase plasma free fraction of these agents. Oral and nasogastric routes are currently used whereas the i.v. route is seldom needed.

In summary, hypertensive patients appear at high risk of haemodynamic instability during the perioperative period.

Therefore we recommend:

- *Preoperatively* to adjust the treatment in order to administer anaesthesia in normotensive stabilized patients.
- *Intraoperatively* to prevent hypovolaemia either for general or medullar anaesthesia. Induction must be progressive in order to avoid hypotension. Nitrous oxide and isoflurane are commonly utilized for maintenance.
- The *postoperative period* is at higher risk as emergence of anaesthesia induces a sympathetic response leading to acute hypertension, particularly in cardiovascular surgery. Monitoring of arterial pressure must be performed during the postoperative hours by trained personnel. I.V. vasodilators are used in order to decrease cardiac preload and afterload. The usual antihypertensive agents are progressively resumed.

References

1. Bristow JD, Honour AJ, Pickering GW et al (1969) Diminished baroreflex sensitivity in high blood pressure. Circulation 39:48-54
2. Gribbin B, Pickering TG, Sleight P, Peto R (1971) Effect of age and high blood pressure on baroreflex sensitivity in man. Circ Respir 29:424-431
3. Abboud FM (1982) The sympathetic system in hypertension. State of the art review. Hypertension 4:208-225
4. Hemming AE, Howell S, Sear JW, Foex P (1978) Admission blood pressure is predictive of silent myocardial ischaemia in treated hypertension. Br J Anaesth 71:760P
5. Caplan LR, Skillman J, Ojemann R et al (1978) Intracerebral hemorrhage following carotid endarterectomy: a hypertensive complication? Stroke 9:457-460
6. Stone JG, Foëx P, Sear JW, Johnson LL, Khabmatta HJ, Triner L (1988) Myocardial ischemia in untreated hypertensive patients: effect of a single dose of a oral beta-blocker. Anesthesiology 68:495-500
7. Braz J, Bertrand M, Coriat P et al (1988) Administration peropératoire de nisoldipine: effets sur l'hémodynamique et les catécholamines plasmatiques. In: 30ème congrès français d'Anesthésie et de Réanimation. Résumé des communications
8. Skarvan K (1983) Preoperative nifedipine treatment and anesthesia in patients with coronary heart disease. Anesthesiology 59:362-363
9. Hess W, Meyer C (1986) Haemodynamic effects of nifedipine in patients undergoing coronary artery bypass surgery. Acta Anaesthesiol Scand 30:614-619
10. Helbo-Hansen S, Fletcher R, Lundberg D, Nordstrom L, Werner O, Stahl E, Norden N (1986) Clonidine and the sympatho-adrenal response to coronary artery bypass surgery. Acta Anaesthesiol Scand 30:235-242
11. Inomata S, Nishikawa T, Kihara S, Akiyoshi Y (1995) Enhancement of pressor response to intravenous phenylephrine following oral clonidine medication in awake and anaesthetized patients. Can J Anaesth 42:119-125
12. Leth A (1970) Changes in plasma and extracellular volumes in patients with essential hypertension during long-term treatment with hydrochlorothiazide. Circulation 42:479-485
13. Chauvin M (1986) Médicaments à poursuivre ou à interrompre avant une anesthésie. Enc Med Chir, Instantanés Médicaux 6:35-37
14. Leone BJ, Lehot JJ, Francis M, Cutfield GR, Foex P (1987) Beta-blockade reverses regional dysfunction in ischemic myocardium. Anesth Analg 66:607-614
15. Dagnino J, Prys-Roberts C (1984) Studies of anaesthesia in relation to hypertension. VI: cardiovascular responses to extradural blockade of treated and untreated hypertensive patients. Br J Aanesth 56:1065-1073
16. Philbin DM, Sosow CE, Schneider RC, Koski G, D'Ambra MN (1990) Fentanyl and sufentanil anesthesia revisited: how much is enough? Anesthesiology 73:5-11
17. Van Haken H, Cottrell JE, Anger C, Puchstein C (1989) Treatment intraoperative hypertensive emergencies in patients with intracranial disease. Am J Cardiol 63:43C-47C
18. Flacke JW, Bloor BC, Wong D et al (1986) Effects of clonidine upon hyperadrenergic responses and narcotic requirements in patients undergoing CABG surgery. Anesthesiology 65:A16

PAIN

Acute Pain Modulation in the Central Nervous System: A Chronological Review

M. Tiengo, C. Benedetti

Introduction

The objective of this presentation is to trace a short historical and philosophical chronology on the neuronal and neurochemical systems that, in the spinal cord and in the brain, modulate the nociceptive information caused by an algogenic stimulus.

Our aim is to present the genealogic line of the experiments that led to the major discoveries of the cerebral spinal systems which modulate acute pain - a line that begins with the anatomical demonstrations of Ramon y Cajal and the physiological discoveries of Charles Sherrington and extend to our time with the research works of Basbaum and Fields.

Obviously, this presentation is not an extensive review but, more modestly, a brief chronicle of the more illustrious researchers whose discoveries contributed in a fundamental manner to the anatomophysiological description of the neurobiological systems subserving the modulation of acute pain.

Nociception, pain and analgesia

Nociception is defined as the responses which occur whenever an organism is exposed to an injurious or potentially injurious stimulus. These responses include, but are not limited to, phenomena such as bioelectric, molecular, ionic, chemical, genetic expression and plasticity of the nervous system.

With the word *pain* we refer to the integration, at the cortical level, of the sensory, cognitive and affective responses triggered by nociception. In other words, pain is the becoming conscious of nociception.

The analgesic system is the entire set of neuronal pathways, nuclei, and neurotransmitters that control nociception and therefore pain. Analgesia is an expression that points out the attainment of an effect, that is, the disappearance of pain, without specifying if this effect is due to the control of the nociception or of pain. The first is mediated by two major mechanisms:

1. The block of nociceptive afferents, either at the periphery or at the spinal cord
2. The enhancement of the antinociceptive systems

The second, the control of pain, inhibits the cognitive, affective and sensory systems at the cerebral level, in other words, the obliteration of consciousness.

If the conscience is not able to receive messages, for physiological causes (suggestions, distraction, hypnosis, placebo, loss of consciousness) or pharmacological intervention (opioids, sedatives, general anesthesia) nociception doesn't evoke the pain (1).

The levels of the pain threshold and pain tolerance depend on the activation of the endogenous modulating systems from the receptor to the brain and the mind. The individual differences are great because they are dependent on many factors which can interact in a multitude of ways. Some of these components are: physiological, psychological, vocational, socioeconomic and multicultural (2, 3).

Theoretic roots

The first description of a nociceptive pathway was made by Rene Descartes, also known as Cartesio (1595-1650) in his book "De Homine".

In the Cartesian sense, pain is a "warning bell", and it is the maximum ally of man, since it warns the organism of stimuli which can cause damage or potential damage. These stimuli, if prolonged in time, intensity and extension, could be deadly. This was unfortunately well known in the past. People knew that a person could die under torture or, before the advent of anesthesia, under surgery. More recently studies have shown that poor control of postoperative pain significantly increases morbidity and most likely mortality especially in high risk patients (4, 5): pain, indeed, can kill. The organism has therefore developed defensive strategies - some aimed at terminating the nociceptive stimuli, others at raising pain threshold by impairing at the first synapse in the spinal cord the transmission of the nociceptive signal. These strategies begin with the segmental reflex arc in the spinal cord, the first of the defensive reflexes of the organism, which causes withdrawal from the injurious stimulus, and it is followed by production of protective substances, such as analgesics and antistress neurochemicals and hormones which cause adaptation of the cardiovascular and respiratory resources. The risk and the danger for the organism rest in an excess of autonomic responses, which are caused, in part, by the intensity of the nociceptive stimuli that reach the spinal cord (6).

All mammals concentrate the first defenses against acute pain in the first laminae of the dorsal horn of the spinal cord, on the cells of origin of the second neurons that forms the spinothalamic pathways and in that area Melzack and Wall discovered in the mid 1960s, the mechanism of the "gate" (7).

The first discoveries

Until the end of the nineteenth century, physiologists lost themselves in speculative disputes since they lacked anatomical evidence. A famous dispute was that between Weber and Muller on the existence of specific pain pathways, which Muller (8) supported, or that the pain was only the result of an "excessive feeling", as Weber had proposed. It is reported that the controversy became so heated that it resulted in a duel.

At the end of the nineteenth century the physiologist Max Von Frey (9) published a long monograph which reported accurate and fundamental studies on sensory and algic threshold. These studies were carried out using a simple and genial instrument that he had invented and that is still used: the hair esthesiometer. The anatomist Ramon y Cajal, using the method of silver impregnation discovered by Camillo Golgi (both received a Nobel Prize in 1909), traced with great precision the tactile and nociceptive pathways. This gave physiologists the morphological evidence which they were missing.

Between the end of the last century and the first decades of this century, Sir Charles Sherrington, a physiologist from Oxford, and unanimously considered the father of modern neurophysiology (Nobel Laureate for Physiology, together with Adrian, in 1932), studied in great detail the reflex caused by noxious stimulation and how this reflex changes when the cerebrum is separated from the spinal cord. With this model, known in physiology as "decerebrated animal" and "spinal animal" depending on the level of the central nervous system where the section is made, he found that the brain can control spinal activity. Sherrington in 1906 (10) introduced the physiological concepts of "integration" and of "modulation" that are of great importance in understanding the functioning of the CNS. His clinical demonstrations were also very helpful in clarifying the pathogenesis of serious neurological illnesses which, up to that time, had been mysterious.

In one of Sherrington's papers (11), the first to report on the inhibition that brain systems have on spinal cord activity, we read "It has not been widely recognized that this bulbar part of the brain stem, in addition, contains a mechanism capable of exerting a general inhibitory influence on motor activity... demonstrated by observing the effect of bulbar stimulation upon reflexes, upon decerebrate rigidity and upon responses evoked from the motor cortex" (11). Sherrington in 1931, in collaboration with his student John Eccles (12), demonstrated that single break-shock applied to the ipsilateral popliteal nerve causes a reflex activation of the tibialis anticus muscle. But, if the reflexogenic stimulus is briefly preceded by an analogous electric stimulus to the contralateral peroneal nerve, a dramatic reduction of both the mechanical and electric reflex activation is observed. Therefore, a clearly inhibitory effect was demonstrated.

Magoun of Northwestern University reported in 1944: "Since Sherrington's discovery of decerebrate rigidity in 1898, it has been known that the bulbar portion of the brain stem exerts an excitatory influence on the neural motor system, particularly those activating the extensor muscles of the body. That this bulbar region, in addition, contains a mechanism capable of exerting a general inhibitory influence on motor activity does not appear to have been recognized. It was with some astonishment, then, that electrical stimulation of the bulbar reticular formation in the cat was found to bring completely to a halt motor activity, whether induced reflexively, by brain stem mechanisms or from the motor cortex" (13).

At the end of the 1940s, Moruzzi and Magoun, working in Sherrington's physiology laboratory at Northwestern University, used the experimental model of the decerebrated animal. They made one of the most resounding discoveries of neurophysiology of our century: the role of the reticular substance in the regulation of the sleep-awake cycle (14).

Hagbarth and Kerr in 1954 published a paper that is universally considered the starting point for the research leading to the discovery of the descending analgesia systems. In this work, the authors, citing the evidence reached in 1952 by Granit and Kaada, state that "These results indicate the existence of descending nervous pathways, the specific task is to regulate and modify character of afferent messages... The results indicate that spinal afferent pathways can be tonically influenced from higher levels of the nervous system. It is concluded that synaptic afferent transmission in the spinal cord can be influenced in a physiological manner by descending pathway from certain structures in the brain". The authors end with this very important statement: "The reticular formation plays an important role in the central regulation of sensory relays in the spinal cord" (15).

These are, in our opinion, the most important neurophysiological discoveries that paved the way to the individualization of the systems of cerebrospinal control of acute pain.

In 1958, Melzack and his collaborators discovered that lesions of the reticular formation in the proximity of the periaqueductal gray matter caused hyperalgesia and hyperesthesia in the cat. This research demonstrated that fibers depart from these structures and maintain a continuous tonic inhibitory effect on the nociceptive afferents. The abolishment of this inhibition causes continuous pain (16).

Many years elapsed before a young psychologist at the Stanford Research Institute, David Reynolds, realized the importance that such research could have for the control of pain. In 1965, Reynolds presented a film at the meeting of the Federation of American Societies of Experimental Biology which showed surgery being performed on a rat under electrical analgesia. That same year at the California State Psychological Association, he reported the data of a preliminary study which showed that electrical brain stimulation in the rat decreased the sensitivity to adverse foot-shock. For several decades anesthesiologists had reported the possibility of obtaining general anesthesia by applying electrodes on the skulls of patients and delivering electrical current. Reynolds performed surgery in rats by stimulating the region of the midbrain central gray matter with chronically implanted electrodes. Exploratory laparotomy was carried out in these animals during continuous brain stimulation without the use of chemical anesthetics. Reynolds concluded that focal brain stimulation in this region can induce analgesia in the absence of diffusely applied "whole brain" stimulation (17).

David Mayer, a collaborator of John Liebeskind of the University of California at Los Angeles, heard one of Reynolds' presentations and, with Liebeskind and Akil, repeated and expanded this line of research (18). Mayer and Liebeskind in 1974 published a paper that was critically important for developments in this field (19). To the phenomenon of analgesia obtained by electrical stimulation of discrete cerebral areas, they added, among others, the following evidence:

1. Only stimulation of the mesencephalic central gray matter greatly reduced or totally abolished responsiveness to all noxious stimuli employed.
2. Stimulation of central and periventral gray matter produced analgesia equal or greater than 10 mg/kg morphine on all tests.
3. They proposed that focal electrical stimulation activated a pain suppressive system concentrated in periaqueductal regions and its activation reduced responsiveness to noxious stimuli, at least in part, by blocking transmission of nociceptive transmission of noxious information through the spinal cord.

In the early 1970s, another group of researchers greatly contributed to the discovery of descending analgesic system. They are G.L. Oliveras, G. Guilbaud and J.M. Besson. Their first important work on this subject was published in 1974 (20).

The rationale for this research has to be found again in the classical work of Reynolds and in the following studies of Mayer. The evidence is that "midbrain stimulation in chronically implanted, awake cats in the vicinity raphe nucleus evoked profound analgesia to peripherally applied noxious stimulus". Furthermore, the induced analgesia varied: at times it involved the entire animal, while on other occasions it involved only the posterior trunk of the animal. It was also noted that the "stimulation of wide regions of midbrain inhibited pain-evoked activity in most lamina V without affecting response of lamina IV cells. In the same lamina V cells, midbrain stimulation inhibited responses to noxious but not innocuous stimuli". This paper is the first that describes the specificity of the bulbo-mesencefalic analgesic controlling system. The research that followed better delineated the role and the understanding of the neurophysiology of the bulbo-mesencephalic-spinal system in controlling acute pain.

In 1978, Basbaum and Fields (21) described for the first time the endogenous modulating systems of the nociceptive afference by extrapolating the concepts from the knowledge on anatomy, physiology, and pharmacology of neuronal networks involved in the transmission of the nociceptive input. The analgesic system, which appeared to be very complex, was triggered by electric stimulation of circumscribed sites of the midbrain. This system appeared to be organized in three levels of the central nervous system: the mesencephalous, the bulb and the spinal cord. Since that first paper, the authors emphasized that, between the numerous centers involved, the important fulcrum of the whole system was represented by the periaqueductal gray (PAG) matter, which can be activated not only by electric stimuli, but also by opioids and possibly psychological stimuli.

John Bonica wrote soon after, "The recently acquired new knowledge on the modulation of pain is considered by some to constitute the most important recent advance in the field of pain research and among the important and exciting in the entire field of biomedical research" (22). More recently, Basbaum and Fields (23) wrote an accurate and extensive review of the neurotransmitter systems involved in pain modulation.

Thalamic integration and thalamocortical interactions

Which cortical and subcortical structures participate in this extremely complex system of homeostasis? (24). Jones and Powell wrote in 1973: "Presently no one believes that painful sensation can become conscious at the thalamic level. Therefore, our attention must concentrate on the thalamo-cortical projections. It is well known that the neospinothalamic tract projects from the nucleus ventro-posterolateral of the thalamus to the area 3 B of the cortex. The fibers of the paleospinothalamic tract, instead, diffusely project from the nucleus ventro anterior of the thalamus to the entire cortex. As the somatic sensory cortex consists of two main subdivisions (SI and SII) each containing a detailed representation of all or half of the surface of the body a reasonable postulate was that each received separate thalamic input" (25).

We wish to emphasize that the thalamus has also an antinociceptive function. On this subject Willis wrote: "It is believed that the reticular neurons of the nucleus serve as inhibitory interneurons. There have been a number of reports that some neurons in the reticular nucleus respond to or are inhibited by noxious somatosensory stimuli. The thalamic reticular nucleus could serve an important function as the source of inhibitory modulation of nociceptive responses in the thalamus" (26). Therefore, the functions of the thalamus are not only that of a simple relay but also of integration and inhibition of pain sensation.

The role of the cerebral cortex

Canavero, Pagni and coworkers (27) studied the effects of noxious stimuli on SI cortical neurons to document the existence and location of neurons in the somatosensory cortex that receive and process nociceptive information. It is proposed that these cortical nociceptive neurons with large receptive fields subserve an arousal function rather than the sensory-discriminative aspects of pain. Therefore, they provide for that awakening of the conscience necessary to accept the nociceptive information. Currently the study of the cortical and subcortical centers involved in the perception of pain and its control can be carried out directly in humans by means of PET and SPECT.

In this excellent article the authors discussed five patients suffering from central pain syndrome (CPS) of different origin. It is a widely held view that this pain is sensed in the thalamus. The role of the cortex, especially the parietal somatosensory areas, is uncertain, so much so that a clinical tenet holds that "stimulation of any cortical areas in normal, alert human beings does not produce pain" (28). Canavero and coworkers formulated a fascinating theory: that a reverbatory circuit exists between cortex and (possibly) thalamus. The role of cortex would be modulatory and, in fact, pain sensation would arise subcortically. Thus, the cortex would act more as an inhibitor (with disinhibition causing pain) rather than as a localizer.

From the brain to the mind

We can say that pain is a complex mental phenomenon evoked by nociception (29).

If the areas of our brain cannot be activated and become refractory to receive neuronal communication, the transition from nociception and pain does not occur. Nociception remains blocked in the thalamus and is not received by the cortex. This happens under general anesthesia or when a person loses consciousness.

There are particular mental states, such as a major distraction caused by events that are of great interest to the individual (the classical example of the soldier in battle) that can alter the level of algic threshold up to analgesia. In contrast, focusing the attention on the algogenic area, as it happens for instance at night, can lower the threshold and therefore cause hypersensitivity to pain.

In 1988, Tiengo during his lecture presented at the symposium "Highlight on Pain and Suffering", which took place in Lugano, Switzerland, proposed the "Mirror Metaphor". An object is reflected in a mirror. The image reflected may appear of a different size than the real object. This is determined by the sense and the curvature of the reflecting surface: the image will appear smaller if the mirror is convex, magnified if concave. In the metaphor, the real object is the nociception. The reflected image is the pain. The factors that determine the sense and the curvature of the mirror (and therefore the dimensions of the reflected image) represent the cognitive, emotional and other general mental factors that influence the level of sensory and algic threshold. Pain, therefore, is metaphorically the reflection of nociception which can be accurate or altered.

What hypothesis could we propose regarding the passage from a CNS event (nociception) to a mental event (pain)? This implicates not only neurophysiological and neurochemical phenomena but also neurophilosophical and psychological (attention, distraction, anxiety, fear, panic, stress) considerations: in a word "mental" activity.

One of the most famous philosophers and scientists of our century, Karl Popper, wrote extensively on the mutual intercourse between brain and mind. His diagram used to represent the dualistic theory (the brain and the mind are not the same thing) which he contrasted to the concept developed by the supporters of the monadic theory (brain and mind are the same "thing") is famous. Based on present knowledge, both hypotheses are admissable.

The neurobiologist, Jean Pierre Changeux, is the promoter of the monadic hypothesis (30). This hypothesis speculates that small local neural circuits unite to form larger and larger networks which become increasingly more complex and reach enormous dimensions (millions of cells) which Changeaux calls neuronal assembly. From their activity more complex functions are generated. In areas of the cortex, for instance in the frontal lobes that in man reach exceptional proportions, the assemblies unite to form an assembly of assemblies (billion of cells). Changeux believes that from the activities of these enormous groups of interactive neurons the higher intellectual functions such as learning, memory, reasoning, and behaviour are born. These activities are the realm of the conscience and the mind.

The prime supporter of the dualistic hypothesis is Sir John Eccles, Nobel Laureate for Physiology and Medicine in 1962. He has proposed a neurophilosophical hypothesis which is derived from solid neurophysiologic bases and that represent the biologic version of Popper's hypothesis. According to Eccles (31), nociceptive impulses enter the pyramidal cells of the somatosensory cortex. Several hundred dendrites of pyramidal cells unite to form a sheaf. This structural unit, which projects toward the most superficial laminae of the cortex, has been called a "dendrone". The function of the pyramidal cells is to modulate the sensory afferents. Eccles further hypothesizes that the dendrone is surrounded by a "psychone" an immaterial (nonanatomical) structure which has the property of modulating the dendrone (32). The interaction between the dendrone and the psychone occurs, according to Eccles, through immaterial fields analogous to the interactions in quantum physics. The dendrone can be identified in Word 1 of Popper's hypothesis; in other words, the brain, while the psychoma would be the biological reality of Word 2 which includes thoughts, recollections, imagination, dreams, emotions, perceptions and even pain. The passage from nociception to pain would occur from the interactive communication between the dendrone and the psychone.

The other side of modulation

Up to this point we have described the research which has contributed to the elucidation of the CNS's endogenous analgesic systems. The nervous system, however, also has another function, which is much more powerful and clinically significant: the ability of amplifying the intensity of a peripheral stimulus. After prolonged noxious stimuli both the peripheral and central nervous system undergo significant changes which lead to the development of allodynia and hyperalgesia. These effects are easily seen during inflammation and tissue trauma, phenomena which occurs routinely in the postoperative period. Postoperative pain is mostly caused by allodynia and hyperalgesia induced by changes which, after tissue damage, occur both at the site of injury (sensitization of nociceptors) and in the CNS. Changes in the CNS are due to its plasticity. Neuroplasticity was first described by George Washington Crile (33), a surgeon who, in 1914, wrote: "The lesion which produces the painful scar is in the brain, not at the site of the wound... a strong traumatic or psychic stimulus produces some changes in the conductivities somewhere in its cerebral arc, the effect of which is to lower the threshold of that arc... and hence from that time on mere trifles become adequate stimuli. Now if an operation be so performed that no strong stimulus reaches the brain, either during or after the operation, then the threshold... will not be lowered... [C]ontact with the scar or any injury to that part will have little more effect than will contact with any other part of the body. Hence we see how painful scars may be minimized or prevented by complete anoci-association". Crile not only described neuroplasticity but devised a technique, which he called anoci-association (meaning free of noxious stimuli), to abort its development. He used a combination of perioperative treatments to prevent not only strong noxious stimuli but also psychic stimuli (such as those produced by severe anxiety and fear) to reach the CNS. They included pre-operative morphine and scopolamine to decrease preoperative pain and anxiety, general anesthesia with nitrous oxide and oxygen to prevent intraoperative apprehension, and infiltration of the skin, muscles and fascia with local anesthetic before surgical incision and manipulation to prevent noxious stimuli to be generated and reach the CNS. To prevent postoperative pain, he infiltrated the perioperative site with a solution which blocked postoperative nociception for 2-3 days. This concept was not espoused by the medical establishment of the time and was completely forgotten for several decades.

Bonica (34) not only reproposed the concept but also emphasized the deleterious effects that intense, unrelieved acute pain has on the organism. These concepts were, again, not accepted by the medical establishment. In the 1960s and 1970s, several basic studies illustrated the general concept of neuroplasticity and, in 1976 Morpurgo and Spinelli (35, 36) described neuroplasticity induced by nociception which was further elucidated by Morpurgo in 1979 (37). Their observations, like Crile's, were made on the brain. Since then, many other basic research papers have substantiated the concepts of neuroplasticity, at least in the spinal cord (38-41).

On the basis of these laboratory studies, several clinical studies have been published which report on simpler forms of Crile's anoci-association techniques, which have recently been called *pre-emptive analgesia*. It is one of authors' (CB) opinion that a more correct term should be *pre-emptive antinociception or anociception* since analgesia refers to the lack of pain sensation, which is a cortical process, while the true effect of the technique is to prevent nociception from reaching the CNS, as rightly described and designated by Crile.

Pre-emptive antinociception

Clinical evidence supporting pre-emptive antinociception started to reappear in the clinical literature in the late 1980s. Bach et al. (42) reported in 1988 that pre-emptive antinociception is very effective in preventing phantom pain. Twenty-five patients with severe, persistent pain in the lower extremities caused by peripheral vascular disease and scheduled for amputation were divided into two groups. One group received continuous lumbar epidural block for 72 h before amputation, while the control group was treated with analgesics on a PRN basis. Amputation was performed under spinal or epidural analgesia. In the control group, phantom pain was present in 38% of the patients 6 months after the amputation, and in 27% after a year, while in the treated group, the incidence was 0% both at 6 and 12 months after amputation. McQuay et al. (43) reported that patients who had undergone orthopedic surgery and had received preoperative analgesic treatment requested postoperative analgesic significantly later than those who had not.

Since these reports, some studies have substantiated the concept of pre-emptive antinociception for decreasing postoperative pain, while others have failed to do so (44-48). We will review several studies with positive results. In 1990, Tzerskoy et al. (49) clearly showed that the infiltration of local anesthetic before the surgical incision dramatically decreases postoperative pain associated with herniorrhaphy. In a similar study, Jebeles et al. (50) reported that the infiltration of bupivacaine, after the induction of general anesthesia, but before tonsillectomy, significantly decreased postoperative pain.

Katz et al. (51) in 1992 compared the effect of pre- vs postincision fentanyl on postoperative pain. Thirty patients undergoing elective thoracic surgery were randomized into two groups of 15 patients each and prospectively studied in a double-blind manner. One group received the fentanyl 15 min before the incision while the other group received it 15 min after the incision. While the pain scores were similar between the two groups, the group which received the epidural fentanyl before the incision used less opioids than the other group. Shir et al. (52) reported in 1994 the effect of epidural block versus general anesthesia on postoperative pain and analgesic requirements in patients undergoing radical prostatectomy. They found that patients under epidural anesthesia needed significantly less intravenous opioids on day 2 and 3 post-surgery and had less postoperative pain than patients receiving general anesthesia.

These represent just a few of several studies that indicate that preoperative analgesic intervention can prevent or at least decrease the changes which occur in the CNS responsible for a hyperalgesic state. It should be noted, however, that pre-emptive antinociception, as described in these and other studies, causes a variable decrease of postoperative pain which, in most cases, is not clinically significant (53). The reasons for this weak response may be multiple. Most important is that these studies attempted to control nociception only during surgery and not during the entire perioperative period and the control, in many cases, was only partial.

Conclusions

The general meaning of the term modulation in neurophysiology is that of a change or alteration of the original impulse generated by a stimulus as it travels from its point of origin to its point of arrival. With regard to nociception, modulation implies not only a decrease or blockage of the nociceptive impulses, but also a sensitization of the nervous system to the point that non-noxious stimuli are transduced as noxious impulses. In looking for practical clinical applications of present neurophysiological knowledge we are learning that we can intervene by altering the modulating system at two different sites. One implies the activation of the endogenous analgesic systems. Presently this is done by using specific medications (opioids, nonsteroidal anti-inflammatory drugs) which carry associated bothersome side effects (54). The other approach consists of inactivating the modulating systems which cause sensitization of the nociceptive system as we have just described. As we learn more about the fine details of the modulation systems subserving acute nociception and pain, new therapeutic modalities will be developed to provide pain relief with no side effects.

Acknowledgment. The author would like to thank Professor Marshall Devor for his helpful suggestions and references.

References

1. Tiengo M (1994) Dolore, analgesia endogena ed il sistema della coscienza, Seminari sul dolore. Ed Mattioli, Parma, vol III;2:3-7
2. Melzack R (1961) The perception of pain. Sci Am 204:41 49
3. Melzack R, Casev KL (1868) Sensory, motivational and central control determinants of pain. A new conceptual model. In: Kenshalol D (ed) The skin senses. Thomas, Springfield
4. Yeager MP, Glass DD, Neff RK, Bronk-Johnson T (1987) Epidural anesthesia and analgesia in high risk surgical patients. Anesthesiology 66:729-736
5. Truman KJ, McCarthy RJ, March RJ et al (1991) Effects of epidural anesthesia and analgesia on coagulation and outcome after major vascular surgery. Anesth Analg 73:696-704
6. Zimmerman M (1995) Fisiopatologia del dolore. In: M Tiengo e M Zoppi, Guarire dal dolore, Biblioteca Universale Rizzoli, BUR, Milano, pp 11-62
7. Melzack R, Wall P (1965) Pain mechanism: a new theory. Science 150:971-978
8. Muller J (1837) Handbuch der Physiology des Menschen für Vorlesungen. In: Buch V, Von den Sinnen, VV Abschmtt. Von Gefühlssinn, Verlag J Hoschler, Coblenz, pp 494-502
9. Von Frey Max (1896) Untersuchungen uber der Menschlichen Haut. Erste Abhandlung Druckempfindung und Schmerz, N° III, S Hirzel, Leipzig
10. Sherrington CS (1906) The integrative action of the nervous system. Scribner, New York
11. Sherrington CS (1898) Decerebrate rigidity and reflex co-ordination of movements. J Physiol 17-211
12. Eccles JC, Sherrington CS (1931) Studies on the flexor reflex, IV. Inhibition. Proc Roy Soc 109,91

13. Magoun HV (1944) Bulbar inhibition and facilitation of motor activity. Science 100:540-550
14. Moruzzi G, Magoun HV (1949) Brain stem reticular formation and activation of EEG, electroenceph. Clin Neurophysiol 1;455
15. Hagbarth KE, Kerr DIB (1954) Central influence on spinal afferent conduction. J Neurophysiol 17:295-307
16. Melzack R, Stotler WA, Livingston WK (1958) Effects of discrete brain stem lesions in cats on perception of noxious stimulation. J Neurophysiol 21:353-357
17. Reynolds DV (1968) Surgery in the rat during electrical analgesia induced by focal brain stimulation. Science 164:444-5
18. Mayer DJ, Wolfe TL, Akil H, Carder B, Liebeskind JC (1971) Analgesia from electrical simulation in the brain stem of the rat. Science 174:1351-1354
19. Mayer DJ, Liebeskind JJ (1974) Pain reduction by focal electrical stimulation of the brain: an anatomical and behavioral analysis. Brain Res 68:73-93
20. Oliveras GL, Guilbaud G, Besson JM, Liebeskind JC (1974) Behavioral and electrophysiological evidence of pain inhibition from midbrain stimulation in the cat. Exp Brain Res 20:32-44
21. Basbaum A, Fields H (1978) Endogenous pain control mechanisms: review and hypothesis. Ann Neurol 4:451-462
22. Bonica J (1981) Achievements of the past and challenge of the future. In: Bonica JJ, Lindbolm U, Iggo A (eds) Proceedings of the Third World Congress on Pain, Advances in Pain Research, vol 5, Edinburgh
23. Basbaum A, Fields H (1996) Meccanismi del Sistema Nervoso Centrale della modulazione del dolore. Masson. In: M Tiengo, C Benedetti (eds) Fisiopatologia e Terapia del Dolore
24. Tiengo M, Agnati LF, Zimmermann M (1991) Pain and analgesia: a homeostatic system. Clin J Pain 7 [Suppl 1]
25. Jones E, Powell TPS (1973) Anatomical organization of the somatosensory cortex. In: Iggo A (ed) Handbook of sensory physiology, somatosensory system, vol 2. Springer, Berlin Heidelberg New York, pp 579-620
26. Willis WD (1985) The pain system. Karger, Basel
27. Canavero S, Pagni CA et al (1993) The role of cortex in central pain syndromes: preliminary results of a long-term technetium-99 hexamethylpropylenaminexima single photon emission computed tomography study. Neurosurgery 185-191
28. Adams RD, Victor M (1989) Principle of neurosurgery. Mc Graw Hill, New York
29. Tiengo M (1995) So human the pain. Pathos 2,1:7-8
30. Changeux J-P, Connes A (1989) Matière à Pensée (ed) Odile Jacob, Paris
31. Eccles J (1991) I meccanismi della percezione del dolore: dai recettori sensoriali, alla corteccia cerebrale e da questa alla mente. Seminari sul dolore, 2:5-26
32. Eccles J (1994) Come l'io controlla il suo cervello. Rizzoli, Milano
33. Crile GW (1910) Anoci-association. Saunders, Philadelphia
34. Bonica JJ (953) The management of pain. Lea and Febiger, Philadelphia, pp 1240-244
35. Morpurgo CV, Spinelli DN (1976) Plasticity of pain perception. Brain Theory. 2:14-15 (newsletter)
36. Morpurgo CV, Spinelli DN (1976) Meccanismo di percezione del dolore: una nuova ipotesi. Anestesia e Rianimazione, 17, 2, pp 133-39
37. Morpurgo CV (1979) The role of cerebral cortex in the pain of cancer. In: Bonica JJ (ed) Advances in pain research and therapy. Raven, New York, pp 77-80
38. Woolf CJ (1983) Evidence for a central component of post-injury pain hypersensitivity. Nature, 306, pp 686-88
39. Wall PD (1988) Editorial: the prevention of postoperative pain. Pain 33:289-290
40. Dubner R (1991) Neuronal plasticity and pain following peripheral tissue inflammation on nerve injury. Proceedings of the VIth World Congress on Pain, pp 263-276
41. Cook AJ, Woolf CJ, McMahon SB (1987) Expansion of cutaneous receptive fields of dorsal hom neurones following C-primary afferent fibre inputs. Nature 325:151-53

42. Bach S, Noreng MF, Tjeliden NU (1988) Phantom limb pain in amputees during the first 12 months following limb amputation, after preoperative lumbar epidural blockade. Pain 33: 297-301
43. McQuay HJ, Carroll D, Moore RA (1988) Postoperative orthopedic pain the effect of opiate premedication and local anesthetic blocks. Pain 33:291-95
44. Rice LS, Pudimat MA, Hannallack RS (1990) Timing of caudal block placement in relation to surgery does not affect duration of postoperative analgesia in paediatric ambulatory patients. Br J Anaesth 70:434-439
45. Dierking G, Dahl JB, Kanstrup J, Dahl AA, Kehiet H (1992) The effect of pre- versus postoperative inguinal field block on postoperative pain after hemiotomy. Br J Anaesth 68: 344-348
46. Gustafsson I, Nystrom E, Quiding H (1983) Effect of preoperative paracetamol on pain after oral surgery. Eur J Clin Pharmacol 24:63-65
47. Sisk AL, Mosley RO, Martin RP (1989) Comparison of preoperative and postoperative diflunisal for suppression of postoperative pain. J Oral Maxillofac Surg 4;7:464-468
48. Murphy DF, Medley C (1993) Preoperative indomethacin for pain relief after thoracotomy: Comparison with postoperative indomethacin. Br J Anesth 70:298-300
49. Tverskoy M, Cozacov C, Ayache M, Bradley Jr EL, Kissin I (1990) Postoperative pain after inguinal hereniorraphy with different types of anesthesia. Anesth Analg 70:29-35
50. Jebeles JA, Reilly JS, Gutierrez JR, Bradley Jr EL, Kissin I (1991) The effect of pre-incisional infiltration of tonsils with bupivacaine on the pain following tonsillectomy under general anesthesia. Pain 47:305-308
51. Katz J, Kavanagh H, Sandier AN, Nierenberg H, Boylan JF, Friedlander M, Shaw BF (1992) Preemptive analgesia: Clinical evidence of neuroplasticity contributing to postoperative pain. Anesthesiology 77:739-746
52. Shir Y, Raja SN, Frank SM (1994) The effect of epidural versus general anesthesia on postoperative pain and analgesic requirements in patients undergoing radical prostatectomy. Anesthesiology 80;1:49-56
53. Dahl JB, Kehlet H (1993) The value of pre-emptive analgesia in the treatment of postoperative pain. Br J Anaesth 70:434-439
54. Benedetti C (1990) Acute pain: a review of its effects and therapy with systemic opioids. In: Benedetti C, Chapman CR, Giron G (eds) Advances in pain research and therapy. Raven, New York, pp 367-424

HOMEOSTASIS

Lactic Acidosis: Diagnosis and Treatment

J.-L. VINCENT

Introduction

Measurements of blood lactate levels can be very useful for detecting the presence of tissue underperfusion and for guiding therapy. Increased blood lactate levels usually reflect an imbalance between the oxygen demand and the oxygen supply to the cells, but other conditions may also be responsible. The present chapter first reviews the biochemistry of blood lactate, then reviews the clinical conditions associated with hyperlactatemia and finally discusses some therapeutic implications.

Lactate metabolism

Lactate can only be transformed into and formed from pyruvate (Eq. 1). Pyruvate, however, has three metabolic pathways: glycolysis or gluconeogenesis; alanine transamination; and the Krebs cycle in mitochondria. In effect, glycolysis accounts for 85% of lactate production and the amino acid metabolism for 15%.

$$lactate + NAD^+ \leftrightarrow pyruvate + NADH + H^+$$

thus
$$lactate = K^+ \cdot [pyruvate] \cdot H^+ \cdot [NADH/NAD^+] \qquad [1]$$

Oxygen supply deficiency blocks the Krebs cycle metabolism and as such is the principal cause of pyruvate accumulation. There are only two molecules of ATP per molecule of glucose in such conditions. In hypoxic states, the constant reoxidation of NADH into NAD in the mitochondria is interrupted, so that the lactate/pyruvate ratio increases.

Lactic acidosis is not the same as hyperlactatemia

While hyperlactatemia refers to elevated blood levels of lactate, lactic acidosis describes metabolic acidosis with accumulation of both lactate and H^+ ions.

Interestingly, the formation of lactate from glucose neither utilizes nor produces H^+, as illustrated:

$$\text{glucose} + 2\text{ ATP} \rightarrow \text{fructose 1, 6 P} + 2\text{ ADP} + 2\text{ H}^+$$
$$\text{fructose 1, 6 P} \rightarrow 2\text{ D-glyceraldehyde-3 P}$$
$$2\text{ D-glyceraldehyde-3P} + 4\text{ ADP} + 2\text{ Pi} + 2\text{ H}^+ \rightarrow 2\text{ lactate} + 4\text{ ATP}$$

$$\text{glucose} + 2\text{ ADP} + 2\text{ Pi} \rightarrow 2\text{ lactate} + 2\text{ ATP} \qquad [2]$$

In the absence of oxygen deficiency, metabolites of ATP are recycled without acidosis. The myokinase (or adenylate kinase) reaction can take part in the formation of acidosis as shown:

$$\text{ADP} + \text{ADP} \rightarrow \text{ATP} + \text{AMP}$$
$$\text{ATP} \rightarrow \text{ADP} + \text{Pi} + \text{H}^+ + \text{energy}$$

hence $\qquad\qquad \text{ADP} \rightarrow \text{AMP} + \text{Pi} + \text{H}^+ + \text{energy} \qquad\qquad [3]$

The lactate/OH^- exchange facilitates metabolic acidosis following lactate production. It is a cellular membrane mechanism in which the cellular entry of OH^- prevents intracellular acidosis while H^+ is simultaneously released from H_2O.

Nevertheless, progressive reduction of blood flow in experiments provokes the onset of hyperlactatemia and the onset of acidosis simultaneously (as revealed by increases in arterio-venous pH and PCO_2 gradients) (1).

The distinction between hyperlactatemia and lactatemia has not been shown to be useful clinically. It can only explain the rather poor relation between the degree of metabolic acidosis (e.g. base deficit) and the blood lactate level.

Acidemia does not necessarily follow from lactate acidosis since hyperventilation often compensates for metabolic acidosis, thereby preventing a decrease in pH. Base deficit is as good a prognostic indicator as lactate in trauma patients, provided that there is no other acid/base disorder. However, the correlation between lactate and base deficit is not very effective in patients who have other complications - especially renal failure.

The anion gap is commonly used as a screening test for hyperlactatemia, but the relation between lactate levels and the anion gap is also quite weak (2). In 56 adult surgical ICU patients, Iberti et al. analyzed the concurrence of anion gaps with peak blood lactate levels $> = 2.5$ mmol/l. In 57% of patients, elevated lactate was not accompanied by a widened anion gap, demonstrating the ineffectiveness of this technique. They proposed, accordingly, that the differential diagnosis of nonanion gap acidosis should also include hyperlactatemia.

The effect of pH on lactate production

One would expect, according to Eq. 1, that intracellular acidosis should increase the lactate/pyruvate ratio and thereby increase the lactate concentration. Nevertheless, several factors prevent this from happening:

1. *The effect of H^+ is only moderate.*
2. *There is a much more marked effect of pH on intracellular enzymes.* As pH decreases, phosphofructokinase, in particular, serves as an important negative feedback on adrenergic glycolysis.
3. *The intracellular content in H^+ can be limited.* H^+ content can be limited by the increased production of lactate via the lactate/OH^- exchange system in the cell membrane.

The origins of hyperlactatemia

For a long time, the Cohen and Woods classification was considered as the "classic" reference for hyperlactatemia. This classification identifies two types:

1. *A-type.* Tissue hypoxia related hyperlactatemia
2. *B-type.* Other mechanisms of hyperlactatemia such as biguanide intoxication or neoplasm

This classification is now outdated: a true B-type is very rare. This is especially the case since biguanide medication was withdrawn, effectively eradicating intoxication of this nature. In addition, hypoxic and metabolic alterations may have mixed origins. Tumors, for example, may induce both increased lactate production and reduced lactate elimination by a metastatic liver.

Consequently, increased lactate levels typically reflect a relative imbalance between the oxygen requirement and supply of the cells. Hyperlactatemia is not readily caused by anemia and hypoxemia because a fall in hemoglobin level can be compensated by an increase in cardiac output or hemoglobin saturation. When oxygen delivery is progressively reduced until a critical level is reached, a classical form of experimental hyperlactatemia is induced (Fig. 1).

Normally, lactate concentration lies in the range 0.8-1.2 mEq/l. During exercise, contracting muscles produce lactate which is then removed by resting muscles (3, 4). Lactate uptake by skeletal muscle is also dependent on blood pH (5, 6). Clearly, blood lactate levels also represent a balance between lactate manufacture and lactate removal.

Manufacture. On average, production is between 15 to 20 mEq/kg/day due to the following main organs: brain, gut, muscle, skin red and blood cells.

Removal. This is mainly due to the liver, primarily through gluconeogenesis (Cori cycle). The kidneys and heart are also responsible, as is hypoxic muscle (7).

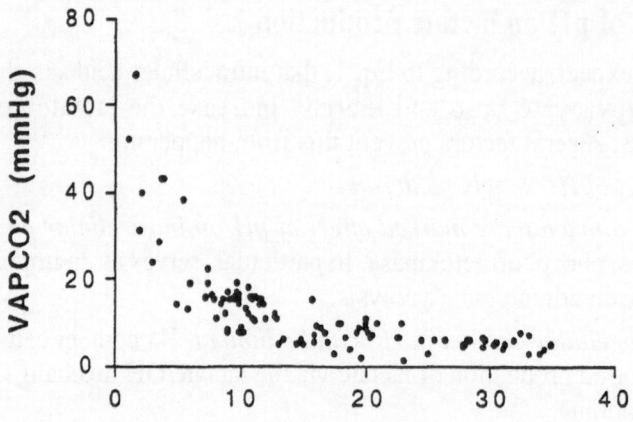

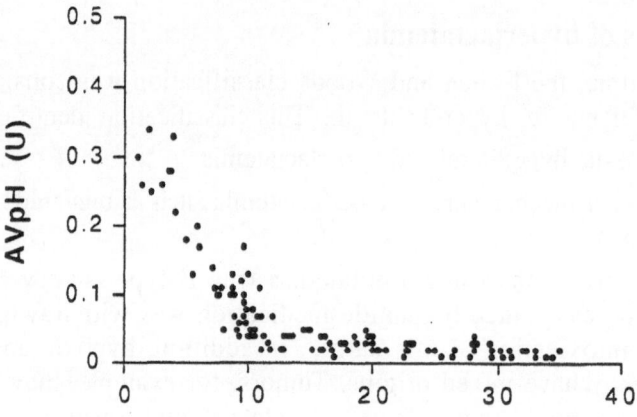

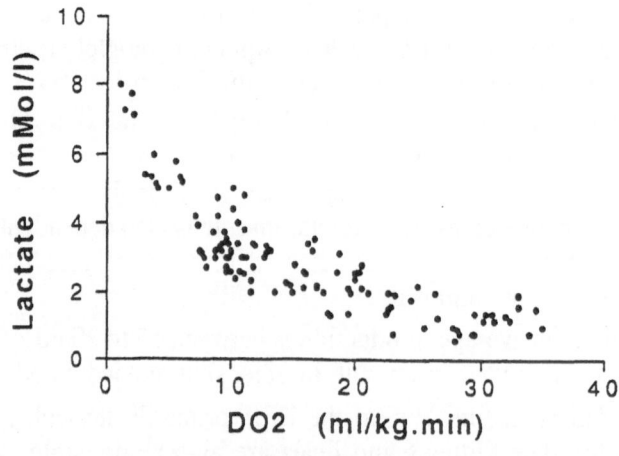

Fig. 1a.

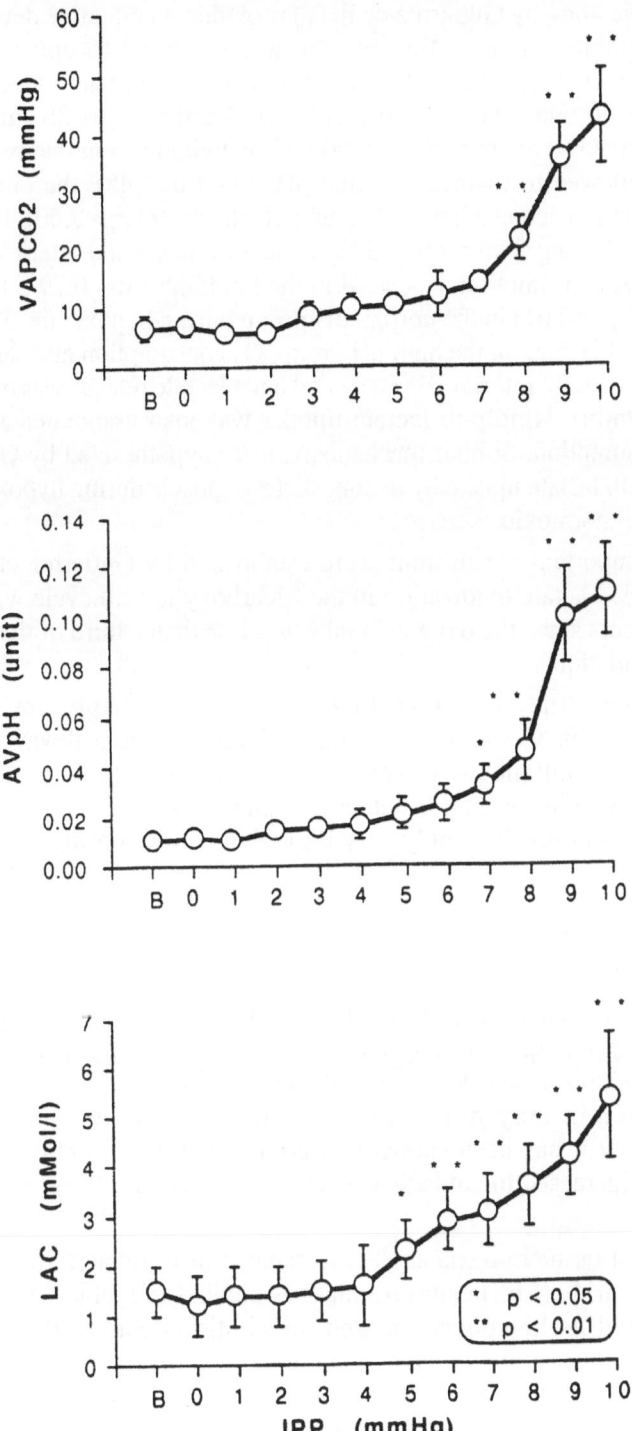

Fig. 1a, b. Relationship between oxygen consumption, oxygen delivery, blood lactate level and venous-arterial PCO_2 differences [from (1)]

The rabbit study by Gutierrez et al. (7) provided an effective demonstration of two major points. First, resting muscle was observed to uptake lactate even during $\dot{V}O_2/DO_2$ dependency. Second, a linear relation was found between pH and glucose uptake. The authors subjected animals to 20 min of arterial hypoxemia (PaO_2 = approx. 20 mmHg) before dividing them into two groups: one group was allowed to maintain normal pH_a (7.40 to 7.45); the other group was hyperventilated to achieve hypocarbia and alkalemia ($pH_a > 7.50$). Lactate uptake was calculated using femoral blood flow measurements and arteriovenous lactate difference. O_2 consumption decreased in the hindlimb from 0.79 ± 0.08 to 0.33 ± 0.06 ml/min ($p < 0.01$) in the normal pH group during hypoxemia. There was also a net uptake of lactate. In the high pH group, O_2 consumption also decreased (0.49 ± 0.06 to 0.24 ± 0.02 ml/min, $p < 0.01$) and a net lactate release was exhibited (1.61 ± 1.0 µmol/min). Hindlimb lactate uptake was also associated with elevated glucose consumption. Similar mechanisms were hypothesized by Gutierrez et al. to explain both lactate uptake by resting skeletal muscle during hypoxia and lactate uptake during normoxic exercise.

Several important conclusions were established by Gutierrez et al. based on their findings. Lactate oxidization in the tricarboxylic acid cycle was discounted by these authors since the oxygen uptake was less than a third of that required for complete oxidation.

Furthermore, they remarked that lactate was probably not converted to glycogen since this would have demanded the glycolytic pathway to operate bi-directionally simultaneously (since the hypoxic hindlimb was shown to be consuming both glucose and lactate at the time). Moreover, glycogen formation requires ATP – available in only very limited quantities during hypoxia.

Lactate levels in sepsis

Investigators (7) have recently challenged the traditional concept that tissue hypoxia is the principal cause of elevated lactate levels in sepsis. Although it is known that blood lactate levels are of good prognostic value in septic shock, hyperlactatemia may not always be due to an anaerobic mechanism. Experimentally it has been shown that administration of endotoxin in animals can result in increased blood lactate levels even preceding $\dot{V}O_2/DO_2$ dependency (8).

The role of tissue hypoxia as the mechanism of lactic acidosis during *E. coli* lipopolysaccharide (LPS) endotoxemia was studied in rabbits by Hurtado et al. who compared its hemodynamic and metabolic effects to those induced by decreasing cardiac output with a balloon inflated in the right ventricle. In skeletal muscle there were no differences in PO_2, as measured with a multiwire surface electrode, nor in the concentrations of high energy phosphates in skeletal and cardiac muscle. As a result, Hurtado et al. (8) hypothesized that higher arterial lactate concentration for the LPS-treated group was a direct effect of LPS or of a mediator as opposed to increased levels of tissue hypoxia. Feasible causal mechanisms include the inhibition of one or several enzymatic reactions, such as the ADP/ATP translocases, the creatine kinase reaction or the pyruvate dehydrogenase (9).

Endotoxin administration in animals can increase blood lactate levels by the deactivation of the pyruvate dehydrogenase (PDH) (9). We (10) and others (11, 12) have shown that dichloroacetate (DCA) administration, which activates the PDH, could decrease levels of lactate following endotoxin administration in sepsis, but without significant hemodynamic effect or effect on $\dot{V}O_2$. In a multicentric study, Stacpoole et al. (12) showed that DCA could reduce lactate levels but that this did not alter the outcome. Hence, where lactic acidosis is extremely severe, DCA may be indicated. Nevertheless, the prognosis is usually very poor in such cases.

Many of these findings do not have a clear clinical application since septic patients do not have elevated lactate levels if they are in shock. In addition, the administration of an endotoxin bolus in animals does not necessarily reproduce a satisfactory representation of the complex septic picture in man.

In severe sepsis, mitochondrial function is either unaltered or even improved in some models (13). Other studies have revealed lower lactate levels in septic shock than in hemorrhagic shock both in animals (5) and in patients (14).

Monitoring of blood lactate levels could provide a supplementary index of severity of shock, aid the evaluation of therapeutic success and provide a prognostic gauge during the early clinical course. Rosenberg and Rush (15) compared equivalent scales of tissue oxygen debt in endotoxic and hemorrhagic shock in dogs and demonstrated lower lactate levels in the endotoxic group. They proposed that there is a lack of correlation between oxygen deficit and lactate values in endotoxic shock and therefore questioned the validity of this as a guide in hypovolemic shock. Nevertheless, Vitek and Cowley (14) showed that lactate measurements can be used as a prognostic guide in septic shock providing the survival probability curve is set at lower lactate levels in sepsis than in hypovolemia. In patients with a rapid reversal of shock due to fluid administration, we showed that a fall in lactate levels reached at least 10% within the first hour of treatment. In nonresponders, however, lactacidemia was not significantly affected (16).

In numerous clinical studies a pathological dependence of $\dot{V}O_2$ on DO_2 has been related to the presence of hyperlactatemia where there was no other cause than tissue hypoxia (17-19). Elevated blood lactate levels were related by Haupt et al. to an increase in $\dot{V}O_2$ in response to an increase in DO_2 following fluid administration. In a later study, the same group of investigators studied 54 septic patients who were separated into two subgroups according to the absence or presence of lactic acidosis. The cut-off point was taken as a lactate value of 2.2 mEq/l. When fluid loading or blood transfusion increased oxygen supply, oxygen consumption increased significantly only in those patients with lactic acidosis. In all of 17 patients treated with various doses of dopamine and dobutamine, they observed an increase in oxygen uptake, although it increased more in patients with lactic acidosis than in those without. The stimulating effect of catecholamines on the cellular metabolism (20) was implicated.

In 73 critically ill patients we (19) tested the hypothesis that a fixed but relatively low dose of 5 mcg/kg/min of dobutamine could facilitate the recognition of an oxygen uptake/supply dependency phenomenon. These patients were separated into four groups based on the nature of their acute illness and also according to their lactate levels. Only those cardiac/septic patients with elevated blood lactate levels exhibited increased $\dot{V}O_2$. This suggests that the $\dot{V}O_2/DO_2$ dependency phenomenon is usually associated with the development of increased blood lactate levels with an anaerobic metabolism.

In patients without lactic acidosis, other studies have not recorded $\dot{V}O_2/DO_2$ dependency (21). These observations, taken together, cast doubt on the hypothesis that $\dot{V}O_2/DO_2$ dependency reflects the use of oxygen by the extramitochondrial or non-ATP producing systems.

Factors altering liver function

Alterations in liver function (either acute or chronic) can delay lactate clearance since lactate is primarily metabolized in the liver. However, it is not unusual for patients with acute or severe chronic liver failure to have a blood lactate level which is either normal or only slightly elevated but still below 2 mEq/l. In fact, extreme damage of the liver is necessary before lactate increases markedly. Patients with liver disease and bilirubin > 2 mg/dl were studied by Kruse et al. (22). In the absence of shock, patients had lactate levels in the range 0.6 to 2.0 mEq/l but patients with shock exhibited increased lactate levels of between 1.2 and 30 mEq/l. Hence, increased lactate levels are indicative in patients with liver impairment, but resolution of hyperlactatemia takes more time in these patients.

The prognostic value of lactate levels

The prognostic value of lactate levels in various forms of circulatory shock has been indicated in many studies (16, 23-26), including in the absence of hypotension (27). Important cut-off values can be identified at 4 mEq/l, where there is 50% survival and at > 8 mEq/l, where the mortality rises to 90%. Increased lactate could, in fact, be a marker of persistent underperfusion even when blood pressure has been restored.

Lactate levels have more prognostic value in septic shock than oxygen derived variables such as oxygen delivery and oxygen consumption (28) (Fig. 2).

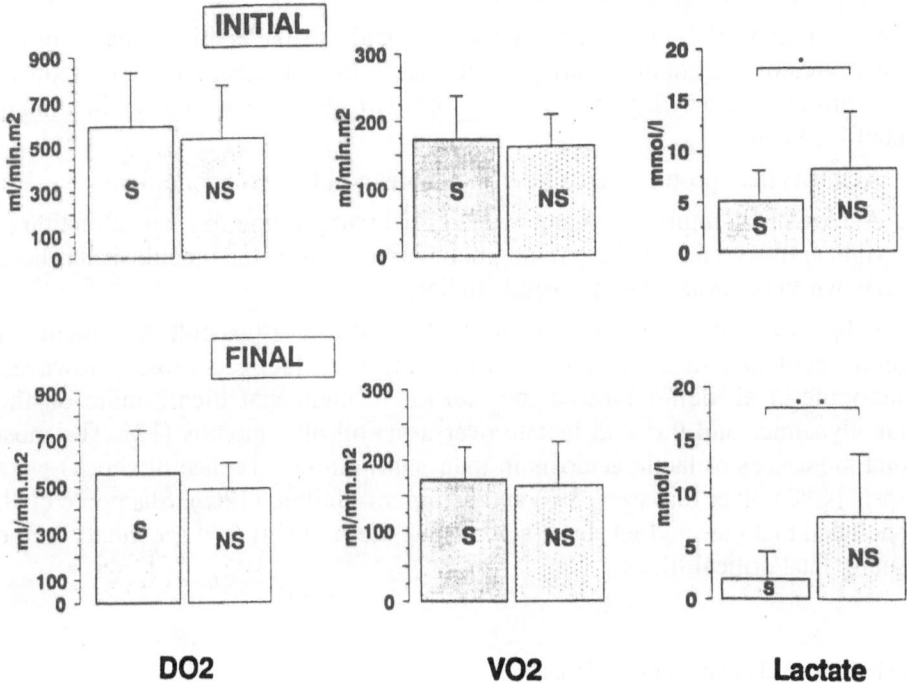

Fig. 2. Values of oxygen consumption ($\dot{V}O_2$), oxygen delivery (DO_2) and blood lactate levels in the survivors and the nonsurvivors from septic shock. Reproduced from (28) with permission

However, it is not only the initial value of lactate which is indicative but also the rate of decline. In those patients who responded well to fluid therapy, we showed that lactate decreased by more than 10% per hour (16). More recently, Bakker et al. (29) demonstrated a link between the time-course of lactate levels and morbidity and mortality. Not only higher initial lactate levels but also more prolonged hyperlactatemia were related to the development of more severe organ dysfunction in their study so that the area under the curve plotted for lactate against time was greater for these patients.

We recommend that in the presence of elevated lactate levels, measurements should be repeated every few hours. If these measurements indicate that there is no rapid decline in lactate, then a more aggressive therapeutic option should be considered. The aim should be to either eradicate the source or to increase the cellular oxygen supply. Further fluid administration and/or dobutamine may be considered as methods of therapy.

Enzymatic techniques offer an easy method for measuring lactate levels using relatively inexpensive material. Lactate levels can be measured together with changes in blood gases using modern technology. Combining these two parameters gives a complete prognostic picture.

When should lactate acidosis be treated?

A worse prognosis is clearly associated with acidosis, but is this the cause or the effect? Acidosis is not necessarily deleterious to the cells, even though it reduces myocardial contractility. Indeed, there are two ways in which acidosis may benefit the cells:

1. Acidosis may protect the cellular metabolism in hypoxic conditions.
2. Acidosis may improve oxygen availability by improving oxygen extraction (a rightshift is seen in the oxyhemoglobin curve). Intracellular acidosis has been shown to be protective in several studies.

It has been suggested that bicarbonate could be a possible treatment for lactate acidosis. In a study of 126 patients with lactic acidosis, however, Stacpoole et al. demonstrated the lack of influence of bicarbonate on the hemodynamics and the acid lactate over a period of 6 months (12). The most common causes of lactic acidosis in their study (in the absence of shock) were sepsis (49%), liver disease (15%) and respiratory failure (12%). Stacpoole et al. concluded that elevated levels of acid lactate are probably just secondary to the usually fatal critical illness.

Table 1. The main causes of hyperlactatemia

Frequent causes
- Circulatory shock/acute circulatory failure:
    * Hypovolemic/traumatic
    * Cardiogenic
    * Obstructive
    * Distributive (sepsis)
- Other forms of oxygen transport deficiency:
    * Acute anemia
    * Severe hypoxemia
    * Cellular hypoxia (e.g., CO intoxication)

Less frequent causes
- Decompensated diabetes
- Intoxications: ethanol, methanol, ethylene-glycol
    * Salicylates
    * Biguanide
    * Cyanide, nitroprussiate
- Expansive malignant tumors, hematologic malignancies
- Fructose or sorbitol-related perfusion abnormalities
- Malnutrition, hypovitaminosis B
- Inherent metabolic deficiencies

N.B.: Hepatic dysfunction can enhance these effects but cannot by itself cause hyperlactatemia.

Conclusion

Frequently observed in critically ill patients, lactic acidosis is associated with a poor prognosis. Severity and persistence are good indicators. Although a number of causes may provoke hyperlactatemia, imbalance between oxygen demand and oxygen supply is by far the most common etiology. Aggressive cardiorespiratory resuscitation is therefore warranted to improve tissue perfusion in lactic acidosis patients. Monitoring of blood lactate levels not only allows evaluation of prognosis but also helps to assess therapeutic effects and to ensure complete cardiorespiratory resuscitation.

References

1. Zhang H, Vincent JL (1993) Arteriovenous differences in PCO_2 and pH are good indicators of critical hypoperfusion. Am Rev Respir Dis 148:867-871
2. Iberti TJ, Leibowitz AB, Papadakos PJ et al (1990) Low sensitivity of the anion gap as a screen to detect hyperlactatemia in critically ill patients. Crit Care Med 18:275-277
3. Poortmans JR, Bossche JD, Leclercq R (1978) Lactate uptake by inactive forearm during progressive leg exercise. J Appl Pysiol 45:835-839
4. Freyschuss U, Strandell T (1967) Limb circulation during arm and leg exercise in supine position. J Appl Physiol 23:163-170
5. Watt PW, MacLennan PA, Hundai HS et al (1988) $L^{(+)}$-Lactate transport in perfused rat skeletal muscle: kinetic characteristics and sensitivity to pH and transport inhibitors. Biochem Biophys Acta 944:213-222
6. Graham TE, Barclay JK, Wilson BA (1986) Skeletal muscle lactate release and glycolytic intermediates during hypercapnia. J Appl Physiol 60:568-575
7. Gutierrez G, Hurtado FJ, Gutierrez AM et al (1993) Net uptake of lactate by rabbit hindlimb during hypoxia. Am Rev Respir Dis 148:1204-1209
8. Hurtado FJ, Gutierrez AM, Silva R et al (1992) Role of tissue hypoxia as the mechanism of lactic acidosis during E. coli endotoxemia. J Appl Physiol 72:1895-1901
9. Vary TC, Siegel JH, Nakatani T et al (1986) Effect of sepsis on activity of pyruvate dehydrogenase complex in skeletal muscle and liver. Am J Physiol 250:E634-E640
10. Preiser JC, Moulart D, Vincent JL (1990) Dichloroacetate administration in the treatment of endotoxin shock. Circ Shock 30:221-228
11. Curtis SE, Cain SM (1992) Regional and systemic oxygen delivery/uptake relations and lactate flux in hyperdynamic endotoxin treated dogs. Am Rev Respir Dis 145:348-354
12. Stacpoole PW, Wright EC, Baumgartner TG et al (1994) Natural history and course of acquired lactic acidosis in adults. Am J Med 97:47-54
13. Mela LM, Miller LD, Nicholas GG (1972) Influence of cellular acidosis and altered cation concentrations on shock-induced mitochondrial damage. Surgery 72:102-110
14. Vitek V, Cowley RA (1971) Blood lactate in the prognosis of various forms of shock. Ann Surg 173:308-313
15. Rosenberg JC, Rush BF (1986) Blood lactic acid levels in irreversible haemorrhagic and lethal endotoxin shock. Surg Gynecol Obstet 126:1247-1250
16. Vincent JL, Dufaye P, Berre J et al (1983) Serial lactate determinations during circulatory shock. Crit Care Med 11:449-451
17. Haupt MT, Gilbert EM, Carlson RW (1985) Fluid loading increases oxygen consumption in septic patients with lactic acidosis. Am Rev Respir Dis 131:912-916
18. Gilbert EM, Haupt MT, Mandanas RY et al (1986) The effect of fluid loading, blood transfusion and catecholamine infusion on oxygen delivery and consumption in patients with sepsis. Am Rev Respir Dis 134:873-878

19. Vincent JL, Roman A, DeBacker D et al (1990) Oxygen uptake/supply dependency: effects of short-term dobutamine infusion. Am Rev Respir Dis 142:2-8
20. Fellows IW, Bennett T, Macdonald IA (1985) The effect of adrenaline upon cardiovascular and metabolic functions in man. Clin Sci 69:215-222
21. Annat G, Viale JP, Percival C et al (1986) Oxygen delivery and uptake in the adult respiratory distress syndrome: lack of relationship when measured independently in patients with normal blood lactate concentrations. Am Rev Respir Dis 133:999-1001
22. Kruse JA, Zaidi SA, Carlson RW (1987) Significance of blood lactate levels in critically ill patients with liver disease. Am J Med 83:77-82
23. Peretz DI, McGregor M, Dosseteur JB (1964) Lactic acidosis: a clinically significant aspect of shock. Can Med Assoc J 90:673-675
24. Peretz DI, Scott HM, Duff J et al (1965) The significance of lactacidemia in the shock syndrome. Ann NY Acad Sci 119:1133-1141
25. Weil MH, Afifi AA (1970) Experimental and clinical studies on lactate and pyruvate as indicators of the severity of acute circulatory failure (shock). Circulation 41:989-1001
26. Bakker J, Leon M, Coffernils M et al (1992) Serial blood lactate levels can predict multiple organ failure in septic shock patients. Crit Care Med 20:S56 (abstr)
27. Aduen J, Bernstein WK, Khastgir T et al (1994) The use and clinical importance of a substrate-specific electrode for rapid determination of blood lactate concentrations. JAMA 272:1678-1685
28. Bakker J, Coffernils M, Leon M et al (1991) Blood lactate levels are superior to oxygen derived variables in predicting outcome in human septic shock. Chest 99:956-962
29. Bakker J, Gris P, Coffernils M et al (1995) Serial blood lactate levels can predict the development of multiple organ failure following septic shock. Am J Surg (in press)

METABOLISM

Immunonutrition - A New Aspect in the Treatment of Critically Ill Patients

S. Bengmark, L. Gianotti

Introduction

The mortality following extensive operations and trauma has decreased considerably during last two decades. The postoperative morbidity remains, however, unacceptably high, especially in burns, after extensive visceral operations, particularly after transplantation, but also in severe liver failure and pancreatitis. A similar development is seen in patients with HIV/AIDS, especially in advanced stages. Infections, sometimes leading to multiple organ failure (MOF), are the dominating cause of postoperative and posttrauma sepsis (POTS). These infections are mainly gram-negative aerobic bacterial, but sometimes of viral, fungal, or protozoal origin.

Most of the septic complications occurring in the visceral organs in POTS relate either to colonization of oropharynx, the tracheobronchial tree, and the whole GI tract, or to translocation of potentially pathogenic microorganisms (PPMs) in the lower GI tract. Microbial translocation is an important etiological factor behind POTS, even in humans. A recent study (1) in donors with a relatively short hospital stay (mean: 1.9 days, range 6 h - 8 days) showed positive cultures in 67%, most often in mesenteric lymph nodes, lungs, liver and spleen. Endotoxin was present in abdominal fluids in approx. 50% of cases, in peripheral blood in approx. 20% and in portal blood in approx. 10%. These changes obviously occurred early and before any light or electron microscopical changes could be demonstrated in the intestinal wall. This is in line with the observations made by McDonald et al. (2) of an increased intestinal permeability as early as 16-20 h after moderate burns. A fourfold increase in lactulose absorbtion and a threefold increase in lactulose/mannitol ratio was reported. The first peak in serum endotoxin has been described to occur as early as 12 h after burns (3). As a single dose of endotoxin to healthy humans immediately and significantly increases intestinal permeability (4), it is likely that the intestinal permeability is increased already at that time.

Incidences of POTS in the groups of patients mentioned above are often reported in the literature to be as high as 25%-50%. For review, see (5). It has been estimated that each year, in the US alone more than one hundred thousand hospitalized patients develop serious gram-negative bacteriemia - some sources claim up to four hundred thousand. It is not unlikely that the numbers are twice as high in Europe, with its twice as large population. In the whole world most probably more that one million patients will die each year due to POTS. For review, see (6). As pointed out by Burd et al., the outcome has not changed much in recent years. "Although a myriad of treatment modalities, including antibiotic therapy have been tried the lethality in this group remains high - more than 10 per cent in immunologically intact individuals and over 30 per cent in immuno-compromized patients" (6). These authors conclude that "it has been increasingly evident that refining the use of currently available therapeutic modalities may not further reduce mortality".

There is an urgent need of new treatment concepts - new treatment modalities.

Early intervention is most important

The presence or absence of gastric intramucosal acidosis during the first 12 h after trauma is predictive of outcome (7); a low pH on admission remaining low at 12 h was associated with an 87% mortality rate, compared to 36% if intramucosal pH had returned to normal after 12 h, and 27% if normal on admission and remaining normal at 12 h. Deranged gastric intramucosal pH reflects poor oxygenation. It can be assumed that what happens to the stomach is representative for the whole GI tract, and most likely also the solid organs, particularly the liver. This will most likely greatly influence the metabolic functions and the resistance to POTS. Splanchnic ischemia is an important etiological factor behind POTS and an important cause of MOF (8).

Before considering active measures to stimulate the immune system of the sick, or potentially sick patient, it is necessary that the present routines of care are reviewed and those with suppressing effects on the immune system reconsidered. These should include measures to guarantee nourishment of the intestinal mucosa early and effectively, and to guarantee an optimal salivation, gastric acidity and splanchnic circulation. These measures are urgent and should be instituted immediately, if possible already before and during surgery, and always immediately after surgery and trauma. *As 12 h postoperation and trauma (POT) seems an important time point they should be instituted effectively and forcefully in good time before this.*

Early mucosal/enteral nutrition

It was shown in experimental animals already in the early 1970s that the intestinal mucosa on starvation loses a large proportion of its structure and function (9). It is likely that this downregulation occurs as early as within 12-18 h of intestinal starvation, e.g. the time of no-eating traditionally practiced for surgical patients before operation. If so, most surgical patients are presently arriving to OR in a condition of "metabolic handicap". As a consequence they are likely to be more susceptible to splanchnic ischemia and microbial translocation already at the time of operation. The liver, which can store only about 500 kcal, is usually devoid of glycogen at this time. The hepatocyte has no capacity to produce and store glycogen during and immediately after anaesthesia (10). Twenty-four hours of fasting increases translocation after hemorrhagic stress (11), an effect which cannot be prevented by parenteral nutrition - enteral feeding is needed. It is thus recommended that the patients receive carbohydrates parenterally (or orally or by enteral tube-feeding) during the 2-3 h before surgery to restore the glycogen stores, which is shown to considerably increase the insulin sensitivity (12, 13). Enteral feeding should also be given *immediately* after operation or trauma in order to increase mucosal and splanchnic blood flow and prevent microbial translocation. McDonald et al. showed in their study of more than 100 burn patients that immediate (within 6 h) nasogastric tube feeding successfully prevents stress ulcer bleedings and *totally eliminates the need for prophylactic antacids or H₂-blockers* (2).

Maintain active salivation

The saliva "possesses a multiplicity of defence systems for antibacterial warfare that Pentagon can envy" (14). Among these are specific antimicrobial proteins like lysozyme, lactoferrin and lactoperoxidase, but also mucin, IgA, and NO-donating substances such as nitrates (see below). The human saliva also contains mucosa-stimulating EGF, although not in the high concentrations as observed in mice and other species (15). In addition, the preventive bacterial flora in the mouth is of the greatest importance for defence against invading microorganisms. Mucus produced by the salivary glands covers the ingested food and follows the food like a mucosa-preventive shield from the mouth and most probably all the way to the colon. It has been shown in experimental animals that extirpation of salivary glands reduces the content of mucus by approx. 80% as far down as presently studied, the lower oesophagus (16). This decrease can, but only partly, be compensated for by local production; stimulation with EGF increases the amount by approx. 50%. This compensatory function is most likely increased in the lower parts of the GI tract as the density of mucus-producing cells, Goblet cells, increases with distance from the mouth and the salivary glands. Salivary mucins possess properties, which enables them to concentrate on mucosal surfaces, and form an effective barrier against environmental insults (17). Eating dietary fibers stimulates the production of intestinal mucus, and prevents potentially pathogenic microorganisms (PPMs) from getting foothold on the mucosal surfaces throughout the GI tract (18).

The amount of saliva produced per day is considerable: 300 ml per hour on food stimulation, and approx. 25 ml per hour during resting conditions. The role of saliva in sepsis prevention should not be neglected. Unfortunately, it is a treatment practice in anesthesiology and intensive care to decrease or inhibit salivation by supply of drugs. Furthermore, apart from antisecratogogues and anticholinergics, also analgetics, antispasmodics, antidiarrheals, antidepressants, antihistamines, antihypertensives, antiparkinsons, antipsychotics and diuretics have profound salivation inhibitory effects. For further information, see (19). It is important to avoid inhibition of salivation. Should the salivation for some reason be inhibited, it should be remembered that the best drug to stimulate salivation is pilocarpine, 5 mg three times per day increases effectively the salivary output (20). This is especially important in patients suffering from xerostomia, associated with salivary gland dysfunction.

Maintain low gastric pH

One of the most important barriers against invading pathogenic microorganisms is low pH of the stomach (21); a pH under 3.5 is usually bactericidal against most species of microorganisms. The clinical practice in the ICU has for decades been to inhibit the gastric acidity in order to prevent stress ulcerations. This is usually done either by alkalization of the gastric contents or decreasing acid production by administration of histamine 2-blocking agents. Uninterrupted tube-feeding directly into the stomach also contributes to breaking the important acid barrier of the stomach. All these measures facilitate colonization of the stomach, overgrowth with PPMs and retrograde colonization of the pharynx with increased risk of bronchopneumonia and other infections. It must be remembered that McDonald et al. found that early tube-feeding totally eliminates the need for stress ulcer prophylaxis (2). It has been recommended to use mucosa-protecting drugs like sucralfate (22), which does not increase gastric pH. This is most likely unnecessary and not without its risk. Studies in experimental animals have shown that aspirated sucralfate mixed with water leads to lung edema, and mixed with hydrochloric acid to severe lung edema (23). Animal studies in our laboratories showed that an oral supply of membrane lipids, surfactants, alone or combined with pectin, offers equally good protection but without side effects. Surfactants occur normally in the respiratory tract and participate in the protection also of the bronchial and alveolar membranes - for review, see (24). The enteral route of tube-feeding has several advantages over the gastric and should be used routinely (see below). However, should for some reason the gastric route be chosen, it seems important to feed intermittently and allow the pH to come down in between the feeding episodes (25).

Supply nitric oxide-donating substances

It is known that inhibition of both the inducible and the constitutive forms of nitric oxide (NO) increases mortality in animal endotoxin models. However, inhibition of only the inducible form has been proven to be protective (26). These observations have led to the most interesting suggestion: that NO released by constitutive enzymes exerts a protective role, at least in septic shock. This favors a vasodilator tone and maintains a good blood flow to the visceral organs, which is clinically important in the management of POT. Methylene blue has been described as a safe option to counteract the malignant effects of NO and to support "the good NO" effects, such as visceral blood flow stimulation, scavenging of free radicals and the most important microbiocidal effects (27-29). The decrease in splanchnic blood flow, regularly seen after burns, can also be pharmacologically improved by supply of another NO-donating substance, nitroprusside, which is shown to prevent microbial translocation (30). It is clear that the different NO actions are highly nutrition-dependent and most often limited by lack of substrates.

Interest has recently been focussed on dietary nitrate as an important NO-donating substance. For many years nitrate in food has been regarded as harmful, due to the risk of producing N-nitroso compounds and the risk of inducing GI cancer. Meat producers, vegetable growers and water companies have been under pressure to reduce the nitrate content. Epidemiological studies in humans have, however, failed to demonstrate an association between nutritional nitrate and gastric cancer (31, 32). Nigel Benjamin and coworkers have in two recent articles in *Nature* and *Nature Medicine* described an important enterosalivary circulation of dietary nitrate. Ingested nitrate (or nitrate produced in the body - nitrate is an important by-product of bacterial fermentation) is secreted by salivary glands. At the surface of the posterior third of the tongue the nitrate is reduced to nitrite by facultative anaerobic bacteria, a function which is not present in germ-free animals and significantly reduced by antibiotic therapy (34). Benjamin et al. (33) showed that nitrite increases tenfold compared to plasma following ingestion of 200 mg of nitrite, e.g. from a mean of 111 nM to 1030 nM. Nitrite, when acidified in the stomach at pH of approx. 2, produces NO to a concentration of about 600 nM, which is several orders of magnitude greater than required for stimulation of mucosal blood flow, mucus formation, to influence motility and for bacteriostasis (35). Another important function of NO is that it stabilizes gastric mucus through increasing its viscosity (36). It is suggested by Benjamin et al. that acidified nitrite is not only effective against *Candida albicans* and *Escherichia coli*, but also against microorganisms such as *Shigella, Salmonella, Helicobacter pylori*, amoebic dysentery and chronic intestinal parasitism. Swallowed food contains significant quantities of nitrate, especially when containing significant amounts of green vegetables such as lettuce, celery and spinach. The formation of NO is enhanced by the presence of vitamin C and iodine, but is inhibited by omeprazole and other H$_2$-blockers. Omeprazole, furthermore, at least under experimental conditions, degrades vitamin C (37). It has been shown that administration of glutathione eliminates the gastric pH-elevating effect of omeprazole (38) - most likely omeprazole also reduces glutathione levels, one of the most important antioxidants in the body. Furthermore, 4 weeks of omeprazole supply in humans significantly increases bacterial concentrations in gastric aspirates (39). All these observations seem to be important reasons to avoid omeprazole and similar products, at least in severely ill patients. There are also reasons to be as restrictive as possible with supply of antibiotics.

If at all possible, one should consider early oral supply of green vegetables or nitrite.

Enteral nutrition - the new standard

It is today well documented that parenteral nutrition (PN) does not meet the requirements to be an effective tool in the nutritive treatment of POT patients. PN is accompanied by a drastic decrease in secretions of saliva, gastric juice, intestinal juice, but also of bile, all important for the GI function and especially for the antimicrobial defense. Furthermore, also the inability of PN to prevent catabolic states, as much as sepsis, is well documented. A study in a group of sick ICU patients receiving aggressive total parenteral nutrition (TPN) consisting in 2750 kcal and 127 amino acid intake per day – considered optimal nutrition – showed that after 10 days of treatment the patients had lost on average 12.5% of the body protein despite a mean gain of 2.2 kg of body fat (40). A rather recent meta-analysis of the effects of perioperative PN showed minimal effects on complication rates, varying from 12.8% better to 2.3% worse (41).

The main reason for ever using PN is for dealing with the problems of gastric stasis, vomiting and diarrhea sometimes seen in POT patients on oral nutrition. The development of devices for enteral tube-feeding has made routine enteral nutrition (EN) possible in almost all POT patients. Feeding directly into the upper jejunum has the potential not only to eliminate the problems of vomiting and diarrhea, but also to prevent microbial translocation and gut origin sepsis. Enteral tube-feeding is metabolically superior to gastric; the metabolic recovery is faster (42) and the risk of aspiration almost ten times less with enteric tube feeding compared to gastric. However, EN by enteric tube feeding should most probably be complemented with smaller quantities of oral or gastric supply, mainly with the aim to stimulate gastric acid secretion and NO production. For such supply chewing green vegetables should be considered, to begin with only in minimal quantities. Simultaneous intragastric supply of pectin and phospholipids has the potential of providing a good mucosal protection. Table 1 summarizes effects of pectin as reported in the literature. The effects of surfactants have been extensively discussed earlier [see (24, 43)]. As an alternative the unripe banana can be considered, known to very rich in pectin and in surfactant lipids. Due to the risk of clogging, pectin should never be applied via any tube.

Fifty years have passed since it was demonstrated for the first time that EN is superior to PN in POT nutrition. Studies in the 1940s by the groups of Mulholland (44) and of Rhoads (45) showed definite advantages with oral/gastric and needle jejunostomy feeding over PN in POT patients. These observations had seemingly no impact on the practice of nutrition for another 25 years. It was not until the relation between lack of enteral nutrition and postoperative/posttrauma sepsis (POTS) came into focus that the interest in EN became more widespread. It was in the year 1980 that four important publications changed the focus of interest from PN to EN. It was, however, to take another 15-20 years before EN became more widely accepted.

Table 1. Pectin

A general intestinal regulator and detoxifying agent
Carrier in many medical preparations
Standard addition in commercial baby food
Known to have high absorbative effects and high metal binding capacity
Delays gastric emptying
Increases intestinal transit time
Modifies intestinal absorption, especially of glucose
Reduces absorption of cholesterol and bile acids
Increases iron absorption
Decreases vitamin B12 absorption
Increases fecal weight and substance, mainly due to its water-binding capacity
Offers mucosal surface protection - antioxidant against all three main types of oxidation damages: peroxy, superoxide and hydroxyl radicals
Increases intestinal barrier and prevents microbial translocation
Increases production of SCFAs, the main nutrient for the colonic mucosa
Prevents disruption of intestinal microflora
Stimulates immune defense
Increases production of hormones and enzymes
Interferes with intestinal and hepatic lipid metabolism
When given to animals, stimulate milk protein synthesis through secretion of prolactin

---

These were the 1980 observations:

1. Early EN increases mesenteric and hepatic circulation [Shephard (46)].

2. Intestinal mucosa is unable to nourish itself from the blood [Roediger (47)].
   EN is needed as half of the demand of the small intestine and more than 80% of the large intestine must be satisfied by luminal nutrition. Mucosal atrophy is an early development in intestinal starvation, even when the most complete PN is given. Later it has been shown that this predisposes for microbial translocation.

3. EN supports a positive nitrogen balance [Hoover et al. (48)]. A positive nitrogen balance (+12%) was found in patients given EN (by jejunostomy) compared to a negative balance (−45%) in PN treated patients.

4. Increasing protein in EN increases survival [Alexander et al. (49)]. Raising the amount of enteral protein supply from 15% to 23% in children with severe burn injuries increased the survival from 56% to 100%.

With time it has become increasingly obvious that EN is a superior modality of treatment to prevent POTS. The impact of this knowledge on clinical practice has not been profound and quick. During the several years after 1980 there remained a hope that the POTS problems would be dealt with successfully using new modalities of antibiotic treatment, such as selective decontamination (SD), most often used in combination with PN or TPN, for which industry – but also scientists – still had the greatest hope. It took more than another decade to realize that both these treatment modalities had failed as instruments for POT infection control. A recent mega-analysis (50) based on eleven studies and about 1500 patients failed to show any major benefits of SD. *Selective decontamination does not address important aspects of POTS, particularly not the immunological and nutritional.*

A new generation of tubes for jejunal feeding

It has been calculated that 90% of all POT nutrition can be satisfied by EN, PN should only be necessary as a complement and in approximately 10% of cases. Jejunal delivery is clearly superior to gastric (see above). In POT patients the routine should be to use jejunal tube feeding as a standard procedure. It is our opinion that this should be practiced in every case, when and wherever possible. In elective patients a jejunal feeding tube can be introduced during the day before surgery. In emergency cases such a tube can be "milked down" during surgery, or – if not subject to a laparotomy – a PEG tube be introduced. It has been calculated that the need for use of this technology is approximately one million patients per year in the US and most probably twice as many in Europe.

The main obstacles to total transfer to this policy has been the poor performance of the existing tubes. *The spontaneous transpyloric passage (STP) has been too low.* Two randomized studies comparing the most popular feeding tubes on the American and European market have demonstrated an SPT of approximately 35% after 1 day (51) and approximately 70% after 3 days (52). Furthermore, expensive endoscopy or X-ray is often needed to manipulate the tip of the tube down into the upper jejunum. The need of extra and expensive technologies and the costs for extra hospital days has discouraged many practicing physicians from routinely using this technology. This was the reason why one of us (SB 53, 54) developed a selfpropelling feeding tube, based on a completely different principle. After introduction into the stomach with the assistance of a guide wire, this tube propels itself down into the jejunum within minutes, or always within 1-4 h. Apart from having a 4-h STP of more than 95%, this tube has never and can never be regurgitated. The tube is likely to be introduced into the American and European markets within 1 year.

Enteral nutrition - the breakthrough

A series of animal studies performed during the 1980s and early 1990s showed a most remarkable superiority of EN over PN, especially with respect to POT infection control. Several clinical studies gave the same results. A mega-analysis of eight different prospective randomized trials published before 1991 (12) showed that septic complications occurred half as often in EN patients (18%), when instituted after 6-72 h, compared to PN (35%). In several of these studies the EN was introduced rather late. If introduced immediately or early, the results would most likely have been even better. From these studies one can conclude that the best results were obtained in trauma patients, e.g. patients immunologically intact, often young, and – before the accident – almost always healthy individuals. It is in these groups of patients that the great breakthrough of EN has come. Another study comparing EN and PN in patients following abdominal trauma (55) showed astonishingly 76% fewer infections in the EN treated patients. It is important to mention that all the above-mentioned results were obtained with standard formulas, without fiber or special immune-stimulating ingredients. This offers the greatest hope for further progress to be made with further improvement of the nutrition formulas.

Immunonutrition - a new concept

Scrimshaw suggested almost 40 years ago a bidirectional interaction between nutrition, immune response and infectious diseases [cited in (56)]. Deficiencies in almost all nutrients can result in impaired host defense (56). Consequently almost every nutrient has the ability to enhance immune defense. Many of these effects are mediated over cytokines but also over the latest known signaling substance - NO. The availability of recombinant cytokines has increased the feasibility of studying the effect of each cytokine on the nutritional status of the host (57). With an increasing knowledge about NO, the use in clinical medicine of NO-donating substances has become increasingly important. Among the NO donating substances are nitrates, nitrites, glyceryltrinitrate, isosorbide dinitrate, nitrothiols, nitroglycerin, methylene blue, nitroprusside, and molsidomine. The most important or at least most studied is, however, l-arginine.

Arginine has long been known to have anabolic effects: increase the plasma growth hormone level (58), revert catabolism (59), reduce nitrogen excretion (60) and improve healing (61). More recent observations show that arginine also has strong immunostimulatory effects (62), improves natural killer cell activity and expression of Il-2 receptors (63) and constitutes an essential substrate for optimal generation of lymphokine-activated killer cells after Il-2 administration (64). It has been shown that arginine is required for cytotoxic effector mechanisms of macrophages (64, 65). Moncada and Higgs have suggested that the l-arginine-NO pathway is the main mechanism of macrophage toxicity for target cells (66). An increased mortality is observed in animals treated with NO inhibitors and subjected to endotoxemia (67) or induced liver damage (68). It has also been shown in animals subjected to cecal ligation and puncture and to burns that arginine supplementation improves survival by modulating bacterial clearance (69). It is most likely that many of these processes depend on the presence of a fermenting probiotic flora. Osborne and Seidel (70) demonstrated a decrease in activity of intraluminal lysine, ornithine and arginine decarboxylase after treatment with nonabsorbable antibiotics, which favors the assumption of a microorganism-mediated production of NO. It is known that microorganisms like lactobacilli can metabolize arginine, sometimes over up to six different pathways (71). Lactobacilli growing during anaerobic storage of meat are known to be entirely dependent on arginine and glucose for their growth (72), and lactobacillus plantarum strains from fish are unable to degrade any other amino acids than tyrosine and arginine (72).

It has also been shown that the omega-3 fatty acids enhance cell-mediated immune responses, inhibit inflammatory diseases and increase the resistance to infection [see Alexander (73)]. Also RNA has been shown to improve natural killer cell activity and increase resistance to infection (74). It was most likely these observations and others that prompted Sandoz to introduce the first immunonutrition formula, IMPACT, an enteral nutrition formula supplemented with l-arginine, omega-3 fatty acids and RNA. Observations made during experimental studies indicated that these substances, like antioxidants and particularly vitamins, and also cytokines work in groups, consortia, and that the presence of several is important for optimal effects: the obtained results are truly multifactorial.

Alexander, Daly and van Buren, respectively, who did several of the underlying experimental studies, have also been the driving forces behind the important clinical trials with immunonutrition. Immunonutrition is without doubt an interesting new concept and IMPACT must be regarded as the first generation of a nutritive pharmaceutical or nutraceutical. There are most certainly more to come. The first clinical study with supplemented immune-stimulatory ingredients was published in 1990 by Gottschlich et al. (75). They reported a significant reduction of nosocomial infectious complications and wound sepsis with a diet enriched with arginine and omega-3 fatty acids. Daly et al. published 2 years later the first study, using IMPACT in its definite version (enteral formula supplemented with arginine, omega-3 fatty acids and arginine) (76). They found in a randomized trial in 85 patients improved lymphocyte mitogenesis, fewer septic complications (11% vs 37%), and shorter hospital stay (15.8 vs 20.2 days) in the IMPACT treated patients. The first European study by Braga et al. (77) fully confirmed these observations, including a shorter hospital stay. However, they could only demonstrate a reduction in severity – *but not in frequency* – of postoperative infections. Recently a large prospective, randomized clinical multicenter trial in ICU patients was published by Bowers et al. (78). This study also verified a significant reduction in hospital stay, *but only in patients stratified as septic*, and a decreased rate of acquired bacteremia and urinary tract infections. No advantages could be observed in the group stratified as having systematic inflammatory response syndrome. The results are reminiscent of and rather similar to what was reported 3-5 years after the introduction of selective decontamination. After an early enthusiasm, more modest results were reported. An important difference is, however, that immunonutrition obviously improves the phagocytic function of monocytes, the release of Il-2, Il-2 receptors, Il-1 beta, IFN gamma, IgM, IgG, the number of CD3+, Cd4+ and beta-lymphocytes, and the response to skin delayed hypersensitivity and reduces the circulating levels of TNF alpha and Il-6 (77, 79, 80). This offers great hope for the concept of immunonutrition when improved immunonutrition formulas have been developed.

Colonic food - important for the outcome

In humans approximately 10% of the caloric demand should be met by colonic feeding. In order to meet this goal food must contain nutrients "destined" for the large intestine, food which cannot be digested or absorbed by the small intestine. The observation of Roediger (46) that colonic mucosa cannot nourish itself from the blood is of outmost importance and explains why patients on PN develop colonic mucosa atrophy within a few days of PN. As most often these patients receive antibiotic treatment it is most likely that also the protective probiotic flora is reduced, allowing PPMs to colonize the colon. The colonic mucosal atrophy and the overgrowth of PPMs are probably the two most important factors behind POTS of gut origin.

Foods, such as fibers and proteinous substances, are destined to the colon and referred to as *prebiotics* or *colonic foods*. In addition sloughed epithelia, pancreatic enzymes and mucus are recycled after bacterial fermentation by bacteria in the colon (81). The amount of epithelium recycled every day has been estimated to near 300 g/day and more in some diseases (82). This is most likely an important source of amino acids, particularly arginine. From this process approximately 80 g of protein and 12-30 g of lipids each day will be obtained. Although some of the need of colonic food can be met by recycling, fiber must be supplied to an amount of 10-30 g/day. When colonic food and other substrates reach the colon, the endogenous microbial flora (probiotic flora) will metabolize these substrates under production of nutrients of special importance for the nourishment and function of the colonic mucosa. Among these substances are short chain fatty acids (SCFAs), amino acids such as arginine, cysteine, glutamine, as well as peptides, polyamines etc. For review see (24, 42, 83, 84). Should the probiotic flora, due to disease or aggressive antibiotic treatment be reduced or eliminated, a resupply of human-specific probiotic bacteria is needed, especially in potential or established MOF patients. Eiseman and Silen (85) and more lately Wilmore (86) have expressed support for such a treatment. In most ICU patients these bacteria are absent, but also in patients with diseases such as ulcerative colitis or HIV/AIDS. Even healthy looking patients can have deficiencies in their probiotic flora. As examples insufficient diet, PN, elemental/fiberfree diet will all lead to a deficient colonic microflora. Astronauts on return to earth showed a very deranged intestinal microflora, a marked increase in enteropathogens and an almost total elimination of *lactobacilli* (87), most likely due to emotional stress and fiber-free diet. IMPACT in its present form does not meet the need of colonic nutrition as does not contain colonic foods, nor does it consider the need of replacement of the flora.

Ecoimmunonutrition - the next generation of formula?

Lactobacilli and *Bifidobacter* play several important roles in the GI tract functions such as:

1. Production of nutrients for the colonic mucosa: acetate, buturate, propionate, other SCFAs, pyruvate, lactate, and amino acids such as arginine, cysteine and glutamine.
2. Production of micronutrients: the B-group and folic acid, antioxidants and polyamines: histamine, 5-hydrooxytryptamine, piperidine, tyramine, cadaverine, pyrrolidine, agmatine, putrescine.
3. Prevention against overgrowth of PPMs.
4. Stimulation of the immune system, especially the so-called GALT system (gut associated lymphoid tissue). NO is produced in the GI tract by bacteria from the mouth to the rectum. It is not yet known whether these bacteria also produce cytokines.
5. Elimination of toxins and "unwanted substances".
6. Regulation of digestive functions: mucus utilization, nutrient absorption, GI motility, blood flow.

We are convinced that the GI probiotic bacteria play a crucial role in the maintenance of health. A library of hundreds of *lactobacilli* has been collected from healthy individuals [for review see (83)]. In order to produce a formula for ecoimmunonutrition it is important to know the fermenting ability of the different *lactobacilli*. It is also important to identify *lactobacilli* which have the ability to survive the acidity of the stomach and the bile acid content of the intestine. Most important is to identify *lactobacilli* with a strong ability to adhere to the colonic mucosa and remain and function there, even when the external supply is stopped. Most of the *lactobacilli* used in the past are of yoghurt nature, which do not fulfill such criteria. The first *lactobacillus* to meet these requirements seems to be *lactobacillus rhamnosus GG*, identified from human feces. Its adherence to human mucosal cells seems, however, to be poor, usually 0.5-2 bacteria per mucosa cell. In sharp contrast, *lactobacillus plantarum 299* has the ability to adhere to a density of approximately 15 bacteria/cell, e.g. the same density as *Escherichia coli*. *Lactobacillus plantarum 299* has been used to produce an ecoimmunonutrition formula. As substrate for fermentation oat was chosen, as it is one of the most complete human foods; has a favorable amino acid pattern, is very rich in fiber, particularly in watersoluble beta-glucans.

Table 2. Nutrient content in 100 ml of nutrition solution

	Standard solutions with fiber (n = 8)	Immunonutrition impact	Ecoimmuno nutrition
Energy (KJ)	429	420	325
Protein (g)	4.0	5.6	2.8
Fat (g)	3.6	2.8	1.1
Linoleic acid (g)	1.7	0.22	0.5
Carbohydrate (g)	13.9	13.2	13.8
Fiber (g)	> 1.0		0.57
Vitamin E (mg)	2.0	6.0 IU	0.23
Thiamine (mg)	0.13	0.20	0.09
Riboflavin (mg)	0.14	0.17	0.02
Vitamin B_6 (mg)	0.16	0.15	0.07
Vitamin B_{12} (mg)	0.4	0.0008	< 0.1
Folic acid (mg)	29	0.04	12
Pantothenic acid (mg)	0.7	0.67	0.09
Sodium (mg)	78.5	110	2.0
Chloride (mg)	126	130	11.3
Potassium (mg)	137	130	55
Calcium (mg)	71	80	10.7
Phosphorus (mg)	70	80	64
Magnesium (mg)	23	27	18.5
Iron (mg)	1.1	1.20	0.72
Zinc (mg)	1.1	1.50	0.62
Iodine (mg)	9.0	0.010	0.13
Copper (mg)	0.12	0.17	0.14
Manganese (mg)	0.3	0.20	0.55
Chromium (mg)	5.0	0.001	0.37
Selenium (mg)	5.0	0.001	0.003
Molybdenum (mg)	10	0.002	20
Arginine (mg)	160	1358 (added)	2500 (added)
Yeast RNA (mg)	0	135	0
Lactobacillus plantarum			1.5 x 10°
Viscosity			0.02 m PaS

However, the most unique feature is its high content of membrane lipids – phospholipids – being one hundred times richer in oat than in any other food known. As a strong synergistic effects between the health promoting effects of *lactobacillus plantarum 299* was found, it was recently decided to supplement the formula with 2.5 g of l-arginine per 100 ml solution. For content, see Table 2. The original formula, without arginine supplementation, has been extensively studied in experimental animals and in humans [for review see (84)]. In summary, these studies have shown pronounced effects both in experimental animals and in very sick patients, such as patients judged as dying of multiple organ failure (MOF). In five consecutive MOF patients all the antibiotic supply was terminated and the patients tubefed with *lactobacilli* and fiber. All the patients recovered and could leave ICU. The Apache II scores fell from a mean of 18.4 before the treatment to 12.2 on the 5th day and 8.8 on the 10th day.

Ecoimmunonutrition, e.g. nutrition containing fermentable fiber and live lactobacilli, has the potential of being the next generation of immunonutrition. The formula is under clinical trials in USA and in Europe in several studies in different patient groups.

Potential indications

Acute: Major trauma, larger operations - especially transplantations such as liver, intestine and bone marrow transplantations.

Chronic: HIV/AIDS (= Chronic MOF), acute pancreatitis, ulcerative colitis, advanced cancer, especially after heavy irradiation and cytostatic treatment.

Addendum

The feeding tube will be manufactured and marketed in Europe by Pfrimmer-Nutricia, Erlangen, Germany, and in the US by Ross/Abbott. The feeding formula is for European use developed for medical nutrition by a leading European producer of enteral nutrition formulas and is presently undergoing controlled clinical trials. A retail version of the formula is presently marketed in Scandinavia under the commercial name of PRO VIVA. The latter product is to be introduced to the markets in several European countries, the US and Japan. PRO VIVA is, in addition to being rich in *Lactobacillus 299V* and oat fiber, also rich in fruit juices.

References

1. van Goor H, Rosman C, Grond J, Kooi K, Wubbels GH, Bleichrodt RP (1994) Translocation of bacteria and endotoxin in organ donors. Arch Surg 129:1063-1066.
2. McDonald WS, Sharp CW, Deitch EA (1991) Immediate enteral feeding in burn patients is safe and effective. Ann Surg 214:177-183
3. Dobke MK, Simoni J, Ninnemann TJ, Garrett J, Hamar TJ (1989) Endotoxin after burn injury: effects of early excision on circulating levels. J Burn Care Rehabil 10:107-111
4. O'Dwyers ST, Michie HR, Ziegler TR, Revhaug A, Smith JR, Wilmore DW (1988) A single dose of endotoxin increases intestinal permeability in healthy humans. Arch Surg 123:1459-1464
5. Bengmark S. Econutrition and health maintenance – a new concept to prevent GI inflammation, ulceration and sepsis – an invited review. J Clin Nutr. Under publication
6. Burd RS, Cody CS, Dunn DL (1992) Immunotherapy of gram-negative bacterial sepsis. Landes, Austin

7. Doglio GR, Pusajo JF, Egurrola MA, Bonfigli G, Parra C, Vetere LM, Hernandez MS, Fernandez S, Palizas F, Gutierrez G (1990) Gastric mucosal pH as a prognostic index of mortality in critically ill patients. Crit Care Med 19:1037-1040

8. Carrico CJ, Meakins JL, Marshall JC, Fry D, Maier RV (1986) Multiple-organ failure syndrome. Arch Surg 121:196-208

9. Levine GM, Deren JJ, Steiger E, Zinno R (1974) Role of oral intake in maintenance of gut mass and disaccharide activity. Gastroenterology 67:975-982

10. Sunzel H (1963) Effects of surgical trauma on the liver glycogen in fasting and in glucose fed patients. Acta Chir Scand 125:118-128

11. Bark T, Katouli M, Ljungquist O, Möllby R, Svenberg T (1995) Glutamine supplementation does not prevent bacterial translocation after non-lethal hemorrhage in rats. Eur J Surg 161: 3-8

12. Moore FA, Feliciano DV, Andrassy RJ, McArdle AH, McL Booth FV, Morgenstein-Wagner TB, Kellum Jr JM, Welling RE, Moore EE (1991) Early enteral feeding, compared with parenteral, reduces postoperative septic complications. Ann Surg 216(2):172-182

13. Ljungquist O, Thorell A, Gutniak M, Häggström T, Efencic S (1994) Glucose infusion instead of preoperative fasting reduces postoperative insulin resistance. Surg Gynecol Obstet 178: 329-335

14. Mandel ID (1987) The function of saliva. J Dent Res 66:623-627

15. Starkey RH, Orth D (1977) Radioimmunoassay of human epidermal growth factor (Urogastrone). Clin Endocrinol Metab 45:1144-1153

16. Sarosiek J, Feng TT, McCallum RW (1991) The interrelationship between salivary epidermal growth factor and the functional integrity of the mucosal barrier in the rat. Am J Med Sci 302:359-363

17. Tabak LA, Levine MJ, Mandel ID, Ellison SA (1982) Role of salivary mucins in the protection of the oral cavity. J Oral Pathol 11:1-17

18. Vahouny GV, Le T, Ifrim I, Satchithanandam S, Cassidy MM (1985) Stimulation of intestinal cytokinetics and mucin turnover in rats fed wheat bran and cellulose. Am J Clin Nutr 41: 895-900.

19. Sreebny LM, Banoczy J, Baum BJ, Edgar WM, Epstein JB, Fox PC, Larmas M (1992) Saliva: its role in health and disease. Int Dent J 42;4 [Suppl 2]:291-304

20. Fox PC, van der Ven PF, Baum BJ, Mandel ID (1986) Pilocarpine for the treatment of xerostomia associated with salivary gland dysfunction Oral Surg 61:243-248

21. Wilder-Smith CH, Spirig C, Krech T, Merki HS (1992) Bactericidal factors in gastric juice. Eur J Gastroenterol Hepatol 4:885-891

22. Driks MR, Craven DE, Celli BR, Manning M, Burke RA, Garvin GM, Kunches LM, Farber HW, Wedel SA, McCabe WR (1987) Nosocomial pneumonia in intubated patients given sucralfate as compared with antacids or histamin type 2 blockers. N Engl J Med 317: 1376-1382

23. Toung TJK, Rosenfeld BA, Yoshiki A, Grayson RF, Traystman RJ (1993) Sucralfate does not reduce the risk of acid aspiration pneumonitis. Crit Care Med 21:1359-1364

24. Bengmark S, Jeppsson B (1995) Gastrointestinal surface protection and mucosa reconditioning. JPEN J Parenter Enteral Nutr (in press)

25. Bonten MJM, Gaillard CA, van Thiel FH, van der Geest S, Stobberingh EE (1994) Continuous enteral feeding counteracts preventive measures for gastric colonization in intensive care patients. Crit Care Med 22:939-944

26. Preiser J-C, Lejeune P, Roman A, Carlier E, De Backer D, Leeman M, Kahn RJ, Vincent J (1995) Methylene blue administration in septic shock: a clinical trial. Crit Care Med 23(2): 259-264

27. Wright CE, Rees DD, Moncada S (1992) Protective and pathological roles of nitric oxide in endotoxin shock. Cardiovasc Res 26:48-57

28. Green SJ (1995) Nitric oxide in mucosal immunity. Nature Med 6:515-517

29. Malawista SE, Montgomery RR, van Blaricom GJ (1992) Evidence for reactive nitrogen intermediates in killing of staphylococci by human neutrophil cytoplasts. A new microbiocidal pathway for polymorphonuclear leukocytes. J Clin Invest 90:631-636

30. Herndon DN, Ziegler ST (1993) Bacterial translocation after thermal injury. Crit Care Med 21:S50-S54
31. Forman D, Al-Dabbagh S, Doll R (1985) Nitrates, nitrites and gastric cancer in Great Britain. Nature 313:620-625
32. Knight TM et al (1990) Nitrate and nitrite exposure in Italian populations with different gastric cancer rates. Int J Epidemiol 19:510
33. Benjamin N, O'Driscoll F, Dougall H, Duncan C, Smith S, Golden M (1994) Stomach NO synthesis. Nature 368:502
34. Duncan C, Dougall H, Johnston P, Green S, Brogan R, Leifert C, Smith L, Golden M, Benjamin N (1995) Chemical generation of nitric oxide in the mouth from the enterosalivary circulation of dietary nitrate. Nature Med 1:546-551
35. Lundberg JON, Weitzberg E, Lundberg JM, Alving K (1994) Intragastric nitric oxide production in humans: measurements in expelled air. Gut 35:1543-1546
36. Brown JF, Hanson PJ, Whittle BJR (1992) Nitric oxide donors increase mucus gel thickness in rat stomach. Eur J Pharmacol 223:103-104
37. Ödum L, Andersson L-P (1995) Investigation of Helicobacter pylori ascorbic oxidation activity. FEMS Immunol Med Microbiol 10(3-4):289-294
38. Fujisaki H, Oketani K, Murakami M, Fujimote M, Wakabayashi T, Yamatsu I, Yamaguchi M, Sakzi H, Takeguchi M (1991) Inhibitions of acid secretion by E 3810 and omeprazole, and their reversal by glutathione. Biochem Pharmacol 42(2):321-328
39. Verdu E, Viani F, Armstrong D, Fraser R, Siegrist HH, Pignatelli B, Idström J-P, Cederberg C, Blum AL, Fried M (1994) Effects of omeprazole on intragastric bacterial counts, nitrates, nitrites and N-nitrose compounds. Gut 35:455-460
40. Streat SJ, Beddoe AH, Hill GL (1987) Aggressive nutritional support does not prevent protein loss despite fat gain in septic intensive care patients. J Trauma 27:262-266
41. Detsky AS, Baker JP, O'Rourke K, Goel V (1987) Perioperative parenteral nutrition: a metaanalysis. Ann Intern Med 107(2):195-203
42. Olivares L, Segovia A, Revuelta R (1974) Tube feeding and lethal aspiration in neurological patients: a review of 720 autopsy cases. Stroke 5:654-657
43. Bengmark S, Larsson K, Molin G (1995) Gut mucosa reconditioning with species-specific lactobacilli, surfactants, pseudomucus and fiber - an invited review. Biotechnol Ther (in press)
44. Mulholland JH, Tui C, Wright AM, Vinci VJ (1943) Nitrogen metabolism, caloric intake and weight loss in postoperative convalescence. Ann Surg 117:512-534
45. Riegel C, Koop CE, Drew J, Stevens LW, Rhoads JE (1947) The nutritional requirements for nitrogen balance in surgical patients during the early postoperative period. J Clin Invest 26: 18-23
46. Shephard AP (1980) Intestinal blood flow autoregulation during foodstuff absorption. Am J Physiol 239:H156-H162
47. Roediger WEW (1980) Role of anaerobic bacteria in the metabolic welfare of the colonic mucosa in man. Gut 21:793-798
48. Hoover HC, Ryan JA, Anderson EJ, Fischer JE (1980) Nutritional benefits of immediate postoperative jejunal feeding of an elemental diet. Am J Surg 139:153-159
49. Alexander JW, MacMillan BG, Stinnett JD et al (1980) Beneficial effects of aggressive protein feeding in severely burned children. Ann Surg 192:505
50. Vandenbroucke-Grauls CMJE, Vandenbroucke JP (1991) Effect of selective decontamination of the digestive tract on respiratory tract infections and mortality in the intensive care unit. Lancet 338:859-862
51. Rees RPG, Payne-James JJ, King C, Silk DBA (1988) Spontaneous transpyloric passage and performance of "Fine Bore" polyurethane feeding tubes: a controlled trial. JPEN J Parenter Enteral Nutr 12(5):469-472
52. Levenson R, Furner Jr WW, Dyson A, Zike L, Reisch J (1988) Do weighted nasoenteric feeding tubes facilitate duodenal intubations? JPEN J Parenter Enteral Nutr 12(2):135-137
53. Bengmark S Swedish patent 8700582, US patent 4 887 996, EU patent PTC/0278937

54. Jeppsson B, Tranberg K-G, Bengmark S (1992) Technical developments. A new self-propelling feeding tube. Clin Nutr 11:373-375
55. Kudsk KA, Croce MA, Fabian TC, Minard G, Tolley EA, Poret HA, Kuhl MR, Brown RO (1992) Enteral versus parenteral feeding: effects on septic morbidity after blunt and penetrating abdominal trauma. Ann Surg 215:503
56. Chandra RK, Baker M, Whang S, Au B (1991) Effect of two feeding formulas on immune responses and mortality in mice challenged with Listeria monocytogenes. Immunol Lett 27:45-48
57. Klasing KC (1989) Nutritional aspects of leukocytic cytokines. J Nutr 118:1436-1446
58. Merimee TJ, Lillecrap DA, Rabinowitz D (1965) Effect of arginine on serum levels of human growth hormone. Lancet 2:668-670
59. Scull CW, Rose WJC (1930) Arginine metabolism: the relation of arginine content of the diet on the increments in tissue arginine during growth. J Biol Chem 39:109-121
60. Elsair J, Poey J, Issad H (1978) Effect of arginine chlorate on nitrogen balance during the three days following routine surgery in healthy human beings. Biomed Expr 29:312-317
61. Seifter E, Rettura G, Barbul A, Levenson SM (1978) Arginine: an essential amino acid for injured rats. Surgery 84:224-230
62. Barbul A, Sisto DA, Wasserkrug HL, Efron G (1981) Arginine stimulates lymphocyte immune response in healthy human beings. Surgery 90:244-251
63. Reynolds JV, Daly JM, Zhang S, Evantash E, Shou J, Sigal R, Ziegler MM (1988) Immunomodulary mechanisms of arginine. Surgery 104:142-151
64. Lieberman MD, Nishioka K, Redmond P, Daly JM (1992) Enhancement of interleukin-2 immunotherapy with l-arginine. Ann Surg 215:157
65. McGhee JR, Mestecky J, Elson CO, Kijono H (1989) Regulation of IgA synthesis and immune response by T cells and interleukins. J Clin Immunol 9:175
66. Moncada S, Higgs EA (1991) Endogenous nitric oxide: physiology, pathology and clinical relevance. Eur J Clin Invest 21:361
67. Nava E, Palmer RM, Moncada S (1991) Inhibition of nitric oxide synthesis in septic shock: how much is beneficial. Lancet 338:1555-1557
68. Billiar TR, Curran RD, Harbrecht BG, Stuehr DJ, Demetris AJ, simmons RL (1990) Modulation of nitrogen oxide synthesis in vivo: NG-monethyl-l-arginine inhibits endo toxin-induced nitrate/nitrite biosynthesis while promoting hepatic damage. J Leukoc Biol 48:565
69. Gianotti L, Alexander JW, Pyles T, Fukushima R (1993) Arginine-supplemented diets improve survival in gut-derived sepsis and peritonitis by modulating bacterial clearance. The role of nitric oxide. Ann Surg 217:644-654
70. Osborne DL, Seidel IR (1989) Microflora-derived polyamines modulate obstruction-induced colonic mucosal hypertrophy. Am J Physiol (Gastrointest Liver Physiol) 19:G1049-1057
71. Montel MC, Champomier M-C (1987) Arginine catabolism in Lactobacillus sake isolated from meat. Appl Environ Microbiol 53:2683-2685
72. Jónsson S, Clausen E, Raa J (1983) Amino acid degradation by a Lactobacillus plantarum strain from fish. System Appl Microbiol 4:148-154
73. Alexander JW (1993) Immunoenhancement in enteral nutrition. Arch Surg 128:1242
74. van Buren CT, Rudolph FB, Kuokarni A, Pizzini R, Fanslow WC, Kumar S (1990) Reversal of immunosuppression induced by protein-free diet: a comparison of nucleotides, fish oil and arginine. Crit Care Med 18:S2114
75. Gottschlick MM, Jenkins M, Warden GD, Baumer T, Havens P, Snook JT, Alexander JW (1990) Differential effects of three enteral dietary regimens on selected outcome variables in burn patients. JPEN J Parenter Enteral Nutr 14:225-236
76. Daly JM, Lieberman MD, Goldfine J, Shou J, Weintraub F, Rosato EF, Lavin Ph (1992) Enteral nutrition with supplemented arginine, RNA, and omega-3 fatty acids in patients after operation: immunologic, metabolic and clinical outcome. Surgery 112:56-67
77. Braga M, Vignali A, Gianotti L et al (1995) Immune and nutritional effects of early enteral nutrition after major abdominal operations. Eur J Surg 221:327-338

78. Bowers RB, Cerra FB, Bershadsky B, Licari JJ, Hoyt DB, Jensen GL, Van Buren CT, Rothkopf MM, Daly JM (1995) Early enteral administration of a formula (Impact) supplemented with arginine, nucleotides, and fish oil in intensive care unit patients: results of a multicenter, prospective, randomized, clinical trial. Crit Care Med 23:436-449
79. Kemen M, Senkal M, Homann HH et al (1995) Early postoperative enteral nutrition with arginine, omega 3-fatty acids and ribonucleic acid-supplemented diet versus placebo in cancer patients: an immunological evaluation of Impact R. Crit Care Med 23:652-659
80. Senkal M, Kemen M, Homann HH et al (1995) Modulation of postoperative response by enteral nutrition with a diet enriched with arginine, RNA, and omega-3 fatty acids in patients with upper gastrointestinal cancer. Eur J Surg 161:115-122
81. Cummings JH (1995) Anatomy and physiology of human colon. Workshop on colonic microflora. Barcelona Spain. Nutr Rev (in press)
82. Croft DN, Cotton PB Gastro-intestinal cell loss in man. Its measurements and significance. Digestion 8:144-166
83. Bengmark S (1995) Eco-nutrition and health maintenance. J Clin Nutr (in press)
84. Bengmark S, Gianotti L (1995) Nutritional support to prevent and treat MOF. World J Surg (in press)
85. Eiseman B, Silen W, Bascom GS, Kauvar AJ (1958) Fecal enema as an adjunct in the treatment of pseudomembranous enterocolitis. Surgery 44:854-859
86. Wilmore DW (1993) The surgeon and intestinal bacteria - reconsideration of our relationship. After Baue A. The role of the gut in the development of multiple organ dysfunction in cardiothoracic patients. Ann Thorac Surg 55:822-829
87. Lencner AA, Lencner ChP, Mikelsaar DR, Thuri ME, Toom MA, Väljaots MW, Silov VM, Liz'ko NN, Legenkov VI, Reznikov IM (1984) Die quantitative Zusammensetzung der Laktoflora des Verdauungstrakts vor und nach kosmischen Flugen unterschiedlicher Dauer. Nahrung 28:607-613

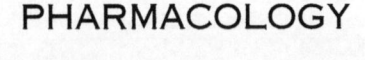

PHARMACOLOGY

Pharmacological Interactions in the Perioperative Period

V.A. PEDUTO, R. D'UVA

Introduction

Considering that patients admitted to a hospital are frequently given regular drug therapy (the incidence being 24%-42% overall and increasing to 70% in patients aged over 70 years) (1, 2), that each patient may receive on average 9.4 drugs during hospitalization (3), and, finally, that another ten or more drugs may be given for a "routine" anesthetic procedure, it is not surprising that the potential for perioperative drug interactions is very significant. Indeed, this risk has been estimated at 7% in patients taking six to ten drugs and 50% in patients taking more than ten drugs (4).

The very essence of a drug interaction is when the spheres of activity of two drugs, administered either concomitantly or sequentially, overlap, so that the action of one drug will modify or affect the behavior of another. Interactions can be either adverse or beneficial: for example, reversal of nondepolarizing neuromuscular blockers is accomplished by giving cholinesterase inhibitors, which increase the concentration of acetylcholine at the nicotinic postjunctional receptors; unfortunately, the concentration of acetylcholine is also increased at the muscarinic receptors, leading to undesirable side-effects such as bradycardia, so an anti-muscarinic agent has to be administered concomitantly to block these unwanted side-effects.

Drug interactions can be classified, according to the mechanism by which they take place, into pharmaceutical, pharmacokinetic and pharmacodynamic. The basic principles of such interactions, illustrated by some examples relevant to the anesthetic practice, are covered in this review.

Pharmaceutical mechanisms

Drug compatibility includes chemical integrity (preservation of active chemical species) and physical integrity (clarity of solution and absence of precipitate). Pharmaceutical incompatibility occurs because one drug reacts chemically or physically with another, usually when they are added to infusion fluids or mixed in the same syringe. The formation of a precipitate or cloudiness following the mixing of drug solutions is definite evidence of pharmaceutical incompatibility, although the absence of a visually detected precipitate does not exclude the possibility that a significant reaction has taken place.

Where the solubility of an agent is pH-dependent, it may be precipitated by changes in the acidity or alkalinity of its solution. Such changes may be brought about by the addition of a solution of markedly different pH or, more simply, by dilution. Examples of solutions with a high pH are acidic drugs (e.g. thiopental, amrinone) and sodium bicarbonate; and those with a low pH include basic drugs (e.g. opioids, muscle relaxants, local anesthetics, midazolam, ketamine, droperidol, sympathetic amines), dextrans, Hartmann's solution, and 5% dextrose. If succinylcholine is injected into i.v. tubing following thiopental, the relaxant is rapidly hydrolyzed and barbituric acid is precipitated, unless the tubing is sufficiently flushed between drugs. When mixed with thiopental or diluted in alkaline solution, atracurium is also rapidly inactivated as a result of the Hofmann reaction, and alcuronium and pancuronium can form dense precipitates. Finally, if thiopental is mixed into a large volume of Hartmann's solution, there will be a significant change in pH as regards thiopental and once again precipitation may result. Mixtures in which a precipitate is formed have the potential to cause vein irritation, embolism and granuloma formation. It is also possible that they are prone to cause histamine release and serious systemic reactions as a result of aggregate anaphylaxis.

Loss of potency or complete inactivation can be expected when amrinone is diluted in dextrose containing solutions or when, during resuscitation from cardiac arrest, epinephrine and sodium bicarbonate are administered into the same i.v. line without sufficient flushing.

The other major group of pharmaceutical interactions involves the physical properties of injectable medications. The osmolality of the infusion fluid provides a familiar example. When mixing hypotonic solution of dextrose and blood, the dextrose can cause clumping of the red blood cells which produces transfusion reactions; similarly, when mixing a hypertonic solution of mannitol and blood, the mannitol can induce agglutination and irreversible crenation of red blood cells. The i.v. infusion set should be changed if administering these solutions consecutively.

Another physical interaction can arise from the solvent system polarity. If the solubility of a drug in aqueous solution is poor (i.e. diazepam), it may be necessary for the drug to be dissolved in a specific solvent (propylene glycol). Subsequent addition of the drug in solvent to an aqueous solution may reduce the solubility of the drug in that mixture and consequently the drug may precipitate out.

Drugs may also interact with the administration sets through which they are given. Absorption is best described in relation to nitrates and their lipophilicity and polarity in the solution. As a result, there is a tendency for them to bind to the matrix of polyvinylchloride (PVC) plastic, the major constituent of most transparent and flexible intravenous fluid containers and tubing (5, 6). This may cause significant changes in the concentration of the drug being administered and, consequently, changes in therapeutic effect (polypropylene syringe and high-density polyethylene tubing connected to a Teflon catheter should be used instead). Similarly, a saturable process of fentanyl sequestration by the cardiopulmonary bypass system appears to create a major alteration in fentanyl kinetics during cardiac surgery (7). Adsorption does not depend on binding of a chemical nature, but rather on adherence to the surface of a drug delivery system, as may occur with insulin in glass or plastic syringes, containers and infusion sets.

Physical drug interaction can also occur in vivo. A common example is the neutralization of heparin with protamine, a base that combines with the strongly acidic heparin molecule to form a stable salt with no anticoagulant activity (8).

Pharmacokinetic mechanisms

Drugs can alter each other's absorption, distribution, metabolism and elimination. Such changes may cause an unexpected clinical response to the drug by affecting its plasma concentration and half-life, or by allowing toxic metabolites to accumulate.

Interactions at the site of the drug's entry into the body can take place in the mouth: disopyramide, for instance, may interfere with the absorption of sublingual preparations such as glyceryl trinitrate, nifedipine and buprenorphine because of its antisialogogue properties (9). The rate of absorption of drugs administered orally is largely dependent on the rate of gastric emptying. The major cause of delayed emptying is the administration of opioids (morphine may decrease emptying by eight- to tenfold) (10) or drugs with anticholinergic effects (atropine) or side-effects (cyclic antidepressants). These drugs can reduce peak blood concentration of other orally administered medications without modifying the total amount of drug absorbed: parenteral morphine has been shown to delay significantly the absorption of oral diazepam and a similar, although less marked, effect was seen following parenteral atropine (11). Drugs which reduce gastric acidity (e.g. H_2-receptor antagonists and antacids) have the capacity to alter the absorption of other weakly acidic or basic drugs by modifying the proportion of ionized/unionized molecules. Therefore, in an environment of reduced acidity, weak bases will be less absorbed and acidic drugs will have enhanced absorption. For parenterally injected drugs absorption rates will be determined by local blood flow. Thus vasoconstrictors such as epinephrine and octapressin are added to local anesthetic solutions to prolong their duration of action at the site of injection and to decrease the risk of systemic toxicity from rapid absorption.

Absorption interactions may also occur in the lungs, an example being the second gas effect where rapid uptake of nitrous oxide concentrates other anesthetic agents, such as isoflurane, resulting in higher alveolar concentrations.

After the administration of the drug it then has to be distributed, and this usually occurs via the blood stream. Many drugs bind avidly to plasma proteins, and only free (unbound) drug molecules are available for distribution and elimination. If there is competition between two drugs for the same binding sites on plasma proteins, one drug may be displaced by another, so that a higher free (and pharmacologically active) drug concentration will exist transiently. However, this will be therapeutically significant only if large numbers of drug molecules are present (approaching or exceeding the molar concentration of binding sites) and if at least one of the drugs is very highly bound. A much quoted example is the prolongation of action of barbiturates by concomitant administration of radiopaque dyes (12), probenecid (13) or certain sulfonamides (14), which compete for albumin binding sites. Also enflurane and its metabolite trifluoroacetic acid, in concentrations relevant to the clinical anesthesia, are able to displace diazepam from binding sites on the serum albumin to such a degree that a temporary potentiation of the pharmacological effect and a more rapid elimination of diazepam could be expected (15). The long-term consequences of these displacement interactions depend on whether the drug's clearance is increased by the increased free fraction (16). For a low extraction drug, the elimination of which is restricted by protein binding, if the free fraction is suddenly increased by a displacement interaction, the resultant increase in the free fraction leads to an increased volume of distribution and, therefore, a decrease in total drug concentration. With continued administration, and re-establishment of a new steady state, the total concentration will tend to recover; however, clearance is also increased by the increase in free fraction, so that the free fraction is reported to predisplacement levels while the total drug concentration decreases. Therefore, after re-establishment of steady state, there is no long-term change in pharmacological effect or toxicity. In contrast, clearance of drugs with high extraction ratios is not restricted to the free fraction and is not affected by changes in binding. Consequently, when the free fraction increases due to displacement, there is a decrease in total concentration due to an increase in volume of distribution, but with continued administration the total concentration eventually returns to its predisplacement levels because the clearance remains unchanged. The increase in free fraction causes a persistent increase in free concentration, and therefore the possibility of increased pharmacological effect and toxicity exists. Clinically important displacement interactions are thus most likely to occur if the displaced drug has high (nonrestrictive) clearance, a small volume of distribution, and is extensively bound to plasma proteins (> 85%). For example, the displacement of bupivacaine by several drugs (e.g. meperidine, diphenylhydantoin, quinidine and desipramine) (17) might enhance the likelihood of local anesthetic toxicity.

Any drug which causes a reduction in cardiac output will modify the distribution of any other drug given concurrently. In particular, the circulation time (and therefore the venous transit time) is increased and the perfusion of large tissue masses, such as muscle, is greatly diminished. Thus negatively inotropic drugs such as halothane and propranolol will delay the distribution and thereby increase the plasma concentrations of other concurrently administered drugs such as intravenous anesthetic agents, muscle relaxants and opioids.

Drugs which reduce (e.g. halothane, propranolol) or increase (e.g. glucagon, isoprenaline, phenobarbital) liver blood flow will reduce or increase the clearance of any other concurrently administered drug which is susceptible to changes in hepatic perfusion (e.g. lidocaine, propofol, fentanyl and, of course, propranolol itself).

Many drugs are metabolized by the liver, and a commonly involved pathway is provided by the mixed oxidase enzyme system found in hepatic microsomes. Drugs such as barbiturates, ethanol, ketamine, inhalation anesthetics, opioids, and many tranquilizers have been found to induce this group of enzymes, so that their own metabolism and the clearances of all drugs which become mixed oxidase substrate are enhanced. The majority of drug interactions associated with enzyme induction do not have major effect on the conduct of anesthesia, but there are definite patients for whom ignoring the potential for anesthetic metabolism could prove dangerous. The first example is halothane hepatitis: animal models have shown one form of direct hepatotoxic effect of halothane which is dependent on enzyme induction either with polychlorinated biphenyls or with phenobarbital pretreatment followed by administration of halothane in a hypoxic environment (18). The proposed mechanism is a change from the normal oxidative pathway to a reductive pathway for halothane metabolism (19). In this example, therefore, the drug interaction is changing qualitatively the type of response, rather than having only a quantitative effect. A second example is provided by isoniazid, which induces enflurane defluorination. There appears to be a bimodal distribution in the response: following enflurane anesthesia only a subgroup of isoniazid-treated patients produces serum fluoride levels reaching the nephrotoxic range (20). This difference may be related to the genetically determined bimodal distribution of slow and rapid acetylation of isoniazid which is known to exist in the normal population. The acetylation of isoniazid results in the formation of hydrazine, which in turn induces formation of cytochrome P451 2E1, which leads to enhanced enflurane defluorination. Thus this example of a drug interaction is the result of biotransformation of the drug, which in turn alters the biotransformation of the other drug. The observation is of interest considering the effects of isoniazid on drug metabolism and should prompt an alternative to enflurane in isoniazid-treated patients.

Just as some drugs induce the mixed oxidase system, others inhibit it. Cimetidine, a histamine H_2 receptor antagonist often used as a premedication to increase gastric fluid pH and for prevention of histamine-related side effects caused by intravenous anesthetics and muscle relaxants, decreases liver blood flow and inhibits microsomal drug metabolism. As a consequence, therapeutic doses of cimetidine impairs the systemic clearance of both flow-limited and capacity-limited drugs, including opioids (21, 22), benzodiazepines (23, 24), propranolol (25), lidocaine (26), and theophylline (27). Cimetidine has been also shown to inhibit pseudocholinesterase activity (28) and to prolong the duration of action of succinylcholine (29). Although this interaction was not seen in a subsequent study (30), caution should be taken when administering succinylcholine to patients on chronic cimetidine therapy. Pseudocholinesterase activity can be inhibited by a variety of other drugs (e.g. echothiophate eye drops, aprotinin, chlorpromazine, cyclophosphamide, glucocorticoids, pancuronium, physostigmine, oral contraceptives, monoamine oxidase inhibitors) (31, 32), the concomitant use of which may prolong the duration of action of succinylcholine. In addition to interactions with sympathetic amines, MAO inhibitors may also interact with opioids (especially meperidine), to cause coma, depressed ventilation and hypotension (33) and with barbiturates, to enhance their sedative and hypnotic effects (34). The mechanism by which these interactions take place seems to be, once again, an inhibition of the liver microsomal enzyme system necessary for opioid and barbiturate detoxification (35).

The excretion of certain drugs may also be affected by drug interactions. If the urine is at a pH at which the drug is present mainly in the ionized form, the possibility of passive reabsorption of the drug in the distal tubule may be considerably reduced, with resulting diminution of drug levels and lowered therapeutic effectiveness. Conversely, if the urine is at a pH at which the drug is unionized, passive reabsorption is enhanced, resulting in higher plasma levels with prolongation of action and increased likelihood of side-effects. The renal clearance of urinary pH-dependent acidic (pKa within a range of 3.5-7.5) and basic (pKa within a range of 7.5-10.5) drugs may be then influenced by changes in the urinary pH: that of barbiturates or salicylate is hastened by administering bicarbonate whereas acidification of the urine with ammonium chloride will increase the renal clearance of meperidine, ephedrine or amphetamine. In contrast, alkaline diuresis reduces the excretion of weak bases as they tend to remain unionized and undergo tubular reabsorption: local anesthetics and anti-arrhythmic drugs can exhibit elevated plasma levels in such a situation.

The action of drugs that depend on the lungs for excretion will be prolonged if alveolar ventilation is depressed. Thus, recovery after inhalation anesthesia is delayed by opioids administration. Still at the end of anesthesia the rapid transit of nitrous oxide (due to its solubility) into the alveolar space may result in effective dilution of the oxygen present there and cause diffusion hypoxia.

Morphine is subjected to conjugation in the gut wall and liver and is excreted into the upper small intestine as the glucuronide metabolite. Breakdown of this conjugate with subsequent release and reuptake of the parent compound occurs after exposure to the intestinal flora (enterohepatic recirculation). Antibacterial agents that inhibit the micro-organisms in the gut may prevent this breakdown and thus reduce the total bioavailability of morphine. A similar mechanism would appear to account for the attenuation of effects of oral contraceptives when tetracyclines are administered concurrently.

Some highly basic and lipophilic opioids (e.g. phenoperidine, meperidine, methadone and fentanyl) may be excreted from the systemic circulation into the acidic environment of the stomach. Their subsequent reuptake from the alkaline medium of the small intestine may result in a secondary increase in plasma concentration sufficient to cause acute respiratory depression or reduced sensitivity of the chemoreceptors to carbon dioxide in the postoperative period (36). This enterosystemic recirculation may be modified by the concurrent administration of antacids (37).

Pharmacodynamic mechanisms

Accounting for the vast majority of drug interactions, both useful and harmful, that are encountered in anesthetic practice, pharmacodynamic interactions involve the enhancement or inhibition of the action of one drug by another, where both agents act at the same receptor or within the same physiological system. Such interactions are usually quite predictable as there is a recognizable pharmacological mechanism underlying them, the effects being antagonistic (competitive or noncompetitive) or agonistic (synergistic or potentiating) in nature without any alteration in drug concentration.

The variety of actual and potential pharmacodynamic drug interactions is limitless, but it is important to distinguish the minority of clinically important interactions from the majority which are mainly of academic interest. Well, most of the important adverse drug interactions which occur in anesthesia involve loss of cardiovascular stability or the prolongation of neuromuscular blockade.

Patients presenting for surgery may be on a variety of directly or indirectly acting sympathomimetic drugs including bronchodilators (beta-adrenergic agonists, phosphodiesterase inhibitors), cyclic antidepressants, MAO inhibitors, levodopa, vasoconstrictor nose drops, decongestant cough mixtures, anorectics and amphetamines. Inhalation anesthetics sensitize the myocardium to the arrhythmogenic effects of these agents: halothane produces the greatest degree of sensitization and isoflurane the least, while the response during enflurane anesthesia is less predictable (38). The likelihood of arrhythmias is increased by hypoxia, marked hypercarbia and thiopental (39), but is decreased by the concomitant administration of lidocaine (40).

Calcium channel blocking drugs are widely used in patients suffering from supraventricular arrhythmias, hypertension, hypertrophic cardiomyopathy, coronary vasospasm and angina pectoris. Verapamil and diltiazem prevalently decrease SA node discharge and increase the AV node conduction time and refractory period. Nifedipine and nicardipine produce major coronary and systemic arteriolar vasodilation. Therefore verapamil and diltiazem produce more myocardial depression than do dihydroperidine blockers, possibly because of a smaller reduction in afterload and more negative chronotropic and dromotropic effects. Since inhalation anesthetics themselves are assumed to alter the voltage-dependent calcium channels by conformational changes (41), a synergistic negative dromotropic (bradyarrhythmias) and inotropic (hypotension) effect can result when both calcium entry blockers and inhalation anesthetics are administered. The negative inotropic effects in this case may be reversed by discontinuation of the inhalation anesthetic, and secondly by calcium salt cautiously administered in small doses. However, calcium is ineffective in conduction disturbances, which may respond to isoprenaline, glucagon and electrostimulation (42). Anyway isoflurane, that appears to more closely resemble the dihydroperidine blockers (e.g. nifedipine and nicardipine), interfere less than halothane and enflurane with the effects of the cardioactive calcium blockers verapamil and diltiazem (43).

Cyclic antidepressants inhibit catecholamine reuptake and have also some anticholinergic effect. Both events may increase the sensitivity of the heart to circulating catecholamine, and the latter may be further increased following pancuronium, which also possess some anticholinergic properties. Therefore the administration of pancuronium during halothane anesthesia of patients taking cyclic antidepressants may precipitate ventricular arrhythmias (44).

Inhalation anesthetics may provoke hypotension and bradyarrhythmias in patients receiving beta-adrenoceptor blocking drugs. The interaction seems to be basically additive or moderately synergistic in nature, depending on the drugs involved. The greater cardiovascular depression results from interactions between pure beta-adrenoceptor antagonists (e.g. atenolol, metoprolol or propranolol) and inhalation anesthetics that produce sympathomimetic stimulation (e.g. diethyl ether, cyclopropane or methoxyflurane). Merely additive cardiovascular effects occur, in contrast, when beta-adrenoceptor antagonists with an intrinsic sympathomimetic (partial agonist) action (e.g. alprenolol, oxprenolol, pindolol or practolol) interact with inhalation anesthetics which maintain cardiac output without stimulating sympathetic discharge (e.g. halothane, enflurane or isoflurane) (45). However, enflurane impairs the ability to respond to blood loss, and in presence of hypercarbia or anemia the combination of propranolol and halothane results in a significant degree of myocardial depression (45). The interaction of isoflurane with the beta-adrenoceptor blockers is less than with any of the other inhalation anesthetics (46), and it would appear to be the anesthetic agent of choice for use with these drugs, especially in the presence of additional stress as anemia, hypovolemia, hypoxia, hypercarbia or depression of left ventricular function.

Severe bradycardia may occur in patients on propranolol following the administration of atropine and neostigmine to reverse neuromuscular blockade (47). This is presumably due to the failure of atropine to exert a positive chronotropic effect in the presence of sympathetic blockade.

Acute ethanol intoxication causes a reduction in anesthetic dose requirements whereas the induction of anesthesia in chronic alcoholics is often prolonged and can be characterized by excitement and an increased anesthetic requirement (48, 49). Tolerance to drug-induced CNS depression in the chronic alcoholic may not apply to the cardiovascular system, so that serious depression may be associated with anesthetic concentrations required for unconsciousness (49).

Stimulation of the cardiovascular system by ketamine is not always desirable, and a number of pharmacological antagonists have been employed to block ketamine-induced tachycardia and systemic hypertension. Perhaps the most useful approach consists in the prior administration of benzodiazepines (50). In contrast, an adverse hemodynamic interaction can occur when diazepam is administered before high-dose fentanyl infusion as part of an anesthetic induction technique for patients undergoing coronary bypass surgery (51). The significant systemic hypotension arising from this interaction is probably due to a decreased adrenergic tone or to enhanced direct systemic vasodilation and can be prevented by small doses of phenylephrine or by increasing intravenous fluid administration.

Cardiac index, stroke index, and systemic blood pressure decrease when ketamine is administered to patients already anesthetized with halothane or enflurane (52). A plausible explanation for this is that the inhalation drug blocks the ketamine-induced sympathetic hyperactivity, which normally antagonizes ketamine's direct myocardial depressant effects.

Muscle relaxants often are combined with narcotic analgesics in anesthesia. Because the narcotics tend to produce vagally mediated bradycardia, one would logically choose a relaxant like pancuronium with an anticholinergic action to prevent or to reverse the bradycardia. Apparently, however, pancuronium not only prevents narcotic-induced bradycardia, but also increases heart rate and perhaps enhances sympathetic responses to noxious surgical stimulation (53). The latter responses may be undesirable in patients with limited coronary vascular reserve.

Inhalation anesthetics produce muscle relaxation in their own right and also potentiate, in a dose-dependent manner, the neuromuscular blockade resulting from the administration of muscle relaxants. Two mechanisms by which this occurs have been proposed (54). First, inhalation anesthetics increase muscle blood flow, enabling a greater concentration of relaxants to reach neuromuscular junction. Second, inhalation anesthetics also desensitize the postjunctional membrane to depolarization. Smaller doses of blocking agents are required for equivalent blockade during enflurane and isoflurane anesthesia than during halothane anesthesia.

Aminoglycoside antibiotics (e.g. amikacin, gentamicin, tobramycin, neomycin, streptomycin, kanamycin) potentiate neuromuscular blockade induced by either depolarizing or nondepolarizing muscle relaxants, but it is only the latter interaction that presents a significant clinical problem. Probably they reduce the influx of calcium presynaptically, thus reducing quantal release of acetylcholine (55). Other antibiotics, including the polymyxins, lincosamides (lyncomycin and clindamycin) and tetracyclines, have been shown to have not only prejunctional, but also postsynaptic effects which, by decreasing the sensitivity of the receptor site to acetylcholine, will potentiate the action of neuromuscular blocking agents (56). The neuromuscular block associated with aminoglycosides can be reversed by calcium, whereas the blockade produced by polymyxins, lincosamides and tetracyclines is often refractory to reversal by calcium salts and may be prolonged by anticholinesterases. The above antibiotics may thus produce different degrees of weakness when used in certain patients (e.g. those with myasthenia gravis), and they potentiate muscle paralysis induced by muscle relaxants. Under these circumstances, calcium salts may be administered to reverse the muscle paralyzing effects of aminoglycosides. However, it may be advisable to continue artificial ventilation and sedation until return of normal muscle function is assured.

Potentiation of the action of muscle relaxants has been reported with a wide range of other drugs. Magnesium can produce muscle weakness and can enhance both depolarizing and nondepolarizing blockade by acting presynaptically as a physiological antagonist to calcium, thus reducing quantal release of acetylcholine (57), and postsynaptically by decreasing both the depolarizing action of acetylcholine and the excitability of the muscle fiber itself (54). Patients presenting for anesthesia who are on magnesium sulfate therapy will therefore require a reduced dose of any neuromuscular blocker. Parenteral calcium will partially reverse magnesium-induced paresis. Lithium, like magnesium, has neuromuscular blocking properties in its own right, due to a prejunctional effect decreasing acetylcholine release. It delays the onset and prolongs the duration of action of succinylcholine and prolongs both the duration of nondepolarizing blockade and the reversal time by anticholinesterases (58). Interaction also occurs between steroids and nondepolarizing muscle relaxants. The acute administration of hydrocortisone decreases endplate sensitivity, thereby potentiating pancuronium, whereas chronic steroid therapy antagonizes pancuronium-induced neuromuscular blockade, probably facilitating calcium transport across the cell membrane (59). An intravenous infusion of nitroglycerin may prolong the duration of pancuronium-induced neuromuscular blockade (60). The reason is unknown but may be due to decreased renal clearance or an increase in affinity of pancuronium for the postjunctional nicotinic receptors in the presence of nitroglycerin. Azathioprine antagonizes the neuromuscular blockade by vecuronium or atracurium (61), whereas cyclosporine enhances it (62). While the mechanism of the latter drug interaction is unknown, that of the former seems to be an inhibition of presynaptic phosphodiesterase, so that the resultant increase in cAMP enhances acetylcholine release at neuromuscular junction. Finally, any drug which acts by depressing the electrical excitability of membranes has the potential to cause muscular weakness and to enhance the effects of muscle relaxants. Thus local anesthetics, antiarrhythmics, antiepileptics, beta-adrenoceptor blockers, calcium channel blockers and a host of related drugs may prolong both depolarizing and nondepolarizing neuromuscular blockade. The most serious interactions reported involve postoperative recurarization following the injection of lidocaine for the control of ventricular arrhythmias secondary to an increase in catecholamines.

Conclusion

This review has attempted to categorize the mechanisms of drug interaction in anesthesia along classic pharmacological lines. In doing so it is obvious that anesthesia comprises a vast array of potential interactions so that, when an anesthetist makes a preanesthetic assessment, not only the clinical status of the patient needs to be determined but also the polypharmacy to which the patient may be subjected. A thorough working knowledge of the anesthetic agents being used should include an awareness of their spheres of activity and where they may overlap with other drugs administered concomitantly. This may help the anesthetist to avoid adverse effects of such a reaction, while exploiting the benefits of others. New drugs are added to our armamentarium and others withdrawn with the passage of time, hence there is a continuing need for periodic reviews of this vast and interesting aspect of pharmacology.

References

1. Duthie DJR, Montgomery JN, Spence AA, Nimmo WS (1987) Concurrent drug therapy in patients undergoing surgery. Anaesthesia 42:305-311
2. Kluger MT, Gale S, Plummer JL, Owen H (1991) Perioperative drug prescribing pattern and manufacturers' guidelines. Anaesthesia 46:456-459
3. Lawson DH, Jick H (1976) Drug prescribing in hospitals: an international comparison. Am J Publ Health 66:644-648
4. Dambro MR, Kallgren MA (1988) Drug interactions in a clinic using costar. Comput Biol Med 18:31-38
5. Yuen IH, Denman SL, Sokoloski TD, Burkman LM (1979) Loss of nitroglycerin from aqueous solution into plastic intravenous delivery systems. J Pharm Sci 68:1163-1166
6. Mutch WAC, Thomson IR (1983) Delivery systems for intravenous nitroglycerin. Can Anaesth Soc J 30:98-99
7. Koren G, Goresky G, Crean P, Klein J, MacLeod SM (1984) Pediatric fentanyl dosing based on pharmacokinetics during cardiac surgery. Anesth Analg 63:577-582
8. Cullen BF, Miller MG (1979) Drug interactions and anesthesia: a review. Anesth Analg 58:413-423
9. Hindle AT, Columb MO, Shah MV (1995) Drug interactions and anaesthesia. Curr Anaesth Crit Care 6:103-112
10. Nimmo WS, Heading RC, Wilson J, Tothill P, Prescott LF (1975) Inhibition of gastric emptying and drug absorption by narcotic analgesics. Br J Clin Pharmacol 2:509-513
11. Gamble JAS, Gaston JH, Nair SG, Dundee JW (1976) Some pharmacological factors influencing the absorption of diazepam following oral administration. Br J Anaesth 48: 1181-1185
12. Lasser EC, Elizondo-Martel G, Granke RC (1963) Potentiation of pentobarbital anaesthesia by competitive protein binding. Anesthesiology 24:665-671
13. Kaukinen S, Eerola M, Ylitalo P (1980) Prolongation of thiopentone anaesthesia by probenecid. Br J Anaesth 52:603-607
14. Csogor SI, Kerek SF (1970) Enhancement of thiopentone anaesthesia by sulphafurazole. Br J Anaesth 42:988-990
15. Dale O, Nilsen OG (1984) Displacement of some basic drugs from human serum proteins by enflurane, halothane and their major metabolites. Br J Anaesth 56:535-542

16. Wood M (1986) Plasma drug binding: implications for anesthesiologists. Anesth Analg 65: 786-804
17. Ghoneim MM, Pandya H (1974) Plasma protein binding of bupivacaine and its interactions with other drugs in man. Br J Anaesth 46:435-438
18. McLain GE, Sipes IG, Brown BR Jr (1979) An animal model of halothane hepatotoxicity: roles of enzyme induction and hypoxia. Anesthesiology 51:321-326
19. Brown BR Jr, Sipes JC (1977) Biotransformation and hepatotoxicity of halothane. Biochem Pharmacol 26:2091-2094
20. Mazze RI, Woodruff RE, Heerdt ME (1982) Isoniazid-induced enflurane defluorination in humans. Anesthesiology 57:5-8
21. Sorkin EM, Ogawa GS (1981) Cimetidine potentiation of narcotic action. Drug Intell Clin Pharm 17:60-61
22. Lam AM (1981) Potentially lethal interaction of cimetidine and morphine. Can Med Assoc J 125:820
23. Klotz U, Reimann I (1980) Delayed clearance of diazepam due to cimetidine. N Engl J Med 302:1012-1014
24. Salonen M, Aantaa E, Aaltonen L (1986) Importance of the interaction of midazolam and cimetidine. Acta Pharmacol Toxicol 56:91-95
25. Freely J, Wilkinson Gr, Wood AJJ (1981) Reduction of liver blood flow and propranolol metabolism by cimetidine. N Engl J Med 304: 692-695
26. Knapp AB, Maguire W, Keren G, Karmen A, Levitt B, Miura DS, Somberg JC (1983) The cimetidine-lidocaine interaction. Ann Intern Med 98:174-177
27. Campbell MA, Plachetka JR, Jackson JE (1981) Cimetidine decreases theophylline clearance. Ann Intern Med 95:68-69
28. Hansen WE, Bertl S (1983) The inhibition of acetylcholinesterase and pseudocholinesterase by cimetidine. Arzneimittelforschung 33:161-163
29. Kambam JR, Dymond R, Krestow M (1987) Effect of cimetidine on duration of action of succinylcholine. Anesth Analg 66:191-192
30. Stirt AJ, Sperry RJ, DiFazio CA (1988) Cimetidine and succinylcholine: potential interactions and effect on neuromuscular blockade in man. Anesthesiology 69:607-608
31. Whittaker M (1980) Plasma cholinesterase variants and the anaesthetist. Anaesthesia 35: 174-197
32. Viby-Mogensen J (1983) Cholinesterase and succinylcholine. Dan Med Bull 30:129-150
33. Rogers KJ, Thornton JA (1969) The interaction between monoamine oxidase inhibitors and narcotic analgesics in mice. Br J Pharmacol 36:470-480
34. Gibb D (1984) Drug interactions in anaesthesia. Clin Anaesthesiol 2:485-512
35. Janowsky EC, Risch SC, Janowsky DS (1986) Psychotropic agents. In: Smith NT, Corbascio AN (eds) Drug interactions in anesthesia. Lea and Febiger, Philadelphia, pp 261-281
36. Stoeckel H, Hengstmann JH, Schuttler J (1979) Pharmacokinetics of fentanyl as a possible explanation for recurrence of respiratory depression. Br J Anaesth 51:741-745
37. Calvey TN, Milne LA, Williams NE, Chan K, Murray GR (1983) Effect of antacids on the plasma concentration of phenoperidine. Br J Anaesth 55:535-539
38. Johnston RR, Eger II EI, Wilson CA (1976) A comparative interaction of epinephrine with enflurane, isoflurane, and halothane in man. Anesth Analg 55:709-712
39. Atlee JL, Roberts FL (1986) Thiopental and epinephrine-induced dysrhythmias in dogs anesthetized with enflurane or isoflurane. Anesth Analg 65:437-443
40. Horrigan RW, Eger II EI, Wilson CW (1978) Epinephrine-induced arrhythmias during enflurane anesthesia in man: a nonlinear dose-response relationship and dose-dependent protection from lidocaine. Anesth Analg 57:547-550
41. Nakao S, Hirata H, Kagawa Y (1989) Effects of volatile anesthetics on cardiac calcium channels. Acta Anaesthesiol Scand 33:326-330
42. Durand PG, Lehot JJ, Foex P (1991) Calcium-channel blockers and anaesthesia. Can J Anaesth 38:75-89

43. Atlee JL, Hamann SR, Brownlee SW, Kreigh C (1988) Conscious state comparisons of the effects of the inhalation anesthetics and diltiazem, nifedipine, or verapamil on specialized atrioventricular conduction times in spontaneously beating dog hearts. Anesthesiology 68: 519-528

44. Quist Christensen L, Bonde J, Kampmann JP (1993) Drug interactions with inhalational anaesthetics. Acta Anaesthesiol Scand 37:231-244

45. Prys-Roberts C (1980) Cardiovascular effects of beta-receptor antagonists during anaesthesia. In: Prys-Roberts C (ed) The circulation in anaesthesia, applied physiology and pharmacology. Blackwell Scientific, Oxford, pp 406-428

46. Philbin DM, Lowenstein E (1976) Lack of beta-adrenergic activity of isoflurane in the dog: a comparison of the circulatory effects of halothane and isoflurane after propranolol administration. Br J Anaesth 48:1165-1170

47. Sprague DH (1975) Severe bradycardia after neostigmine in a patient taking propranolol to control paroxysmal atrial tachycardia. Anesthesiology 42:208-210

48. Wolfson B, Freed B (1980) Influence of alcohol on anesthetic requirements and acute toxicity. Anesth Analg 59:826-830

49. Bruce DL (1983) Alcoholism and anesthesia. Anesth Analg 62:84-96

50. White PF (1982) Comparative evaluation of intravenous agents for rapid sequence induction - thiopental, ketamine, and midazolam. Anesthesiology 57:279-284

51. Tomicheck RC, Rosow CE, Philbin DM, Moss J, Teplick RS, Schneider RC (1983) Diazepam-fentanyl interaction. Hemodynamic and hormonal effects in coronary artery surgery. Anesth Analg 62:881-884

52. Bidwai AV, Stanley TH, Graves CL, Kawamura R, Sentker CR (1975) The effects of ketamine on cardiovascular dynamics during halothane and enflurane anesthesia. Anesth Analg 54: 588-592

53. Salmenpera M, Peltola K, Takkunen O, Heinonen J (1983) Cardiovascular effects of pancuronium and vecuronium during high-dose fentanyl anesthesia. Anesth Analg 62: 1059-1064

54. Ostergaard D, Engbaek J, Viby-Mogensen J (1989) Adverse reactions and interactions of the neuromuscular blocking drugs. Med Toxicol Adverse Drug Exp 4:351-368

55. Fiekers JF (1983) Effects of the aminoglycoside antibiotics, streptomycin and neomycin, on neuromuscular transmission. J Pharmacol Exp Ther 225:487-495

56. Singh YN, Marshall IG, Harvey AL (1982) Pre- and post-junctional blocking effects of aminoglycoside, polymyxin, tetracycline and lincosamide antibiotics. Br J Anaesth 54: 1295-1306

57. Ghoneim MM, Long JP (1970) The interaction between magnesium and other neuromuscular blocking agents. Anesthesiology 32: 23-27

58. Hill GE, Wong KC, Hodges MR (1977) Lithium carbonate and neuromuscular blocking agents. Anesthesiology 46:122-126

59. Laflin MJ (1977) Interaction of pancuronium and corticosteroids. Anesthesiology 47:471-472

60. Glisson SN, El-Etr A, Lim R (1979) Prolongation of pancuronium-induced neuromuscular blockade by intravenous infusion of nitroglycerin. Anesthesiology 51:47-49

61. Dretchen KL, Morgenroth III VH, Standaert FG, Walts LF (1976) Azathioprine: effects on neuromuscular transmission. Anesthesiology 45:604-609

62. Gramstad L, Gjerlow JA, Hysing ES, Rugstad HE (1986) Interaction of cyclosporin and its solvent, cremophor, with atracurium and vecuronium. Studies in the cat. Br J Anaesth 58: 1149-1155

INJURY AND TISSUE DAMAGE

Cellular and Humoral Markers of Tissue Damage

W. URACZ, R.J. GRYGLEWSKI

Introduction

Patients with sepsis who are hospitalized in intensive care units frequently develop multiple organ dysfunction failure syndrome (MODFS) with a poor prognosis (1-3). It is believed that injury in MOFDS is brought about by factors which under normal conditions play a regulatory role in homeostatic mechanisms (Table 1).

Table 1. Factors involved in septic shock

Cytokines
Growth factors
Adhesins
CD antigens
Lipid mediators
Gas mediators
Transcription factors
Oncogenes
Genes

Some of these factors are humoral like cytokines, growth factors, lipid and gas mediators while others like oncogenes and their protein products, transcription factors (i.e. nuclear factor kappa B, NFκB) or DNA nuclear material are widely recognized as cellular ones. Adhesins might be viewed both as cellular (or membrane-bound) and soluble (humoral) factors. The distinction between cellular and humoral factors tends to be more and more vague.

A widely used classification for the cluster of differentiation (CD) antigens involves not only cellular markers but also some cytokines and their receptors in membrane-bound and soluble forms (4). The best example of the dual role of cellular markers is class I major histocompatibility antigens (MHC or HLA) (5). These were first recognized as membrane-bound molecules on all nucleated cells, and the existence of soluble HLA antigens has also been reported. HLA antigens are known markers of severe brain damage or of the onset of transplant rejection (5, 6).

Many of the mediators associated with MODFS are generated by macrophages which being maximally stimulated already escaped physiological regulatory mechanisms and are genetically recoded to their death. This state is known as programmed cell death or apoptosis (7, 8). At a cellular level apoptosis and necrosis are responsible for the release of cellular markers to the body fluids. Apoptosis regulates cell number and eliminates damaged or infected cells. Also shedding off the cell-bound molecules from macrophages, or from other cells with the fast membrane turnover might be a source of soluble forms of cellular markers.

Baue and Faist suggested the following stages of development of MODFS: infection, increased permeability of intestinal mucosa, involvement of immune system (macrophages, cytokines, antibodies, receptors); generalized inflammation associated with a damage to endothelium, oedema and impaired oxygen availability; and finally ischaemia with reduced microcirculatory flow, necrosis and eventually MODFS (2).

This systemic inflammatory response syndrome (SIRS) caused by infection is characterized by the exacerbation of the production of pro- and anti-inflammatory mediators (9). The cascade of cellular and humoral factors (Table 1) released by endotoxin (LPS) includes thromboxane A_2 (TXA_2), nitric oxide (NO), oxygen free radicals (O_2-, OH'), lipid peroxides (LOO'), leukotrienes (LTB_4-E_4), platelet-activating factor (PAF), tumour necrosis factor ($TNF\alpha$), interleukins (IL-1, IL-4, IL-6, IL-8, IL-10, IL-12, IL-13), interferons α and γ ($IFN\alpha$, $IFN\gamma$), cytoadhesins (ELAM, ICAM, sPAGEM), soluble TNF (sTNF R) and IL-1 (IL-1ra) receptors, transforming growth factor β ($TGF\beta$) and many others.

Although in many animal models of septic shock removal of the above mediators has conferred successful protection, so far very poor results have been achieved in humans. Current understanding of the setting of an anti-inflammatory response by the host seems to indicate that the host organism is responsible for putting into motion most of the necessary regulatory processes. Indeed, both pro- and anti-inflammatory mediators appear to be markers of the severity of the disease. However, after exhaustion of adaptive mechanisms, therapeutic help in SIRS is required.

Various therapeutic approaches have been proposed to interfere with the development of SIRS (9-11). These include antibodies to: endotoxin (LPS), anti-IL-1, anti-IL-8, anti-IL-12, anti-CD14, anti-73kDa LPS receptor, anti-IFNγ, monoclonal antibodies to TNFα, macrophage migration inhibitory factor (MIF) and lymphocyte migration inhibitory factor (LIF), anti-CD11b, anti-ICAM-1, anti-ELAM-1, anti-superoxide dismutase, IL-1 receptor antagonists, sTNF R, IL-1β converting enzyme inhibitors (ICE), aprotinin, hirudin, heparin, platelet activating factor (PAF) antagonists, cyclooxygenases (COX-1 and COX-2) inhibitors (nonsteroidal anti-inflammatory drugs, NSAID), steroid hormones, lipooxygenase inhibitors and NO synthase (NOS) inhibitors, prostacyclin analogues, tyrosine kinase inhibitors, lipid X, lipoaminoacids, as well as infusions of various electrolytes or buffers containing catecholamines, vasopressin, angiotensin Il or sometimes phenoxybenzamine (10, 12-22). A relapse of time between an infection and administration of a putative drug is crucial for its efficacy. Lack of success in the treatment of MODFS with curative molecules which were effective in the experimental models of septic shock might be explained, at least partially, by a late stage of SIRS at which the therapy is usually implemented (9).

Out of a broad scope of tissue damage markers which are important in MODFS we will focus on: i) LPS/ceramide CD14 system in the induction of septic shock, ii) cytokines - inhibition of their production and cytokine-binding proteins, iii) serum HLA class I antigens, iv) lipid mediators, v) NO as a marker of septic shock and vi) apoptosis.

LPS/ceramide CD14 system

Most cases of sepsis and septic shock are secondary to infections with Gram-negative bacteria (23, 24). The Gram-negative bacterial cell wall consists of inner and outer membranes, the latter portion of which contains proteins as well as LPS (14, 25). It is useful to review briefly the structure of LPS. LPSs are complex molecules composed of three major parts: a polysaccharide side chain (O-antigen), which is attached via a bridging (core) polysaccharide to a glucosamine-based phospholipid (lipid A). The most variable part of the LPS structure is the O antigen. In contrast, the lipid A and to some extend also core region are more conserved (26). This is why antibodies are produced which may cross-react.

Endotoxin is measured utilizing the haemolymph of amoebocytes from the Limus horseshoe crab (27). This substance contains a proenzyme which is directly activated by endotoxin leading to visible gelling of the mixture. Spectrophotometric modification of the Limus amoebocyte lysate (LAL) assay detects endotoxin to less than 10 pg/dl. Unfortunately, the accuracy of the LAL assay is affected by numerous circulating plasma proteins (i.e. antithrombin III, anti-endotoxic antibodies, etc.) and it can be positive in patients with Gram-positive bacterial and fungal infections (28). This may be related to the gut leak which accompanies these infections. Measurement of LPS levels in diagnostic practice shows that endotoxin is often present in sepsis; its presence might correlate with the severity of clinical manifestations and end-organ dysfunction. However, the same literature consistently finds out that endotoxaemia, as detected by LAL assay, is not invariably present in clinical sepsis as the results of LAL assay must be viewed with scepticism (14). In clinical practice, useful markers that may indicate the presence of Gram-negative bacteria sepsis are: blood culture for Gram-negative microbe or culture or Gram stain positive for a Gram-negative microbe at a local site of infection (26).

It has been shown that nerve growth factor (NGF), TNFα, IL-1β or Fas ligand after binding to their specific CD40 transmembrane receptors stimulate cells by releasing the intracellular messenger ceramide (29-32). This stimulation is completed through activating neutral sphingomyelinases. Agonist-induced hydrolysis of sphingomyelin puts in motion the sphingomyelin cycle analogous to the signal transduction by the phosphatidyloinositol and glycerophospholipid system (33).

Recent studies on the composition of the outer leaflet of the outer membrane of some Gram-negative bacteria emphasize the presence of a glycosphingolipid but not the LPS. This bacterium has been named *Sphingomonas* (34). The substitution of sphingolipids for LPS in this bacterium confirms that the physical properties of sphingolipids may be interchangeable with those of LPS. Indeed, the examination of the structure of LPS and ceramide have revealed a strong similarity between their molecules. Computer molecular modelling and conformational dynamics yielded a solution structure for the acylated glucosamine I of LPS with a strong similarity to that of ceramide (35). Identical chirality at two optical active carbon centres and approximately similar lengths of the hydrocarbon chains make the molecules of LPS and ceramide very much alike. LPS along with TNF and IL-1 cause common events in cells such as: (i) mitogen-activated protein kinase activation; (ii) NF-κB translocation; (iii) activator protein 1 stimulation; (iv) phospholipase A_2 activation and (v) TNF gene expression (35).

For recognition of endotoxin, a binding protein/receptor system involving LPS-binding protein (LBP) and CD14 molecule has been postulated. However, effects of LPS occur also in CD14-negative cells, and not all of them depend on the presence of LPB. This is why not all pathways in recognition of endotoxin are already defined. Several cellular structures have been found to bind LPS. For instance, the scavenger receptor or CD11/CD18 are involved in the detoxification of LPS (36). Several not well characterized membrane proteins with 18, 25, 38, 55, and 65 kDa were found to bind LPS. Also, 40- and 80 kDa, as well as 70- to 80 kDa proteins have been postulated in LPS recognition by various cell types (25). The CD14 molecule, however, has been unequivocally established to be a LPS receptor (37). CD14 is found as a 53 kDa glycoprotein on the cell surface (mCD14) of all mature myeloid cells. The gene for CD14 is located on the fifth chromosome in a region known to encode several cytokines including granulocyte/macrophage colony stimulating factor (GM-CSF), CSF-1, IL-3, endothelial cell growth factor (ECGF), as well as receptors like CSF-1 receptor, platelet-derived growth factor receptor, FMS (c-fms photooncogen) and β-adrenergic receptor. The 32 identified amino acid residues have 40 kDa and almost completely match the amino acid sequence deduced from the CD14 cDNA. In the plasma of healthy adults 4-6 µg/ml of soluble CD14 (sCD14) are found and sCD14 is highly elevated up to 200 µg/ml in the plasma of septic patients. Two slightly different soluble forms of CD14 molecules exist which can be found in normal serum, most likely due to shedding of mCD14 as it was shown for endothelial cells (38).

Endotoxins or LPS are undoubtedly the molecules responsible for most of the pathophysiological phenomena associated with Gram-negative infections. Experimental and clinical observations indicate that endotoxin may exert its deleterious effects upon the host to a large part by provoking the release of a variety of endogenous mediators, although direct toxicity may also occur. In 1968, Chedid et al. proposed and used an antibody capable of neutralizing endotoxins. In 1982, Ziegler et al. used antiserum prepared in healthy volunteers injected with J5 LPS of rough mutant of *Escherichia coli* and substantially reduced deaths from bacteraemia (10, 11, 14). Modern technology has enabled researchers to prepare monoclonal antibodies (mAb). Many mAbs have been generated and studied. The most well known are those which reached the stage of clinical studies. E5 mAb from Xoma Corporation and HA.1A mAb from Centocor were reported to be effective for patients with sepsis and Gram-negative bacteraemia (39, 40). The neutralizing therapy is extremely expensive and the results of double blind randomized placebo controlled multicentre trials are indicative but not conclusive. The current limitations of treatment of septic patients with anti-LPS antibodies, beside the not trivial financial impact, are connected with the fact that an increasing proportion of cases of sepsis are related to infection with Gram-positive bacteria; it is difficult to demonstrate cross-reactivity against rough mutants and so far neutralization of the effect of endotoxin by antibodies has not been described. The theoretical premise that LPS antibodies are cross-protective is attractive but requires further investigation (14).

Soluble CD14 can act as an inhibitor at the monocyte/macrophage level. In contrast, sCD14 is involved in the activation of endothelial cells by LPS (41). This observation limits the therapeutic use of sCD14 but leaves room for the use of anti-CD14 antibodies. It was reported that the anti-CD14 strategy reduced hypotension, lowered cytokine production and prevented pulmonary oedema.

Proinflammatory cytokine in sepsis

While the initiating event in sepsis may be the release of endotoxin, many of the clinical symptoms of sepsis result from the release of endogenous mediators such as TNF, IL-1, IL-6, IL-8, PAF etc., mononuclear phagocytes and other cells, including endothelial cells. Each of these mediators stimulates both its own release and the release of other mediators and acts in concert to produce symptoms of sepsis. The proinflammatory cytokines TNFα and IL-1β have been studied extensively. It is generally accepted that these cytokines play a central role in the pathogenesis of sepsis (13, 19, 20, 42).

Plasma levels of TNF are a marker of sepsis and depend on the severity of disease. After bolus injection of endotoxin, blood levels of TNFα typically increase at 30 min and peak at 90 min (9, 19, 20). TNF is known to stimulate not only the release of several other cytokines (e.g. IL-1, IL-6, PAF), but also the production of endothelial adhesion molecules which promote neutrophil-endothelial cell adherences. Likewise, TNF enhances neutrophil phagocytosis and injures endothelial cells as manifested by an increase of endothelial cell permeability. TNF is rapidly cleared from the systemic circulation due to its short half-life (14-18 min in humans) and returns to base levels within a few hours (43). This is why plasma TNF activity alone is not a reliable prognostic factor in septicaemia and supports the concept that TNFα is an early mediator that initiates the changes that lead to the extensive cellular injury (44). However, the strongest evidence supporting the role of the TNF in the pathogenesis of septic shock, SIRS and MODFS comes from studies that employed anti-TNF antibodies (10). The favourable effect of anti-TNF antibodies in experimental septic shock were most prominent when antibody was administered prior to the infusion of LPS. Based on these observations, it is clear that for TNF antibodies to be effective, the antibody must be given before or very soon after the onset of bacterial infection (14).

The polypeptide hormone IL-1 is another important factor in host defence and exists in two forms: IL-1α and IL-1β. Both are potent proinflammatory monokines with biological effects that include endothelial cell activation and increase of adhesion molecule receptor expression. In addition, IL-1 promotes the release of other cytokines (TNF, IL-6, PAF) and acts synergistically with TNF in the production of many of its biological and inflammatory effects such as hypotension, endothelial cell injury, increased vascular permeability and, finally, death (45). Like TNF, serum levels of IL-1 rise after endotoxin infusion. However, in contrast with TNF, serum levels of IL-1 reach their peak 3-4 h after LPS challenge (20).

IL-6 is another cytokine in the inflammatory network. Expression of IL-6 is induced in many cells, including mononuclear phagocytes and endothelial cells, after stimulation with LPS, IL-1 and TNF. IL-6 is thought to promote neutrophil activation and accumulation at sites of inflammation (46). In keeping with these properties of IL-6, increased plasma concentrations of IL-6 have been detected in patients with sepsis and are associated with increased mortality. For that reason, most authors now agree that IL-6 is a marker of the severity of the infection (45, 47, 48).

IL-8 is a recently described peptide that is secreted by a variety of cells such as alveolar macrophages, monocytes, endothelial cells in response to endotoxin, IL-1 and TNF (15, 49). IL-8 causes chemoattraction and activation of neutrophils and is believed to mediate neutrophil recruitment in host defence and disease (50-52). It was also demonstrated that IL-8 enhances binding affinity of adhesion molecules on human neutrophils (53, 54). The accumulation of activated neutrophils in lungs and other organs is felt to play a key role in the pathogenesis of SIRS and MODFS (55, 56).

An important first step in the process of neutrophil-mediated organ injury involves the binding of neutrophils to endothelial cells (57, 58). This interaction is largely regulated by complementary adherence molecules that are present on these cells and expressed in increasing numbers in response to endotoxin, TNF, IL-1, and IL-8. Endothelial and neutrophil cell activation by these cytokines is accompanied by enhanced expression of adhesin molecules such as ELAM1, VCAM1, ICAM1 (59). Anti-CD18 antibodies, in contrast to anti-CD11 antibodies, are able to reduce LPS-induced neutrophil sequestration in tissue and organ injury (59, 60). This antibody worsened endotoxaemia, acidosis and cardiovascular function in a canine model of LPS shock and in the baboon model of sepsis. In the same model, anti-ELAM1 therapy was beneficial. The contribution of the adhesion molecule and the interaction between endothelial and circulating cells play a major role in tissue damage and organ dysfunction. However, the use of antibodies to interfere in this process remains controversial (13).

Cytokine-binding proteins

Cytokine-binding proteins (CBPs), such as cytokine receptors and antibodies, mostly monoclonal, impair interactions of cytokines with their cellular receptors and so these agents can potentially provide a means for treating pathological conditions that have a significant cytokine involvement as is the case in septic shock. Indeed, the efficacy of such treatment was demonstrated for the first time a decade ago whereby experimental shock was prevented by antibodies against TNFα (61, 62). The cloning of genes encoding cytokine receptor chains, and the characterization of their soluble forms, has opened the way to new strategies in anticytokine therapy. These molecules clearly act as antagonists of their respective ligands through competition with the membrane receptors that transduce the biological signal into the target cell. As anticipated, the injection of sIL-1R modulate the allogenic response in vitro and prevent allograft rejection (63). Cerami's group and many others have confirmed the protective activities of anti-TNF antibodies in various models. Also in humans, anti-TNF antibodies were effective when combined with antibiotics (10, 14, 61). Counteracting the effect of another proinflammatory cytokine, IL-1 has been investigated with the IL-1 receptor antagonist (IL-1-ra) (64-66). This natural IL-1-like molecule binds to the same receptors as IL-1, but fails to transmit any signal (61). A second phase III study of IL-1ra was dropped after an interim analysis had failed to show any evidence of benefit (10). Another possibility for containing IL-1 is the use of IL-1β converting enzyme (ICE) inhibitors. ICE is responsible for cleaving a biologically inactive IL-1 precursor into the mature IL-1 active form (67). The results of the INTERSEPT placebo-controlled trial of anti-TNF mAb

(Bayx1351) in 563 patients with severe sepsis shows lack of significantly altered mortality between the studied groups (68).

In contrast, the results of the Immunex study of p75 sTNFR-Fc which have now been reported indicate an increase of mortality among patients in the treated group. In patients with sepsis, plasma levels of both sTNFR p55 and p75 are markedly increased and highly correlate with simultaneously obtained APACHE II and MODFS scores. Since the degree of increased sTNFR levels correlated poorly with patient survival, elevated sTNFR levels represent a good marker for severity of sepsis and predict an outcome (69).

However, exceptions do exist: soluble IL-6 receptor and cilliary neurotrophic factor act as agonists (70). A potential advantage of soluble receptors over high affinity mAbs is that they are of human origin and, accordingly, the problem of patient immunization is obviated. There are two drawbacks of soluble receptors: (i) their usually lower affinity than that of mAb and (ii) their shorter half-life in vivo because they are molecules smaller than antibodies. To overcome these problems, for instance, immunoadhesins have been generated that comprise two soluble receptor fragments linked genetically to a human immunoglobulin constant region (i.e. sTNFR-Fc) (71-74). Additionally, this procedure decreases the therapeutic dose of soluble CBPs in vivo. However, the major drawback of using CBPs relates to the fact that they stabilize the cytokine in the form of a cytokine-CBP complex in vivo (61). The first demonstration that CBPs are capable of stabilizing cytokines was provided by treatment with anti-IL-6 mAbs. The longer in vivo half-life of IL-6-anti-IL-6 complexes (3.5 days) provides a pharmacokinetic explanation for the accumulation of cytokine (the half-life of free IL-6 is as low as 20 min) and for their potential action as agonists (62). However, when CBPs are present in excess over the cytokine-membrane receptor, they seem to act as antagonists.

Inhibition of proinflammatory cytokine production

Rather than counteracting cytokines already generated, inhibition of their production may prevent these mediators from becoming involved in the immunoinflammatory cascade. Glucocorticoids were thought to do it; however, using them in sepsis has not been successful (13). Pentoxyphylline, a phosphodiesterase inhibitor, limits the synthesis of TNF (75). Various drugs which reduced TNF and/or IL-1 production (e.g. linomide, prostacyclin analogues or chlorpromazine) also had beneficial effects in experimental models of septic shock (76-78). More recently, it has been shown that tyrosine kinase inhibitors block LPS-induced TNF and NO production (79).

Cytokines such as IL-4, IL-10, IL-13 and TGFβ possess anti-inflammatory properties because they inhibit the generation of the most of proinflammatory cytokines in monocytes/macrophages. Moreover, these particular cytokines also induce IL-1-ra (13). Among other putative beneficial cytokines is IFNα (80). Its usefulness in septic shock is still controversial. Maybe the natural balance between pro- and anti-inflammatory cytokines is not sufficient to slow down the running inflammatory cascade.

Serum HLA class I antigens

More than 20 years ago, MHC class I antigens were reported to be present in serum. The development of anti-HLA mAbs had a significant impact on the analysis of serum HLA class I antigens. Similar to their cell-membrane associated counterpart, the serum HLA class I molecular complex comprises a polymorphic heavy α-chain noncovalently associated with β_2 microglobulin. The level of serum HLA class I antigens markedly increases in the course of viral infections caused by cytomegalovirus, hepatitis B virus, hepatitis C virus, varicella-zostervirus, and human immunodeficiency-1 virus. During HIV-1 infection, the level of serum HLA class I antigens correlates with stages of disease and represents a good prognostic marker of the disease progression. An increase in the level of total serum HLA class I antigens has also been observed in recipients of heart, kidney or liver transplants. The rapid decrease in the level of serum HLA antigens observed following immunosuppressive therapy of acute episodes of graft rejection suggests that their level may be the result of immune system activation. The elevation of donor-derived serum HLA class I allospecificities precedes the clinical evidence of a graft rejection episode. It means that measurement of donor-derived serum HLA antigens may represent a test to diagnose graft rejection episodes (5, 6, 81, 82).

Lipid mediators

Many other mediators produced by activated cells contribute to the inflammatory syndrome. Some may be directly induced by LPS while others may be induced following target cell activation by proinflammatory cytokines. As a consequence, prostaglandins (PGs), thromboxane, leukotrienes and PAF are other potential targets for therapeutic approach (13, 21). Inhibition of PG formation by COX-2 rather than COX-1 inhibitors (e.g. ibuprofen) attenuate many alterations associated with LPS injection in animal models of endotoxin shock and inhibit TNF production. However, the experiments in human volunteers show that an injection of ibuprofen immediately before administration of endotoxin caused a significant increase in the level of circulating TNF. Prostaglandin E_1 (PGE_1) has several properties that could be beneficial for the treatment of severe sepsis. It is a potent vasodilator of the pulmonary and systemic circulation. Like prostacyclin, it has also important anti-inflammatory effects by blocking macrophage activation. It can influence coagulation by inhibiting platelet aggregation and by inducing fibrynolysis. In dogs, PGE$_1$ almost entirely restored tissue oxygen extraction after endotoxin challenge (83). PAF antagonists have led to successful protection in various septic shock models induced by LPS. Recent study in patients with sepsis has shown that BN52021 (a PAF inhibitor) offered an improvement (10, 13). Another PAF antagonist, TCV-309, inhibited cytokine production in experimental endotoxaemia in chimpanzees (84).

Nitric oxide as a marker of septic shock

The free radical of NO is synthesized from L-arginine by a family of enzymes - NO synthases (NOS) (85). The continuous biosynthesis of NO by the constitutive endothelial isoform of NOS (eNOS) keeps the vasculature in active vasodilatation and reduces platelets and polymorphonuclear cell adhesion to the endothelium. The inducible isoform of NOS (iNOS) is expressed in response to immunological stimuli. iNOS produces NO at nanomolar amounts and then acts as a cytostatic and cytotoxic agent.

The role of NO in septic shock will be presented in a separate contribution and this is why only a very short summary of available data will be presented here. It has been suggested that the overproduction of NO is responsible for death during endotoxic shock or sepsis (86-91). In 1989, Vallance et al. showed that inhibition of NO synthesis by N^G-monomethyl-L-arginine (L-NMMA) had elevated blood pressure in rats (92). Furthermore, it was demonstrated that local infusion of L-NAME into brachial artery of healthy volunteers caused a dose-dependent fall in resting forearm blood flow and attenuated the dilator response to acetylcholine. The effect of L-NAME was stereospecific (D-NAME was ineffective) and reversed by supplying an excess of L-arginine (93). Ochoa et al. found elevated nitrite/nitrate levels (stable breakdown products of NO) in patients with septic shock but these levels were decreased in patients with trauma (94, 95). Recently, Wang and Chaudry pointed out the complexity of the alteration in NO production with the progression of sepsis (91). They hypothesized that NO inhibition under some septic conditions might be detrimental. We also observed ambiguous effects of NOS inhibitors in rats with LPS-induced shock. When NOS inhibitors had been administered before LPS was given, the removal of NO potentiated LPS-induced shock. Administration of NO inhibitors in the second hour after injection of LPS caused a temporary improvement. The activity of eNOS is regulated by calmodulin and changes in intracellular calcium. The enhanced formation of NO in the early stage of shock is due to the activation of eNOS. We observed the induction of iNOS mRNA in the lungs, spleen and heart of LPS-treated rats as early as 1 h after endotoxin administration. This is why we postulate that in early and late stages of shock, differential effects of nonselective NOS inhibitors might account for their action on different isoforms of NOS. So far, the role of NOS inhibitors in the treatment of sepsis remains to be defined. The availability of specific inhibitors of iNOS would help to answer the relevant questions. Such agents are in the early stages of development but they have not as yet been studied in humans (96, 97).

Programmed cell death - apoptosis

Apoptosis constitutes an efficient system in cell biology designed to eliminate superfluous, unwanted, altered, aged, or transformed cells without eliciting damage to adjacent normal cells or surrounding tissues. The mechanism of apoptosis has long been neglected in clinical research and in clinical thinking. Nevertheless, apoptosis offers understanding of a number of pathological syndromes and clinical observations which otherwise cannot be explained by well-known biological processes. Leucocytes, monocytes and macrophages are selectively eliminated from inflammatory tissues by the occurrence of programmed cell death. The therapeutic regulation of apoptosis during and after an inflammation offers a new approach for promoting rapid healing and reduction of unwanted pathological sequelae of inflammation processes (7, 8, 98, 99).

Necrosis, or accidental cell death, occurs in response to harmful insults such as physical damage, hypoxia, hyperthermia, complement attack or chemical injury. Table 2 shows the differences between apoptosis and necrosis.

Analysis of the mechanism that prevents cell death, such as activation of the bcl-2 gene, addition of growth factors and the use of protein synthesis inhibitors or calcium entry blockers, might aid in the development of new treatment strategies. Drug and therapy designs directed at the modulation of apoptotic process will offer new opportunities for the treatment and control of tissue damage in the coming years. If these goals can be accomplished, we may finally see a reduction in the morbidity and mortality associated with MODFS.

Conclusion

Comprehension of the basic mechanisms involved in the host inflammatory response is necessary for clinicians to make educated choices and decisions regarding therapies. The discovery of the sphingomyelin cycle as a target of LPS action that mimics natural mediator ceramide promoted progress in our understanding of the events during the development of septic shock. Advances in molecular biology and in the cytokine network led to the development of novel approaches to the treatment of septic shock, SIRS and MODFS. As noted in this review, therapies are directed to distinct levels: the initiating event (i.e. endotoxin), to various mediators, and the effector cells (i.e. macrophages, endothelial cells). These factors are not merely markers of sepsis and its severity,

Table 2

	Apoptosis	Necrosis
Origin	Lack of growth factors, hormonal factors, mild toxic stimuli	Anoxia, starvation, physical and chemical damage
Occult phase	Minutes to hours	None
First manifestation	Shrinking	Swelling
Nuclear changes	Pyknosis, condensation, internucleosome cleavage, DNA laddering	Karyolysis
Chromatin	Segmentation and margination	Nuclear folding
Nucleolar changes	Intact	Granulated
Membrane integrity	Persists	Failure
Surface	Smoothing	Lysis, blebbing
Cytoskeleton	Formation of apoptotic bodies	Fragmentation
Mitochondria	Unaffected	Swelling
Endoplasmic reticulum and Golgi apparatus	Unaffected	Dilated
Organelles	Intact	Swollen, leaky
Gene expression	p53 ↑, bcl-2 ↓, c-myc ↑	No change
Protein synthesis	Blocked by cycloheximide and actinomycin D	Not affected by antibiotics
Cytoplasmic changes	Endonuclease activity ↑, transglutaminase ↑	Release of lysosome content
Cells affected	Dispersed cells	Diffuse degradation
Cell elimination	Engulfment by macrophages and endothelial cells	Inflammatory response in adjacent tissues

but play an important role in the pathophysiological mechanisms. The era of cytokine response modification in patients with severe sepsis has evolved rapidly. These therapies if they prove effective in clinical trials are in progress and it should be stressed that current interventional capacities are far ahead of our comprehension of the mechanisms involved. Moreover, we should remember that these therapies are enormously expensive. Finally, taking into account that apoptosis is a natural route of macrophage elimination, some present therapies might be ineffective because they act on cells already programmed to their death, no matter how much effort is engaged to keep them alive.

References

1. Barton R, Cerra FB (1989) The hypermetabolism. Multiple organ failure syndrome. Chest 96:1153-1160
2. Baue AE (1994) Organ dysfunction (MODS), organ failure (MOF) and therapeutic conundrums in injured and septic patients. In: Gullo A (ed) Sepsis and organ failure. Fogliazza editore, Trieste, pp 9-39
3. Baue AE (1992) The horror autotoxicus and multiple-organ failure. Arch Surg 127:1451-1462
4. Schlossman SF, Boumsell L, Gilks W, Harlan JM, Kishimoto T, Morimoto C, Ritz J, Shaw S, Silverstein RL, Springer TA, Tedder TF, Todd RF (1993) CD antigens 1993. Immonol Today 15:98-99
5. Puppo F, Scudeletti M, Indiveri F, Ferrone S (1995) Serum class I antigens: markers and modulators of an immune response? Immonol Today 16:124-127
6. Ferrone S, Yamamura M, Grosse-Wilde H, Pouletty P (1992) Summary of serum-soluble HLA class I antigen component. In: Kimiyoshi Tsuji MA (ed) HLA 1991. Oxford, New York, pp 1057-1061
7. Haanen C, Vermes I (1995) Apoptosis and inflammation. Mediators of Inflammation 4:5-15
8. Vermes I, Haanen C (1994) Apoptosis and programmed cell death in health and disease. Adv Clin Chem 31:177-246
9. Darville T, Giroir B, Jacobs R (1993) The systemic inflammatory response syndrome (SIRS): immunology and potential immunotherapy. Infection 21:279-290
10. Lynn WA, Cohen J (1995) Adjunctive therapy for septic shock: a review of experimental approaches. CID 20:143-158
11. Manthous CA, Hall JB, Samsel RW (1993) Endotoxin in human disease. Part 2: Biologic effects and clinical evaluations of anti-endotoxin therapies. Chest 104:1872-1881
12. Gawaz M, Fateh-Moghadam S, Pilz G, Gurland H-J, Werdan K (1995) Severity of multiple organ failure (MOF) but not of sepsis correlates with irreversible platelet degranulation. Infection 1:16-23
13. Cavaillon J-M (1995) Controversies surrounding current therapies for sepsis syndrome. Bull Inst Pasteur 93:21-41
14. Talan DA (1993) Recent developments in our understanding of sepsis: evaluation of anti-endotoxin antibodies and biological response modifiers. Ann Emerg Med 22:1871-1890
15. St. John RC, Dorinsky PM (1993) Immunologic therapy for ARDS, septic shock, and multiple-organ failure. Chest 103:932-943
16. Bar Natan MF, Wilson MA, Spain DA, Garrison RN (1995) Platelet-activating factor and sepsis-induced small intestinal microvascular hypoperfusion. J Surg Res 58:38-45
17. Lin RY, Astiz ME, Saxon JC, Rackow EC (1993) Altered leukocyte immunophenotypes in septic shock. Studies of HLA-DR, CD11b, CD14, and IL-2R expression. Chest 104:847-853
18. Lin RY, Astiz ME, Saxon JC, Saha DC, Rackow EC (1993) Alterations in C3, C4, factor B, and related metabolites in septic shock [see comments]. Clin Immunol Immunopathol 69:136-142
19. Busund R, Lindsetmo RO, Rasmussen LT, Rokke O, Rekvig OP, Revhaug A (1991) Tumor necrosis factor and interleukin 1 appearance in experimental gram-negative septic shock. The effects of plasma exchange with albumin and plasma infusion. Arch Surg 126:591-597
20. van Deuren M, van der Ven Jongekrijg J, Demacker PN, Bartelink AK, van Dalen R, Sauerwein RW, Gallati H, Vannice JL, van der Meer JW (1994) Differential expression of proinflammatory cytokines and their inhibitors during the course of meningococcal infections. J Infect Dis 169:157-161
21. Korbut R, Warner TD, Gryglewski RJ, Vane JR (1994) The effect of nitric oxide synthase inhibition on the plasma fibrinolytic system in septic shock in rats. Br J Pharmacol 112:289-291
22. Smith MFJ, Eidlen D, Arend WP, Gutierrez Hartmann A (1994) LPS-induced expression of the human IL-1 receptor antagonist gene is controlled by multiple interacting promoter elements. J Immunol 153:3584-3593

23. Glauser MP, Heumann D, Baumgartner JD, Cohen J (1994) Pathogenesis and potential strategies for prevention and treatment of septic shock: an update. Clin Infect Dis 18 (Suppl 2):S205-S216
24. Parrillo JE (1993) Pathogenetic mechanisms of septic shock [see comments]. N Engl J Med 328:1471-1477
25. Schumann RR, Rietschel ET, Loppnow H (1994) The role of CD14 and lipopolysaccharide-binding protein (LBP) in the activation of different cell types by endotoxin. Med Microbiol Immunol 183:279-297
26. Manthous CA, Hall JB, Samsel RW (1993) Endotoxin in human disease. Part 1: Biochemistry, assay, and possible role in diverse disease states. Chest 104:1572-1581
27. Levin J, Tomasulo PA, Oser RJ (1970) Detection of endotoxin in blood and demonstration of an inhibitor. J Lab Clin Med 75:903-911
28. Danner RL, Elin RJ, Hosseini JM, Wesley RA, Reilly JM, Parillo JE (1991) Endotoxemia in human septic shock. Chest 99:169-175
29. Bagasra O, Wright SD, Seshamma T, Oakes JW, Pomerantz RJ (1992) CD14 is involved in control of human immunodeficiency virus type 1 expression in latently infected cells by lipopolysaccharide. Proc Natl Acad Sci USA 89:6285-6289
30. Machleidt T, Wiegmann K, Henkel T, Schutze S, Baeuerle P, Kronke M (1994) Sphingomyelinase activates proteolytic I kappa B-alpha degradation in a cell-free system. J Biol Chem 269:13760-13765
31. Mohri M, Spriggs DR, Kufe D (1990) Effects of lipopolysaccharide on phospholipase A2 activity and tumor necrosis factor expression in HL-60 cells. J Immunol 144:2678-2682
32. Raines MA, Kolesnick RN, Golde DW (1993) Sphingomyelinase and ceramide activate mitogen-activated protein kinase in myeloid HL-60 cells. J Biol Chem 268:14572-14575
33. Pushkavera M, Obdeid LM, Hannun YA (1995) Ceramide: an endogenous regulator of apoptosis and growth suppression. Immonol Today 16:294-297
34. Kawasaki S, Moriguchi R, Sekiya K, Nakai T, Ono E, Kume K, Kawahara K (1994) The cell envelope structure of the lipopolysaccharide-lacking gram-negative bacterium Sphingomonas paucimobilis. J Bacteriol 176:284-290
35. Wright SD, Kolesnick RN (1995) Does endotoxin stimulate cells by mimicking ceramide? Immonol Today 16:297-302
36. Hampton RY, Golenbock DT, Penman M, Krieger M, Raetz CR (1991) Recognition and plasma clearance of endotoxin by scavenger receptors. Nature 352:342-344
37. Ziegler-Heitbrock HWL, Ulevitch RJ (1993) CD14: cell surface receptor and differentiation marker. Immonol Today 14:121-125
38. Goyer DT, Ferrero E, Retting WJ, Yenamandra AK, Obata F, LeBeau MM (1988) The CD14 monocyte differentiation antigen maps to a region encoding growth factors and receptors. Science 239:497-500
39. Greenman RL, Schein RM, Martin MA, Wenzel RP, MacIntyre NR, Emmanuel G, Chmel H, Kohler RB, McCarthy M, Plouffe J et al (1991) A controlled clinical trial of E5 murine monoclonal IgM antibody to endotoxin in the treatment of gram-negative sepsis. The XOMA Sepsis Study Group [see comments]. JAMA 266:1097-1102
40. Teng NNH, Kaplan HS, Herbert JM (1985) Protection against Gram-negative bacteremia and endotoxemia with human monoclonal IgM antibodies. Proc Natl Acad Sci USA 82:1790-1794
41. Frey EA, Miller DS, Jahr TG, Sundan A, Bazil V, Espevik T, Finlay BB, Wright SD (1992) Soluble CD14 participates in the response of cells to lipopolysaccharide. J Exp Med 176:1665-1671
42. Simpson SQ, Casey LC (1989) Role of tumor necrosis factor in sepsis and acute lung injury. Crit Care Clin 5:27-47
43. Champan PB, Lester TJ, Casper ES, Gabrolove JL, Wong GY, Kempin SJ, Gold PJ, Welt S, Warren RS, Starnes F, Sherwin SA, Old LJ, Oettgen HF (1987) Clinical pharmacology of recombinant human tumour necrosis factor in patients with advanced cancer. J Clin Oncol 5:1942-1951

44. Bone RC (1991) The pathogenesis of sepsis. Ann Intern Med 115:457-469
45. Waage A, Brandtzaeg P, Halstensen A, Kierulf P, Espevik T (1989) The complex pattern of cytokines in serum from patients with meningococcal septic shock. Association between interleukin 6, interleukin 1, and fatal outcome. J Exp Med 169:333-338
46. Wong GC, Clark SC (1988) Multiple actions of interleukin 6 within a cytokine network. Immonol Today 9:137-139
47. Hack CE, De Groot ER, Felt Bersma RJ, Nuijens JH, Strack Van Schijndel RJ, Eerenberg Belmer AJ, Thijs LG, Aarden LA (1989) Increased plasma levels of interleukin-6 in sepsis [see comments]. Blood 74:1704-1710
48. van der Poll T, Levi M, Hack CE, ten Cate H, van Deventer SJ, Eerenberg AJ, De Groot ER, Jansen J, Gallati H, Buller HR et al (1994) Elimination of interleukin 6 attenuates coagulation activation in experimental endotoxemia in chimpanzees. J Exp Med 179:1253-1259
49. Martich GD, Danner RL, Ceska M, Suffredini AF (1991) Detection of interleukin 8 and tumor necrosis factor in normal humans after intravenous endotoxin: the effect of antiinflammatory agents. J Exp Med 173:1021-1024
50. Baggiolini M, Walz A, Kunkel SL (1989) Neutrophil-activating peptide-1/interleukin 8, a novel cytokine that activates neutrophils. J Clin Invest 84:1045-1049
51. Leonard EJ, Yoshimura T (1990) Neutrophil attractant/activation protein-1 (NAP-1 [interleukin-8]). Am J Respir Cell Mol Biol 2:479-486
52. Leonard EJ, Yoshimura T (1990) Human monocyte chemoattractant protein-1 (MCP-1). Immunol Today 11:97-101
53. Carveth HJ, Bohnsack JF, McIntyre TM, Baggiolini M, Prescott SM, Zimmerman GA (1989) Neutrophil activating factor (NAF) induces polymorphonuclear leukocyte adherence to endothelial cells and to subendothelial matrix proteins. Biochem Biophys Res Commun 162:387-393
54. Detmers PA, Lo SK, Olsen Egbert E, Walz A, Baggiolini M, Cohn ZA (1990) Neutrophil-activating protein 1/interleukin 8 stimulates the binding activity of the leukocyte adhesion receptor CD11b/CD18 on human neutrophils. J Exp Med 171:1155-1162
55. Mizer LA, Weisbrode SE, Dorinsky PM (1989) Neutrophil accumulation and structural changes in nonpulmonary organs after acute lung injury induced by phorbol myristate acetate. Am Rev Respir Dis 139:1017-1026
56. Weiss SJ (1989) Tissue destruction by neutrophils [see comments]. N Engl J Med 320: 365-376
57. Argenbright LW, Letts LG, Rothlein R (1991) Monoclonal antibodies to the leukocyte membrane CD18 glycoprotein complex and to intercellular adhesion molecule-1 inhibit leukocyte-endothelial adhesion in rabbits. J Leukoc Biol 49:253-257
58. Chang HR, Vesin C, Grau GE, Pointaire P, Arsenijevic D, Strath M, Pechere JC, Piguet PF (1993) Respective role of polymorphonuclear leukocytes and their integrins (CD11/118) in the local or systemic toxicity of lypopolysaccharide. J Leukoc Biol 53:636-639
59. Morisaki T, Goya T, Toh H, Nishihara K, Torisu M (1991) The anti Mac-1 monoclonal antibody inhibits neutrophil sequestration in lung and liver in a septic murine model. Clin Immunol Immunopathol 61:365-375
60. Burch RM, Noronha Blob L, Bator JM, Lowe VC, Sullivan JP (1993) Mice treated with a leumedin or antibody to Mac-1 to inhibit leukocyte sequestration survive endotoxin challenge. J Immunol 150:3397-3403
61. Klein B, Brailly H (1995) Cytokine-binding proteins: stimulating antagonist. Immonol Today 16:216-220
62. Klein B, Wijdenes J, Zhang XG, Jourdan M, Boiron JM, Brochier J, Liautard J, Merlin M, Clement C, Morel Fournier B et al (1991) Murine anti-interleukin-6 monoclonal antibody therapy for a patient with plasma cell leukemia. Blood 78:1198-1204
63. Franslow WC, Sims JE, Sassenfeld H, Morrissey PJ, Gillis S, Dower SK, Widmer MB (1990) Regulation of alloreactivity in vivo by a soluble form of the interleukin-1 receptor. Science 248:739-742

64. Fischer E, Van Zee KJ, Marano MA, Rock CS, Kenney JS, Poutsiaka DD, Dinarello CA, Lowry SF, Moldawer LL (1992) Interleukin-1 receptor antagonist circulates in experimental inflammation and in human disease. Blood 79:2196-2200
65. Granowitz EV, Porat R, Mier JW, Orencole SF, Callahan MV, Cannon JG, Lynch EA, Ye K, Poutsiaka DD, Vannier E et al (1993) Hematologic and immunomodulatory effects of an interleukin-1 receptor antagonist coinfusion during low-dose endotoxemia in healthy humans. Blood 82:2985-2990
66. Rogy MA, Moldawer LL, Oldenburg HS, Thompson WA, Montegut WJ, Stackpole SA, Kumar A, Palladino MA, Marra MN, Lowry SF (1994) Anti-endotoxin therapy in primate bacteremia with HA-1A and BPI. Ann Surg 220:77-85
67. Dinarello CA (1993) Modalities for reducing interleukin-1 activity in disease. Immonol Today 14:260-264
68. Carlet J, Cohen J, Andersson J (1994) INTERSEPT: an international efficacy and safety study of monoclonal antibody to human TNF in patients with sepsis syndrome. In: Program and Abstracts of the 34th Interscience Conference on Antimicrobial Agents and Chemotherapy, American Society for Microbiology, Washington DC
69. Ertel W, Scholl FA, Gallati H, Bonaccio M, Schildberg FW, Trentz O (1994) Increased release of soluble tumor necrosis factor receptors into blood during clinical sepsis. Arch Surg 129:1330-1336
70. Rose John S, Heinrich PC (1994) Soluble receptors for cytokines and growth factors: generation and biological function. Biochem J 300:281-290
71. Ashkenazi A, Marsters SA, Capon DJ, Chamow SM, Figari IS, Pennica D, Goeddel DV, Palladino MA, Smith DH (1991) Protection against endotoxic shock by a tumor necrosis factor receptor immunoadhesin. Proc Natl Acad Sci USA 88:10535-10539
72. Kurschner C, Ozmen L, Garotta G, Dembic Z (1992) IFN-gamma receptor-Ig fusion proteins. Half-life, immunogenicity, and in vivo activity. J Immunol 149:4096-4100
73. Lesslauer W, Tabuchi H, Gentz R, Brockhaus M, Schlaeger EJ, Grau G, Piguet PF, Pointaire P, Vassalli P, Loetscher H (1991) Recombinant soluble tumor necrosis factor receptor proteins protect mice from lipopolysaccharide-induced lethality. Eur J Immunol 21:2883-2886
74. Peppel K, Crawford D, Beutler B (1991) A tumor necrosis factor (TNF) receptor-IgG heavy chain chimeric protein as a bivalent antagonist of TNF activity. J Exp Med 174:1483-1489
75. Schade UF (1990) Pentoxifylline increases survival in murine endotoxin shock and decreases formation of tumor necrosis factor. Circ Shock 31:171-181
76. Gadina M, Bertini R, Mengozzi M, Zandalasini M, Mantovani A, Ghezzi P (1991) Protective effect of chlorpromazine on endotoxin toxicity and TNF production in glucocorticoid-sensitive and glucocorticoid-resistant models of endotoxic shock. J Exp Med 173:1305-1310
77. Gonzalo JA, Gonzalez Garcia A, Kalland T, Hedlund G, Martinez C, Kroemer G (1993) Linomide, a novel immunomodulator that prevents death in four models of septic shock. Eur J Immunol 23:2372-2374
78. Grundmann HJ, Hahnle U, Hegenscheid B, Sahlmuller G, Bienzle U, Blitstein Willinger E (1992) Inhibition of endotoxin-induced macrophage tumor necrosis factor expression by a prostacyclin analogue and its beneficial effect in experimental lipopolysaccharide intoxication. J Infect Dis 165:501-505
79. Novogrodsky A, Vanichkin A, Patya M, Gazit A, Osherov N, Levitzki A (1994) Prevention of lipopolysaccharide-induced lethal toxicity by tyrosine kinase inhibitors. Science 264:1319-1322
80. Tzung SP, Mahl TC, Lance P, Andersen V, Cohen SA (1992) Interferon-alpha prevents endotoxin-induced mortality in mice. Eur J Immunol 22:3097-3101
81. Rhynes VK, McDonald JC, Gelder FB, Aultman DF, Hayes JM, McMillan RW, Mancini MC (1993) Soluble HLA class I in the serum of transplant recipients. Ann Surg 217:485-489
82. Zavazava N, Bottcher H, Ruchholtz WM (1993) Soluble MHC class I antigens (sHLA) and anti-HLA antibodies in heart and kidney allograft recipients. Tissue Antigens 42:20-26
83. Zhang H, Benlabed M, Spapen H, Nguyen DN, Vincent JL (1994) Prostaglandin E1 increases oxygen extraction capabilities in experimental sepsis. J Surg Res 57:470-479

84. Kuipers B, van der Poll T, Levi M, van Deventer SJ, ten Cate H, Imai Y, Hack CE, ten Cate JW (1994) Platelet-activating factor antagonist TCV-309 attenuates the induction of the cytokine network in experimental endotoxemia in chimpanzees. J Immunol 152:2438-2446

85. Moncada S, Higgs A (1993) The L-arginine-nitric oxide pathway. N Engl J Med 329: 2002-2012

86. Szabo C, Thiemermann C (1995) Invited opinion: role of nitric oxide in hemorrhagic, traumatic, and anaphylactic shock and thermal injury. Shock 2:145-155

87. Szabo C, Southan GJ, Thiemermann C (1994) Beneficial effects and improved survival in rodent models of septic shock with S-methylisothiourea sulfate, a potent and selective inhibitor of inducible nitric oxide synthase. Proc Natl Acad Sci USA 91:12472-12476

88. Vallance P, Moncada S (1994) Nitric oxide-from mediator to medicines. J R Coll Physicians Lond 28:209-219

89. Vallance P, Moncada S (1994) Drugs that alter nitric oxide homeostasis: a reply [letter; comment]. Cardiovasc Res 28:284

90. Vallance P (1994) Nitric oxide in clinical arena. Biochemist 16:23-28

91. Wang P, Ba ZF, Chaudry IH (1994) Nitric oxide. To block or enhance its production during sepsis? Arch Surg 129:1137-1142

92. Vallance P, Collier J, Moncada S (1989) Effects of endothelium-derived nitric oxide on peripheral arteriolar tone in man [see comments]. Lancet 2:997-1000

93. Vallance P (1989) The interplay between platelet and vessel-wall mediators in coronary artery occlusion. Biomed Pharmacother 43:113-119

94. Benjamin N, Vallance P (1994) Plasma nitrite as a marker of nitric oxide production [letter]. Lancet 344:960

95. Lin PJ, Chang C-H, Chang J-P (1994) Reversal of refractory hypotension in septic shock by inhibitor of nitric oxide synthase. Chest 106:626-629

96. Petros A, Lamb G, Leone A, Moncada S, Bennett D, Vallance P (1994) Effects of a nitric oxide synthase inhibitor in humans with septic shock. Cardiovasc Res 28:34-39

97. Southan GJ, Szabo C, Thiemermann C (1995) Isothioureas: potent inhibitors of nitric oxide synthases with variable isoform selectivity. Br J Pharmacol 114:510-516

98. Earnshaw WC (1995) Apoptosis: lessons from in vitro systems. Trends Cell Biol 5:217-220

99. Hawkins CJ, Vaux DL (1994) Analysis of the role of bcl-2 in apoptosis. Immunol Rev 142: 127-139

Role of Free Radicals in Critical Illness

G.P. Novelli, A. Di Filippo, C. Adembri

The essentials of oxygen radicals (OR°) and the biochemical consequences of their generation are well known. It's well known also that the oxidative stress and the consequent tissue damage and/or diseases are due to an imbalance between OR° and biological defenses against them (1-4).

The putative sources of OR° are a) the incomplete reduction of molecular oxygen in mitochondrial respiratory chains during deprivation of energy, b) the metabolic pathway of arachidonic acid overactivated by phospholipases, c) the xanthine-oxidase activated by proteases, and d) the so-called "respiratory burst" of polymorphonucleate granulocytes activated by complement, bacteria, endotoxin, proteases, lysosomal enzymes, etc.

The biological defenses against OR° and their actions include the scavenging molecules that are a) enzymes such as superoxide-dismutases, catalase, peroxidases, b) lipophilic substances, such as vitamin E that protect cell membranes by a "quenching" mechanism, c) hydrophilic substances, such as vitamin C, methionine, d) other endogenous molecules, such as glutathione or cysteine that exert their antioxidant action through various mechanisms that could be peroxidase-like or protecting thiol groups from oxidative damage, and e) finally there are many exogenous substances that are active as antioxidants through various mechanisms. In this group the nitrones (5, 6) and the salycilic acid and NSAIDs are included too (7). Such drugs act by trapping and chemically inactivating OR°. Other drugs exert an antioxidant effect by inhibiting some OR° generating events, such as local anesthetics, steroids and aminosteroids that stabilize the PMN membranes and prevent the production of secondary radicals.

The most relevant molecular targets of OR° are:

1. Polyunsaturated fatty acids of plasma membranes and intracellular organelles which undergo a process of lipid peroxidation, a chain reaction inducing chaotic structural changes until formation of hydroperoxides and cytotoxic and mutagenic hydroxyalkenyls

2. Proteins which undergo fragmentation or denaturation which in turn enhance susceptibility to proteolysis (one of the inactivated proteins is the inhibitor of circulating alpha-1-protease) (8)

3. Amino acids which undergo oxidation (those containing thiol groups being mostly susceptible)

4. Polysaccharides which undergo a process of depolimerization

5. Nucleic acids which are modified by oxidation, so acting on the genome and form the basis of mutagenesis and carcinogenesis.

Based on the biochemical damages summarized above, it is not surprising that OR° lead to perturbations of cells, of tissues and of organs (9). The list might be endless.

In relation to critical illnesses it must be remembered that cell membranes become more rigid and permeable, that the intracellular matrix becomes fluid, that the endothelium and capillary walls become more and more permeable, that the synthetic activity of alveolar type II cells is inhibited, that calcium moves into the neurons and that microcirculatory flow is hampered etc.

The list of the diseases accepted as OR° derived diseases is very long (see Table 1) and extends from senescence to exhaustion of muscle exercise (10), from cataract to acute liver necrosis and brain ischemia (11, 12). However, the aim of this paper is to discuss the role of OR° in sepsis, septic shock and MODS.

Table 1. Oxygen radical derived diseases

Brain:	trauma, stroke dementia hyperoxia ischemia, reperfusion	Gastrointestinal:	infarction endotoxin translocation
Heart:	infarction angioplasty	Vessels:	atherosclerosis
Lung:	ARDS asthma hyperoxia	Multiorgan:	radiation aging transplantation ischemia-reperfusion muscle fatigue autoimmune diseases
Skin:	dermatitis, psoriasis burn		
Kidney:	glomerulonephritis		
Eye:	cataract		

Oxygen radicals in sepsis and septic shock

The discussion on the putative role of OR° in sepsis and septic shock is not a recent one and was initiated by ourselves in 1983 in a presentation held at the constitutive meeting of the European Shock Society in Sweden (13).

During the course of all these years the topic has been more and more explored and antioxidants have been included into the soup of treatments proposed for therapy of septic shock. Unfortunately all the discussions concerning OR° derived diseases are difficult due to the impossibility to directly observe and quantitate the OR° themselves in vivo. Therefore all the data are almost indirect and derived from antioxidants or from byproducts of peroxidative reactions.

In our laboratory the spin trapping nitrones were suggested and used as the most selective scavengers (14). In fact they don't affect the pathophysiology of OR° but simply "capture" the primary and secondary free radicals before they achieve their molecular targets without any known biological effect [for the pharmacology of spin trapping nitrones see (15, 16, 6)].

To discuss the role of OR° in the pathogenesis of sepsis and septic shock some questions must be addressed.

Relationships between OR° and sepsis/septic shock

The demonstrations of the relationship between OR° and sepsis/septic shock are numerous and obtained mostly by the use of scavengers or spin trappers deprived of action on other putative mediators of shock.

In our laboratory a lot of experiments were performed with the above quoted nitrones. They gave the opportunity to demonstrate that in rats submitted to injection of a lethal dose of endotoxin, the inactivation of OR° increases survival, improves microcirculation, prevents stiffening of cell membranes and prevents exhalation of ethane, a marker of lipid peroxidation (5).

However, prevention of experimental shock has been also observed in experiments using inhibitors of radical-generating systems [i.e. allopurinol (17, 18)], physiological enzymatic scavengers [i.e. superoxide-dismutase and catalase (19-23, 18)], physiological antioxidants [i.e. tocopherol or glutathione (13) or nitrones (24, 25)].

However, it must be noted that in all the experiments the antioxidant drugs were effective when given before the shock inducing maneuvers or within 30-60 min but not after a longer interval. In fact, inactivation of OR° blocks only the first phase of shock, that is, the phase where the reactions against the aggression to the body homeostasis are more prominent and where the OR° generating mechanisms are more active. That is the SIRS phase.

OR° production endotoxin

The response to this question was given by Brackett et al. (24) who demonstrated by electron spin resonance an OR° signal appearing in the liver and the heart of rats 20-30 min after endotoxin. The interval within endotoxin and appearance of OR° suggests a role of some intermediate events (PNM activation).

Other experiments were presented by Lloyd (26) on baboons during infusion of live gram-negative bacteria. Electron spin resonance spectra demonstrated the presence of OR° in the liver of septic animals.

The production of an electron spin resonance signal attributable to OR° was also observed from macrophages challenged with endotoxin (27) and from granulocytes taken from septic rats (28).

In a series of septic shock patients neutrophil respiratory burst function was observed to be significantly depressed in the earliest phases of shock and to recover as patients improved (29). The depression of production of OR° by neutrophils is a sign of exhaustion after massive stimulation during the early phases of SIRS preceding the appearance of septic shock. In the same study critically ill patients without signs of infection or sepsis showed normal neutrophil function.

OR° overgeneration during established septic shock

In animal experiments the peroxidative generalized damage was demonstrated by measuring byproducts of lipid peroxidation (30, 31), chemiluminescence (32) alkanes in exhaled air (5, 33), and consumption of physiological scavengers (9, 30, 32, 34).

A model of sepsis in guinea pigs showed evidence of pulmonary interstitial edema, increased albumin leakage and accumulation of neutrophils well correlated with tissue and alveolar concentration of products of lipid peroxidation (35). In a lethal model of sepsis in the dog there was a 200% rise in fluorescent lipid peroxidation products that was prevented by antioxidants (36).

In man also a lot of data confirm the presence of OR° damage during sepsis and septic shock. In fact hydroperoxides and alkanes have been found in exhaled air (37, 38), increased rigidity was observed in red cell membranes (39), and physiological scavengers were consumed. In septic human patients lipid peroxidation products were evaluated with an extremely sensitive test of hydroperoxides (40). The same test was adopted to differentiate arterial and venous concentrations in blood going/coming from a septic focus.

In septic humans, α-tocopherol consumption has been shown to correlate inversely with plasma peroxidation products (41). However, the sole administration of antioxidants during severe clinical septic shock was never completely effective by itself.

Pathways from OR° to sepsis/septic shock

The main step of OR° seems to be located in the first phase of bodily reaction to the aggression that is SIRS, whose main characteristics are hypotension, decreased cardiac output and increased capillary permeability. The enhancement of capillary permeability induced by endotoxin and its preventability by antioxidant was demonstrated (42). It must be noted that a 10 to 20-min interval was present between endotoxin and the first sign of change in permeability: endotoxin activates PMN to produce OR°.

In a clinical study also on volunteers injected with a low dose of endotoxin pulmonary capillary permeability increased after some 10 min after endotoxin (43).

The increase in capillary permeability might be accepted as the initiating mechanism leading to tissue hypoperfusion through microcirculatory maldistribution and cell dysoxia.

Oxygen radicals in multiple organ failure

To discuss the role of OR° in multiple organ dysfunction syndrome (MODS) the work of Goris and his coworkers (44) must be considered. They demonstrated that a model of MODS was provoked by injection of sterile zymosan under aseptic conditions in germ-free rats. Zymosan being a complement activator, it is evident that MODS is consequent to complement activation alone, not to bacteria that remain efficient activators of complement anyway. However, activated complement is an activator of neutrophils and of other phagocytic cells.

The main characteristics of MODS are tissue hypoperfusion, increased capillary permeability, interstitial edema, endothelial damage and finally phlogosis. In this picture the role of OR° generation by phagocytic cells and by other mechanisms is obvious as it is that of xanthine-oxidase and of OR° produced in xanthine metabolism.

Moreover, the role of the gut must be taken in account, considering that during the first phase of response to a bodily aggression the intestinal permeability increases and bacteria/endotoxins translocate into the systemic circulation. Bacterial translocation is an OR° mediated damage (45) and it is adequate to continuously maintain activation of complement, production of mediators etc. so as to maintain the continuous production of OR°.

In our laboratory, a model of experimental MODS in rats has been developed, based on the intraperitoneal injection of zymosan (a complement activator) in paraffin under sterile conditions. Rats showed mucosal hemorrhage, diarrhea, tachypnea, and piloerection; mortality was maximal in the first 3 days and at the twelfth day. These peak points corresponded to the moment of peak activity of superoxide production and of products of lipid peroxidation in plasma as reported by Van Bebber et al. (46).

On our model – confirmed by tomography of the liver and the lung (47) – the role of OR° has been demonstrated by a relationship between severity of the disease and ethane exhalation (48).

Many other data support the role of OR° in MODS. Plasma levels of elastase – an enzyme released by activated granulocytes together with OR° – give good indication about the evolution and severity of organ failure in man (49, 50). The role of granulocytes as OR° generating factors was demonstrated in neutrophil-depleted guinea pigs challenged with TNF (51).

Other reports confirm the role of OR° in the appearance and worsening of MOFS by measuring consumption of physiological scavengers (52).

The reciprocal roles of OR° and other mediators in sepsis, septic shock and MODS

Many data support the hypothesis that OR° are the molecular cause of septic shock. However, there is much criticism of this theory and also many other mechanisms have been proposed, each one confirmed by adequate proofs. Some of the criticisms are based on incomplete results (53), species variations, and impossibility of quantitating OR° (54). However, the OR° damage has also been demonstrated to be responsible for many particular aspects of sepsis such as gastric mucosal lesions, pancreatitis (55), intestinal bacterial translocation (56), and skeletal muscle dysfunction (57).

When we look at other pathogenic hypotheses for sepsis septic shock and to other putative mediators we see that all of them involve phagocytic cells and their stimulus to produce OR°.

Endothelin 1 is a potent constrictor of vascular smooth muscles produced by the endothelium in response to endotoxin, ischemia, and hypoxia: it is an activator of OR° production by neutrophils, probably via a mechanism involving IL-8 (58).

Nitric oxide – whose production contributes to maintaining tissue perfusion during endotoxemia (59, 60) – might inactivate superoxide, so forming the radical peroxynitrite. The cytokine TNF – that is increased during severe sepsis in man – increases neutrophil margination and activates the OR production by neutrophil margination and activates the OR production by neutrophils and other phagocytic cells (61-63). Granulocyte depletion protects against multiple organ damage provoked by TNF (51). IL_1 is accepted as a shock-provoking mediator: it stimulates granulocytes and fibroblasts to produce OR° (63). Another cytokine, the IL_2, is claimed to be causative of acute lung injury through an OR° overgeneration (64).

The action of spin-trapping nitrones has been attributed to a down-regulation of the cytokine network and therefore to a diminished stimulus to the generation of OR° (65).

The platelet activating factor is linked to the OR generating systems by thrombin, kinins and neutrophils (66) whose activity has a central position in the whole problem of SIRS, sepsis, septic shock and multiple organ failure.

The complement activation (by bacteria, by hypoxia, by endotoxin, by proteases, by thrombin, by platelet aggregation etc.) and the consequent activation of phagocytic cells (exposed also to the stimulus by cytokines etc.) provokes OR° generation and initiates the chain reaction, leading to sepsis/septic shock (67, 68) (Fig. 1).

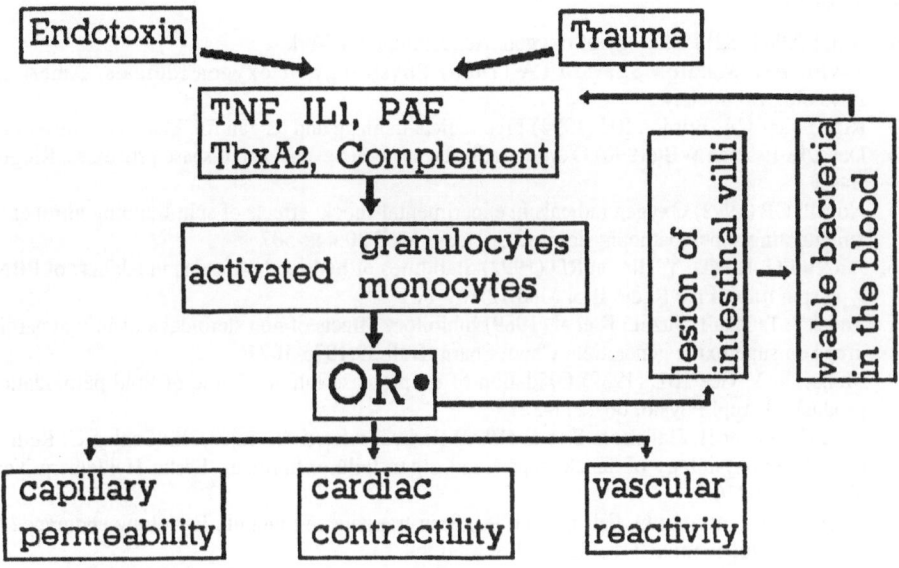

Fig. 1. The chain reaction leading to septic shock

The endothelium exposed to the action of OR° produced by neutrophils and other phagocytic cells or producing OR° by itself (69) develops a lot of reactions, including production of vasoactive mediators such as endothelium and nitric oxide. One of the immediate reactions is the expression of adhesion proteins such as ELAM and ICAM (70, 71) whose action is to promote the adherence of leukocytes to capillaries and postcapillary veins.

In summary, widespread endothelial destruction leading to vascular hyperpermeability is one of the key derangements underlying sepsis/septic shock/MODS. A number of inflammatory mediators have been claimed to be involved in these illnesses, including endotoxin, cytokines, lipokines, and lysosomal enzymes. Although each of these mediators has individual effects, all of them share the ability to recruit and activate neutrophils and phagocytic cells to produce OR°. Several of them (most notably endotoxin and TNF) also activate the complement, thereby further intensifying the effects on neutrophils so as to make the lethal vicious circle stronger.

Certainly, not all the doubts and the perplexities have been solved; however, OR° appear to be the final step common to many different ways, so that it should be therapeutically more effective to inactivate them than to try to inactivate each one of the other mediators.

References

1. Autor AP (1982) Pathology of oxygen. Academic, New York
2. Taylor AE, Matalon S, Ward PA (1986) Physiology of oxygen radicals. American Physiological Society
3. Rice-Evans CA, Burdon RH (1994) Free radical damage and its control. Elsevier, Amsterdam
4. Das DK, Essman WB (1990) Oxygen radicals: systemic events and disease processes. Karger, Basel
5. Novelli GP (1992) Oxygen radicals in experimental shock: effects of spin-trapping nitrones in ameliorating shock pathophysiology. Crit Care Med 20:449-507
6. Janzen EG, Kotake Y, Hinton RD (1992) Stabilities of hydroxyl radical spin adducts of PBN-type spin traps. Free Radic Biol Med 12:169-173
7. Yudai Y, Tanaka J, Suzuki K et al (1989) Inhibitory effects of non steroidal anti-inflammatory drugs on superoxide generation. Chem Pharm Bull 39:1075-1077
8. Mohsenin V, Gee JBL (1989) Oxidation of α_1-protease inhibitor: role of lipid peroxidation products. J Appl Physiol 66:2211-2215
9. Redl H, Gasser H, Hallstrom S et al (1993) Radical related cell injury. In: Schlag G, Redl H (eds) Pathophysiology of shock, sepsis and organ failure. Springer, Berlin Heidelberg New York, pp 92-110
10. Novelli GP, Bracciotti G, Falsini S (1990) Spin-trappers and vitamin E prolong endurance to muscle fatigue in mice. Free Radic Biol Med 8:9-13
11. Novelli GP, De Gaudio AR, Paternostro E et al (1993) Il significato dei radicali liberi dell'ossigeno nel trauma del sistema nervoso centrale. Minerva Anestesiol 59:719-731
12. Zini I, Tomasi A, Grimaldi R et al (1989) Detection of free radicals during brain ischemia and reperfusion by spin trapping and microdialysis. Neurosci Lett 138:279-282
13. Novelli GP, De Gaudio AR (1983) Oxygen free radicals in shock states. In: Lewis and Haglund (eds) Shock research. Elsevier, Amsterdam, pp 31-42
14. Novelli GP, Angiolini P, Tani R et al (1986) Phenyl-t-butyl-nitrone is active against traumatic shock in rats. Free Radic Res Commun 1:321-327
15. Cheng HY, Liu T, Feuerstein G et al (1993) Distribution of spin-trapping compounds in rat blood and brain: in vivo microdialysis determination. Free Radic Biol Med 14:243-250
16. Buettner GR (1987) Spin trapping: ESR parameters of spin adducts. Free Radic Biol Med 3: 159-203
17. Demling RH, Lalonde C (1990) Early postburn lipid peroxidation. Effect of ibuprofen and allopurinol. Surgery 107:85-93
18. Kunimoto F, Morita T, Ogawa R et al (1987) Inhibition of lipid peroxidation improves survival rate of endotoxic rats. Circ Shock 21:15-22
19. Bond RF, Haines GA, Johnson G (1988) The effect of allopurinol and catalase on cardiovascular hemodynamics during hemorrhagic shock. Circ Shock 25:139-151
20. McKechnie K, Furman BL, Parratt JR (1986) Modification by oxygen free radical scavengers of the metabolic and cardiovascular effects of endotoxin infusion in conscious rats. Circ Shock 19:429-439
21. Saez JC, Ward PH, Gunther B et al (1984) Superoxide radical involvement in the pathogenesis of burn shock. Circ Shock 12:229-239
22. Broner CW, Shenep JL, Stidham GL et al (1989) Effect of antioxidants in experimental Escherichia coli septicemia. Circ Shock 29:77-92

23. Bitterman H, Aoki N, Lefer AM (1988) Anti-shock effects of human superoxide dismutase in splanchnic artery occlusion shock. Proc Soc Exp Biol Med 188:265-271

24. Brackett DJ, Lai EK, Lerner MR et al (1989) Spin trapping of free radicals produced "in vivo" in heart and liver during endotoxemia. Free Radic Res Commun 7:315-324

25. Hamburger SA, McCay PB (1989) Endotoxin-induced mortality in rats is reduced by nitrones. Circ Shock 29:329-334

26. Lloyd SS, Chang AK, Taylor FB et al (1993) Free radicals and septic shock in primates: the role of tumor necrosis factor. Free Radic Biol Med 14:223-242

27. Jackson SK, Stark JM, Rowlands CC et al (1989) Electron spin resonance detection of oxygen-centred radicals in murine macrophages stimulated with bacterial endotoxin. Free Radic Biol Med 7:165-170

28. Simons RK, Maier RV, Lennard ES (1987) Neutrophil function in a rat model of endotoxin-induced lung injury. Arch Surg 122:197-203

29. Vespasiano MC, Lewandoski JR, Zimmerman JJ (1993) Longitudinal analysis of neutrophil superoxide anion generation in patients with septic shock. Crit Care Med 21:666-672

30. Yoshikawa T, Takano H, Takahashi S et al (1994) Changes in tissue antioxidant enzyme activities and lipid peroxides in endotoxin-induced multiple organ failure. Circ Shock 42:53-58

31. Demling R, Nayak U, Ikenami K et al (1994) Comparison between lung and liver lipid peroxidation and mortality after zymosan peritonitis in the rat. Shock 2:222-227

32. Llesuy S, Evelson P, Gonzales-Flecha B et al (1994) Oxidative stress in muscle and liver of rats with septic syndrome. Free Radic Biol Med 16:445-451

33. Peavy DL, Fairchild EJ (1986) Evidence for lipid peroxidation in endotoxin poisoned mice. Infect Immunol 52:613-616

34. Keller GA, Barke R, Harty JT et al (1985) Decreased hepatic glutathione levels in septic shock. Arch Surg 120:941-945

35. Ishizaka A, Stephens K, Takelaar K et al (1988) Pulmonary edema after Escherichia coli peritonitis correlates with thiobarbituric acid reactive materials in bronchoalveolar lavage fluid. Am Rev Respir Dis 137:783-789

36. Morgan RA, Manning PB, Coran AG et al (1988) Oxygen free radical activity during live E. coli septic shock in the dog. Circ Shock 25:319-323

37. Ortolani O, Parlato V, Gravino E et al (1990) The monitorage of the perioxidative damage in patients undergoing cardiac surgery. Acta Anaesth Ital 41 [Suppl 2]:127-130

38. Weitz ZW, Birnbaum AJ, Sobotka PA et al (1991) High breath pentane concentration during acute myocardial infarction. Lancet 337:933-935

39. Poli G, Biasi F, Chiarpotto E et al (1989) Lipid peroxidation in human disease: evidence of red cell oxidative stress after circulatory shock. Free Radic Biol Med 6:167-170

40. Keen RR, Stella L, Flanigan DP et al (1989) Differential detection of plasma hydroperoxides in sepsis. Crit Care Med 19:1114-1119

41. Takeda K, Shimada Y, Amano M et al (1984) Plasma lipid peroxides and alpha tocopherol in critically ill patients. Crit Care Med 12:957-959

42. Novelli GP, Casali R, Bonizzoli M et al (1993) Aumento della permeabilità capillare provocato dall'endotossina: protezione con antiossidanti e glutatione. Minerva Anestesiol 59:211-216

43. Suffredini AF, Shelhamer JH, Neumann RD et al (1992) Pulmonary and oxygen transport effects of intravenously administered endotoxin in normal humans. Am Rev Respir Dis 145:1398-1403

44. Goris RJA, Boekoltz WKF, Ignas PT et al (1986) Multiple organ failure and sepsis without bacteria. Arch Surg 121:897-901

45. Deitch EA, Specian RD, Berg RD (1991) Endotoxin-induced bacterial translocation and mucosal permeability: role of xanthine oxidase, complement activation and macrophage products. Crit Care Med 19:785-791

46. Van Bebber IPT, Boekholz WKF, Goris RJA et al (1989) Neutrophil function and lipid peroxidation in a rat model of multiple organ failure. J Surg Res 47:471-475

47. Di Filippo A, Scardi S, Consalvo M et al (1994) Valutazione di un modello sperimentale di disfunzione multipla di organo (MODS). Minerva Anestesiol 60:157-164
48. Di Filippo A, Scardi S, Consalvo M et al (1994) L'etano espirato come marker non invasivo della evoluzione della Multiple Organ Dysfunction Syndrome (MODS) sperimentale. Minerva Anestesiol 60:295-303
49. Pacher R, Redl H, Frass M et al (1989) Relationship between neopterin and granulocyte plasma levels and the severity of multiple organ failure. Crit Care Med 17:221-226
50. Tanaka H, Sugimoto H, Yoshioka T et al (1991) Role of granulocyte elastase in tissue injury in patients with septic shock complicated by multiple organ failure. Ann Surg 213:81-85
51. Mallick AA, Ishizaka A, Stephens KE et al (1989) Multiple organ damage caused by tumor necrosis factor and prevented by neutrophil depletion. Chest 95:1114-1120
52. Maderazo EG, Woronick CL, Hickhin Bothan N et al (1990) Additional evidence of antioxidation as a possible mechanism of neutrophil locomotory dysfunction in blunt trauma. Crit Care Med 18:141-147
53. Mainous MR, Xu D, Deitch EA (1993) Role of xanthine oxidase and prostaglandins in inflammatory-induced bacterial translocation. Circ Shock 40:99-104
54. Haglund U, Gerdin B (1991) Oxygen-free radicals (OFR) and circulatory shock. Circ Shock 34:405-411
55. Nonaka A, Manabe T, Kyogoku T et al (1990) Changes in lipid peroxide and oxygen radical scavengers in cerulein-induced acute pancreatitis. Digestion 47:130-137
56. Deitch EA, Kemper AC, Specian RD et al (1992) A study of the relationship among survival, gut-origin sepsis, and bacterial translocation in a model of systemic inflammation. J Trauma 32:141-147
57. Walden DL, McCutchan HJ, Enquist EG et al (1990) Neutrophils accumulate and contribute to skeletal muscle dysfunction after ischemia-reperfusion. Am J Physiol 259:H1809-H1812
58. Huribal M, Kumar R, Cunningham ME et al (1994) Endothelin-stimulated monocyte supernatants enhance neutrophil superoxide production. Shock 1:184-187
59. Spain DA, Wilson MA, Bar-Natan MF et al (1994) Role of nitric oxide in the small intestinal microcirculation during bacteremia. Shock 2:41-46
60. Novelli GP, Livi P, Melani AM et al (1994) Il nitrossido nell'insufficienza circolatoria. Minerva Anestesiol 60 [Suppl 1]:201-208
61. Tracey KJ, Lowry SF, Cerami A (1988) Cachectin/TNF in septic shock and septic adult respiratory distress syndrome. Am Rev Respir Dis 138:1377-1379
62. Ward PA, Warren JS, Johnson KJ (1988) Oxygen radicals, inflammation and tissue injury. Free Radic Biol Med 5:403-408
63. Meier B, Radeke HH, Selle S et al (1989) Human fibroblast release reactive oxygen species in response to interleukin-1 or tumor necrosis factor-α. Biochem J 263:539-545
64. Klausner JM, Paterson IS, Goldman G et al (1991) Interleukin-2-induced lung injury is mediated by oxygen free radicals. Surgery 109:169-175
65. Pogrenbniak HW, Merino MJ, Hahn SM et al (1992) Spin trap salvage from endotoxemia: the role of cytokine down-regulation. Surgery 112:130-139
66. Feuerstein G, Siren AL (1988) Platelet-activating factor and shock. Prog Biochem Pharmacol 22:181-190
67. Bengtsson A, Redl H, Paul E et al (1993) Complement and leukocyte activation in septic baboon. Circ Shock 39:83-88
68. Schirmer WJ, Schirmer JM, Naff GB et al (1988) Systemic complement activation produces hemodynamic changes characteristic of sepsis. Arch Surg 123:316-318
69. Reilly PM, Schiller HJ, Bulkley GB (1991) Pharmacologic approach to tissue injury mediated by free radicals and other active oxygen metabolites. Am J Surg 161:488-501
70. Suzuki M, Asako H, Kubes P et al (1991) Neutrophil-derived oxidants promote leukocyte adherence in postcapillary venules. Microvasc Res 42:125-138
71. Formigli L, Ibba-Manneschi L, Adembri C (1995) Expression of E-selectin in ischemic and reperfused human skeletal muscle. Ultrastruct Pathol 19:193-200

Pathophysiology and Therapy of End-Organ Failure in Critical Illness

M.R. PINSKY

Introduction

The pattern of death of critically ill patients aggressively treated with life-sustaining therapies following the initial resuscitative effort is remarkably similar across patient groups (1). Most of the critically ill patients who eventually go on to die during that hospitalization in whom initial resuscitative efforts are successful do so because of progressive multi-system deterioration often punctuated by infectious episodes and a non-specific septic state. The clinical expression of this initial process a sepsis or sepsis syndrome has been termed the systemic inflammatory response syndrome or SIRS by a recent consensus conference (2). The deterioration of these patients over time with progressive failure of multiple often unrelated organ systems is referred to a multiple organ dysfunction syndrome or MODS to underscore the continuum of tissue injury which may develop rather than by defining a threshold level to indicate the presence of organ failure. Patients usually first express SIRS and then MODS, progressing along a clinical pathway from initial partial recovery following resuscitation, though relapses and septic episodes to death. Diverse disease states such as infection, trauma and burns, pancreatitis and organ rejection share this common process (1). It is our hypothesis that MODS represents the phenomenological process of progressive and cumulative organ system dysfunction that may occur after a variety of diseases characterized by continual intravascular inflammation (3). According to this hypothesis, specific organ dysfunction is less important to outcome than the cumulative tissue burden of SIRS. The relative importance of global organ dysfunction and lack of importance of specific organ dysfunction was recently underscored by the studies of Knaus et al. (4) who showed that survival from trauma was closely correlated only to global organ performance. It follows from this logic that treatments which support the physiologic function of failing organs, such as hemodialysis and artificial ventilation, although important in maintaining patient viability, will do little to reverse the complex processes that either initiated organ dysfunction in the first place or account for subsequent impairment of organ systems. Thus, their impact on long term patient survival from critical illness may be much less than would be expected if single organ failure were the primary process determining outcome (5, 6).

The systemic inflammatory response: malignant intravascular inflammation

Conceptually, SIRS and its offspring MODS can be thought of as the product of a system wide process termed *malignant intravascular inflammation* (7): *Malignant*, because it is uncontrolled, rather than overwhelming in its unregulated and self-sustaining nature; *intravascular*, because it represents the blood-borne spread of what is usually a cell-cell interaction in the interstitial space; and *inflammation*, because all the primary processes that characterize the response are part of the host's normal inflammatory response. The normal process of inflammation describes a cellular immune effector mechanism designed to localize, suppress and clear foreign and toxic compounds and processes. This inflammatory process is characterized by cytokine up-regulation and initiation of the inflammatory cascade leading to both activation of immune effector cells and vascular endothelium (8). This results in adhesion of polymorphonuclear leukocytes and platelets to vascular endothelium, with subsequent transcapillary migration of immune effector cells and scavenging of inflammatory species (9).

The impact of this inflammatory process can be considered relative to the proximity of the cytokine pro-inflammatory mediator action. Using the endotoxin activated macrophage model it has been shown that activation of tissue macrophages induces an up-regulation of tumor necrosis factor-alpha (TNF-α) gene transcription and release of TNF-α into the micro-environment around the cell (10). This initiator pro-inflammatory cytokine can then stimulate itself through cell surface TNF-α receptors in an *autocrine* fashion helping to maintain its level of activation of both TNF-α and IL-1β synthesis (11, 12). The secreted TNF-α and IL-1β can also stimulate adjacent cells with TNF-α and IL-1β receptors in a *paracrine* fashion (13). This stimulation amplifies the inflammatory signal locally and aids in recruitment of circulating immune effector cells into the site of inflammation. If the TNF-α and other pro-inflammatory cytokines gain access to the circulation, they can stimulate immune effector cells and endothelial surfaces remote to the site of inflammation in an *endocrine* fashion (14). Conceptually SIRS can be thought of as the inflammatory process exceeding the level of paracrine activation. If endocrine activation is sustained, according to this model, MODS will follow.

Several lines of reasoning suggest that the manifestations of SIRS and MODS are due to host-derived damage of vascular endothelial cells and parenchymal cells through activation of the effector limb of the inflammatory cascade ending in cell mediated cytotoxic and complement mediated cell injury: a truly malignant intravascular inflammation. First, elevated levels of TNF-α and IL-6 are seen in the blood of subjects challenged with endotoxin (14). The elevated levels of TNF-α pre-date systemic responses, such as fever and malaise. Furthermore, suppression of fever by cyclooxygenase inhibition does not preclude either cytokine release or leukocytosis in human experimental endotoxemia. Second, binding of TNF-α with anti-TNF-α antibodies inhibits the effects of endotoxin infusion (15). Third, elevated levels of TNF-α and IL-6 are commonly seen in the blood of patients with sepsis (16). Fourth, absolute levels of TNF-α and IL-6 are crudely predicative or mortality in septic patients (17, 18). Finally, persistence of TNF-α and IL-6 in the blood and not their absolute levels is highly predictive of those patients would will ultimately go on to develop MODS and/or die (19). Subsequent clinical and laboratory studies have subsequently identified numerous interrelated pro- and anti-inflammatory pathways which operate at several levels of autocrine, paracrine and endocrine function (8, 13).

In its simplest terms, some initiating process, such as trauma, infection, burn or toxemia induces the binding of a pro-inflammatory ligand the cell surface of a competent immune effector cell in the micro-environment. It is impressive the variety of toxins which are capable of inducing this initial activation. The cell surface receptor CD-14 plays a pivotal role in the recognition of many microbiological toxins (20). Endotoxin, for example, through binding to the soluble acute phase reactant protein, referred to in lipopolysaccharide binding protein (LBP), complexes with the cell surface receptor CD-14 to induce intracellular signal transduction for the synthesis of new TNF-α and other pro-inflammatory cytokines. These pro-inflammatory cytokines stimulate the same macrophage (autocrine) and neighbor cells (paracrine) to synthesize and release TNF-α and IL-1 (11, 12, 16). This amplification also activates the vascular endothelium to up-regulate pro-adhesion cell surface receptors (selectins). If endothelial activation continues due to local stimulation, the endothelium expresses integrin receptors (ICAMs) to firmly bind circulating immune effector cells as well as releasing IL-8, a potent polymorphonuclear leukocyte (PMN) chemo-attractant, into its own micro-environment (13). As the inflammatory system is activated, it is also being suppressed through the synthesis of acute phase reactants, which are the body's endogenous anti-inflammatory agents, prostaglandin E1, another anti-inflammatory agent, IL-4 and IL-10, selective inhibitors of T cell activation, and possibly nitric oxide (NO) which may prevent thrombosis and leukocyte adhesiveness in the appropriate settings (21-27). If systemic release of pro-inflammatory cytokines occurs then a generalized toxemic phenotype develops, characterized by fever, malaise, tachycardia, and hypotension (14). This process is referred to as SIRS (2). If the stimulus is either sustained or of sufficient enough strength to overwhelm the anti-inflammatory autoregulatory mechanisms normally in place, then propagation of the pro-inflammatory stimulus from these proximal sites to more remote ones will occur resulting in parenchymal cell dysfunction (28). If the systemic inflammatory process is sustained then remote organ system dysfunction will become more pronounced leading to MODS (2).

Thus, one can consider inflammation as a cytokine-regulated process which is both essential for normal host defense and detrimental to bodily function. The normal host-derived inflammatory response is a highly integrated process of inflammation which operates within a restricted environment, such as a tissue plane or an alveolus, to contain, suppress, and eliminate infecting organisms, and then to clear damaged tissues of cell debris and foreign material. The final act of the inflammatory process is the remolding of the old inflammatory site by the deposition of fibrous tissue derived from local fibroblasts. Inflammation mobilizes numerous powerful immune effector cells and alters local micro-vasculature resulting in the containment of the inflammatory process into a lethal pool or abscess. With rapid clearance of inflammatory mediators and toxic products of trauma and infection, a nonspecific inflammatory response or SIRS-like process develops. If SIRS is sustained, remote organ system dysfunction or MODS ensues.

The cytokine paradigm of sepsis

Several lines of evidence suggest that cytokines are integral in the expression of SIRS and MODS. Most hypotheses about SIRS are based on the principle that TNF-α elaboration is an essential initial step for subsequent cellular damage (13). Support for this opinion comes from three seminal studies which support the Koch Hypothesis. First, C3H/HeJ mice which are genetically deficient in the ability to produce TNF-α tolerate otherwise lethal doses of endotoxin with minimal effects (15). Second, exogenously administered TNF-α reproduces the clinical syndrome observed in SIRS (10). Finally, the metabolic abnormalities seen during experimental endotoxic shock are prevented by anti-TNF-α antibodies (15).

TNF-α has direct effects on cellular function and indirect effects mediated by other cytokine and lipid inflammatory molecules (11, 13). By inducing the production of numerous additional mediators of inflammation, the inflammatory response is amplified and extended. Such effects include biosynthesis and release of IL-1 (11), platelet activating factor, IL-2, IL-6, IL-8, IL-10, γ-interferon, eicosionoids, and activation of PMN, tissue macrophages, and lymphocytes (12, 21, 22). The cytokines induce immune effector cell and endothelial cell activation and alter parenchymal cell metabolism (29). Impressively, the overall immuno-response is characterized by multitude of redundant pathways producing direct cell toxicity, and perpetuating the inflammatory process through activation of the complement, coagulation, and fibrinolytic systems, and increased synthesis of kinin (23). The endothelium becomes procoagulant due to expression of new adhesion molecules which attract activated platelets and PMNs which first roll along their surfaces as the immune effector cell and vascular endothelium weakly bind (selectin-specific) (13). If the PMNs find an appropriate endothelial receptor (integrin) they then bind more firmly and stop rolling (13). Platelets are consumed in the formation of microthrombi within multiple organs, which together with increased adhesiveness of activated PMNs to endothelial cells, decrease local nutritive blood flow by mechanical obstruction (25) and by damage of the endothelium by oxygen free radicals released by the now activated and adherent PMNs (26, 27). Together with microthrombosis, the associated loss of normal vasodilatation responses mediated by NO through up-regulation of vascular endothelial indelible nitric oxide synthase (24), can result in paradoxical co-existence of vasoconstriction and vasodilatation leading to both shunting of blood through the microvasculature and tissue ischemia (25, 28). In short, it is a mess. Hopefully though, the process is contained or suppressed minimizing injury of non-offending tissues.

If the inflammatory response is not contained at some local site or nidus, a generalized activation of inflammatory effector cells, including PMNs, macrophages, and lymphocytes ensues. This malignant intravascular inflammation is the result of systemic release of local inflammatory mediators leading to a viscous cycle of remote tissue damage by these processes, which through their injury further stimulate additional inflammation.

Failure of molecular therapies for SIRS and MODS

Based on the assumption that uncontrolled up-regulation of the pro-inflammatory cascade induces SIRS and MODS several immunosuppressive therapies have been proposed to mitigate the negative aspects of this systemic process. Schematically, these approaches can be grouped into those that either block mediator-receptor interactions, inhibit signal transduction, or inhibit the effects of pro-inflammatory mediators once released. Examples of receptor blockade therapy for sepsis include the systemic infusion of monoclonal antibodies to endotoxin. Initial uncontrolled studies with pooled antisera to endotoxin showed increased survival in septic patients (30). Two different monoclonal anti-endotoxins antibodies, HA-1A (31) and E-5 (32), have been studied in large multi-center clinical trials; both have proven to be less than beneficial in all patients. Although post hoc subgroup analysis suggested that some patients would benefit from HA-1A whereas other sub-groups would benefit from E-5 therapy, optimism for these therapies is diminishing. HA-1A was found to have no beneficial effects in a repeat study targeting their patient sub-population thought to have benefited from the initial clinical trial (33). The final clinical trial of E-5 is on-going, but probably will not show much differences from those already done with this agent. Inhibition of signal transduction has been tried using a variety of anti-inflammatory agents. In theory, since corticosteroids are excellent anti-inflammatory agents they should be of benefit to patients with SIRS (34). Similar arguments could be made for prostaglandin E1 and prostacyclin (35). However, neither high dose corticosteroid therapy (36, 37) nor prostaglandin E1 have been proposed to minimize inflammation. Although both agents are excellent anti-inflammatory agents when given prior to insult (34, 35), neither therapy improved survival in septic patients when studied prospectively in a randomized clinical trial. Corticosteroids actually increased mortality due to increased incidence of serious bacterial infections. Ibuprofen trials for human sepsis and ARDS are on-going and results are not available. Receptor blockade therapy has been studied by infusion of the naturally occurring IL-1 receptor antagonist (IL-1ra) (38) and murine monoclonal antibodies to TNF-α (39). IL-1ra proved to be ineffective in reducing mortality in sepsis whereas anti-TNF-α antibody trials are still ongoing.

Clearly, a theme is developing in these clinical trials of sepsis (40). Initial non-randomized clinical trials suggest benefit of therapy across all patient groups. Subsequent prospective randomized clinical trials demonstrate no overall benefit but by post hoc analysis suggest a benefit of therapy for selected sub-groups of patients. This last glimmer of hope is then destroyed by a final randomized clinical trial. Based on the uniformly negative results of these clinical studies it seems reasonable to assume that at the present none of the available immunomodulating agents tried will measurably reduce mortality from severe SIRS and MODS. Although new agents and older ones not yet tried await clinical trials (41-43), the optimism that once permeated medicine regarding finding a "magic bullet" cure for sepsis and septic shock analogous to antibiotic for infection is decreasing. Considering the redundant and reciprocating nature of the inflammatory response, interindividual differences in host response, and variable time during the process of SIRS and MODS that patients present for treatment, it seems reasonable to conclude that mono-therapies for SIRS and MODS are doomed to failure as non-specific therapies for all patients (3).

Conventional therapies as catalysts for MODS

If one assumes that remote organ dysfunction or MODS is a manifestation of an uncontrolled and persistent systemic inflammatory process (19), then therapies which only support vital organ-system function without reversing the systemic inflammatory response should only prolong the dying process, not prevent it. Since persistence of intravascular inflammation rather than peak levels of pro-inflammatory mediators in the circulation appear predicative of the development of MODS and death (19), we hypothesize that MODS is a disease created by modern technology (3). The syndrome is created by our ability to artificially support patients with critical illness no matter how severe the insult without eradicating the primary process. The associated continual diffuse intravascular inflammatory process would induce over time progressive failure of multiple organs, alter cellular metabolism, and eventually lead to death. In essence, MODS can be thought of as an iatrogenic disease created by our technology which supports the patients physiological needs but does not cure the disease.

Although single system organ failure often represents isolated organ system dysfunction, it also occurs as part of a system-wide response to an insult (28, 44, 45). If single organ failure is due to an isolated event then the mortality associated with it is usually low, whereas if it is due to a generalized process, then its mortality rate is much higher. For example, aspiration-induced acute lung injury or viral pneumonia can produce ARDS. Furthermore, acute hypovolemia which is easily correctable can induce acute renal failure (ARF). All these forms of single organ failure have a relatively good prognosis with mortality rates below 10%. However, when either ARDS or ARF occur within the setting of severe SIRS or MODS the mortality rate approaches 50% (5). As clinicians we often focus our attention of pulmonary and renal function because their status can be easily monitored. With the advent of gastric tonometry, we now realize that many organs, like the gut, can express ischemic dysfunction in the setting of what would otherwise be considered adequate resuscitation and hemodynamic status (46). In support of this concept that ARDS and ARF reflect an isolated organ's response to a generalized process, the mortality rates for all patients with ARDS and ARF have not decreased much over the past 30 years despite marked improvements in ventilatory and dialactic techniques (5, 45) and patients with end-stage liver failure who subsequently develop ARDS have a mortality rate approaching 100% (47).

Our support of critically ill patients may be even more dangerous than merely sustaining life and allowing the disease process to continue. Artificial organ support can also induce organ-system dysfunction. An appreciation of this aspect of intensive support is now emerging as a potentially major cause of increased morbidity and mortality in critically ill patients. Artificial ventilation, renal dialysis and parenteral nutrition represent three common clinical examples of this process. Positive-pressure ventilation can damage lung tissue, induce barotrauma, and induce acute lung injury by several processes. First, by supplying a high F_IO_2 (> 0.6) oxygen toxicity can develop which over time will promote surfactant destruction, alveolar membrane rupture and alveolar capillary leak (48). Repetitive expansion and overdistention of aerated alveoli will induce alveolar epithelial and endothelial rupture inducing both barotrauma and acute lung injury, which if sustained will progress to fulminate respiratory failure (49, 50). Hemodialysis commonly decreases urine output and may convert low output renal failure into anuric renal failure by reducing intravascular blood volume. Finally, parental alimentation by placing the bowel to rest induces intestinal mucosal atrophy which decreases the barrier function of the gut to translocation of toxic species from the gut lumen (51). Furthermore, bacterial colonization of the stomach with gram-negative bacilli commonly occurs with gastric acid neutralization therapy as gastric stasis (52).

Regrettably, not only do these therapies potentially damage the very organs they aim to support, but they may induce organ damage remote from their primary site of action. Positive-pressure ventilation by increasing intrathoracic pressure will impede systemic venous return and left ventricular filling (53). This is the most common complication of artificial ventilation and can markedly reduce steady state cardiac output in patients with functional hypovolemia (volume loss or loss of vasomotor tone). Furthermore, ventilation-induced barotrauma, by exposing the circulating blood to collagen, activated Hagerman's factor (Factor XII) which results in the systemic release of TNF-α and remote organ dysfunction (50, 54). Dialysis may induce remote bleeding, especially from the gastrointestinal tract if anti-coagulation is not localized. Dialysis-induced disequilibrium syndrome is also possible when large quantities of solute is removed over a short interval. Furthermore, PMNs in the blood passing over dialysis membranes can become activated and will then impact on the capillary of the lung, which is the next organ in the system (55). Finally, based on the "gut hypothesis" toxic substances from the gut and proinflammatory and inflammatory substances released from the liver in response to these stimulants may directly damage the lung endothelium (51). According to this scenario, pulmonary endothelial injury may occur as a complication of intra-abdominal inflammation (intra-abdominal sepsis and pancreatitis) even in the absence of documented bacteremia (3, 5, 45). Abnormal liver performance appears to be important in the development of acute lung injury (28, 47) and the subsequent development of MSOF (19). The lung is also susceptible to nosocomial infection in the critically ill, owing to a greater occurrence of tracheal colonization with Gram-negative bacteria and the common need for endotracheal intubation (56).

Novel organ-specific supportive therapies which minimize the inflammatory response

Inherent in the practice of medicine is the assumption that by close monitoring and titration of therapy, complications of acute, episodic illness can be minimized, progressive organ system dysfunction prevented, and mortality in the critically ill reduced. Unfortunately, the above data question this approach and logic. Although both immunomodulating therapies and conventional artificial organ supporting therapies appear to not decrease morbidity and mortality from critical illness, the present day therapy of critically ill patients is not without novel and potentially useful therapeutic approaches.

Such novel therapies include pressure-limited ventilation (57), continuous high-flow venovenous hemofiltration (CVVH) (58, 59) and selective decontamination of the digestive tract (SDD) (52, 56, 60). They address fundamental aspects of organ protection and the propagation of pro-inflammatory mediators. These therapies are based on strong physiologic principals, have supporting clinical studies but have not yet either passed the scrutiny of randomized clinical trials. However, it would be unreasonable to assume that these therapies, like the immunotherapies described above would be universally effective in reducing mortality in all critically ill patients. These therapies have, however, two primary advantages over both immunotherapy and conventional therapies: first, they do not increase morbidity while adequately supporting organ function, and, second, they are inexpensive relative to the cost of both immunomodulating therapies and treating patients once they develop MODS.

Several pressure-limited ventilatory strategies have been developed and are presently being tested. Pressure-limited ventilation strategies assume that regional inhomogeneties of lung consolidation exist and that repetitive overdistention of aerated lung units will induce local and systemic endothelial damage. To minimize these effects, pressure-limited ventilation halts positive-pressure inspiration once airway pressure reaches some preset upper limit. Since oxygenation is more a function of F_IO_2 and mean alveolar pressure, whereas barotrauma is more a function of peak airway pressure, the rate of change in lung volume, and repetitive re-inflation of collapsed lung units, these types of ventilatory support should minimize lung injury without compromising arterial oxygenation. Recent data in animal models support this assumption (54) and a non-randomized clinical trial showed significant reductions in mortality from ARDS from expected levels (57). Regrettably, minute alveolar ventilation is usually reduced in patients with ARDS receiving pressure-limited ventilation, and has given rise to the term "permissive hypercapnia" which means that the co-existent hypercapnia is accepted as a necessary consequence of this change in ventilatory support priorities. To date only one study has been done using this technique in a comparison with more conventional modes of ventilation, and that study found that morbidity was increased in patients receiving pressure-limited ventilation (61). Thus, this form of ventilation, though physiologically sound may not turn out to be the savior of lung function in the initial phase of acute lung injury. Further studies are on-going and we await their answers.

Hemodialysis can activate PMNs as they pass over the dialysis membrane (6). Furthermore, the absolute amount of filtrate cleared by hemodialysis is limited. Since SIRS and MODS are associated with sustained levels of pro-inflammatory mediators in the blood if one could increase clearance of these inflammatory substances from the blood then the systemic inflammatory process may lessen. Along these lines, CVVH has been used to treat patients in septic shock with acute renal failure (58). Unlike conventional hemodialysis, it does not result in a disequilibrium syndrome or episodic hypotension, but allows for titration of fluid and electrolyte therapy, including hyperalimentation (59). That larger molecules are filtered during CVVH than during hemodialysis suggests that metabolically active substances, such as toxic amines, are also cleared from the circulation (55). The hemodynamic status of endotoxemic pigs was improved by high-flow CVVH but not low-flow CVVH (62). Furthermore, infusion of ultrafiltrate from endotoxic pigs into normal animals induced a similar septic response (63). Thus, the term *hemopurification* has been proposed to describe this process. However, based on the data from previous studies many remain to be convinced, awaiting the results of prospective randomized clinical trials (64).

Although SDD is not effective in reducing mortality in the treatment of all critically ill patients (13), it does reduce the incidence of nosocomial infections in all studies (13, 52) and in certain subgroups studied prospectively, has been proven effective at reducing mortality (65). Patients in whom a known insult is planned and in whom immune status will be compromised would seem ideal candidates for SDD. Indeed, the one patient subgroup that was found to benefit from SDD when studied in a prospective randomized trial was pediatric orthotopic liver transplant recipients, if treated with SDD preoperatively (65). As a prototype for this model, patients undergoing other forms of transplantation, bone marrow suppression and other types of immuno-suppression may benefit from SDD. It appears, however, that to reduce mortality, decontamination of the gut of gram-negative organisms must be achieved (66). This end-point of therapy occurs in approximately 60% of patients treated for one week or less. Again, additional clinical trials of other specific sub-groups of patients need to be done to define more clearly who should receive SDD and how its effectiveness should be monitored.

These data, however, suggest that in the future, benefit of specific therapies in the treatment of critically ill patients will need to be studied in well defined diagnostic patient groups rather than in all patients with either SIRS or MODS since these two syndromes are neither specific disease entities nor reflect a common initiating or sustaining process.

References

1. Carrico CJ, Meakins JL, Marshall JC, Fry D, Maier RV (1986) Multiple-Organ-Failure Syndrome. Arch Surg 121:196-200
2. American College of Chest Physicians/Society of Critical Care Medicine Consensus Conference (1992) Definitions for sepsis and organ failure and guidelines for the use of innovative therapies in sepsis. Crit Care Med 20:864-874
3. Pinsky MR, Matuschak GM (1990) Multiple systems organ failure: a unifying hypothesis. J Crit Care 5:108-114
4. Knaus WA, Draper EA, Wagner DP, Zimmerman JE (1985) Prognosis in acute organ-system failure. Ann Surg 202:685-693
5. Montgomery AB, Stager MA, Carrico CJ, Hudson LD (1985) Causes of mortality in patients with the adult respiratory distress syndrome. Am Rev Resp Dis 132:485-489
6. Butkus DE (1983) Persistent high mortality in acute renal failure. Arch Intern Med 143: 209-212
7. Pinsky MR (1989) Multiple systems organ failure: Malignant intravascular inflammation. In: Pinsky MR and Matuschak GM (eds.) Multiple systems organ failure. Clin Crit Care 5(2): 195-198
8. Movat HZ, Cybulsky MI, Colditz IG, Chan MK, Dinarillo CA (1987) Acute inflammation in Gram-negative infection: endotoxin, interleukin-1, tumor necrosis factor, and neutrophils. Fed Proc 46:97-104
9. Korthuis RJ, Anderson DC, Granger DN (1994) Role of neutrophil-endothelial cell adhesion in inflammatory disorders. J Crit Care 9:47-71
10. Tracy KJ, Beutler B, Lowery SF et al (1986) Shock and tissue injury induced by recombinant human cachectin. Science 234:470-474
11. Dinarello CA, Cannon JG, Wolff SM et al (1986) Tumor necrosis factor (cachectin) is an endogenous pyrogen and induces production of interleukin-1. J Exp Med 163:1433-1450
12. Cybulsky MI, Colditz IG, Movat HZ (1986) The role of interleukin-1 in neutrophil leukocyte migration induced by endotoxin. Am J Pathol 124:367-372
13. Tracy KJ, Cerami A (1993) Tumor necrosis factor: an updated review of its biology. Crit Care Med 21:S415-S422

14. Michie HR, Manogue KR, Spriggs DR, Revhaug A, O'Dwyer S, Dinarello CA et al (1988) Detection of circulating tumor necrosis factor after endotoxin administration. N Engl J Med 318:1481-1486
15. Beutler B, Milsark IW, Cerami A (1985) Passive immunization against cachectin/tumor necrosis factor protects mice from lethal effect of endotoxin. Science 229:869-871
16. Waage A, Brandtzaeg P, Halsteusen A, Kierulf P, Espevik T (1989) The complex pattern of cytokines in the serum of patients with meningococcal septic shock. J Exp Med 169:333-338
17. Waage A, Halstensen A, Espevik T (1987) Association between tumor necrosis factor in serum and fatal outcome in patients with meningococcal disease. Lancet 1:355-357
18. Hack CE, DeGroot ER, Felt-Bersma RJF, Nuijens JH, Strack van Schijundel RS, Eerenberg-Belmer AJ et al (1989) Increased plasma levels of interleukin-6 in sepsis. Blood 74:1704-1710
19. Pinsky MR, Vincent JL, Deviere J, Alegre M, Kahn R, Dupont E (1993) Serum cytokine levels in human septic shock: Relation to multiple systems organ failure and mortality. Chest 103:565-575
20. Wright SD, Ramos RA, Tobias PS et al (1990) CD14, a receptor for complexes of lipopolysaccharide (LPS) and LPS binding protein. Science 249:1431-1433
21. Chouaib S, Welte K, Mertelsmann R, DuPont B (1985) Prostaglandin E_2 acts at two distinct pathways of T lymphocyte activation: inhibition of interleukin 2 production and down regulation of transferrin receptor expression. J Immunol 135:1172-1179
22. Beutler B, Tkacenko V, Milsark I et al (1986) Effect of gamma interferon on cachectin expression by mononuclear phagocytes. J Exp Med 164:1791-1796
23. Stotman GJ, Burchard KW, Williams JJ, D'Anezzo A, Yellin SA (1986) Interaction of prostaglandins, activated complement, and granulocytes in clinical sepsis and hypotension. Surgery 99:744-751
24. Palmer RMJ, Ferrige AG, Moncada S (1987) Nitric oxide release accounts for the biological activity of endothelium-derived relaxation factor. Nature 327:524-526
25. Altura BM, Gegrewold A, Burton RW (1985) Failure of microscopic metarterioles to elicit vasodilator responses to acetylcholine, bradykinin, histamine, and substance P after ischemic shock, endotoxemia, and trauma: possible role of endothelial cells. Microcirc Endothelium Lymphatics 2:121-129
26. Buckley G (1983) The role of oxygen free radicals in human disease processes. Surgery 94: 407-414
27. Morgan RA, Manning PB, Coran AG et al (1988) Oxygen free radical activity during live E. coli septic shock in the dog. Circ Shock 25:319-323
28. Matuschak GM, Rinaldo JE (1988) Organ interactions in the adult respiratory distress syndrome during sepsis. Role of the liver in host defense. Chest 94:400-406
29. Weksler BB, Goldstein IM (1980) Prostaglandins: interactions with platelets and polymorphonuclear leukocytes in hemostasis and inflammation. Am J Med 68:419-428
30. Ziegler EJ, McCutchan JA, Fierer J et al (1982) Treatment of Gram-negative bacteremia and shock with human antiserum to a mutant E. coli. N Engl J Med 307:1225-1230
31. Ziegler EJ and the HA-1A Sepsis Study Group (1991) Treatment of gram negative bacteremia and septic shock with HA-1A human monoclonal antibody against endotoxin: a randomized, double-blind, placebo-controlled trial. N Engl J Med 324:429-436
32. Greenman RL, Schein RMH, Martin MA et al (1991) A controlled clinical trial of E5 murine monoclonal IgM antibody to endotoxin in the treatment of gram-negative sepsis. JAMA 266: 1097-1102
33. McCloskey RV, Straube RC, Sanders C, Smith SM, Smith CR and the CHESS Trail Study Group (1994) Treatment of septic shock with human monoclonal antibody HA-1A: A randomized, double-blind, placebo-controlled trial. Ann Intern Med 121:1-5
34. Hinchaw LB, Beller BK, Chang ACK et al (1986) Effect of prior administration of steroids upon recovery from lethal sepsis. Surg Gynecol Obstet 163:335-344
35. Lefer AM, Tabas J, Smith EF (1980) Salutory effects of prostacyclin in endotoxic shock. Pharmacology 21:206-212

36. Sprung CL, Caralis PV, Marcial EH et al (1984) The effects of high-dose corticosteroids in patients with septic shock. A prospective, controlled study. N Engl J Med 311:1137-1143

37. Bone RC, Fisher CJ, Clemmer TP et al (1987) A controlled clinical trial of high-dose methylprednisolone in the treatment of severe sepsis and septic shock. N Engl J Med 317: 653-659

38. Fisher CJ Jr, Dhainaut JF, Opal SM, Pribble JP, Balk RA, Slotman GJ, Iberti TJ, Rackow EC, Shapiro MJ, Greenman RL et al (1994) Recombinant human interleukin-1 receptor antagonist in the treatment of patients with sepsis syndrome. Results from a randomized, double-blind, placebo-controlled trial. JAMA 271:1836-1843

39. Abraham E, Wunderink R, Silverman H, Perl TM, Nasraway S, Levy H, Bone R, Wenzel RP, Balk R, Alfred R, Pennington JE, Wherry JC et al (1995) Efficacy and safety of monoclonal antibody to human tumor necrosis factor α in patients with sepsis syndrome. JAMA 273: 934-941

40. Luce JM (1993) Introduction to new technology into critical care practice: a history of HA-1A human monoclonal antibody against endotoxin. Crit Care Med 21:1233-1241

41. Gnidec AC, Sibbald WJ, Cheung H, Metz CA (1988) Ibuprofen reduces the progression of permeability edema in an animal model of hyperdynamic sepsis. J Appl Physiol 65:1024-1032

42. Fink MP, Morrissey PE, Stein KL et al (1988) Systemic and regional hemodynamic effects of cyclo-oxygenase and thromboxane synthetase inhibition in normal and hyperdynamic endotoxic rabbits. Circ Shock 26:41-57

43. Kilbourn RO, Gross SS, Jubran A et al (1990) N-methyl-L-arginine inhibits tumor necrosis factor-induced hypotension: implications for the involvement of nitric oxide. Proc Natl Acad Sci USA 87:3629-3632

44. Bell R, Coalson J, Smith J et al (1983) Multiple organ system failure and infection and the adult respiratory distress syndrome. Ann Intern Med 99:293-298

45. Fry D, Pearlstein L, Fulton R et al (1980) Multiple system organ failure. The role of uncontrolled infection. Arch Surg 115:136-140

46. Gutierrez G, Palizas F, Doglio G et al (1992) Gastric intramucosal pH as a therapeutic index of tissue oxygenation in critically ill patients. Lancet 339:195-199

47. Matuschak GM, Rinaldo JE, Pinsky MR, Gavaler JS, Van Thiel DH (1987) Effect of end-stage liver failure on the incidence and resolution of the adult respiratory distress syndrome. J Crit Care 2:162-173

48. Lamy M, Fallat RJ, Koeniger E et al (1976) Pathologic features and mechanisms of hypoxemia in adult respiratory distress syndrome. Am Rev Respir Dis 114:267-284

49. Gattinoni L, Persenti A, Avalli L, Rossi F, Bombino M (1987) Pressure-volume curve of total respiratory system in acute respiratory failure. Computed tomographic scan study. Am Rev Respir Dis 136:730-736

50. Dreyfuss D, Bassett G, Soler P, Saumon G (1985) Intermittent positive-pressure hyperventilation with high inflation pressures produces pulmonary microvascular injury in rats. Am Rev Respir Dis 132:880-884

51. Deitch EA, Winterton J, Bey R (1987) The gut as the portal of entry for bacteremia. Ann Surg 205:681-692

52. Ledingham IMcA, Allcock SR, Eastaway AT et al (1988) Triple regimen of selective decontamination of the digestive tract, systemic cefotaxime, and microbiological surveillance for prevention of acquired infection in intensive care. Lancet 1:785-790

53. Pinsky MR (1990) Hemodynamic Effects of Mechanical Ventilation. Appl Cardiopulm Pathophysiol 3:219-227

54. Valenza F, Ribeiro SP, Slutsky AS (1995) High volume low pressure mechanical ventilation up-regulates IL-1ß production in an ex vivo lung model. [abstract] Am J Respir Crit Care Med 151:A552

55. Bergstrom J (1978) Ultrafiltration without dialysis for removal of fluid and solutes in uremia. Clin Nephrol 9:156-164

56. Pugin J, Auckenthaler R, Lew DP, Suter PM (1991) Oropharyngeal decontamination decreases incidence of ventilator-associated pneumonia. JAMA 265:2704-2710

57. Hickling KG, Walsh J, Henderson S et al (1994) Low mortality rate in adult respiratory distress syndrome using low-volume, pressure-limited ventilation with permissive hypercapnia: A prospective study. Crit Care Med 22:1568-1578
58. Ossenkoppele GJ, van der Meulen J, Bronsveld W, Thijs LG (1985) Continuous arteriovenous hemofiltration as an adjuctive therapy for septic shock. Crit Care Med 13:102-104
59. Kaplan AA, Longnecker RE, Folkert VW (1984) Continuous arteriovenous hemofiltration: a report on six months' experience. Ann Intern Med 100:358-367
60. Reidy JJ, Ramsay G (1990) Clinical trials of selective decontamination of the digestive tract: review. Crit Care Med 18:1449-1456
61. Blanch L, Fernandez R, Valle J, Sole J, Roussos Ch, Artegas A (1994) Effect of two tidal volumes on oxygenation and respiratory system mechanics during the early stage of adult respiratory distress syndrome. J Crit Care 9:151-158
62. Grootendorst AF, Van Bommel EF, Van Leengoed LA et al (1994) High volume hemofiltration improves hemodynamics and survival in pigs exposed to gut ischemia and reperfusion. Shock 2:72-78
63. Grootendorst AF, Van Bommel EF, Van Leengoed LA et al (1993) Infusion of ultrafiltrate from endotoxemic pigs depresses myocardial performance in normal pigs. J Care Med 8: 161-169
64. Vincent J-L, Tielemans C (1995) Continuous hemofiltration in severe sepsis: is it beneficial? J Crit Care 10:27-32
65. Smith SD, Jackson RJ, Hannakan CJ et al (1993) Selective decontamination in pediatric liver transplants. A randomized prospective study. Transplantation 55:1306-1309
66. Tetteroo GW, Wagenvoort JH, Mulder PG, Ince C, Bruining HA (1993) Decreased mortality rate and length of stay in surgical intensive care patients with successful decontamination of the gut. Crit Care Med 21:1692-1698

ORGAN PERFUSION

Research Studies on Organ Perfusion: From the Lab to the Clinic

J.-L. VINCENT, P. VAN DER LINDEN, H. ZHANG

A number of important medical questions cannot be addressed in patients for several reasons. First, the population is often too heterogeneous, with intricate underlying problems. Second, patients are usually seen when the disease state is already established so that the mechanisms of its development cannot be adequately studied and early interventions are impossible. Third, the methods necessary to the study may be too mutilating to be used in patients. In other words, the risk/benefit ratio is often too high for human application.

The substantial medical progress which has been facilitated by experimental animal studies cannot be denied. In Aristotle's day, animals were dissected for study and teaching purposes. Later, many anatomists, among whom Galen (second century) and Vesalius (sixteenth century) are notable examples, made great contributions to our medical knowledge, primarily through their use of live animal experimentation. In the last century, Claude Bernard's animal experiments were very important to our improved understanding of physiology. The extremely complicated nature of the cardiovascular system, interacting as it does with all the other organs, cannot be modelled without animals; such experiments have a fundamental role to play in investigations in the fields of the cardiovascular physiology and pathophysiology.

An example of one of the questions which cannot be directly addressed in patients is the nature of shock. The word "shock" was used first by the French surgeon Henry-Francis Le Dran in 1743, when he referred to the effects of acute injury (1). His views about therapy were quite approximate, however:

"Can there be any Remedy more efficacious and expeditious, than frequent Bleedings in the Beginning? By these Means, both the general Plethory of the whole Body, and that peculiar to the Part affected, are diminished; by this Means the Parts are no more distended by too great a Weight of Fluids, and therefore recover their natural Elasticity; which Elasticity accelerates the Circulation through those Parts where it was checked before, and is even capable of removing many slight Obstructions" (2).

Although the latter comments about microvascular obstructions may be quite accurate (one would refer today to the activation of the leukocytes and their interactions with the endothelial cells), the former comments about the removal of fluids as part of the treatment are certainly unacceptable! Medicine had to wait for another 200 years before Wiggers described, with the aid of his elegant and fundamental animals studies, the alterations observed in hemorrhagic shock, thus making effective treatment possible at last.

Clearly, clinical studies, although invaluable, are not sufficient when considering therapies for the critically ill. For example, the heterogeneity of the critically ill population (medical, surgical or traumatized) presents significant problems. Another difficulty with clinical studies is that the previous health status of the patients is usually impaired: arteriosclerosis or chronic hypertension, chronic heart failure or coronary heart disease, chronic lung disease, diabetes, and cancer are common features of patients' histories, and these elements may confound the issues under study.

The animals used in experimental studies represent a much more homogenous group (Table 1). One must be ready to answer the criticism that studies on animals with normal underlying health status may not always be applicable to humans with underlying impairments to their health (Fig. 1). There is some validity in this criticism, which underlines the importance of establishing representative models.

Table 1. Differences between animal and clinical studies

Feature	Animal	Patient
Underlying disease	None (or single)	Multiple
Pathogenesis	Single	Multiple
Type of intervention	Well-controlled	Not well-controlled
Timing of intervention	Early	Late
Outcome	Related to insult	May be related to numerous factors

Septic patients provide a good example of those patients who are difficult to study, since they are certainly a heterogeneous group. Indeed, in many septic patients an infectious process cannot be demonstrated. Even if a study is limited to documented infections, these may be pneumonia, peritonitis, simple urinary tract infections or more specific diseases such as meningitis or endocarditis. There are so many factors that can influence the outcome of septic patients that to evaluate the effects of a new therapeutic intervention is just too difficult (3) (Fig. 2).

The fact that patients present with established disease means that the way the disease state developed cannot be adequately studied. Furthermore, early interventions are often impossible. Patients in the intensive care unit (ICU), for example, are often observed with full-blown symptoms. This is true in particular for septic shock. Only exceptionally can the patient be studied using a high risk

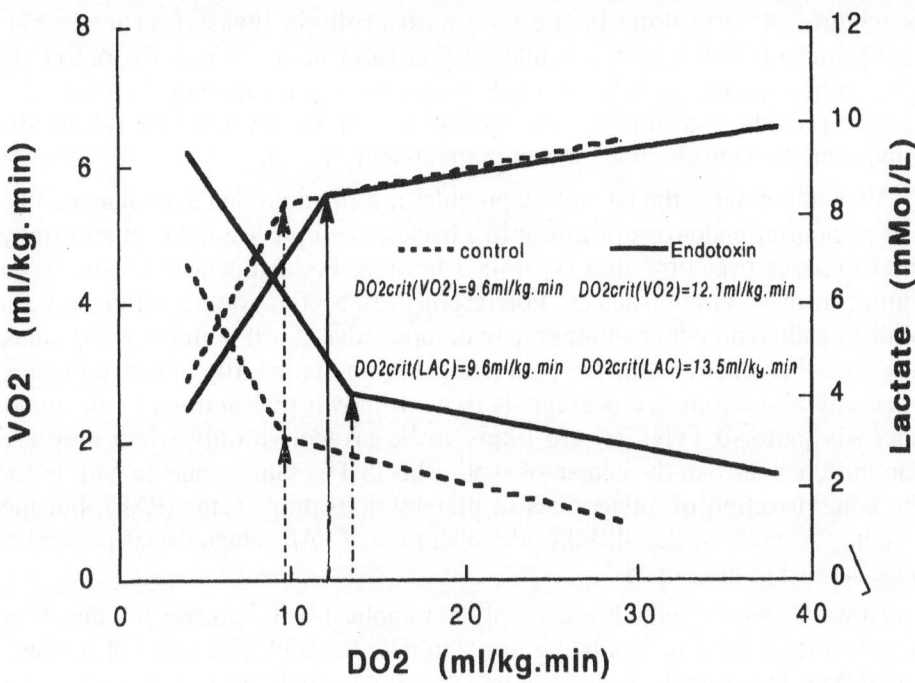

Fig. 1. Changes in oxygen consumption ($\dot{V}O_2$) during an acute reduction in cardiac output and oxygen delivery (DO_2) induced by tamponade, in control conditions and in the presence of endotoxin. Such a relation could hardly be obtained in humans. (From [12], with permission)

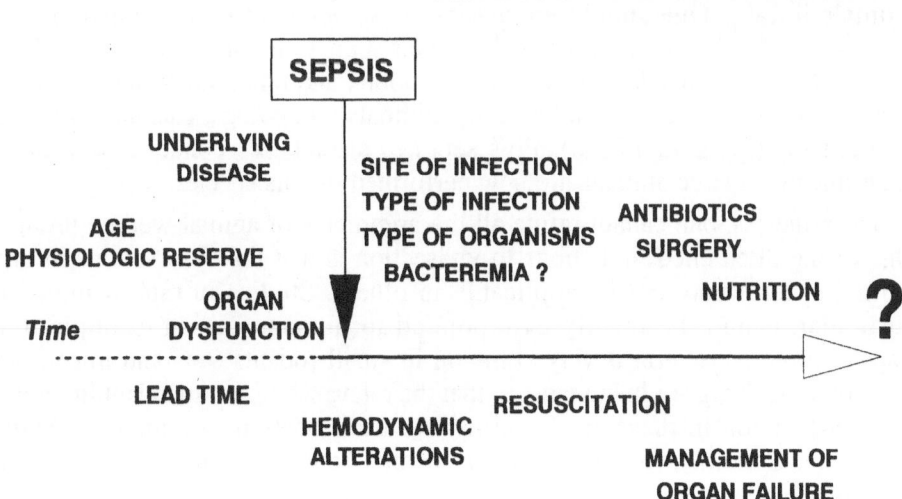

Fig. 2. Illustration of the heterogeneity of the patient population, based on studies in the field of sepsis

procedure (as was done in the past with urologic invasive procedures). Pretreatment is also seldom possible. As pretreatment of septic shock, one could give corticosteroids, as it has been demonstrated clearly in animal studies that steroids provide protection against septic shock (4). However, we rarely have the opportunity to consider this form of pretreatment, if at all.

Very importantly, the laboratory provides a well-controlled environment: one can administer endotoxin or infuse live bacteria at a precise moment and study the responses over time in a controlled fashion. Pretreatment is obviously an option in these circumstances. For instance, N-acetylcysteine administration prior to endotoxin administration may be protective (5). It is important to note, however, that what is effective pretreatment is not necessarily effective therapy once any alterations are present. It is well known that antibodies to tumor necrosis factor-α (TNF-α) are likely to be protective only when they are administered early in the course of septic shock. The same seems to be true for the administration of antagonists to platelet activating factor (PAF), but the evidence is much weaker that the administration of PAF antagonists is protective once sepsis has developed.

However, some methods are simply not applicable in humans, because they may be too invasive or mutilating or potentially harmful. The study of regional blood flow, for example, is difficult and thus limited in humans, but much easier in animals using electromagnetic methods or Doppler studies. Using these techniques, we were recently able to document some increase in blood flow to the mesenteric region by interventions such as 21-aminosteroids, strong antioxidant substances (6) or methylene blue, a substance acting principally by reducing the effects of nitric oxide on guanylate cyclase (7).

For several centuries, animal welfare groups have fought against the use of animals in labs. One should emphasize, however, that their campaigns are somewhat selective, concentrating particularly on some large animals such as dogs, cats, and primates. In fact, rodents, rabbits and other small, purpose-bred animals account for 88% of all research animals while dogs, cats and primates account for less than 1% (8). Pigs seem to attract less concern, and many experiments on large animals are now performed on this species.

Nevertheless, one cannot refute all the arguments of animal welfare groups. One of the often cited limitations to vivisection is that the observations in one animal species may not be applicable in others. Studies in rats or mice, in particular, cannot be readily extrapolated to humans. As an example, the translocation of bacteria is very common in small rodents (rats and mice), but less common in pigs or in humans, so that the relevance of the abundant literature on translocation in these small animals to translocation in humans remains debatable. Certainly, one animal study cannot reproduce all the aspects of a particular human pathological condition, but it can serve as a model to address specific questions. In this way, several animal experiments may be needed in the course of an investigation. The general rule is that several species should be studied before human studies are started. A transition is usually made from small animals to larger ones, and then to humans (other primates are sometimes required in between).

In practice, the choice of animal species are often influenced by logistic considerations, financial restraints, emotional and political issues. To study the effects of endotoxin, for example, the horse may be the best choice: it is sensitive to low doses of endotoxin, develops a hyperdynamic state, and is easy to instrument and to study regionally. However, horses are very rarely used due to restrictions such as the size of the laboratory, costs and emotional issues. At the other end of the extreme, rats are easily handled, cheap and stir much less emotion.

It is generally agreed that efforts should be concentrated more on avoiding animal suffering than on preventing animal deaths (most are sacrificed). It is important, therefore, that animal research is controlled to avoid excessive experimentation. Table 2 presents a list of fundamental questions that should be asked before beginning an animal experiment. It is important first to ask a specific and original question; all vague ideas based on an incomplete review of the literature are likely to result in a waste of resources and animals. It is important also to avoid animal studies for which the question could be addressed in man. As an example, it would hardly be justifiable to set up a series of experiments only to obtain blood samples that could be obtained in patients.

Table 2. The 10 essential questions (of equal importance) to be asked before an animal study is conducted

---

1. Is a specific question asked?
2. Is the question original?
   (Are we avoiding duplication?)
3. Have we established that there is no substitute?
   (Cell cultures, in vitro assays, computer modeling...)
4. Are we sure that this question cannot be addressed in humans?
5. Is the species properly chosen?
   (Are we sure that a smaller/cheaper species cannot be used?)
6. Is the model appropriate?
7. Is the number of animals kept as minimal?
   (Is there a proper statistical plan?)
8. Is the experimental protocol complete enough to yield sufficient information?
9. Is animal suffering avoided during the procedure and following it?
   (If the animal is not sacrificed)
10. Is the environment adequate to conduct this experiments?
    (Trained team, established facilities...)

In exceptional conditions, certain procedures can induce some alterations that may be related to some of the features of severe sepsis. Immunotherapy for organ transplants using OKT3, for example, can trigger the release of cytokines. Furthermore, the use of hemodialysis or cardiopulmonary bypass (CPB) can activate the complement system and induce the release of cytokines (9). CPB can trigger a proinflammatory response (TNF, IL-8) and also an anti-inflammatory response (IL-10) (10, 11). This response may be proportional to the duration of the CPB (11), and endotoxin release from the gut may be implicated. Pretreatment is possible in many such cases: the administration of corticosteroids prior to CPB, for instance, can reduce the proinflammatory mediators and also promote the release of IL-10 (10). This is a good example of a situation that can be studied in humans to provide substantial information.

Vivisection is a topic which sometimes becomes so emotional that some people would like to ban it in all its forms. Others have even proposed to replace animals by prisoners! It is important that scientists inform lay people about the necessity of animals for biomedical research and of its benefits to humans. It should be underlined that biomedical research uses less than 50% of all animals destined for laboratory research (8).

The issue of pound animals is a frequent topic of debate. It is estimated that today less than 5% of animals are released by pounds for biomedical use (8). Animal welfare groups often pretend that pets suffer more than specially bred animals when exposed to experiments, so that only the latter should be used. In fact, this is a claim which is difficult to justify and one might reasonably suspect that many of its supporters are just attempting to make animal research more difficult and more expensive.

Animal research must obviously avoid cruelty and waste. The number of animals should be kept to a minimum but at the same time, the methods used should be complete and adequate to obtain as much information as possible from the experiments. There should be adequate anesthesia and analgesia during the experiment and also after the experiment, if the animal is not sacrificed during the experiment. Guidelines exist for animal experimentation (such as those of the National Institute of Health in the U.S.) and it is important that researchers declare adherence to them. It is also important that animal experiments should be monitored (as is the case in university laboratories).

Of course, suffering is unpleasant in any species. However, the medical community has a commitment to improve the quality of medical care and to develop new and more effective therapeutic options. It would be unethical to expose patients to excessive risks if the study of a given intervention does not have enough chance of being effective, or if it carries an excessive risk of deleterious effects. Animal research needs to be promoted because it is sometimes the only reasonable option to obtain improvements in our health and thus our welfare.

References

1. Stevenson GW, Hall SC, Rudnick S, Seleny FL, Stevenson HC (1990) The effect of anesthetic agents on the human immune response. Anesthesiology 72:542-552
2. Friedman G, Gomez J, Shahla M, Vincent JL (1995) Mortality from septic shock: have we made progress? Am J Respir Crit Care Med 151:A494 (Abstr)
3. Sibbald WJ, Vincent JL (1995) Round table conference: clinical trials in sepsis. Crit Care Med 23:294-399
4. Lefering R, Neugebauer EA (1995) Steroid controversy in sepsis and septic shock: a meta-analysis. Crit Care Med 23:1294-1303
5. Zhang H, Spapen H, Nguyen DN, Benlabed M, Buurman WA, Vincent JL (1994) Protective effects of N-acetylcysteine in endotoxemia. Am J Physiol 266:H1746-H1754
6. Zhang H, Spapen H, Manikis P et al (1995) Tirilazad mesylate (U74006F) inhibits the effects of endotoxin in dogs. Am J Physiol 268:H1847-H1855
7. Zhang H, Rogiers P, Preiser JC, Spapen H, Manikis P, Vincent JL (1995) Effects of methylene blue on oxygen availability and regional blood flow during endotoxic shock. Crit Care Med (in press)
8. Range SP, Knox AJ (1995) rhDNase in cystic fibrosis (editorial). Thorax 50:321-322
9. Pradier O, Gerard C, Delvaux A et al (1993) Interleukin-10 inhibits the induction of monocyte procoagulant activity by bacterial lipopolysaccharide. Eur J Immunol 23:2700-2703
10. Mark DB, Naylor CD, Hlatky MA et al (1994) Use of medical resources and quality of life after acute myocardial infarction in Canada and the United States. N Engl J Med 331: 1130-1135
11. Pingleton SK (1994) The efficacy/cost ratio of new therapy: what is the physician's fiduciary responsibility? (editorial). Chest 105:329-330
12. Zhang H, Vincent JL (1993) Oxygen extraction is altered by endotoxin during tamponade-induced stagnant hypoxia in the dog. Circ Shock 40:168-176

Ischemic Microvascular Failure in Severe Head Injury

S. COTEV, L.A. EIDELMAN, Y.G. WEISS

It is becoming increasingly evident that cerebral dysfunction and outcome after severe (i.e., Glasgow Coma Scale - GCS ≤ 8) head injury (SHI) are related, as a rule, not only to the initial structural injury to the brain, but also to a variety of secondary pathophysiological mechanisms, the common denominator of which is ischemia. The ischemic insult apparently initiates several known (and probably many others yet unknown) metabolic/biochemical cascades that are often interacting, and may also, in themselves additionally contribute to the ischemic insult. Many pathways of the injurious pattern had been described and recently reviewed (1-3). Accordingly, reports of improved animal outcome have often appeared which were related to employment of various specific antagonists/competitors/inhibitors to either block, blunt or treat steps in these injurious pathways. The reports from the laboratories leave little doubt as to the relevance of these cascades to the clinical equivalent following SHI in man. Several recent reports have now come from studies in humans that tend to reinforce the evidence from the laboratory. The use of pharmacological agents to prevent, or treat the results of these cascades in humans must still be viewed as experimental at the time these lines are being written. It is not the intention of this presentation to review the extensive research that we and many others had published on the chain of very important events associated with the secondary ischemic injury following SHI. Rather, we aim to briefly touch on evidence that CNS ischemia indeed occurs with SHI, on the possible etiological elements that may lead to ischemia, and on preventive and therapeutic means that attempt to reduce the ischemic insult.

The role of ischemia

Already in 1970, Zupping (4) measured CSF pH and lactate concentration very soon after admission to the hospital of patients with SHI. The degree of CSF lactacidosis was directly related to the estimated severity of injury, as well as to eventual poor outcome, suggesting that cerebral ischemic anaerobic metabolism may be involved. Several years later, others (5, 6) had demonstrated that brains of casualties dying after SHI contained gross, as well as microscopic evidence of an ischemic injury, the extent of which was correlated to ante-mortem episodes of arterial hypoxemia and hypotension, as well as the occurrence of raised intracranial pressure (ICP). Ischemia predominated in brain regions where blood supply is more vulnerable (i.e., boundary zones between perfusion territories of major arterial vessels), or regions where metabolic demands for O_2 are greatest (i.e., hippocampus, basal ganglia), suggesting the detrimental occurrence of O_2 supply/demand imbalance after SHI. Thus, Miller, a central investigator of CNS trauma, suggests that "brain ischaemia may therefore be the single most important mechanism in the production of secondary brain dysfunction and damage after SHI" (7). What, then, may be the etiological mechanisms that contribute to the development of CNS ischemia during, or soon after SHI? As previously suggested, these are related to either decreased O_2 delivery (i.e., decreased cerebral blood flow - CBF, anemia, arterial hypoxemia and increased ICP), or increased consumption (e.g., pyrexia, seizures). Both categories may manifest either globally, or regionally. Compensatory protective mechanisms exist such that decreased O_2 delivery after SHI is generally accompanied by decreased O_2 demand; or, increased oxidative metabolism, as it occurs in seizure activity, triggers (pH-mediated) increased CBF. The presence of ischemic injury after SHI may be seen as absence or dysfunction of these compensatory mechanisms.

Hypotension

Many studies have now demonstrated the prime importance of systemic hypotension, whether at the site of injury (8), upon admission to the neurosurgical facility (9-11), or even in the early ICU period (12), on outcome determination after SHI. The presumption in most of these studies is that systemic hypotension results in decreased global, hemispheric or regional CBF, depending on the mode of CNS injury (i.e., diffuse or focal) and ICP. This assumption is even more obvious after SHI, when CBF so often becomes pressure-dependent due to loss of the autoregulative function. In infants and children, even solitary head injury may result in hypovolemia and hypotension because of extensive bleeding from the vascular scalp; in adults with blunt SHI, significant hypovolemia is more likely to be the result of an associated extracranial injury (e.g., abdominal, chest, thigh). The work of Siegel et al. (11) clearly demonstrates this point. Recent studies from Edinburgh (12), using PC-based minute-to-minute monitoring of 14 physiological variables in the ICU after SHI, have emphasized the devastating role of hypotension (MBP $\leq$ 70 mmHg) on outcome, also when it occurs after presumed stabilization, following injury.

Cerebral hypoperfusion

While the effect on outcome of systemic hypotension, as an indirect measure of decreased CBF, had been amply demonstrated, recent data shed more direct light on the role of decreased CBF per se.

Measurements of regional or global CBF after SHI were in the past generally performed at least 1-2 days after the injury (13). These studies demonstrated hemispheric and regional CBF patterns to be quite different between SHI patients of similar severity of coma. Only recently were we exposed to data on CBF during the first 4-8 h after injury (14-16). In the clinical setting, however, circumstances dictate that such early measurements can only be obtained in patients who had stabilized early after injury, and who do not require surgery. Thus, the studies were performed on a preselected patient population. Nevertheless, the results of these studies are quite revolutionary, and may shed light on the pathogenesis of CNS ischemia after SHI, independent of systemic hypoperfusion. The studies (on adult patients) show, in many of these preselected patients, that cerebral oligemia occurs in the early (i.e., first 8h) post-injury period, but subsides within 24 h of injury. This early oligemia was quite severe in some patients (CBF reaching ischemic thresholds - below 18 ml/100 g/min), and was statistically correlated to both severity of injury (i.e., motor GCS) and Glasgow Outcome Score (GOS). The pathophysiological mechanism leading to this temporary, early oligemia is unclear at this time. One possible explanation (probably able to account for only a fraction of cases demonstrating oligemia) may stem from recent publications (17, 18), using bed-side transcranial Doppler (TCD) sonography, and showing evidence of arterial vasospasm, mostly in patients exhibiting subarachnoid hemorrhage in the initial CT scan. Regional and/or global ischemia may also be iatrogenically induced by over-zealous hyperventilation (19) (see subsequent discussion).

Intracranial hypertension

Raised ICP has long been recognized as a major predictor of poor outcome after SHI (11, 12, 20, 21). Its incidence, degree of elevation, as well as duration, have all been correlated to poor outcome. Intracranial hypertension may contribute to the ischemic injury either globally, or focally, by exerting extravascular pressure opposing the intravascular hydrostatic pressure. Thus, cerebral perfusion pressure (CPP) = mean systemic pressure - ICP; its level, relative to O_2 demand of the brain, is the determinant of the ischemic injury. Many, therefore, consider the control of CPP to be the central goal in the management of SHI.

Anemia

Hypovolemic anemia (independent of hypoperfusion) was mentioned earlier, and requires no further discussion. It may become a significant contributor to cerebral ischemia after SHI in the relatively rare circumstance of inadequate, or late correction of traumatic hemorrhage.

Hypoxemia

Like hypotension, hypoxemia, and its duration has been identified as a factor that when it occurs in the peri-injury period increases the chances of poor outcome from SHI (9, 12, 22). Presumably, one of the venues by which early hypoxemia affects outcome is by contributing to the CNS ischemic injury. From the studies coming from Edinburgh (12) it seems that hypoxemic insults in the ICU (their ICU!) are not frequent, though significantly affecting outcome. Early, pre-hospital hypoxemia has been recorded in some 65% of patients, and is related to either associated chest injury, gastric contents aspiration, neurogenic pulmonary edema, upper airway obstruction, or even prolonged apnea.

Pyrexia and seizures

Both pyrexia and seizure activity after SHI are considered as factors affecting outcome (12, 23). In fact, both the occurrence and duration of pyrexia were found out to be highly significant predictors of poor outcome one year after SHI in the Edinburgh study (12). When they occur in injured patients, with compromised global or regional circulation, these conditions of increased metabolic demand are likely to tip the delicate O_2 balance towards ischemic injury.

Newer management considerations

In the previous discussion, an attempt was made to emphasize and focus on recent information regarding the impact that some pathophysiological deviations may have on the creation of the formidably important secondary ischemic injury associated with SHI. Based on these considerations, efforts must be implemented to augment monitoring, and as a result manage SHI patients so as to minimize and shorten insults that may lead to CNS ischemia.

Advancing SHI management to the site of injury

There is no universal agreement as to the value of advancing SHI management to the site of injury. We suggest to the reader that SHI is a unique injury, with a very narrow "golden hour" window during which every effort should be invested to establish a safe airway (i.e., intubation), ventilation and oxygenation, and to stabilize cardiac output and cerebral perfusion (24-26). Sedation of the restless patient, as cerebral demand for O_2 is being reduced, at the site of injury and during transport to the nearest neurosurgical facility, is also recommended, as long as hemodynamic stability is not compromised due to associated injury. Thus, the principle of "scoop and run" in this injured population should be adhered to only in situations where the injury occurs relatively close to a neurosurgical facility, or when the attending help providers are not sufficiently qualified. The study by Klauber et al. (27) seems to support these conclusions when they demonstrated reduced mortality from SHI after introducing county-wide, dedicated emergency medical services (EMS).

Adequately monitored hyperventilation

Routine hyperventilation (HV) during the acute/immediate phase following SHI had been universally practiced for over 25 years, with the major aim to control ICP and reverse CSF acidosis. Obrist in 1984 (13) and Cold in 1989 (19), and their colleagues, as well as others, offered reservations from this universal practice after recording regional CBF before and after HV. It became obvious that cerebrovascular behavior after SHI is unpredictable, especially in response to HV (to what was considered to be acceptable levels of hypocapnia, i.e., 25-30 mmHg). Focal CBF often fell during routine HV to "ischemic values" (i.e., ≤ 18 ml/100g/min) while total hemispheric CBF remained adequate. Even more recently, a prospective controlled study of the use of "prophylactic" HV in SHI (28) suggested that its use had no salutary effect on outcome 1 year after injury. Most clinical facilities caring for SHI patients, however, are not equipped with the sophisticated means to measure CBF at the bedside. General guidelines may be suggested, therefore, according to which HV can be used. In children and young adults, for example, who are more likely to incur diffuse brain swelling or congestion, rather than a focal, asymmetric structural injury. HV is less apt to lead to focal ischemia than in elderly adults with an asymmetric injury. Furthermore, HV will be most effective in patients demonstrating preserved CO_2-vascular responsiveness and electrical activity. It is likely to have a devastating effect, however, in hypovolemic patients because of its exaggerated effect on venous return, cardiac output, cerebral perfusion and presumably CNS ischemia under such circumstances. In the absence of CBF measurements to guide the risk/effectiveness of HV in reducing ICP, the use of TCD and continuous monitoring of jugular venous oxygen saturation ($SjvO_2$) may be advantageous (29, 30).

Calcium channel blockers

The suggestion that cerebral arterial vasospasm may be incriminated in early cerebral oligemia and ischemia in certain subgroups of SHI patients raises the possibility of using specific therapeutic means to relieve it. Induced systemic hypertension, hemodilution, hypervolemia and Ca ion blockers may be considered, but cannot be safely recommended at this point. In an anecdotal report Kostron et al. (31) described excellent outcome in six of eight patients, with very severe SHI (i.e., initial GCS 3-5), who demonstrated angiographic evidence of subarachnoid hemorrhage, and were treated with nimodipine. In two placebo-controlled, prospective multi-center European studies, the same calcium channel blocker had only a non-statistical tendency to improve long-term outcome when started several hours after SHI (32, 33). In a subgroup of 41 patients of the second study, however, with proven subarachnoid hemorrhage, nimodipine had a significantly improved outcome as compared to 72 placebo-treated patients (i.e., 44% as compared to 61% of patients with poor outcome, respectively). Nimodipine may therefore be recommended only in SHI patients with proven subarachnoid hemorrhage. This treatment may be accompanied by a tendency to hypotension, and should therefore be extremely well-controlled.

Conclusions

In this chapter we have attempted to focus on the role of CNS ischemia in determining outcome after SHI, and the various known risk factors that may contribute to the creation of the ischemic injury. Based on the identification of these factors, it is the authors' opinion that the most promising approach to reduce the secondary ischemic injury, and improve outcome, is the advancement of expert CNS resuscitation teams and means to the site of injury in an effort to take maximal advantage of the all too short "golden hour" after SHI. We risk presenting this opinion even though direct scientific data to back it is unavailable. We have purposely not dealt with the voluminous new data appearing on the role of the various metabolic cascades induced by ischemia, and the experimental means to block them. The impact of these must await wider universal confirmation.

References

1. Siesjo BK (1992) Pathophysiology and treatment of focal cerebral ischemia. Part I: pathophysiology. J Neurosurg 77:169-184
2. Siesjo BK (1992) Pathophysiology and treatment of focal cerebral ischemia. Part II: mechanisms of damage and treatment. J Neurosurg 77:337-354
3. Hans P (1995) Acute management of the head-trauma patient. Curr Opin Anaesth 8:163-167
4. Zupping R (1970) Cerebral acid-base and gas metabolism in brain injury. J Neurosurg 33: 498-505
5. Graham DI, Adams JH, Doyle D (1978) Ischaemic brain damage in fatal non-missile head injuries. J Neurol Sci 39:213-234
6. Graham DI, Ford I, Adams JH et al (1989) Ischaemic brain damage is still common in fatal non-missile head injury. J Neurol Neurosurg Psychiatry 52:346-350
7. Miller JD (1985) Head injury and brain ischaemia-implications for therapy. Br J Anaesth 57:120-129
8. Chesnut RM, Marshall LF, Klauber MR et al (1993) The role of secondary brain injury in determining outcome from severe head injury. J Trauma 34:216-222
9. Miller JD, Sweet RC, Narayan R et al (1978) Early insults to the injured brain. JAMA 240:439-442
10. Pietropaoli JA, Rogers FB, Shackford SR et al (1992) The deleterious effects of intraoperative hypotension on outcome in patients with severe head injuries. J Trauma 33:403-407
11. Siegel JH, Gens DR, Mamanov T et al (1991) Effect of associated injuries and blood volume replacement on death, rehabilitation needs, and disability in blunt traumatic brain injury. Crit Care Med 19:1252-1265
12. Jones PA, Andrews PJD, Midgley S et al (1994) Measuring the burden of secondary insults in head-injured patients during intensive care. J Neurosurg Anesth 6:4-14
13. Obrist WD, Langfitt TW, Jaggi JL et al (1984) Cerebral blood flow and metabolism in comatose patients with acute head injury. Relationship to intracranial hypertension. J Neurosurg 61:241-253

14. Marion DW, Darby J, Yonas H (1991) Acute regional cerebral blood flow changes caused by severe head injuries. J Neurosurg 74:407-414

15. Bouma GJ, Muizelaar JP, Choi SC et al (1991) Cerebral circulation and metabolism after severe traumatic brain injury: the elusive role of ischemia. J Neurosurg 75:685-693

16. Bouma GJ, Muizelaar JP, Stringer WA et al (1992) Ultra-early evaluation of regional cerebral blood flow in severely head-injured patients using xenon-enhanced computerized tomography. J Neurosurg 77:360-368

17. Martin NA, Doberstein C, Zane C et al (1992) Posttraumatic cerebral arterial spasm: transcranial Doppler ultrasound, cerebral blood flow, and angiographic findings. J Neurosurg 77:573-583

18. Steiger HJ, Aaslid R, Stooss R et al (1994) Transcranial Doppler monitoring in head injury: relations between type of injury, flow velocities, vasoreactivity, and outcome. Neurosurgery 34:79-86

19. Cold GE (1989) Does acute hyperventilation provoke cerebral oligaemia in comatose patients after acute head injury? Acta Neurochir 96:100-106

20. Miller JD, Becker DP, Ward JD et al (1977) Significance of intracranial hypertension in severe head injury. J Neurosurg 47:503-516

21. Marmarou A, Anderson RL, Ward JD et al (1991) Impact of ICP instability and hypotension on outcome in patients with severe head trauma. J Neurosurg 75:S59-S66

22. Price DJE, Murray A (1972) The influence of hypoxia and hypotension on recovery from head injury. Injury 3:218-224

23. Tsementzis SA, Gillingham FJ, Hitchcock ER (1979) The effect of focal twitching on the intracranial pressure during paralysis and mechanical ventilation. Ann Clin Res 11:253-257

24. Richards P (1986) Severe head injury: the first hour. Br Med J 293:643

25. Wilden JN (1993) Rapid resuscitation in severe head injury. Lancet 342:1378

26. Gentleman D, Dearden M, Midgley S et al (1993) Guidelines for resuscitation and transfer of patients with serious head injury. Br Med J 307:547-552

27. Klauber MR, Marshall LF, Toole BM et al (1985) Cause of decline in head-injury mortality rate in San Diego County, California. J Neurosurg 62:528-531

28. Muizelaar JP, Marmarou A, Ward JD et al (1991) Adverse effects of prolonged hyperventilation in patients with severe head injury: a randomized clinical trial. J Neurosurg 75:731-739

29. Sheinberg M, Kanter MJ, Robertson CS et al (1992) Continuous monitoring of jugular venous oxygen saturation in head-injured patients. J Neurosurg 76:212-217

30. Chan KH, Miller JD, Dearden NM et al (1992) The effect of changes in cerebral perfusion pressure upon middle cerebral artery blood flow velocity and jugular bulb venous oxygen saturation after severe brain injury. J Neurosurg 77:55-61

31. Kostron H, Rumpl E, Stampfl G et al (1985) Treatment of cerebral vasospasm following severe head injury with the calcium influx blocker nimodipine. Neurochirurgia 28:103-109

32. Bailey I, Bell A, Gray J et al (1991) A trial of the effect of nimodipine on outcome after head injury. Acta Neurochir 110:97-105

33. The European Study Group on Nimodipine in Severe Head Injury (1994) A multicenter trial of the efficacy of nimodipine on outcome after severe head injury. J Neurosurg 80:797-804

Intestinal Microvascular Injury

U. HAGLUND

Inadequate microcirculation in sepsis and shock causes tissue injury. In this chapter the small intestinal circulation will be used as an example of such tissue injury. The selection of the small intestine as an example is made for two reasons: this organ represents those that early suffer from inadequate microcirculation in critical illness and, moreover, the consequences of gut tissue injury are thought to be of significant importance for the further development into multiple organ dysfunction.

Small intestinal mucosal injury develops very rapidly in critical illness and reduced intramucosal pH. Initially there is increased permeability of the intestinal mucosa. Morphologically detectable injury with loss of the epithelial lining of the villi is found following 20 min of near total ischemia or 60 min of sepsis/hemorrhagic shock. After successful resuscitation complete restoration takes place within 4 h. The pathophysiology of this injury has an ischemic and a reperfusion component (1) (Table 1).

Table 1. Pathophysiology of small intestinal mucosal injury

I. Ischemia
Reduced oxygen delivery
Reduced blood flow
Short-circuiting of oxygen in the mucosal counter-current exchanger
Increased demand for oxygen
Decreased ability for extraction/utilisation
II. Reperfusion injury
Increased generation of oxygen free radicals

In this chapter the different pathophysiological mechanisms illustrated in Table 1 will be discussed briefly.

Ischemic injury

Oxygen delivery is decreased with decreased blood flow as in hemorrhage. However, the extraction of oxygen increases simultaneously and the small intestine can in this way compensate for blood losses up to one third of the total blood volume (2). The oxygen consumption is thus maintained in the normal range down to an intestinal blood flow of 50% of control. The sympathetic nerve system seems to play only a minor role in the vascular adjustments during hemorrhage and instead there is evidence that the renin-angiotensin system is very important for intestinal vascular control during hemorrhage (3). Microvascular disturbances that generally occur during shock states, such as increased sticking of white blood cells to the endothelium and injury to endothelial cells, further impairs the situation also as regards oxygen delivery in the small intestine.

As a consequence to the increased oxygen extraction the O_2 content of the portal venous blood becomes very low and hepatic ischemia is the price to be paid for maintaining intestinal oxygenation following hemorrhage.

The intestinal blood flow in sepsis seems to follow cardiac output fairly well. It is therefore often maintained in septic states. In addition, intraintestinal redistribution of blood flow occurs and favors the superficial mucosa. Still, it is this portion of the mucosa that is highly vulnerable in critical illness. To further add to the confusion, intralumenal supply of oxygen may prevent intramucosal acidosis as well as mucosal injury during sepsis (4, 5). This paradox with maintained blood supply and hypoxic injury is explained by the anatomical arrangement of the villous vascular supply which creates the prerequisites for a counter-current exchanger between the central arterial vessel and the subepithelial network of capillaries and venulae. The distance between the two sets of vessels with mainly opposite direction of flow is small enough to allow diffusion of easily diffusible substances, such as oxygen. There is direct experimental support for such short-circuiting of oxygen at the base of the villi and this process becomes much more effective at hypotension (6). This system explains significant hypoxia at the villous tip despite the mainly unchanged supply of blood to this region (7).

Sepsis seems to add at least one dimension to this problem. Intestinal blood flow follows the changes in cardiac output and unproportionate intestinal vasoconstriction does not seem to occur in sepsis. Intestinal oxygen consumption is increased in sepsis (8, 9) (approximately 75% in a severe model of sepsis induced in pigs by fecal peritonitis) (9). The cause of the increased demand for oxygen remains unclear. One hypothesis put forward is that invasion of inflammatory cells (mainly polymorphonuclear leukocytes) and activation of the high number of resident macrophages and lymphocytes by the infammatory process could account for the increase. However, in recent experiments IB4, a monoclonal antibody to the CD11/CD18 complex thus preventing white blood cells from sticking to the endothelial layer (and later penetrating into the tissue), failed to prevent the increased oxygen consumption (10) as well as to prevent mucosal injury. It is still possible that resident cells play a dominating role, however.

Despite the increased consumption of oxygen in this experimental septic model there are signs of intestinal mucosal ischemia as revealed by intramucosal acidosis (11) (Table 2), increased mucosal permeability and microscopically

Table 2. Oxygen delivery (DO_2), oxygen consumption ($\dot{V}O_2$), and intramucosal pH (pHi) in pigs made septic from peritonitis at time 0 hour [Data from Rasmussen et al. 1992, (11)]

Time, hours	DO_2	$\dot{V}O_2$	pHi
0	7.5/0.5	1.4/0.1	7.30/0.05
1	8.1/0.8	2.4/0.3	7.19/0.07
2	5.6/0.4	2.2/0.3	7.07/0.05
3	4.8/0.2	2.2/0.3	7.06/0.07
4	4.3/0.3	2.0/0.2	7.04/0.09
5	3.5/0.2	1.8/0.2	7.05/0.10

DO_2 and $\dot{V}O_2$ are expressed in ml/minxkg - mean values ± SE

detectable mucosal injury. Furthermore, the intramucosal acidosis occurs with a much lower intestinal oxygen extraction rate as compared with the situation in hemorrhage (12). Tonometrically measured intramucosal pO_2 indicates that the reduction in intramucosal pH (pHi) occurs with a high amount of oxygen present in the tissue (12). Thus, it seems as if the problem in sepsis is *not* inadequate delivery of oxygen to the tissue but inadequate tissue metabolism of the oxygen delivered. Sepsis causes a change at the mitochondrial level blocking the adequate utilization of available oxygen, causing the tissue to produce increased amounts of carbon dioxide. The reason as well as the mechanisms for this change is yet unknown. On the other hand, increasing the amount of oxygen delivered to the intestine by increasing cardiac output by means of dextran infusions and dobutamine, may prevent the reduction of pHi (13). However, this does not necessarily mean a normalization of the metabolic situation since increased wash out of carbon dioxide alone may explain the normalization of pHi. On the other hand, Fink and coworkers have recently demonstrated that sepsis causes a much more marked increase in mucosal permeability than what is caused by similar reductions in sup. mesenteric artery blood flow alone. Reduced pHi rapidly causes permeability increase of the small intestinal mucosa and shoud be regarded as potentially harmful by itself (14, 15).

In summary, the small intestinal oxygen metabolism has a good capacity to compensate for decreased blood flow, caused by hemorrhage or mechanical constriction of the supplying artery, by increased extraction of oxygen. However, even a less pronounced reduction in blood flow caused by sepsis creates significant changes in the small intestinal oxygen metabolism since in sepsis the capacity to increase oxygen extraction is less, the metabolism of the oxygen present becomes inadequate and at the same time the needs for oxygen consumption increase.

Reperfusion injury

This component of the ischemic injury was first described by Granger et al. 1981 (16). These authors also hypothesized the underlying mechanisms which largely have been verified in the following experiments from their own and other laboratories (17, 1). The reperfusion component has attracted considerable interest because of its general biological implications and not because of a verified important role in sepsis. On the contrary, it is not likely that the reperfusion component is important in sepsis and critical illness as we recognise these conditions clinically.

The reperfusion component is caused by increased generation of oxygen free radicals. During ischemia the break down of ATP stops at hypoxanthine, since the further metabolism to xanthine and urea demands the presence of oxygen. As a consequence, hypoxanthine accumulates in the ischemic tissue. The converting enzyme, xanthine hydroxylase (XD), is simultaneously changed by a proteolytic process initiated by ischemia to xanthine oxidase (XO). XD uses NAD as a electron acceptor while XO creates superoxide anion - an oxygen derived free radical. At reperfusion oxygen is available in high amounts, the substrate has been accumulated and the radical forming enzyme is there and activated. The resulting radical formation may exceed the defense capacity of the tissue and oxygen free radicals may then initially cause endothelial cell injury. In addition, radicals may activate leukocytes to cause microvascular impairment resulting in tissue injury. Polomorphonuclear leukocytes may become activated to cause oxygen free radicals by other mechanisms than the XO pathway during the septic process mainly by activated white blood cells, causing endothelial cell damage. Oxygen free radicals may by this effect promote microvascular disturbances (reduced oxygen delivery), tissue injury and multiple organ dysfunction during sepsis.

References

1. Haglund U, Bulkley GB, Granger DN (1987) On the pathophysiology of intestinal ischemic injury. Acta Chir Scand 153:321-324
2. Kvietys PR, Granger DN (1982) Relation between intestinal blood flow and oxygen uptake. Am J Physiol 242:G202-G208
3. Bailey RW, Bulkey GB, Hamilton SR, Morris JB, Haglund U (1987) Protection of small intestine from nonocclusive mesenteric ischemic injury due to cardiogenic shock. Am J Surg 153:108-116

4. Falk A, Redfors S, Myrvold H, Haglund U (1985) Small intestinal mucosal lesions in feline septic shock: a study on the pathogenesis. Circ Shock 17:327-337
5. Haglund U (1993) Therapeutic potential of intraluminal oxygenation. Crit Care Med 21: S69-S71
6. Lundgren O, Haglund U (1978) The pathophysiology of the intestinal countercurrent exchanger. Life Sci 23:1411-1422
7. Haglund U, Jodal M, Lundgren O (1984) The small bowel in arterial hypotension and shock. In: Sheperd AP, Granger DN (eds) Physiology of intestinal circulation. Raven, New York, pp 305-319
8. Dahn MS, Lange P, Lobdell K, Hans B, Jacobs LA, Mitchell RA (1987) Splanchnic and total body consumption differences in septic and injured patients. Surgery 101:69-80
9. Arvidsson D, Rasmussen I, Almqvist P, Niklasson F, Haglund U (1991) Splanchnic oxygen consumption in septic and hemorrhagic shock. Surgery 109:190-197
10. Wollert S, Rasmussen I, Lundberg C, Gerdin B, Arvidsson D, Haglund U (1993) Inhibition of CD 18-dependent adherence of polymorphonuclear leukocytes does not affect liver oxygen consumption in fecal peritonitis in pigs. Circ Shock 41:230-238
11. Rasmussen I, Haglund U (1992) Early gut ischemia in experimental fecal peritonitis. Circ Shock 38:22-28
12. Antonsson JB, Haglund UH (in press) Gut intramucosal pH and intraluminal pO_2 in a porcine model of peritonitis or hemorrhage. Gut (in press)
13. Ljungdahl M, Rasmussen I, Haglund U (1995) Flow dependency of gastro-intestinal mucosal acidosis in sepsis (Abstrac). Shock 3 [Suppl 2]:22
14. Fink MP, Kaups KL, Wang H, Rothschild HR (1991) Maintenance of superior mesenteric arterial perfusion prevents increased intestinal mucosal permeability in endotoxic pigs. Surgery 110:154-161
15. Fink MP, Cohn SM, Lee PC, Rothschild HR, Deniz YF, Wang H, Fiddian-Green RG (1989) Effect of lipopolysaccharide on intestinal intramucosal hydrogen ion concentration in pigs: Evidence of gut ischemia in a normodynamic model of septic shock. Crit Care Med 17: 641-646
16. Granger DN, Rutili G, McCord JM (1981) Superoxide radicals in feline intestinal ischemia. Gastroenterology 81:22-29
17. Parks DA, Bulkley GB, Granger DN, Hamilton SR, McCord JM (1982) Ischemic injury in the cat small intestine: role of superoxide radicals. Gastroenterology 82:9-15

Vasoactive Drugs and Splanchnic Perfusion

J. TAKALA

Vasoactive drugs, especially sympathomimetic amines, are often needed to support tissue perfusion in circulatory failure. The effects of sympathomimetic drugs on splanchnic circulation and metabolism have not been well documented in humans. Based on the available data, it seems evident that the regional hemodynamic effects of various vasoactive drugs in intensive care patients can neither be predicted from their pharmacological characteristics alone nor extrapolated from experimental models. Inadequate splanchnic tissue perfusion may contribute to the development of multiple organ failure and ultimately death in critically ill patients. The catecholamines used to support the circulatory functions may markedly modify the activity of various metabolic pathways in the liver and simultaneously alter the splanchnic blood flow and its distribution. Accordingly, catecholamines may induce regional perfusion abnormalities and alter the balance between regional oxygen delivery and tissue metabolic demands. Due to these interactions, the effects of vasoactive drugs on splanchnic oxygen transport and substrate metabolism should be evaluated in intensive care patients.

Traditionally, the potential effects of adrenergic agents on regional perfusion have been interpreted in terms of their relative adrenergic receptor activity. In critically ill patients, the effects may be modified, e.g., due to receptor downregulation. In experimental studies, alpha-adrenergic stimulation by dopamine, norepinephrine and epinephrine increases renal and visceral vascular resistance and reduces renal and visceral blood flow (1). The effects of dobutamine depend on the balance between its alpha-mediated vasoconstriction and beta-mediated vasodilation (2). Dopexamine with beta$_2$- and dopaminergic properties and without alpha-stimulation may have beneficial effects on splanchnic blood flow (3). The effects of a vasoactive drug may not be uniform in different parts of the splanchnic region: e.g., in an endotoxin shock model, vasopressor therapy with dopamine or norepinephrine increases regional vascular resistance of the colon, while the perfusion in the other parts of splanchnic region is well maintained (4). In addition, the effects of vasoactive drugs on the microcirculation may be different despite similar effects on blood flow distribution in major vessels. Observations in experimental peritonitis support this concept: treatment with dobutamine produced more hepatocellular damage as compared to dopexamine (5).

Recently, the effects of adrenergic agents on splanchnic perfusion have been studied in septic patients. In ten patients with septic shock, correction of hypotension by administration of vasopressor doses of dopamine increased splanchnic blood flow, whereas the effects of norepinephrine were more variable (6). In contrast, dopamine worsened gastric mucosal acidosis in septic shock, while norepinephrine resulted in increased gastric mucosal pH despite identical effects on systemic hemodynamics (7). These findings support the view that sympathomimetic drugs may induce a mismatch between splanchnic oxygen delivery and demand.

Low cardiac output syndrome with tissue hypoperfusion is an infrequent but serious complication of cardiac surgery. Regional tissue hypoxia may develop despite apparently stable systemic hemodynamics, as suggested by episodes of gastric mucosal acidosis in up to 50% of patients after cardiac operation (8). The metabolic demands increase during the immediate postoperative period and this increases the risk of tissue hypoxia if any compromise of hemodynamics occurs (9). Using techniques of regional catheterization and dye dilution, we have recently demonstrated that immediately after coronary artery by-pass operation, the enhanced metabolic demand is compensated by a combination of increased oxygen extraction and blood flow both in the whole body and in the splanchnic region and that the regional oxygen extraction capability is well preserved (10). The gastric mucosal pH_i continues to decrease and reaches its minimum several hours postoperatively (11). This suggests that a regional mismatch between oxygen delivery and demand may persist or develop after the stabilization of systemic hemodynamics.

The effects of various vasoactive drugs on regional blood flow have previously been studied in patients with chronic congestive heart failure, and these results have been extrapolated to intensive care patients. Neither dopamine nor dobutamine had an effect whereas dopexamine increased the splanchnic blood flow (12, 13). Based on recent studies, extrapolation of these data to the critically ill is clearly not justified. In contrast, we have recently demonstrated that immediately after coronary artery by-pass operation both dobutamine and dopexamine consistently increased splanchnic blood flow (10, 14, 15). Despite the major increases in total splanchnic blood flow in response to both dobutamine and dopexamine, gastric mucosal acidosis persisted and in patients with no mucosal acidosis, the gastric mucosal pH decreased. These effects were observed even more prominently in patients with low cardiac output (15). It is evident that the underlying disease modifies the responses to vasoactive drugs and the responses of patients with acute postoperative circulatory failure and acutely septic patients may not be similar.

References

1. Ruffolo RR Jr, Fondacaro JD, Levitt B, Edwards RM, Kinter LB (1987) Pharmacologic manipulation of regional blood flow. In: Snyder JV, Pinsky MR (eds) Oxygen transport in critically ill, 1st edn, Year Book Medical, Chicago, pp 450-474
2. Vernon DD, Garret JS, Banner W Jr, Dean JM (1992) Hemodynamic effects of dobutamine in an intact animal model. Crit Care Med 20:1322-1329
3. Lokhandwala MF, Jandhyala BS (1992) Effects of dopaminergic agonists on organ blood flow and function. Clin Intensive Care [Suppl] 3:12-15
4. Breslow MJ, Miller CF, Parker SD, Walman AT, Traystman RJ (1987) Effect of vasopressors on organ blood flow during endotoxin shock in pigs. Am J Physiol H291-H300
5. Webb AR, Moss RF, Tighe D, Al-Saady N, Bennet ED (1991) The effects of dobutamine, dopexamine and fluid on hepatic histological responses to porcine faecal peritonitis. Intensive Care Med 17:487-493
6. Ruokonen E, Takala J, Kari A, Saxén H, Mertsola J, Hansen EJ (1993) Regional blood flow and oxygen transport in septic shock. Crit Care Med 21:1296-1303
7. Marik PE, Mohedin M (1994) The contrasting effects of dopamine and norepinephrine on systemic and splanchnic oxygen utilization in hyperdynamic sepsis. JAMA 272:1354-1357
8. Fiddian-Green RG, Baker S (1987) Predictive value of the stomach wall pH for complications after cardiac operations: comparison with other monitoring. Crit Care Med 15:153-156
9. Chiara O, Giomarelli PP, Biagioli B, Rosi R, Gattinoni L (1987) Hypermetabolic response after hypothermic cardiopulmonary bypass. Crit Care Med 15:995-1000
10. Ruokonen E, Takala J, Kari A (1993) Regional blood flow and oxygen transport in low cardiac output syndrome after cardiac surgery. Crit Care Med 21:1304-1311
11. Kuttila K, Niinikoski J, Haglund U (1990) Visceral and peripheral tissue perfusion after cardiac surgery. Scand J Thor Cardiovasc Surg 25:57-62
12. Leier CV, Heban BT, Huss P, Bush CA, Lewis RP (1978) Comparative systemic and regional hemodynamic effects of dopamine and dobutamine in patients with cardiomyopathic heart failure. Circulation 58:466-475
13. Leier CV, Binkley PF, Carpenter J, Randolph PH, Unverferth DV (1988) Cardiovascular pharmacology of dopexamine in low output congestive heart failure. Am J Cardiol 62:94-99
14. Parviainen I, Ruokonen E, Takala J (1995) Dobutamine-induced dissociation between changes in splanchnic blood flow and gastric intramucosal pH after cardiac surgery. Br J Anaesth 74:277-282
15. Uusaro A, Ruokonen E, Takala J (1995) Gastric mucosal pH does not reflect changes in splanchnic blood flow after cardiac surgery. Br J Anaesth 74:149-154

Perfusion in Renal Dysfunction

G. BERLOT

Introduction

In normal conditions, the kidney receives 20%-25% of the cardiac output (VB). Thus, it not surprising that several blood-borne endogenous or exogenous nephrotoxic substances (radiocontrast media, amynoglycosides, pigments, immunocomplexes etc.) can cause a disturbance of the renal function, which is principally be related to the damage of the renal microvascular network and possibly leading to acute renal failure (ARF). However, the term "renal vascular injury" usually indicates the pathophysiologic consequences of the shortage of renal blood supply occurring in many clinical settings, including trauma and hemorrhage, surgical interventions and burns, ultimately leading to the occurrence of the prerenal ARF. Due to several pathophysiological factors, the renal medulla is particularly at risk of ischemic damage (1), and the occurrence of ARF is usually associated to extensive anatomofunctional damage of the deepest region of the kidney.

Due to the high mortality rate associated with the occurrence of ARF in critically ill patients, a thorough knowledge of the pathophysiologic mechanism underlying the onset of the medullary ischemia/hypoxia is essential in order to avoid, to limit and possibly to prevent the noxious factors which jeopardize the blood flow to the more vulnerable regions of the kidney. However, in the clinical setting, several factors cooperate to damage this particularly vulnerable tract of the nephron, and it can be difficult to separate the action exerted by each of them.

Pathophysiologic considerations

A description of the basic mechanism underlying the control of renal perfusion is essential in order to understand the pathophysiologic alterations occurring in critical conditions.

The renal blood flow is regulated by a dual mechanism. The first, under extra-renal neurohormonal influences, controls the amount of blood flowing into the renal arteries and their main ramifications, whereas the second is responsible for to the intrinsic fine-tuning of the intrarenal microvascular network (renal autoregulation) (2, 3).

Catecholamines are mainly responsible for the variations of the renal blood flow, particularly in the cortex. In normal conditions, the administration of high doses of epinephrine and norepinephrine is associated with the reduction of the renal blood flow. Also angiotensins II and III, which are produced and released under ischemic conditions via the renin-angiotensinogen pathway, are powerful vasoconstrictors. The secretion and the release of angiotensins is regulated by many factors, including hypoxia, the sodium content of the tubular fluid, the sympathetic discharge and the intravascular pressure of the afferent arterioles.

Renal autoregulation plays a major role in the maintenance of the perfusion under conditions of reduced renal blood flow. Actually, renal blood flow remains relatively constant in face of wide variations of systemic arterial pressure. Several mechanisms are implicated in the autoregulation, which is ultimately aimed to match the oxygen availability with the metabolic needs. First, afferent arterioles can vary their width in response to changes of the arterial pressure, so maintaining the intraglomerular blood flow and pressure. Second, the glomerular blood flow can be reduced by the tubuloglomerular feedback mechanism, consisting in the macula densa-mediated vasoconstriction of the afferent artery in response to an increased sodium content in the distal tubular fluid: the ensuing reduced filtration decreases the tubular workload and, consequently, the metabolic needs. Third, many substances with either vasodilating and/or vasoconstricting properties have been so far identified as biochemical mediators of the renal autoregulation. The maintenance and restoration of the medullary blood flow is ultimately given by the balance between vasodilating and vasoconstricting influences. Besides their action on the blood flow, some of these substances can modulate the reabsorption of solutes, thus modifying the metabolic requests. Prostaglandin E_2 (PGE_2) dilates medullary vessels and reduces the medullary oxygen consumption ($\dot{V}O_2$) – also other lipidic mediators, such as cytochrome P-450-dependent arachidonate derivates and platelet activating factor (PAF). Nitric oxide (NO), which exerts a strong local vasodilating action, is synthetized in the cells of the medullary thick limb (4). Adenosine, produced during the breakdown of ATP, can induce cortical vasoconstriction associated with medullary vasodilation, so promoting the redistribution of blood flow toward the less perfused areas (5). Among vasoconstrictors, endothelin-1 is implicated in the pathogenesis of many renal vascular disorders as well as in cyclosporin-associated nephrotoxicity (6). Many others substances, including tumor necrosis factor (TNF), epithelial growth factor and insulin-like growth factor 1 play a role in the regulation of the medullary perfusion (3).

Despite the relatively high blood flow directed to the kidney, and the sophisticated regulatory mechanisms, the renal medulla is at risk of hypoxia even in normal conditions. Several mechanisms can account for its sensitivity to the ischemic damage. First, the bulk of the renal blood flow is mainly directed toward the cortex, with the aim to optimize the flow-dependent renal functions (glomerular filtration and reabsorption of the solutes in the proximal tubules).

Second, in the renal medulla a low blood flow and, consequently, a relatively reduced pressure of oxygen (pO_2) is required in order to maintain the osmotic gradient necessary for the urine concentration. Actually, in normal subjects, the medullary pO_2 is 10-20 mmHg (2), sharply contrasting with the cortical pO_2 which is around 50 mmHg (3). Last, in clinical conditions, the restoration of renal blood flow obtained with volume resuscitation or inotropic and vasodilating agents is followed by the production of free radicals of oxygen, further amplifying the initial ischemic insult (7). Thus, it appears that the outer medulla, the medullary thick ascendent limb (TAL) and the distal portion of the distal tubule (S3) can be considered a target either for hypoxic-ischemic injuries, including those derived by the reperfusion, or for nephrotoxic agents (3).

Clinical considerations

In general terms, every circumstance characterized by a normal or increased medullary workload associated with a reduced regional perfusion can lead to the development of ARF. Conversely, pharmacologic interventions aimed to reduce the O_2 needs or to increase its availability are supposed to exert a protective effect, particularly at the S3 and TAL level.

Experimentally, the administration of furosemide and ouabain, which reduce the medullary $\dot{V}O_2$ by inhibiting the medullary Na+/K+ pumps, prevents, in vivo and in vitro, the onset of medullary alterations (8). In contrast, amphotericin B exerts its nephrotoxic action by enhancing the membrane pump activity and vasoconstricting the medullary vessels, thus causing a mismatch in the regional $\dot{V}O_2/DO_2$ relationship (9). This effect is inhibited by the administration of ouabain (10).

Furhermore, many other insults can disrupt the precise regulation of the medullary perfusion, including shortage of blood flow due to a reduced cardiac output or to its redistribution toward other vascular beds, drugs and radiocontrast media. The block of the vasodilating PGE_2 synthesis associated with the administration of nonsteroidal anti-inflammatory drugs (NSAID) can exert an hypoxic effect by reducing the medullary blood flow and, at the same time, by increasing the tubular reabsorption (11). A similar mechanism has been proposed also for radiocontrast media-induced nephrotoxicity (3, 12).

Even if some techniques able to measure renal blood flow at the bedside have been recently described (13, 14), at the present time the detection of renal hypoxic injury relies on indirect signs. The loss of urinary concentration (isosthenuria) represents the first sign of established medullary ischemic or cytotoxic damage (12). During hypovolemic or low-cardiac output states, the loss of the renal concentrating ability indicates the border between prerenal and renal ARF. In some circumstances (i.e. the administration of nephrotoxic agents such as aminoglycosides or certain antineoplastic agents), a mild-to-moderate reduction of glomerular blood flow associated with polyuria is the predominant clinical feature (3). The appearance in the urine of brown granular casts, mainly constituted by the Tamm-Horsfall protein, is considered a marker of a hypoxic injury somewhat limited to the TAL. Frank ischemic necrosis of the papillae reflects deep medullary ischemia, possibly associated with the effects of other aggravating conditions, such as sickle cell disease, analgesic abuse etc., which are able to jeopardize the blood flow directed toward the deepest medullary areas (3).

Besides ischemia and/or hypoxia, the TAL and the renal medulla are exposed to other potentially harmful factors. According to Garcia-Perez et al. (15), the continuous shifts of osmolality of the medullary fluid causes a hydrostatic stress on the tubular cells, which must up- or downregulate their internal osmolality in response to changes of the surrounding environment. Other substances normally present in relatively high concentrations in the medulla, including calcium and ammonium, can exert toxic effects on the cells either directly or through the activation of the complement cascade, respectively (3).

Theoretically, conditions known to be associated with the risk of medullary ischemic/hypoxic damage could be prevented with the restoration and maintenance of euvolemia and with the avoidance (or limitation) of potentially nephrotoxic agents. However, we recognize that these goals might not be easily accomplished in every patients. Then, in the presence of persisting risk factors or once the damage is already established, the main therapeutic goal of renal medullary hypoxia and consequent ARF consists in the reduction of the workload and/or on the improvement of perfusion, not dissimilarly from what is usually indicated in conditions characterized by an imbalance between oxygen needs and oxygen availability (i.e. acute myocardial infarction, heart failure etc.).

The reduction of the workload can be obtained by the administration of normal saline, with the aim to reduce the concentration in the TAL and in the medulla, and with the administration of loop diuretics, which reduce the $\dot{V}O_2$ of the tubular cells by inhibiting the energy-dependent membrane reabsorption of chloride (8). The use of mannitol is controversial: several studies indicated that it was effective in the prevention of ARF associated with profound jaundice (16) myoglobinuria and abdominal aortic surgery (17). However, its administration has been also associated with the onset of ARF, probably due to the increased osmotic workload (see above) imposed upon an already damaged medulla (18).

The administration of low dose dopamine (1-4 mcg/kg/min), alone or in combination with furosemide, has been advocated the prevention and the treatment of ARF (19). The rationale of its use consists in the dopamine-induced increase of cortical blood flow, which has been shown to be reduced in ARF and in the activation of dopaminergic receptors in the proximal tubule (20). Even if low-dose dopamine is widely used, its efficacy has been recently questioned (21). Other substances, such as Ca++ antagonists, ACE inhibitors and amino acids are currently under investigation (3).

The improvement of medullary blood flow can be obtained by the increase in cardiac output, which is accomplished by the administration of fluids, inotropics and vasodilators, alone or in combination, or by the increase of the renal perfusion pressure, obtained through the use of vasopressors. Despite the widespread concern regarding the effects of vasoconstricting agents on the kidney, several investigators were able to demonstrate both experimentally and clinically an increase of urine output associated with an increase of the mean arterial pressure after the administration of catecholamines (22-24).

References

1. Symon Z, Brezis M (1995) Pathophysiology of acute renal failure. In: Bellomo R, Ronco C (eds) Acute renal failure in the critically ill. Springer, Berlin Heidelberg New York, pp 58-63
2. Leonhardt KO, Landes RR (1963) Oxygen tension of the urine and renal structures. New Engl J Med 269:115-121
3. Brezis M, Rosen S (1995) Hypoxia of the renal medulla: its implications for disease. New Engl J Med 332:647-655
4. Morissey JJ, McCracken R, Kaneto H, Vehaskari M, Montani D, Khlar S (1994) Location of an inducible nitric oxide synthase mRNA in the normal kidney. Kidney Int 45:998-1005
5. Dinour D, Brezis M (1991) Effects of adenosine on intrarenal oxygenation. Am J Physiol 261:F787-F791
6. Levin ER (1995) Mechanisms of disease: endothelins. New Engl J Med 333:356-363
7. Odeh M (1991) Mechanisms of diseases: the role of reperfusion-induced injury in the pathogenesis of the crush syndrome. New Engl J Med 324:1417-1422
8. Bonventre JV (1993) Mechanisms of ischemic acute renal failure. Kidney Int 43:1160-1178
9. Brezis M, Rosen S, Silva P, Spokes K, Epstein FH (1984) Polyene toxicity in renal medulla: injury mediated by transport activity. Science 224:66-8
10. Heyman SN, Stillmn IE, Brezis M, Epstein FH, Spokes K, Rosen S (1993) Chronic amphotericin nephropathy: morphometric, electron microscopic and functional studies. J Am Soc Nephrol 4:69-80
11. Agmon Y, Brezis M (1993) Effects of nonsteroidal anti-inflammatory drugs upon intrarenal blood flow: selective medullary hypoperfusion. Exp Nephrol 1:357-363
12. Brezis M, Rosen S, Epstein FH (1991) Acute renal failure. In: Brenner BM, Rector FC (eds) The kidney, 4th edn. Saunders, Philadelphia, pp 993-1061
13. Brenner M, Schaer GL, Mallory D, Suffredini A, Parrillo JE (1990) Detection of renal blood flow abnormalities in septic and critically ill patients using a newly designed indwelling thermodilution renal vein catheter. Chest 98:170-179
14. Haywood GA, Stewart JT, Counihan PJ et al (1992) Validation of bedside measurements of absolute human renal blood flow by a continuous thermodilution technique. Crit Care Med 20: 659-664
15. Garcia-Perez A, Burg MB (1991) Renal medullary organic osmolytes? Physiol Rev 71: 1081-1115
16. Dawson JL (1965) Postoperative renal function in obstructive jaundice: effect of a mannitol diuresis. Br Med J 1:82-86
17. Eneas JF, Shoenfeld PJ, Humphreys MH (1979) The effect of infusion of mannitol-sodium bicarbonate on the clinical course of myoglobinuria. Arch Intern Med 139:801-805
18. Heyman SN, Brezis M, Epstein FH, Spokes K, Silva P, Rosen S (1991) Early renal medullary hypoxic injury from radiocontrast and indomethacin. Kidney Int 40:632-642

19. Davis RD, Lappas DG, Kirklin JK, Buckley MJ, Lowenstein (1982) Acute oliguria after cardiopulmonary bypass: renal functional improvement with low-dose dopamine infusion. Crit Care Med 10,12:852-856
20. Lee MR (1993) Dopamine and the kidney: ten years on. Clin Sci 84:357-375
21. Swigert TH, Clayton Roberts L, Valek TR et al (1991) Effect of intraoperative low-dose dopamine on renal function in liver transplant recipients. Anesthesiology 75:571-576
22. Desjars P, Pinaud M, Potel G et al (1987) A reappraisal of norepinephrine therapy in human septic shock. Crit Care Med 15:134-137
23. Hesselvik JF, Brodin B (1989) Low dose norepinephrine in patients with septic shock and oliguria: effects on afterload, urine flow, and oxygen transport. Crit Care Med 17:179-180
24. Redl-Wenzl EM, Armbruster C, Edelmann G et al (1993) The effects of norepinephrine on hemodynamics and renal function in severe septic shock. Crit Care Med 19:151-154

Oxygen Supply Dependency - Fact or Artifact?

K. Reinhart

Historical background

Intensive care specialists became interested in this topic following a paper of Danek et al. (1) that appeared 15 years ago. Their observation was that oxygen uptake ($\dot{V}O_2$) varied directly and linearly with any change in DO_2 in ARDS patients. This was not the case in a comparable group of ventilator patients who did not have ARDS. The apparent dependence of $\dot{V}O_2$ upon DO_2 in ARDS patients was seen at relative high levels of DO_2, well above those that were thought to be critical. From experiments on anesthetized animals, $\dot{V}O_2$ was known to remain unchanged over a wide range of DO_2, by altering O_2 extraction appropriately. When the limit of compensatory changes was reached as DO_2 was progressively lowered, $\dot{V}O_2$ would then change linearly with DO_2. The term "physiologic O_2 supply dependency" was first introduced by Cain for this phenomenon in contrast to the feature that was strikingly different in ARDS and sepsis patients which was called "pathologic supply dependency" (2).

There was further evidence for the existance of such a pathologic O_2 supply dependency by clinical studies from the 1980s, in which DO_2 was altered by various means including fluid loading and use of catecholamines (3-7). The general results of these studies were that $\dot{V}O_2$ increased when DO_2 increased. Further evidence in this direction was provided by a prospective study of Bihari et al. (8) who used the vasodilator prostacyclin to increase DO_2 in critically ill patients. Those patients who showed a positive response (increase in $\dot{V}O_2$) all died, whereas the patients who showed independence of $\dot{V}O_2$ from DO_2 survived.

The conclusion that evolved from these observations was that pathologic supply dependency and the tissue hypoxia that it was thought to represent plays an important role in the pathogenesis of multiple systems organ failure, which is the major cause of death in sepsis and ARDS patients (8). It was further shown that high risk surgical patients with higher values for DO_2 and $\dot{V}O_2$ had better outcome than patients with only normal values for cardiac output and the oxygen transport related variables (9). Thus, hyperresuscitation levels of oxygen delivery were thought to prevent tissue hypoxia, organ dysfunction, and hence improve patient outcome (9).

The data to apply this hypothesis to critically ill patients, especially those with sepsis or ARDS, are not convincing and such studies have been criticized for weak design and subgroup analysis (9-11). One recent well-performed study even reported worse outcome for high risk patients who were treated with dobutamine up to 200 mg/kg/min when volume loading failed to achieve a cardiac index > 3.5 l/min/m^2, in comparison to patients that were treated conventionally (12). This and other observations (13) have prompted strong doubts about the clinical validity of the concept of pathologic O_2 supply dependency (14). The challenges for this concept are the following:

1. The apparent dependence of $\dot{V}O_2$ upon DO_2, when it does occur, is actually a normal response that is initiated by a primary increase in O_2 demand and does not result from an O_2 extraction deficit by peripheral tissues. This view is supported by several studies that showed O_2 supply dependency in many non-ARDS and nonsepsis patients, too (15, 16).

2. Pathologic O_2 supply dependency does not exist in reality but can be attributed to an artifactual $\dot{V}O_2/DO_2$ relationship caused by mathematical coupling as described and illustrated by Archie (17). Indeed most of the clinical studies used a thermodilution cardiac output to calculate both DO_2 and $\dot{V}O_2$. Several groups have reexamined pathologic O_2 supply dependency while avoiding a coupling error by using $\dot{V}O_2$ obtained from expired gas analysis and DO_2 as a product of thermodilution cardiac output and arterial O_2 content. These studies were unable to confirm supply dependency in patients with sepsis and ARDS (18). Some of these studies have been also criticized, however, due to methodological problems (19).

These conflicting data give rise to questions that may have impact on our daily practice at the bedside.

1. Do tissue hypoxia and an O_2 extraction deficit really exist in patients with sepsis and ARDS?

2. Is tissue hypoxia really an important cofactor in the pathogenesis of sepsis and multiple systems organ failure?

3. Is it necessary to aim for supranormal levels of DO_2 and $\dot{V}O_2$ in patients with sepsis and ARDS?

There is a broad body of evidence from animal studies that the microcirculation is disturbed and O_2 extraction is impaired in the peripheral tissues by sepsis. The gut was shown to be particularly susceptible to the effects of endotoxin whereas resting skeletal muscle was quite resistant (20, 21).

This goes along with clinical studies which demonstrated that lowered gastric mucosal pH may exist in critically ill patients despite normal or even supranormal O_2 delivery, whereas muscle tissue pO_2 remains normal (22).

Tissue hypoxia therefore, at least in "nonvital" organs like the gut or the kidney, is likely to exist. Gastric mucosal pH has been shown to be correlated with patient outcome (23), and there is at least one study that indicates that when therapy is guided by pHi in an attempt to keep it normal, patient outcome is better than in control patients in whom the responsible physician was not aware of the actual pHi (24).

As to the question of whether it is necessary to aim for supranormal levels for DO_2:

1. There is good evidence both from animal experiments and human studies that sepsis in adequately volume-resuscitated animals or patients elicits a hyperdynamic circulatory response. This response may be interpreted as an attempt by the body to compensate an O_2 extraction deficit and to meet the increased metabolic demands.

2. There is also good evidence that septic animals without adequate volume therapy rapidly die in hypodynamic shock. It has been demonstrated in several studies that patients who are unable to achieve a supranormal cardiac output due to preexisting cardiac disease or other reasons have poorer outcome (25). The proposal to "aim" for supranormal levels for DO_2 and $\dot{V}O_2$ is somewhat misleading in this context because it directs our thinking too much towards active measures to stimulate or even overstimulate the cardiovascular system beyond its physiological reserves. We should keep in mind that many patients achieve the hemodynamic goals proposed by Shoemaker and colleagues with fluid administration alone. In one study this was the case in two thirds of the patients, suggesting that the improved outcome in this study may have been largely related to more aggressive volume replacement (25).

There is one study, however, of high risk surgical patients whose treatment was aimed at achieving a level of oxygen delivery higher than 600 ml/min/m², instituted preoperatively by adequate volume resuscitation and dopexamine (26). The 28-day mortality rate was reduced by 75%, and a second multicenter study is currently trying to confirm this striking result. Regional rather than global effects of dopexamine and the fact that therapy was already instituted preoperatively might account for the differences between that study and the one of Hayes et al. who used dobutamine in the postoperative and ICU setting only (12). In that study the patients who reached a cardiac index > 5.5 l/min/m² by adequate volume loading alone together with the patients who did so by additional inotropic support with dobutamine had a significantly higher survival rate than those patients whose cardiac output remained below this target value despite all therapeutic efforts, including the use of inotropes. This led the authors to the conclusion that the ability to achieve supranormal levels of oxygen delivery and oxygen consumption indicates a larger physiologic reserve, less severe illness, and, consequently, a better prognosis (12). Due to their larger physiologic reserves these patients seem to be better able to compensate for the myocardial depression, peripheral vasodilation and the O_2 extraction defect due to the alterations of the microcirculation.

Increasing DO_2 may not be the complete answer to preventing tissue hypoxia because the main problem with tissue oxygenation in sepsis may be a disturbed nutritive blood flow, especially in the gut (20, 21). Approaches to improve the O_2 extraction capability by drugs such as prostacyclin (27) or N-acetylcysteine have been shown to be effective in both experimental and clinical studies (28).

There is some evidence that regional indicators of tissue oxygenation such as pHi better reflect changes in tissue O_2 supply than global measures like $\dot{V}O_2$ (27, 29). In the future therefore therapy might be more guided by indicators of regional tissue oxygenation than by global measures such as DO_2 and $\dot{V}O_2$.

Coming back to the initial question of whether O_2 supply dependency really exists in patients with ARDS and sepsis – in view of the existing data my answer is yes, however, only under certain circumstances. For the whole body it is very likely in underresuscitated patients in the early phase of septic shock when DO_2 is only say 400 ml/min/m² (3-6). It is ever more likely when serum lactate levels are elevated. Global O_2 supply dependency seems unlikely to exist in adequately volume resuscitated patients under inotropic and vasopressor support. We could find no increase in $\dot{V}O_2$ after augmenting DO_2 from ~ 700 ml/min/m² to ~ 830 ml/min/m² by different approaches, including the administration of prostacyclin (30), dopexamine, and hypertonic saline.

However, despite the lack of a demonstrable O_2 supply dependency by the whole body measurements, tissue hypoxia with O_2 supply dependency may be persistent on the organ level, especially for the gut (21, 29). Both an increase in cardiac output and in the O_2 extraction capabilities have been demonstrated in the clinical setting to be effective in improving regional perfusion as indicated by an increase in pHi (27, 28).

Summary and clinical implications:

1. Global oxygen supply dependency may exist in underresuscitated patients and in patients with limited cardiovascular reserves due to underlying cardiovascular diseases or an overwhelming septic insult.

2. Regional tissue hypoxia may exist despite the achievement of "optimal goals" for cardiac output, O_2 delivery and O_2 consumption.

3. Increases in O_2 delivery and/or improvement of nutritive blood flow may improve regional perfusion, which is not necessarily reflected in increases in whole body O_2 consumption.

4. Testing for global O_2 supply dependency in the clinical setting is not very helpful due to methodological problems, spontaneous fluctuations of O_2 consumption by patient movements, changes in body temperature and the potential effects of metabolically active drugs such as catecholamines.

5. Rather than aiming for the achievement of arbitrary target values, therapy should be based on the individual patient whose optimal values may vary over a wide range. Global hemodynamic measurements should be combined with other measurements of tissue perfusion such as base deficit, blood lactate levels, gastric intramucosal pH or arteriovenous CO_2 difference.

6. Use of excessive doses of adrenergic agents in an attempt to optimize DO_2 and tissue oxygenation may result in the contrary, i.e., deterioration of tissue function and increased mortality.

7. Tissue hypoxia and oxygen debt should be corrected early because it may become refractory in the later stages of critical illness and shock.

References

1. Danek S, Lynch JP, Weg JG, Dantzker DR (1980) The dependence of oxygen uptake on oxygen delivery in the adult respiratory distress syndrome. Am Rev Respir Dis 122:387-395
2. Cain SM (1984) Supply dependency of oxygen uptake in ARDS: myth or reality? Am J Med Sci 288:119-124
3. Kaufmann BS, Rackow EC, Falk JL (1984) The relationship between oxygen delivery and consumption during fluid resuscitation of hypovolemic and septic shock. Chest 85: 336-340
4. Haupt MT, Gilbert EM, Carlson RW (1985) Fluid loading increases oxygen consumption in septic patients with lactic acidosis. Am Rev Respir Dis 131:912-916
5. Gilbert EM, Haupt MT, Mandanas RY, Huaringa AJ, Carlson RW (1986) The effect of fluid loading, blood transfusion, and catecholamine infusion on oxygen delivery and consumption in patients with sepsis. Am Rev Respir Dis 134:873-878
6. Astiz ME, Rackow EC, Falk JL, Kaufmann BS, Weil MH (1987) Oxygen delivery and consumption in patients with hyperdynamic septic shock. Crit Care Med 15:26-28
7. Mohsenifar Z, Amin D, Jasper AC, Shah PK, Koerner SK (1987) Dependence of oxygen consumption on oxygen delivery in patients with chronic congestive heart failure. Chest 92: 447-450
8. Bihari D, Smithies M, Gimson A, Tinker J (1987) The effects of vasodilation with prostacyclin on oxygen delivery and uptake in critically ill patients. N Engl Med 317:397-403
9. Shoemaker WC, Appel PL, Kram HB (1988) Prospective trial of supranormal values as therapeutic goals in high risk surgical patients. Chest 94:1176-86
10. Yu M, Levy MM, Takiguchi SA, Miyasaki A, Myers SA (1993) Effect of maximizing oxygen delivery on morbidity and mortality rates in critically ill patients: a prospective, randomized, controlled study. Crit Care Med 21:830-8
11. Tuchschmidt J, Fried J, Astiz M, Rackow E (1992) Elevation of cardiac output and oxygen delivery improves outcome in septic shock. Chest 102:216-220
12. Hayes MA, Timmins AC, Yau EHS et al (1994) Elevation of systemic delivery in the treatment of critically ill patients. N Engl J Med 330:1717-1722
13. Mira JP, Fabre JE, Baigorri F et al (1994) Lack of oxygen supply dependency in patients with severe sepsis. Chest 106:1524-1531
14. Dantzker DR, Foresman B, Guiterrez G (1991) Oxygen supply and utilization relationships. A reevaluation. Am Rev Respir Dis 143:675-679
15. Albert RK, Schrijen F, Poincelot F (1986) Oxygen consumption and transport in stable patients with chronic obstructive pulmonary disease. Am Rev Respir Dis 134:678-682
16. Boyd O, Grounds M, Bennett D (1992) The dependency of oxygen consumption on oxygen delivery in critically ill postoperative patients is mimicked by variations in sedation. Chest 101:1619-1624
17. Archie JP (1981) Mathematic coupling of data – a common source of error. Ann Surg 193: 296-303
18. Ronco JJ, Phang PT, Walley KR, Wiggs B et al (1991) Oxygen consumption is independent of changes in oxygen delivery in severe adult respiratory distress syndrome. Am Rev Respir Dis 143:1267-1273

19. Cain SM (1994) A current view of oxygen supply dependency. In: Reinhart K, Eyrich K, Srung C (ed) Sepsis-current perspectives in pathophysiology and therapy. Springer, Berlin Heidelberg New York, pp 150-162 (Update in intensive care and emergency medicine)
20. Nelson DP, Samsel RW, Wood LDH, Schumacker PT (1988) Pathological supply dependence of systemic and intestinal O2 uptake during endotoxemia. J Appl Physiol 64:2410-2419
21. Vallet B, Lund N, Curtis SE, Kelly DR, Cain SM (1993) Gut and muscle tissue PO_2 in endotoxemic dogs during shock and resuscitation. Am Rev Respir Dis 147:A618
22. Reinhart K, Hannemann L, Meier-Hellmann A, Specht M (1994) Monitoring of O_2 transport and tissue oxygenation in septic shock. In: Reinhart K, Eyrich K, Sprung C (ed) Sepsis-current perspectives in pathophysiology and therapy. Springer, Berlin Heidelberg New York, pp 193-213 (Update in intensive care and emergency medicine)
23. Fiddian-Green RG, Baker S (1987) Predictive value of the stomach wall pH and PO_2 for complications after cardiac operations: comparison with other monitoring. Crit Care Med 15:153-156
24. Guiterrez G, Palizas F, Doglio G et al (1992) Gastric intramucosal pH as a therapeutic index of tissue oxygenation in critically ill patients. Lancet 339:195-199
25. Shoemaker WC, Kram HB, Appel PL, Fleming AW (1990) The efficacy of central venous and pulmonary artery catheters and therapy based upon them in reducing mortality and morbidity. Arch Surg 125:1332-8
26. Boyd O, Grounds RM, Bennett ED (1993) A randomized clinical trial of the effect of deliberate perioperative increase of oxygen delivery on mortality in high-risk surgical patients. JAMA 270:2699-707
27. Rademacher P, Buhl R, Santak B (1993) Prostacyclin improves gastric intramucosal pH in patients with septic shock. Clin Intensive Care 4 [Suppl 12]:7
28. Spies CD, Reinhart K, Witt I et al (1994) Influence of N-acetylcysteine on indirect indicators of tissue oxygenation in septic shock patients: results from a prospective, randomized, double-blind study. Crit Care Med 11:1738-1746
29. Hannemann L, Meier-Hellmann A, Specht M, Spies C, Reinhart K (1993) O_2-Angebot, O_2-Verbrauch und Mukosa pH-Wert des Magens. Indikatoren der Gewebeoxygenierung. Anaesthesist 42:11-14
30. Hannemann L, Reinhart K, Meier-Hellmann A, Bredle DL (1994) Prostacyclin in septic shock. Chest 105:1504-1510

Debate on $DO_2/\dot{V}O_2$ Dependency During Inotropic Treatment

G. GUTIERREZ

The relationship of oxygen transport to oxygen consumption

Few topics in critical care medicine are as controversial as the clinical significance of the systemic DO_2-$\dot{V}O_2$ relationship (1, 2). Even the definition of these variables has been a subject of debate, as some investigators maintain that the term O_2 delivery should be reserved to denote the rate of oxygen reaching the cell mitochondria, whereas the term O_2 transport is more indicative of the rate of oxygen carried by arterial blood to tissue capillaries (3). The phrase "oxygen offering" has been proposed to define the product of the cardiac output and the arterial O_2 content, since it emphasizes the intrinsic degree of control that tissues have over their rate of O_2 utilization (4). Similarly, the term O_2 uptake has been used in lieu of O_2 consumption, since an unspecified amount of oxygen extracted from capillary blood is used for nonoxidative cellular functions, including the synthesis of nitric oxide and the generation of O_2 free radical species. For the purposes of this paper, the term O_2 delivery (DO_2) refers to the rate of O_2 carried by arterial blood to the tissue capillaries and the term O_2 consumption ($\dot{V}O_2$) denotes the rate of oxygen uptake from arterial blood by the tissues.

Experimental studies

In animal experiments (5-7), the DO_2-$\dot{V}O_2$ relationship is best described as a nonlinear function encompassing two regions: a supply independent region, characterized by aerobic metabolism, and a supply dependent region, in which anaerobic metabolism predominates (Fig. 1). Under physiologic conditions, the supply of O_2 to the tissues is in excess of cellular O_2 demand as the tissues extract only $_20\%$-$_25\%$ of DO_2 (point A). Here $\dot{V}O_2$ is determined primarily by the cellular requirements for ATP and a rough equivalence exists between $\dot{V}O_2$ and cellular energy requirements. If $\dot{V}O_2$ remains constant with decreases in DO_2 the fraction of O_2 extracted from capillary blood increases (point B). With progressive reductions in DO_2, a "critical" DO_2 is reached (point C) where DO_2 barely suffices to sustain aerobic metabolism. The value of the critical DO_2 is remarkably, regardless of the method used to decrease DO_2, i.e. anemia, hypoxemia, or hypovolemia (8), approximately 10 ml/kg/min. Additional decreases in DO_2 below the critical point result in proportional decreases in $\dot{V}O_2$. Since cellular energy requirements remain constant, or may even increase as the result of circulating catecholamines, anaerobic sources of ATP production are recruited below the critical point to complement mitochondrial ATP production. This results in lactate production, intracellular acidosis, the accumulation of inorganic phosphate, and eventually in cellular death (point D).

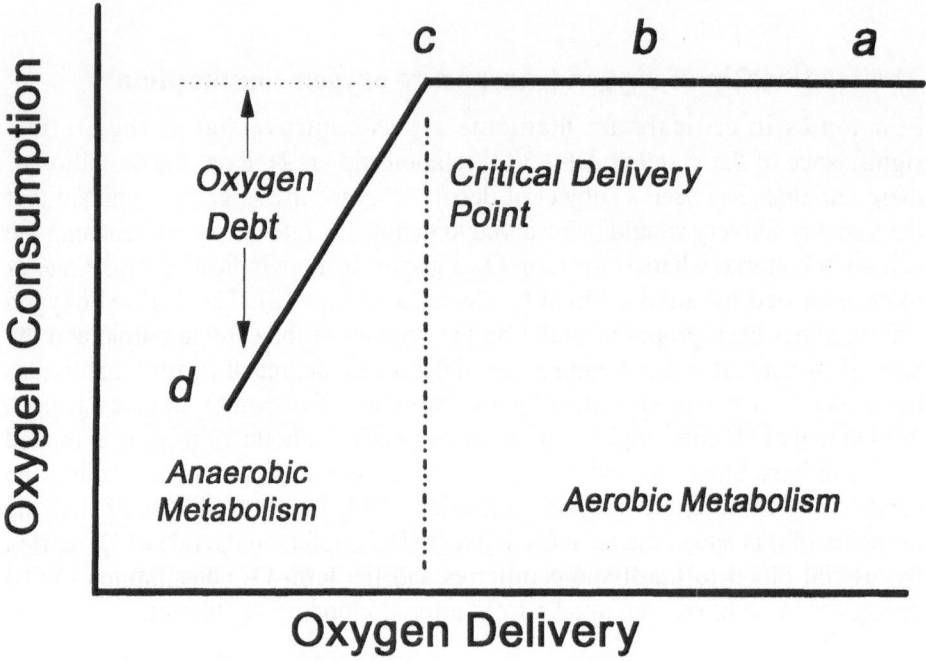

Fig. 1. Schematic representation of the relationship between O_2 delivery and O_2 consumption, as derived from animal experiments

The DO_2-$\dot{V}O_2$ relationship - clinical studies

Among the earliest clinical studies on the DO_2-$\dot{V}O_2$ relationship are those of Lutch and Murray (9) and of McMahon et al. (10). These investigators found no changes in systemic $\dot{V}O_2$ when small decreases in DO_2 were produced by the application of PEEP in mechanically ventilated patients. Conversely, Powers et al. (11) noted linear decreases in $\dot{V}O_2$ in 33 patients with ARDS when declines in cardiac output were produced by PEEP. This finding was supported by the study of Rhodes at al. (12) who measured the effect of increasing DO_2 by i.v. infusions of mannitol and also noted linear increases in $\dot{V}O_2$. The proportional relationship of $\dot{V}O_2$ to decreases in DO_2 was firmly established in the clinical literature by the now classic work of Danek et al. (13) who subjected 11 patients with ARDS to decreases in cardiac output produced by PEEP. O_2 supply dependency also has been demonstrated in patients with septic shock, hypovolemia, and with respiratory failure from causes other than ARDS (14).

Gutierrez and Pohil (15) measured DO_2 and $\dot{V}O_2$ at 6 hour intervals in a group of 30 critically ill patients. They noted that patients could be segregated according to their ability to increase O_2 extraction in response to decreases in DO_2, although both groups had linear DO_2-$\dot{V}O_2$ functions. The group unable to increase ERO_2 was composed mostly of patients with sepsis, ARDS, and acute gastro-intestinal bleeding (80%). This group showed marked $\dot{V}O_2$ dependency on DO_2 and had a mortality rate of 70%. The group able to increase ERO_2, and in which $\dot{V}O_2$ was independent of DO_2, had a significantly lower mortality rate (30%). The latter group also had fewer patients with sepsis or ARDS (30%) and required significantly lesser use of vasopressor agents. These data suggest that diseases that affect the microcirculation, such as sepsis, are characterized by a loss of O_2 extraction capacity resulting in O_2 supply dependency.

Cain (16) proposed the term pathologic O_2 supply dependency to explain the finding of a linear DO_2-$\dot{V}O_2$ function in patients with sepsis or ARDS, as opposed to the non-linear DO_2-$\dot{V}O_2$ curve observed in animal studies (Fig. 2). According to this concept, critically ill patients have greater energy needs for resulting in a higher $\dot{V}O_2$ plateau. Their microvascular control also may be affected, impairing their ability to increase ERO_2. The combination of a higher $\dot{V}O_2$ plateau and impaired O_2 extracting mechanisms result in a greater critical DO_2. A reasonable corollary to this hypothesis is that patients with pathologic O_2 supply dependency will reach supply independency when subjected to pharmacologic increases in DO_2 (17).

In my opinion, much of the debate revolving around the concept of O_2 supply dependency and the use of inotropes to increase DO_2 is the consequence of applying the wrong physiological model to the clinical data. Therefore, it is worthwhile to review the experimental conditions used in these studies. Experimental studies employ anesthetized, paralyzed, healthy animals subjected to decreases in DO_2 in a relatively short length of time, usually 3-6 h. Most of these animal preparations have intact microvascular control mechanisms and their energy requirements remain constant during the experiment. In contrast, clinical studies include patients with varying degrees of microvascular dysfunction, having fluctuating energy requirements, and take place over a longer time period, sometimes spanning several days. It is not surprising, therefore, that controversy exists regarding the different responses to reductions in TO_2 in humans and in animals (18).

The linear DO_2-$\dot{V}O_2$ relationship noted in critically ill patients most likely represents the normal physiologic response of the peripheral gas exchange system, instead of an abnormal manifestation of impaired oxygen extraction. In experimental preparations $\dot{V}O_2$ is clearly the dependent variable as a healthy animal is subjected to reductions in DO_2. This is not the case in the clinical setting, where variations in DO_2 occur spontaneously in response to changes in the patient's metabolic rate. A linear DO_2-$\dot{V}O_2$ relationship is the manifestation of time related changes in O_2 demand. That is, increases $\dot{V}O_2$ in response to agitation, fever, work of breathing, etc., results in appropriate increases in DO_2. This physiologic response of DO_2 to increases in $\dot{V}O_2$ is akin to that of exercise. A proportional DO_2-$\dot{V}O_2$ relationship resulting from this adaptive response does not represent tissue hypoxia or "O_2 supply dependency". On the contrary, it represents the dependency of O_2 supply on O_2 demand, a normal physiological state.

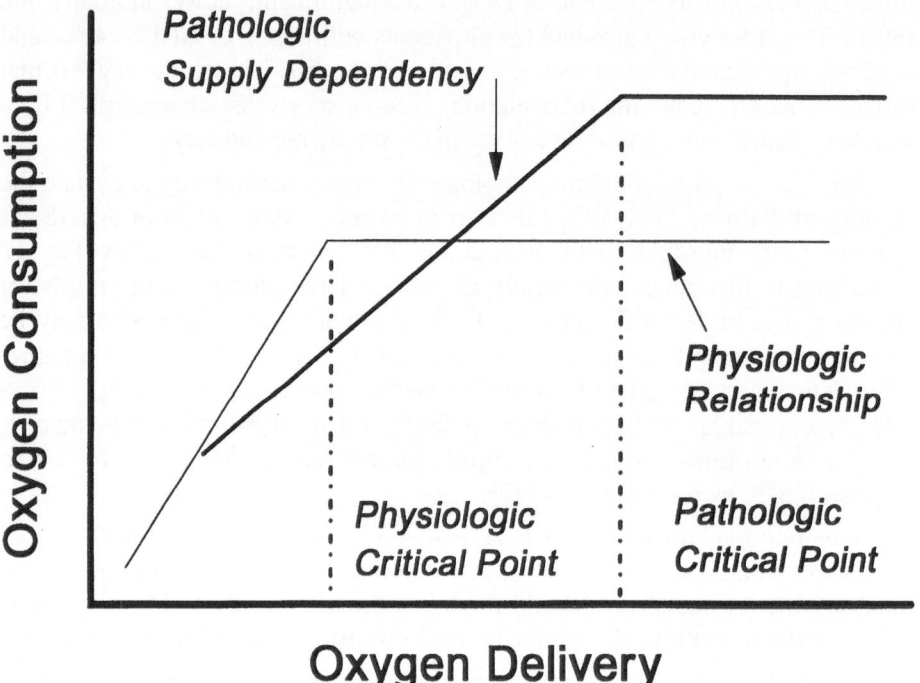

Fig. 2. The concept of "pathologic supply dependency" is characterized by a higher aerobic $\dot{V}O_2$ plateau and a shift of the DO_2-$\dot{V}O_2$ relationship to the right. This results in a greater than normal critical DO_2

Is O_2 supply dependency a pathologic condition?

Many studies dispute the existence of "pathologic supply dependency". These studies have as a common denominator the measurement of $\dot{V}O_2$ by analysis of the expired gases. A recent study (19) measured changes in $\dot{V}O_2$ in a small group of critically ill patients in whom life support was withdrawn according to the request of the patient's immediate family. The results from this study support the concept that the biphasic DO_2-$\dot{V}O_2$ relationship found in animals also may be an accurate representation of human physiology. These investigators found that septic and nonseptic patients alike exhibited a supply independent plateau at normal or high levels of DO_2. DO_2 decreased over an average of 4 h with a DO_{2crit} of 4 mL.kg^{-1} for both groups, a value considerably lower than previously reported in humans from pooled group data (20). Of note, increases in blood lactate in these patients were not associated with greater DO_{2crit} or impaired tissue O_2 extraction.

Several studies support the notion that O_2 supply dependency is a measuring artifact, the result of mathematical coupling of data yielding a linear DO_2-$\dot{V}O_2$ function. Since both DO_2 and $\dot{V}O_2$ are calculated from common variables, C_aO_2 and cardiac output, random errors in the measurement of these variables could result in a factitious spread of values for DO_2 and $\dot{V}O_2$ along a straight line. This problem was analyzed by Moreno et al. (21), who concluded that mathematical coupling, although present when determinations of DO_2 and $\dot{V}O_2$ share a common variable, probably plays a minor role in the genesis of the linear DO_2-$\dot{V}O_2$ function, as long as changes in DO_2 are sufficiently large. This may not be the case for data from individual patients are analyzed. Both Archie (22) and Stratton et al. (23) proposed measuring $\dot{V}O_2$ independently of DO_2 using the expired gases method to avoid the possibility of mathematical coupling.

Hanique et al. (24) made simultaneous measures of $\dot{V}O_2$ using the expired gases method and Fick's Principle in 32 patients subjected to increases in DO_2 by colloid infusion. Oxygen supply dependency was present when $\dot{V}O_2$ was calculated by Fick's principle, whereas directly measured $\dot{V}O_2$ did not change with changes in DO_2. In a companion article (25), these authors used statistical methods to analyze the mathematical relationship of $\dot{V}O_2$ to DO_2 and found that Fick's principle and the direct measurement of $\dot{V}O_2$ using calorimetry yield different results. They concluded that direct measurements of $\dot{V}O_2$ are more reliable and should be used in preference to calculating $\dot{V}O_2$ by Fick's principle. Other studies in which $\dot{V}O_2$ consumption was measured from the expired gases by indirect calorimetry also have failed to show sepsis associated "pathological O_2 supply dependency" (26, 27).

Effects of pharmacologic increases of DO_2 on $\dot{V}O_2$

Several investigators have attempted to combine information derived from the DO_2-$\dot{V}O_2$ relationship and elevations in blood lactate to test for the existence of covert tissue hypoxia in critically ill patients. Haupt et al. (28) noted that the infusion of colloidal fluids increased $\dot{V}O_2$ in septic patients with concurrent lactic acidosis. In a subsequent study (29), these investigators found that the infusion of fluids or blood increased $\dot{V}O_2$ in patients with sepsis who also had blood lactate > 2.2 mM. In contrast, dobutamine raised $\dot{V}O_2$ in septic patients with or without lactic acidosis. They concluded that fluid or blood infusion could be used to predict the presence of anaerobic metabolism in sepsis, whereas dobutamine was not as useful, since this catecholamine appeared to exert a direct positive effect on metabolic rate. Similar findings have been noted in studies using fluids (30) and red blood cell transfusions (31) to increase DO_2.

The results from a study by Bihari et al. (32) also support the notion that many critically ill patients suffer from inadequate tissue oxygenation. They increased DO_2 in critically ill patients by infusing prostacyclin, a potent vasodilator. $\dot{V}O_2$ increased with prostagladin in a group of patients that uniformly died. In another group who survived their stay in the ICU, prostaglandin administration increased DO_2 but $\dot{V}O_2$ remained constant. Bihari and coworkers concluded that patients who had increases in $\dot{V}O_2$ had a substantial oxygen deficit. The results of this study have been criticized by the finding that these patients were relatively hypovolemic. A subsequent study by De Backer et al. (33) failed to show a difference in the response to prostacyclin in survivors and non-survivors in 17 patients with sepsis. Further, when $\dot{V}O_2$ was measured from the expired gases in 15 patients with post-operative septic shock (34), the infusion of prostacyclin did not produce an increase in $\dot{V}O_2$, although DO_2 increased 14%.

Vincent et al. (35) proposed a short term trial of dobutamine to disclose an oxygen uptake/supply dependency condition in sepsis. They found increased $\dot{V}O_2$ in response to a dobutamine infusion of 5 µg/kg/min in a septic group of patients with lactic acidosis. There were no increases in $\dot{V}O_2$ in another group of septic patients with normal lactate. Based on these results, these investigators concluded that, at the dose used, dobutamine does not increase $\dot{V}O_2$ in critically ill patients, unless there is coexisting tissue hypoxia evidenced by lactic acidosis.

The prognostic value of the dobutamine test was tested by Vallet et al. (36) in 50 patients with sepsis syndrome. They excluded patients in shock and those with lactate concentrations > 2.0 mM. They found 23 responders in whom DO_2 and $\dot{V}O_2$ increased 39% and 41%, respectively. The mortality rate was significantly greater in the non-responders (44% vs. 9%). Vallet et al. concluded that increases in $\dot{V}O_2$ in the responders were related to the calorigenic effect of dobutamine, given that these were patients without shock or hyperlactatemia.

Increases in systemic oxygen transport as a therapeutic option: an ongoing debate

The effect of increasing O_2 transport to supernormal levels with fluid, catecholamines, and blood transfusions on patient outcome is not known, but recent data suggests that indiscriminate increases in DO_2 do not improve survival, in fact, a recent study suggests that this approach may be associated with increased mortality.

The concept that increasing DO_2 to supranormal values in critically ill patients improves survival originated with the work of Shoemaker et al. (37), who found significantly greater postoperative survival rates in nonseptic patients in whom pulmonary artery catheters (PA) were used to maximize cardiac output, $\dot{V}O_2$, and DO_2. This prospective, randomized study compared three groups: one treated according to the information derived from central venous lines (CVP-control), another using pulmonary artery catheters to achieve normal values of oxygenation parameters as therapeutic goals (PA-control), and a protocol group, where patients with PA catheters were treated with fluids and catecholamines (mainly dobutamine) in efforts to reach supranormal levels of $\dot{V}O_2$ and DO_2 as therapeutic end points (PA-protocol). Hospital mortality rates were 38%, 23%, and 4% for the CVP-control, PA-control, and PA-protocol groups, respectively, suggesting that prevention of an oxygen debt improved mortality in this group of patients. The results of this study were confirmed by Boyd et al. (38) in a prospective, randomized trial testing the effect of deliberate increases in DO_2 during the perioperative period on morbidity and mortality. A control group of patients classified as "high-risk" ($n = 38$) received standard perioperative care and were compared to a protocol group ($n = 43$) in whom DO_2 was maintained ≥ 600 ml/min/m^2 during surgery and post-operatively until arterial lactate concentration was < 1.5 mM. Dopexamine hydrochloride was used to augment cardiac output in the protocol group. The protocol group achieved higher DO_2 than the control group, but significantly, there were no differences in $\dot{V}O_2$. The 28 day mortality in the protocol group was significantly lower than that for the control group (7.0% vs. 23.7%; $p = 0.04$).

The studies of Shoemaker et al. and Boyd et al. suggest that maintenance of adequate O_2 transport during the perioperative period improves survival. However, their results should be interpreted in the context of patients who presumably have intact microvascular control and whose tissues are adequately oxygenated prior to sustaining the insult of surgery. Preventing tissue hypoxia under those conditions appears to be a beneficial therapeutic intervention.

Conversely, the application of the "supranormal" DO_2 concept to a heterogeneous population of critically ill patients, many of whom have already sustained irreversible cellular damage, has met with little success. The few studies in the literature in which a consistent effort has been applied to maintain greater than normal values of DO_2 in critically ill patients show disappointing results. In a randomized, double blind trial for treatment of ARDS (39, 40), a study group ($n = 50$) was randomized to receive prostaglandin E_1 (PGE_1) for seven days. This group was compared to an equal number of patients given placebo. An unexpected finding of the trial was a significantly greater DO_2 and $\dot{V}O_2$ for the study group, probably related to the vasodilator effect of PGE_1. Survival, however, was similar for both groups (60% for the PGE_1 vs. 48% for placebo). Tuchschmidt et al. (41) studied a group of patients with septic shock ($n = 26$) in whom cardiac index was increased to 6.0 l/min/m^2 for 72 h using dobutamine. This group was compared to a normal treatment control with cardiac indices averaging 3.6 $l/min/m^2$. They found no difference in mortality between the groups ($p < 0.14$), although their sample may not have had sufficient power to detect a significant difference.

A recent study by Hayes et al. (42) showed increased mortality when dobutamine was used to raise DO_2 in a group of critically ill patients. This was a randomized, prospective study in which a treatment group ($n = 50$) was given dobutamine until the following goals were achieved simultaneously: cardiac index > 4.5 $l/min/m^2$, DO_2 values > 600 $ml/kg/m^2$, and $\dot{V}O_2$ > 170 $ml/kg/m^2$. A control group ($n = 50$) was given dobutamine only if the cardiac index was below 2.8 $l/min/m^2$. Patients in whom the treatment goals were achieved with fluid replacement alone were not included in the study. Treatment was continued until death or apparent resolution of the acute illness. ICU mortality rates were 50% for the treatment group and 30% for the control group ($p = 0.04$). It is not clear why the treatment group had greater mortality, although the very high doses of dobutamine used (up to 200 $\mu g/kg/min$) may have been responsible for the worse outcome. As acknowledged by the investigators, perhaps the larger doses of dobutamine exacerbated the maldistribution of blood flow in the microcirculation, resulting in impaired perfusion of vital organs, such as the gastrointestinal tract.

The possibility that increases in DO_2 guided by changes in regional oxygenation may improve survival in critically ill patients was tested in a multicenter, prospective, randomized study (43) in which gastric pHi was measured at 6-h intervals in 260 patients admitted to the ICU with APACHE II scores between 15 and 25. Decreases in pHi below 7.35 were treated with therapy aimed at increasing DO_2, including fluids, blood transfusions, and the infusion of dobutamine. Patients admitted with pH_i < 7.35 did not benefit from this resuscitation protocol. On the other hand, patients admitted with $pH_i \geq 7.35$, in whom pH_i guided resuscitation was actively pursued whenever pH_i decreased below 7.35, had a 58% survival rate, compared to 42% for the control group. A possible interpretation of these data is that increases in systemic DO_2 may not be efficacious in a subpopulation of patients who have sustained irreversible cellular damage prior to their admission to the ICU. On the other hand, there are patients admitted to the ICU who have adequate regional oxygenation, in whom aggressive treatment aimed at preventing episodes of regional hypoxia may result in improved outcome.

Optimization of tissue oxygenation in the critically ill patient

The successful treatment of patients suffering from derangement in tissue gas should be guided by broad guidelines revolving around the principle of adequate regional tissue oxygenation (44-46). It is important to insure adequate ventilation of the lungs by establishing a patent airway. Given the hemodynamic instability of these patients, as well as the frequency with which respiratory failure associated with critical illness, many of these patients will require mechanical ventilation. The smooth coupling of the patient's respiratory efforts to ventilator driven breaths cannot be overemphasized, since this will minimize the amount blood diverted from hypoperfused organs to the respiratory muscles (47).

Hemodynamic and oxygenation parameters should be monitored regularly, at least every 6 h in acutely ill patients. From the point of view of insuring appropriate systemic O_2 transport, I support the use of pulmonary catheters to assess cardiac function, pulse oximetry to measure arterial blood oxygenation, and gastric tonometry to assess the adequacy of tissue oxygenation in a sentinel organ. The placement of an arterial line should be considered, since it allows continuous monitoring of systemic blood pressure and also serves to sample arterial blood for blood gases. Serial measurements of DO_2, $\dot{V}O_2$, ERO_2, and gastric mucosal pH provide valuable information regarding the oxygenation-metabolic state of the patient. Alterations in regional tissue oxygenation and metabolism usually do not result in hemodynamic alterations or in end organ function for several hours. This provides the clinician with an early warning period that should be used judiciously if organ failure is to be avoided. Important questions that must be answered during that time are: what are the causes of inadequate oxygenation? Are the data correct? Is it a local or a global phenomenon? Is the cardiac output adequate? Is the patient bleeding? Is there a continuing source of cytokine release, such as an abscess, resulting in impaired microvascular control?

Conclusions

There is little argument that assuring adequate tissue oxygenation to all organs is a successful strategy for survival. However, the key concept is to prevent hypoxic tissue damage by assuring the appropriate level of tissue oxygenation at all times during the patient's illness. It is an unlikely proposition that increasing oxygen delivery to a dying cell will improve its metabolic function.

I think that enough time and effort has been expended in proving the existence of "pathologic O_2 supply dependency". In my opinion, the controversy regarding the clinical significance of the DO_2-$\dot{V}O_2$ relationship is largely academic. This argument is the result of mistakenly applying a physiological concept, one that is valid within a narrow range of experimental conditions, to interpret a highly complex clinical situation characterized by changing bioenergetic parameters, circulating cytokines and inflammatory agents, and deranged vascular control mechanisms. It appears to me that knowledge of the DO_2-$\dot{V}O_2$ relationship in a critically ill patient has little practical value, since we are unable to distinguish dependent from independent variable. In other words, how should we interpret decreases in $\dot{V}O_2$? As inadequate tissue O_2 supply? Or as the resolution of a hypermetabolic inflammatory state?

Unless new studies prove otherwise, increases in DO_2 to supranormal levels should not be attempted in every patient. Instead, the judicious interpretation of changes in cardiac output, arterial blood pressure, lactate levels, and gastric mucosal pH, should be used to guide therapy directed at improving tissue oxygenation in these patients. Provided that control of the microvasculature is not impaired, many patients will have perfectly adequate tissue perfusion at relatively low levels of DO_2 (48). Instead of indiscriminately raising DO_2 to a preassigned value, the therapeutic goal should be to achieve a systemic DO_2 high enough to satisfy the O_2 requirements of all organs, no more, no less. In my opinion, only in response to rapid increases in arterial lactate concentration, decreases in gastric pH_i, or changes in organ function, such as rapidly deteriorating renal or hepatic function, should one attempt to increase DO_2 in critically ill patients.

References

1. Russell JA, Phang PT (1994) The oxygen delivery/consumption controversy. Approaches to management of the critically ill. Am J Respir Crit Care Med 1994;149:533-537
2. Gutierrez G (1991) Summary of the round table conference on tissue utilization. Int Care Med 17:67-68
3. Smithies M, Bihari DJ (1993) Delivery dependent oxygen consumption: Asking the wrong questions and not getting any answers. Crit Care Med 21:1622-1625
4. Honig C personal communication
5. Pappenheimer JR (1941) Blood flow, arterial oxygen saturation, and oxygen consumption in the isolated perfused hindlimb of the dog. J Physiol (Lond) 99:283-303
6. Cain SM (1978) O_2 extraction by hindlimb versus whole dog during anemic hypoxia. J Appl Physiol 45:966-970
7. Cain SM (1978) Effects of time and vasoconstrictor tone on O_2 extraction during hypoxic hypoxia. J Appl Physiol 45:219-224
8. Schwartz S, Frantz RA, Shoemaker WC (1981) Sequential hemodynamic and oxygen transport responses in hypovolemia, anemia, and hypoxia. Am J Physiol 241:H864-H871
9. Lutch JC, Murray JF (1972) Continuous positive-pressure ventilation: effects of systemic oxygen transport and tissue oxygenation. Ann Intern Med 76:193-202
10. McMahon SM, Halprin GM, Sieker HO (1973) Positive end-expiratory airway pressure in severe arterial hypoxemia. Am Rev Respir Dis 108:526-535
11. Powers SR, Mannal R, Neclerio M et al (1973) Physiological consequences of positive-end expiratory pressure (PEEP) ventilation. Ann Surg 178:265-272
12. Rhodes GR, Newell JC, Shah D et al (1978) Increased oxygen consumption accompanying increased oxygen delivery with hypertonic mannitol in adult respiratory distress syndrome. Surgery 84:490-497
13. Danek SJ, Lynch JP, Weg JG et al (1980) The dependence of oxygen uptake on oxygen delivery in the adult respiratory distress syndrome. Am Rev Respir Dis 122:387-395
14. Dorinsky PM, Costello JL, Gadek JE (1988) Relationship of oxygen uptake and oxygen delivery in respiratory failure not due to the adult respiratory distress syndrome. Chest 93: 1013-1019
15. Gutierrez G, Pohil R (1986) Oxygen consumption is linearly related to O_2 supply in critically ill patients. J Crit Care 1:45-53
16. Cain SM (1984) Supply dependency of oxygen uptake in ARDS: myth or reality? Am J Med Sci 288:119-124.70

17. Edwards JD, Clarke C (1991) Therapeutic implications of oxygen transport in critically ill patients. In: Gutierrez G, Vincent JL (eds) Tissue oxygen utilization. Springer, Berlin Heidelberg New York, pp 286-299 (Update in intensive care and emergency medicine, vol 12).

18. Schlichtig R, Pinsky MR (1991) Defining the hypoxic threshold. Crit Care Med 19:147-149

19. Ronco JJ, Fenwick JC, Tweeddale MG et al (1993) Identification of the critical oxygen delivery for anaerobic metabolism in critically ill septic and nonseptic humans. JAMA 270: 1724-1730

20. Shibutani K, Komatsu T, Kubal K et al (1983) Critical level of oxygen delivery in man. Crit Care Med 11:640-643

21. Moreno LF, Stratton HH, Newell JC et al (1986) Mathematical coupling of data: correction of a common error for linear calculations. J Appl Physiol 60:335

22. Archie JP Jr (1981) Mathematical coupling of data: a common source of error. Ann Surg 193: 296-303

23. Stratton HH, Feustel PJ, Newells JC (1987) Regression of calculated variables in the presence of shared measurement error. J Appl Physiol 62:2083-2093

24. Hanique G, Dugernier T, Laterre PF et al (1994) Significance of pathologic oxygen supply dependency in critically ill patients: comparison between measured and calculated methods. Int Care Med 20:12-18

25. Hanique G, Dugernier T, Laterre PF et al (1994) Evaluation of oxygen uptake and delivery in critically ill patients: a statistical reappraisal. Int Care Med 20:19-26

26. Ronco JJ, Fenwick JC, Wiggs BR et al (1993) Oxygen consumption is independent of increases in oxygen delivery by dobutamine in septic patients who have normal or increased plasma lactate. Am Rev Respir Dis 147:25

27. Manthous CA, Schumacker PT, Pohlman A et al (1993) Absence of supply dependence of oxygen consumption in patients with septic shock. J Crit Care 8:203-211

28. Haupt M, Gilbert E, Carlson R (1985) Fluid loading increases oxygen consumption in septic patients with lactic acidosis. Am Rev Respir Dis 131:912-916

29. Gilbert E, Haupt M, Mandanas R et al (1986) The effect of fluid loading, blood transfusion, and catecholamine infusion on oxygen delivery and consumption in patients with sepsis. Am Rev Respir Dis 134:873-878

30. Wolf YG, Cotev S, Perel A et al (1987) Dependence of oxygen consumption on cardiac output in sepsis. Crit Care Med 15:198-203

31. Lucking SE, Williams TM, Chaten FC et al (1990) Dependence of oxygen consumption on oxygen delivery in children with hyperdynamic septic shock and low oxygen extraction. Crit Care Med 18:1316-1319

32. Bihari D, Smithies M, Gimson A, Tinker J (1987) The effects of vasodilation with prostacyclin on oxygen delivery and uptake in critically ill patients. New Engl J Med 317:397-403

33. De Backer D, Berre J, Zhang H et al (1993) Relationship between oxygen uptake and oxygen delivery in septic patients: Effects of prostacyclin versus dobutamine. Crit Care Med 21: 1658-1664

34. Hannemann L, Reinhart K, Meier-Hellmann A et al (1994) Prostacyclin in septic shock. Chest 105:1504-1510

35. Vincent JL, Roman A, De Backer D et al (1990) Oxygen uptake/supply dependency. Effect of short-term dobutamine infusion. Am Rev Respir Dis 142:2-7

36. Vallet B, Chopin C, Curtis SE et al (1993) Prognostic value of the dobutamine test in patients with sepsis syndrome and normal lactate values: a prospective, multicenter study. Crit Care Med 21:1868-1820

37. Shoemaker W, Appel P, Kram H et al (1988) Prospective trial of supranormal values of survivors as therapeutic goals in high risk surgical patients. Chest 94:1176-1186

38. Boyd O, Grounds RM, Bennett ED (1993) A randomized clinical trial of the effect of deliberate perioperative increase of oxygen delivery on mortality in high-risk surgical patients. JAMA 270:2699-2707

39. Bone RC, Slotman G, Maunder RJ et al (1989) Randomized double-blind, multicenter study of prostaglandin E_1 in patients with the adult respiratory distress syndrome. Chest 96:114-119
40. Silverman HJ, Slotman G, Bone RC et al (1990) Effects of prostaglandin E_1 on oxygen delivery and consumption in patients with the adult respiratory distress syndrome. Chest 98: 405-410
41. Tuchschmidt J, Fried J, Swinnery R et al (1989) Early hemodynamic correlates of survival in patients with septic shock. Crit Care Med 17:719-723
42. Hayes MA, Timmins AC, Yau EHS et al (1994) Elevation of systemic oxygen delivery in the treatment of critically ill patients. New Engl J Med 330:1717-1722
43. Gutierrez G, Palizas F, Doglio G et al (1992) Gastric intramucosal pH as a therapeutic index of tissue oxygenation in critically ill patients. Lancet 339:195-199
44. American College of Chest Physicians/Society of Critical Care Medicine Consensus Conference (1992) Definitions for sepsis and organ failure and guidelines for the use of innovative therapies in sepsis. Crit Care Med 20:864-874
45. Society of Critical Care Medicine Guidelines Committee (1992) Guidelines for the care of patients with hemodynamic instability associated with sepsis. Crit Care Med 20:1057
46. Fiddian-Green RG, Haglund U, Gutierrez G et al (1993) Goals for the resuscitation of shock. Crit Care Med 21:S25
47. Mohsenifar Z, Hay A, Hay J et al (1993) Gastric intramural pH as a predictor of success or failure in weaning patients from mechanical ventilation. Ann Intern Med 119:794-798
48. Silverman HJ, Tuma P (1992) Gastric tonometry in patients with sepsis. Effects of dobutamine infusions and packed red blood cell transfusions. Chest 102:184-188

CELLULAR AND HUMORAL ACTIVITY IN TRAUMA AND SEPSIS

The Endothelium: A New Secretory Organ Target or Promoter of Pathophysiological Derangements in ICU Patients

R.J. GRYGLEWSKI

Introduction

The vascular endothelium constitutes an interface between the blood and the rest of the tissues. It occupies a good strategic position for fulfilling its metabolic and endocrine functions. The former include removal and inactivation of biogenic amines, nucleotides, eicosanoids, lipoproteins, kinins or conversion of angiotensin I to angiotensin II, whereas the secretory activities comprise generation of prostacyclin (PGI_2), nitric oxide (NO), endothelins (ET 1-3), plasminogen activators (t-PA), plasminogen activator inhibitor (PAI-1), thrombomodulin (TRM), platelet-derived growth factor ß (PDGF-ß), von-Willebrandt factor (v-WF), vascular cell adhesion molecule-1 (VCAM-1) and many others.

Endothelial biosynthesis of the above factors depends on the local availability and activity of corresponding enzymes. The best known of them are the key enzymes for the biosynthesis of NO and PGI_2, namely, endothelial constitutive nitric oxide synthase (ecNOS) and endothelial constitutive prostaglandin H synthase 1 (PGHS-1), better known as cyclooxygenase 1 (COX-1). These enzymes are activated by a rise in cytoplasmic calcium $[Ca^{2+}]i$, which triggers a coupled release of NO and PGI_2. A rise in $[Ca^{2+}]i$ is brought about by stimulation of kinin, muscarinic, purinergic and other receptors on endothelial cells.

Molecular mechanisms underlying the regulation of transcription of ecNOS and PGHS-1 are the subject of thorough studies. The structures of their genes which encode corresponding mRNAs are known. The multiplicity of potential regulatory elements in their putative promoter regions speak for an assumption that the expression of these enzymes may be regulated at the transcriptional step as it is the case with their inducible isoforms. Indeed, the steady-state levels of ecNOS mRNA seem to be modulated by tumour necrosis factor α (TNFα), shear stress or oestrogens.

In this paper our attention will be focused on the role of endothelial and non-endothelial sources of NO in ICU patients, while other factors involved with MODFS are reviewed in the accompanying paper (1).

Nitric oxide synthases (NOSs)

NOSs (EC 1.14.13.39) are homodimers (≈ 300 kDa) that require three substrates, L-arginine, NADPH and oxygen, to make two products, NO and citrulline with a help of five cofactors, FAD, FMN, calmodulin, tetrahydrobiopterin (BH4) and haeme (2-4). An important intermediate in the NO synthesis is N^G-hydroxy-L-arginine (3), which like L-arginine is a substrate for NOSs (5); however, in their absence N^G-hydroxy-L-arginine can be converted to NO by a cytochrome P 450-dependent enzyme (6). The Strasbourg group (7) considers this finding to be an important hint in understanding pathomechanism and treatment of septic shock.

Three prototype isoforms of NOS, endothelial constitutive (ecNOS), neuronal constitutive (ncNOS), and inducible (iNOS) are derived from separate genes located on various chromosomes and are regulated by diverse signalling pathways (8). Originally the induction of iNOS has been described in murine macrophages. There were difficulties in spotting it in human monocytes and macrophages. Recently, however, the presence of iNOS mRNA and cNOS mRNA has been clearly demonstrated in human monocytes and macrophages (9). Moreover, activation of these human cells with LPS and INF-γ was associated with an increased expression of iNOS mRNA and suppression of the cNOS signal (9). There exists a silent antagonism between the product made by cNOS and the product made by iNOS, although both of them are expected to be NO. This enigmatic behaviour of products of cNOS and iNOS may find its explanation either in different sites of their generation or in different amounts produced by the constitutive and inducible enzymes or finally in different structures of the products, perhaps *NO free radicals* versus *S-nitrosothiols* or *NO complexes*. iNOS can be expressed not only in myeloid but also in mesenchymal cells such as smooth muscle, fibroblasts, neurons or astrocytes and in epithelial cells such as hepatocytes or even in endothelial cells (2, 10).

The main switch for activity of ecNOS and ncNOS is the level of $(Ca^{2+})i$, while the main switch for iNOS is the level of its mRNA (iNOS mRNA) (10). iNOS activity hardly depends on $(Ca^{2+})i$ since it forms a very tight complex with calmodulin, the formation of which cannot be controlled by $(Ca^{2+})i$ like in the case of constitutive NOSs. (2, 3). In this way iNOS remains under prevailing transcriptional control. The best known inducers of iNOS are lipopolysaccharide (LPS) acting synergically with interferon-γ (INF-γ) and interleukin 1ß (IL-1ß), while transforming growth factor ß (TGFß) inhibits the induction of iNOS. In cultured macrophages the induction of iNOS occurs after 2-4 h of lag period, and the production of NO may last 5 days provided L-arginine is supplied (2).

Cultured endothelial cells express both ecNOS and iNOS. In these cells LPS or INF-γ regulate their activities differentially by inhibiting the generation of NO via ecNOS and by stimulating its production by iNOS (11). It may not be the case in vivo. For example, in rats endotoxin stimulates sequentially both ecNOS and iNOS. During the first phase of action LPS seems to support beneficial *NO tone* that controls vascular patency and prevents a decrease in tissue blood flow, ischaemia and necrosis. Only after a few hours, endotoxin acts as an inducer of detrimental *NO surge* that is responsible for tissue damage, and therefore LPS is a toxin [see the discussion on papers (45, 46)].

Stability of m-RNA is a major posttranscriptional control point in regulating NOSs. For example, TGFß destabilizes and cyclic-AMP stabilizes iNOS mRNA (12) while TNFα destabilizes and oestrogens stabilize ecNOS mRNA.

Many agents push NOS mRNA levels up or down, but the mechanism of their action, especially in vivo, is not always clear (10, 13). For example, extracellular ATP via P_{2y} receptors on macrophages potentiates the LPS-induced iNOS expression (14). In the lungs of rats challenged with LPS the induction of iNOS leads to an increase of the generation of PGI_2. This speaks for the in vivo activation of PGHS by NO (15). One may consider it as a feedback mechanism that limits the cytotoxic action of iNOS-derived NO by pushing the synthesis of cytoprotective PGI_2, which is the major prostanoid made by the lung. Phosphatidyl serine (PS) isolated from tumour cells (the same PS, the translocation of which in platelet membrane is responsible for their procoagulant properties) is a potent inhibitor of iNOS in macrophages (16). Finally, iNOS may be also subject to negative feedback by NO, its own product, either by binding of the surplus of NO with the enzymic haeme moiety (17) or by posttranscriptional regulation of iNOS gene expression (2).

Functions of nitric oxide

Biological activities of NO depend on the site and amount of generated NO (2, 18, 19). One should keep in mind that NO acts as a double-edged sword. The versatility of interactions of NO with biomolecules depends on the richness of redox chemistry of NO. Both, covalent modifications of protein molecules as well as oxidation events that do not involve attachment of the NO group to the substrate have been acquired as signalling mechanisms for this mediator (20). Nitroxyl and nitroxonium ions, S-nitrosocysteine, mono- and dinitroxy-glutathione, nitrosoalbumin, complexes of NO with haeme and with non-iron structures are analysed as possible forms of storage of NO or stabilizing its biological activity.

NO when generated at low amounts by ecNOS exerts its action through cyclic-GMP-dependent and cyclic-GMP-independent transductional pathways. The former pathway mediates actions of NO in smooth muscle and platelets via oxidizing the active haeme centre of soluble guanylate cyclase (4). The cyclic-GMP-independent mechanisms comprise S-nitrosylation of proteins and amino acids, and ADP-ribosylation reactions (21). Via cyclic-GMP NO is responsible for maintaining vascular tone, arterial resistance, nutritional blood flow, also through the heart, and the above in association with negative inotropic effect of cyclic-GMP may offer cardioprotection. The NO-induced prevention of ischaemic events, thrombosis, migration and proliferation of vascular smooth muscle is considered as a preventive measure against atherogenesis. The activity of ncNOS promotes synaptogenesis, synaptic plasticity, neuroendocrine secretion, visual transduction, olfaction while ncNOS in non-adrenergic non-cholinergic (NANC) nerve endings is responsible for bronchodilation, erection of the penis, pancreatic and intestinal secretion and peristalsis. Even the generation of NO at relatively high concentrations by iNOS plays an important defensive role in fighting the invasion of viruses, bacteria, fungi, protozoa and helminths.

In contrast, NO made by iNOS may override a barrier of the host defence and become autotoxic to the host cells. There is a long list of sins of NO. Excessive production of NO and superoxide anion (O_2-) with a subsequent generation of peroxynitrite $(ONOO^-)$ (22) is responsible for many symptoms of septic shock, with a special reference to the lung injury (23), ARDS, reperfusion damage, microvascular leakage, glomerulonephritis, allograft rejection, mutagenesis, mucosal damage and diseases from autoaggression including ulcerative colitis and type I diabetes. Actually, NO made by macrophages induces selective damage to ß cells in the Langerhans islets. NO is also generated by rat islet capillary endothelial cells by both ecNOS and iNOS, the activities of which are regulated by glucose concentrations (24).

In liver not only Kupffer cells but also hepatocytes are capable of generating NO in response to LPS. In hepatocytes LPS stimulates the synthesis of TNFα and IL-6 but only the former triggers the release of NO (25). Unlike in the lung, in liver the role of NO during septic shock is not clear. It is true that in vivo TNFα acts as a signal for induction of hepatic iNOS; however, TNFα seems to be responsible also for mediation of the LPS hepatotoxicity without collaboration with NO in this respect. If anything, NO seems to be rather hepatoprotective than hepatotoxic during endotoxaemia (13). Endogenous NO attenuates also ethanol-induced hepatic damage, probably opposing ethanol-induced hepatic vasoconstriction (26).

Endotoxic shock and NO

The systemic inflammatory response syndrome (SIRS) in patients with sepsis involves the immune system, mobilizes inflammatory mediators and free radicals, and eventually leads to damage to endothelium, oedema, disseminated intravascular coagulation, impaired tissue perfusion and oxygen availability, ischaemia, necrosis and multiple organ dysfunction failure syndrome (MODFS). Experimental models of septic shock (perforation of gut) (27) are used less frequently than neat models of endotoxin shock induced by administration of lipopolysaccharides (LPS) from Gram negative bacteria (1, 28). It is true that LPS plays a major role in the development of septic shock, yet endotoxic shock differs considerably from septic shock, from SIRS or MODFS. With that precaution in mind let us inspect the information concerning the role of endothelium in endotoxic shock.

Experimental endotoxic shock is most frequently studied in rodents, although cats and dogs are also used. Intravenous injection of LPS to anaesthetized rats elicits an immediate fall in the arterial blood pressure which soon levels off, and after the next 2-3 h develops a late phase of hypotension with a concomitant loss of reactivity to pressor responses to noradrenaline, while endogenous noradrenaline is released by LPS from the peripheral nerve endings and from the adrenal medulla (29). Depending on a dose of LPS this late phase might be reversible or fatal. Microvascular perfusion is impaired in a rat model of normotensive sepsis (27). It is proposed that the acute phase of hypotension by LPS results from activation of ecNOS whereas the delayed phase of hypotension is associated with the induction of iNOS by LPS and with the simultaneous suppression of ecNOS activity (28). Recently, it has been proposed that formation of endogenous bradykinin contributes primarily to the acute but not to the delayed fall in blood pressure elicited by LPS. In contrast, the formation of endogenous platelet activating factor (PAF) contributes to both the acute and the delayed hypotension produced by LPS (30). The mechanisms of haemodynamic effects of LPS are still disputed. For instance, in septic normotensive and hyperdynamic rats with high cardiac output and low systemic vascular resistance the unfavourable redistribution of blood flow between organs does not seem to depend on overproduction of NO since pharmacological blockade of NOSs does not correct faulty organ blood flow redistribution, and other haemodynamic effects (decrease in cardiac output, rise in peripheral resistance and mean arterial blood pressure) are the same in control and septic animals (31).

In rats LPS induces iNOS in many organs including lung, heart, spleen, gut, liver, kidney, and blood vessels. Two hours after intravenous injection of LPS at a dose of 5 mg/kg the intensity of appearance of iNOS mRNA decreases in the indicated sequence of organs (our unpublished data). Cellular localization of iNOS in endotoxic shock in the rat shows its expression in monocytes, macrophages, in epithelial cells of respiratory and gastrointestinal tracts and in hepatocytes. iNOS expression peaked at 5 h after administration of LPS and returned to normal after 12 h except in spleen macrophages (32). The mechanism of the iNOS induction by LPS is still under study. The participation of various components of LPS in this process is analysed, and mediation by TNFα is generally accepted (13), while involvement of tyrosine kinase has recently been proposed (33). It is obvious that NO might be only one of many factors which mediate endotoxic shock. For example, LPS-induced adhesion of neutrophils to endothelial cells occurs owing to an increased expression of adhesion glycoproteins ICAM-1, CD11/CD18 as well as generation of PAF and superoxide anions (34), while biphasic hypotensive response to LPS is associated also with endogenous formation of kinins and PAF (30). Nonetheless, a general opinion on a major role of NO in endotoxic shock is supported by recent studies on the in vivo mechanism of tolerance to endotoxin (35). Cardiovascular tolerance to endotoxin develops after repeated administration of small doses of LPS to rats. The phenomenon can be explained by attenuated induction of iNOS to each next dose of LPS which occurs owing to LPS-induced elevation of endogenous glucocorticoid levels. These in turn suppress the induction of iNOS by LPS.

Lungs, heart, liver, kidneys and gut are the main organs to suffer from MODFS. Over 40 types of cells reside in the lung, and many of them express ecNOS, ncNOS and iNOS. The richest source of this last isoenzyme are alveolar macrophages, whereas human alveolar and bronchial epithelial cells are capable of expressing not only cytokines, growth factors (e.g. EGF) and cytoadhesins but also NOSs. In epithelial cells iNOS and cNOS coexist. This shows molecular identity with ncNOS while iNOS is identical with that in macrophages and its induction is achieved by LPS, ILß, INF-γ and TNFα (36). The same ncNOS found in epithelial cells is also found in NANC nerve endings, which are abundantly distributed in the lung.

Hearts of rats produced NO via cNOS; however, after treatment of rats with LPS a (Ca^{2+})i-independent cardiac generation of NO, accumulation of cyclic-GMP and suppression of cardiac contractility did occur. These events were blocked by pretreatment with dexamethasone or with cyclohexamide (37). Cardiomyocytes seem to be a rich source of iNOS of macrophage-like type. 1L-ß induces iNOS mRNA expression in cultured rat neonatal cardiomyocytes, and subsequent de novo synthesis of enzymic protein leads to massive production of NO by cardiac cells (38). Along with IL-ß LPS also stimulates massive generation of NO by cardiac myocytes and it is associated with a rise in cyclic-GMP. Pretreatment with TGFß or with N^G-mono-methyl-L-arginine inhibited both events (39). Cyclic-GMP is known to antagonize the effects of cyclic-AMP in the heart. NO at high concentrations is likely to be cardiotoxic; however, it is not the only route by which LPS can influence cardiac function. In patients with catecholamine-refractory septic shock an increase in myocardial inhibitory G-protein (Giα) was observed (40). Not only endotoxic shock but also myocardial infarction might be associated with the upregulation of cardiac iNOS, and glucocorticoids inhibit the expression of iNOS in infarcted myocardium (41) as anywhere else. It has been predicted (37) that the enhanced cardiac production of NO by iNOS may account for cardiovascular disturbances in septic shock. Indeed, not only myocardium but also endocardium, after appropriate induction (TNFα or IL-1ß), is capable of expressing iNOS (42).

As discussed earlier, the significance of induction of iNOS in Kupffer cells and hepatocytes by LPS and TNFα awaits its appreciation, and a hepatoprotective rather than hepatotoxic role of NO is argued (13, 25, 26). In contrast, renal glomeruli, but not mesangial cells, generated NO and this production could be enhanced by LPS. It appears that renal NO may play a pathogenic role in the mechanism of glomerular injury in nephrotoxic nephritis and in pathological glomerular haemodynamics (43).

A pathogenic role of NO was proposed in the delayed phase of endotoxin-induced damage to the jejunum and colon of the rat (44). Colonic and jejunal vascular permeability increased after a lag period of 3-5 h following administration of LPS. An unusual behaviour of NOS inhibitors was recorded. When NOS inhibitors were administered concurrently with LPS they enhanced the endotoxin-induced intestinal vascular injury. In contrast with the above, when NOS inhibitors were injected 3 h after LPS, a dose-dependent reduction in the LPS-provoked vascular damage was observed (45). In other words, an early administration of nonselective NOS inhibitors aggravated symptoms of endotoxin shock, probably in consequence of blocking of the activity of ecNOS, whereas a delayed administration of NOS inhibitors provided protection against the damage to intestinal vasculature elicited by NO which had been made by iNOS.

The detrimental involvement of endogenous TXA_2 and PAF in the early response to LPS + L-NMMA was proposed, and the protective role of NO formed by ecNOS in modulation of microvascular integrity at the early stage of sepsis established (46).

NOS inhibitors in endotoxic shock

The group of Moncada proposed a pathogenetic role for iNOS in septic shock, and subsequently the efficacy of NOS inhibitors was studied both in experimental models of endotoxic shock and in patients with septic shock (47, 48). Recently, a prospective study on the relationship between NO production, endotoxaemia and haemodynamic disturbances in patients with septic shock has been reported (49). In septic patients evidence for such a relationship consisted of increased plasma nitrite and nitrate levels which correlated directly with endotoxin concentration and cardiac output, and inversely with systolic blood pressure.

Three classic NOS inhibitors: N^G-monomethy-L-arginine (L-NMMA), N-iminoethyl-L-ornithine (L-NIO) and N^G-nitro-L-arginine methyl ester (L-NAME) evoke hypertension and blunt hypotensive responses to acetylcholine and bradykinin (50). Studies with NOS inhibitors demonstrated the significance of basal endothelial NO release for defending against arterial hypertension. Recently, it has been put forward that NOS inhibitors merely unmask a physiological tonic pressor influence of endothelins (51). On the other hand, during septic shock NOS inhibitors reverse arteriolar hyporesponsiveness to catecholamines (52). L-NMMA, L-NIO and L-NAME are nonselective inhibitors of constitutive and inducible isoforms of the enzyme, and this is why objections have been put forward (53) that their use in septic shock could be detrimental because of inhibition of physiologically required ecNOS parallel to inhibition of pathologically activated iNOS. Indeed, as it has been already discussed the beneficial or deleterious effects of NOS inhibitors in rats with endotoxic shock depend on dosage and time of the drug administration (45, 46). In patients with septic shock who are treated with L-NMMA, apart from the desired rise in blood pressure and recovery of responsiveness to noradrenaline, a significant fall in cardiac output also occurs, and it may worsen tissue perfusion (48, 49).

The conception of a selective iNOS inhibitor as a prospective drug for the treatment of septic shock is finding its way. A search for selective iNOS inhibitors brings new representatives of this class of agents. For example, L-N^6-(1-iminoethyl)lysine (l-NIL) is a 28 times stronger inhibitor of iNOS than of ecNOS (54). S-Methyl-isothiourea (SMT) selectively inhibits iNOS and improves survival in the rodent model of septic shock (55).

Other approaches include scavenging of the surplus of NO made by iNOS during septic shock. For example, imidazolineoxyl-N-oxides scavenge toxic NO free radicals (56), while leaving the genuine mediator, i.e. S-nitrosocysteine or any low molecular S-nitrosothiol (20) untouched. Glibenclamide, an inhibitor of ATP-sensitive potassium channels (57) as well as the aldehyde metabolites of spermine (58) suppress the induction but not the activity of iNOS in vitro and in vivo. In contrast with them NO gas suppresses the action but not the induction of iNOS (59). NO from S-nitroso-N-acetylpenicillamine (SNAP) protects against the jejunal damage induced by the combined administration of LPS and L-NMMA (60), most likely because of replacement by SNAP of endogenous ecNOS-derived NO. Perhaps, in septic shock the selective removal of iNOS-derived NO is beneficial whereas removal of ec-NOS-derived NO or S-nitroso thiols is deleterious.

Still another approach to combat the induction of iNOS is desensitization to endotoxin with monophosphoryl lipid A (MLA), which is a relatively non-toxic fragment of the structure of lipid A in LPS (61).

Conclusion

Septic shock induces multivarious changes in metabolic, haemostatic and endocrine functions of the vascular endothelium. Increased expression of cytoadhesions, suppressed generation of t-PA, thrombomodulin and PGI$_2$ are responsible for the disseminated intravascular coagulation syndrome. On the other hand, the impaired tissue perfusion with subsequent injury of vital organs, fall in blood pressure, loss of pressor response to catecholamines and depression of cardiac output are largely associated with disturbances in the production of nitric oxide by various cells, including endothelium. It seems that the initial endotoxin-induced activation of endothelial constitutive NO synthase is a desirable defensive reaction which must not be deleted. Only the delayed induction by endotoxin of inducible NO synthase is harmful. Rectification of this complex involvement of NO in septic shock is a challenge for pharmacologists and molecular biologists.

References

1. Uracz W, Gryglewski RJ (1995) Cellular and humoral markers of tissue damage. This volume pp 109-125
2. Xie Q, Nathan C (1994) The high-output nitric oxide pathway: role and regulation. J Leukocyte Biol 56:576-582
3. Marletta MA (1994) Nitric oxide synthase: aspects concerning structure and catalysis. Cell 78: 927-930
4. Mayer B (1994) Regulation of nitric oxide synthase and soluble guanyl cyclase. Cell Biochem Funct 12:167-177
5. Korth HG, Sustman R, Thater C, Butler AR, Ingold KU (1994) On the mechanism of the nitric oxide synthase - catalyzed conversion of N^{ω}-hydroxy-L-arginine to citrulline and nitric oxide. J Biol Chem 269:17776-17779
6. Schott CA, Bogen CM, Vetrovsky P, Berton CC, Stocklet JC (1994) Exogenous N^G-hydroxy-L-arginine causes nitrite production in vascular smooth muscle cells in the absence of nitric oxide synthase activity. FEBS Lett 341:203-207
7. Stocklet JC, Fleming I, Gray G, Julon-Schaeffer G, Schneider F, Schott C, Parratt JR (1993) Nitric oxide and endotoxemia. Circulation 87:V77-V80
8. Sessa WC (1994) The nitric oxide synthase family of proteins. J Vasc Res 31:131-143
9. Reiling N, Ulmer AJ, Duchrow M, Ernst M, Flad HD, Hauschildt S (1994) Nitric oxide synthase: mRNA expression of different isoforms in human monocytes/macrophages. Eur J Immunol 24:1941-1944
10. Nathan C, Xie Q (1994) Nitric oxide synthases: roles, tolls, and controls. Cell 78:915-918
11. Walter R, Schaffner A, Schoedon G (1994) Differential regulation of constitutive and inducible nitric oxide production by inflammatory stimuli in murine endothelial cells. Biochem Biophys Res Commun 202:450-455
12. Imai T, Hirate Y, Kanno K, Marumo F (1994) Induction of nitric oxide synthase by cyclic AMP in rat vascular smooth muscle cells. J Clin Invest 93:543-549
13. Harbrecht BG, DiSilvio M, Demetris AJ, Simmons RL, Billar TR (1994) Tumor necrosis factor-α regulates in vivo nitric oxide synthesis and induces liver injury during endotoxemia. Hepatology 20:1055-1060
14. Tonetti M, Sturla L, Bistolfi T, Benatti U, DeFlora A (1994) Extracellular ATP potentiates nitric oxide synthase expression induced by lipopolysaccharide in RAW 264,7 murine macrophages. Biochem Biophys Res Commun 203:430-435
15. Sautebin L, DiRosa M (1994) Nitric oxide modulates prostacyclin biosynthesis in the lung of endotoxin-treated rats. Eur J Pharmacol 262:193-196
16. Calderon C, Huang ZH, Gage DA, Sotomayor EM, Lopez DM (1994) Isolation of nitric oxide inhibitor from mammary tumor cells and its characterization as phosphatidyl serine. J Exp Med 180:945-958
17. Wang J, Rouseau DL, Abu-Soud HM, Stuehr DJ (1994) Heme coordination of NO in NO synthase. Proc Natl Acad Sci USA 91:10512-10516
18. Schmidt HHHW, Walter U (1994) NO at work. Cell 78:919-925
19. Lowenstein CJ, Dinerman JL, Snyder SH (1994) Nitric oxide: a physiologic messenger. Ann Intern Med 120:227-237
20. Stamler JS (1994) Redox signaling: nitrosylation and related target interactions of nitric oxide. Cell 78:931-936
21. Mohr S, Stamler JS, Brüne B (1994) Mechanism of covalent modification of glyceralaldehyde-3-phosphate dehydrogenase at its active site thiol by nitric oxide, peroxynitrite and relating nitrosating agents. FEBS Lett 348:223-227
22. Beckman J, Tsai JH (1994) Reactions and diffusion of nitric oxide and peroxynitrite. Biochemist 16:8-10
23. Haddad IY, Patakig HP, Galliani C, Beckman JS, Matalon S (1994) Quantitation of nitrotyrosine levels in lung sections of patients and animals with acute lung injury. J Clin Invest 94:2407-2413

24. Suschek C, Fehsel K, Kröncke KD, Sommer A, Kolb-Bachhofen V (1994) Primary cultures of rat islet capillary endothelial cells. Constitutive and cytokine-inducible macrophagelike nitric oxide synthases are expressed and activities regulated by glucose concentration. Am J Pathol 145:685-695

25. Saad B, Frei K, Scholl FA, Fontano A, Maier P (1995) Hepatocyte-derived interleukin-6 and tumor necrosis factor α mediate the liposaccharide-induced acute-phase response and nitric oxide release by cultured rat cells. Eur J Biochem 229:349-355

26. Oshita M, Takei Y, Kwano S (1994) Endogenous nitric oxide attenuates ethanol-induced perturbation of hepatic circulation in the isolated perfused rat liver. Hepatology 20:961-965

27. Lam C, Tymi K, Martin C, Sibbald W (1994) Microvascular perfusion is impaired in a rat model of normotensive sepis. J Clin Invest 94:2077-2083

28. Szabó C, Thiemermann C (1994) Role of nitric oxide in hemorrhagic, traumatic, and anaphylactic shock and thermal injury. Shock 2:145-155

29. Jones SB, Kotsonis P, Majewski H (1994) Endotoxin enhances norepinephrine release in the rat by peripheral mechanism. Shock 2:370-375

30. Ueno A, Ishida H, Ohishi S (1995) Comparative study of endotoxin-induced hypotension in kininogen-deficient rats with that in normal rats. Br J Pharmacol 114:1250-1256

31. Martin CM, Sibbald WJ (1994) Modulation of hemodynamics and organ blood flow by nitric oxide synthase inhibition is not altered in normotensive, septic rats. Ann J Respir Crit Care Med 150:1539-1544

32. Cook HT, Bune AJ, Jansen AS, Taylor GM, Loi RK, Cattell V (1994) Cellular localization of inducible nitric oxide synthase in experimental endotoxic shock in the rat. Clin Sc 87:179-186

33. Akarasereenont P, Mitchell JA, Appetton I, Thiemermann C, Vane JR (1994) Involvement of tyrosine kinase in the induction of nitric oxide synthase by endotoxin in cultured cells. Br J Pharmacol 113:1522-1528

34. Harris NR, Russell JM, Granger DN (1994) Mediators of endotoxin-induced leukocyte adhesion in mesenteric postcapillary venules. Circ Shock 43:155-160

35. Szabó C, Thiemermann C, Wu CC, Perretti M, Vane JR (1994) Attenuation of the induction of nitric oxide synthase by endogenous glucocorticoids accounts for endotoxin tolerance in vivo. Proc Natl Acad Sci USA 91:271-275

36. Asano K, Chee CBE, Gaston B, Lilly CM, Gerard C, Drazen JM, Stamler JS (1994) Constitutive and inducible nitric oxide synthase gene expression regulation and activity in human lung epithelial cells. Proc Natl Acad Sci USA 91:10089-10093

37. Schulz R, Nava E, Moncada S (1992) Induction and potential biological relevance of a Ca^{2+}-independent nitric oxide synthase in the myocardium. Br J Pharmacol 105575-580

38. Tsujino H, Hirata Y, Imai T, Kanno K, Eguchi S, Ito H, Marumo F (1994) Induction of nitric oxide synthase gene by interleukin-1ß in cultured rat cardiocytes. Circulation 90:375-383

39. Shinado T, Ikeda U, Ohkawa F, Takahashi H (1994) Nitric oxide synthesis in rat cardiac myocytes. Life Sci 55:1101-1108

40. Böhm M, Kirchmayer R, Gierschlik C, Erdmann E (1995) Increase of myocardial inhibitory G-proteins in catecholamine-refractory septic shock or in septic multiorgan failure. Am J Med 98:183-186

41. Dudek RR, Wildhirt S, Pinto V, Giesler G, Bing RJ (1994) Dexamethasone inhibits the expression of an inducible nitric oxide synthase in infarcted rabbit myocardium. Biochem Biophys Res Commun 202:1120-1126

42. Smith JA, Radomski MW, Schulz R, Moncada S, Lewis MJ (1993) Porcine ventricular endocardial cells in culture express the inducible form of nitric oxide synthase. Br J Pharmacol 108:1107-1110

43. Cattel V, Cook T, Moncada S (1990) Glomeruli synthesize nitrite in experimental nephrotoxic nephritis. Kidney Int 38:1056-1060

44. Boughton-Smith NK, Evans SM, Laszlo F, Whittle BJ, Moncada S (1993) The induction of nitric oxide synthase and intestinal vascular permeability by endotoxin in the rat. Br J Pharmacol 110:1189-1195

45. Laszlo F, Whittle BJ, Moncada S (1994) Time-dependent enhancement or inhibition of endotoxin-induced vascular injury in rat intestine by nitric oxide synthase inhibitors. Br J Pharmacol 111:1309-1315

46. Laszlo F, Whittle BJ, Moncada S (1994) Interactions of constitutive nitric oxide with PAF and thromboxane on rat intestinal vascular integrity in acute endotoxaemia. Br J Pharmacol 113: 1131-1136

47. Petros A, Lamb G, Leone A, Moncada S, Bennett D, Vallance P (1994) Effects of nitric oxide synthase inhibitor in humans with septic shock. Cardiovasc Res 28:34-39

48. Vallance P (1994) Nitric oxide in the clinical arena. Biochemist 16:23-27

49. Gomez-Jimenez J, Solgado A, Mourelle M, Martin MC, Segura RM, Peracaula R, Moncada S (1995) L-arginine: nitric oxide pathway in endotoxaemia and human septic shock. Crit Care Med 23:253-258

50. Rees DD, Palmer RMJ, Schulz R, Hodson HF, Moncada S (1990) Characterization of three inhibitors of endothelial nitric oxide synthase in vitro and in vivo. Br J Pharmacol 101: 746-752

51. Richard V, Hogie M, Clozel M, Löffer BM, Thuillez C (1995) In vivo evidence of an endothelin-induced vasopressor tone after inhibition of nitric oxide synthesis in rats. Circulation 91:771-775

52. Hollenberg SM, Cunnion RE, Zimmerberg J (1993) Nitric oxide synthase inhibition reverses arteriolar hyporesponsiveness to catecholamines in septic rats. Am J Physiol 264:H660-H663

53. Bouskela E, Rubanyi G (1994) Effects of Nω - L-arginine and dexamethasone on early events following lipopolysaccharide injection: observations in the hamster check pouch microcirculation. Shock 1:347-353

54. Moore WM, Webber RK, Jerome GM, Tjoeng FS, Misko TP, Currie MG (1994) L- N^6 - (1-iminoethyl) lysine: a selective inhibitor of inducible nitric oxide synthase. J Med Chem 37: 3886-3888

55. Southan GJ, Szabó C, Thiemermann C (1995) Isothioureas: potent inhibitors of nitric oxide synthases with variable isoform selectivity. Br J Pharmacol 114:510-516

56. Yoshida H, Akaike T, Wada Y, Sato K, Ikeda K, Ueda S, Maeda H (1994) Therapeutic effects of imidazolineoxyl N-oxide against endotoxic shock through its direct nitric oxide-scavenging activity. Biochem Biophys Res Commun 202:923-930

57. Wu CC, Thiemermann C, Vane JR (1995) Glibenclamide-induced inhibition of the expression of inducible nitric oxide synthase in cultured macrophages and in the anaesthetized rats. Br J Pharmacol 114:1273-1281

58. Szabó C, Southan GJ, Thiemermann C, Vane JR (1994) The mechanism of the inhibitory effect of polyamines on the induction of nitric oxide synthase: role of aldehyde metabolites. Br J Pharmacol 113:757-766

59. Kiff RJ, Moss DW, Moncada S (1994) Effect of nitric oxide gas on the generation of nitric oxide by isolated blood vessels: implication for inhalation therapy. Br J Pharmacol 113: 496-498

60. Boughton-Smith NK, Hutcheson IR, Deakin AM, Whittle BJ, Moncada S (1990) Protective effect of S-nitroso-N-acetylpenicillamine in endotoxin-induced acute intestinal damage in the rat. Eur J Pharmacol 191:485-488

61. Yao Z, Foster PA, Gross GJ (1994) Monophosphoryl lipid A protects against endotoxic shock via inhibiting neutrophil infiltration and preventing disseminated infravascular coagulation. Circ Shock 43:107-114

Antioxidant Activity in the Therapy of Sepsis: From Experimental Data to Clinical Practice

G.P. NOVELLI, R. CASALI, S. FALSINI, E. PIERACCIOLI

An antioxidant is defined as any substance which delays or prevents the oxidation of a substrate when it is present in small amounts relative to the amount of the substrate itself. Antioxidants are active at several levels of the oxidative sequence and their mechanism of action may be unique.

In the living organisms the first line of antioxidant protection involves enzymes (i.e. SOD, CAT, PERx), the activity of which depends on trace amounts of Mn, Se, Cu and consist in the control of formation of OR°. The second line involves vitamins E and C, methyonine, and cysteine which all are concerned with the proliferation and diffusion of secondary radicals. The third line consists mostly of exogenous substances that are active at various levels of the oxidative process; sometimes pharmacological interventions directed to suppress OR° generating conditions have been classified as antioxidants.

The most widely known exogenous antioxidants are listed in Table 1.

Table 1. Exogenous antioxidants

Superoxide dismutase	Catalase
Native SOD	Native CAT
PEG-SOD	PEG-CAT
Liposome-SOD	Liposime CAT
Xanthine-oxidase inhibitors	Protease inhibitors
Allopurinol	Soybean trypsin inhibitor
Oxypurinol	Protease inhibitors
Folic acid	Gabesate mesylate
Tungsten	
NADPH-oxidase inhibitors	Scavengers
Adenosine	Nitrones
Local anesthetics	
NSAIDS	Lazaroids
Steroids	Mannitol
Inhibitors of iron	Augmentation of endogenous antioxidants
Deferoxamine	Tocopherols
Ceruloplasmin	Glutathione
	N-acetylcysteine

The aim of this paper is to discuss the possibilities and the limitations of the use of antioxidants as therapy of acute critical illnesses and mainly of sepsis, septic shock, ARDS and MODS.

The difficulty of this argument is to keep apart antioxidants as tools to demonstrate the role of OR° in the investigated disease from antioxidants as therapy of the disease itself. Literature data concerning the administration of antioxidants to reverse an already developed sepsis, septic shock or MODS (i.e. "therapy") are very few.

The earliest experiments were performed administering endogenous enzymatic scavengers to animals submitted to various kinds of shock. The first report was that of Lefer and his coworkers on traumatic shock (1).

In our laboratory a highly significant protection against endotoxin and trauma shock was observed in rats injected with vitamin E or glutathione (2). Inhibition of the scavenging enzymes by diethylthiocarbamate increased lethality (3). Injection of superoxide dismutase was adopted to demonstrate a role of OR° in burn shock as well (4). Experiments performed in our laboratory during many years using the spin trapping nitrones to prevent experimental shock and its particulate aspects (microcirculation, cell membranes, etc.) were directed only to confirm the role of OR° (5).

However, one such experiment resembled the first attempt of antioxidant therapy of shock: in fact the nitrone phenyl-butyl-nitrone reverted a developed traumatic shock in rats (6). Therapy was successful only when nitrone was administered no later than 30 min after trauma, that is, before irreversible damage appeared.

In very recent years, the concept of antioxidant therapy has slowly developed up and some papers have been published on this topic (7-11).

The concrete possibilities of a clinically oriented antioxidant therapy are (Table 1):

Blockade of OR° generation

Being impractical to use SOD, CAT and PERx (adverse reactions, brief half-life), the blockade of OR° overgeneration can be obtained by:

1. Inhibition of xanthine-oxidase activity by allopurinol or oxypurinol; however, all these ways need a long time and never have been practiced as therapy of sepsis/septic shock (12). A study has been published in stress-induced gastric mucosal hemorrhagic ulcers in men treated with allopurinol with beneficial effects (13).

2. Prevention of formation of xanthine-oxidase by action of proteolytic enzymes and calcium on dehydrogenase. In fact the role of protease inhibitors in the therapy of shock has long been known (14) although based on more classic pharmacologic interpretation. Recently the wide-spectrum protease inhibitor gabexate mesylate has been used in therapy of severe

shock in man (15) and also in acute pancreatitis, i.e. in a typical OR° derived disease (16). The antioxidant activity of gabexate mesylate on the endotoxin-induced microcirculatory overpermeability has been demonstrated in our laboratory (17).

3. Prevention of activation of PMN granulocytes and other phagocytic cells that are potent OR° generators. Granulocyte activation is consequent to complement activation and this, in turn, is consequent to bacteria, endotoxin etc. but also to several circulating mediators and to proteases. The previously quoted protease inhibitors prevent complement activation through the alternative pathway and suppress the respiratory burst of granulocytes (18). Steroids also inhibit complement activation and, in this way they are active on shock.

4. Another way to block OR° production from granulocytes is to stabilize their membrane and to inhibit the membrane bound enzyme NADPH-oxidase. Adenosine, local anesthetics, nonsteroid anti-inflammatory analgesic drugs and glucoactive steroids are typically active in this direction and, in fact, their use as antishock agents is known.

5. Prevention of increase in the production of OR° is obviously relevant in every therapeutic program: abolishing all the forms of hyperoxia (19) and ensuring tissue perfusion are the cardinal point in preventing OR° production.

Scavenging of OR°

Scavenging enzymes are clinically useless due to their adverse side effects and to their very brief half-life. The iron chelator deferoxamine has an intrinsic toxicity and its use has been restricted to the laboratory (20). The nitrone PBN was the first antioxidant to be used as "therapy" in a strict sense, as quoted before (6), but this datum remained isolated and restricted to animal experiments.

The "lazaroids" are a class of 21-amino steroids related to methylprednisolone that protect the cells from oxidative damage induced by OR° in a variety of in vitro and in vivo test systems and also in man. The most recent studies (21, 22) indicate that these new compounds are scavengers of primary and secondary free radicals by their in vivo inhibition of lipid peroxidation and of protection against neurologic consequences of CNS focal lesions. No data are available concerning lazaroids in sepsis and septic shock although some are available about other shock models (23).

Augmentation of endogenous antioxidants

The antioxidant power of plasma has epidemiological relationships with several diseases such as atherosclerosis, stroke, ischemic heart attacks, carcinoma, etc. (8, 9). It is based on enzymes and their related oligo-elements (Mn, Cu, Se) but also on the tissue reserves of tocopherols, carotenoids, glutathione and cysteine.

Vitamin E is the main physiologic antioxidant that is located in cell membranes and quenches OR°. However, vitamin E is a lipophilic drug that cannot be injected intravenously so that its use is possible in many OR° derived diseases but not in the acute ones.

There are two compounds that can be used to acutely increase antioxidant tissue levels also in man: reduced glutathione (GSH) and acetyl-cysteine.

GSH, a tripeptide consisting of glutamate, cysteine and glycine is a potent endogenous antioxidant that serves as one of the body's most important defenses against OR°. Many studies strongly indicate that depletion of tissue stores of GSH is likely to occur in critical illness. Because such patients are exposed to increased oxidant stresses, GSH deficiency predispose them to a vicious circle of widespread OR°-mediated tissue damage and possibly MODS.

The sites of action of GSH are extracellular and intracellular. The extracellular action consists in protecting plasma proteins and cell surface thiols are protected from oxidative stress and to maintain the redox state (24). The intracellular action is consistent with the role of GSH as the substrate of peroxidases. The intracellular level depends on an active process of resynthesis from the constitutive amino acids (glutamate, glycine and cysteine) by the enzyme gamma-glutamyl-transpeptidase (25, 26). Glutathione monoester quickly enhances tissue antioxidant stores (27).

An active transport of GSH from plasma to the cytoplasma has been demonstrated in isolated cells (28).

In our laboratory we have demonstrated that GSH exert a potent protective action against endotoxin or traumatic shock (3) that is due mostly to an intracellular action and is evident within a few minutes after injection of very large doses of the tripeptide (29). The physiological kinetics of increase of the intracellular level of GSH are quite slow but the intravenous injection of a very large dose makes them sufficiently rapid to satisfy the needs of an acute oxidative stress. In fact, experiments on endurance to muscle effort in mice showed the antioxidant action of GSH to be present 10 min after an intraperitoneal injection of 500 mg/kg or more of GSH (30).

Adverse effects of very large doses of GSH have never been reported even if they have been demonstrated to be effective in a) preventing lipid peroxidation during aortic surgery in man as expressed by ethane exhalation (31), b) preventing the increase of extravascular lung water during ischemia and reperfusion in man (32), and c) preventing lipid peroxidative stress during hyperoxia in man (33). Moreover, large doses of GSH acutely administered provoke a) protection against endotoxin and trauma shock in rats (29), b) protection against the increase in capillary permeability provoked by endotoxin in rats (34), c) protection against experimental multiorgan failure (35), d) amelioration of the neurologic consequences of spinal trauma in rats (36), and e) improvement of acute lung injury in man (preliminary data in 37).

N-acetylcysteine (NAC) has been frequently reported as an antioxidant in critical illnesses as a drug favoring an increase of glutathione within the cells so as to replace an impaired antioxidant defense system. In fact in our experiments on traumatized rats, cysteine was as effective in preventing shock as GSH (29).

NAC is a thiol donor and has an established efficacy on at least one human OR°-derived disease, i.e., paracetamol overdose. NAC has been demonstrated to directly scavenge hydroxyl peroxide and hydroxyl radicals (38).

A randomized trial was performed on ARDS patients receiving high doses of intravenous NAC. Cardiopulmonary status was favorably affected by NAC (39).

Recently, another randomized double-blind study was performed on 58 septic shock patients given 150 mg/kg NAC as a bolus followed by 12.5 mg/kg/h over 90 min. NAC provided a significant improvement in tissue oxygenation in about half of the septic patients; however, the results were not so definite (40).

Conclusions

Antioxidant therapy of acute critical diseases has been recently discussed in many papers (7-11) and many arguments in favor have been reported. However, randomized controlled clinical studies are lacking, probably as a consequence of the lack of the ideal drug.

Zimmerman in an editorial published on critical care medicine in 1992 (41) noted that it would be easier to manufacture a small molecular weight compound like nitrone as an antioxidant therapeutic agent compared to the great scientific and industrial efforts to manufacture a recombinant superoxide dismutase. Anyway various interventions to abolish, to control or at least to modulate oxygen radical production will likely have major therapeutic implications in a variety of critical illnesses.

The points to be stressed, however, are: 1) the effectiveness of every antioxidant therapy is strictly linked with its timing, being the effectiveness linked to the precocity; 2) the antioxidants are active at the final point of the whole chain of the mediators of sepsis/septic shock because they inactivate OR° produced activity of cytokines, PAF, PMN's etc. (42). Currently, glutathione seems to be the antioxidant most likely to be used in clinical conditions.

References

1. Lefer AM, Araki H, Okamatsu S (1981) Beneficial actions of a free radical scavenger in traumatic shock and myocardial ischemia. Circ Shock 8:273-282
2. Novelli GP, De Gaudio AR (1983) Oxygen free-radicals in shock states. Elsevier, Amsterdam
3. De Gaudio AR, Sarti A, Palmarini M et al (1983) Prevenzione dello shock sperimentale mediante uno scavenger di radicali liberi: il glutatione ridotto. Acta Anaesth Ital 34:501-507
4. Saez JC, Ward PH, Gunther B et al (1984) Superoxide radical involvement in the pathogenesis of burn shock. Circ Shock 12:229-233
5. Novelli GP (1992) Oxygen radicals in experimental shock: effects of spin-trapping nitrones in ameliorating shock pathophysiology. Crit Care Med 20:499-507
6. Novelli GP, Angiolini P, Tani R et al (1985) Phenyl-t-butyl-nitrone is active against traumatic shock in rats. Free Radic Res Commun 1:321-327

7. Goode HF, Webster NR (1993) Free radicals and antioxidants in sepsis. Crit Care Med 21: 1770-1776
8. Schiller HJ, Reilly PM, Bulkley GB (1993) Antioxidant therapy. Crit Care Med 21:S92-102
9. Rice-Evans CA, Diplock AT (1993) Current status of antioxidant therapy. Free Radic Biol Med 15:77-96
10. Bone RC (1992) Inhibitors of complement and neutrophils: a critical evaluation of their role in the treatment of sepsis. Crit Care Med 20:891-898
11. Youn YK, Lalonde C, Demling R (1991) Use of antioxidant therapy in shock and trauma. Circ Shock 35:245-249
12. Mannion D, Fitzpatrick GJ, Feeley M (1994) Role of xanthine oxidase inhibition in survival from hemorrhagic shock. Circ Shock 42:39-43
13. Salim AS (1991) Protection against stress-induced acute gastric mucosal injury by free-radical scavengers. Intensive Care Med 17:455-460
14. Tani T, Aoki H, Yoshioka T (1993) Treatment of septic shock with a protease inhibitor in a canine model: a prospective, randomized, controlled trial. Crit Care Med 21:925-930
15. Novelli GP, Innocenti P, Livi P (1993) Il gabesato mesilato (Foy) nuovo antiproteasico sintetico nel trattamento dello shock. Studio multicentrico italiano. Minerva Anestesiol 58: 247-253
16. Novelli GP, Casali R, Bonizzoli M et al (1995) Azione antiossidante del gabesato mesilato (Foy) in un modello sperimentale di shock. Minerva Anestesiol 60 (in press)
17. Sanfey H, Bulkley GB, Cameron JL (1985) The pathogenesis of acute pancreatitis. The source and the role of oxygen-derived free radicals in three different experimental models. Ann Surg 201:633-639
18. Fujishima S, Aikawa N (1995) Neutrophil-mediated tissue injury and its modulation. Intensive Care Med 21:277-285
19. Wolbarsht ML, Fridovich I (1989) Hyperoxia during reperfusion is a factor in reperfusion injury. Free Radic Biol Med 6:61-62
20. Drugas GT, Paidas CN, Yahanda AM et al (1991) Conjugated desferoxamine attenuates hepatic microvascular injury following ischemia-reperfusion. Circ Shock 34:278-283
21. Fleckenstein AE, Smith SL, Linseman KL et al (1991) Comparison of the efficacy of mechanistically different antioxidants in the rat hemorrhagic shock model. Circ Shock 35: 223-230
22. Zhao W, Richardson JS, Mombourquette MJ et al (1995) An in vitro EPR study of the free radical scavenging actions of the lazaroid antioxidants U-74500 A and U-78517 F. Free Radic Biol Med 19:21-30
23. Johnson G, Lefer AM (1990) Protective effects of a novel 21-aminosteroid during splanchnic artery occlusion shock. Circ Shock 30:155-164
24. Inove M, Saito Y, Hirata E et al (1987) Regulation of redox states of plasma proteins by metabolism and transport of glutathione and related compounds. J Prot Chem 6:207-225
25. Meister A (1988) Glutathione metabolism and its selective modification. J Biol Chem 263: 17205-17208
26. Robinson MK, Ahn MS, Rounds JD (1992) Parenteral glutathione monoester enhaucas tissue antioxidant stores. JPEN J Parenter Enteral Nutr 16:413-418
27. Griffith OW, Meister A (1985) Origin and turnover of mitochondrial glutathione. Proc Natl Acad Sci USA 82:4668-4672
28. Hagen TM, Yee AWT, Jones DP (1988) Glutathione uptake and protection against oxidative injury in isolated kidney cells. Kidney Int 34:74-81
29. Falsini S, Cellai MP, Angiolini P et al (1994) Glutatione ridotto e L-cisteina nello shock endotossinico nel ratto. Minerva Anestesiol 60:413-418
30. Novelli GP, Falsini S, Bracciotti G (1991) Exogenous glutathione increases endurance to muscle effort in mice. Pharmacol Res 23:149-155
31. Scardi S, Rossi R, Pieraccioli E et al (1993) Reduced glutathione prevents lipid peroxidation as expressed by ethane exhalation during aortic surgery in man. Minerva Anestesiol 59:S2-215

32. Mediati RD, Girardi G, Rossi R et al (1993) Glutathione administration prevents the increase of extravascular lung water during ischemia and reperfusion in man. Minerva Anestesiol 59: S2-214

33. Paternostro E, Scardi S, Pellegrini G (1993) Lung lipoperoxidative stress during hyperoxic anaesthesia: protective effects of reduced glutathione. Minerva Anestesiol 59:S2-213

34. Novelli GP, Casali R, Bonizzoli M et al (1993) Aumento della permeabilità capillare provocato dall'endotossina: protezione con antiossidanti e glutatione. Minerva Anestesiol 59: 211-216

35. Di Filippo A, Paternostro E, Scardi S et al (1992) Insufficienza multipla d'organo sperimentale nel ratto: effetti protettivi del glutatione ridotto. Acta Anaesth Ital 43:358-369

36. Novelli GP, Melani AM, Consales G et al (1994) Antioxidant drugs in cerebral and spinal ischemia. Minerva Anestesiol 60:543-546

37. Novelli GP (1990) I radicali liberi nello shock e in alcuni quadri ad esso correlati. In Albano et al (eds): Radicali liberi in patologia - nuovi orientamenti patogenetici e strategie cliniche. Prag 6-9 December 1990

38. Aruoma OI, Halliwell B, Hoey BM (1989) The antioxidant properties of n-acetyl-cysteine. Free Radic Biol Med 6:593-597

39. Bernard GR (1991) N-acetylcysteine in experimental and clinical acute lung injury. Am J Med 91:S3 54-59

40. Spies CD, Reinahart K, Witt I et al (1994) Influence of n-acetylcysteine on indirect indicators of tissue oxygenation in septic shock patients: results from a prospective, randomized, double-blind study. Crit Care Med 22:1738-1746

41. Zimmerman JJ (1992) Radical viewpoints in critical illness. Crit Care Med 20:448-449

42. Yamauchi N, Watanabe N, Kuriyama H et al (1990) Suppressive effects of intracellular glutathione on hydroxyl radical production induced by tumor necrosis factor. Int J Cancer 46: 884-888

Posttrauma Oxygen Debt and Its Metabolic Consequences

J.H. Siegel

Oxygen debt and metabolic acidosis as the consequence of hypovolemic ischemic shock

Oxygen is the critical carbon acceptor in the generation of energy from metabolic fuel substrates. Consequently, oxygen consumption is a closely regulated phenomenon in all animal cells and more complex higher organisms. Following injury, or during severe sepsis, oxygen consumption increases, especially when these conditions are associated with an increase in body temperature. Moreover, the host-defense response consequent on these conditions changes both the quality and the quantity of the metabolic response. Over the years, evidence has been accumulated that the host-defense response pattern can be initiated by a number of different etiologic agents. These range from sterile inflammatory mediators or tissue injury, anamestic immunologic challenges, bacterial endotoxin administration and/or sepsis, and hypovolemic ischemic shock produced either by blood loss, third space fluid dislocations from the circulatory system, or cardiac failure. In these latter conditions, oxygen delivery is restricted by a decreased flow. As a consequence, oxygen consumption decreases, falling below the oxidative requirement of various organ metabolic processes (Fig. 1). In this concept, a decrease in oxygen consumption occurring after the loss of perfusion to metabolic tissues, which reduces delivery below the baseline level of oxygen consumption, produces a *deficit* in oxygen consumption, which is the accumulating difference over time between the organism's oxygen demand and the actual oxygen consumption permitted. This deficit is known as the *oxygen debt* (O_2 debt).

In this presentation, we will deal with the specific circumstance in which oxygen debt accumulates during hemorrhagic hypovolemic ischemic shock associated with posttraumatic blood loss. Both human and experimental hypovolemic shock have been studied extensively as functions of volume loss and the consequent reduction in arterial perfusion pressure (mean arterial blood pressure). Only recently have animal models and human studies been carried out which attempt to quantify this process in terms of oxygen debt (1-3). An example of the manner in which oxygen debt accumulates during hemorrhagic hypovolemic ischemic shock is shown in Fig. 2.

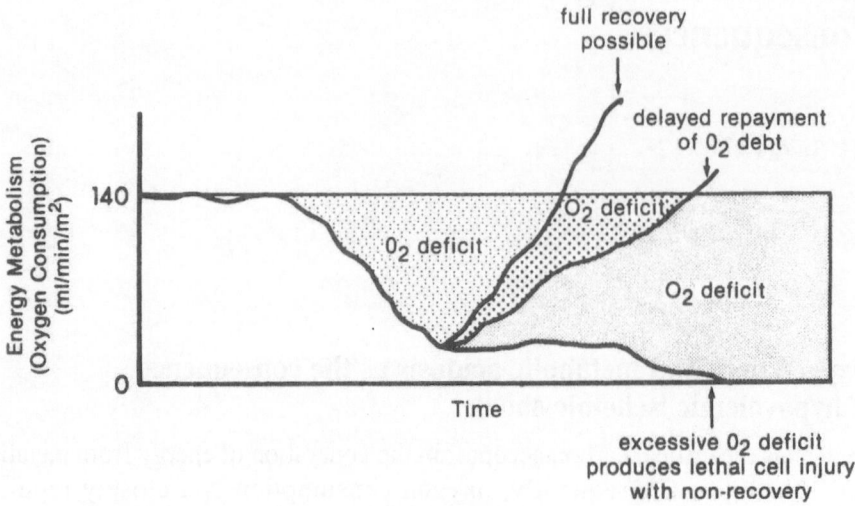

Fig. 1. Diagram of concept of oxygen debt and its consequences. From (2)

#32801 blood pressure, heart rate, debt during hemorrhage 01-17-95
(colloid/blood resuscitation)

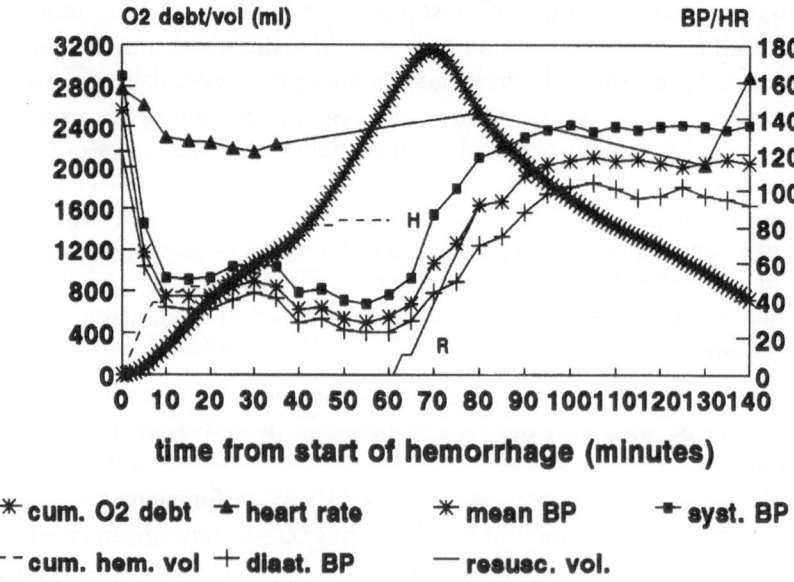

Fig. 2. Accumulation of oxygen debt in experimental hypovolemic hemorrhagic shock as a function of blood loss over a 60 min period, with repayment of O_2 debt as resuscitation is carried out with colloid (plasmanate) at 60% of the shed blood volume (first 10 min) followed by return 60% the shed blood (second 10 min). From (13)

This example, taken from a canine model of progressive blood volume loss, shows the increase in oxygen debt which is associated with hemorrhage of 66% of the total estimated blood volume over a 60-min period. In this figure, the initial rapid hemorrhage occurring in the first 10 min, withdrew approximately 30% of the blood volume and was associated with a fall in blood pressure to shock levels. Hemorrhage then continued over the remaining 50 minutes, at a slower rate, so that by 60 min just prior to resuscitation, the blood pressure was 45/30 mmHg. At 60 min, the resuscitation was begun using a clinically relevant protocol to a total volume of 120% of the 60-min shed blood volume. The first half of resuscitation equal to 60% of the total shed blood volume was given over a 10-min period with a nonhemoglobin containing solution of plasmanate; in the second half of the resuscitation 60% of the shed blood volume was returned. The blood also was infused over a 10-min period, for a total of 20 min of volume resuscitation (begun at 60 min posthemorrhage and lasting until 80 min posthemorrhage).

The important point demonstrated by this example of hypovolemic hemorrhagic shock is that during the entire period of hemorrhage, once perfusion has dropped below a critical level, there is a net deficit between oxygen delivery and metabolic demands. As a result, the oxygen debt continues to rise in a progressive fashion, reaching a maximum debt of 2.941 ml O_2 (106 ml O_2 per kilogram of body weight) at the time of hemorrhage cessation. It is important to note that even though blood withdrawal is episodic, *once a critical level of perfusion deficit has been reached, the oxygen debt continues to rise*. Equally important is that during the initial 10-min period of resuscitation with *non-blood* containing solution, during a time when 60% of the shed volume is returned and while blood pressure is rising, *the oxygen debt continues to rise* to nearly 3200 ml O_2 (117 ml O_2 per kg of body weight) in spite of the fact more than half of the total volume loss has been repaid. Only during the second 10 min of resuscitation, when oxygen carrying red cell mass is being returned and effective perfusion of the previously ischemic body tissues is achieved, does the oxygen debt fall as the blood pressure returns to adequate levels. Moreover, once perfusion has been restored to an adequate level by blood volume restitution, to a maximum of 120% of the total shed blood volume, oxygen debt continues to fall without further transfusion (if there is no further blood loss). Restoration of this level of blood volume with oxygen carrying capabilities permits the animal to repay 65% of the maximum oxygen debt by 80 min after the initiation of postshock blood volume resuscitation and to survive without organ failure sequalae, without further volume being given.

The reduction in oxygen metabolism induced by reduction in oxygen delivery below the level of mandatory oxygen consumption (the oxygen debt) is associated with a rise in those metabolic parameters of ischemia most directly related to induction of anaerobic metabolism (1). Since glucose cannot be effectively metabolized in the absence of oxygen, there is a rise in the arterial blood lactic acid (lactate) which occurs when hypoperfusion of muscle beds and liver and kidney reaches a critical level (Fig. 3). This forced anaerobic metabolism also reduces the oxidation of substrates other than glucose, and amino acids and other metabolic acids also accumulate in the plasma, together with phosphoric acid due to the breakdown of adenosine triphosphate (ATP) and its degradation products. The increase in total metabolic acids in the plasma resulting from the oxygen debt produces a net metabolic acidosis known as the base deficit.

As shown in Fig. 3, the base deficit (negative base excess) rises at a more rapid rate to a higher level than does the lactic acid. It appears to be a somewhat more sensitive index of the total magnitude of the oxygen debt-induced acute ischemic metabolic acidosis. When the oxygen debt is repaid with reperfusion of ischemic tissue, there is a fall in both the extracellular base deficit as well as the blood lactate, which parallels the reduction in oxygen debt and quantifies this debt repayment.

Finally, as shown conceptually in Fig. 1, to repay the ischemia-induced oxygen debt, the total metabolism of the host during the shock resuscitation period must increase not only to the preinjury level, but must also rise above this level in order to permit oxidation of unmetabolized substrates (1, 2). This produces an overshoot in oxygen consumption during the initial O_2 debt repayment phase, which is accompanied by a mandatory increase in the cardiovascular response so that there is a rise in cardiac output associated with a fall in peripheral vascular resistance due to shock mediator-induced arterial relaxation during the repayment period. This cardiovascular and metabolic response is known as the posttrauma hyperdynamic state (4).

If the cardiovascular mediated repayment in oxygen debt is achieved before the O_2 deficit has induced mechanisms leading to cell death, the anoxic cellular dysfunction is reversible, and the ischemia does not induce activation of destructive intracellular mechanisms such as the liberation of intracellular lysozymes. Under these circumstances, complete repayment of the oxygen debt during the hyperdynamic period occurs with an increase in oxygen consumption above the baseline and full recovery is possible (Fig. 1). If the oxygen debt progresses to the point where irreversible lethal cell injury has occurred to a preponderance of body cells, or to the cells of a critical organ required for the maintenance of the circulatory hyperdynamic state such as the heart, recovery is not possible. Consequently, oxygen consumption does not rise to repay the oxygen debt, since there are no longer viable cells and death of the organism occurs. In many cases, especially under clinical circumstances, there is delayed repayment of oxygen debt because of a failure to adequately restore oxygen delivery. Consequently, some cells in various organs are either irreversibly injured, or damaged to the point where their critical energy producing substrate metabolism and protein synthetic and detoxification mechanisms are altered, or anoxic brain injury occurs. This circumstance initiates a sequence of critical host defense mechanisms which leads to late organ failures as a sequela of the

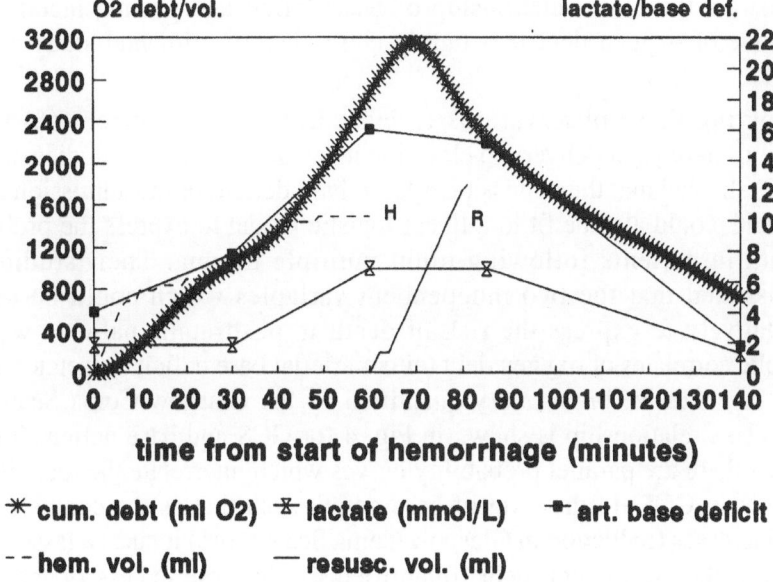

Fig. 3. Relationship of metabolic parameters of oxygen debt, lactic acid and base deficit (negative base excess) in experimental hypovolemic hemorrhagic shock and subsequent volume resuscitation. Legend as in Fig. 2

hypovolemic ischemic process, even though a hyperdynamic cardiovascular response may occur.

Clinical quantification of oxygen debt and its implications with regard to outcome and complications

Crowell and Smith (5) were the first individuals to demonstrate that a lethal dose (LD) curve could be constructed for oxygen debt and that the LD_{50} occurred at 120 ml/kg of oxygen debt. These studies were recently repeated in a more quantitative way by Dunham et al. (1) and showed a similar LD_{50} occurring at 113.5 ml/kg, or approximately the same level noted earlier by Crowell and Smith. However, the Dunham et al. studies (1) also showed that an accurate prediction of the probability of death (*P Death*) could be made from the magnitude of the oxygen debt. This probability of death increased in an exponential fashion as the oxygen debt rose, such that the LD_{25} occurred at 95.5

ml/kg, the LD_{50} at 113.5 ml/kg and the LD_{75} at 126.5 ml/kg. These data also showed that if the quantity of oxygen debt could be estimated and the rate of increasing O_2 ascertained, then at any given oxygen debt, the time remaining until the estimated LD_{50} would be reached could be approximated as a guide to the urgency of resuscitation. The second important aspect of this study was to demonstrate the close relationship of base deficit and plasma lactate to the magnitude of oxygen debt in a tightly controlled experimental study environment (1).

Applying these observations to man, Bakker and Vincent (6) related limitations in oxygen delivery to elevation in lactate. The earlier studies of Siegel et al. (7) showed that the admission arterial base deficit, or the admission arterial lactic acid, could also be fit to a linear logistic model to express the probability of death in patients following blunt multiple trauma. Their studies also demonstrated that the two independent variables which could be utilized quantitatively to express the risk of death in posttrauma patients were the metabolic correlates of oxygen debt (either arterial base deficit or lactate) and the degree of contusive brain injury quantified by the Glasgow Coma Scale score (GCS). This relationship is shown in Fig. 4 for GCS and base deficit. It can be seen that there are parallel probability curves which interrelate the magnitude of brain injury (GCS) to the level of base deficit such that as the contusive brain injury increases (reduction in Glasgow Coma Scale score) it takes a lesser shock-induced ischemic oxygen debt (quantified by the base excess or lactate) to produce a lethal effect. Thus, it would appear, both in animals and in man, that the use of the metabolic correlates of ischemic metabolism can be used to closely monitor the total body oxygen debt and to provide a means of hypovolemic shock *severity* prediction based on the *probability of death* which enables a quantitative estimate of the physiologic magnitude of the trauma insult to be made.

These studies have been further amplified by the observations of Rixen and Siegel (8), who demonstrated that the lowest level of base deficit or the highest level of lactic acid achieved during the immediate posttrauma period, which includes the admission or posttrauma surgical resuscitative events, was statistically significantly correlated with the likelihood of death. More important, they showed that the subsequent development of the more severe complications of the posttrauma organ failure sequence, i.e., the development of the adult respiratory distress syndrome (ARDS), or the later occurrence of severe septic metabolic complications could also be associated with the initial magnitude of oxygen debt, as reflected in its metabolic correlates. These data are further reinforced by the clinical studies of Siegel et al. (2, 4) and Shoemaker and associates (3) which have shown the need for a hyperdynamic response following posttrauma shock. The studies of Shoemaker et al. (3) are particularly important in this regard since they demonstrate a better outcome in a broad class of surgical patients in whom a hyperdynamic state was prospectively achieved compared to those in whom volume infusion and cardiovascular inotropic support were used

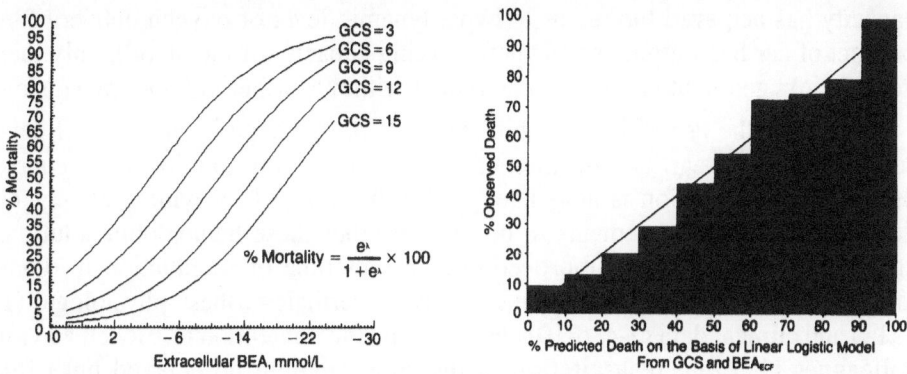

Fig. 4. Linear logistic model of the *probability of death (P Death)* in 185 patients following blunt trauma showing relationship of metabolic ischemic, indicated by base deficit *(BEA)*, and brain injury, indicated by Glasgow Coma Scale (GCS) score to *P Death*. Also shown is the accuracy of the *observed death rate* compared to the *predicted death rate* using this logistic model. From (7)

to maximize the hyperdynamic response only after signs of circulatory inadequacy became evident.

The current studies of Rixen et al. (8-10) have shown that the magnitude of the oxygen debt quantified by its metabolic parameters can also be correlated with the magnitude of the cytokine, histamine and nitric oxide responses seen in posttrauma patients. These data suggest that *the predisposing factor which sets the magnitude of the subsequent shock mediator response is the magnitude of the oxygen debt achieved during the immediate posttrauma period of hypovolemic ischemic shock.*

Therapeutic implications of oxygen debt

These data, both clinical and experimental, strongly suggest that it is not only the final magnitude of the postinjury hypovolemic ischemia-induced oxygen debt which is achieved, but it is also the rate of recovery from the oxygen debt which are the critical factors that predicate the incidence of severe organ failure complications, as well as the ultimate outcome of survival. A re-examination of the sequence of oxygen debt accumulation as shown in Fig. 2 demonstrates that once a critical level of hypoperfusion has been induced by withdrawal of blood volume the oxygen debt then proceeds *even though no further blood loss occurs,* or when the blood loss continues at only a very minimal rate. It can also be seen from this figure that even after total the blood hemorrhage has been stopped and resuscitation begun, the oxygen debt continues to rise. Only when a critical level of organ perfusion and oxygen delivery has been achieved, utilizing either blood or blood substitutes, does oxygen debt cease and O_2 debt repayment occur. Moreover, once a critical level of volume restitution and oxygen carrying capacity has achieved the requisite hyperdynamic level of oxygen delivery (the product of cardiac output and oxygen carrying capacity of the blood), only then does the oxygen debt continue to be repaid without further volume transfusion.

Studies of the use of hemoglobin solutions in this experimental model have suggested that the earlier utilization of an oxygen carrying solution in the course of volume resuscitation is associated with a more rapid repayment of oxygen debt (13). However, it remains to be seen whether these hemoglobin solutions can be shown to have an improved clinical outcome or a reduction in organ failure complications after traumatic shock. Nevertheless, these physiologic (1, 5, 13) and clinical data (2-4, 6-10) clearly refute the contention of Bickell and his colleagues (11) that resuscitation of the shock patient be delayed until full surgical control of hemorrhage is possible. Indeed, their own data when stratified by patient severity shows no statistically significant differences between their immediate and delayed resuscitation groups (12). While the clinical and experimental data cited earlier in this review do not imply that full volume restitution must be achieved, they do demonstrate that a critical level of reperfusion must occur if the rate of oxygen debt increase is to be arrested, especially if even a slow rate of recovery from oxygen debt is to be achieved. Continuing oxygen debt in the presence of hypovolemia following injury will continue to increase the degree of ischemia as reflected in its metabolic parameters of base deficit and lactate acidemia. Once a critical threshold for oxygen debt has been passed, then the *probability of death* appears to rise in an exponential fashion (1, 7). The specific relationship between oxygen debt and metabolic failure can be modified by ambient conditions such as a reduction in body temperature and perhaps may be beneficially influenced by agents which can protect against cellular anoxic injury or reperfusion superoxide production. *However, the ultimate relationship between oxygen debt and cell, tissue, organ and patient death appears to be one of the iron rules of life, which can be violated by the physician or surgeon only at great peril to the patient.*

References

1. Dunham CM, Siegel JH, Weireter L et al (1991) Oxygen debt and metabolic acidemia as quantitative predictors of mortality and the severity of the ischemic insult in hemorrhagic shock. Crit Care Med 19:1-14
2. Siegel JH, Linberg S, Wiles III CE (1987) Therapy of low-flow shock states. In: Siegel JH (ed) Trauma: emergency surgery and critical care. Churchill-Livingston, New York, pp 201-284
3. Showmaker WC, Apple PL, Kram HB et al (1988) Prospective trial of supranormal values of survivors as therapeutic goals in high-risk surgical patients. Chest 94:1176-1186
4. Siegel JH, Farrell EJ, Miller et al (1973) Cardiorespiratory interactions as determinants of survival and the need for respiratory support in human shock states. J Trauma 13:602-619
5. Crowell JW, Smith EE (1964) Oxygen deficit and irreversible hemorrhagic shock. Am J Physiol 206:313-316
6. Bakker J, Vincent JL (1991) The oxygen supply dependency phenomenon is associated with increasing lactate levels. J Crit Care 6:152-159

7. Siegel JH, Rivkind AC, Dalal SA, Goodarzi S (1990) Early physiologic predictors of injury severity and death in blunt multiple trauma. Arch Surg 125:498-508
8. Rixen D, Siegel JH (1995) Oxygen debt as the precursor stimulus to posttrauma organ failure syndromes and sepsis (work in progress)
9. Rixen D, Siegel JH, Abu-Salih A et al (1995) Physiologic state severity classification as an indicator of posttrauma cytokine response. Shock 4:27-36
10. Rixen D, Siegel JH, Bertolini M, Espina N (1995) Histamine, cytokine and metabolic relationships in posttrauma critical illness. Surgery (submitted for publication)
11. Bickell WH, Wall MJ, Pepe PE et al (1995) Immediate versus delayed fluid resuscitation for hypotensive patients with penetrating torso injuries. N Engl J Med 331:1105-1109
12. Siegel JH (1995) Immediate versus delayed fluid resuscitation in patients with trauma. Letter to the Editor. N Engl J Med 332:681
13. Siegel JH, Fabian M, Smith JA, Costantino D (1995) The use of a recombinant hemoglobin solution in reversing lethal hemorrhagic, hypovolemic, oxygen debt ischemic shock. J Trauma

CHEST IMAGING IN THE ICU

Lung Disease in the ICU:
A Difficult Diagnostic Challenge

L.R. GOODMAN

Introduction

Determining the cause of lung disease in the critically ill is often a frustrating task. Numerous primary diseases may affect the lung and systemic disorder (e.g. sepsis, ARDS) may affect the lung independently or may superimpose on a pre-existing lung disorder. Evaluation is also made more difficult by various therapeutic maneuvers (e.g. artificial ventilation, tracheal bronchial toilet) which alter the appearance of the radiograph. Despite these problems, an understanding of both the timing, radiographic appearance, and progression of these lesions is extremely helpful in sorting out the various etiologies. A constant dialogue between the radiologist and clinical team is required to maximize information and minimize the number of imaging procedures (1).

The portable radiograph, for all its shortcomings, remains the mainstay of ICU imaging (2). However, fast CT scanners (< 2 s/scan) provide images that are often very helpful in difficult diagnostic cases.

Aspiration pneumonitis

The varied appearance of aspiration syndromes is best understood by knowledge of the substance aspirated. Toxic fluids, bland fluids and particles, and infected secretions may all be aspirated by the obtunded patient but each presents a different clinical and radiological course (3, 4).

The prototype for toxic fluid aspiration is the inhalation of gastric fluid with a pH of < 2.5 (Mendelsohn's syndrome). Within a matter of seconds, the aspirated acid crosses both the alveolar epithelium and the capillary endothelium, causing a capillary permeability edema. Symptoms are present within minutes and radiographic evidence of consolidation is usually present within a few hours. Consolidation usually progresses for the first twenty-four hours, followed by a brief period of stability. By 48 to 72 h, there is usually evidence of some clearing. Depending on the severity of the pneumonitis, total clearing may take a week or two. The lung pattern may vary from diffuse interstitial thickening to focal dense airspace consolidation. Although the right lower lobe is most frequently affected, distribution is variable. Following massive aspiration, the pneumonitis may progress to a full-blown ARDS.

Approximately a quarter of patients with aspiration pneumonitis develop secondary infection, usually with aerobic gram negative bacilli or staphylococcus. This is usually evidenced by an area of worsening consolidation, 3 to 7 days after injury, at a time when the radiograph should be improving. Pleural effusions associated with post aspiration pneumonias are often infected and may require tube drainage. If the infection does not show evidence of clearing within a few days of antibiotic administration, an abscess or loculated empyema should be sought by CT scan.

The aspiration of neutral pH gastric contents (food, blood, etc.) usually causes some tracheobronchial irritation but does not cause a chemical pneumonitis. The lungs may be normal or show evidence of some consolidation due to flooding. Particles or clot may cause focal atelectasis. In general, with prompt removal of the obstructing material, the lung returns to normal rapidly.

Infected secretions may be aspirated from the sinuses, the pharynx, or the tracheobronchial tree. The radiographic appearance may vary from a focal indolent basilar consolidation to rapidly progressive bilateral symmetrical, consolidation often mimicking pulmonary edema in both its distribution, its pattern, and its rapidity. This diffuse pattern is most frequently associated with pseudomonas and other aerobic gram negative organisms. (see "Pneumonia", below).

The sinuses may be a source of aspirated secretions in patients with prolonged naso *or* orotracheal intubation. Nosocomial pneumonia is four times more common in intubated patients with proven purulent sinusitis. Sinus CT's are considerably more sensitive than facial radiography in demonstrating mucosal thickening and fluid. However, aspiration and culture of the sinus secretions are necessary because the majority of cultures do not grow significant organisms (5).

It is a common misconception that patients with endotracheal tubes, tracheostomy tubes, and nasogastric tubes are protected from aspiration. In fact, tracheal intubation interferes with glottic and nasogastric intubation interferes with the gastroesophageal closure. Patients with tracheostomies have twice the incidence of aspiration as patients with endotracheal tubes (6).

Atelectasis

This is by far the most common cause of parenchymal consolidation in the ICU. Linear, subsegmental, or segmental, consolidation and volume loss usually presents no diagnostic difficulty. Patchy airspace consolidation without obvious volume loss is frequently confused with more important causes of consolidation such as pneumonia or infarction. Primary atelectasis usually appears rapidly and may change rapidly from film to film, especially following physical therapy. It should be suspected in any patient with recent abdominal or thoracic surgery, obtundation, thoracic trauma, or a neuromuscular disorder such as myasthenia gravis. Atelectasis, of course, may be associated with many more significant lung diseases (e.g. pulmonary embolism, pneumonia, etc.) (1).

In the bedridden patient, atelectasis is most frequent in the dorsal, dependent segments. The gravitational force of the more ventral lung diminishes dependent aeration and secretions tend to pool dorsally. Retrocardiac atelectasis is particularly difficult to evaluate through the opacity of the heart. Clues to diagnosis include loss of the diaphragmatic and descending aortic shadow, a homogeneous opacification behind the heart obscuring the pulmonary vessels, and depression of the left hilum or left main stem bronchus. Cephalad angulation of the X-ray beam may give a false impression of lower lobe consolidation. CT scans are considerably more sensitive in diagnosing dependent atelectasis. In everyday practice, one should assume that every bedridden and postoperative patient has dependent atelectasis, whether visible or not. CT is not usually required.

The presence or absence of an air bronchogram may predict the cause of atelectasis, the approximate site of obstruction, and the appropriate course of therapy. If an air bronchogram is clearly seen within a focal area of consolidation, this strongly suggests that the atelectasis or consolidation is not due to obstruction of a major bronchus. Conversely, the absence of an air bronchogram in an area of consolidation suggests mucous filling the bronchus. The latter will benefit markedly form tracheobronchial sectioning or bronchoscopy whereas the former will show minimal benefit.

Pneumonia

Hospital acquired or nosocomial infection is an infection that appears beyond the third day of hospitalization. Infection occurs in approximately 10% of ICU patients and approximately 30%-60% of patients with ARDS. This is generally associated with a mortality of approximately 25% in the general ICU population, a mortality rate of approximately 50% in the ARDS population, and a mortality rate of approximately 90% when multiple organ failure is present. Staphylococcus and aerobic gram negative bacilli are most frequent. Polymicrobial infection is very frequent.

Even the most basic of pulmonary disease, pneumonia, is not easily diagnosed in the ICU patient (7-9). The hallmarks of pneumonia such as fever, pathogens in the sputum, altered white blood cell count, and X-ray evidence of consolidation may be present for multiple other reasons and lead to the inappropriate diagnosis of pneumonia. A fever may be present from pneumonia, atelectasis, aspiration, or numerous extrathoracic causes. Pathogens in the sputum are almost universal following prolonged hospitalization or intubation. A heavy growth of pathogens, plus bacteria within the white blood cells on smear, is required to document intrapulmonary infection. Bronchoscopy using protected brushes greatly improves the accuracy of diagnosis. An elevated or depressed white count may have multiple nonpulmonary etiologies. Similarly, parenchymal consolidation is most often due to a noninfectious cause such as atelectasis, aspiration pneumonitis, pulmonary edema, or infarction. Although infectious pulmonary infiltrates may worsen rapidly over several days, their progression is seldom as rapid as atelectasis, aspiration pneumonitis, or pulmonary edema.

In patients with ARDS, a diagnosis of superimposed pneumonia is even more difficult. Fever, altered white blood cell count, and positive sputum cultures for pathogens is present in the vast majority of both infected and noninfected patients. A markedly asymmetrical chest X-ray is a modest predictor of the presence of pneumonia.

Pleural effusion associated with hospital acquired pneumonias present additional diagnostic problems. There are many etiologies other than the infection that may be responsible for the effusion. However, effusions due to nosocomial infection are potentially serious problems since empyemas and bronchopleural fistulas are common. On portable radiographs, it is often difficult to differentiate pulmonary consolidation from loculated pleural effusions or to document the presence or absence of lung abscesses. CT is an invaluable adjunct in both diagnosing the various components and planning therapy.

Pulmonary edema and ARDS

Both diseases will be reviewed in depth elsewhere. However, because of pre-existing lung disease, many patients with cardiac and noncardiac edema, present with unilateral or asymmetrical edema patterns that are more suggestive of a focal pulmonary inflammatory process than edema (10). The possibility of edema should always remain in one's differential diagnosis whenever there is diffuse pulmonary disease.

Pleural disease

The detection of pneumothorax may be difficult. On the supine radiograph, air in the pleural space may be visible along the lateral chest wall, along the diaphragm, or along the medial lung surface, simulating a pneumomediastinum. Air collecting anterolaterally causes the lateral diaphragmatic area over the liver or spleen to appear radiolucent (deep sulcus sign) (11). A lateral decubitus film with the side in question elevated is often helpful when upright radiographs cannot be obtained (12).

Pleural effusions are very difficult to detect and quantitate on portable radiographs. Approximately 30% of patients believed to have effusions have no demonstrable effusion on decubitus radiographs and about 30% of radiographs without signs of effusion have demonstrable effusions on decubitus films. The most sensitive but least specific signs include blunting of the costophrenic angle and indistinct diaphragmatic shadow (13). Decubitus radiographs, ultrasound, or CT all provide better detection and quantitation when clinically important.

Pulmonary insufficiency and the normal chest radiograph

Acute respiratory failure is the sudden inability of the respiratory system to provide adequate arterial oxygenation and adequate carbon dioxide elimination for the patient's metabolic level. Although seldom seen as completely separate disorders, carbon dioxide retention is most frequently due to inadequate ventilation, whereas hypoxia is usually secondary to impaired gas exchange. Respiratory insufficiency is frequently associated with underlying cardiopulmonary disease (e.g. COPD, fibrosis) which further complicates diagnosis and treatment and increases both mortality and morbidity.

Potentially life-threatening pulmonary insufficiency may be present in the face of a normal radiograph. This combination suggests several diagnostic possibilities. In patients with central nervous system disease, neuromuscular disorders, and most drug overdoses, the initial and subsequent radiographs remain normal unless a secondary complication, such as atelectasis, aspiration or pneumonia, develops. Patients with severe COPD frequently have potentially fatal pulmonary insufficiency with little or no radiographic evidence of an acute process superimposed. Subtle pulmonary edema is often enough to cause great distress in these already compromised patients but is often difficult to detect radiographically. Careful examination of the radiographs and comparison with multiple previously radiographs will often allow one to diagnose subtle edema. Edema patterns are often atypical but tend to repeat in a given patient. In other disorders, such as pulmonary embolus, sepsis, smoke inhalation, and respiratory distress syndrome, the speed at which the radiograph turns "positive" may help confirm or refute the initial impression.

References

1. Goodman LR, Putman C (eds) (1992) Critical care imaging, 3rd edn. Saunders, Philadelphia
2. Wandtke JC (1994) Bedside chest radiography. Radiology 190:1
3. Bartlett JG, Gorbach SL (1975) The triple threat of aspiration pneumonia. Chest 68:560-566
4. Shifrin R, Choplin R (1996) Aspiration in patients in critical care units. In: Goodman LR, Kuzo RS (eds). Radiol Clin North Am (in press)
5. Holzapfel L, Chevret S, Madinier G, Ohen F, Demingeon G, Coupry A, Chaudet M (1993) Influence of long-term oro- or nasotracheal intubation on nosocomial maxillary sinusitis and pneumonia: results of a prospective, randomized, clinical trial. Crit Care Med 21(8): 1132-1138

6. Elpern H, Jacobs ER, Bone RC (1987) Incidence of aspiration in tracheally intubated adults. Heart Lung 26:527-531
7. Lefcoe MS, Fox GA, Leasa DJ et al (1994) Accuracy of portable chest radiography in the critical care setting: diagnosis of pneumonia based on quantitative cultures obtained from protected brush catheter. Radiology 192:882
8. Pingleton S (1988) Complications of acute respiratory failure. Am Rev Resp Dis 137: 1463-1493
9. Winer-Muram HT, Rubin SA, Ellis JV, Jennings SG, Arheart KL, Wunderink RG, Leeper KV, Meduri GU (1993) Pneumonia and ARDS in patients receiving mechanical ventilation: diagnostic accuracy of chest radiography. Radiology 188:479
10. Morgan PW, Goodman LR (1991) Pulmonary edema and adult respiratory distress syndrome. In: Müller NL (ed). Radiol Clin North Am 29(5):943-963
11. Tocino I, Westcott, J (1996) Barotrauma. In: Goodman LR, Kuzo RS (eds). Radiol Clin North Am (in press)
12. Beres RA, Goodman LR (1993) Pneumothorax: detection with upright versus decubitus radiography. Radiology 186:19-26
13. Ruskin JA, Gurney JW, Thorsen MK, Goodman LR (1987) Detection of pleural effusions on supine chest radiographs. AJR 148:681-683

PULMONARY OEDEMA

A Window with a View of the Water

E.N.C. MILNE

All organs in the body – with one singular exception, the lungs – are radiodense and their intra and extravascular fluid content cannot be visualized on plain films. Conventional angiograms, and CT or MRI angiography can reveal the *intra*vascular volume in all organs but none of these techniques can differentiate between intra and extravascular water. In contrast, the air content of the lungs outlines with excellent clarity, not only the pulmonary vascular bed (from which we can derive pulmonary blood volume), but also the largest systemic vessels in the body (the "vascular pedicle" described below), from which we derive the intravascular systemic blood volume and the vascular and bronchial walls (from which we can derive the pulmonary extravascular volume). The lungs therefore act as a translucent window through which we have an excellent view of

1. Pulmonary intravascular water (pulmonary blood volume)
2. Pulmonary extravascular water (pulmonary oedema, pleural effusions)
3. Systemic intravascular water (systemic blood volume)
4. Systemic extravascular water (soft tissue oedema, ascites)

The chest radiograph is the best available tool for detecting and quantifying intra and extravascular water and for determining the etiology of excess water (oedema). Since pulmonary oedema can *only* be detected at its earliest stages by the chest radiograph (not by auscultation or by indicator dilution techniques) (1) oedema should be defined in radiologic terms, i.e. as "a general or regional excess of extravascular water detected on the chest radiograph". There are only three categories of pulmonary oedema: 1) hydrostatic, 2) "injury" oedema, and 3) allergic oedema. The phrase "injury" oedema is preferable to the more commonly used term "capillary permeability oedema" because it is normal for all capillaries to be permeable and this permeability varies greatly according to their histologic structure, e.g. glomerular capillaries are very permeable and brain capillaries quite impermeable. The term "non-cardiac oedema" is also very frequently used to mean injury oedema and this has caused (and is still causing) great confusion in the world literature because there are many causes of non-cardiac oedema which are *not* due to injury oedema, e.g. renal failure, overhydration, near-drowning, high altitude, reexpansion oedema, negative pressure oedema from croup, and laryngospasm, etc. (several of these are purely hydrostatic and others, such as high altitude and neurogenic oedema are mixed hydrostatic and injury). It is therefore inappropriate and very confusing to use the phrase "non-cardiac oedema" as if this implied only injury oedema. The desirable terms to use are: 1) hydrostatic oedema, 2) injury oedema, 3) allergic oedema, and 4) mixed oedemas.

The chest radiograph is now the "gold standard" for detecting and quantifying pulmonary oedema and for measuring changes in systemic blood volume (2).

Our "window" on body water can be used:

1. For detecting and quantifying pulmonary oedema
2. For detecting changes in circulating (systemic and pulmonary) blood volume
3. For detecting increased systemic extravascular water
4. For differentiating between hydrostatic and injury oedema
5. For determining the etiology of hydrostatic oedema

We will take the above tasks in sequence and illustrate how each can be done.

Detection and quantification of pulmonary oedema (hydrostatic)

Excess water passing out of the "loose" junctions of the pulmonary capillaries, secondary to increased transmural pressure (hydrostatic and/or oncotic), flows immediately into the interstitium of the lung. Since hydrostatic oedema is non-viscous it flows freely a) medially, into the peribronchovascular sheaths to cause vessel marginal blurring and peribronchial "cuffs", and b) laterally to cause septal lines (less frequent) (Fig. 1). Because hydrostatic oedema flows freely, it follows any gravitational gradient and accumulates increasingly in the dependent portion of the lungs. When the oedema reaches the pleura, the increased fluid pressure within the lung interstitium causes it to pass through the visceral pleura (which has very high hydraulic conductivity) resulting in pleural effusions (3). If the interstitial fluid continues to accumulate, the interstitial "sump" will be filled to a point at which pressure will rise abruptly (interstitial tamponade) and the oedema will then pass through the "tight" alveolar junction cells to cause alveolar oedema (4). From this behavior derive the four simple factors we need, to quantify lung water: a) the sharpness of the hila and large vessels, b) the presence of peribronchial cuffs, c) the lucency of the lungs, d) the ability to see small background vessels (at the bases) (Table 1). In order to remove subjectivity from the quantification process, the table is in the form of questions to be answered (e.g. concerning the hilum and large vessels, are they "excessively sharp," – is there "definite blurring" – or a "whiteout", etc.). Observers can be taught to use this table accurately within only minutes - it does not require extensive radiologic experience. We have correlated the results of these assessments with the most sophisticated indicator dilution technique and the correlation coefficient is .82, $p < .0001$ (5). The radiograph consistently detects

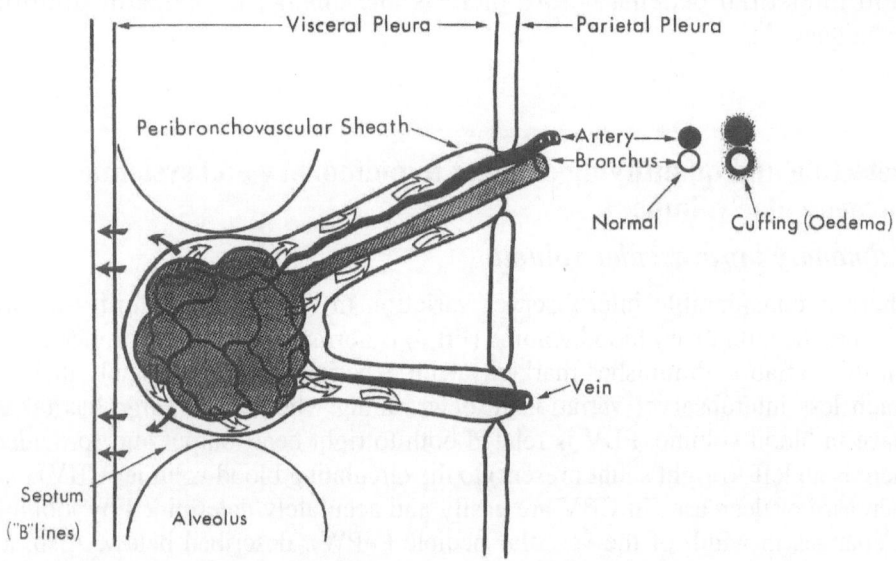

Fig. 1. *Open arrows*, water passing medially from the pulmonary capillaries into the peribronchovascular sheath causing cuffing and blurred vessel margins (see end-on view of artery and bronchus). *Closed curved arrows*, water passing laterally to form septal ('B' lines) and crossing the visceral pleura (*straight arrows*) to form pleural effusions

Table 1. Table for quantifying oedema

EVLW ml/ liter lung at T.L.C.			Border-line Inter-stitial Edema	Mild Inter-stitial Edema	Moderate Inter-stitial Edema	Severe Inter-stitial Edema	Question-able Alveolar Edema	Mild Alveolar Edema	Moder-ately Severe Alveolar Edema	Severe Alveolar Edema	Fulmi-nating Alveolar Edema
	20–40	40–50	50–60	60–70	70–80	80–90	90–100	100–120	120–140	140–180	180 plus
Hilum and Large Vessels	Excess-ively sharp	Normal defini-tion	Question-able blurring	Definite blurring (mild degree)	Definite blurring (mild degree)	Definite blurring (moderate degree)	Definite blurring (moderate to severe)	Definite blurring (severe)	Becoming obscured by alveolar filling	Only larger vessels and hilum seen	Hilum and large vessels obscured ("white-out")
Cuffing	Defin-itely none	Defin-itely none	Defin-itely none	Question-able	Defin-itely present	Definite	Definite	Becoming obscured by alveolar filling	Becoming obscured by alveolar filling	Obscured. Question-able Air Bron-chograms	"White-out"
Lung Lucence	Excess-ively black	Normal black	Question-able loss of blackness	Definite minimal greying	Changed from black to dark grey	Grey	Grey/ white	Grey/ white	White (regional)	White (exten-sive)	"White-out"
Small (subseg-mental) Vessels	Excess-ively well seen but sparse	Well-seen normal	Well-seen	Question-able loss of visi-bility	Definite early loss of visi-bility	Vessels difficult to make out	Vessels very difficult to make out	Vessels obscured at bases	Vessels obscured at bases	Vessels obscured through-out lung	"White-out"

mild interstitial oedema before there is any change in indicator dilution techniques (1).

Detecting and quantifying changes in pulmonary and systemic intravascular volume

Pulmonary intravascular volume

There is considerable interobserver variation in film readers' ability to say whether the pulmonary blood volume (PBV) is normal, diminished, or increased, but this variation diminishes markedly with experience (6). Fortunately there is much less interobserver variation in determining whether a *change* has taken place in blood volume. PBV is related both to right heart output and (provided there is no left-to-right shunt present) to the circulating blood volume (CBV) (7). Increases or decreases in CBV are easily and accurately determined by looking at changes in width of the vascular pedicle (VPW), described below. Also, as PBV increases the usual gravitationally determined ratio between the size of the upper and lower lobe vessels progressively increases from approximately .6 in an oligemic lung, to .8 in a normovolemic lung to 1.0 in a hyperemic lung with a large pulmonary blood volume (4). The PBV and systemic blood volume usually increase or decrease concomitantly and any discrepancy between them indicates a pathologic dissociation between systemic and pulmonary blood volume, e.g. by a left-to-right shunt or by pericardial tamponade (8).

Systemic intravascular volume

Our "window" allows us to distinguish clearly the vascular pedicle of the heart (the leash of vessels entering the thoracic inlet, from which the heart virtually hangs, the "vascular pedicle"). These are the largest systemic veins and arteries in the body (Fig. 2). The width of the pedicle is closely related to the patient's build, i.e. large obese patients have wide pedicles and small thin patients have narrow pedicles (9); however, the most valuable relationship is between *change* in width of the vascular pedicle and change in the systemic blood volume (Fig. 3). This has a very high correlation (.93, $p < .001$) (8). A useful number to remember is that a change of 1.0 cm in VPW equals a change of 2.0 l in circulating blood volume.

Detecting increased systemic extravascular water

On most chest radiographs one or both chest walls can be clearly seen. The chest wall thickness, measured from the maximum outer convexity of the rib cage to the skin surface, is closely related to the quantity of systemic extravascular water.

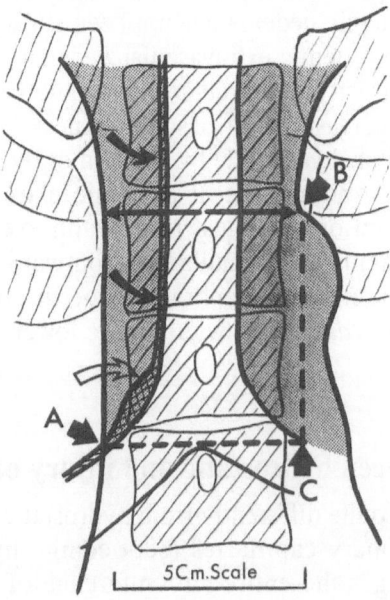

Fig. 2. The vascular pedicle: the right-hand border is all venous (right brachiocephalic vein and superior vena cava) and the left, all arterial (aorta and left subclavian artery). In the erect position, the distance from the midline to the right and left borders (*long arrows*) is equal, but in the supine position or with increasing blood volume the much more compliant left venous side will enlarge much more than the right. Note "golf-club" appearance: the "shaft" (*curved black arrows*) is the paratracheal stripe and the "head" (*open curved arrow*) is the vena azygos. Pedicle width is measured by placing the edge of a sheet of paper against A (where the right main bronchus crosses the SVC) and marking its upper border at B, where the left subclavian artery arises from the aorta

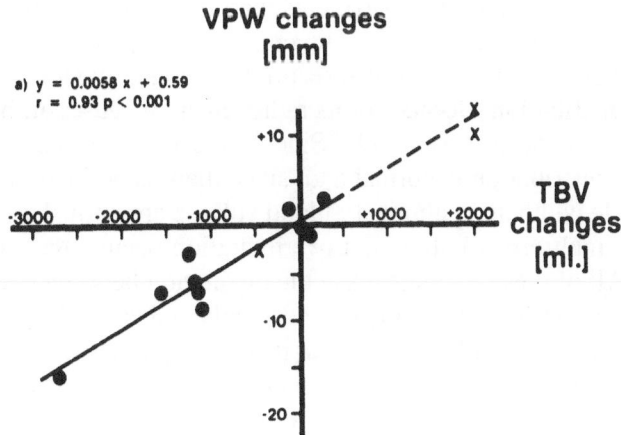

Fig. 3. Correlation between change in vascular pedicle width (*VPW*) measured on chest X-rays with change in total blood volume (*TBV*) measured radioisotopically. [A 1.0 cm change in VPW = a 2.0 l change in TBV. The two positive X^s indicate two volunteers given 2.0 l of saline in 20 min and the *minus X* indicates a volunteer who donated 0.5 l of blood]

These changes are frequently not looked for since the importance of the soft tissues in assessing systemic oedema has not been sufficiently emphasized. The first sign of developing systemic extravascular oedema is loss of the clear tissue density differences between the muscular planes and overlying fat in the chest wall, and the second, increasing soft tissue thickness (4). The thickness of the chest wall tissues is affected very little by rotation or by changing from the erect to the supine position. Another site of systemic extravascular fluid increase (ascites) can be detected on the chest radiograph even at an early stage by elevation of the diaphragms with simultaneous outward flaring of the lower rib cage - note that elevation of the diaphragms due to poor inspiratory effort is always accompanied by *reduction* in width of the lower rib cage.

Differentiating between hydrostatic and injury oedema

Injury oedema behaves quite differently from hydrostatic oedema - whatever it is that injures the pulmonary capillaries (septicemia, hypovolemic shock, fat embolism, etc.), damages the entire circumference of the capillary (the side facing the interstitial space - the thick side, and the thin side where the capillary endothelial and alveolar epithelial basement membranes are fused) - as a result, fluid will pass *simultaneously* into the interstitium and the alveolus and, unlike hydrostatic oedema, there will be no purely interstitial phase (4) (Fig. 4). The material exuded from the damaged vessels contains protein, cellular debris, red cells and actin molecules, and is quite viscid - as a result it cannot flow from the point at which it is generated and cannot therefore cause peribronchial cuffing, septal lines or pleural effusions (4). Prior claims that pleural effusions *are* found in injury lung oedema stem from somewhat artificial experiments in dogs and from observations made in ARDS patients who not only had injury oedema but were also overhydrated (10). CT scans confirm that pleural effusions do not occur in pure injury oedema. Because injury oedema cannot flow it has no gravitational distribution. Because of its radiodensity it causes air bronchograms very frequently (85% of cases) (11). Since there is no elevation of left atrial pressure, flow distribution is normal and, since there is no increase in CBV, the vascular pedicle width and pulmonary blood volume are normal, and in the early stages, before multiorgan failure and overhydration occurs, the soft tissues are also normal. All of these findings make the distinction between pure hydrostatic oedema and pure injury oedema easy and highly reliable (95% accuracy) (11) (Fig. 5). Injury oedema will not change in its intensity or its distribution once the initial damage has occurred and if the patient survives, will remain unchanged for *weeks* while it is being organized and the lung is being restructured. Any *new* superimposed changes are therefore not due to the injury oedema. This is a very simple but clinically very useful rule. The commonest superimposed change is the addition of *hydrostatic* oedema due to "optimization" of the patient's hydration. These mixed oedemas are very common but their etiology can often

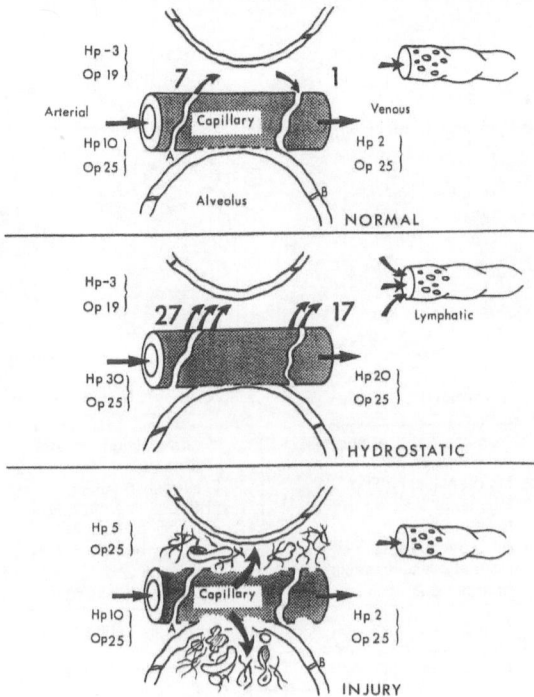

Fig. 4. Comparison of normal lung water, hydrostatic injury lung oedema. *Upper diagram:* in the normal subject the balance of Starling forces (*Hp*, hydrostatic pressure; *Op*, oncotic pressure) results in a small continual transudation of water (*black curved arrows*) from the arterial end of the capillary, into the interstitium. The water is reabsorbed partly at the venous end of the capillaries and partly by the lymphatics. *Middle diagram:* elevating left atrial pressure from 2 to 20 increases the outward driving force for water from 6 (7-1) to 44 (27 + 17). The lymphatics cannot handle the increase in water and interstitial oedema develops, but the alveoli will remain dry until the interstitial space "sump" is completely filled - at this point interstitial pressure rises and oedema is now pushed through the tight alveolar epithelial junctions (B) into the alveolus. *Lower diagram:* injury affects the capillaries circumferentially and water, containing protein, red cells, debris and actin molecules flows out into the interstitium and alveolus *simultaneously*. The very viscid fluid cannot flow freely and there is little increase in lymph flow

be sorted out by studying sequential films, e.g. if a patient on day 1 or 2 has pure injury oedema and then begins to develop peribronchial cuffing, increased vascular pedicle width and increased soft tissue thickness, he clearly has superimposed hydrostatic oedema (12).

Determining the etiology of hydrostatic oedema

Every type of hydrostatic oedema has its own distinguishing characteristics, e.g. in high altitude oedema the oedema only occurs in regions of *increased*

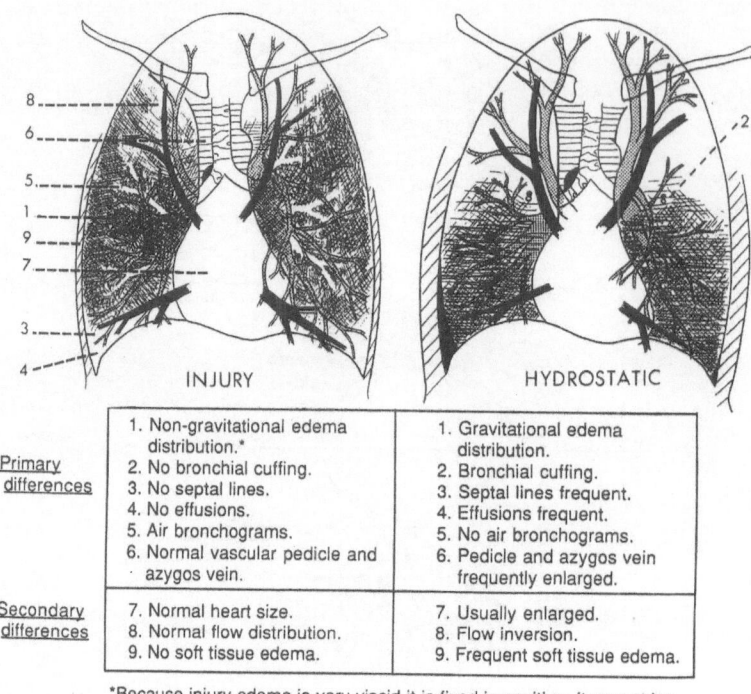

	INJURY	HYDROSTATIC
Primary differences	1. Non-gravitational edema distribution.* 2. No bronchial cuffing. 3. No septal lines. 4. No effusions. 5. Air bronchograms. 6. Normal vascular pedicle and azygos vein.	1. Gravitational edema distribution. 2. Bronchial cuffing. 3. Septal lines frequent. 4. Effusions frequent. 5. No air bronchograms. 6. Pedicle and azygos vein frequently enlarged.
Secondary differences	7. Normal heart size. 8. Normal flow distribution. 9. No soft tissue edema.	7. Usually enlarged. 8. Flow inversion. 9. Frequent soft tissue edema.

*Because injury edema is very viscid it is fixed in position, it cannot be affected by gravity and since it cannot flow through the interstitium it does not produce cuffing, septal lines or effusions

Fig. 5.

pulmonary blood flow – in neurogenic oedema abrupt evidence of pulmonary arterial hypertension develops – in oncotic oedema all of the signs of hydrostatic oedema are present (cuffing, septal lines, gravitational distribution, effusions, etc.). But the CBV, PBV and cardiac size are all normal and there is frequently evidence of ascites (11, 12). However, the etiologies that the clinician is usually interested in are cardiac failure vs renal failure or overhydration. The principal differentiating points are shown in Fig. 6. However, it is common in chronic cardiac failure for the kidneys to be involved (secondary to hypoperfusion), causing an increased circulating blood volume, and in these cases the separation of cardiac oedema from renal oedema is difficult (11). One useful differentiating point is that renal oedema frequently has a rather nodular/acinar appearance which is not seen in the pure hydrostatic oedema of cardiac failure or overhydration (12). Note also that while overhydration oedema is always accompanied by a wide vascular pedicle and large azygos vein, in late stage renal failure vasomotor tone is so high that the vascular pedicle does not enlarge. Therefore, when one sees a constellation of radiologic criteria which indicate overhydration or renal failure, but the pedicle is narrow, chronic renal failure is usually the aetiology (12).

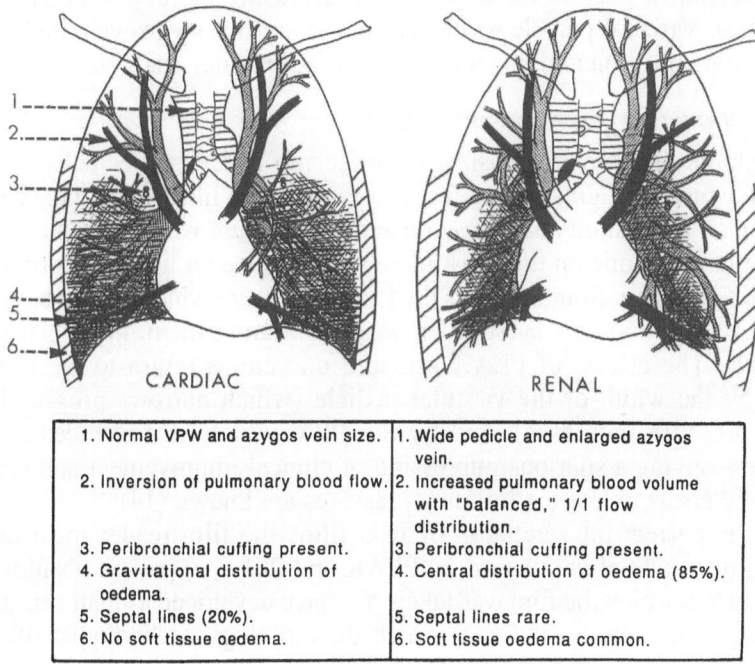

1. Normal VPW and azygos vein size.	1. Wide pedicle and enlarged azygos vein.
2. Inversion of pulmonary blood flow.	2. Increased pulmonary blood volume with "balanced," 1/1 flow distribution.
3. Peribronchial cuffing present.	3. Peribronchial cuffing present.
4. Gravitational distribution of oedema.	4. Central distribution of oedema (85%).
5. Septal lines (20%).	5. Septal lines rare.
6. No soft tissue oedema.	6. Soft tissue oedema common.

Fig. 6.

Since all of the above radiologic analyses are being made in the ICU where patients are frequently supine or partially supine and are very frequently on positive pressure ventilation, the effects of these factors must be known.

Effects of position

On oedema

In the supine position hydrostatic oedema will migrate to the dorsum of the lungs – but since the AP diameter of the lungs is much greater at the bases than at the apices there will still be much more oedema visible at the bases – just as in the erect position. Gravity has no effect on injury lung oedema which therefore does not change from the erect to the supine position.

On systemic and pulmonary blood volumes

If there is an *inversion* of pulmonary blood flow on the erect film (caused by elevated left atrial pressure), this inversion will *not* disappear in the supine position and can sometimes be exaggerated (13) because there is a 30% (approximate) increase in pulmonary blood volume in the supine position, which goes wherever the pulmonary vascular resistance is lowest, i.e. in the presence of flow inversion it goes to the upper lobes increasing the upper lobe/lower lobe flow ratios. Vascular pedicle width and the size of the azygos vein both increase in the supine position and this must be factored into our analyses.

Effects of positive pressure ventilation

Although the literature emphasizes the effects of PEEP, it is actually the PEAK pressure which is of greatest interest and value to the film reader, i.e. chest films are taken on inspiration not expiration and the pressure which must be correlated with the lung volume on the chest radiograph to give an index of compliance is the PEAK pressure. Similarly, it is the PEAK pressure which causes barotrauma, not PEEP (e.g. balloons burst when we are inflating them, not when they are deflated!). The effects of PEAK pressure on venous return to the thorax are shown by the width of the vascular pedicle (which narrows progressively as PEAK pressure increases), and by the PBV which also reduces as PEAK increases - giving a spurious impression of clinical improvement and leading to diagnostic errors unless the inflating pressures are known (14).

For the correct interpretation of ICU films the film reader must therefore know a) the mode of ventilation, b) PEAK and PEEP, c) patient position, d) the kV and mA at which the film was taken. We have developed a small self-adhesive label (approximately 6 x 2.5 cm) which the radiologic technologist fills in and attaches to the processed film (Fig. 7) (14). Without these data accurate interpretation of ICU films cannot be made.

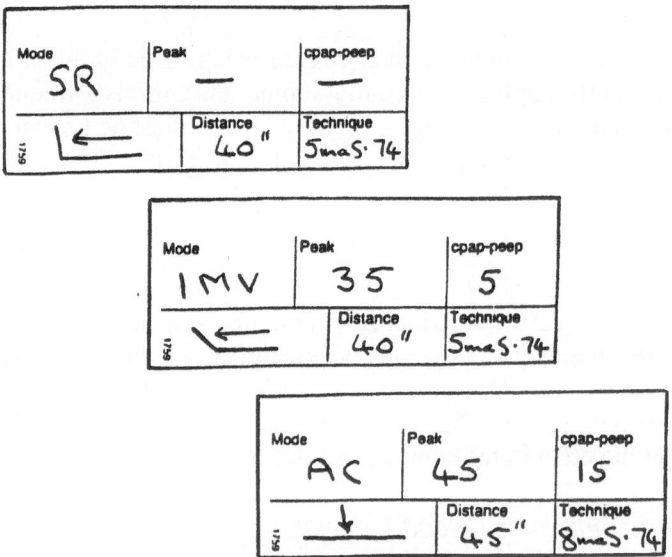

Fig. 7. Label attached to all ICU films. Three successive labels show a patient progressing from spontaneous respiration [SR] - sitting upright with a horizontal X-ray beam [⬑] to intermittent mandatory ventilation [IMV] at a PEAK of 35 and PEEP of 5 - now partially erect but beam still horizontal [⬑] to assist-control ventilation (AC) with a PEAK of 45 andPEEP of 15. Patient is now supine and the X-ray beam vertical [↓]

References

1. Pistolesi M, Giuntini C (1978) Assessment of extravascular lung water. Rad Clin North Arn 16(3):551-574
2. Staub NC, Hogg JC (1980) Conference report of a workshop on the measurement of lung water. Crit Care Med 8:752-759
3. Pistolesi M, Miniati M, Giuntini C (1989) State of the art: pleural liquid and solute exchange. Am Rev Respir Dis 140:825
4. Milne ENC, Pistolesi M (1993) Appearances of pulmonary oedema (anatomic and physiologic basis). Chapter 2, In: Reading the chest radiograph - a physiologic approach. Mosby, St. Louis
5. Pistolesi M, Miniati M, Milne ENC, Giuntini C (1991) Measurement of extravascular lung water. Intensive Care World 8(1):16-21
6. Weitzman S, Pocock WA, Hawkins DM, Barlow JB (1974) Observer variation in radiological assessment of pulmonary vasculature. Br Heart J 36:280-290
7. Milne ENC (Dec 1978) Some new concepts of pulmonary blood flow and volume. Rad Clin J North Am 16(3):515-536
8. Pistolesi M, Milne ENC, Miniati M (1984) The vascular pedicle of the heart, and the vena azygos. Part II. Acquired heart disease. Radiology 152(1):9-17
9. Milne ENC, Pistolesi M, Miniati M, Giuntini C (1984) The vascular pedicle of the heart and the vena azygos. Part I. The normal subject. Radiology 152(1):1-8
10. Aberle DR, Wiener-Kronish JP, Webb WR, Matthay MA (1988) Hydrostatic versus increased permeability edema: diagnosis based on criteria in critically ill patients. Radiology 168:73-79
11. Milne ENC, Pistolesi M, Miniati M, Giuntini C (1985) The radiologic distinction of cardiogenic and non-cardiogenic oedema. Am J Roentgenol 144:879-894
12. Milne ENC, Pistolesi M (1990) Pulmonary oedema - cardiac and noncardiac. In: Putman CE (ed) Diagnostic imaging of the lung. Dekker, New York (Lung biology in health and disease, vol 46)
13. Anderson CG (1964) Large upper lobe veins. J Coll Radiol Aust 8(3):214-219
14. Milne ENC (1986) A physiological approach to reading critical care unit films. J Thorac Imag 1(3):60-90

For anyone interested in a much fuller discussion of how physiologic data can be abstracted from the plain chest film we would recommend the book, "Reading the Chest Film - A Physiologic Approach" - authors Eric N.C. Milne and Massimo Pistolesi, published by Mosby Year Book, Inc., 1993.

Radiological Monitoring of Pulmonary Edema

M. Maffessanti, G. Berlot, P. Bortolotto

Introduction

The reliability of the radiograph of the chest (CXR) in assessing pulmonary edema remains a controversial matter (1-8). The assessment of edema on radiographs is usually obtained through a score based upon the presence and/or the degree of peculiar radiological signs (1-4, 6, 9).

The "gold standard" most widely used in the literature on humans to compare the radiological score with, is the double indicator-thermal dye technique (TDT) (1, 3, 4, 8, 10); the latter is reported to correlate well with gravimetric measurements both in animal and cadaver studies (8).

While it is universally accepted that CXR has a definite capacity to detect extravascular lung water (EVLW) (11, 12), several studies have pointed out its inability to quantitatively predict the exact amount of edema (1, 4), or its variations over time (1, 3, 10). Pulmonary overinflation due to mechanical ventilation with PEEP is reported as the main reason for radiological underestimation of EVLW; hypoinflation of the lungs, bronchial infection, and pleural effusion as reasons for overestimation (4, 10).

Other papers, however, show fair correlation between CXR and either TDT and other physiological parameters (5, 6, 9). They suggest that the usage of poor systems of scoring the radiographs together with limitations pertinent to the TDT itself may be responsible for some of the unsatisfying comparisons between the two, and that the radiographs are a reliable and highly cost-efficient tool in the clinical practice (2, 5, 9).

In this study we report the influence that different scoring systems have on the correlation between chest X-ray and thermal green dye technique of measuring lung water, and at the same time we try to analyze some of the aforementioned problems in further detail.

Material and methods

The study was done retrospectively on 34 patients admitted to the Critical Care Trauma Unit of Victoria Hospital, London, Western Ontario, Canada, for various non-cardiac (n = 24) or cardiac (n = 10) reasons requiring invasive hemodynamic monitoring. The 34 subjects (19 màles and 15 females) had a mean age of 60 ± 15 years (min 25, max 82) and belonged to a group of patients previously reported (13).

The choice of the patients for the present study depended upon the availability of three or more radiographs performed on different days *and* of contemporary measures of EVLW by the double-indicator dilution technique using indocyanine green as a nondiffusible indicator and heat as the diffusible indicator (TDT) (8). A total of 159 matching studies (CXR *and* TDT) were available at the end in the 34 patients, the first study and the subsequent controls were undertaken over a period variable between 1 and 30 days from the first (mean 6 ± 7 days). All the radiographs were bedside films of good quality performed in the standard AP projection within 1.8 ± 2.4 h of each measurement of EVLW.

The CXR was independently scored without any knowledge of the patient's status, clinical course or any other related parameter by two radiologists. One of them used the scoring system more commonly reported in the literature in comparison with the TDT (1, 4, 8, 10) and which attributes a single edema score to the whole chest, from 0 to 4, with 0 being normal, 1 representing mild interstitial edema, 2 definite interstitial, 3 patchy alveolar and 4 diffuse bilateral alveolar edema (Syst. 1).

The other radiologist used a different scoring system (Syst. 2). For each radiograph, the pulmonary fields were divided into three parts (upper, middle and lower) on both sides, so that six different regions were separately evaluated for each film. Each area received a score on the basis of a 5 points scale, 0 being normal, 1 indicating interstitial edema (vascular haze, peribronchial cuffing, Kerley lines); 2, 3 and 4 indicating alveolar edema, vessels well recognizable in 2, patchy recognizable in 3 and not recognizable in 4; finally, 5 indicated complete opacification of the examined area. The edema score of the whole chest was the summation of scores from the six areas and could therefore range from 0 (absence of abnormalities) to (theoretically) 30 points (complete opacification of both lungs). The variability of the reading with Syst. 2, either within and between observers, was previously tested using a sample of 18 randomly selected radiographs, independently read three times at different hours of different days by three different radiologists with experience in pulmonary radiology and statistically computed obtaining an overall intraclass coefficient of reliability = .9247.

Inflation of the lungs was also assessed multiplying a) the hemism of the height of the two lung fields (h), as measured from the posterior portion of the first rib to the dome of the corresponding emidiaphragm, and b) the maximum transverse thoracic diameter (w), as measured on the frontal film across the inner thoracic cage at the level of the maximum pulmonary width (usually at the level of the 8th or 9th ribs).

Details of the TDT in a group of patients to which the present group belongs have been described in a previous study (13).

The radiological edema scores, both with Syst. 1 and Syst. 2, were then correlated using simple linear regression analysis with the corresponding TDT values in 3 different ways:

1. Absolute scores (159 measurements).
2. Changes (∂) in the scores [the difference between each measurement from the second on (CXR_i) *and* the first observed in each patient (CXR_0) used as a baseline] (159 – 34 = 125 measurements).
3. As in b), but correcting the score of each radiograph from the second on (CXR_i) with the changes in lung volume from the first (CXR_0) (159 – 34 = 125 measurements). Actually, the heights (h) and the widths (w) of the lungs were used for correcting the scores, according to the formula:

$$CXR_i \ (corrected) \ = \ CXR_i * \frac{h_i}{h_0} * \frac{w_i}{w_0}$$

where (h_0) is the height and (w_0) the width of the lungs on the first (baseline) radiograph (CXR_0) and (h_i) and (w_i) the height and the width on each subsequent film (CXR_i).

Other physiological parameters were recorded at the time of the TDT measurements; among them, the pulmonary artery pressure (PAP), the pulmonary capillary wedge pressure (PCWP), the cardiac index (CI), the pulmonary shunt (Qs/Qt) and the amount of positive end-expiratory pressure (PEEP) have been also tested together with water in a regression analysis vs the radiological score, because they were reported to have an effect on results of the radiological reading (4, 14-20) or on the precision of TDT measurements (5, 21), and we wished to verify if their sequential addition modified the strength of the correlation in our group of subjects.

To evaluate with a frugal solution the most efficient regression with the smallest number of variables, the stepwise regression analysis was used setting the radiological absolute score (only Syst. 2) as the dependent variable and TDT EVLW, PEEP, PAP, PCWP, CI and Qs/Qt absolute values as independent variables. One hundred forty-one sets of data were available, and the critical F value that must be exceeded for significance was set to correspond to *n-2* degrees of freedom.

The results of all statistical analysis were considered to achieve significance when the *p* values were less than 0.01.

Results

Table 1 lists mean, SD and range of the radiological scores, TDT EVLW values and other physiologic measurements.

Table 1. Measured and calculated variables

	n	Mean	SD	Min	Max
CXR (Syst. 1)	158	2.4	1.2	0	4
CXR (Syst. 2)		13.9	7.8	0	27
TDT EVLW, ml/kg	158	12.3	6.5	2.3	42.5
PEEP, cm H_2O	152	10.6	5.8	5	26
PAP, mmHg	157	32.4	8.9	10	57
PWP, mmHg	151	15	6.1	1	35
CI, L/min/m^2	158	3.9	1.2	1.8	7
Qs/Qt, percent	150	20.9	10.5	4.8	83
∂ CXR (Syst. 1)	124	0.14	0.76	– 2	4
∂ CXR (Syst. 1) corrected	124	0.21	0.87	– 2	4.29
∂ CXR (Syst. 2)	124	1.19	4.09	–14	12
∂ CXR (Syst. 2) corrected	124	1.71	4.83	–15.3	15.11
∂ TDT EVLW, ml/kg	124	–0.82	8.07	–23.02	31.5
∂ PEEP, cm H_2O	119	1.9	6	– 7	19
∂ PAP, mmHg	123	4.05	9.77	–15	35
∂ PVP, mmHg	117	–0.15	6.48	–14	20
∂ CI, L/min/m^2	158	0.44	1.08	– 3.04	2.86
∂ Qs/Qt, percent	117	1.6	11.9	–27.8	64.2

A positive correlation was found between TDT EVLW and radiological score, either with Syst. 1 (n = 158; r = 0.38) and with Syst. 2 (n = 158; r = 0.53). The difference between the two "r" resulted significant at the 0.05 level (1 tailed p-value). The details of the relative regression equations are shown with the scattergram in Fig. 1a and b.

A positive correlation was also found between ∂ TDT EVLW and ∂ CXR score, but only for Syst. 2 (n = 124; r = 0.36). However, when the correcting factor for pulmonary volumes was introduced, the correlation improved becoming significant for the Syst. 1 (n = 124; r = 0.27) and rising up for the Syst. 2 (n = 124; r = 0.53). The details of the relative regression equations are shown with the scattergram in Fig. 2a and b only for Syst. 2.

Stepwise regression analysis between radiological score (Syst. 2, absolute values) as the dependent variable and TDT EVLW, PEEP, PAP, PWP, CI and Qs/Qt (absolute values) as the dependent variables showed the highest partial correlation for water, that was introduced in the first step (r = 0.546), then for CI in the second step, with the "r" of correlation rising up to r = 0.674, then for Qs/Qt (r = 0.691) and finally for PAP in the last step, with a final r = 0.701, the regression equation being:

$$\text{CXR score (Absolute values, System 2)} =$$
$$= 8.138 + 0.538 \text{ TDT EVLW} + 0.113 \text{ PAP} + 2.407 \text{ CI} + 11.71 \text{ Qs/Qt}$$

The scattergram of regression is plotted in Fig. 3.

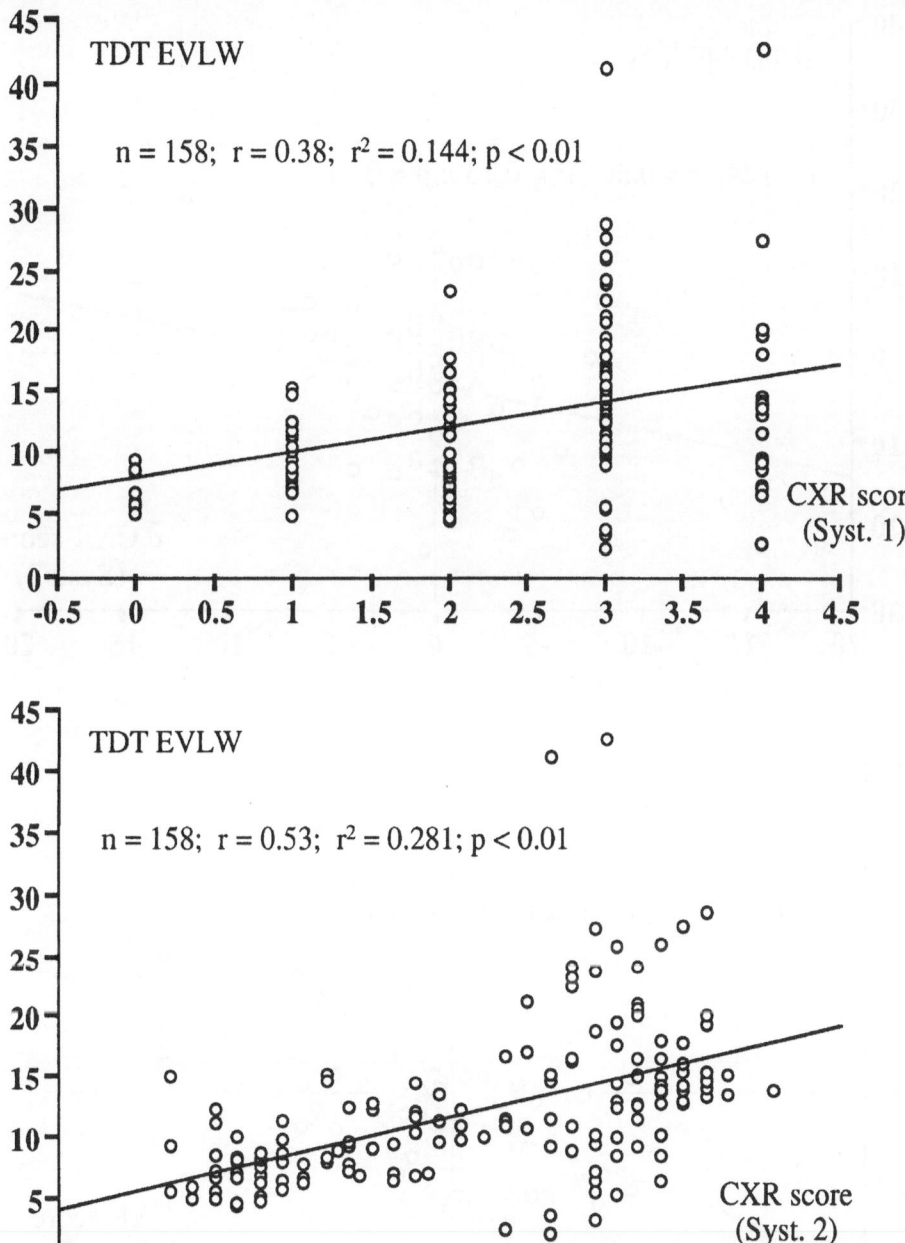

Fig. 1. a) CXR score (Syst. 1) and contemporary TD measures of EVLW. b) Same as in a), but using Syst. 2 for reading the radiographs

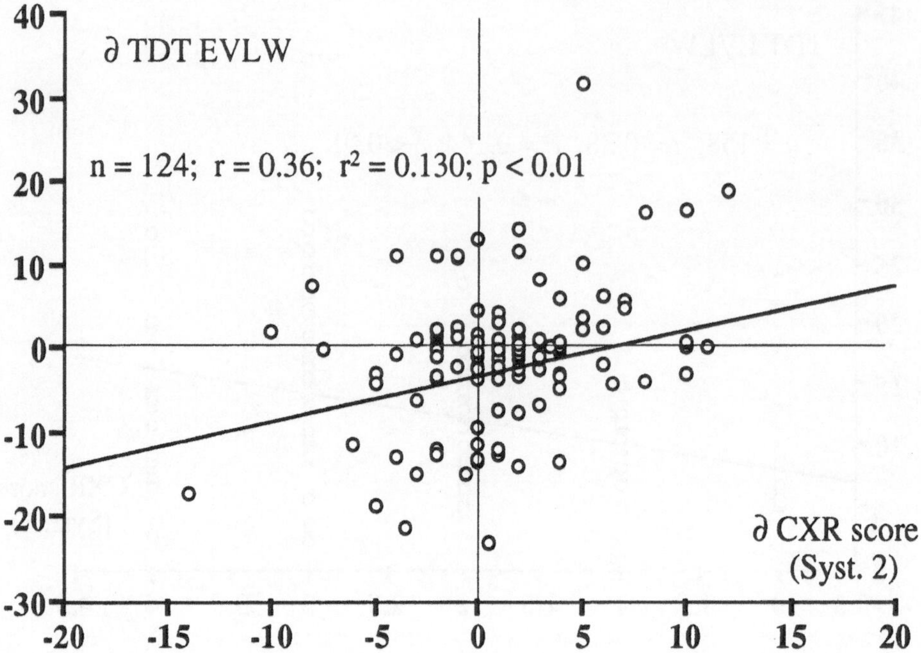

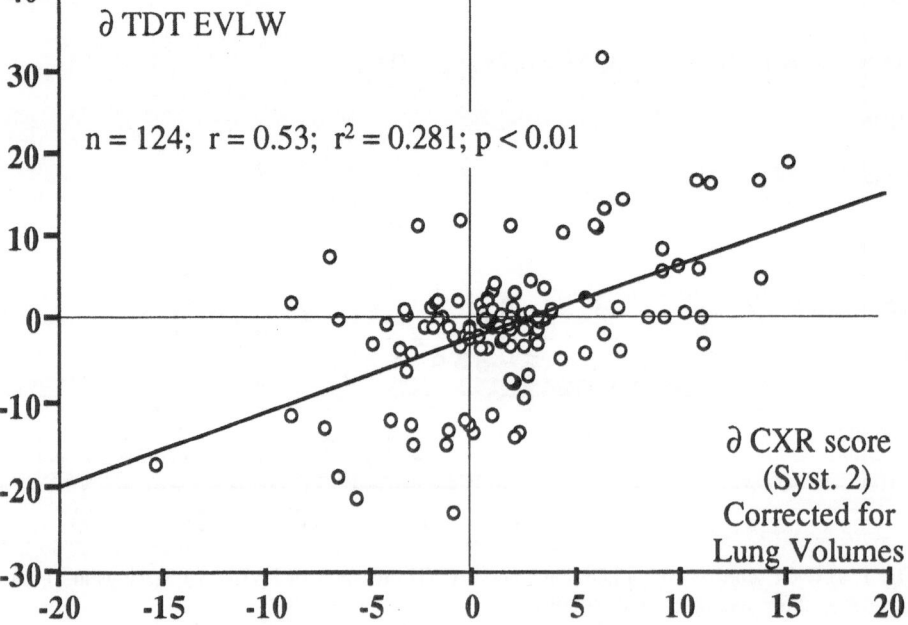

Fig. 2. a) Change in the radiological edema – ∂ CXR score (Syst. 2) – and change in the TD measured values of EVLW, ml/kg –∂ TDT EVLW – in repeated controls on 34 patients. b) As in a), but after correction of the radiological score for the changes of the pulmonary volumes

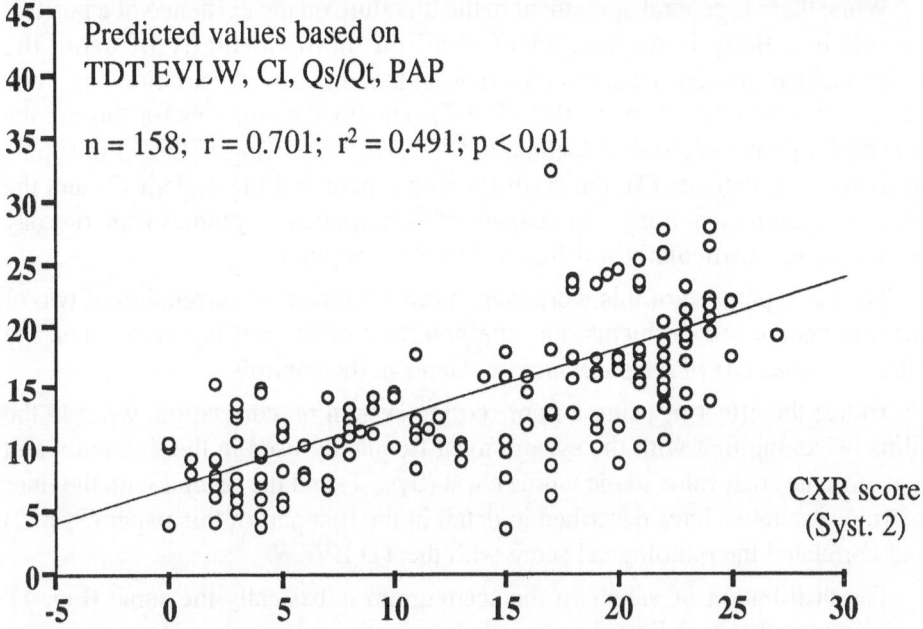

Fig. 3. Scattergram of stepwise regression analysis between Radiological score of edema – CXR score (Syst. 2) – as the dependent variable and TDT EVLW, PEEP, PAP, PWP, CI and Qs/Qt as independent variables

Discussion

Chest radiographs are widely used in clinical practice at the bedside of patients with pulmonary edema. Their popularity is mainly based upon the practicability, non invasiveness, nearly ubiquitous availability, reproducibility and, last but not least, low cost (11, 12).

From the clinical point of view, CXR helps indicating edema as the reason for a respiratory distress and, according to some authors (22), in particular clinical settings, suggesting its origins (cardiac, non cardiac, etc.). An assessment of the amount of fluid in the lung, and of its changes over time following therapy is also theoretically possible scoring the presence and/or the intensity of specific radiological signs.

Different scoring systems have been suggested in the literature, from the more simple (1, 4, 8, 10), very easy to use in the clinical setting, to others more detailed (3, 6, 9) and probably harder to manage in the every day practice, still useful for research purposes.

All the above mentioned papers have compared the radiological score in a certain number of patients with the "real" EVLW as measured by other means. One of the most used is the thermal dye technique, which has been repeatedly tested by very rigorous experimental and clinical work (14).

While there is general agreement in the literature on the existence of a positive correlation, there is no agreement at all on the opportunity of using the radiographs to predict the amount of fluid in the lungs, or its variation over time because of a low "r" of correlation (1, 3-8). The invoked reasons for this are the usage of a poor radiological technique (10), the films being obtained in supine uncooperative patients (3), the readings with a poor scoring system (7) and the effect on radiological images of changes of the pulmonary volumes from one day to another (4), particularly if different PEEP are applied.

The basic purpose of this work was to test the effect on correlation of two of the aforementioned problems, i.e., the *precision of the scoring system* and the *effect of variations of the pulmonary volumes* in the controls.

To test the effect of using a poor scoring system on correlation, we read the films twice, the first with the system most frequently used in the literature, and that attributes one value to the whole chest (Syst. 1) and the second with the finer scoring system we have described in detail in the first part of this paper (Syst. 2) and correlated the radiological score with the TD EVLW.

The distribution of values in the scattergram is basically the same (Fig. 1), which means that both Syst. 1 and Syst. 2 depict the same reality. However, using Syst. 2, the correlation increases, and the improvement is statistically significant.

This is even more evident when looking at the changes of the opacities over time: using Syst. 1, the correlation between ∂ CXR and ∂ TD EVLW is not significant; on the contrary, the correlation is significant using the Syst. 2. Our results suggest that the lack of correlation reported by some authors (1) when looking at the differences can really be motivated by a poor scoring system used to read the radiographs. In our experience, edema may change from day to day selectively in restricted thoracic areas, so that the assessment of its variations can be quite imprecise when evaluating the lungs as a whole. Halperin and coworkers (3) divided the lungs in different areas, as we did, and used a detailed system of scoring to compare the radiographs with TDT (both absolute values and changes), and indeed their "r" of correlation for absolute values is r = 0.51, which is very similar to ours, r = 0.53 for Syst. 2. The general form of the plot is very similar to ours, perhaps with some more stretching of the radiological values at the foot of the curve (it should be reminded that nearly 70% of their scoring system depended as signs such as vascular congestion, vessel blurring and septal lines, that are the very early manifestations of edema). However, Halperin did not find a significant correlation when looking at the differences (changes of water over time). These modifications are probably more important to be known than the absolute values for the clinician testing the outcome of his patient and the effect of the therapy.

On the contrary, in our study a positive significant correlation was found also for the changes. Actually, the correlation shows quite a loose connection (r = 0.36) (Fig. 2a); however, the correction for changes in lung height and lung width, that somehow express from one day to another the modifications of the lung volumes that are so important in determining the radiological images (4, 20) proved helpful, increasing the tightness of the correlation significantly (r = 0.53).

We suggest that our Syst. 2, that mediates the recommendations of the International Labor Office (ILO) on pneumoconiosis to increase the reproducibility of reading, may work better than Halperin's because it is *based on detecting the presence of a sign* (interstitial or alveolar, vessels recognizable or not) *more than on evaluating the intensity of a given set* of signs, which is less precise and thereafter less reproducible. The study of reproducibility we did on Syst. 2 gave a very high overall accuracy within and between independent readers.

The stepwise regression analysis showed TD EVLW, PAP, CI and Qs/Qt among the physiological parameters we considered getting into the final correlation with the radiological score. PEEP and PCWP, on the contrary, did not. But for extravascular lung water, as far as we know, the others have no effect on the films while they are reported to affect the TDT measurements.

A low PAP may result in underestimation of TD EVLW because significant areas of the lung can be converted to Zone 1 regions, particularly when positive end-expiration pressures are needed (15, 17).

The influence of CI is controversial. There are several evidences that when there is an important shortening of the transit times at the high flows characteristic of burned and other critically ill patients with hyperdinamic circulation, TD technique may underestimate the amount of measured EVLW (15, 16, 18). However, not all the authors agree (19). Finally, a high Qs/Qt may also cause an analogous underestimation, because it is proportional to the cardiac output at any given level of lung dysfunction (23).

Our data would confirm that TD EVLW, PAP, CI and Qs/Qt are somehow connected in having an effect on the radiological "water"; indeed, the correlation with the latter increases when these variables are introduced in the equations. Beyond EVLW, the most important is CI; after introducing this variable into the equations, the correlation strengthens from an r = 0.520 to an r = 0.684.

TDT is reported to be a reliable and precise tool to measure EVLW in several experimental and clinical conditions. However, as we have pointed out in this discussion, there are also evidences of some clinical limitations of the technique depending upon the clinical status of the patient. Moreover, technical limitations due to distortions of the TD dilution curve due to the position of the arterial thermistor (17) or to measures performed at random times during the respiratory cycle (24) are also possible.

Our study would support the evidence that TD measurements might underevaluate the real amount of EVLW in patients with high CI and high Qs/Qt, because we cannot think of an influence of these parameters on radiographic opacification.

Conclusions

A comparison between the amount of chest opacification in the radiographs of a group of ICU patients and contemporary measurements of extra vascular lung water through the double indicator thermal green-dye technique shows correlation significantly higher using a finer system of scoring than the one more commonly used in the literature.

The system we used divides each lung in 3 areas and attributes to each of them a score based on the *existence* of radiological signs. With this system the correlation with EVLW are significant not only for the absolute values but for the changes in the amount of water over time as well.

When looking at the changes, a correction of the radiological score for variations in height and width of the lungs further improves the correlation, possibly compensating the inverse effect of PEEP on the amount of pulmonary opacification.

The introduction of other physiological variables in the equation of regression would support the assumptions of some literature, i.e., TDT tends to underestimate the EV volume in patients with high cardiac output.

The suggested system of reading the radiographs of patients with pulmonary edema is simple and easy to use in everyday practice and showed to be highly reproducible.

Acknowledgments. The present study has been partially supported by 60% Funds of research of the University. We wish to thank Dr. Michael Lefcoe (Director, Department of Radiology, Victoria Hospital, London, Ontario, Canada) for his cooperation in doing the research, and Dr. William J. Sibbald (Coordinator, Critical Care Trauma Centre, Victoria Hospital, London, Ontario, Canada) for having allowed the collection of the clinical data on his patients, provided secretarial and statistical support to the research and given detailed review and useful suggestions to the manuscript.

References

1. Baudendistel L, Shields JB, Kaminski DL (1982) Comparison of double indicator thermodilution measurements of extravascular lung water (EVLW) with radiographic estimation of lung water in trauma patients. J Trauma 12:983-988
2. Böck JC, Keske U, Lewis FR, Felix R (1993) Korrelation des Lungenödemgrades mit der Thorax-aufnahme und Lungenfunktionsparametern bei Patienten mit adultem respiratorischen Distress-Syndrom. Radiologia Diagnostica vol 34 5:354-357
3. Halperin BD, Feeley TW, Minh FG, Chiles C, Guthaner DF, Blank NE (1985) Evaluation of the portable chest roentgenogram for quantitating extravascular lung water in critically ill adults. Chest 88:649-652

4. Laggner A, Kleinberger G, Haller J, Lenz K, Sommer G, Druml W (1984) Bedside estimation of extravascular lung water in critically ill patients: comparison of the chest radiograph and the thermal dye technique. Intensive Care Med 10:309-313
5. Miniati M, Pistolesi M, Milne ENC, Giuntini C (1987) Detection of lung edema. Crit Care Med vol 15 12:1146-1155
6. Pistolesi M, Giuntini C (1978) Assessment of extravascular lung water. Radiol Clin N Am XVI:551-574
7. Pistolesi M, Milne ENC, Miniati M, Giuntini C (1986) Detection and measurement of pulmonary edema: the chest radiographic approach. Intensive and Critical Care Digest 5: 34-36
8. Sibbald WJ, Warshawski FJ, Short AK, Harris J, Lefcoe MS, Holliday RL (1983) Clinical studies of measuring extravascular lung water by the thermal dye technique in critically ill patients. Chest 83:725-731
9. Pistolesi M, Miniati M, Milne ENC, Giuntini C (1985) The chest roentgenogram in pulmonary edema. Clinics in Chest Med 6:315-344
10. Sivak ED, Richmond BJ, O'Donovan PB, Borkowski GP (1983) Value of extravascular lung water measurement vs portable chest X-ray in the management of pulmonary edema. Crit Care Med 11:498-501
11. Staub NC, Hogg JC (1980) Conference report of a workshop on the measurement of lung water. Crit Care Med 8:752-759
12. Staub NC (1986) Clinical use of lung water measurements: report of a workshop. Chest 90:588-594
13. Sibbald WJ, Short AK, Warshawski FJ, Cunningham DG, Cheung H (1985) Thermal dye measurements of extravascular lung water in critically ill patients. Chest 87:585-592
14. Allison RC, Carlile PV, Gray BA (1985) Thermodilution measurement of lung water. Clinics in Chest Med 3:439-457
15. Effros RM (1985) Lung water measurements with the mean transit time approach. J Appl Physiol 59:673-683
16. Goodwin CW Jr, Pruitt BA Jr (1982) Underestimation of thermal lung water volume in patients with high cardiac output. Surgery 92:401-408
17. Gray BA, Beckett RC, Allison RC, McCaffree DR, Smith RM, Sivak ED, Carlile PV Jr (1984) Effect of edema and hemodynamic changes on extravascular thermal volume of the lung. J Appl Physiol 56:878-890
18. Hill SL, Elings VB, Lewis F (1981) Effect of cardiac output on extravascular lung water. Am Surg 47:522-528
19. Lewis FR, Elings VB, Hill SL, Christensen JM (1982) The measurement of extravascular lung water by thermal-green dye indicator dilution. Ann NY Acad Sci 384:394-410
20. Enderson BL, Rice CL, Moss GS (1985) Effect of positive end-expiratory pressure on accuracy of thermal-dye measurements of lung water. J Surg Res 38:224-230
21. Milne ENC, Pistolesi M, Miniati M, Giuntini C (1985) The radiologic distinction of cardiogenic and noncardiogenic edema. AJR 144:879-894
22. Zimmerman JE, Goodman LR, Shahvari MGB (1979) Effect of mechanical ventilation and positive end-expiratory pressure (PEEP) on chest radiograph. AJR 133:811-815
23. Bongard FS, Matthay M, Mackersie RC, Lewis FR (1984) Morphologic and physiologic correlates of increased extravascular lung water. Surgery 96:395-402
24. Stevens JH, Raffin TA, Mihm FG, Rosenthal MH, Stetz CW (1985) Thermodilution cardiac output measurement. JAMA vol 253 15:2240-2242

PULMONARY EMBOLISM

MR Imaging in Venous Thromboembolism

H.D. Sostman

Introduction

Effective therapy is available for venous thromboembolism, but can itself produce significant morbidity. Thus, an accurate diagnosis is mandatory. The clinical presentation and laboratory findings in pulmonary embolism (PE) are nonspecific; therefore, additional evaluation with imaging studies is essential. However, the most accurate imaging test (pulmonary angiography) is invasive, while noninvasive imaging tests (such as the ventilation-perfusion [V-Q] scan) have limited accuracy. Accordingly, there have been persistent attempts to develop a less invasive, more accurate imaging procedure which could replace either the V-Q scan or the pulmonary angiogram. In addition, the use of noninvasive lower extremity venous imaging to evaluate patients who present with respiratory symptoms has become widespread.

Venous imaging

In some patients it may be more appropriate to look for thrombus in the venous system than for a pulmonary embolus, particularly if venous interruption is contemplated. There is, of course, a strong correlation between pulmonary embolism and venous thrombosis. In one study, 71% of PE suspect patients with positive pulmonary angiograms, and 33% with negative pulmonary angiograms had DVT on bilateral venography (1). Conversely, in another study, 76% of patients with proven DVT had abnormal lung scans, including 35% who had "high probability of PE" interpretations (2).

In a patient with respiratory symptoms, imaging evaluation for possible PE should first be directed to the chest and a chest film followed by a lung scan should be obtained. If a diagnosis of PE is established, venous imaging should be considered if there is reason to believe that recurrent venous disease could develop or that venous thrombosis could persist despite therapy, since venous imaging would be important in follow-up and venous interruption may be considered as therapy. If the diagnosis remains in doubt after the scintigraphic study, venous imaging can be considered as an alternative to pulmonary angiography. Venous imaging is generally safer and more pleasant for the patient than arteriography and requires less technical expertise than arteriography (therefore, it is more widely available). It is generally less expensive than arteriography, as well. On the other hand, there is a substantial negative rate in venous studies of patients with PE as indicated above and arteriography may still be needed if the venous imaging is negative. Finally, if arteriography is negative but DVT is still suspected clinically, venous imaging is indicated.

Radiologic venous imaging techniques

Contrast venography is the diagnostic "gold standard" for DVT. Extensive experience has shown that identification of well-defined filling defects in fully opacified veins is accurate for detection of DVT, while negative conventional venography has been shown to exclude clinically significant DVT (3). However, venography does have limitations. These include difficulties in venous cannulation, incomplete filling and other technical problems in as many as 5% of cases (4); discomfort in up to 18% of patients even with nonionic contrast (5, 6); and a variety of local and systemic reactions to contrast material, including induced DVT in as many as 8% of cases even with nonionic contrast (5, 6).

Such limitations of conventional venography have led to development of alternative, noninvasive tests for DVT. Compression ultrasound and its refinements have been investigated extensively in patients with proof by venogram (7) and outcome analysis (8). The sensitivity and specificity of ultrasound for femoropopliteal DVT have been shown in these and many other studies to exceed 90%. Accordingly, ultrasound has been widely adopted as a cost-effective, noninvasive method for screening patients suspected of DVT. However, ultrasound also has limitations. Its accuracy in calf DVT is variable (7, 9); it is less accurate in recurrent DVT (10-12), although follow-up studies after acute episodes can improve accuracy in subsequent diagnostic encounters; it is operator-dependent; and its accuracy in pelvic DVT has not been investigated extensively. Of concern, it appears that asymptomatic DVT is detected by ultrasound with significantly reduced sensitivity (13). A recent meta-analysis (14) found a sensitivity for ultrasound of only 39% in a study of six publications (including 1015 patients) when compared with sensitivity of 97% for detecting DVT in symptomatic patients. Moreover, it is physically impossible to examine the peripheral pulmonary arteries with ultrasound to detect PE.

Preliminary reports described the use of venous imaging with MR for detecting DVT (15-17) in a total of 111 patients with correlative conventional venograms. In two series (62 patients with conventional venogram correlation), sensitivities of 90% and 100% and specificities of 100% and 93% were reported (15, 16). We have recently performed two prospective trials of MR for DVT in a total of 136 patients. In a prospective blinded trial comparing MR and venography in 61 patients (18), MR was better (sensitivity 100%, specificity 95%) in the pelvis than venography (sensitivity 78%, specificity 100%); the two tests were completely concordant in the thigh (the sensitivity and specificity of both considered to be 100%), and venography was better than MR (sensitivity 87%, specificity 97%) in the calf. In a second study (unpublished, 1993), 75 patients referred clinically for ultrasound were imaged on a research basis with MR. When there was disagreement between ultrasound and MR, either repeat ultrasound or venography was performed. Although it was not possible to document the true status of the patient in all cases of minor disagreement, almost all cases with major disagreement (one test showing DVT and the other negative) could be resolved. Preliminary analysis of the results shows MR to be more sensitive than ultrasound in areas which are known to be difficult to image with ultrasound (pelvis, adductor canal, calf) while the specificity of the two techniques appears to be equivalent. For detection of proximal (above-knee) DVT, we found that MR (sensitivity 96%, specificity 100%) was more accurate than ultrasound (sensitivity 70%, specificity 98%). Other reports have indicated that MRV can detect venous thrombi accurately in other body regions (19). The current clinical role of MR for DVT at our hospital is as follows. MR is recommended as the best test for DVT in: 1) asymptomatic patients being screened for DVT because of suspected PE; 2) suspected pelvic DVT; 3) nondiagnostic ultrasound or conventional venography; 4) clinical suspicion of DVT vs non-vascular disease (e.g., cellulitis, ruptured Baker cyst). About 250 MR exams are done for suspected DVT per year at Duke (with routine on-call coverage), compared with about 750 ultrasound studies and 50 venograms.

Radionuclide venous imaging techniques

Several radionuclide techniques have been studied for the detection of DVT, including radionuclide venography and radiolabeled fibrinogen (together with impedance plethysmography), platelets and monoclonal antibodies (20). None of these methods are currently in widespread clinical use.

Pulmonary imaging

Noninvasive techniques for imaging PE

Thrombus-specific scintigraphy (20), dynamic high-speed CT (21-26) and MRI (27-29) have been investigated for their accuracy in diagnosing PE and there has been some preliminary work using intravascular ultrasound (30). PE can be demonstrated in patients by all of these methods, but none of them has been sufficiently well validated to be generally applicable to clinical work.

Perhaps the most theoretically attractive of these methods are thrombus-specific radiopharmaceuticals and MRI, due to their ability to scan the whole body, but experience with these modalities for PE is quite limited. Thrombus-specific radiopharmaceuticals have been interesting in animal models and some clinical pilot studies, but have not yet stood the test of extensive clinical application. As described above, MR, in experienced hands, has proven to be extremely accurate for detecting DVT. In a few early clinical trials, MR has yielded sensitivities and specificities in the 65%-95% range. It has several technical problems which, in theory, can be overcome. Whether they will be solved in practice remains to be seen.

The experience to date with high speed (helical or electron beam) CT has yielded the highest accuracy for detecting PE. Very promising results have been obtained with electron beam CT; however, the small number of these instruments in clinical installations limits the impact of this technique. Helical CT is widely available and a number of preliminary studies have been done. Various techniques have been proposed, but most workers are using 5-mm collimation, pitch close to 1, and the equivalent of 80-100 ml of 30% contrast injected at 2 ml/sec. In the 1992 report by Remy-Jardin and colleagues (21), 41/42 patients had technically satisfactory CT examinations. Of these, 23/23 patients with normal CT had normal pulmonary angiograms, one patient had a false positive CT and 17 had true positive CT scans. In the positive cases, eight main pulmonary artery emboli, 28 lobar and 76 segmental emboli were seen on CT and angiography. However, nine intersegmental lymph nodes were erroneously considered to be emboli on CT. In another study of 44 patients, sensitivity of helical CT was 96% and specificity was 100% (22). However, not all studies have reported such excellent results; a recent study of 25 patients suggested that the sensitivity of CT was 91% and the specificity 86% when only emboli in major vessels were considered, but that the sensitivity fell to 77% and the specificity to 79% when all emboli were evaluated (24). Accordingly, larger prospective studies are needed to ascertain definitely the accuracy of CT for PE in unselected patient populations. Finally, helical CT is not likely in the near future to be able to evaluate the lower extremity venous system and the chest in a single examination.

Only when the cost, accuracy and patient management implications of such new tests are well characterized will it be possible to formulate rational guidelines for their use in routine clinical practice. It is probably even too early to determine if such methods are likely to replace the V-Q scan or the pulmonary angiogram.

Preliminary results with MR imaging of PE

We recently compared the accuracy of helical CT and MR for detecting PE in a canine model (31). Seven dogs who received experimental pulmonary emboli and one control were imaged with helical CT, and with 2D and 3D time-of-flight (TOF) MR. Blinded, independent evaluations of the CT and MR images by two MR radiologists and two chest radiologists were compared to the location of emboli as determined by subsequent pathologic evaluation of the excised lungs. Embolus: blood contrast: noise ratio (CNR) was determined on both MR and CT images for pulmonary emboli which could be identified on them. Fifty emboli ranging from 1.0 to 5.5 mm (mean = 2.7 ± 0.14 SE) in diameter and from 3.0 to 60 mm (28.1 ± 1.9) in length were found in the seven embolized dogs on pathologic examination. With detailed knowledge of the pathology findings, an unblinded observer was able to identify 90% of the emboli imaged by CT, 91% of emboli imaged by transaxial FMPVAS, 68% of emboli imaged by sagittal FMPVAS, and 64% of emboli imaged by sagittal contrast-enhanced 3D TOF. Three of the four radiologists identified more emboli on CT images than they did on the best MR pulse sequence and with greater confidence. The fourth radiologist identified an equal fraction of emboli on CT and MR images. The two MR radiologists had significantly greater accuracy in interpreting the MR images than did the other two observers. Combining retrospectively the data from different MR techniques improved the percentage of emboli detected. Combining the results of the two MR radiologists for FMPVAS in the sagittal and axial planes, average percent of emboli identified rose to 51% (95% CI, 39%-63%), compared to the 21% of emboli (95% CI, 11%-31%) which they identified on the sagittal images and the 40% of emboli (95% CI, 28%-52%) which they identified on the transaxial images, and comparable to the 56% (95% CI, 46%-66%) of emboli which these two readers detected on helical CT. The average embolus: blood CNR was greater for all MR techniques than for CT. Accordingly, we considered that a clinical trial comparing multiplanar FMPVAS MR imaging with helical CT was warranted.

Such a clinical trial is now in progress in our hospital. Its purpose is to compare the sensitivity and specificity of helical CT and MR imaging for detecting pulmonary embolism (PE) in patients in whom the diagnosis was suspected clinically. Patients who are suspected of having PE and who have no medical contraindications potentially are eligible for enrollment into the study. Patients in whom the presence or absence of PE can not be established with confidence are excluded. Enrolled patients are randomly assigned to undergo either CT or MR. If one modality is contraindicated medically, the patient is assigned to the other. Patients are considered to have PE if they have either: 1) high-probability V-Q scan and high clinical probability of PE by a study clinician; or 2) conventional pulmonary angiogram positive for PE. Patients are considered not to have PE if they have either: 1) normal V-Q scan; 2) low probability V-Q scan and low clinical probability of PE by a study clinician; or 3) conventional pulmonary angiogram negative for PE. Patients undergo helical contrast-enhanced CT or FMPVAS gradient-echo MR. The CT and MR images are read randomly and independently by five radiologists. Two are experienced with contrast-enhanced CT and with vascular MR. Two are experienced with contrast-enhanced CT but not with vascular MR. One is a radiology resident. In this way we hope to evaluate the effect of reader experience on diagnostic accuracy. Patients are categorized on MR or CT as having or not having PE.

Fifty-three patients have been studied thus far. Of these, 28 underwent CT and 25 MR. A total of 21 patients underwent pulmonary angiography (six had PE, 15 did not have PE). Of the other 32 patients, 15 had high probability scan/high clinical probability and 17 had low probability scan/low clinical probability. For the five observers, the average sensitivity of CT was 75% and of MR 46%. The average specificity of CT was 89% and of MR 90%. Experience with vascular MR and enhanced CT was influential upon diagnostic accuracy. For the two vascular MR experts, average sensitivity and specificity of MR were 71% and 97%, and of CT 73% and 97%. For the two non-MR experts, average sensitivity and specificity of MR were 21% and 94%, and of CT 69% and 90%. Therefore, the vascular MR experts had higher sensitivity on MR without reduction in specificity. The preliminary results in this pilot study suggest that, when CT and MR were interpreted with comparable expertise, they have similar accuracy for detecting pulmonary embolism. We feel that, with further observer training, the accuracy of both modalities can be improved.

Results of conventional pulmonary angiography

In the PIOPED study (32), the accuracy of arteriography for the diagnosis of acute PE was not investigated specifically. However, the interobserver variability and the relationship of the arteriographic diagnosis to patient outcome were investigated and bear an obvious relationship to the clinical value of pulmonary arteriography. The agreement between pairs of blinded observers as to the presence of emboli in the main pulmonary artery or lobar pulmonary artery was greater than 97%. When the embolus was in a segmental artery, the interobserver agreement was only 80%. When the embolus was in a more peripheral pulmonary artery segment, the independent reader agreement was only 40%. Thus, even with the superb spatial resolution of pulmonary angiography, small peripheral emboli are difficult to diagnose with confidence even for acknowledged experts. However, review of clinical outcomes rarely changed angiographic diagnoses in this study. Thus, it is unlikely that clinically significant pulmonary emboli will be missed by good quality pulmonary arteriography. How many clinically insignificant, small emboli or normal patients are subjected to unnecessary treatment on the basis of angiography is unknown.

In addition, the occurrence and distribution of solitary pulmonary emboli was investigated in the PIOPED study. Fifty-eight patients within the PIOPED investigation had only one embolus demonstrated by pulmonary arteriography. Four (7%) were in the main pulmonary artery, 10 (17%) were in a lobar pulmonary artery, 30 (52%) were in a segmental pulmonary artery, and an additional 14 (24%) were in a peripheral pulmonary artery. This distribution underscores the necessity for excellent quality pulmonary arteriography including magnification technique. It also suggests a mechanism by which some patients with PE could be missed by V-Q scanning. Fortunately, in the overall study only 14/251 (5.6%) of patients with PE had only a solitary peripheral embolus.

References

1. Hull RD, Hirsch J et al (1983) Pulmonary angiography, ventilation lung scanning and venography for clinically suspected pulmonary embolism with abnormal perfusion lung scan. Ann Intern Med 98:891-899
2. Dorfman GS, Cronan JJ, Tupper TB et al (1987) Occult pulmonary embolism: a common occurrence in deep venous thrombosis. AJR 148:263-266
3. Hull R, Hirsh J, Sackett DL et al (1981) Clinical validity of a negative venogram in patients with clinically suspected venous thrombosis. Circulation 64:622-625
4. Redman HC (1988) Deep venous thrombosis: is contrast venography still the diagnostic "gold standard"? Radiology 168:277-278
5. Bettmann MA, Robbins A, Braun SD, Wetzner S, Dunnick NR, Finkelstein J (1987) Contrast venography of the leg: diagnostic efficacy, tolerance and complication rates with ionic and nonionic contrast media. Radiology 165:113-116
6. Lensing AWA, Prandoni P, Buller HR, Casara D, Cogo A, Wouter ten Cate J (1990) Lower extremity venography with iohexol: results and complications. Radiology 177:503-505
7. Lensing AWA, Prandoni P, Brandjes D et al (1989) Detection of deep-vein thrombosis by real-time B-mode ultrasonography. N Engl J Med 320:342-345
8. Vaccaro JP, Cronan JC, Dorfman GS (1990) Outcome analysis of patients with normal compression US examinations. Radiology 175:645-649
9. Yucel EK, Fisher JS, Egglin TK, Geller SC, Waltman AC (1991) Isolated calf venous thrombosis: diagnosis with compression US. Radiology 179:443-446
10. Murphy TP, Cronan JJ (1990) Evolution of deep venous thrombosis: a prospective evaluation with US. Radiology 177:543-548
11. Cronan JJ, Leen V (1989). Recurrent deep venous thrombosis: limitations of US. Radiology 170:739-742
12. Murphy TP, Cronan JJ (1990) Evolution of deep venous thrombosis: a prospective evaluation with US. Radiology 77:543-548
13. Ginsberg JS, Caco CC, Brill-Edwards PA et al (1991) Venous thrombosis in patients who have undergone major hip or knee surgery: detection with compression US and impedance plethysmography. Radiology 181:651-654
14. Khaitan L, Midgette AS, Taylor CL, Zwolak RM, Stukel TA (1993) A meta-analysis of the use of color flow Doppler ultrasound in assessing proximal deep vein thrombosis in symptomatic compared to asymptomatic high-risk patients. Presented at the 15th Annual Meeting, Society for Medical Decision Making, Research Triangle, NC
15. Spritzer CE, Sostman HD, Wilkes DC, Coleman RE (1990) Deep venous thrombosis: experience with gradient-echo MR imaging in 66 patients. Radiology 177:235-241
16. Erdman WA, Jayson HT, Redman HC, Miller GL, Parkey RW, Peshock RW (1990) Deep venous thrombosis of the extremities role of MR imaging in the diagnosis. Radiology 174:425-431
17. Vukov LF, Berquist TH, King BF (1991) Magnetic resonance imaging for calf deep venous thrombosis. Ann Emerg Med 20:497-499
18. Evans AJ, Sostman HD, Knelson MH, Spritzer CE, Newman GE, Paine SS, Beam CA (1993) Detection of deep venous thrombosis: prospective comparison of MR imaging with contrast venography. AJR 161:131-139
19. Hansen ME, Spritzer CE, Sostman HD (1990) Assessing the patency of mediastinal and thoracic inlet veins: value of MR imaging. AJR 155:1177-1182
20. Knight LC (1993) Scintigraphic methods for detecting vascular thrombus. J Nucl Med 34:554-561
21. Remy-Jardin M, Remy J, Wattine L, Giraud F (1992) Central pulmonary thromboembolism: diagnosis with spiral volumetric CT with the single-breath-hold technique – comparison with pulmonary angiography. Radiology 185:381-387

22. Chintapolli K, Thorsen MK, Olsen DL, Goodman LR, Gurney J (1988) Computed tomography of pulmonry thromboembolism and infarction. J Comput Assist Tomogr 2: 553-559
23. Rossum AV, Kieft G, Treurniet F, Schepers-Bok R, Smith S (1994) Spiral volumetric CT in patients with clinical suspicion of pulmonary embolism. Radiology 193(P):262 (abstr)
24. Goodman LR, Curtin JJ, Foley WD, Lipchik RJ, Mewissen MW, Sagar KB (1994) Helical CT of patients with "unresolved suspicion" of pulmonary embolism. Radiology 19(P):262 (abstr)
25. Stanford W, Reiners TJ, Thompson BH, Landas SK, Galvin JR (1994) Contrast-enhanced thin slice ultrafast computed tomography for the detection of small pulmonary emboli. Invest Radiol 29:184-187
26. Teigen CL, Maus TP, Sheedy PF, Johnson TM, Stanson AW, Welch TJ (1993) Pulmonary embolism: diagnosis with electron-beam CT. Radiology 188:839-845
27. Grist TM, Sostman HD, MacFall JR, Foo TKF, Spritzer CE, Witty L, Newman GE, Debatin JF, Tapson V, Saltzman HA (1993) Pulmonary angiography using MRI: initial clinical experience. Radiology 189:528-530
28. Schiebler ML, Holland GA, Hatabu H, Listerud J, Foo T, Palevsky H, Edmunds H, Gefter WB (1993) Suspected pulmonary embolism: prospective evaluation with pulmonary MR angiography. Radiology 189:125-131
29. Erdman WA, Peshock RM, Redman HC et al (1994) Pulmonary embolism: comparison of MR images with radionuclide and angiographic studies. Radiology 190:499-508
30. Porter TR, Mohanty PK, Pandian NG (1994) Intravascular ultrasound imaging of pulmonary arteries. Chest 106:1551-1557
31. Woodard PK, Sostman HD, MacFall JR et al (1995) Detection of pulmonary embolism: comparison of contrast-enhanced spiral CT and time-of-flight MR techniques. J Thorac Imaging 10:59-72
32. The PIOPED Investigators (1990) Value of the ventilation/perfusion scan in acute pulmonary embolism. JAMA 263:2753-2759

Pulmonary Embolism: Role of Spiral CT

L. BONOMO

Spiral computed tomography (CT) also referred to as helical or volume-acquisition CT, is a newly introduced technique which allows continuous scanning of large volumes during a single acquisition (1). Use of the spiral technique has improved established CT applications by the reduction of motion artifacts, the elimination of respiratory misregistration artifacts and the production of overlapping images without additional X-ray exposure (2, 3). Moreover, high-quality multiplanar and three-dimensional (3D) images can be obtained from multiple transaxial images acquired in a single breath-hold (3-6).

Whereas conventional CT is based on a section-by-section principle that leads to intervals between single scans due to the time needed for table feed and breathing commands, spiral CT involves continuous movement of the patient through the gantry during continuous rotation of the tube-detector assembly (1-3, 7, 8). As a result, the X-ray focus performs a spiral or helical path relative to the patient, which led to defining the new technique spiral CT.

As a matter of fact, spiral CT represents a new way of thinking about acquisition: don't think of single scan slices, but think of imaged volumes.

After acquisition of the raw projection data set, transaxial planar images can be reconstructed at any level within the scanned volume (1, 7). Image reconstruction is the same, in principle, as in conventional CT, and the same algorithms and reconstruction kernels are used (8). However, an additional step of data processing is necessary before image reconstruction can be started. In fact, direct reconstruction of image from any segment of a spiral CT acquisition would result in motion artifacts due to patient transport (2, 3, 7). To avoid such artifacts, planar data sets must be calculated from the volume data set. The simplest approach is linear interpolation between the two neighboring points measured at the same angle of rotation (i.e., points separated by a full 360° rotation of the X-ray tube). This results in axial images quite similar to those obtained with conventional CT (2); however, 360° linear interpolation (360° LI) diminishes longitudinal resolution (2, 3). Therefore, new reconstruction algorithms, performing interpolation between points that are only 180° apart, have been developed (9, 10).

The performance of spiral CT scans requires several scanning and reconstruction parameters, including slice thickness, table speed, total scanning time, and image reconstruction intervals. Since the scanned volume is determined by the table feed and the scanning time, the higher the table feed and the scanning time, the larger the volume scanned. However, the selection of scanning parameters largely depends on two factors:

– The clinical indication and diagnostic task
– The image quality

As with conventional CT, the study of small structures, such as pulmonary nodules or renal arteries, may require 2-3 mm collimation, whereas collimation of 8-10 mm is usually employed in routine examination of the chest or abdomen (2, 3, 5).

According to the patient's ability to hold the breath and the scanner capabilities, scanning time can range from less than 10 to as long as 50 (3).

In order to allow the mathematical reconstruction be correct, a table feed equal to the collimation is generally recommended (2, 3, 9, 10) so that the pitch is 1 (pitch is defined as the table feed distance per 360° rotation divided by the nominal slice thickness). A pitch greater than 1, and up to 2, is also possible. It offers potential advantages like scanning the largest possible volume in a short time and reduction in mean organ dose radiation, but causes increase of volume averaging effect and requires a 180° data processing algorithm (2, 3, 9).

It has been demonstrated that the image quality of spiral scanning is equivalent to that of conventional CT with respect to most parameters (7-9). In particular, there is no difference between the two techniques as regards spatial resolution in the axial plane when the table feed is less than or equal to the nominal slice thickness.

Only the pixel noise and the shape of the section sensitivity profile are changed (3, 9, 10). Pixel noise is slightly reduced in spiral CT thanks to the linear interpolation; however, with 180° linear interpolation noise is increased when compared with conventional CT (8, 9).

The section sensitivity profile (SSP) describes how thick a section is imaged and to what extent details within the section contribute to the signal. In spiral CT, SSP is broadened because of patient transport (8-10); this causes a decrease in spatial resolution along the longitudinal axis but not in the axial plane. The effect of continuous translation on longitudinal resolution can be reduced by using a table feed less than the nominal slice thickness or by the introduction of 180° reconstruction algorithms.

A decrease in contrast resolution is sometimes observed, due to the low dose employed in spiral CT (7).

Many advantages have made spiral CT a welcome tool used in everyday practice of whole-body CT. The primary advantage is that the volume of interest is scanned continuously, in a short time, providing real section contiguity. This feature is helpful in scanning organs subject to respiratory motions where misregistration may occur if the patient is not able to reproduce his or her respiratory levels during conventional scanning (3, 4). By avoiding any gap or overlapping set of images, spiral CT allows the detection of small lesions that might otherwise be missed (11, 12). Moreover, multiplanar and 3D reconstructions are improved with spiral CT due to the absence of motion artifacts (3, 7).

Because of the short scanning time available, spiral CT enables the optimal use of a contrast medium bolus, allowing volume scanning during the phase of maximum vascular enhancement, using smaller volumes of i.v. contrast medium (3, 7, 13). Volume scanning in a short time allows the examination of patients in uncomfortable positions, needed for some orthopedic studies, and can improve evaluation in pediatric and traumatized patients (7).

As compared to conventional CT, patient dose is reduced with spiral CT for two main reasons: the first is that scan repetitions due to respiratory or other patient motion are excluded; the second reason is the limited capacity of the X-ray tube which implies low mA values (7, 8).

The heat capacity of the X-ray tube is the major limit of spiral CT. In fact there are limitations on the available mA, and these become more marked as the acquisition time increases (14). As we discussed before, in spiral scanning there is an increase of partial volume averaging but this effect can hardly be noticed in axial CT slices (9).

Another disadvantage of spiral CT is the time required for planar image reconstruction at the end of the acquisition so that the number of CT examinations doesn't increase although the scanning time is reduced (3).

The patient's co-operation, such as apnea, is not a real problem as most of the patients are able to hold their breath during the acquisition. Sometimes a preparation of the patient by means of a short period of hyperventilation can be useful.

The entire thorax can be scanned during a single breath-hold thus avoiding motion artifacts and variation in respiratory levels. This way, spiral CT can be successfully applied to the detection of pulmonary nodules, contrast enhanced studies or multiplanar reconstructions.

Recent interest has been focused on a preliminary study showing the use of spiral CT in the detection of pulmonary thromboemboli. The study compared selective pulmonary angiography and spiral CT in 42 patients and showed that spiral CT can depict thromboemboli in second- to fourth-division pulmonary arteries (15). Central pulmonary emboli are readily demonstrated by spiral CT and although spiral CT may not replace pulmonary angiography, it may be considered a useful imaging alternative for the detection of pulmonary emboli, particularly in patients in whom a rapid, noninvasive way of detecting acute thromboemboli is required.

Although spiral CT cannot replace pulmonary angiography, it represents a noninvasive and fast way to detect acute thromboembolic disease.

References

1. Kalender WA, Seissler W, Klotz E, Vock P (1990) Spiral volumetric CT with single-breath-hold technique, continuous transport, and continuous scanner rotation. Radiology 176: 181-183
2. Brink JA, Heiken JP, Wang G, McEnery KW, Schlueter FJ, Vannier MW (1994) Helical CT: principles and technical considerations. RadioGraphics 14:887-893
3. Heiken JP, Brink JA, Vannier MW (1993) Spiral (helical) CT. Radiology 189:647-656
4. Soucek M, Vock P, Daepp M, Kalender WA (1990) Spiral CT: a new volume scanning technique. II. Clinical applications. Roentgenpraxis 43:365-375
5. Kalender WA, Polacin A, Suss C (1994) A comparison of conventional and spiral CT: an experimental study on the detection of spherical lesions. JCAT 18:167-176
6. Kuhlman JE, Ney DR, Fishman EK (1994) Two-dimensional and three-dimensional imaging of the in vivo lung: combining spiral computed tomography with multiplanar and volumetric rendering techniques. J Digital Imaging 7:42-47
7. Kalender WA, Vock P, Polacin A, Soucek M (1990) Spiral CT: a new volume scanning technique. I. Principles and methodology. Rontgenpraxis 43:323-330
8. Kalender WA (1994) Technical foundation of spiral CT. Semin US, CT, MRI 15:81-89
9. Polacin A, Kalender WA, Marchal G (1992) Evaluation of section sensitivity profiles and image noise in spiral CT. Radiology 185:29-35
10. Brink JA, Heiken JP, Balfe DM, Sagel SS, Di Croce J, Vannier MW (1992) Spiral CT: decreased spatial resolution in vivo due to broadening of section-sensitivity profile. Radiology 185:469-474
11. Remy-Jardin M, Remy J, Giraud F, Marquette CH (1993) Pulmonary nodules: detection with thick-section spiral CT versus conventional CT. Radiology 18:513-520
12. Urban BA, Fishman EK, Kuhlman JE, Kawashima A, Hennessey JG, Siegelman SS (1993) Detection of focal hepatic lesions with spiral CT: comparison of 4-and 8-mm interscan spacing. AJR 160:783-785
13. Costello P, Dupuy DE, Ecker CP, Tello R (1192) Spiral CT of the thorax with reduced volume of contrast material: a comparative study. Radiology 183:663-666
14. Hacking JC, Dixon Ak (1992) Spiral versus dynamic incremental CT. In: Felix R, Langer M (eds) Advances in CT. II. Springer, Berlin Heidelberg New York, pp 101-107
15. Remy-Jardin M, Remy J, Wattinne L, Giraud F (1992) Central pulmonary thromboembolism: diagnosis with spiral volumetric CT with the single-breath-hold technique - comparison with pulmonary angiography. Radiology 185:381-387

Vascular Techniques in Pulmonary Embolism

C. Fava, M. Grosso, A. Veltri, J. Galli

Introduction

Pulmonary embolism (PE) is a frequent event, especially in certain patient groups, and carries a high mortality rate in affected individuals (1). It has been estimated that early diagnosis and start of an adequate therapeutic regimen is responsible for a 50% reduction of immediate mortality (2). Acute PE, untreated, causes approximately 30% mortality, of which about one third of deaths occurring within the first hour. Immediate death is essentially due to massive embolism causing critical obstruction of the pulmonary arterial bed.

The entity of embolization is the guiding criterion in classifying PE, which is usually (3) divided into three types:

1) Massive thromboembolism: corresponds to occlusion of at least 40% of the pulmonary arterial bed and is clinically the most severe form, responsible for about 30% of all cases of PE

2) Sub-massive thromboembolism: corresponds to occlusion of less than 40% of the pulmonary arterial bed and is the most frequent form (60% of cases) and often clinically misdiagnosed

3) Chronic, recurring thromboembolism: characterized by repetitive, moderate embolic events associated with vague symptoms and, therefore, difficult to diagnose. In this last form, repetition of embolism leads to a progressive reduction of the pulmonary vascular bed and, in advanced stage, pulmonary hypertension.

Establishment of a diagnosis of PE is important because in many patients there is a tendency for the embolic event to recur, potentially in a more severe or fatal form. There is a general consensus that PE remains a widely underdiagnosed condition. The probability of establishing the correct diagnosis increases with the extension of embolism in the pulmonary vasculature. The greater is the clinical severity of the patient, the greater is the clinician's probability of suspecting PE. Clinical suspicion of PE is the essential condition in initiating the diagnostic work-up. However, the number of clinically suspected cases with a negative diagnostic work-up is high (4).

It has been estimated that in patients surviving a pulmonary thromboembolic event, only in 30% was the diagnosis suspected (2). It is, therefore, evident that the clinical suspicion of PE must be kept higher in the clinician's mind, above all when dealing with certain patient groups (orthopedic surgery, obstetrics). However, objective diagnosis is important, especially when clinical suspicion is great, in avoiding the over-treating condition: a high percentage of patients treated with fibrinolytics or anticoagulants have therapeutic complications (5).

Having established the correct diagnosis and starting, if necessary, therapy for acute PE, it is important to determine the necessity of a strategy for the prevention of new embolic episodes. Most pulmonary emboli arise from thrombi in the lower extremities due to venous phlebothrombosis and thrombophlebitis. Instrumental exams allow detection of thrombotic disease and eventual vascular lesions (varicosities, etc...) which sustain it. Such findings, as well as the patient's clinical history, can orient towards the use of medical prophylaxis or mechanical devices in preventing PE.

In each step of the diagnostic-therapeutic work-up, the vascular radiologist can offer significant, at times decisive, contributions. Although non-invasive techniques have evolved, the importance of invasive studies using catheters remains great and that of interventional radiology is increasing. The role of different techniques, based on the use of catheters, in the various phases of the diagnostic work-up shall be taken into consideration separately.

Diagnosis

Imaging diagnosis of PE is based, above all, on the comparative evaluation of the chest X-ray and the lung scintiscan. A higher yield of information can be obtained from the lung scintiscan if the perfusion lung scintiscan is associated with a ventilation lung scintiscan. The role of the perfusion lung scintiscan is to detect non-vascularized areas whereas the ventilation lung scintiscan, in association with chest X-ray, can establish if the defects seen on the perfusion scan are due to other causes.

Diagnosis based on these exams has a wide margin of uncertainty, as demonstrated by the multicenter PIOPED study (6), especially in cases of moderate pulmonary thromboembolism. It is, therefore, justified if we turn to a more objective diagnostic test which can directly demonstrate the presence of emboli in the pulmonary arterial bed. Apart from the possibility of detecting voluminous thrombi in large caliber arterial vessels using CT (especially spiral CT), direct demonstration of PE is possible only using pulmonary angiography (7), during which a catheter is advanced into the pulmonary artery and radiopaque material is injected.

The most frequently used venous access for pulmonary angiography is the femoral vein. Jugular access or access through an arm vein (above all, the basilic vein) can be considered (8) when patency of the inferior vena cava or lower extremity veins has not been confirmed.

The exam should be performed selectively (injecting first one pulmonary artery and then the other) and a series of images in at least two projections should be obtained (9). The current diffusion of digital subtraction angiography (DSA) does not allow alternative techniques. It should be remembered that, although large quantities of contrast material are used, conventional serial-film angiography can give superior images with lesser occurrence of movement artifacts than DSA. With DSA, however, the quality of the images can be modest due to such artifacts, especially when the patient is in critical condition, dispneic, or tachycardic (10).

Catheterization of the pulmonary artery and its branches can be performed using many types of catheters. Currently, the most frequently used is the pigtail catheter, which comes in a model specifically designated for the pulmonary circulation. This model, which does not permit greater selectivity, has the advantage of preventing recoil of the catheter tip during high flow injection of contrast material.

Once high quality images are obtained, it is possible to reach an accurate diagnosis. The sensitivity and specificity of pulmonary angiography for PE are very high (8). Specificity can reach 100% using optimal technique and considering the direct vascular signs of pulmonary thromboembolism: abrupt "cut-off" (occlusion) of an arterial vessel and demonstration of filling defects within the lumen of a vessel (11). A certain percentage of false negatives occurs and renders the sensitivity less elevated, in part due to sub-optimal technique and in part due to delay in performing the exam (9). Spontaneous thrombolysis begins within 48 h after the acute embolic event and can rapidly dissolve the embolic material, thereby limiting the diagnostic value of pulmonary angiography.

Complications of pulmonary angiography are not rare and occur in 3.5% of cases (12). Mortality is approximately 0.2%: this is relatively high, but the clinical condition of patients affected by important thromboembolic events is sometimes very critical. The refusal to reach a precise diagnosis can be no less risky than the invasive vascular study. The diffusion of DSA, which requires injection of much less contrast material, and the systematic used non-ionic contrast material have reduced the incidence of complications in recent years.

It must be remembered that the potential role of spiral CT, whose characteristics include rapid execution and study of poorly collaborative patients, must be determined in the preliminary study of critical patients suspected of having massive proximal embolization. This technique, which is less invasive than pulmonary angiography, can easily detect large thrombi in the right and left branches of the pulmonary artery and, sometimes, in the segmental branches (13). Spiral CT may provide the objective diagnostic confirmation of PE in such critical patients, who should then be started on a treatment regimen without delay. Performance of pulmonary angiography, which is a more complex, costly and invasive exam, could be done when CT results are negative.

Regarding cost, it must be underlined that the high specificity of pulmonary angiography permits avoidance of potentially useless thrombolytic therapy when diagnosis of PE is uncertain. Such therapy is always expensive and carries certain risks (14).

In conclusion, pulmonary angiography remains the "gold standard" for diagnosing PE. Its infrequent use can be explained by difficulty in access to the procedure (few hospitals have an experienced and efficient angiography service) and by the diffident attitude many clinicians have toward the procedure, overestimating its risks. In cases with dubious chest X-ray and radionuclide scans (and eventual negative or dubious spiral CT findings), pulmonary angiography, whose greatest yield of diagnostic information is near the time of the acute embolic episode, is indicated.

Treatment of acute pulmonary embolism

Once the diagnosis of PE is confirmed, the clinician must evaluate the treatment choices, which are mainly medical and consist of the administration of thrombolytics and/or anticoagulants. The risk is the inherent danger associated with thrombolytic therapy; in fact, this treatment is reserved only for patients with a severe clinical presentation. In these patients, who frequently have a large proximal embolus, the vascular radiologist also has a role in treatment. The vascular radiologist can position a catheter, through which the thrombolytic agent is infused, immediately upstream from the embolus. Such selective thrombolytic treatment allows a reduction of the total dose of thrombolytic agent administered while maintaining its local concentration high (15). In reality, there is not yet a general consensus regarding the effectiveness of this type of selective treatment, which some consider to have no advantages over the general systemic administration of thrombolytics. Local infusion can be considered in patients whose clinical condition contraindicates the use of high doses of thrombolytic agents (16).

Fragmentation of the embolus can also be attempted using the same angiographic catheter employed for the diagnostic pulmonary angiography (17, 18). Recently, new mechanical devices called atherotomes have become available to the vascular radiologist. They consist of a rotating cutter mounted on the tip of catheters of modest caliber (19). These devices can fragment or pulverize the embolic material and re-establish vessel patency directly or else indirectly by increasing the area of contact of the embolus with the circulating blood, thereby favouring spontaneous thrombolysis.

Overall, the role of the vascular radiologist in treating acute PE appears modest. Consideration of such invasive techniques, currently sporadic, could increase in the future with improvements and simplification of fragmentation devices, which also have an elevated cost.

Prevention of pulmonary embolism

Having diagnosed PE and instituted effective treatment of the acute embolic event, the clinician must decide on the need for prophylaxis of recurrent embolism. It must be remembered that over 90% of cases of PE follow disattachment of thrombotic material from a vein in the lower extremity and migrating along the femoro-iliac axis to the inferior vena cava and then through the right heart to the pulmonary circulation.

Prophylaxis of recurrent pulmonary embolism can be oriented along two directions:

1) Prevention of formation of new thrombi and

2) Prevention of already formed thrombi from migrating to the pulmonary circulation.

The first prophylactic method is medical and uses administration of antiaggregants and/or anticoagulants (20). The second method can be achieved with surgical intervention or employing interventional radiology techniques. Due to their simplicity, interventional radiology techniques are playing an increasing important role in preventing PE, in part due to continuous development of new materials.

There is a consensus that the best prevention of PE is medical prophylaxis, which eliminates the cause, namely, thrombus formation. However, there are many morbid conditions which do not allow institution or adequate maintenance of a prophylactic regimen; above all, pathologic conditions with a high probability of hemorrhagic complications (gastroduodenal ulcers, etc...) are a contraindication to this type of preventive treatment (16).

There are certain situations, which are easily detected using current imaging techniques, which require urgent preventive treatment of PE. Detection of floating thrombi, above all in the inferior vena cava and iliac veins, represent a therapeutic emergency (Fig. 1). In these cases, in which a large thrombus has already formed, institution of medical thrombolysis is ineffective and may be dangerous by accelerating disattachment of a fragment of thrombus (causing pulmonary embolism). The only beneficial treatment in these patients is caval interruption, which can be accomplished surgically or, more recently, with interventional radiology procedures. It should be underlined that this particular indication (floating thrombi) for prophylactic treatment can occur in patients who never had an embolic event: it is a typical, casual finding in patients who have undergone surgery, especially orthopedic surgery (21), in whom subcutaneous heparin prophylaxis has been ineffective. It also occurs in patients with clinical signs of phlebothrombosis or thrombophlebitis in whom eventual endovascular thrombi are detected. In these subjects, it is necessary to immediately apply a mechanical caval interruption, preferably with interventional radiology procedures (faster to perform and less invasive than surgical interruption). Radiologically, a device called a filter can be positioned in the inferior vena cava, whose purpose is to block migration of thrombotic

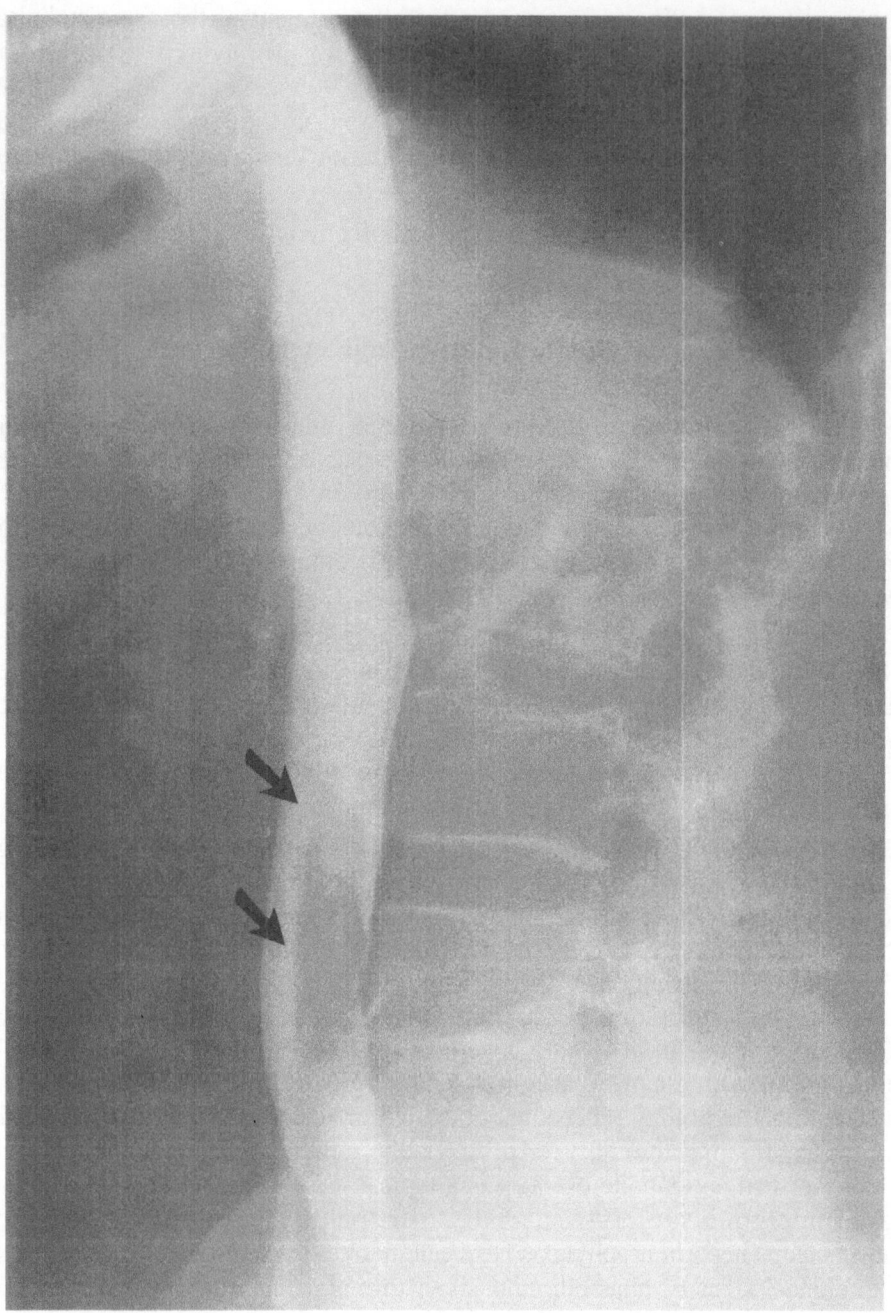

Fig. 1. Floating thrombus in the inferior vena cava (arrows): detection of this type of pathology is an absolute indication for emergency placement of a caval filter. In the case presented, placement of the filter requires a cranial venous access (usually, the right jugular veins) since the femoral route is not usable

material while permitting blood flow through the inferior vena cava. Such filters, which are introduced into the inferior vena cava via femoral or jugular vein access, have undergone considerable development recently (22). The filter is mounted in non-distended form within the tip of a catheter and automatically expands once outside of the catheter.

Two types of filters exist: temporary and permanent. Temporary filters can be removed after a brief period of use (not more than 7-10 days); they remain connected to the outside by a catheter or wire which anchors the filter and permits its retrieval. Permanent filters are more frequently used and cannot be removed once positioned in the inferior vena cava. They have a system of anchoring hooks by which embed themselves into the walls of the vessel (Fig. 2); after about 10 days, the hooks undergo endothelization which permanently stabilizes the filter.

Improvements have brought about a simplification of the filters, which are currently introduced using moderate caliber catheters (7-8F) (23-25). Even Greenfield filters, the oldest type still in use today, have been modified to allow introduction through such catheters (in the past, placement of a Greenfield filter required surgical exposure of the vein) (26). All filters are now available in kits which provide everything necessary for their placement, depending on the venous access (femoral or jugular) chosen. Some filters are symmetrical and can be positioned using either access route. Other than their shape, filters have seen improvements in the materials used for their fabrication. Non-ferrous alloys are now used which are less subject to corrosive phenomena and more resistant to mechanical stress.

A permanent filter is usually positioned in the inferior vena cava below the level of the renal veins in order to reduce the risk of renal vein thrombosis and consequent damage to the kidneys. If necessary, due to absence of sufficient space or to origin of emboli from the pelvic veins (typically, although rare, from a pelvic varicocele), the filter can be placed above the renal veins.

The indications unequivocally accepted as requiring the placement of a permanent caval filter are:

1) Contraindications to medical prophylaxis
2) Recurrent pulmonary thromboembolism in patients on a correct and adequate medical prophylaxis, and
3) Presence of floating femoro-iliac or caval thrombi (24). The indications, therefore, include all clinical types of pulmonary thromboembolism as well as recurrent forms.

The indications for temporary filter placement are less well defined. There is a consensus on its use in young subjects who are at a temporary high risk of PE (orthopedic surgical interventions) or as a protection during thrombolytic therapy of documented large thrombi. However, its use is still controversial (27). Contraindications to temporary filters are not numerous and are, in general,

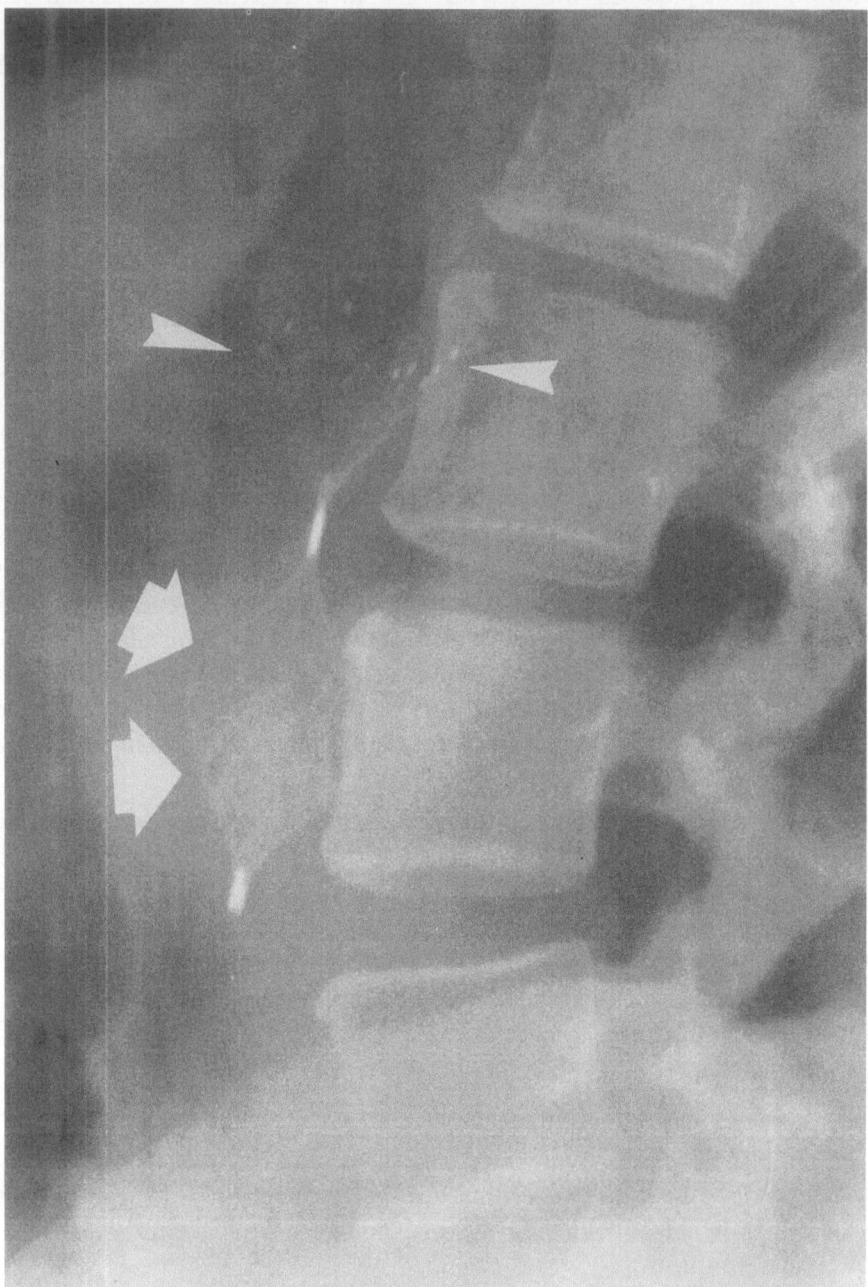

Fig. 2. Caval filter (Gunther) seen on a plain abdominal X-ray in lateral projection. In this case, the filtering element ("basket") is an oval structure composed of 12 metallic filaments placed in a helical arrangement (large arrows). The basket is mounted on an anchoring system made of 12 "legs" with hooked extremities which embed themselves inside the caval wall, solidly anchoring the filter to the vessel wall

relative: hemorrhagic coagulation disorders, non-patency of the route of placement... No absolute contraindications exist.

Various complications are known to occur during and after placement of a filter. Complications are divided into minor (hematoma at percutaneous access site...) and major types 29. Of these, the worst is the cranial migration of the filter, usually into the chambers of the right heart. This usually happens early because once endothelization occurs, the filter is solidly anchored to the vessel wall. Breakage of the filter from mechanical stress can be responsible for a late migration (28).

Caval thrombosis is another possible complication (2%-8% with current filters; originally greater than 50% with Mobin-Uddin filters, the first type of caval filter produced commercially) which, if progressive, can develop with modest symptoms. Retroperitoneal hematoma (2%) and arteriovenous fistula (> 1%) are rare (26, 30).

Recurrence of PE has greater clinical importance and implies failure of treatment. It occurs in 2%-5% of cases, varying according to the type of filter used (31). It is tied to the width of the mesh and the geometric shape of the filter. However, it must be pointed out that the finer is the filter's mesh, the greater is its capture of embolic particles with consequent decreased blood flow and greater risk of caval thrombosis. Conversely, when the filter has a wider mesh there is better blood flow through the filter with less risk of caval thrombosis, but there is less capture of embolic particles, especially small ones (26, 32). This implies that the choice of filter can be conditioned by the type of thromboembolic pathology encountered: in recurrent microembolism, it is better to use fine mesh filters. The vast experience which has, by now, matured in this field confirms the usefulness of such devices, which continuously undergo improvements.

Conclusions

Vascular radiology is now able to offer a wide range of diagnostic and therapeutic options in pulmonary thromboembolism. In both fields it may play a primary role: diagnostically, pulmonary angiography is the "gold standard" to turn to in the numerous cases of uncertain diagnosis in order to avoid useless thrombolytic therapy with its non-insignificant risks. In treating acute PE, interventional radiology has a promising future due to the development of new devices designed to fragment or pulverize the embolus and thereby rapidly resolving the problems of pulmonary perfusion and oxygenation of blood.

In prevention of recurrent PE, the role of interventional radiology is primary in creating a caval interruption, given its advantages in comparison to surgical interruption. Caval filters, which are percutaneously positioned by the vascular radiologist with minimal invasiveness, are very effective devices able to rapidly resolve very risky clinical situations for the patient.

References

1. Bell MR, Smith TL (1982) Current status of pulmonary thromboembolic disease: pathophysiology, diagnosis, prevention and treatment. Am Heart J 103:239-244
2. Dalen JE, Alpert JS (1975) Natural history of pulmonary embolism. Prog Cardiovasc Dis 17: 259-272
3. Dalla Volta S (1988) La tromboembolia polmonare. Giornale di Clinica Medica 12:723-731
4. Lilienfeld DE, Chan E, Ehland J, Godbold JH, Landrigan PJ, Marsh G (1990) Mortality from pulmonary embolism in the United States: 1962 to 1984. Chest 98:1067-1072
5. Mant MJ, Thong KL, Kirtwhistle RV et al (1977) Hemorrhagic complications of heparin therapy. Lancet 1:1133-1139
6. PIOPED investigators (1990) Value of ventilation-perfusion scan in acute pulmonary embolism. JAMA 263:2753-2759
7. Feltrin GP, Torraco A, Savastano S, Chiesura-Corona M, Miotto D (1993) Diagnostic imaging of pulmonary embolism. Rays 18:272-286
8. Newman GE (1989) Pulmonary angiography in pulmonary embolic disease. J Thorac Imag 4: 28-35
9. Quinn HF, Lundell CJ, Klotz TA et al (1987) Reliability of selective pulmonary arteriography in the diagnosis of pulmonary embolism. AJR 149:469-471
10. Musset D, Rosso J, Petitpretz P et al (1988) Acute pulmonary embolism: diagnostic value of digital subtraction angiography. Radiology 166:455-459
11. Bookstein JJ, Silver TM (1974) The angiographic differential diagnosis of acute pulmonary embolis. Radiology 110:25-33
12. Mills SR, Jackson DC, Older RA et al (1980) The incidence, etiologies and avoidance of complications of pulmonary angiography in a large series. Radiology 136:295-297
13. Remy-Jardin M, Remy J, Wattinne L, Giraud F (1992) Central pulmonary thromboembolism: diagnosis with spiral volumetric TC with the single-breath-hold technique. Comparison with pulmonary angiography. Radiology 185:381-387
14. Hyers TM, Hull RD, Weg JG (1989) Antithrombotic therapy for thromboembolic disease. Chest 95(S):375-381
15. Leeper KV, Popovich J, Lesser BA et al (1988) Treatment of massive acute pulmonary embolism. Chest 93:234-240
16. Vujic I, Young JR, Gobien RP et al (1983) Massive pulmonary embolism: treatment with full heparinization and topical low-dose streptokinase. Radiology 148:671-675
17. Feltrin GP, Pramstraller C, Fiore D et al (1980) Frammentazione degli emboli polmonari. Radiol Med 66:793-798
18. McCowan TC, Eidt JF, Ferris EJ (1989) Interventions in pulmonary embolism. J Thorac Imag 4:67-74
19. Schmitz-Rode T, Gunther RW (1991) New device for percutaneous fragmentation of pulmonary emboli. Radiology 180:135-137
20. Harrison's (1988) Principles of internal medicine. McGraw Hill, New York
21. Vaughn BK, Knezevich S, Lombardi AV, Mallory TH (1989) Use of the Greenfield filter to prevent fatal pulmonary embolism associated with total hip and knee arthroplasty. J Bone and Joint Surg 71A:1542-1547
22. Pais SO, Mirvis SE, De Orchis DF (1987) Percutaneous insertion of the Kimray-Greenfield filter: technical considerations and problems. Radiology 165:377-381
23. Millward SF, Marsh JI, Peterson RA et al (1991) LGM (Vena Tech) vena cava filter: clinical experience in 64 patients. JVIR 2:429-435
24. Jones TK, Barnes RW, Greenfield LJ (1986) Greenfield vena caval filter: rationale and current indications. Ann Thorac Surg 42 [Suppl]:S48-S55
25. Mobbin-Uddin K, McLean R, Bolooki H, Jude J (1969) Caval interruption for prevention of pulmonary embolism. Arch Surg 99:711-715
26. Yune HY (1989) Inferior vena cava filter: search for an ideal device. Radiology 172:15-16

27. Epstein DH, Darcy MD, Hunter DW, Coleman CC, Tadavarthy SM, Murray PD, Castaneda-Zuniga WR (1989) Experience with the Amplatz retrievable vena cava filter. Radiology 172: 105-110
28. Castaneda F, Herrera M, Cragg AH, Salamonowitz E, Lund G, Castaneda-Zuniga WR, Amplatz K (1983) Migration of a Kimray-Greenfield filter to the right ventricle. Radiology 149:690
29. Roehm F, Gianturco H, Barth C, Wright (1984) Percutaneous transcatheter filter for the inferior vena cava. Radiology 150:255-257
30. Messmer JM, Greenfield (1985) Greenfield caval filters: long-term radiographic follow-up study. Radiology 156:613-618
31. Geisinger MA, Zelch MG, Risius B (1987) Recurrent pulmonary embolism after Greenfield filter placement. Radiology 165:383-384
32. Thompson BH, Cragg AH, Smith TP, Bareniewski H, Barnhart WH, De Jong SC (1989) Thrombus-trapping efficiency of the Greenfield filter in vivo. Radiology 172:979-981

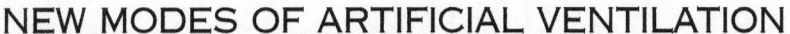

NEW MODES OF ARTIFICIAL VENTILATION

Proportional Assist Ventilation (PAV): Physiologic Rationale and Clinical Advantages

M. Ranieri, S. Grasso, L. Mascia, R. Giuliani

Considerable interest has recently developed in pressure-assisted methods of ventilatory support. Two of these have been so far described, pressure support ventilation (PSV) (1, 2) and the more recent proportional assist ventilation (PAV) (3, 4). The intent of these methods is to assist each spontaneous breath by providing positive pressure at the airway (Paw) during the period of spontaneous inspiration. During PSV and PAV, Paw is the ventilator controlled variable while inspiratory flow and tidal volume are determined by the combined action of the pressure generated by the respiratory muscles (P_{mus}) and the pressure generated by the ventilator (P_{appl}). Because the ventilatory consequences of these methods are essentially the result of patient-ventilator interaction, the patient retains considerable control over breathing pattern, flow pattern and ventilation, and this is expected to result in greater patient comfort (5).

The main theoretical difference between PSV and PAV is the function that P_{appl} is designed to follow during inspiration (6). With PSV, the ventilator causes P_{appl} to rise to a preset level that remains at that level until the cycle-off criteria are reached. The magnitude of ventilator applied pressure should therefore not be affected by the course of patient effort (1, 2). By contrast, with PAV, the time course of P_{appl} is linked to the time course of patient effort. P_{appl} rises as long as inspiratory muscle effort is produced by the patient. What is preset is not a target pressure, but the proportionality between Paw and inspiratory muscle effort, i.e. how much will P_{appl} rise for a given increase in P_{mus} during inspiration (3, 4).

PAV is actually provided through the Winnipeg ventilator (University of Manitoba, Winnipeg, Canada). This is an experimental prototype designed to provide PAV. It is also capable of delivering all conventional modes of ventilation. The design and operation of this unit are similar to those previously described (3, 4). The gas delivery system consists of a freely moving piston reciprocating within a chamber. The electronics control a motor which moves a piston from left to right. As the patient pulls, the piston moves freely into the cylinder providing an initial flow and volume when the velocity of the piston movement (i.e. inspiratory flow) reaches a preset threshold value, the motor starts to assist the movement of the piston. The flow level required to trigger the motor is variable, and in the present study was set at 0.05 l/s (4). When the piston is activated it creates a pressure in the piston chamber and the forward movement of the piston produces air flow. This air is directed to the patient through a one-way valve, the inspiratory line and the humidifier. The difference between the chamber pressure and the proximal airway pressure creates a trigger or assist signal. This signal in turn switches the three-way solenoid valve connecting the pump pressure to the exhalation valve line. This causes the exhalation valve to close. Gas transfer is terminated when the patient makes an expiratory effort and stops flow. This creates a positive pressure in reference to the chamber pressure. When patient pressure exceeds chamber pressure the trigger signal goes off, causing the exhalation valve line to open. This allows passive deflation through the exhalation valve. The piston returns to the starting position, thus intaking gas from the ventilator input because of the backward movement of the piston. An external demand blended gas system is attached to the input opening. When the piston has returned to the starting position, the machine is reset and is ready for the next inspiration. PEEP can be applied by adding a PEEP valve on the exhalation line of the ventilator circuit. The motor applies force to the piston according to different command signals relative to the operating ventilatory mode. During PSV, the control denotes the level of pressure assistance for a patient initiated breath. The changeover from inspiration to expiration can be set as different absolute flow values or as different percentage values of the initial peak flow. In this study, cycling between inspiration and expiration occurred when the flow rate fell to 5 l/min. Inspiratory time (Ti) can not exceed 3 s or the machine will reset for the next inspiration. During PAV, the command signals are instantaneous inspired flow (derived from the rate of forward motion of the piston) and instaneous inspired volume (derived from piston displacement since onset of inspiration). Once flow begins, pressure in the chamber raises in proportion to ongoing flow and volume, thereby augmenting the pressure gradient for chest expansion. The magnitudes of assistance for flow and volume can be set as varying percentage values of the patient's total resistance and elastance of the total respiratory system through external controls. When they are set below patient's resistance and elastance, chamber pressure increases only if the patient effort increases. When inspiratory effort decreases at end-inspiration, inspiratory flow decreases and then stops, causing the integrator to reset and the assist to terminate.

Substantial differences between PSV and PAV on patient-ventilator interaction are expected to occur consequently to variations of ventilatory requirement. We studied differences between PSV and PAV and evaluated their physiologic relevance during acute variations of ventilatory requirement induced by hypercapnic stimulation of the respiratory drive in mechanically ventilated patients (7, 8).

In order to induce acute hypercapnia with a consequent variation of patient's ventilatory requirement a fixed dead space of 150 ml was applied between the pneumotachograph and the y-piece of the ventilator circuit. Measurements were obtained before (dead space off) and after (dead space on) application of dead space. During "dead space on" condition an increase in $ETCO_2$ of −30% of its baseline value was considered as the target value.

Our data show that, in mechanically ventilated patients during the weaning phase, the strategy used to compensate for increased ventilatory requirements due to CO_2 stimulation substantially differs during PSV and PAV. During PSV, the increase in V_E due to acute hypercapnia is obtained through an increase in respiratory rate, remaining V_T and inspiratory muscle effort per breath unchanged. In contrast, during PAV, the increase in V_E is obtained through an increase in V_T due to the larger inspiratory muscle effort with remaining respiratory rate unchanged. When the energy cost (evaluated as PTP/min and PTP/l) of such different strategies is compared, our data show that, to increase V_E in response to the hypercapnic stimulation, a larger amount of inspiratory muscle effort is required during PSV than during PAV. Besides, patient discomfort during CO_2 stimulation seems lower during PAV than during PSV (7, 8).

In order to evaluate the efficacy of the neuroventilatory coupling during PSV, the PTI/b vs V_T, PTI/b vs peak flow and PTI/b vs P_{appl} relationships for each individual patient were constructed at both levels of PSV by plotting values obtained from 15-20 consecutive breaths during "dead space off" and "dead space on" conditions. As expected, changes in inspiratory muscle effort were neither correlated with V_T nor with ventilator applied pressure, while a significant positive correlation was found only between PTP/b and peak flow. It follows that with PSV, patient's ability to modulate V_T according to the ventilatory requirements by varying inspiratory muscle effort is limited and a discrepancy between the respiratory rates of patient and ventilator likely occurs. Besides, duration and peak value of inspiratory flow seems more sensitive than V_T, as indicators of changes in intensity of patient effort.

In conclusion, in mechanically ventilated patients in whom ventilatory requirements are acutely increased by causing hypercapnia through application of a dead space, the physiological capability to increase V_E through changes in V_T modulated by variations in inspiratory muscle effort was preserved only during PAV. In contrast, during PSV, the increase in V_E due to the higher ventilatory requirements was obtained through an increase in respiratory rate, with substantially unchanged V_T and inspiratory muscle effort. The compensatory strategy used to increase V_E during PSV had a higher energy cost for the respiratory muscles and caused a more pronounced patient discomfort than the one used during PAV (7, 8). It remains to be confirmed whether such physiological differences between PSV and PAV during the weaning phase have significant clinical implications. Besides, the presence of spontaneous variations of ventilatory requirements as large as the one experimentally produced in our study remains to be proved.

References

1. Brochard L, Harf A, Lorino H, Lemaire F (1989) Inspiratory pressure support prevents diaphragmatic fatigue during weaning from mechanical ventilation. Am Rev Respir Dis 139:513-521
2. Macintyre NR, Leatherman NE (1990) Ventilatory muscle loads and the frequency-tidal volume pattern during inspiratory pressure-assisted (pressure supported) ventilation. Am Rev Respir Dis 141:327-331
3. Younes M (1992) Proportional assist ventilation, a new approach to ventilatory support. Am Rev Respir Dis 145:114-120
4. Younes M, Puddy A, Roberts D, Light RB, Quesada A, Taylor K, Oppenheimer L, Cramp H (1992) Proportional assist ventilation. Results of an initial clinical trial. Am Rev Respir Dis 145:121-129
5. Brochard L (1994) Pressure support ventilation. In: Tobin MJ (ed) Principles and practice of mechanical ventilation. McGraw-Hill, New York, pp 239-257
6. Younes M (1991) Proportional assist ventilation and pressure support ventilation: similarities and differences. In Marini JJ, Roussos C (eds) Ventilatory failure. Springer, Berlin Heidelberg New York, pp 361-380
7. Mascia L, Grasso S, Giuliani R, Caracciolo A, Brienza A, Bruno F, Fiore T, Ranieri VM (1995) Patient-ventilator interaction following sudden changes in respiratory drive: pressure support ventilation (PSV) vs proportional assist ventilation (PAV). Am J Respir Crit Care Med (in press)
8. Grasso S, Mascia L, Giuliani R, Lagioia V, Spagnolo A, Pugliese V, De Tullio R, Ranieri VM (1995) Ventilatory support in COPD during Proportional Assist Ventilation (PAV): Effects on breathing pattern and inspiratory effort. Am J Respir Crit Care Med (in press)

Airway Pressure Release Ventilation

J. RÄSÄNEN

Traditionally mechanical ventilatory support has relied on increasing airway pressure above ambient to inflate the lungs. Mechanical inflation of the lungs with positive pressure causes fundamental alterations in cardiopulmonary mechanics which frequently lead to pulmonary and circulatory complications (1). Moreover, high airway and intrathoracic pressure during positive pressure breaths may not allow use of adequate continuous positive airway pressure (CPAP) to restore expiratory lung volume and, consequently, prevents optimization of lung mechanics and gas exchange (2, 3). Even when the ventilator is adjusted carefully, positive pressure ventilation will elevate mean intrathoracic pressure and result in cardiovascular compromise in patients with normal or low intravascular volume. Periodic alveolar overinflation may cause structural lung injury, or may impair healing of the already injured lung.

Airway pressure release ventilation (APRV) was developed to provide ventilatory support to a patient with acute lung injury with minimal airway pressure and hyperinflation. Airway pressure release ventilation is based on intermittent decrease, rather than increase, in airway pressure and lung volume. The ensuing effects on cardiopulmonary mechanics differ markedly from those of previously used techniques.

Technical considerations

In its simplest form an APRV ventilator consists of a high-flow CPAP circuit with an electrically or pneumatically driven release valve which directs expiratory flow alternately through two CPAP-valves that have different opening pressures (Fig. 1) (4). As the release valve opens the gas flow to the CPAP-valve with lower pressure threshold, the circuit pressure falls abruptly, allowing outflow of gas from the lungs. The transient fall in airway pressure is used to decrease lung volume below the initial level by a desired amount. When CPAP is re-established, the lungs are reinflated with fresh gas to the previous volume. The CPAP-valves must be true threshold resistors that are capable of maintaining opening pressure unchanged despite alterations in flow (5). The pressure release valve must have minimal resistance to gas flow to effect a sharp, nearly instantaneous drop in airway pressure that allows sufficient time for reduction in lung volume and augmentation of carbon dioxide removal during the APRV cycle. The flow resistance of the release pathway is also critical; a single 90 angle may effect sufficient flow resistance to significantly delay pressure release and impair proper functioning of the circuit.

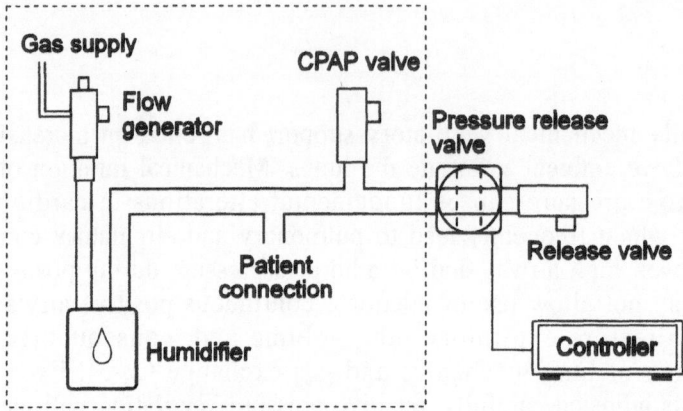

Fig. 1. A high-flow CPAP-system (*dotted box*) modified to provide APRV by adding a timer-controlled airway pressure release valve and a second threshold resistor valve to the circuit

Tidal volume of the APRV breath depends on lung compliance, airway resistance, the magnitude of airway pressure release, and the duration of pressure release. The contribution of the APRV breaths to total minute ventilation and carbon dioxide elimination further depends on the frequency of the APRV breaths.

Airway pressure release ventilation differs conceptually from all other ventilatory modalities, because it effects movement of gas by decreasing airway pressure below that which has been established to produce optimum resting lung volume in a given patient. If alveolar ventilation is increased sufficiently to abolish the patient's spontaneous breathing, the airway and intrathoracic pressure patterns become indistinguishable from those seen during pressure-controlled inverse inspiratory:expiratory time ratio ventilation. However, inverse ratio ventilation was originally designed only to deliver controlled ventilation to patients who have been rendered apneic using hyperventilation, deep sedation, or neuromuscular blockade, and weaning from inverse ratio ventilation requires changeover to another mode of mechanical ventilation. Therefore, traditional pressure-limited inverse ratio ventilation can be viewed as a special case of APRV, and the relationship between inverse ratio ventilation and APRV resembles that between conventional controlled positive pressure ventilation and intermittent mandatory ventilation.

Advantages of APRV

Since mechanical ventilation during APRV is accomplished by decreasing airway pressure from the level of CPAP considered optimal for the patient, peak airway pressure equals the CPAP level (Fig. 2). Augmentation of alveolar ventilation with low peak airway pressure and without overdistention of the lung parenchyma appears to be a consistent major advantage of APRV. Changeover from positive pressure ventilation to APRV has been shown to allow a 30 to 75 percent reduction in peak airway pressure both in experimental and clinical studies (6, 7). The extent of peak airway pressure reduction depends on lung mechanics and on whether APRV and positive pressure ventilation have been adjusted to a similar mean airway pressure or to a similar level of CPAP. When peak airway pressure is maintained at a low level and lung volume is not increased from the level assumed to optimize gas exchange and lung mechanics, the risk of ventilator-induced lung injury should be at its minimum. However, the clinical significance of this theoretical advantage of APRV has not yet been demonstrated scientifically.

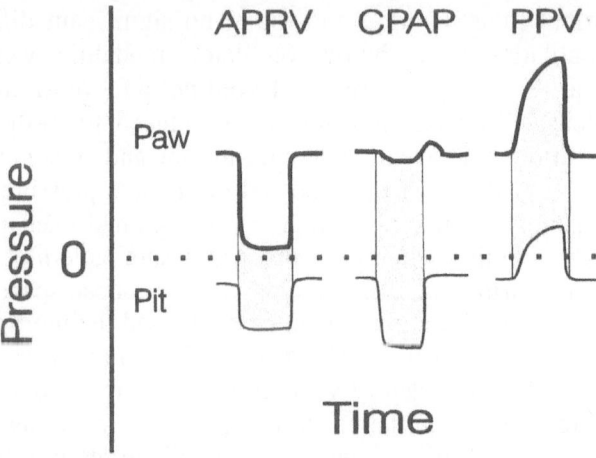

Fig. 2. Changes in airway pressure (*Paw*), intrathoracic pressure (*Pit*), and transpulmonary pressure (*shaded*) during APRV, during spontaneous breathing with CPAP, and during conventional positive pressure ventilation (*PPV*)

The intrathoracic pressure pattern during APRV resembles that recorded during a spontaneous breath with CPAP (Fig. 2). When APRV is started in a subject who is breathing spontaneously with CPAP, mean airway pressure decreases while peak airway pressure and mean intrathoracic pressure remain largely unchanged. An increase in APRV rate in an apneic subject decreases both mean airway pressure and intrathoracic pressure. This is in contrast with conventional positive pressure ventilation during which an increase in mechanical ventilatory support always increases airway and intrathoracic pressure. Since intrathoracic pressure is not elevated by APRV, initiation of mechanical ventilation using APRV should not depress cardiovascular performance in a patient with normal myocardial function.

Whether or not hemodynamic differences exist between APRV and positive pressure ventilation depends on the design of the study. Most comparisons between positive pressure ventilation and APRV have been made with equivalent mean airway pressure (6, 8). If the spontaneous minute ventilation is also similar between the two modalities, intrathoracic pressure does not change upon changeover from one modality to another and, consequently, no change in circulatory function would be expected. On the other hand, in two experimental studies comparing the cardiovascular effects of spontaneous breathing, positive pressure ventilation and APRV using equivalent levels of continuous positive airway pressure, stroke volume, cardiac output and oxygen delivery were similar during spontaneous breathing and APRV but significantly depressed during positive pressure ventilation (7, 9).

Stock et al. compared APRV and conventional positive pressure ventilation in animals with normal lung function and found no significant differences in oxygenation or ventilation, when the two ventilatory modalities were delivered using similar mean airway pressure, tidal volume, and ventilator rate (6). However, when oleic acid-induced lung injury was induced, the authors observed significantly lower arterial blood carbon dioxide tension and higher arterial blood oxygen tension during APRV when compared to positive pressure ventilation even though mechanical minute ventilation was maintained unchanged. These results suggested that in injured lungs the airway pressure pattern of APRV may effect more uniform distribution of inspired gas with less dead space ventilation than positive pressure lung inflation. Valentine et al. used the multiple inert gas elimination technique to compare matching of ventilation and perfusion during synchronized intermittent mandatory ventilation, pressure support ventilation and airway pressure release ventilation in nine patients recovering from open-heart operations performed under hypothermic cardiopulmonary bypass (10). The results showed that dead space ventilation was indeed significantly lower during APRV than during the other ventilatory modalities. The reduction in dead space is believed to result primarily from low peak airway pressure which minimizes distention of conducting airways and generation of West zone I conditions in the lungs.

Disadvantages of APRV

Tidal volume is accomplished during APRV with a primary alteration of airway pressure. Under these conditions, and assuming adequate inspiratory and expiratory time, the magnitude of tidal volume depends on the pressure-volume characteristics of the lungs. Therefore, a change in lung compliance will alter the tidal volume if the ventilator settings are not adjusted. This limitation is not specific to APRV but applies to all pressure-controlled or pressure-limited ventilation. Since APRV typically involves some spontaneous breathing, reduction or increase in mechanical ventilation probably will be at least temporarily compensated for by a change in spontaneous ventilation. Cane et al. reported the development of lobar atelectasis during ventilation with APRV in two of 16 patients with severe acute lung injury. This complication was attributed to the volume-variable nature of APRV (11).

In addition to pressure-volume characteristics of the lungs, tidal volume during an APRV breath depends on adequate airway pressure release time to allow sufficient emptying of the lung. The traditional airway pressure release time during APRV in adults has been 1.5 s, which will allow complete cessation of expiratory flow in normal subjects. However, in patients with pulmonary disease a release time of 1.5 s may not be ideal. Since the essential derangement in lung mechanics in most patients with acute lung injury is a reduction in lung compliance, the standard 1.5-s release time should be adequate for these patients, and it has been successfully used in all published human studies. However, in patients with significant airway obstruction, a longer release time may be required. Extention of the release time decreases the maximum frequency of airway pressure release and, consequently, the mechanical minute ventilation, that can be achieved with APRV. Theoretically, one should use the shortest release time that allows expiratory flow to stop by the end of pressure release. This adjustment would allow maximum tidal volume and minimum time at low airway and transpulmonary pressure. The variability of "optimum" release time among patients requiring ventilatory support for acute lung injury has not yet been defined.

The fall in airway pressure during APRV effects ventilation by decreasing transpulmonary pressure and lung volume. Since average lung volume is a major determinant of ventilation/perfusion relationships, and the lung volume at CPAP is optimum for the patient, ventilation with APRV could theoretically impair oxygenation. When comparing spontaneous breathing, APRV, and positive pressure ventilation using a similar level of expiratory airway pressure in dogs with oleic acid-induced lung injury we found that while ventilatory failure and hypoxemia that existed during spontaneous breathing could be corrected equally effectively with APRV or positive pressure ventilation, the use of APRV resulted in significantly lower arterial blood oxygen tension and higher venous admixture than positive pressure ventilation (8). The differences in oxygenation may have reflected the lower mean transpulmonary pressure during APRV, or it may have resulted from reduction and redistribution of pulmonary blood flow during positive pressure ventilation. Nevertheless, systemic oxygen delivery was far superior during APRV, and comparable to values measured during spontaneous breathing, because the use of APRV did not depress circulatory function even when ventilation was controlled by hyperventilating the animal. A similar study in pigs by Smith et al. revealed a 5 mmHg average fall in PaO_2, but no statistically significant change in venous admixture, during changeover from positive pressure ventilation to APRV (12). Both of these studies compared the two ventilatory modalities with similar levels of CPAP, a design which always results in lower average transpulmonary pressure during APRV.

All clinical studies of APRV have compared this ventilatory modality and conventional positive pressure ventilation with similar mean airway pressure, and have not shown a detrimental effect of APRV on oxygenation of arterial blood. Valentine et al. observed a slight, inconsequential increase in intrapulmonary shunt measured with the inert gas elimination technique during APRV, when compared with synchronized intermittent mandatory ventilation and pressure support ventilation (10). This difference was attributed to microatelectasis in the absence of periodic hyperinflation of the lungs.

Theoretically, an airway pressure release during spontaneous inspiration and restoration of CPAP during spontaneous exhalation could conflict, causing an increase in the work of spontaneous breathing and discomfort to the patient. Such potential for interference exists in other ventilatory modalities as well, particularly during ventilation with non-synchronized intermittent mandatory ventilation. With APRV conflict between spontaneous and mechanical ventilation has been demonstrated in studies conducted in a lung analog (13) but it has not been reported to be a problem in patients ventilated with APRV (8, 11, 14). It is likely that when APRV is used in a subject with intact respiratory feedback mechanisms the problem of dyssynchrony will remain theoretical as it did with intermittent mandatory ventilation (15).

Clinical experience with APRV

Results from four published clinical studies are available to evaluate the use of APRV in patients requiring mechanical ventilatory support. In the first human study of APRV, Garner et al. compared APRV and positive pressure ventilation in patients with mild acute lung injury following cardiopulmonary bypass (8). The comparisons were made using similar mean airway pressures for both ventilatory modalities. The results of this study were similar to those obtained in the laboratory under comparable conditions. APRV and positive pressure ventilation provided equally effective ventilation and oxygenation for all patients in the study. Peak airway pressure, however, was significantly reduced during APRV. No differences in circulatory function were detected between the two ventilatory modalities. All patients were weaned successfully from ventilatory support using APRV, and no complications were reported.

A prospective multi-institutional investigation evaluated APRV as a primary ventilatory support modality in adults with mode rate to severe acute respiratory failure of variable etiology (14). All except one of the 50 patients included in the study required mechanical ventilatory support and positive end-expiratory airway pressure therapy based on clinical assessment. Development of respiratory acidemia upon reduction of mechanical ventilatory support could be demonstrated in 13 of the 50 patients. In 47 of the 50 patients, including 11 of the 13 patients with respiratory acidemia, adequate alveolar ventilation could be maintained with APRV. Average relative reduction in peak airway pressure upon initiating APRV was $55 \pm 17\%$. Institution of APRV did not have a significant effect on variables reflecting oxygenation of arterial blood or circulatory function. Apart from inadequate alveolar ventilation in three of the 50 patients, no complications related to the use of APRV were reported. The failure to achieve adequate ventilation in three patients likely resulted from inadequate adjustment of airway pressures and release rate. Data regarding use of APRV after the initial cardiopulmonary measurements were not reported.

Cane et al. reported data from 18 adult patients with severe acute respiratory failure, who were sequentially ventilated with continuous positive pressure ventilation and APRV (11). APRV provided effective ventilatory support to 17 of the 18 patients with an average peak airway pressure (39 ± 10 cmH$_2$O) that was significantly lower than that during positive pressure ventilation (64 ± 15 cmH$_2$O). One patient developed cardiopulmonary decompensation after initiation of APRV for unexplained reasons, despite being adequately ventilated with positive pressure ventilation. Six of the remaining 17 patients who initially responded well to APRV were later returned to positive pressure ventilation because of lobar atelectasis (two patients), hypoxemia (two patients) and alveolar hypoventilation (two patients). The deterioration of pulmonary function could be reversed in five of these six patients after reinstitution of positive pressure ventilation. The authors attributed the development of atelectasis to the volume-variable nature of APRV.

Valentine et al. compared APRV, synchronized IMV and pressure support ventilation in a short-term study of eight patients recovering from open-heart operations performed under hypothermic cardiopulmonary bypass (10). APRV provided adequate alveolar ventilation with lower peak airway pressure and lower dead space ventilation than the other modalities. A slight increase in intrapulmonary shunting of blood was observed during APRV, but it did not affect oxygenation of arterial blood. Hemodynamic, respiratory or technical complications were not seen during APRV. However, this study was focused on short-term effects on gas exchange, and did not encompass the entire duration of postoperative ventilatory support.

Available experimental and clinical data indicate that a marked lowering of peak airway pressure is a major advantage of APRV. Depending on the method of application, mean airway and mean intrathoracic pressure may be reduced as well. Therefore, use of APRV may lower the incidence of pulmonary barotrauma and the severity of circulatory impairment associated with mechanical ventilatory support. Furthermore, APRV may allow delivery of effective ventilatory support to some patients without tracheal intubation. Results of clinical trials published so far do not yet allow one to define a role for APRV in clinical practice of critical care. In particular, insufficient data is available to assess the effect of APRV on cardiopulmonary function over several days of ventilatory support. More information is also needed to more clearly define the optimum procedure in adjusting the pressure levels and the duration of pressure release during ventilation with APRV. However, available data do indicate that APRV may offer clinically important advantages that have the potential to improve the care of patients requiring ventilatory support.

References

1. Montgomery AB, Stager MA, Carrico CJ, Hudson LD (1985) Causes of mortality in patients with the adult respiratory distress syndrome. Am Rev Respir Dis 132:485-489
2. Katz JA, Marks JD (1985) Inspiratory work with and without continuous positive airway pressure in patients with acute respiratory failure. Anesthesiology 63:598-607
3. Kirby RR, Downs JB, Civetta JM, Modell JH, Dannemiller FJ, Klein EF, Hodges M (1975) High level positive end-expiratory pressure (PEEP) in acute respiratory insufficiency. Chest 67:156-163
4. Downs JB, Stock MC (1987) Airway pressure release ventilation: a new concept in ventilatory support. Crit Care Med 15:459-461
5. Banner MJ, Downs JB, Kirby RR, Smith RA, Boysen PG, Lampotang S (1988) Effects of expiratory flow resistance on inspiratory work of breathing. Chest 93:795-799
6. Stock MC, Downs JB, Frolicher DA (1987) Airway pressure release ventilation. Crit Care Med 15:462-466
7. Martin L, Wetzel RV, Bilenki AL (1991) Airway pressure release ventilation in a neonatal lamb model of acute lung injury. Crit Care Med 19:373-378
8. Garner W, Downs JB, Stock MC, Räsänen J (1988) Airway pressure release ventilation (APRV): a human trial. Chest 94:779-781
9. Räsänen J, Downs JB, Stock MC (1988) Cardiovascular effects of conventional positive pressure ventilation and airway pressure release ventilation. Chest 93:911-915
10. Valentine DD, Hammond MD, Downs JB, Sears NJ, Sims WR (1991) Distribution of ventilation and perfusion with different modes of mechanical ventilation. Am Rev Respir Dis 143:1262-1266
11. Cane RD, Peruzzi WT, Shapiro BA (1991) Airway pressure release ventilation in severe acute respiratory failure. Chest 100:460-463
12. Smith D, Leon M, Mann M, Rubin M (1991) Does airway pressure release ventilation alter lung function during acute lung injury? Crit Care Med 19.S51
13. Putensen Ch, Putensen-Himmer G, Leon M (1992) Synchronization of the release during airway pressure release ventilation. Anesthesiology 77:A1207
14. Räsänen J, Cane RD, Downs JB, Hurst JM, Jousela IT, Kirby RR, Togove HJ, Stock MC (1991) Airway pressure release ventilation during acute lung injury: a prospective multicenter trial. Crit Care Med 19:1234-1241
15. Heenan TJ, Downs JB, Douglas ME, Ruiz BC, Jumper L (1980) Intermittent mandatory ventilation: is synchronization important? Chest 77:598-602

High Frequency Positive Pressure Ventilation

U.H. Sjöstrand

Introduction

The prototype for high frequency ventilation is found in nature - the respiration of hummingbirds and insects is synchronous with the beat of their wings. In 1915 Henderson et al. (1) commented on the rapid, shallow breathing in dogs during heat polypnea: "There may easily be a gaseous exchange sufficient to support life even when tidal volume is considerably less than the dead space". Briscoe et al. (2) confirmed Henderson's observations, and demonstrated in a patient with a dead space of 170 ml that tidal volumes as small as 60 ml provided alveolar gas exchange. A similar principle was first applied by Jack Emerson, who called his US patent application in 1959 an "apparatus for vibrating portions of a patient's airway".

High frequency positive pressure ventilation (HFPPV) (3) was primarily developed in an attempt to provide positive-pressure ventilation free of circulatory effects synchronous with respiration (U.H. Sjöstrand and P.Å. Öberg, unpublished observations 1967). The original rationale was that a reduction in dead space produced by means of endotracheal insufflation would make it possible to provide adequate ventilation with relatively small tidal volumes at frequencies of 60-100 bpm. To compensate for the increased dead space to tidal volume ratio (VD/VT) during high frequency ventilation, a ventilator system with almost insignificant compressible volume and internal compliance was required. In the first experiments gas was supplied through an insufflation catheter inserted into the endotracheal tube with its tip just above the carina. Anesthetized dogs were adequately ventilated and oxygenated with small tidal volumes and very low airway pressures. By means of a simple expiratory resistance positive end-expiratory airway pressure (PEEP) of 2.5-5 cm H_2O was guaranteed, giving moderate but continuous expansion of the lungs. When air was intermittently supplied by endotracheal insufflation at a frequency of 60-80 bpm, spontaneous breathing ceased almost instantaneously (4). As this suppressive effect occurred even during eucapnia ventilation, it was assumed that it most probably resulted from suppression of the reflexogenic spontaneous respiratory rhythm.

Experimental and clinical studies of HFPPV

Initial studies

Initially HFPPV was compared with spontaneous ventilation in anesthetized dogs. Subsequent comparisons (Fig. 1) were made between spontaneous breathing, HFPPV and IPPV (Engström "volume-cycled" respirator, ER). HFPPV provided adequate ventilation at ventilatory frequencies (f) of 60-100 bpm with inspiratory times relative to the ventilatory cycle (t%) of 14%-35% and expiratory tidal volumes within the range of 90-190 ml. In healthy dogs HFPPV produced eucapnia ventilation and arterial oxygenation with *negative* intrapleural pressure (Fig. 1) – i.e., with low transpulmonary pressures – and without any ventilation-synchronous circulatory or any negative systemic effects (3). In 1971, the accumulated experimental experience with HFPPV justified a study in 15 patients scheduled for elective surgery under general anesthesia (5): adequate oxygenation and ventilation were achieved with HFPPV of 60-110 bpm and t% of 15%-30%, and with expiratory tidal volumes which notably approximated anatomical dead space.

The pneumatic valve principle

Flowing gas has a tendency to adhere to walls - the *wall effect* (= Coanda effect). By application of the pneumatic valve principle (6, 7), a ventilator system for HFPPV without an insufflation catheter or a consequent increase in compliance[1] was developed. This is illustrated in the left part of Fig. 2 (A): there is no gas entrainment. However – due to their open characteristics – ventilator systems and techniques for HFPPV using an insufflation catheter, or a pneumatic valve, lacked the capacity to provide volume-controlled ventilation. This motivated further technical and functional development in order to provide volume-controlled ventilation during routine clinical management (see *Volume-Controlled Ventilation*).

High frequency ventilation - HFV

High frequency ventilation (HFV) actually represents a heterogeneous group of ventilatory techniques which differ in system design, cycle frequency, and method of gas delivery. This also explains much of the conflict and confusion in the literature concerning high frequency ventilation - it arises from attempts to compare experimental results of studies in which methods of high and

---

[1] The internal volume at ambient pressure (IVA, in ml) of the patient circuit is known as compressible volume, and the internal static compliance (ISC, in ml per cmH_2O) of the patient circuit (below positive pressures of 50 cmH_2O) is known simply as internal compliance (13, 14). Compression volume (Vc) equals internal pressure (IP) at end-insufflation multiplied by ISC (Vc = IP x ISP).

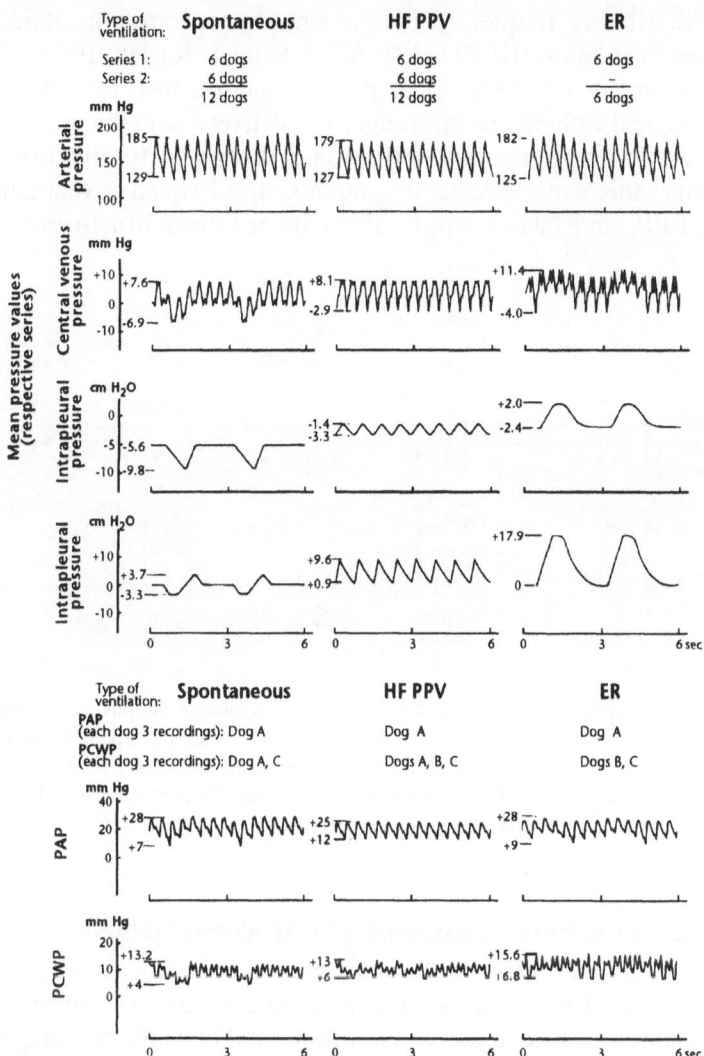

Fig. 1. Intrathoracic, circulatory, and ventilatory pressure conditions during spontaneous breathing and with the two compared types of positive pressure ventilation - HFPPV and IPPV (IPPV-ER, Engström ventilator). When the two types of positive pressure ventilation are compared, the differences in airway and intrapleural pressures are substantial. Pulmonary arterial pressure (*PAP*) and pulmonary capillary wedge pressure (*PCWP*) were obtained in three dogs. Reproduced with permission from Jonzon et al. (3)

conventional frequency ventilation differ. For instance, *the major functional difference between the injector and pneumatic valve techniques is gas entrainment* (7, 9-11): the injector technique *mixes two gases*, injector and entrained gas, whereas the pneumatic valve technique delivers *all gas* via a side-arm in a fashion similar to most conventional ventilators. Techniques that work with high ventilatory frequency and gas entrainment are considered as high frequency jet ventilation (HFJV) (12). All techniques for HFPPV work without gas/air entrainment, i.e., they either involve endotracheal insufflation with a specially designed catheter, or inspiratory gas delivery with the pneumatic valve principle. As high frequency oscillation (HFO) will be discussed by Dr. Lunkenheimer, this overview mainly presents high frequency ventilation in the form of HFPP, and (when applicable) its relationship to conventional ventilation.[2]

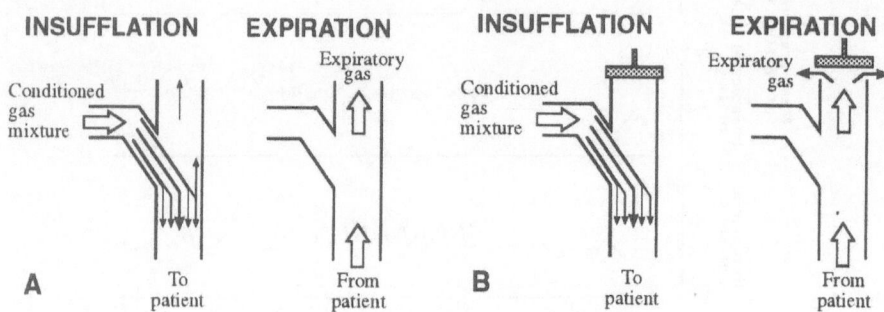

Fig. 2. A Schematic illustration of the construction and function of the pneumatic valve: a pneumatic valve is obtained when gas is supplied to the side-arm of the pneumatic valve connector. It instantly ceases when the gas supply is interrupted, leaving the expiratory pathway open, as seen on the right side of the figure. **B** Patient curcuit for pressure/flow-generated volume-controlled ventilation (system H). Reproduced by permission from Sjöstrand (8, 14, 16)

HFPPV for broncho/laryngoscopy and tracheal stenosis

In 1973, the need for efficient methods of ventilation during endoscopy led to the elaboration of HFPPV techniques for bronchoscopy and laryngoscopy (8, 15, 16). A ventilator with low compressible volume and low internal compliance was developed (AGA Bronchovent, Siemens-Elema AB, Solna, Sweden). Based on experimental studies ventilatory frequency was set to 60 bpm, and t% to 22% (6-10, 16), and the safety features of the Bronchovent were settled (8-11).

Bronchoscopic HFPPV

Ventilation by the fixed side-arm of the bronchoscope was first described by Carden et al. (17) and utilizes the Coanda effect, i.e. ventilation is directly by the

[2] Results of experimental and clinical evaluations during HFPPV, including some technical modifications between the years 1972-77, are presented collectively in a special issue of Acta Anaesthesiologica Scandinavica, Supplementum in 1977 (13). The development of HFV (HFPPV, HFO and HFJV), including experimental and clinical results, is also described in a special issue of International Anesthesiology Clinics in 1983 (14).

side-arm of the bronchoscope. This has several advantages over the injector technique as it is much less sensitive to instruments placed within the lumen of the bronchoscope (8-11). *Bronchoscopic HFPPV* combines HFPPV with the side-arm technique. Experimental and clinical evaluations of HFPPV during bronchoscopy under general anesthesia (9) have shown that there is no gas entrainment. Even when instruments of reasonable size are introduced through the bronchoscope no significant change in ventilation or oxygenation occurs. This is in contrast to the injector technique in which the introduction of instruments through the bronchoscope usually impairs gas entrainment severely and unpredictably reducing ventilation and thereby increasing inspired oxygen concentration. Based on clinical experience gained from 800 bronchoscopies (10) ventilation nomograms have been designed for bronchoscopic HFPPV to standardize the procedure and increase its safety (9, 10): ventilation is regulated by the magnitude of ventilator gas output, whereas inspired oxygen concentration is adjusted by means of the oxygen concentration delivered by the ventilator.

Laryngoscopic HFPPV

Laryngoscopic HFPPV combines HFPPV with an endotracheal insufflation catheter for ventilation (15). The naso/orotracheal insufflation catheter is supplied with side-holes close to its tip which functionally abolish the injector effects (10, 11, 16), i.e. with this technique no entrainment of gas occurs through the airways during ventilation. Absence of air entrainment means that a controlled mixture of gas can be provided for ventilation, and the continuous upward stream of gas through the larynx prevents blood or tissue from being sucked into the trachea. This is particularly important when the technique is used for ventilation during laser surgery. A ventilation nomogram for laryngoscopic HFPPV, based on clinical experience yielded by 500 laryngoscopies (10) shows the appropriate ventilator gas output to be used. This makes it possible to standardize the procedure to increase its safety.

HFPPV during resection of tracheal stenosis

A combination of bronchoscopic and laryngoscopic HFPPV has been used (10, 18) during tracheal stenosis resection without the interference of an endotracheal tube. Because of the continuous positive airway pressure before, during, and after resection of the tracheal stenosis, the risk of atelectasis formation with an open thorax is reduced. Similar experience has been reported using HFJV during tracheal surgery (19).

Volume-controlled ventilation

In volume-controlled ventilation the patient circuit should have minimal compressible volume and minimal internal compliance - ideally the compression volume (Vc) of the patient circuit should be much less than the tidal volume (V_T) (16, 20). A pneumatic valve principle for volume-controlled ventilation requires the addition of a valve (Fig. 2B) closing the expiratory port during the inspiratory phase (6, 8, 16, 20, 21). A prototype system (Fig. 3) for pressure/flow-generated volume-controlled ventilation has an internal compliance of 0.06 ml/cmH$_2$O of the patient circuit (8). During early inspiration the initial accelerating flow rapidly turns into decelerating flow during the major part of the inspiratory phase (22). Drive gas pressure of the ventilator is set to provide the desired tidal volume, which is the primary (independent) parameter, with airway pressure being the dependent variable (8). With present technical and clinical requirements for respirators most modern low-compression ventilator systems can be used both for volume-controlled and for pressure-controlled ventilation. Pressure-controlled ventilation provides early delivery of the major part of the tidal breath (see *Combined Pressure-Volume-Controlled Ventilation*).

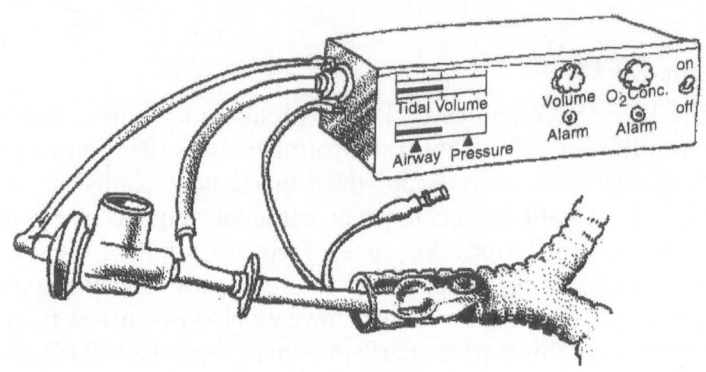

Fig. 3. System H with the pneumatic valve connector and an expiratory valve for pressure/flow-generated volume-controlled ventilation. Reproduced with permission from Sjöstrand et al. (21)

Comparative studies in dogs

Initial studies were made in healthy dogs with normal lungs (23) and the ventilatory patterns of a conventional volume-controlled ventilator at 20 bpm and volume-controlled HFPPV at 60 bpm were compared. It was anticipated that a system with negligible compressible volume and decelerating inspiratory flow may induce more efficient intrapulmonary mixing of gas (8, 20). In dogs with normal lungs (24) further comparisons were therefore made between the ventilatory pattern of Servo Ventilator 900 (SV900, Siemens-Elema) and a prototype system (H) for volume-controlled ventilation. During ventilation with decelerating inspiratory flow (system H) intrapulmonary gas distribution was improved, both at 20 and 60 bpm relative to ventilation with constant inspiratory flow (SV900).

Intrapulmonary distribution during bronchoscopy

In nine patients scheduled for diagnostic bronchoscopy, FRC and intrapulmonary gas distribution were evaluated by a nitrogen washout technique (25) with the patients in the supine position (first awake during spontaneous breathing, then under general anesthesia and HFPPV via a pneumatic valve connector). In terms of lung clearance index and nitrogen washout delay (25) gas distribution improved during HFPPV (f 60 bpm, t% 22%).

IPPV and HFPPV during thoracic surgery

In nine patients scheduled for open chest surgery, intrapleural pressure measurements were made (26). Volume-controlled HFPPV produced normocapnia and adequate oxygenation despite low mean airway pressure (P_{aw}). There were significant differences between intrapleural pressure during HFPPV (60 bpm) relative to conventional volume-controlled IPPV (20 bpm). In some patients, HFPPV with tidal volumes approximately 25% lower than the estimated anatomic dead space resulted in normocapnia.

Regional organ blood flow during IPPV and HFPPV

Effects of HFPPV on cerebral blood flow at normal and elevated intracranial pressure (ICP) were compared with those of IPPV in the same conditions in six mongrel dogs (27). Cerebral blood flow during HFPPV was comparable to that during IPPV. Ventilator-synchronous fluctuations in ICP observed during IPPV were reduced during HFPPV when ICP was normal. In relation to the mode of ventilation, no differences were found in mean organ blood flow in lungs (bronchial artery supply), kidneys and heart.

Comparative studies in pigs

The premise that collateral ventilation normally occurs in the human and the dog lung has led to the suggestion that it might contribute to the successful experimental and/or clinical effects of HFPPV. As the pig has poor collateral ventilation, a study was conducted in nine pigs anesthetized with ketamine hydrochloride (28). Comparisons were made between the ventilatory patterns provided by a conventional ventilator (Servo Ventilator 900C, Siemens-Elema AB, Sweden) and a prototype system (H) for volume-controlled ventilation. A ventilatory frequency of 20 bpm with SV900C (SV-20) and system H (H-20) and of 60 bpm with system H (H-60) were used. PEEP was set to maintain the same mean airway pressure with the three modes of ventilation. There were no differences in circulatory and oxygen transport variables. Measurements of airway pressure and intrapleural liquid surface pressure demonstrated that the distending pressure (at end-inspiration) was lower with the low-compression system (H-20 vs. SV-20), especially at a high ventilatory frequency (H-60 *vs.* H-20). To achieve the same alveolar ventilation and arterial oxygenation H-20 and, especially H-60 (= HFPPV), provided ventilation with the lowest distending pressures. In an additional investigation (29) intrapulmonary gas distribution was studied with the nitrogen washout technique in nine piglets under general anesthesia. Clearance of N_2 during washout was most efficient with H-60 and least efficient with SV-20.

Volume-controlled IPPV and HFPPV during surgery

Seventy-four patients undergoing biliary tract surgery (30) were intubated with Hi-Lo Jet Mallinckrodt tracheal tubes (National Catheter Corp., Argyle, NY) with an inspiratory:expiratory lumen ratio of 1:10 (31). Patients were first ventilated by IPPV from a conventional ventilator with tidal volumes and frequency adjusted to produce a $PaCO_2$ within the normal range (FIO_2 of 0.4). After the abdominal retractors had been positioned, volume-controlled HFPPV (of 60 bpm) was started using the small lumen inspiratory line for inspiration, and the expiratory lumen adapted with an expiratory valve. In all patients a PEEP of 7 cmH_2O was maintained by adjusting the PEEP valve of the ventilator systems. Airway pressures (P_{aw}) were monitored by a transducer using a water-filled tubing connected to the pressure monitoring port of the tracheal tube. Smaller tidal volumes produced lower airway pressures during volume-controlled HFPPV.

In ten patients who underwent coronary artery bypass grafting, conventional IPPV (Airshields Anesthesia Ventilator, Air-Shields Inc., Hatboro, PA) and volume-controlled HFPPV were studied immediately before and after surgery (32). All patients were adequately ventilated with HFPPV or IPPV. Direct and indirect hemodynamic and respiratory variables were recorded and calculated. No significant differences in hemodynamic stability were noted either before or after coronary bypass, although both peak and mean airway pressures were significantly lower during HFPPV than during IPPV.

HFPPV and HFJV in acute respiratory failure

The ability to ventilate patients with smaller tidal volumes and at lower airway pressures has served as the major justification for the use of HFPPV and HFJV in the intensive care setting. A number of studies have focused on acute respiratory failure (ARF) and adult respiratory distress syndrome (ARDS), but as yet very few investigations have demonstrated any major or convincing advantages of HFPPV or HFJV over conventional volume- or pressure-controlled ventilation. A brief review seems justified.[3]

Long-term treatment of two patients with respiratory insufficiency with IPPV/PEEP and HFPPV/PEEP was described by Bjerager et al. (34) in 1977. During HFPPV with ventilatory frequencies of 60 bpm an inhibitory effect on spontaneous respiration occurred. In the early 1980s a study of 17 patients with ARF/ARDS by Wattwil et al. (22, 35) compared volume-controlled ventilation (Servo Ventilator 900B) at a ventilatory frequency of 20 bpm (SV-20) with a low-compression system (system H) at two ventilatory frequencies, 20 and 60 bpm (H-20 and H-60). PEEP was used to reduce airway closure and ventilation/perfusion mismatch. The linear velocity of gas during H-60 (= HFPPV) was calculated to be 2500-3000 cm/s, corresponding to peak Reynold's numbers of well above 10000 and therefore turbulent flow (36). During H-60, normoventilation was achieved with smaller tidal volumes and lower mean intratracheal pressures than during SV-20 and H-20. Cardiac index and oxygen transport were not affected by changes in ventilatory pattern. In most patients, arterial oxygenation was related to mean airway pressure during all three modes of ventilation. In ten patients intrapulmonary gas distribution was measured as nitrogen washout delay percent (NOWOD%) and showed improvement from 106% during SV-20 to 74% with H-60 ($p < 0.05$) (35). H-60 also increased carbon dioxide elimination in the two patients with the most severe pulmonary dysfunction. Compared with conventional ventilation (SV-20), volume-controlled HFPPV (H-60) was equally efficient and accepted by the patients.

The only prospective, controlled large scale study of conventional ventilation and HFJV was published in 1983 by Carlon and co-workers (37) and did not show any significant differences in overall patient survival, duration of intensive care stay, or occurrence of pulmonary barotrauma in adults with ARF. In 1986, 19 critically ill patients with acute respiratory failure were studied by Fusciardi et al. (38) with the aim of comparing the hemodynamic effects of continuous positive pressure ventilation (CPPV) and HFJV at comparable levels of alveolar ventilation. In all patients comparable levels of arterial PCO_2 were obtained with CPPV and HFJV. The authors concluded that patients with circulatory shock and acute respiratory failure had a more favorable hemodynamic profile during HFJV than during CPPV at identical levels of mean airway pressure. In 1987 Wetzel and Gioia (39) also reported mixed results in 12 patients with severe ARDS in infants and children treated with conventional ventilation vs. HFJV. Most patients experienced temporary improvement in oxygenation with HFJV. While there were only three survivors, this group represented the most extreme cases of respiratory failure encountered in which high mortality was expected. The authors claimed that survivors "tend to display progressive improvement in

---

[3] A more detailed review was presented in *Problems in Respiratory Care* in 1989 (33).

oxygenation following initiation of HFJV". In 1989, based on many years of experience with HFJV in the intensive care setting, Rouby and Viars (40) claimed that there are indications for HFJV in critically ill patients, such as ARF with circulatory shock, acute cardiac failure, bronchopleural fistula with large air leaks, and tracheal lesions secondary to tracheostomy or intubation. Contraindications for the use of HFJV are patients with chronic obstructive pulmonary disease or asthma (absolute) and unilateral acute lung disease (relative).

Current characteristics and applications of HFPPV

Mandatory in all forms of HFPPV is careful, accurate monitoring and qualified supervision. In the healthy lung normocarbia is produced with smaller tidal volumes and lower airway pressures with volume-controlled HFPPV (= constant inspiratory pressure with decelerating inspiratory flow) than with conventional volume-controlled ventilation (= constant inspiratory flow with increasing inspiratory pressure) (34, 41). Pressure-volume-controlled HFPPV generates a ventilatory pattern with an inspiratory flow, i.e. initially rapidly accelerating and then of a decelerating character (see above, *volume-controlled ventilation*). Clinically HFPPV is an established procedure during anesthesia in airway endoscopy. For thoracic and laryngo-tracheal surgery this technique has also gained some merits. Provided mean airway pressure (and lung volumes) are similar, oxygenation in critical care patients during HFPPV seems to be equivalent to conventional IPPV (22, 35). Major differences in the clinical applicability of low-compression and conventional ventilatory systems were described by Smith et al. (42), and by Sjöstrand (33) also listing "Characteristics and functions related to differences between HFPPV and IPPV documented in experimental and/or clinical investigations" (43).

The open lung concept in acute respiratory failure

The "Open up the lung and keep it open" concept will be presented by Dr. Lachmann. It originates from experimental and clinical results obtained by Lachmann et al. (44) regarding arterial oxygenation and oxygen transport which indicate that evolution of pulmonary damage in ARDS is closely related to airway pressures required to recruit, or to allow reopening of, collapsed alveoli. In the maintenance of alveolar patency (without overdistension of compliant lung units) sufficient airway pressure is necessary to keep different lung units open. In this context, inverse ratio, pressure-controlled ventilation has been advocated (44, 45).

Although the role of HFPPV in the management of pulmonary diseases still remains to be clarified, it has at least been a stimulus for research and for development of new technologies, procedures and ventilatory strategies (3, 5, 7-16, 18-43, 45-48) which provide ventilation in patients requiring advanced ventilatory support. It has been emphasized (45-48) that controlled animal and clinical studies must be accomplished before recommendations can be made regarding general clinical use in the intensive care setting.

Combined pressure-volume-controlled ventilation

In ARF the present ideology is that the ventilatory mode should recruit ("open") and maintain the patency of the airways (44-48). Since 1987 this justified some of our group's experimental studies of induced acute respiratory distress in the pig under general anesthesia (46-48). We have employed an animal experimental model of acute pulmonary dysfunction induced by bronchoalveolar lavage ad modum Lachmann and collaborators (44-47) by which surfactant deficiency is achieved. The result is low-compliant (stiff) lungs, a threefold increase of extravascular lung water (EVLW), and reduced FRC. A pronounced liability for alveolar collapse arises unless the ventilatory pattern provided by the respirator offers an adequate pressure-volume ratio (44-48). The bronchoalveolar lavage model has proven to be reproducible and stable (46, 47) and functionally it is a simplified model of the very complex condition found in acute respiratory failure (ARF). The stability of the animal model is demonstrated by constant O_2 consumption and CO_2 production. Morphologically, the lung model has also been studied with light and electron transmission and scanning electron microscopy (46, 48), but also with computed tomography (CT) scans (Fig. 4) (48).

Since the end of the 1980s volume-controlled (VC) and a modified form of pressure-controlled (PC) ventilation, combined pressure-volume-controlled ventilation (PVC), has been studied in the above-mentioned pig model of induced acute respiratory failure (46, 47). Pressure regulated volume controlled (PRVC) ventilation has been developed by Siemens-Elema AB (Solna, Sweden) and it is inherent in the Servo Ventilator 300. PRVC has been used in studies of different ventilatory modes keeping the lung "open" with tidal volumes which maintain normoventilation (48; unpublished results). Recent experimental studies (unpublished results) confirm earlier findings (46, 47) that PRVC keeps the airways open at a low inspiratory drive gas pressure of the ventilator and provides adequate oxygen transport. The low driving gas pressure produces low peak inspiratory (PIP) and end-inspiratory ($PAW_{endinsp}$) airway pressures and appropriate end-inspiratory lung volumes - important prerequisites for reduced baro/volutrauma. Studies using CT (Fig. 4) demonstrate how the lung can be kept open (45, 48), but also shows that when the lungs are deficient of surfactant there may easily be pronounced pulmonary collapse if ventilation is maintained without PEEP. Morphologically this has also been illustrated with scanning electron microscopy (48) (Fig. 4).

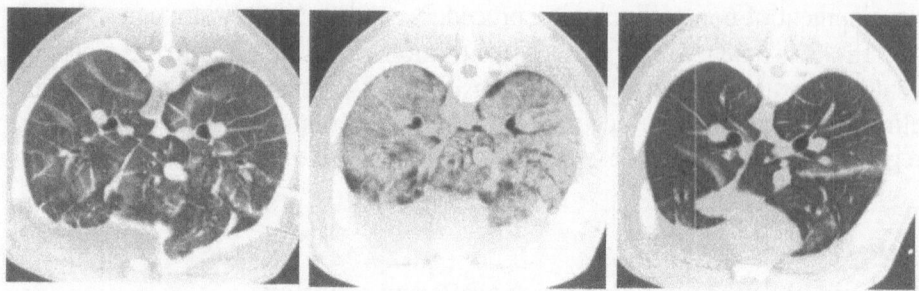

Fig. 4. Computed tomography (CT) scans of the chest during "Pause hold Exp." of the Servo Ventilator 300 in one of the piglets in a study by Sjöstrand et al. (48). The time sequence between the different settings is 5 min. Based on a previous study (47) mean airway pressure was set to be 25 cmH$_2$O for "open lung" ventilation (*left*): note normal aeration of the lung parenchyma with dependent densities representing pleural effusion; fluid is also present in interlobar and segmental fissures. Mean airway pressure was 8 cmH$_2$O during ventilation with zero PEEP (*center*): note extensive and widespread densities compatible with reduced aeration ("alveolar collapse") and probably some alveolar edema. Mean airway pressure returned to 25 cmH$_2$O (by addition of the same PEEP as with the initial open lung ventilation), reopened lung (*right*): note the almost immediate restoration of aeration of the lung parenchyma. Reproduced by permission from Sjöstrand et al. (48)

For the past few years our clinical strategy has followed the above principles, often resulting in clinical effects (unpublished data) similar to those obtained experimentally.

References

1. Henderson Y, Chillingworth FP, Whitney JL (1915) The respiratory dead space. Am J Physiol 38:1
2. Briscoe WA, Forster RE, Comroe JH (1954) Alveolar ventilation at very low tidal volumes. J Appl Physiol 7:27-30
3. Jonzon A, Öberg PÅ, Sedin G, Sjöstrand U (1971) High-frequency positive-pressure ventilation by endotracheal insufflation. Acta Anaesthesiol Scand 15 [Suppl 43]:1-43
4. Öberg PÅ, Sjöstrand U (1971) Studies of blood-pressure on carotid-sinus nerve stimulation. Acta Physiol Scand 81:96-109
5. Heijman K, Heijman L, Jonzon A et al (1972) High frequency positive pressure ventilation during anaesthesia and routine surgery in man. Acta Anaesthesiol Scand 16:176-187
6. Sjöstrand U (1975) High-frequency positive-pressure ventilation (HFPPV) technique for artifical ventilation. In: Stembera ZK, Polácek K, Sabata V (eds) Pernatal medicine Thieme, Stuttgart, pp 333-335
7. Eriksson I, Heijman L, Sjöstrand U (1974) High-frequency positive-pressure ventilation (HFPPV) in bronchoscopy during anesthesia. Opuscula Medica (Stockholm) 19:14-24
8. Sjöstrand U (1980) High-frequency positive-pressure ventilation (HFPPV): a review. Crit Care Med 8:345-364

9. Eriksson I, Sjöstrand U (1977) Experimental and clinical evaluation of high-frequency positive-pressure ventilation (HFPPV) and the pneumatic valve principle in bronchoscopy under genaral anaesthesia. Acta Anaesthesiol Scand 21 [Suppl 64]:83-100

10. Borg U, Eriksson I, Sjöstrand U (1980) High-frequency positive-pressure ventilation (HFPPV). A review based upon its use during bronchoscopy and for laryngoscopy and microlaryngeal surgery under general anesthesia. Anesth Analg 59:594-603

11. Eriksson I, Sjöstrand U (1977) A clinical evaluation of high-frequency positive-pressure ventilation (HFPPV) in laryngoscopy under general anaesthesia. Acta Anaesthesiol Scand 21 [Suppl 64]:101-110

12. Klain M, Smith RB (1977) High frequency percutaneous transtracheal jet ventilation. Crit Care Med 5:280-287

13. Sjöstrand U (1977) Experimental and clinical evaluation of high-frequency positive-pressure ventilation - HFPPV: Introduction. Acta Anaesthesiol Scand 21 [Suppl 64]:5

14. Smith RB, Sjöstrand UH (1983) High frequency ventilation. Development of high frequency positive pressure low-compression ventilation. Int Anesthesiol Clin 21:11-32

15. Eriksson I, Sjöstrand U (1974) High-frequency positive-pressure ventilation (HFPPV) during laryngoscopy. Opuscula Medica (Stockholm) 19:278-286

16. Sjöstrand U (1977) Review of the physiological rationale for and development of high-frequency positive-pressure ventilation - HFPPV. Acta Anaesthesiol Scand 21 [Suppl 64]:7-27

17. Carden E, Trapp WG, Oulton J (1970) A new and simple method for ventilating patients undergoing bronchoscopy. Anesthesiology 33:454-458

18. Eriksson I, Nilsson L-G, Nordström S et al (1975) High-frequency positive-pressure ventilation (HFPPV) during transthoracic resection of tracheal stenosis and during peroperative bronchoscopic examination. Acta Anaesthesiol Scand 19:113-119

19. Carlon GC, Turnbull AD, Alexander JD et al (1981) High frequency jet ventilation during tracheal surgery. Crit Care Med 9:163-167

20. Sjöstrand U (1977) Pneumatic systems facilitating treatment of respiratory insufficiency with alternative use of IPPV/PEEP, HFPPV/PEEP, CPPB or CPAP. Acta Anaesthesiol Scand 21 [Suppl 64]:123-147

21. Sjöstrand UH, Wattwil LM, Borg UR et al (1982) Volume-controlled high-frequency positive-pressure ventilation as a useful mode of ventilation during open-chest surgery - a report of three cases. Resp Care 27:1380-1385

22. Wattwil LM, Sjöstrand UH, Borg UR, et al (1983) Comparative studies of IPPV and HFPPV with PEEP in critical care patients. II: studies on intrapulmonary gas distribution. Crit Care Med 11:38-43

23. Eriksson I, Jonzon A, Sedin G, Sjöstrand U (1977) The influence of the ventilatory pattern on ventilation, circulation and oxygen transport during continuous positive-pressure ventilation - an experimental study. Acta Anaesthesiol Scand 21 [Suppl 64]:149-163

24. Borg U, Eriksson I, Sjöstrand U et al (1981) Experimental studies of continuous positive-pressure ventilation (CPPV) and high-frequency positive-pressure ventilation (HFPPV). Resuscitation 9:1-21

25. Eriksson I, Sjöstrand U (1980) Effects of high-frequency positive-pressure ventilation (HFPPV) and general anesthesia on intrapulmonary gas distribution in patients undergoing diagnostic bronchoscopy. Anesth Analg 59:585-593

26. Malina JR, Nordström SG, Sjöstrand UH et al (1981) A clinical evalution of high-frequency positive-pressure ventilation (HFPPV) in patients scheduled for open-chest surgery. Anesth Analg 60:324-330

27. Bunegin L, Smith RB, Sjöstrand UH et al (1984) Regional organ blood flow during high frequency positive pressure ventilation (HFPPV) and intermittent positive pressure ventilation (IPPV). Anesthesiology 61:416-419

28. Sjöstrand UH, Smith RB, Bunegein L et al (1987) Gas exchange in low-compression HFPPV is maintained at low distending pressures in the pig. Acta Anaesthesiol Scand 31:417-422

29. Nielsen JB, Sjöstrand UH, Henneberg SW (1991) An experimental randomized study of six different ventilatory modes in a piglet model with normal lungs. Intensive Care Med 17: 169-174

30. Babinski MF, Smith RB, Sjöstrand UH (1985) Volume-controlled high frequency positive pressure ventilation for upper abdominal surgery. A clinical report. Anaesthesia 40:619-623

31. Sjöstrand UH, Bunegin L, Smith RB et al (1983) Development and clinical application of high frequency ventilation. In: Scheck PA, Sjöstrand UH, Smith RB (eds) Perspectives in high frequency ventilation. Marinus Nijhoff, The Hague, pp 12-38

32. Smith RB, Swartzman S, Sjöstrand UH et al (1988) Low-compliance, volume-controlled HFPPV and conventional IPPV in coronary artery bypass grafting. J Cardiothorac Anesth 2:627-632

33. Sjöstrand UH (1989) High frequency positive pressure ventilation. In: Branson RD, Hurst JM, Davis K Jr (eds) Alternative modes of ventilatory support. Problems in Respiratory Care 2(1). Lippincott, Philadelphia, pp 1-15

34. Bjerager K, Sjöstrand U, Wattwil M (1977) Long-term treatment of two patients with respiratory insufficiency with IPPV/PEEP and HFPPV/PEEP. Acta Anaesthesiol Scand 21 [Suppl 64]:55-68

35. Wattwil LM, Sjöstrand UH, Borg UR (1983) Comparative studies of IPPV and HFPPV with PEEP in critical care patients. I: a clinical evaluation. Crit Care Med 11:30-37

36. Eriksson I (1982) The role of the conducting airways in the process of gas exchange during high-frequency ventilation - a clinical and theoretical analysis. Anesth Analg 61:483-489

37. Carlon GC, Howland WS, Ray C et al (1983) High-frequency jet ventilation: a prospective randomized evaluation. Chest 84:551-559

38. Fusciardi J, Rouby JJ, Barakat T et al (1986) Hemodynamic effects of high-frequency jet ventilation in patients with and without circulatory shock. Anesthesiology 65:485

39. Wetzel RC, Gioia FR (1987) High frequency ventilation. Pediatr Clin North Am 34:15-38

40. Rouby J, Viars P (1989) Clinical use of high frequency ventilation. Acta Anaesthesiol Scand 33 [Suppl 90]:134-139

41. Sjöstrand UH (1985) The low-compression approach for ventilatory support - not just a matter of ventilatory frequency. Intensive Crit Care Digest 4:5-8

42. Smith RB, Sjöstrand UH, Babinski MF (1983) Technical considerations using high frequency positive pressure ventilation and high frequency jet ventilation. Int Anesthesiol Clin 21: 183-200

43. Sjöstrand UH (1989) In what respect does high frequency positive pressure ventilation differ from conventional ventilation? Acta Anaesthesiol Scand 33 [Suppl 90]:5-12

44. Lachmann B, Danzmann E, Heandly B et al (1982) Ventilator setting and gas exchange in respiratory distress syndrome. In: Prakash O (ed) Applied physiology in clinical respiratory care. Martinus Nijhoff, The Hague, pp 141-176

45. Lachmann B (1992) Open up the lung and keep the lung open. Intensive Care Med 18: 319-321

46. Nielsen JB, Sjöstrand UH, Edgren EL et al (1991) An experimental study of different ventilatory modes in piglets in severe respiratory distress induced by surfactant depletion. Intensive Care Med 17:225-233

47. Lichtwarck-Aschoff M, Nielsen JB, Sjöstrand UH, Edgren EL (1992) An experimental randomized study of five different ventilatory modes in a piglet model of severe respiratory distress. Intensive Care Med 18:339-347

48. Sjöstrand UH, Lichtwarck-Aschoff M, Nielsen JB et al (1995) Different ventilatory approaches to keep the lung open. Intensive Care Med 21:310-318

High Frequency Oscillation

K. Redmann, P.P. Lunkenheimer, G. Meurer, S. Fischer

Summary

Controversy exists as to whether limitations in high-frequency oscillation efficiency are caused by the size and shape of the bronchial system, by the lack of low impedant intersegmental gas flow in lung parenchyma, or by inappropriate high-frequency ventilators and ancillary hardware. Our objective in this study using the adult pig as a model of the adult patient was to test whether the adult airway system is suited to the use of high-frequency oscillatory ventilation.

We evaluated the ventilatory effect of a wide range of oscillation frequencies (10-15 to 35-45 Hz), tidal volumes (0.5 to 22.2 ml/kg), and bias flow volumes (10 to 70 l/min) at a mean airway pressure of 12 ± 1 cm H_2O in anesthetized and relaxed pigs who did not have lung injury.

Arterial blood gases are mainly dependent on tidal volume, frequency, and mean airway pressure. A threshold bias flow volume of 35 ± 5 l/min is required to prevent CO_2 rebreathing. In the group of light-weight animals (65 to 99 kg), the most efficient frequency band for CO_2 elimination was ~ 25 Hz. The most efficient frequency band for arterial oxygenation was found to vary between individuals more than the most efficient frequency band for CO_2 elimination. In the group of heavy animals (100 to 140 kg), no most efficient mean frequency could be assessed, probably because the excitation system was limited. We confirmed that tidal volume on its own had an effect on CO_2 elimination ("tidal-volume effect"), although CO_2 elimination was mainly determined by the product of tidal volume and oscillation frequency.

Conclusions: Adult pigs with a body weight in the range of the weight of clinical adult patients can be ventilated by high-frequency oscillation at tidal volumes smaller than, equal to, or slightly more than anatomical deadspace. The most efficient frequency for gas exchange varied between individuals. Tidal volume had an enhancing effect on CO_2 elimination. Failure of adequate ventilation by high-frequency oscillation is caused by a) CO_2 rebreathing, b) the avoidance of an appropriate alveolar recruitment strategy, and c) an underpowered, high-frequency ventilatory system (oscillator) that is unable to deliver appropriate pressure oscillations.

Introduction

Emerson (1) conceived high-frequency oscillation from an engineering standpoint in 1952, designing a high-frequency oscillator without ever proving the ventilatory efficiency of the principle. In 1967, Sanders (2) used jets of air to ventilate patients during bronchoscopy. In 1968, Sjöstrand (3) used high frequency ventilation during neurophysiologic animal experiments; at frequencies up to 2.5 Hz, ventilatory efficiency was preserved. In 1974 Klain and Smith (4) took up Sjöstrand's basic idea. Jet ventilation has since become the most extensively studied mode of high-frequency ventilation. In otorhinolaryngology and bronchial surgery, advantage has been taken of the small tube necessary to apply jet ventilation when the field of operation is narrow. Unresolved problems remain: an inadequate power output in currently used jet ventilators, and uncontrolled gas flow that depends on lung compliance and resistance to the lungs.

The discovery of high-frequency oscillation ventilation was a by-product of our investigations into myocardial impedance in experimental animals (5). We were using pericardial pressure oscillations to measure transmyocardial pressure transmission and feeding in energy via the bronchial system to excite the heart (6). The oscillated gas volume was less than the deadspace volume. Nevertheless, the arterial blood gas values were kept within the limits of normoventilation.

Thanks to the vision of Butler et al. (7), high-frequency oscillation proceeded to broader experimental and, ultimately, clinical validation. Butler and co-wokers launched the necessary methodologic improvements by adoption of the "bias flow" system and the "volume recruitment" strategy (8, 9). The clinical use of high-frequency oscillatory ventilation in adults has been investigated by Rehder and Didier (10) at the Mayo Clinic, who ultimately concluded that there was no advantage of high-frequency oscillation over conventional ventilation.

Unfortunately, almost all of the experimental work was done on small animals weighing up to 20 kg. As for our own experience, we repeatedly complained about the capriciousness of high-frequency oscillation when applied to animals weighing > 40 kg. We ultimately learned that our early work on large dogs was limited because of CO_2 rebreathing due to a low-flow bias flow system, an underpowered exciting system, an insufficient alveolar recruitment strategy (8) (i.e., a partially atelectatic lung), and too small a range of frequencies available to adapt the oscillation pattern to individual requirements.

The goals of all forms of high-frequency ventilation are to improve gas exchange and reduce the adverse effects of assisted ventilation. The distribution of alveolar ventilation during conventional mechanical ventilation is determined by focal airway closure and reopening dynamics and by local compliances. Alveolar recruitment during conventional mechanical ventilation is achieved by increasing positive end-expiratory pressure and/or mean or peak airway pressure, which may injure lung tissue by inhomogeneous overdistention during long-term use (see 28). High-frequency oscillatory ventilation has been recommended for increasing the efficiency of gas exchange by recruitment of alveolar compartments with less risk of alveolar injury by barotrauma (9, 11-13).

The failure of high-frequency oscillatory ventilation on pigs was explained by lack of sufficiently low impedant intersegmental communications in the porcine lung. However, in most but not in all experiments on dogs (up to 80 kg), goats and sheep, high-frequency oscillatory ventilation was efficient. These inconsistencies have not been resolved and efficiency of high-frequency oscillatory ventilation on large animals and adult humans has not yet been established.

Many endobronchial aerodynamic mechanisms are related to, and developed from, the fundamental process of shear dispersion, which was first recognized by Taylor in 1953 (14). In this process, an initially planar interface between two gases is drawn out into an ever-lengthening shape by the shear in the underlying velocity distribution. Longitudinal transport is greater than by molecular diffusion alone. Mixing is achieved by transverse diffusion, so the greater the molecular diffusivity, the less the interface is stretched longitudinally and the lower is the effective longitudinal transport (15). Physical and mathematical investigations in basic mechanisms in high-frequency oscillatory ventilation have concentrated on the airways to the exclusion of the gas exchange parenchyma. This fact is mainly due to the absolute lack of any measuring approach to the alveolar compartment. Thus, mathematical models still start from the idea that there is no movement of gas within the alveoli. Of the three effects – bronchial curvature, taper, and flexibility – the axial curvature is most important for gas transport in many oscillatory flow situations, and transport is always less with flexible airway walls than with a rigid tube (15).

High-frequency oscillatory ventilation promises to bring at least two additional degrees of freedom to mechanical ventilation: a smaller magnitude of phasic tissue distention, and some control over its regional distribution. According to Venegas et al., the pressure cost of ventilation increases greatly at high positive end-expiratory pressure levels because, with increasing lung volume, the parenchyma becomes less compliant, and because the anatomical deadspace increases with lung volume (16). The flow cost decreases when fresh gas is delivered closer to the trachea. The optimal frequency, requiring the lowest pressure cost of ventilation, shifts to higher frequency as compliance is reduced and to lower frequency as resistance is increased.

Humidification of the bias-flow has a narrow zone of efficiency between foam formation in the bronchi, on the one hand, and mucosal damage by desiccation, on the other. Foam within the airways cuts high-frequency ventilatory efficiency to zero for as long as it persists (17). Mucosal desiccation appears to be an irreversible, ultimately lethal complication of any type of ventilation.

There is no oscillatory device ready for clinical use in adult patients, but there is increased knowledge about the creation of an adult ventilator. High-frequency oscillatory ventilation is safe and efficient in the "defined volume mode" (i.e., when volume is delivered by a piston pump), whereas tidal volumes delivered by a membrane pump or by a bi-directional gas flow interrupter critically vary with airway impedance and lung compliance.

The minute bias flow related to body weight is efficient in large subjects at < 1 l/kg of body weight. Efficiency is closely related to the configuration of the bias flow system, i.e., the position of the inflow with respect to the outflow opening. A coaxial, lungward fresh gas flow over a long enough distance is a particularly effective arrangement (17). However, the "high impedance bias flows system" (18) runs the risk of the outflow opening becoming obstructed by mucus.

The explosive proliferation of clinical and experimental use of high-frequency ventilation in Europe within the last 5 years has shown that high-frequency oscillatory ventilation is an efficient method in neonatology (19, 20) and in large animals with weights exceeding the weights of any adult patient (17). The boundary conditions for efficient use of high-frequency oscillatory ventilation in adults have been defined, assuming extremely unfavorable, prospective, clinical conditions (17).

High-frequency oscillatory ventilation remains a dangerous method when used by unskilled physicians. Safe and efficient use of the method is determined by experience. Clinicians cannot become acquainted with it by reading handbooks or introductory reviews, because there is no specific monitoring for lung volume over functional residual capacity. Distal airway pressure, delivered oscillated volume, inhomogeneities in alveolar ventilation, although critical variables, cannot be quantitatively surveyed.

Airway impedance measured by the pressure oscillation method gives insight into the function of the conductive system of the lung. However, the method seems to be insensitive to changes in the mechanical properties of the lung parenchyma. Even interstitial water accumulation remains undetected (21).

In clinical use, high-frequency oscillatory ventilation is labor intensive. In babies, the pressure can be measured only at the tube's entrance. In adults, continuous monitoring of the mean airway pressure and PCO_2 beyond the tracheal end of the endotracheal tube is feasible. Blood gas controls are needed in adults to adjust the ventilatory variables. Pulse oximetry may serve to detect and quickly treat complications such as pneumothorax or foam formation. Further efforts are needed to develop monitoring systems assessing mean alveolar distention and segmental lung dynamics.

We wanted to know whether inefficient gas exchange with high-frequency oscillatory ventilation was related to the adult patient's lung structure and dimensions, to the oscillatory devices used, or to the management of high-frequency oscillatory ventilation. Thus, we focussed on the boundary conditions and requirements for the use of high-frequency oscillation on large animals, corresponding in size and shape to adult humans.

Material and methods

All procedures for animal care and experimentation followed the guidelines of the American Physiological Society and the German Law of Animal Protection. This protocol was approved by the University of Münster Institutional Animal Care and Use Committee and adhered to National Institutes of Health and Prevention guidelines for the use of laboratory animals (Der Regierungsprasident Münster, Genehmigungsbescheide 36/91 [20.12.1991] and 31/93 [16.8.1993]).

Eighteen pigs, weighing 65-140 kg (mean 98 ± 20 kg) were anesthetized with 10 to 15 mg/kg i.m. ketamine, followed by 0.2 to 0.3 g i.v. pentobarbital and 0.1 to 0.2 mg i.v. fentanyl. Supplemental pentobarbital and fentanyl were administered, as requested, to maintain anesthesia. The animals were intubated after tracheostomy with a metal tube (21 cm long, 16 mm inner diameter). The right carotid artery was isolated by cutdown and cannulated with a polyethylene catheter (internal diameter 1.7 mm). The right internal jugular vein was isolated and cannulated by cutdown for drug and fluid administration.

The oscillator used in our experiments consisted of a hydropulse system (hydraulic actuator, Series 208 MTS Systems GmbH, Berlin, FRG) as a driving system, a pneumatic piston pump as the high-frequency ventilator, a high-flow bias flow system, and a metal endotracheal tube (31 cm long, 16 mm wide). The hydropulse device was operated by an internal signal for monofrequent ventilation (e.g., by frequencies between 10 and 45 Hz sine wave). Expired gas was aspirated from near the entrance of the airways at a steady flow rate through two 5-mm catheters connected to a vacuum pump. Compressed air mixed with oxygen (FIO_2 0.35; 10 to 70 l/min) was flushed through the bias-flow system, purging the tube from its proximal entrance to near its distal tip. Endotracheal pressure was measured with a 16-gauge catheter (length 60 cm), protruding 8 cm from the tip of the endotracheal tube to obtain the mean airway pressure. Blood gases were measured (Acid-Base Analyzer, ABL 30, Radiometer, Copenhagen, Denmark) every 15 min and at shorter intervals when the ventilatory pattern was changed. The central venous pressure was measured intermittently and was adjusted to 14 ± 2 cm H_2O by volume infusion. Before the initiation of high-frequency oscillatory ventilation 1000-1500 ml of hydroxyethyl starch solution (6% HES, Fresenius) was administered intravenously during continuous control of the central venous pressure.

Initial oscillatory settings were standardized as follows: a) FIO_2 0.35; b) frequency 25 Hz; c) mean airway pressure 18 ± 2 cm H_2O for 60 to 90 s, then mean airway pressure was gradually decreased in 2-cm increments to a minimum of 12 ± 1 cm H_2O; d) bias flow $\geq$ 45 l/min; and e) set tidal volume 68 and 103 ml, corresponding to a delivered tidal volume of 0.52 to 2.23 ml/kg.

The target $PaCO_2$ was between 40 and 45 torr (5.3 and 6.0 kPa). If adequate mechanical ventilation was not achieved with the initial setting of variables, the oscillatory frequency was incrementally changed to a minimum of 10 to 15 Hz and a maximum of 45 Hz. Tidal volume was increased stepwise (75, 110, and

140 ml) at the most efficient frequency. In three animals, the effect of bias flow was investigated. Minute flow varied between 10 and 70 l/min at frequencies of 7, 15, 25, and 35 Hz. The total of 18 animals were divided into two groups according to their body weight [small animals ($n = 11$) 65 to 98 kg; large animals ($n = 7$) 100 to 140 kg]. The highest tidal volume (140 ml) was only applied in one subject of the small group (96 kg) and in two subjects in the large group (102 and 140 kg).

Results

Hemodynamic variables did not show persistent deviations from control values during high frequency oscillation, provided central venous pressure was maintained at a higher level than mean central airway pressure. This was always the case except for the short periods of time (60-90 s) during the alveolar recruitment maneuver which was sometimes paralleled by a transient fall in mean airway pressure.

CO_2 elimination and arterial oxygenation obeyed an individual setting of high frequency oscillation variables: at rising oscillation frequency from 10 to 45 Hz in the group of 11 small animals, $PaCO_2$ varied along a biphasic characteristic, which ultimately yielded the most efficient individual frequency range where $PaCO_2$ was minimal. This most efficient frequency range was centered around 25 Hz, with some scatter across the individuals. When tidal volume was increased from 75 to 110 ml, a most efficient frequency range was even more obvious (less scatter between individuals). At a tidal volume of 140 ml PCO_2 decreased further. Within the limitations of frequency dependency, a stepwise increase in tidal volume by ~ 30 ml yielded a decrease of the mean minimal $PaCO_2$ by ~10 torr (~ 1.3 kPa).

PaO_2 also followed an individual frequency characteristic that yielded a most efficient frequency where PaO_2 was highest. However, the range of interindividual variations was broader than for $PaCO_2$.

In the group of small animals the mean highest PaO_2 did not essentially increase when tidal volume increased from 75 to 110 ml. The interindividual scatter was more marked at low tidal volumes than at 110 ml. In this group the very high tidal volume of 137-145 ml was applied only in one subject, which also showed frequency-dependent variations in gas exchange.

In the cohort of eight large animals gas exchange was found to be less markedly frequency determined. Arterial PO_2 continued to vary with the oscillation frequency. However, no reliable, mean, most efficient frequency could be assessed. Some animals showed a slight trend towards increasing PaO_2 with an increasing frequency up to 45 Hz.

$PaCO_2$ showed a trend towards a reduction with rising oscillation frequency, at least at a tidal volume of 75 ml. At higher tidal volumes the effect was less obvious.

When separately plotting blood gas data vs. the oscillated minute volume (tidal x frequency) at all tidal volumes for PaO_2 and for the two groups of animals, the effect of the tidal volume in addition to the effect of the oscillated minute volume becomes obvious. This "tidal-volume effect" (see 26) is particularly marked in the $PaCO_2$ values of the small animals, but is less marked in the group of large animals. The "tidal-volume effect" also interferes with oxygenation, at least in the group of large animals.

PaO_2 and $PaCO_2$ varied with the oscillated minute volume, with oscillation frequency, tidal volume, and with the bias flow volume per minute. Arterial blood gas values confirmed a threshold bias flow required for adequate CO_2 elimination. Any further augmentation of the bias flow had only a moderate effect on PCO_2. However, the effect of the oscillation frequency on $PaCO_2$ (7, 15, 25 and 35 Hz) was definitely more pronounced than the effect of the bias flow on $PaCO_2$. PaO_2 was scarcely modulated by changes in bias flow as long as the oscillation frequency was sufficiently high.

The initial alveolar recruitment maneuver was extremely efficient regarding oxygenation with virtually no effect on CO_2 elimination.

Discussion

The aim of the present study was to find out if there is a geometrical limitation to the effective use of high-frequency oscillatory ventilation or if there are methodological, in particular hardware, requirements, which have to be handled in an individual way when applying high frequency oscillation to the adult airway system.

The important findings of this study are that adult pigs, which are comparable with adult humans in body weight, definitely can be ventilated by high-frequency oscillation, provided hardware and high-frequency oscillation handling are adapted to particular adult requirements. These requirements include (1) high bias flow (> 35 l/min), (2) broad frequency range (15 to 35 Hz) with (3) large enough tidal volumes (0.8 tol.4 ml/kg b.w.), (4) an endotracheal tube that is not essentially smaller in diameter than the diameter of the patient's trachea, and (5) an efficient alveolar recruitment strategy by a widely variable and securely controllable mean airway pressure (> 19 cm H_2O). Contrary to daily experience with high-frequency oscillatory ventilation in neonates, the excitation frequency is an individual variable that has to be continuously tuned up to changes in lung function over the period of evolving lung injury and during recovery.

We were concerned about the required tracheal tube dimension (22) and rigidity, and the particular configuration of our bias flow system, which made CO_2 elimination so efficient, but which required a tracheostomy. Some large subjects demonstrated the need for frequencies of > 25 Hz. However, from 35 Hz on, the tube started to heat up. As a result, the mean and the lowest individual

$PaCO_2$ values were higher in the cohort of large animals than those values in small animals. The system (namely, the tube's dimension) reached its limits.

We found that tidal volume, oscillation frequency, mean airway pressure, and the bias flow are variables requiring monitoring and repeated correction, not only between individuals but also in the same animal when lung function changes over time. These high standards of patient-related activities may frighten the user because they render the use of high-frequency oscillation difficult to handle in the adult patient.

However, we assume that the determinants of efficient high-frequency oscillation reported earlier (23-25) were partially derived from observations on excitation systems that were too small. According to Slutsky et al. (25), frequencies of > 20 Hz do not improve gas exchange as much as frequencies between 10 and 20 Hz. The oscillatory requirements of the individual airway system become evident when a powerful system such as ours is used and when essential energy loss on the transfer link (tube) is omitted, and thus, when an adequate tidal volume at high-enough frequencies to the lung is conveyed. Otherwise, the patient is most likely to be ventilated by the oscillation pattern that is optimal to the device's capacity rather than at a setting that unconditionally covers patient requirements.

In 1984 Khoo and co-workers (26) published model calculations that might be helpful in explaining the dependency of gas exchange on the oscillation frequency. Their model predicts that the cycle-averaged CO_2 elimination rate depends most strongly on the product of frequency and tidal volume. However, tidal volume has an effect on its own, denoted "tidal-volume effect". It means that at a given frequency x tidal volume, an increase in tidal volume enhances the rate of CO_2 elimination.

Given a carefully controlled oscillation pattern, we found in the group of small animals an individual frequency range response for CO_2 elimination, less for O_2 uptake. Using a powerful oscillation system, adult pigs (65 to 98 kg) on the average required a frequency of ~ 25 Hz for the most efficient CO_2 elimination. At lower and higher frequencies, $PaCO_2$ was higher in most animals. Smaller animals needed lower frequencies. Larger animals needed higher frequencies. PaO_2 reached its maximum at an individual frequency, too. However, the most efficient frequency varied among individuals.

$PaCO_2$ decreased at a given tidal volume with increasing oscillation frequency up to 25-35 Hz, which means that the rate of CO_2 elimination increased with the product of the oscillation frequency and tidal volume. This finding is in accordance with findings published previously by Khoo et al. (26), except for the high range of the most efficient frequencies, which we found. Our results demonstrate that the body weight of the subjects interferes with gas exchange during high-frequency oscillation. In the group of small animals, $PaCO_2$ was definitely lower at the same tidal volume and frequency than in the group of large subjects. So the particularly high frequencies required to ventilate our animals are likely to be related to the extraordinary size of their airway system. The limitation of CO_2 elimination to a critical frequency between 25 and 35 Hz can be partially explained as a result of the frequency-dependent mechanical properties of the lung, so that the upper airway walls act as a shunt compliance, which decreases the gas flow to the periphery of the lung (27). Any further increase in the oscillation frequency was accompanied by increased heat of the metal tube, with an imminent thermal trauma of the airways. Because of increased tube heat, higher frequency efficiency could not be assessed in the group of large animals.

Efficiency of arterial oxygenation depends essentially on the efficiency of the initial alveolar recruitment maneuver (8, 9, 11, 13) and on the extent to which alveolar opening can be maintained over the duration of high-frequency oscillation. The mean airway pressure (and thus lung volume over functional residual capacity) obtained by an initial and intermittently repeated alveolar recruitment maneuver accounts for arterial oxygenation.

Large variations in gas exchange during high-frequency oscillatory ventilation comply with predictions from the model calculations (26), where alveolar ventilation during high-frequency oscillation depends on individual airway geometry. Because we investigated a wide range of body weights (65-140 kg) and the animals were not pure bred (different breeds from different farmers), we assume that there were variations in airway dimensions and geometry across the population we studied.

There are arguments supporting the idea that, at least in the large experimental animal (~ 70 kg), high-frequency oscillatory ventilation is accompanied by frequency-dependent, segmental oscillations which, more or less, differ between areas (17). The global ventilatory effect may then be understood as the synthesis of a segmentally variable, frequency dependent gas exchange pattern. In that case, the mean airway pressure is not a reliable index with which to describe the remodeling process within the airway structure, in particular when inhomogeneous changes in segmental compliance develop over the time of the experiment.

References

1. Emerson JH (1959) Apparatus for vibrating portions of a patient's airway. United States Patent Office, 1959, Serial No. 491, 699, patented Dec. 29
2. Sanders RD (1980) Two ventilatory attachments for bronchoscopes. Del Med J 8:39-71
3. Sjöstrand U (1980) High-frequency positive pressure ventilation. Crit Care Med 8:345-364
4. Klain M, Smith RB (1977) High-frequency percutaneous transtracheal jet ventilation. Crit Care Med 5:280-287
5. Lunkenheimer PP, W Rafflenbeul H, Keller I, Frank HH, Dickuth C (1972) Fuhrmann application of transtracheal pressure-oscillations as a modification of "diffusion respiration". Br J Anaesth 33:627

6. Lunkenheimer PP, Keller H, Wallner F et al (1972) Ein Versuch der Messung der Myokardkonsistenz mit Hilfe trans-trachealer Schwingungsanregung des Herzens durch Druckschwankungen. Arch Kreislaufforsch 67:73-83

7. Butler WJ, Bohn DJ, Bryan AC, Froese AB (1980) Ventilation by high-frequency oscillation in humans. Anesth Analg 59:577-584

8. Froese AB, Bryan AC (1987) High-frequency ventilation. Am Rev Respir Dis 135:1365-1374

9. Froese AB (1989) Role of lung volume in lung injury: HFO in the atelectasis-prone lung. Acta Anaesthesiol Scand Suppl 33:126-130

10. Rehder K, Didier P (1984) Gas transport and pulmonary perfusion during high-frequency ventilation in humans. J Appl Physiol 54:1231-1237

11. Bond DM, Froese AB (1993) Volume recruitment manoeuvres are less deleterious than persistent low lung volumes in the atelectasis-prone rabbit lung during high-frequency-oscillation. Crit Care Med 21:402-412

12. Kolton M, Cattran CB, Kent G (1982) Oxygenation during high-frequency ventilation compared with conventional mechanical ventilation in two models of lung injury. Anesth Analg 61:323-332

13. McCulloch PR, Farkert PG, Froese AB (1988) Lung volume maintenance prevents lung injury during high frequency oscillatory ventilation in surfactant-deficient rabbits. Am Rev Respir Dis 137:1185-1192

14. Taylor GJ (1953) Dispersion of soluble matter in solvent flowing slowly through a tube. Proc R Soc Lond 205:186-203

15. Pedley TJ, Corieri P, Kamm RD et al (1994) Gas flow and mixing in the airways. Crit Care Med 22 [Suppl]:S24-S36

16. Venegas JG, Fredberg JJ (1994) Understanding the pressure cost of ventilation: why does high-frequency ventilation work? Crit Care Med 22 [Suppl]:S49-S57

17. Lunkenheimer PP, Redmann K, Stroh N et al (1994) High-frequency oscillation in an adult porcine model. Crit Care Med 22 [Suppl]:S37-S48

18. Slutsky AS, Drazen JM, Kamm RD et al (1980) Effective pulmonary ventilation with small-volume oscillations at high frequency. Science 209:609-611

19. Clark R, Gerstmanan DR, Null DM et al (1992) Prospective randomized comparison of high-frequency oscillatory and conventional ventilation in respiratory distress syndrome. Pediatrics 99:5-12

20. Miguet D, Claris O, Lapillonne A et al (1994) Preoperative stabilization using high-frequency oscillatory ventilation in the management of congenital diaphragmatic hernia. Crit Care Med 22 [Suppl]:S77-S82

21. Sipinkova I, Koller EA, Buess C et al (1994) Mechanical respiratory system input impedance during high-frequency oscillatory ventilation in rabbits. Crit Care Med 22 [Suppl]:S66-S70

22. Bush EH, Spahn DR, Niederer PF et al (1989) Flow separation, an important mechanism during high-frequency oscillation. J Biomech Eng 111:17-23

23. Brusasco vT, Knopp J, Schmid ER et al (1984) Ventilation-perfusion relationship during high-frequency ventilation. J Appl Physiol 56:454-458

24. deLemos RA, Yoder B, McCuring D et al (1992) The use of high-frequency oscillatory ventilation (HFOV) and extracorporeal membrane oxygenation (ECMO) in the management of the term/near term infant with respiratory failure. Early Hum Dev 29:299-303

25. Slutsky AS, Kamm RD, Rossing TH et al (1981) Effects of frequency, tidal volume and lung volume on CO_2-elimination in dogs by high frequency (2-30 Hz), low tidal volume ventilation. J Clin Invest 68:1475-1484

26. Khoo MCK, Slutsky AS, Drazen JM et al (1984) Gas mixing during high-frequency ventilation: an improved model. J Appl Physiol 57:493-506

27. Mead J (1981) Contribution of compliance of airways to frequency-dependent behaviour of the lungs. J Appl Physiol 51:1507-1514

28. Tsuno K, Prater P, Kolobow T (1990) Acute lung injury from mechanical ventilation at moderately high airway pressure. J Appl Physiol 69:956-961

Insufflation of Air / Oxygen into the Trachea: An Old Principle with New Perspectives

E. MÜLLER

The insufflation of fresh gas or oxygen into the trachea is an old therapeutic approach with fascinating new perspectives. Originally developed to support just oxygenation, current research activities focus on the potential to use this technique also to augment alveolar ventilation and to reduce dead space ventilation.

This article will focus on current research activities and clinical applications of intratracheal gas insufflation under the following three aspects and indications:

– Apneic oxygenation
– Continuous flow apneic ventilation
– Dead space reduction

Apneic oxygenation and continuous flow apneic ventilation

Robert Hooke in 1667 (1) was the first to describe the possibility to sustain life in an animal without any motion of the lungs by just providing a continuous intratracheal flow of "fresh air". Volhard in 1908 (2) demonstrated that apneic animals could survive for more than 1 h with a continuous intratracheal stream of oxygen. Draper and Whitehead in 1944 (3) were able to maintain oxygenation with this technique for up to 90 min, before the animals died from profound respiratory acidosis. To describe the physiological principle behind oxygen uptake they coined the term "diffusion respiration". This term was somewhat misleading since during apnea the vast majority of metabolically produced CO_2 is stored in the tissue; therefore, per time unit more oxygen diffuses from the alveoli to the blood than CO_2 from the blood into the alveoli. This results in a subatmospheric alveolar pressure, causing oxygen to flow from the large airways to the alveoli by convection and not diffusion.

Comroe and Dripps in 1946 (4) were possibly the first who used continuous intratracheal oxygen insufflation clinically; with a flow rate of 6 l/min arterial saturation after 3 h could be maintained between 65%-75% in their apneic and comatose patients; $PaCO_2$ reached values of up to 314 mmHg. Unfortunately, adverse effects and outcome were not reported. Enghoff and colleagues in 1951 (5) were the first to use this technique in anesthetized patients. They described the beneficial effects of prior denitrogenation on oxygenation, when they ventilated the patients with pure oxygen for 30 min prior to the apneic period.

Nahas and L'Allemand in 1956 (6) finally coined the term "apneic oxygenation". Frumin and coworkers in 1959 (7) studied the effects of apneic oxygenation in healthy paralyzed patients. After 55 min arterial saturation was still 98%, but $PaCO_2$ had reached values of up to 250 mmHg with pH < 6.8; increased plasma catecholamine levels led to a 26% increase of mean arterial pressure without any other major adverse effects.

Eger and Severinghaus in 1961 (8) demonstrated the beneficial effects of hyperventilation prior to the apneic period on $PaCO_2$. Without hyperventilation $PaCO_2$ increased at a rate of 13.4 mmHg in the first minute with a relatively constant increase of 4.2 mmHg/min thereafter; hyperventilation prior to the apneic period resulted in a much slower increase of $PaCO_2$ (9.6 mmHg in the first minute 3 mmHg/min thereafter, respectively). Heller and colleagues in 1965 (9) demonstrated a much slower decrease of arterial oxygen saturation if during the apneic period a source of oxygen was connected to the endotracheal tube instead of leaving the tube open to room air.

A transtracheal catheter to supply oxygen was first used by Jacoby and coworkers in 1951 (10); with a flow of 15 l/min they could maintain oxygenation, but also provide some CO_2 elimination. Gattinoni and colleagues in 1980 (11) started to use apneic oxygenation in patients with severe ARDS during extracorporeal CO_2 removal ($ECCO_2$-R); it is interesting to note that at flow rates between 0.5-1.5 l/min they could provide total body oxygenation via the natural severely diseased lungs.

Slutsky and coworkers in 1985 (12) reevaluated these techniques and coined the term "tracheal insufflation of oxygen (TRIO)". They advanced the catheter tip to the level of the carina; with a flow of only 0.2-3 l/min oxygenation could be maintained throughout a 5-h period, even without prior hyperventilation or denitrogenation. They demonstrated that even these low flows contributed with up to 25% to alveolar ventilation; as a result, $PaCO_2$ reached a plateau between 100-200 mmHg with no further increase.

Lehnert and coworkers (13) looked at other possibilities to provide not only oxygenation but also ventilation (CO_2 elimination) with a continuous intratracheal stream of oxygen. Their approach (continuous flow apneic ventilation, CFAV) was certainly more invasive, since they advanced insufflation catheters into each main-stem bronchus bronchoscopically.

With two catheters in place and huge flow rates between 1.5-2.5 l/kg/min they were able to provide total gas exchange in healthy animals. Others (14) could also provide total gas exchange in an animal model for 5 h at flow rates of 1 l/kg/min with endobronchial catheters; if the catheter tip rested above the carina, this technique resulted in an impairment of gas exchange (possibly because of creation of a carinal "high pressure zone" with dynamic hyperinflation).

Up to now the clinical application of CFAV had only limited success. Oxygenation could be provided, but $PaCO_2$ values continued to rise between 0.6 and 1.1 mmHg/min at endobronchial flow rates between 0.6 and 1 l/kg/min (15, 16). Several factors may contribute to this lack of clinical success. Clearly, in this setting, CO_2 elimination is flow dependent.

Proper flow adjustment as well as correct endobronchial placement of the insufflation catheters is obligatory. In addition, gas exchange physiology may be, at least in part, different between humans and animals. During CFAV gas exchange may be facilitated by several factors: turbulences generated at the catheter tip with bidirectional streaming, convective gas movement, cardiogenic oscillations, molecular diffusion, and, in particular, collateral ventilation may play a role. A higher resistance to collateral ventilation in humans than in dogs may in part explain these disappointing clinical results (17, 18).

In conclusion, clinical application of apneic oxygenation, TRIO and CFAV is presently limited to the following indications:

1. In patients with severe advanced chronic obstructive or restrictive lung diseases oxygenation can be supported with continuous oxygen insufflation via nasal cannulas or even transtracheal catheters. Those may be advantageous in regard to (exercise) tolerance, decrease of dyspnea and work of breathing, but especially and probably most important in regard to quality of life.
2. Apneic oxygenation for apnea test during brain death assessment (19).
3. To support oxygenation during extracorporeal membrane oxygenation (ECMO) or $ECCO_2$-R (11, 20-22).
4. CFAV techniques are occasionally used for limited time periods in anesthesia for surgery of the larynx or major airways in order to keep the surgical field free and motionless. Closed heart surgery as well as nuclear magnetic resonance scanning are possible other indications for CFAV.
5. In patients with (unexpected) extremely difficult airway management or in mass casualties oxygenation may be provided temporarily by insufflation of oxygen through endo- or transtracheal catheters.
6. In patients on mechanical ventilation (MV) hypoxia during endotracheal suctioning may be avoided by insufflating oxygen during disconnection. Oxygen can be supplied using a mechanical clamp on the suction catheter, which allows alternatively either suction or oxygen insufflation (23). Another option to maintain positive airway pressures, functional residual capacity (FRC) and hence oxygenation during disconnection and suctioning are modified endotracheal tubes with lateral holes at the tip, through which oxygen can be blown (24).

Intratracheal gas insufflation for dead space reduction in patients on mechanical ventilation

Recently, scientific and clinical interest refocused on techniques of intratracheal gas insufflation due to their potential to reduce dead space. This new interest is clearly linked to the improvement in understanding more of the pathophysiology not only of acute respiratory failure and ARDS, but also of the potential detrimental effects of mechanical ventilation.

It is now accepted that mechanical ventilator settings beyond certain limits may additionally injure healthy lungs, or healthy parts of otherwise diffusely diseased lungs (25-29). Today, the term "barotrauma" is not only defined as extraalveolar air with subcutaneous emphysema, pneumothorax, pneumomediastinum, or even systemic air embolism, for example, but also as severe microvascular injury to the lung. It is accepted that not the pressure itself, but the related volume changes (barotrauma = volutrauma) cause transalveolar shear stress and iatrogenic lung injury. Inadequate end-expiratory lung volume with repeated opening and collapse of unstable (surfactant deficient) alveoli as well as the end-inspiratory lung volume may play a crucial role in creating shear stress and ventilator – induced lung injury (30). Especially the remaining healthy parts ("baby lung" according to Gattinoni) in otherwise diffusely diseased lungs are prone to injury from either continuous or repeated overinflation due to their almost normal compliance; they are inadvertently subjected to pressures and volumes applied with the intention to reopen or ventilate the most diseased parts of those lungs. Therefore, aggressive mechanical ventilation may at least contribute to (if not even being responsible for) the progression from mild forms of respiratory failure to even severest forms (ARDS).

Since neither regional volumes nor transalveolar shear forces can be measured clinically at present, one has to pay careful attention to all factors contributing not only to end-expiratory, but especially to end-inspiratory lung volume.

The peak inspiratory pressure (PIP) is one of the main determinants of this volume; it is accepted today that a PIP above 25-30 cm H_2O may induce or, at least, contribute to iatrogenic injury (25-27, 30, 31). Any higher pressures should, therefore, be avoided.

One recent promising approach is the strict limitation of PIP to safe limits, thereby accepting inadequate alveolar ventilation with a controlled rise in $PaCO_2$ and corresponding drop in pH (permissive hypercapnia) (32-35). This strategy, even if not scientifically evaluated as yet, appears to be beneficial and safe, if certain limits are obeyed.

Another approach to protect diseased lungs against additional iatrogenic injury from aggressive MV is to improve the efficiency of each tidal breath (volume) through reduction of dead space. This may allow the use of lower tidal volumes (VT) and, hence, reduction of PIP to possibly safe limits, as well as the increase of respiratory rates beyond the "normal" range, but with normal $PaCO_2$

and pH. If the fresh gas is delivered via an intratracheal catheter directly to the level of the carina, a large portion of the anatomical dead space is bypassed and any VT becomes more "effective" in regard to alveolar ventilation. Sznajder and coworkers in 1989 (36) were able to achieve a significant reduction of VT and intrathoracic pressure by using a continuous intratracheal gas stream of up to 36 l/min as an adjunct to conventional MV in a canine model of oleic acid-induced lung injury. Müller and coworkers in 1991 (37-39) inaugurated the technique of intratracheal pulmonary ventilation (ITPV) (Fig. 1); briefly, a continuous intratracheal gas stream combined with only a time-cycled expiratory valve provided inspiration (valve closed) and expiration (valve opened) with measurable VT without conventional MV. Oxygenation and alveolar ventilation could be sustained in an animal model of a "small lung", where 88% of the (healthy) lung was surgically resected, without any iatrogenic damage from MV to the remaining parts. ITPV was used as the sole mode of respiratory support, and also, but less efficiently, as an adjunct to any form of mechanical ventilation (hybrid ITPV) at any inspiration / expiration (I:E) ratio.

Considerable subsequent work on this issue of dead space reduction by intratracheal gas insufflation has been done by the group of J. Marini in Minneapolis, USA (40-45). To describe their technique, they coined the term "tracheal gas insufflation TGI". They demonstrated the ability of their technique not only to reduce dead space in healthy animals, but also to result in some improvement in venous admixture and PaO_2. They confirmed that a continuous intratracheal gas stream is superior to only phasic flow either during inspiration (inspiratory bypass of the upper airways) or only during expiration (washout of residing CO_2 from anatomic and apparatus dead space) (42). They also confirmed the findings from other groups that efficiency increases with the magnitude of intratracheal gas flow through the catheter (41). The closer the catheter tip to the carina, the more efficient the technique was. They explored different design variants of the catheter tip: neither a diffuser (Fig. 2) nor an inverted catheter design showed any advantage over the normal straight catheter with an open tip. Here, the turbulences generated at the tip may contribute to improved alveolar ventilation. Dependent on the flow they observed an increase in end-expiratory lung volume (with dynamic hyperinflation) which may contribute to improved ventilation - perfusion matching with decrease in venous admixture and increase of PaO_2 (44).

With the reverse-thrust insufflation catheter designed by Kolobow and coworkers (46) (Figs. 2, 3) the situation may be different: all gas exits in an oral direction, thereby avoiding dynamic hyperinflation at the level of the carina with possible consequences on gas exchange and hemodynamics. Entrainment of air from the distal airways during expiration may even decrease carinal end-expiratory pressure with possible impact on FRC and arterial oxygenation. Carinal pressure should, therefore, be continuously measured and, if necessary, adjusted by external PEEP.

Intratracheal gas insufflation techniques (ITPV/TGI) are clearly able to reduce dead space by 40%-80% in experimental studies (40-46). As a

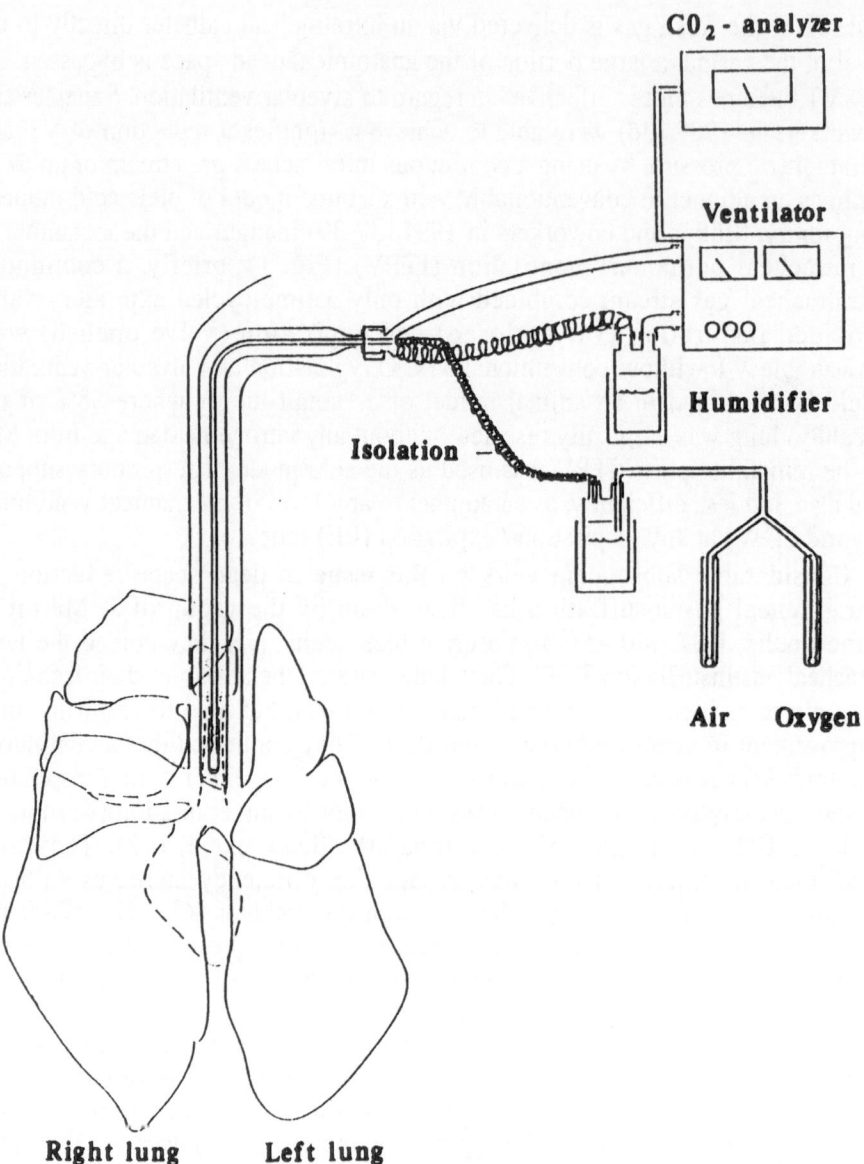

Fig. 1. Schematic of the intratracheal pulmonary ventilation (ITPV) system as applied in a sheep model. A continuous flow of humidified air/oxygen is delivered through a catheter with a reverse-thrust - tip (see text for details). The air and oxygen lines of the Siemens Servo ventilator 900C are disconnected; only the expiratory valve is active in determining the I:E ratio and respiratory rate; otherwise the ventilator delivers no air to the animal, but the control function is used to record only the data from the ITPV system

consequence, the same alveolar ventilation can be achieved with much lower VT and hence PIP at unchanged respiratory rates; with effective dead space reduction

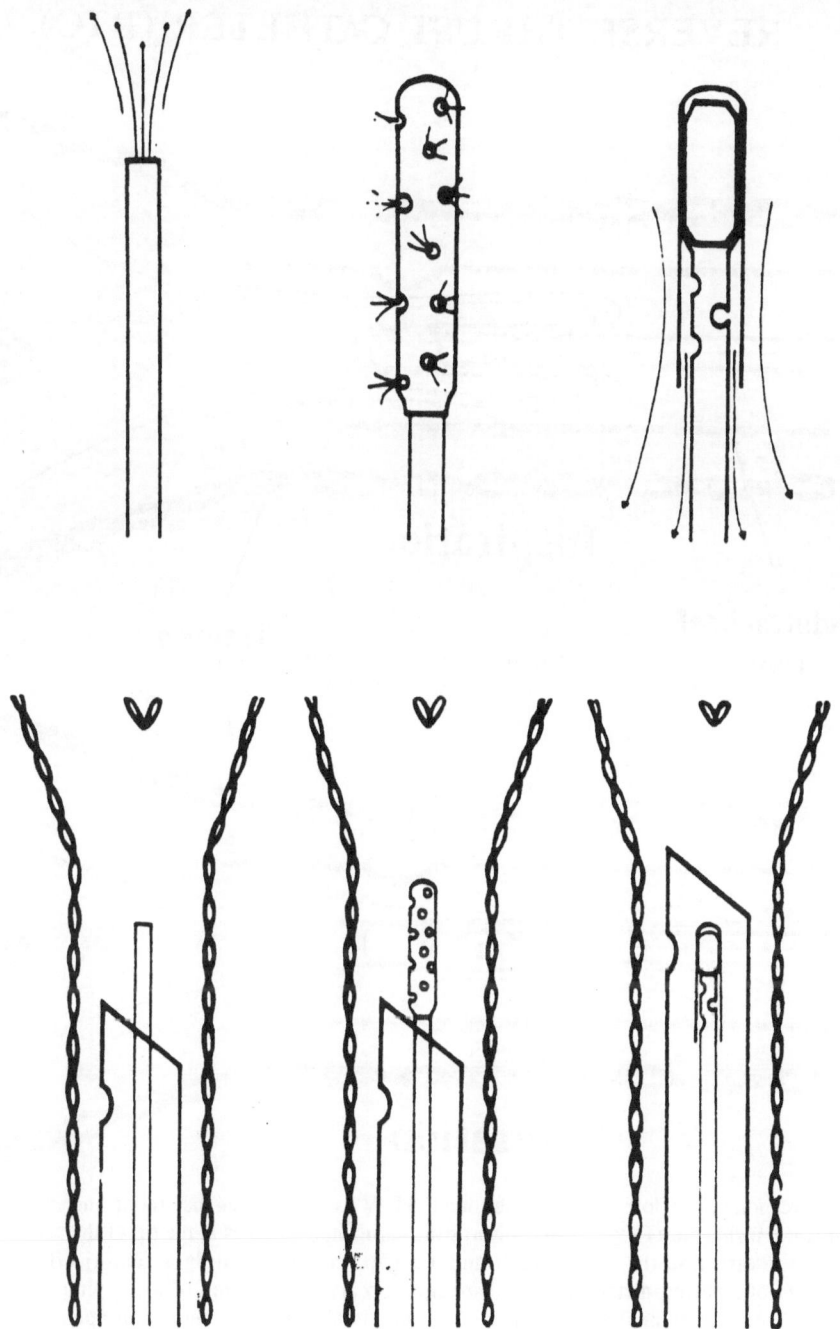

Fig. 2. Possible design variants of the tip of the insufflation catheter [straight open tip, diffuser, or reverse thrust design (on the *right side*) with the tip closed]. Note that the straight open and the diffuser tip is advanced beyond the tip of the endotracheal tube, whereas the RTC tip remains within the ET tube

REVERSE THRUST CATHETER (RTC)

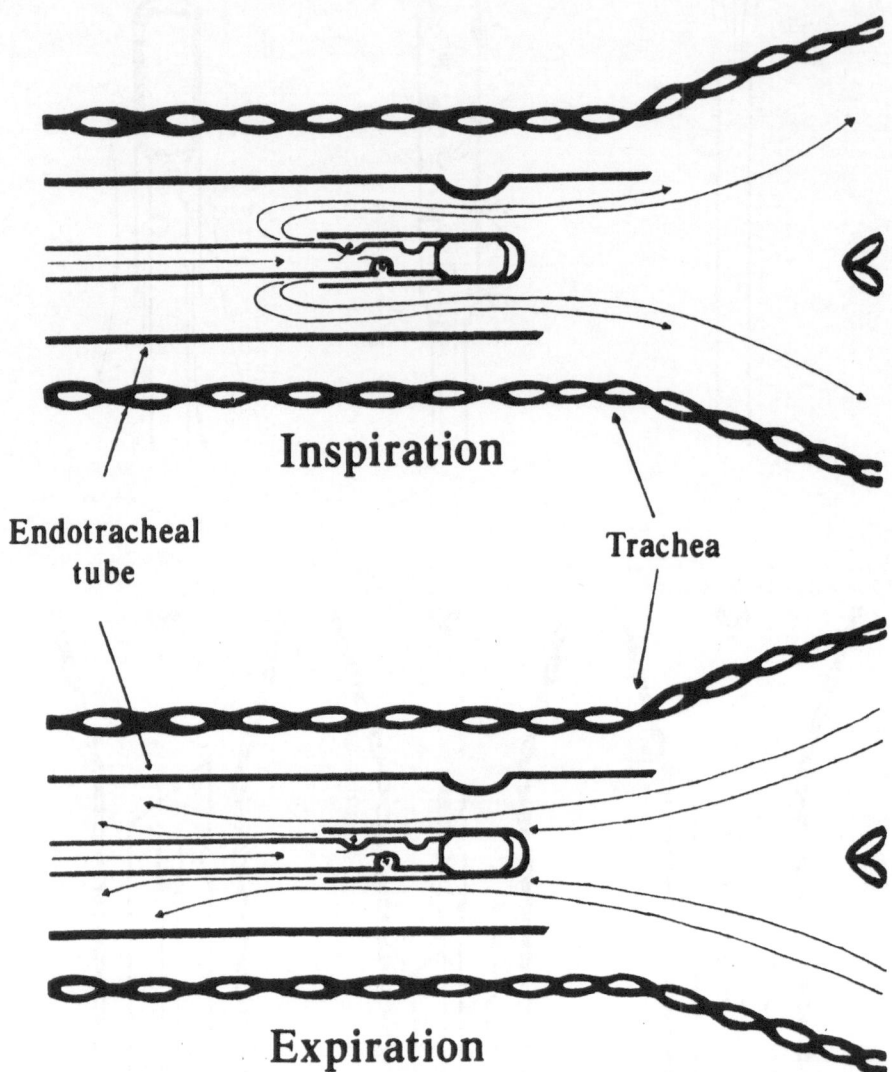

Fig. 3. Direction of gas flow in the reverse-thrust - ITPV catheter during inspiration and expiration. All air flows inside the ITPV catheter towards the carina and emerges at the tip of the catheter in the opposite direction through a small annular gap, thereby creating a venturi effect with entrainment of air from distal airways. Inspiration occurs after closing of the expiratory valve; expiration with entrainment and flushing of the proximal airways occurs upon opening of the expiratory valve

even higher frequencies may be used to lower PIP yet further. Sznajder et al. (36) could reduce VT by 65%, and hence PIP by 30% in their animal studies.

Kolobow and coworkers (46) could reduce dead space by some 75% at different I:E ratios; at certain respiratory and flow rates dead space may even become negative, when the reverse-thrust catheter is used (Fig. 4); they could accomplish normal alveolar ventilation at PIP only 3 cm above PEEP level. Nahum and colleagues (45) demonstrated a significant reduction of $PaCO_2$ and total physiologic dead space with an increase of alveolar ventilation by 25% at both low and high end-expiratory volumes. With a constant end-expiratory lung volume TGI had no effect on oxygenation. It is worthwhile to note that TGI with a flow of 10 l/min could reduce the total physiologic dead space fraction from 58% to only 14% in healthy animals; with injured lungs efficiency was much lower with a reduction of only about 10% at the same settings (43, 45). Giocomini and coworkers (47) recently reported that animals with severe inhomogeneous lung injury sustained gas exchange and finally recovered, while

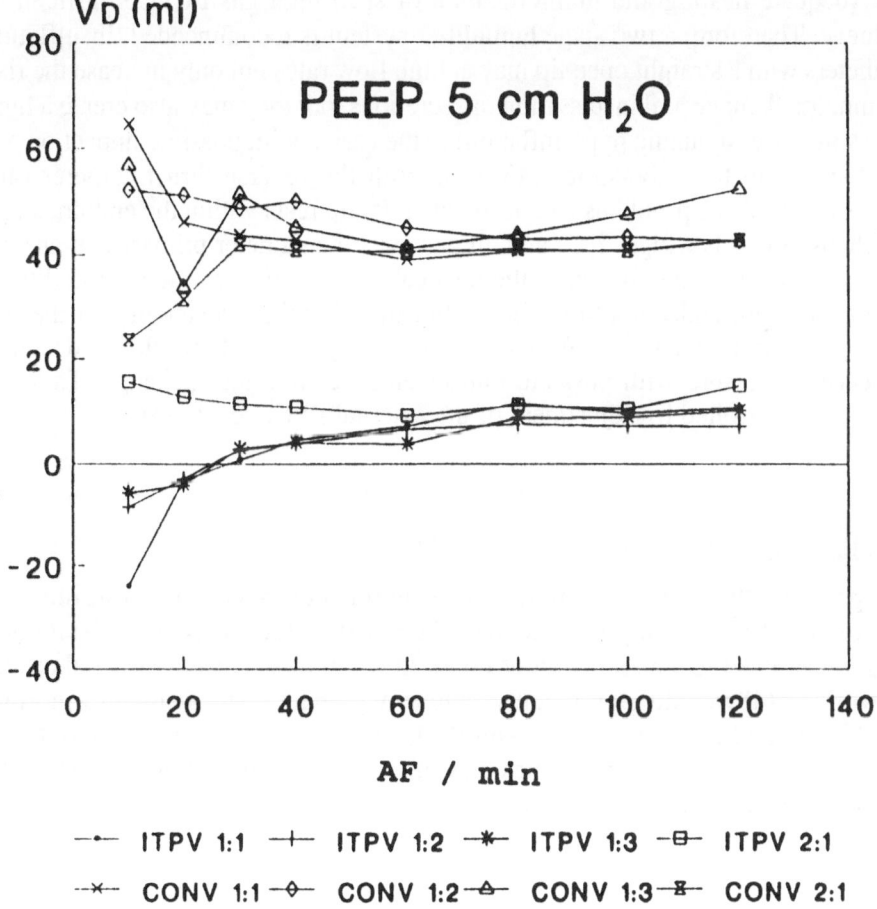

Fig. 4. Dead space with conventional (*conv*) mechanical ventilation and intratracheal pulmonary ventilation at different inspiration/expiration - ratios in a 18 kg sheep (constant VCO_2 of 4.3 ml/kg/min). (Courtesy of T. Kolobow, NIH, Bethesda, Md, USA)

breathing spontaneously (at high respiratory rates) on a newly developed CPAP system with ITPV; in the control group without ITPV all animals died from respiratory failure.

Potential risks of ITPV/TGI

Clear benefits in regard to dead space reduction may be inadvertently counterbalanced by risks related to the continuous intratracheal gas stream of up to 15 l/min (in adults). Therefore, continuous clinical observation of the patient on ITPV/TGI is obligatory, since in case of outflow obstruction airway pressures will increase rapidly with the risk of potentially life threatening barotrauma. This potential for severe injury requires the integration of a pressure release valve into the ITPV/TGI circuit for safety reasons.

Adequate heating and humidification of such high gas flows is difficult to achieve. Therefore, a two stage humidifier system is recommended. Insufflation catheters with a straight open tip may at high flow rates not only increase the risk of mucosa damage and inspissation of secretions, but they may also create a high pressure zone (dynamic hyperinflation) at the carina with possible impact on gas exchange and hemodynamics (43, 44). With the reverse-thrust catheter (46) almost all of these problems can be avoided. Its tip rests within the endotracheal/tracheostomy tube (Figs. 2, 3) and all gas exits the catheter primarily in an oral direction without any contact to the tracheal mucosa, but with the possibility of further heating and humidification within the ET tube. Depending on the gas flow rate, entrainment of air from the distal airways can only result in a decrease of carinal pressure with possible impact on FRC and gas exchange. This can easily be controlled by adjustment of the external PEEP level (46).

Preliminary clinical results of ITPV/TGI

At present, the clinical experience in using ITPV/TGI as an adjunct to conventional MV is very limited. With TGI at flow rates between 4-10 l/min a significant dead space reduction of up to 25% can be achieved (44). Nakos and coworkers (48) could significantly reduce VT and PIP to maintain a normal $PaCO_2$ without any adverse effect on PaO_2, but with some increase in systemic oxygen delivery. At high flow rates they observed a significant increase in PaO_2, possibly related to a decrease in $PaCO_2$, or to dynamic hyperinflation with some alveolar recruitment.

Preliminary reports (49, 50) about the clinical use of ITPV are also very encouraging. Neonatal and adult patients, who could not be weaned off ECMO, were able to sustain gas exchange and finally survived when ITPV was used as an adjunct to conventional MV. We were also able to substantially reduce dead space and hence airway pressures by using ITPV with the reverse-thrust catheter as an adjunct to MV (Fig. 5, unpublished data).

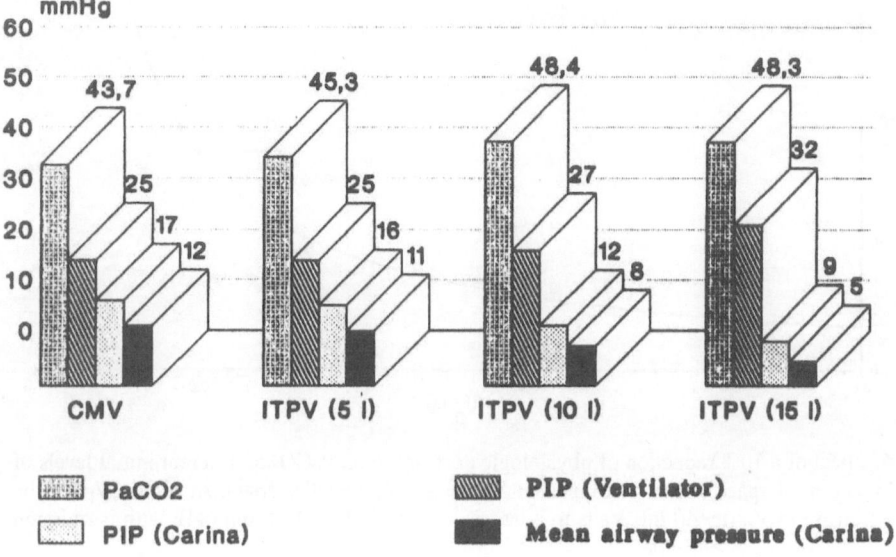

Fig. 5. Arterial $PaCO_2$ and airway pressures under conventional mechanical ventilation (*CMV*) alone and in combination with intratracheal pulmonary ventilation (*ITPV*) at different gas flows in an 80 kg patient (constant VCO_2). In proportion to the magnitude of the ITPV gas flow the reverse thrust design will result in entrainment of air from the distal airways with a decrease of peak and mean airway pressure at the carina (control of the carinal pressure is possible by adjustment of the external PEEP level). Note also that with increasing ITPV gas flow the pressures measured at the ventilator side differ substantially from true carinal pressures

Outlook

Experimental and preliminary clinical studies have shown that ITPV/TGI can reduce dead space and therefore allow the reduction of airway pressures possibly to safe limits during any form of respiratory support. In the clinical setting of severe acute respiratory failure one can expect that efficiency will be less in comparison to the animal studies because of the increased alveolar dead space which may not be affected in the same magnitude as the anatomical and apparatus dead space. ITPV/TGI may be combined with other new lung protective approaches such as permissive hypercapnia (32-35). The higher the $PaCO_2$, the greater the impact of a for example 10% dead space reduction on CO_2 elimination (and hence PIP) (Fig. 6).

Both catheter designs may adversely affect (in different directions) the carinal pressure which should, therefore, be measured continuously during ITPV/TGI.

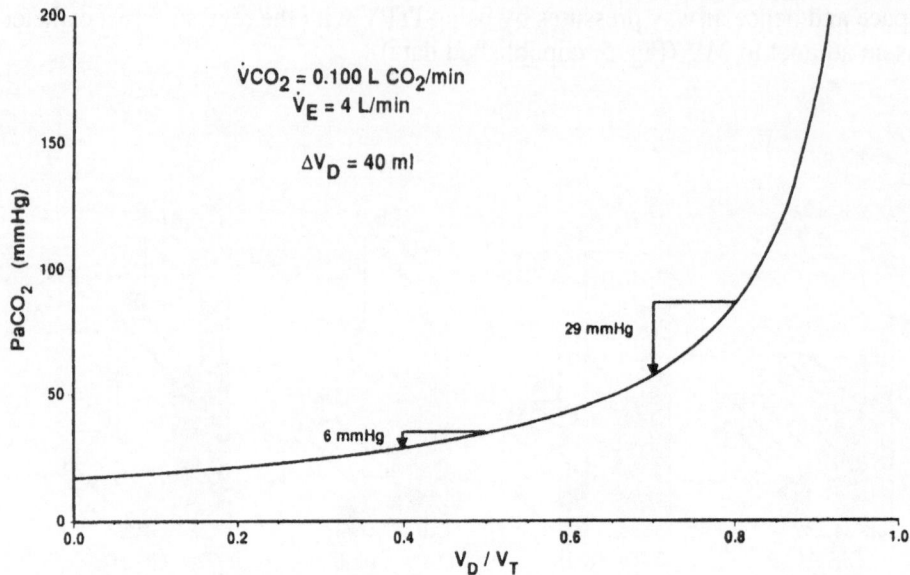

Fig. 6. Effect of a 10% reduction of physiologic dead space on $PaCO_2$ at different initial levels of physiologic dead space (V_D/V_T) at constant $\dot{V}CO_2$ and V_E (healthy dogs). At higher V_D/V_T the same decrease in V_D (by 40 ml) leads to a larger decrease in $PaCO_2$. From (44), with permission

This can be accomplished through additional endotracheal catheters advanced beyond the tip of the insufflation catheter. In the long run it may be desirable to integrate electronic pressure sensors into the (outside) wall of (new kinds of) endotracheal tubes.

At present, a substantial part of the observed dynamic hyperinflation during TGI is related to outflow obstruction, caused by the endotracheal tubes. Additional pressure monitoring devices may even exaggerate this problem, especially, when small endotracheal tubes have to be used, as in neonatology. Double lumen endotracheal tubes with separate lumens for inspiration and for TGI (and expiration) (51) may have an even higher outflow resistance; despite the inverted TGI flow and some entrainment the risk of dynamic hyperinflation with impairment of gas exchange and hemodynamics is obvious. This design may increase the work of breathing to an extent that (desirable) spontaneous breathing is not possible at all. Newly designed ultrathin-walled endotracheal tubes (52) in combination with the reverse-thrust catheter may overcome the problems of heating, humidification, dynamic hyperinflation and increase in work of breathing due to outflow resistance. With the newly developed, ultralow resistance CPAP system (47) we may be able to keep many of the patients, currently subjected to different forms of assisted or controlled MV, just on CPAP/ITPV throughout their whole disease process. Pure ITPV (all gas for ventilation comes from the catheter) is clearly superior to any hybrid form, since it allows the use of very high, but still effective respiratory rates (e.g., 30-120 l/min) at lowest PIP (39). But, clinically, ITPV/TGI will very likely be used in the majority of cases as an adjunct to CPAP, MV, or as the sole mode to (transtracheally) support oxyenation and ventilation in patients with severe chronic obstructive lung disease.

Interesting to note that TGI has as yet only been tested at normal respiratory rates; it remains to be elucidated whether TGI has the same excellent performance characteristics at high respiratory rates, since this is one of the major advantages of using ITPV. The TGI catheter design may inadvertently create a high pressure zone with dynamic hyperinflation at high rates, thereby compromising not only gas exchange, but also hemodynamics, as we have seen in our studies using a straight catheter tip (unpublished data).

Further controlled clinical studies should, therefore, address questions of optimal catheter design (open tip or reverse-thrust), adverse effects, impact on work of breathing, efficiency at different disease stages and settings in neonatal, pediatric, and adult intensive care medicine. We might come to a point, where we start with ITPV/TGI already at the time of intubation.

References

1. Hooke R (1667) Account on an experiment, made by Robert Hooke, of preserving animals alive by blowing through their lungs with bellows. Philos Trans R Soc Lond 2:539-540
2. Volhard F (1908) Über künstliche Atmung durch Ventilation der Trachea und eine einfache Vorrichtung zur rhythmischen künstlichen Atmung. Munchner Med Wochenschr 55:209-211
3. Draper WP, Whitehead RW (1944) Diffusion respiration in the dog anesthetized with pentothal sodium. Anesthesiology 5:262-263
4. Comroe JH Jr, Dripps RD (1946) Artificial respiration. JAMA 130:381-383
5. Enghoff H, Holmdahl MH, Risholm L (1951) Diffusion respiration in man. Nature 168:830
6. Nahas GG, L'Allemand H (1956) Circulation in dogs after respiratory arrest by curare. J Appl Physiol 89:368-372
7. Frumin MJ, Epstein RM, Cohen G (1959) Apneic oxygenation in man. Anesthesiology 20:789-798
8. Eger EI, Severinghaus JW (1961) The rate of rise of $PaCO_2$ in the apneic anesthetized patient. Anesthesiology 22:419-425
9. Heller ML, Watson TR Jr, Imredy DS (1964) Apneic oxygenation in man: polarographic arterial oxygen tension study. Anesthesiology 25:25-30
10. Jacoby JJ, Reed JP, Hamelberg W et al (1951) Simple method of artificial respiration. Am J Physiol 167:798-799
11. Gattinoni L, Agostoni A, Pesenti A et al (1980) Treatment of acute respiratory failure with low-frequency positive pressure ventilation and extracorporeal removal of CO_2. Lancet 2: 292-294
12. Slutsky AS, Watson J, Leith DE, Brown R (1985) Tracheal insufflation of O_2 (TRIO) at low flow rates sustains life for several hours. Anesthesiology 63:278-286
13. Lehnert BE, Oberdorster G, Slutsky AS (1982) Constant flow ventilation in apneic dogs. J Appl Phsyiol 52:483-489
14. Smith RB, Babinski M, Bunegin L et al (1984) Continuous flow apneic ventilation. Acta Anaesth Scand 28:631-639

15. Babinski MF, Sierra OG, Smith RB et al (1985) Clinical application of continuous apneic ventilation. Acta Anaesth Scand 29:750-752
16. Breen PH, Sznajder JF, Morrison P et al (1986) Constant flow ventilation in anesthetized patients: efficacy and safety. Anesth Analg 65:1161-1169
17. Villar J, Slutsky AS (1994) Apneic oxygenation and other nonconventional techniques of ventilatory support. In: Tobin MJ (ed) Principles and practice of mechanical ventilation. McGraw Hill, New York, pp 499-509
18. Smith RB (1992) Continuous flow apneic ventilation. In: Perel A, Stock MC (eds) Handbook of mechanical ventilatory support. Williams and Wilkins, Baltimore, pp 175-184
19. Marks SJ, Zisfein J (1990) Apneic oxygenation in apnea test for brain death. A controlled trial. Arch Neurol 47:1066-1068
20. Müller E, Kolobow T, Knoch M, Höltermann W (1992) Akutes Lungenversagen - Unterstützung des Gasaustausches mittels extrakorporaler oder implantierter Oxygenatoren. Gegenwärtiger Stand und zukünftige Entwicklung. Anästhesiol Intensivmed Notfallmed Schmerzther 27:259-273.
21. Chevalier JY, Couprie C, Larraquet M, Renolleau S, Durandy Y, Costil J (1993) Venovenous single lumen cannula extracorporeal support in neonates. A five year experience. ASAIO Trans 39:M654-658
22. Kolobow T, Tsuno K (1994) Extracorporeal membrane oxygenation and intravascular membrane oxygenation. In: Tobin MJ (ed) Principles and practice of mechanical ventilation. McGraw Hill, New York, pp 461-482
23. Graff M, France J, Hiatt M, Hegyi T (1987) Prevention of hypoxia and hyperoxia during endotracheal suctioning. Crit Care Med 15:1133-1135
24. Brochard L, Mion G, Isabey D et al (1991) Constant-flow insufflation prevents arterial oxygen desaturation during endotracheal suctioning. Am Rev Respir Dis 144:395-400
25. Kolobow T (1988) Acute respiratory failure: on how to injure healthy lungs (and prevent sick lungs from recovering). ASAIO Trans 34:31-34
26. Müller E (1992) Searching for the cause of the adult respiratory distress syndrome (ARDS) Int J Artif Organs 15:197-199
27. Parker JC, Hernandez LA, Peevy KJ (1993) Mechanisms of ventilator-induced lung injury. Crit Care Med 21:131-43.
28. Pingleton SK (1995) Barotrauma in acute lung injury: is it important? Crit Care Med 23: 223-224
29. Dreyfuss D, Soler P, Saumon G (1995) Mechanical ventilation-induced pulmonary edema. Interaction with previous lung alterations. Am J Respir Crit Care Med 151:1568-1575
30. Lachmann B (1992) Open the lung and keep it open. Intensive Care Med 18:319-321
31. Marini JJ (1994) Ventilation of the acute respiratory distress syndrome. Looking for Mr. Goodmode. Anesthesiology 80:972-975
32. Hickling KG, Henderson SJ, Jackson R (1990) Low mortality associated with low volume pressure limited ventilation with permissive hypercapnia in severe adult respiratory distress syndrome. Intensive Care Med 16:372-377
33. Hickling KG, Walsh J, Henderson S, Jackson R (1994) Low mortality rate in adult respiratory distress syndrome using low-volume, pressure-limited ventilation with permissive hypercapnia. A prospective study. Crit Care Med 22:1568-1578
34. Tuxen DV (1994) Permissive hypercapnic ventilation. Am J Respir Crit Care Med 150: 870-874
35. Feihl F, Perret C (1994) Permissive hypercapnia. How permissive should we be? Am J Respir Crit Care Med 150:1722-1737
36. Sznajder JI, Becker CJ, Crawford GP et al (1989) Combination of constant-flow and continuous positive-pressure ventilation in canine pulmonary edema. J Appl Physiol 67: 817-823
37. Müller E, Kolobow T, Mandava S et al (1991) On how to ventilate lungs as small as 12% of normal. Intratracheal pulmonary ventilation (ITPV) - one mode of pulmonary ventilation. Am Rev Resp Dis 143:A693 (abstr)

38. Kolobow T, Müller E, Mandava S et al (1991) Intratracheal pulmonary ventilation (ITPV). A new technique. Am Rev Resp Dis 143:A602 (abstr)
39. Müller E, Kolobow T, Mandava S et al (1993) How to ventilate lungs as small as 12% of normal. The new technique of intratracheal pulmonary ventilation (ITPV). Pediatr Res 34:606-610
40. Nahum A, Burke WC, Ravenscraft SA et al (1992) Lung mechanics and gas exchange during pressure controlled ventilation in dogs: augmentation of CO_2 elimination by an intratracheal catheter. Am Rev Respir Dis 146:965-973
41. Nahum A, Ravenscraft SA, Nakos G et al (1992) Tracheal gas insufflation during pressure controlled ventilation: effect of catheter position, diameter, and flow rate. Am Rev Respir Dis 146:1411-1418
42. Burke WC, Nahum A, Ravenscraft SA et al (1993) Modes of tracheal gas insufflation: comparison of continuous and phase specific gas injection in normal dogs. Am Rev Respir Dis 148:562-568
43. Nahum A, Ravenscraft SA, Nakos G, Adams AB, Burke WC, Marini JJ (1993) Effect of catheter flow direction on CO_2 removal during tracheal gas insufflation. J Appl Physiol 75:1238-1246
44. Nahum A, Marini JJ (1994) Tracheal gas insufflation as an adjunct to conventional ventilation. In: Vincent JL (ed) (1994) Yearbook of intensive care and emergency medicine. Springer, Berlin Heidelberg New York, pp 511-523
45. Nahum A, Chandra A, Nikman J, Ravenscraft S, Adams AB, Marini JJ (1995) Effect of tracheal gas insufflation on gas exchange in canine oleic acid-induced lung injury. Crit Care Med 23:348-356
46. Kolobow T, Powers T, Mandava S, Aprigliano M, Kawaguchi A, Tsuno K, Müller E (1994) Intratracheal pulmonary ventilation (ITPV): control of positive end-expiratory pressure (PEEP) at the level of the carina through the use of a novel ITPV catheter design. Anesth Analg 78:455-461
47. Giocomini M, Kolobow T, Reali-Foster C (1995) Intratracheal pulmonary ventilation (ITPV) combined with CPAP in the treatment of severe ARF - a controlled study. Cardiol Young 5 [Suppl 2]:A31 (abst)
48. Nakos G, Zakinthinos S, Kotanidou A, Tsagaris H, Roussos C (1994) Tracheal gas insufflation reduces the tidal volume while $PaCO_2$ is maintained constant. Intensive Care Med 20:407-413
49. Wilson JM, Thompsen JR, Schnitzer JJ et al (1993) Intratracheal pulmonary ventilation and congenital diaphragmatic hernia; a report of two cases. J Pediatr Surg 28:484-487
50. Raszynski A, Hultquist KA, Latif H et al (1993) Rescue from pediatric ECMO with prolonged hybrid intratracheal pulmonary ventilation. A technique for reducing dead space ventilation and preventing ventilator induced lung injury. ASAIO Trans 39:M681-685
51. Mang H (1995) Tracheale Gas - Insufflation und intratracheale Ventilation. Anaesthesist 44 [Suppl 1]:S41
52. Kolobow T, Tsuno K, Rossi N, Aprigliano M (1994) Design and development of ultrathin-walled nonkinking endotracheal tubes of a new "no pressure" laryngeal seal design. A preliminary report. Anesthesiology 81:1061-1067

Concept: Open Up the Lung and Keep the Lung Open

B. LACHMANN

After more than 40 years of clinical use, artificial ventilation has proven to be a life-saving method or therapy in intensive care. Yet, it has remained a topic of much discussion and controversy because artificial ventilation involves a disturbance to normal respiratory and cardiovascular function.

It is well established that artificial ventilation, especially with large tidal volumes and high peak inspiratory pressures, leads to a decrease in lung compliance and dysfunction of gas exchange. Of even greater importance is the realization that ventilation itself can lead to formation of atelectasis, pulmonary edema, pneumonitis and fibrosis (for review see 1-4); that is why the adult respiratory distress syndrome (ARDS) may be, in part, a product of our therapy - rather than the progression of the underlying disease.

To date no adequate explanation of the pathophysiologic basis of these changes caused by artificial ventilation has been documented. The main contributing factors which emerge from almost all the above-mentioned references seem to be the ventilatory modes which fail to prevent partial (or complete) end-expiratory lung collapse combined with high peak inspiratory pressures.

Why use the smallest possible pressure amplitude?

More than twenty years ago Mead et al. stated that: "at a transpulmonary pressure of 30 cmH$_2$O, the pressure tending to expand an atelectatic region surrounded by a fully expanded lung would be approximately 140 cmH$_2$O" (5). Such forces may well be the major cause of structural damage (especially to bronchiolar epithelium, alveolar epithelium and capillary endothelium) and may not only be the basis for formation of hyaline membranes but may also cause the release of mediators from the disrupted parenchyma - triggering the pathophysiological mechanisms of ARDS (6).

During ventilation of patients with ARDS, who almost always have atelectatic lung regions, pressure differences of 30 cmH$_2$O or higher are quite common. We have to understand, however, that it is not the 30 cmH$_2$O pressure difference that damages the lungs but rather the resulting shear forces of more than 140 cmH_2O which are responsible for the barotrauma.

Data from experiments related to different modes of artificial ventilation in ARDS lungs (see referred reviews) clearly demonstrated that lungs ventilated with modes which did not prevent end-expiratory alveolar collapse, thus creating shear forces, showed more severe morphologic damage (and lower arterial PaO_2) compared to modes which kept the entire lungs open during the whole respiratory cycle.

It must be concluded that in order to prevent lung damage due to high shear forces between open and closed lung units only ventilation modes which result in the smallest possible pressure amplitude should be used.

Why open up the lung and keep it open?

As demonstrated in an experimental study using five different ventilatory modes (7), if one opens the lungs (by applying a peak inspiratory pressure of 55 cmH_2O with an end-expiratory alveolar pressure of 16 cmH_2O for about 10 min) only about 20 cmH_2O (range 16-23 cmH_2O) pressure amplitude is required in all the ventilatory modes which create an intrinsic PEEP to achieve optimal gas exchange in animals suffering from severe ARDS. This is an important finding and confirms earlier experimental and clinical data showing that if the right modes of ventilation are chosen, dangerous high shear forces can be avoided (1).

The LaPlace law ($P = 2\gamma/r$, where P = pressure to stabilize a bubble/alveoli; γ = surface tension at the air-liquid interface; r = radius of the bubble/alveolus) may offer an explanation why surfactant-depleted ARDS-like lungs with a high and constant surface tension at the air-liquid interface could be adequately ventilated with a pressure amplitude of only 20 H_2O (which is half the pressure necessary to open up the lung).

Since the critical opening pressure is inversely proportional to alveolar unit size, it follows that progressive recruitment of air spaces requires a continuously increasing pressure during inflation which translates to high peak inspiratory pressure. The pressure necessary to induce volume changes depends on the initial radius. In other words, to get a certain volume change in larger alveoli, the necessary pressure changes are much smaller compared to alveoli which are collapsed or have a lower volume. It can further be derived from the law of LaPlace that the pressure necessary to keep the alveoli open is smaller at a high FRC level. Therefore, the PEEP necessary to stabilize the end-expiratory volume can be minimized if the lungs are totally opened to an FRC level of a healthy lung.

Another reason why the lung should be kept open is the fact that under certain circumstances artificial ventilation affects the pulmonary surfactant system (8). In normal healthy lungs, during end-expiration the surfactant molecules are compressed on the small alveolar area (leading to a low surface tension or a high surface pressure) thus preventing the alveoli from collapse. If the surface of the alveolus becomes smaller than the total surface of the surfactant molecules, the molecules are squeezed out of the surface and forced towards the airways and thus lost for the alveoli. During the following inflation of alveoli, the surface is replenished with surfactant molecules that were in the hypophase. During the next expiration, the same mechanism continues to work and again surfactant molecules are forced into the airways; this is a continuing cycle (9). With large tidal volume and/or high rates, surfactant molecules are lost into the airways rather rapidly, as demonstrated by Faridy (10).

This mechanism explains how loss of surfactant by artificial ventilation can be caused by the rhythmic compression (expiration) and decompression (inspiration) of the alveolar lining, especially when the compression is far below (or extremely below if alveolar collapse occurs) the static state of the surfactant layer, which is normally equal to or just above the FRC level (11). Thus to prevent loss of surfactant by artificial ventilation one should maintain aeration of as large parts of the lung as possible without allowing either hyperdistention or lung collapse.

Keeping the lung open by the appropriate ventilatory modes not only prevents lung damage due to high shear forces, but may also prevent alveolar flooding (i.e. preventing alveolar edema) (12). In general, alveolar flooding will not occur as long as the negative force in the pulmonary interstitium exceeds the pressure gradient generated by surface tension in the alveolar air-liquid interface. Since the pressure gradient is inversely related to the radius of the alveolar curvature there is, for each combination of interstitial resorptive force and average surface tension, a critical value for surface tension and alveolar radius below which alveolar flooding occurs. In other words a disturbed surfactant system, which in itself leads to alveolar collapse together with smaller alveoli, promotes intra-alveolar lung edema.

Why is intrinsic PEEP at pressure controlled ventilation superior to external PEEP at volume controlled ventilation?

In an ARDS lung there is non-homogeneous distribution of damage over the whole lung. If one applies an external (static) PEEP to a patient with ARDS at volume controlled ventilation with a frequency of 10-15 per minute, the following changes may be observed:

1. The set PEEP will only balance the increased retractive forces of parts of the damaged lung so that only these parts of the lung will not collapse during the expiratory phase and thus gas exchange will continue during the whole respiratory cycle leading to improved blood gases.

2. The applied external PEEP, however, will not be sufficient to keep all parts of the lungs open. Highly damaged lung regions will be reaerated only at the end of the inspiratory phase; due to the high intra-alveolar pressure at end-inspiration, perfusion will be decreased limiting the contribution of these lung regions to gas exchange.

3. There may also be some healthy regions of the lungs for which the applied external PEEP already leads to capillary compression and a ventilation/perfusion mismatching. This will be even more prominent during the inspiratory phase, causing a dramatic over-distension of these parts.

This may be the scenario for volume controlled PEEP ventilation as it is used in clinical routine. One has to point out, however, that if one does not consider high peak airway pressures as causing lung damage almost every stiff lung can be kept open by a large external PEEP (7).

In contrast, at pressure controlled ventilation, if the pre-set peak inspiratory pressure is set to a value which just compensates for the retractive forces of the whole lung, dangerous over-distension of the alveoli can never occur. If one then either increases the I/E ratio at a constant frequency, or increases the frequency at a constant I/E ratio (or both) to establish an expiratory time which will be too short to allow emptying of the lung to the ambient pressure, an intrinsic PEEP will be created. If one chooses the absolute time of the expiratory phase so short that even the stiffest parts of the lung have no time for collapse, the lungs will be kept open and can then be ventilated with a significantly smaller pressure amplitude compared to volume controlled PEEP ventilation.

It should be stressed, however, that one should never try to get intrinsic PEEP with volume controlled ventilation, due to the danger of a permanent increase of lung volume resulting finally in barotrauma. In other words, intrinsic PEEP at volume controlled ventilation should be considered as a professional error.

Another finding is that if one just balances the retractive forces by the right pre-set peak pressures at pressure controlled ventilation in combination with proper fluid management, this mode will not lead to additional cardiocirculatory depression compared with volume controlled PEEP ventilation.

In summary, an optimal ventilatory mode should produce minimal pressure swings during the ventilatory cycle and keep the lung volume equal to or just above the FRC level – this to prevent a significant depletion of surface active material. If one follows this concept which, in fact, is not new (1) and if it is once proven to be the right way for any form of respiratory support, the diversity of ventilatory modes may no longer cause confusion for the practitioner as there is only one rational concept to preserve lung integrity: open up the whole lung and keep it totally open, with the least influence on the cardiocirculatory system.

References

1. Lachmann B, Danzmann E, Haendly B, Jonson B (1982) Ventilator settings and gas exchange in respiratory distress syndrome. In: Prakash O (ed) Applied physiology in clinical respiratory care. Martinus Nijhoff, The Hague, pp 141-176
2. Froese AB (1989) Role of lung volume in lung injury: HFO in the atelectasis-prone lung. Acta Anaesthesiol Scand 33 [Suppl 90]:126-130
3. Sykes MK (1991) Does mechanical ventilation damage the lung? Acta Anaesthesiol Scand 35 [Suppl 95]:35-39
4. Hickling KG (1990) Ventilatory management of ARDS: can it affect the outcome? Intensive Care Med 16:219-226
5. Mead J, Takishima T (1970) Leith. Stress distribution in lungs: a model of pulmonary elasticity. J Appl Physiol 128:596-608
6. Spragg RG, Smith RM (1991) Biology of acute lung injury. In: Crystal RG, West JB, et al (eds) The lung: scientific foundation. Raven, New York, pp 2003-2017
7. Lichtwarck-Aschoff M, Nielsen JB, Sjöstrand UH, Edgren EL (1992) An experimental randomized study of five different ventilatory modes in a piglet model of severe respiratory distress. Intensive Care Med 18:339-347
8. Houmes RJM, Bos JAH, Lachmann B (1994) Effect of different ventilator settings on lung mechanics: with special reference to the surfactant system. Appl Cardiopulm Pathophysiol 5:117-127
9. Bos JAH, Lachmann B (1992) Effects of artificial ventilation on surfactant function. In: Rügheimer E (ed) New aspects on respiratory failure, Springer, Berlin Heidelberg New York, pp 194-208
10. Faridy EE (1976) Effect of distension on release of surfactant in excised dogs' lungs. Respir Physiol 27:99-114
11. Benzer H (1969) Respiratorbeatmung und Oberflächenspannung in der Lunge. In: Frey R, Kern F, Mayrhofer O (eds) Anaesthesiologie und Wiederbelebung, vol 38. Springer, Berlin Heidelberg New York
12. Guyton AC, Moffat DS, Adair TA (1980) Role of alveolar surface tension in transepithelial movement of fluid. In: Robertson B, Van Golde LMG, Batenburg JJ (eds) Pulmonary surfactant. Elsevier, Amsterdam, pp 171-185

Computer Supported Ventilation

S. Böhm, B. Lachmann

History

The first widespread use of long-term artificial ventilation, despite experimental attempts for more than a century, was during the poliomyelitis epidemic of 1952 in Copenhagen (1). The alveolar ventilation of patients suffering from this neuromuscular deficiency was assured by the means of iron lungs. These devices were huge, since they had to cover almost the entire body, and did not allow for precise measurement of respiratory volume and transpulmonary pressure. No reliable alarms were available and thus many patients succumbed due to technical failures. The routine nursing and medical care of a patient in the iron lung was highly demanding, if not sometimes almost impossible. This form of respiratory therapy was not likely to become the standard future treatment for respiratory insufficiency.

With the clinical acceptance of endotracheal intubation as the access to the airway for prolonged periods of time, positive pressure ventilation became feasible as a treatment of impaired pulmonary function. Mechanical ventilators became popular during the late 1950s and had a major impact on the fast development of intensive care medicine. Most ventilators at that time were operating purely mechanically and allowed only the most basic parameters to be adjusted. Generally, they provided one single mode of ventilation delivering either a preset pressure or a predetermined tidal volume. The measurement of volumes and pressures delivered by the respirator was purely mechanical, no feed-back control existed. Alarms and safety features, if available at all, were minimal and unreliable. Adequate patient safety could therefore not always be assured. Most PEEP valves could only be added to the systems externally. In 1969 Ashbaugh and coworkers reported that the use of continuous positive pressure ventilation using positive end-expiratory pressure improved gas exchange in patients with acute lung injury (2).

The introduction of the microcomputer in the 1970s dramatically increased the availability of computers (3). It was during that decade that computers began to be routinely used in hospitals, ICUs and, especially, in ventilators. There are few devices in health care that are as complex, data intensive, and associated with well-defined repetitive tasks (delivering constant breaths repeatedly), as a ventilator. These features made ventilators the ideal target for the rapid introduction of the newly developed computer technology which was designed to help the human mind deal with large amounts of information, complex data manipulations and to automate repetitive tasks. An increasing number of analog and hardware operations were turned over to microprocessor controls. Even though many of the more modern ventilators of that time already had some excellent analog electronic controls incorporated, digital close loop control of respiratory valves was not implemented until the late 1970s (4). In a feed-back manner electronically measured pressure or flow signals from the ventilatory circuit were used by a microprocessor to control the valve's performance to maintain a desired pressure or flow.

Microprocessor systems provided an excellent platform upon which to build ventilators that could easily be modified and updated, because:

1. It was no longer necessary to change expensive physical components.
2. Alarm functions could now easily be realized.
3. More extended displays of ventilatory parameters were accomplished.
4. The miniature size of the computer components enabled more than one single electronic circuit to be built into a ventilator.

This redundance ("watch dog principle") in the monitoring and control of the ventilator's performance enhanced the reliability of the devices and, together with multiple alarm systems, also dramatically improved patient safety. The servo-controlled valves were the key to the explosion of a vast number of diverse new ventilatory modes (i.e. VC, SIMV, flow by CPAP, PS, ASB, BIPAP, PRVC, etc.).

Today

Many of the technical problems confronted during the development from the first clinically used mechanical ventilator to the computerized machines of today, have now been solved. There is now an abundant number of possible modes of artificial ventilation which technically perform well. Multiple safety options ensure that transgressions of safe limits either do not happen, or at least activate alarms when they occur. However, with the complexity of the ventilators also the number of variables that need to be adjusted in a particular mode of ventilation increased.

Physiologic monitoring

In addition to the improvements of the mechanical ventilators towards the end of the 1970s on-line measurements of the respiratory gas composition became available. The signal from capnography together with the measured respiratory volumes helped to assess the patient's pulmonary gas exchange. In the 1980s, with the introduction of pulsoximetry, a parameter for tissue oxygenation became available. The combination of these variables with easier measurements of the blood gases made a more sophisticated titration of the ventilatory mode possible. Today, computerized systems for the continuous measurement of arterial blood gases via a small indwelling catheter are available. The patient's response to the ventilatory treatment can thus be monitored more closely and more directly. Yet again, the number of available data has increased dramatically.

Decision making in general

The ventilatory management of patients on an intensive care unit is an uninterrupted process which is highly demanding for the clinical staff. Around-the-clock decisions need to be made and implemented on the ventilator. Fortunately many patients can be treated successfully with only a few simple adjustments of the respirator. However, there remains a considerable number of patients that challenge all the knowledge, experience and time of experts in intensive care medicine. Then, simple solutions for the respiratory problem do not exist. To make proper decisions a huge amount of data are being collected. All these data need to be considered and many have to be integrated for a clinical decision (5). This complex decision making, however, may be insufficient due to the limited capacity of the human mind to assimilate information (6). It has been shown that the average human can consider no more than seven simple variables at the same time when making a simple decision (7). If the variables become more complex (such as during artificial ventilation) four of them are the maximum that an unaided mind can take into account simultaneously. Furthermore, the decision process itself is highly influenced by the selectivity of the human memory for new, important data and for data that support one's own opinion. In the presence of a theoretical concept for a possible relatedness of variables the empirical causative relationship is regularly overestimated; in the absence of such a concept, humans tend to underestimate such a relationship. It may be concluded, therefore, that for daily routine decision making, no reproducible conditions exist which would ensure the highest quality and thus the best possible outcome for the patients.

Additional factors negatively influencing the quality of the process of clinical decision making include:

1. Unrepresentative data.
2. Nonergonomical user-unfriendly data representation.
3. Different stages of training of physicians and respiratory therapists.
4. a) Working in shifts (human performance is decreased during nights); b) High turnover of personnel.

5. Short presence of highly trained and experienced critical care physicians at the bedside.

Especially when relying on an automated data collection system the question always arises whether the data are valid (3, 8). Artifacts with no clinical implications (i.e. patient movement, O_2 flushing, suctioning, etc.) have to be distinguished from true technical events (i.e. disconnection, ventilator malperformance, etc.) and changes in the patient's actual clinical condition (i.e. worsening of pulmonary condition, pneumothorax, etc.). These latter conditions represent serious clinical situations that need to be considered and treated. The quality of the raw data can be enhanced successfully by suppressing artifacts using various filtering methods. Some of these methods are computationally highly demanding because they use complicated mathematical algorithms for identifying artifacts and significant events. Others use less complex filtering functions such as the moving median value of the particular parameter derived from a defined time period (i.e. 1 or 3 min).

People are poor processors of numerical or digital data. Most frequently they use mental models and pattern recognition in making decisions. None of the traditional and available graphic options of modern ventilators meet these needs. Therefore ways of graphical or, even better, of intuitive data representation have to be found (9). One way is to create graphical objects that are metaphors for the data set. These metaphor graphics can easily be interpreted and the user can ask for a display of the numerical values if needed. High performance video features may also help the process of making competent clinical decisions.

Unfortunately the other factors – the human resources – that have an even greater impact on the quality of the patient care cannot be optimized effortlessly. Computers may offer a variety of solutions to this problem; the idea being that the clinical performance of the medical staff, and thus the outcome for the patients, can be significantly improved with the help of modern computer systems and artificial intelligence techniques (10, 11).

Computerized decision support for artificial ventilation

The amount of data generated by a modern ventilator exceeds the limits of effective comprehension of the human mind. Therefore, despite the achieved technical perfection of the devices, their use has not become simpler but rather more difficult. The titration of artificial ventilation is usually based on a patho-physiologically derived therapy concept. The realization of such a concept in the clinical practice is usually impaired by the deficiencies of human decision making, as mentioned above.

A computer system, due to its ability to handle huge amounts of data in a standardized and timely correct sequential manner, is capable of avoiding some of the inherent deficiencies of the human brain. When a computer system is programmed with the knowledge of experts in the domain of artificial ventilation it does not only theoretically improve respiratory therapy. It has been shown in first clinical trials that the standardized application of expert knowledge by a 24-h available computer system is very successful in guiding ventilatory care and may even reduce mortality of acute respiratory failure (5, 12). Due to the uniformity of care, learning as well as teaching of artificial ventilation are enhanced, especially when interactive teaching material and literature are provided with the expert system. Early expert systems functioned without a direct data link between the ventilator and the computer. The ventilatory data had to be manually charted into the computer database. The active knowledge system would then draw inferences from the updated data and the knowledge base and generate case-specific advice.

All the following more modern realizations require a hardware connection between the ventilator and the computer system. Therapy suggestions generated by a computer system can be realized in various ways (12, 13):

1. The system displays verbal or graphical directions for the treatment. They have to be manually implemented or dismissed by the medical personnel (open loop system).

2. Optimal settings for the ventilator are proposed. In case of compliance with these suggestions a key on the keyboard is pressed. This confirmation will make the computer set the desired values on the ventilator (open loop system with automated therapy implementation).

3. Other systems operate within a precisely defined therapeutic interval automatically requiring no further human input. Only when the boundaries are reached the system requires interactions with the medical personnel (full close loop system).

Such decision support systems are not designed to replace the physician at the bedside. Their purpose is to aid and guide the clinician during the demanding process of clinical decision making in an environment of overwhelming amount of data. Decision support systems should be designed to make the best use of the enormous technical potential of modern ventilators to assure a treatment that is optimally tailored to the patient's pulmonary status.

Another important advantage of such decision support systems is the reproducibility of their clinical performance. This implies that the computer will always suggest the identical optimized ventilator settings under the same pulmonary circumstances, represented by an identical set of data, regardless of the time of the day, the clinicians involved, or the multiple other influences of an ICU treatment. This unique feature of a computerized decision support system also ensures that the treatment of patients in the different limbs of a randomized clinical trial will be highly reproducible (5). Because of the multiple influences of intensive care treatment in general (the noise) on the result of a clinical trial, this reproducibility is an important prerequisite for establishing causative relationships between therapy on the one hand (the signal) and the outcome on the other. Standardization considerably reduces the unwanted noise of therapeutic interventions to be studied, so that a better quality of the final signal, the outcome variables is obtained. Only by applying those rigid rules, new therapeutical concepts can be tested against standard therapies. Better quality of patient care at lower cost will be the results.

References

1. Colice GL (1994) Historical perspective on the development of mechanical ventilation. In: Tobin MJ (ed) Principles and practice of mechanical ventilation. McGraw-Hill, New York, pp 1-36
2. Ashbaugh DG, Petty TL, Bigelow DB et al (1969) Continuous positive pressure breathing (CPPB) in the adult respiratory distress syndrome. J Thorac Cardiovasc Surg 57:31
3. East TD (1994) Role of the computer in delivery of mechanical ventilation. In: Tobin MJ (ed) Principles and practice of mechanical ventilation. McGraw-Hill, New York, pp 1005-1038
4. Sanborn WG (1993) Microprocessor-based mechanical ventilation. Respir Care 38:72-109
5. Eddy DM (1990) Clinical decision making. JAMA 263:1265-1275
6. Morris AH (1993) Protocol management of adult respiratory distress syndrome. New Horizons 1:593-602
7. Miller G (1956) The magic number seven, plus or minus two: some limits on our capacity for processing information. Psychol Rev 53:81-97
8. Brunner JX, Thompson JD (1993) Computerized ventilation monitoring. Respir Care 38: 110-124
9. Cole WG, Stewart JG (1993) Metaphor graphics to support integrated decision making with respiratory data. Int J Clin Monit Comput 10:91-100
10. Johnston ME, Langton KB, Hayes RB Mathieu A (1994) Effect of computer-based clinical decision support systems on clinician performance and patient outcome. Ann Intern Med 120:135-142
11. Uckun S (1994) Intelligent systems in patient monitoring and therapy management. Int J Clin Monit Comput 11:241-253
12. East TD, Bhm SH, Wallace CJ et al (1992) A successful computerized protocol for clinical management of pressure control inverse ratio ventilation in ARDS patients. Chest 101: 697-710
13. Laubscher TP, Frutiger A, Fanconi S, Jutzi H, Brunner JX (1994) Automatic selection of tidal volume, respiratory frequency and minute ventilation in intubated ICU patients as startup procedure for close-loop controlled ventilation. Int J Clin Monit Comput 11:19-30

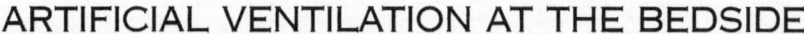

ARTIFICIAL VENTILATION AT THE BEDSIDE

The Problem of Weaning in COPD Patients

R. Brandolese, U. Andreose

When we consider diseases of the respiratory system from the point of view of mechanics, we can divide them into obstructive and restrictive disorders, which can be diagnosed readily by spirometry (1). We discuss, here, the problems inherent to obstructive pulmonary disease because they are, in clinical practice, more important and there are many speculative studies. Lung disease characterized by breathlessness and a slowing lung emptying are very common in our intensive respiratory units.

Chronic obstructive lung disease can be defined as a disorder whose feature is an abnormal test of expiratory flow that does not change, significantly, over periods of several months. We know that the expiratory flow limitation is due to both structural and functional abnormalities. Moreover, a bronchial hiperreactivity may be present in patients affected by COPD, and we can speculate that, in general, there are two types of COPD: chronic bronchitis and emphysema (3-5).

Chronic bronchitis is defined as a condition asssociated with a large amount of tracheobronchial mucus sufficient to cause cough and expectoration for at least 3 months in a year for more than two consecutive ones. The major pathological features include, moreover, gland hyperplasia, muscle hypertrophy that, all together, narrow the lumen of the tracheobronchial tree, leading to airflow obstruction (2).

Emphysema is defined as a disorder of the lung characterized by a distension of the air spaces distal to the terminal bronchiole with destruction of alveolar septa. In emphysema the main mechanism that leads to flow limitation is the loss of elastic recoil of the lung (2).

In other words, the driving pressure of the expiration is decreased because the static lung compliance is enhanced. There is a condition of static hyperinflation, and the elastic equilibrium volume of total respiratory system is in a higher position in the relaxation curve of the total respiratory system in comparison with normal subjects (6, 7).

In established chronic obstructive lung disease standard test results of lung mechanics are quite abnormal, such FEV1 and airway resistances. There is, also, an increase of both RV and FRC (functional residual capacity). The changes in respiratory mechanics are distributed unevenly and the presence of frequency dependence of compliance and of resistance is evident (7). Moreover, the increase in FRC because of static hyperinflation places the inspiratory muscles in a disadvantageous position with regard to their force-length relationship (9, 10).

Airway function

As COPD progresses, maximum flow is reduced both during inspiration and expiration. In addition the conductance (G) of airways is reduced at all lung volumes because of the reduction of $\Delta G/\Delta V$ ratio (11). This increased airway resistance and airflow limitation are predominantly in the intrapulmonary airways and in the air spaces. The dynamic narrowing of airways during forced expiratory maneuvers is increased too. In COPD patients the reduction in elastic recoil pressure which causes a decrease in extra airway distending pressure, and airway narrowing (the pressure loss is greater down the airway), both increase dynamic compression of large intrathoracic airways during the expiration phase (12). The site of increased respiratory resistance was in the peripheral airways with a diameter of less than 2-3 mm.

Alteration in lung mechanics in COPD

The main characteristic change in respiratory mechanics in emphysema is a marked loss of the elastic recoil pressure of the lung which is related to the severity of the inflammatory process involving the airways. Patients with severe airflow limitation develop chronic hypercapnia, show low values of dynamic compliance, have an increased respiratory resistance, and ventilate a small tidal volume during resting breathing (13, 14).

Consider, therefore, the following equation:

$$WOB = 1/2\ Vt^2/Cdyn + 1/4\ \pi^2\ R\ f\ Vt^2 \qquad [1]$$

WOB is work of breathing expressed in kgm
Cdyn is dynamic compliance of total respiratory system
R is respiratory resistance
Vt is tidal volume.

In the Eq. 1 Vt has a maximum exponent '2' and, if Vt doubles WOB becomes four times: then COPD patients adopt a strategy of rapid shallow breathing.

Although in CAO patients minute ventilation is usually normal at rest, this is achieved by considerable adjustment in respiratory muscle activity quite different from the normal pattern. Consequently there is an increased swing in pleural pressure in order to overcome the increased workload (due to increased resistance and decreased dynamic compliance). Any increase in metabolic demand is accomplished by an increase in minute ventilation obtained by increasing respiratory rate rather than Vt.

Because of increased airflow resistance, decreased dynamic compliance, and increased FRC, the inspiratory muscles in COPD patients must generate considerable pressure to ventilate the lungs. Pulmonary dynamic hyperinflation, by decreasing the optimal resting length of inspiratory muscles, reduces their capability as pressure generators (15). Inspiratory muscles work chronically at a higher proportion of their total capacity than in normal subjects (16) and WOB calculated by the Campbell diagram is underestimated because it takes no account of extra work due to distortion of the chest wall and hysteresis (17). The result of all these altered mechanical properties is that the oxygen consumption of respiratory muscles is greatly increased out of proportion to the mechanical work done (18). The performance of the inspiratory muscles becomes a limiting factor in determining the development of acute respiratory failure in COPD patients. By contrast because of hyperinflation the expiratory muscles are lengthened and their capability as pressure generators is well preserved.

The respiratory system can be divided in two parts: the lungs and the pump that ventilates the lungs. The lung, when compromised by an infection and/or an ARDS, determines an alteration in causes ventilatory failure with hypercapnia. Ventilatory failure is sustained by alteration of neuromuscular transmission, by depression of respiratory centers, by alteration of geometry of the rib cage as results in patients with flail chest and/or kyphoscoliosis and, finally by respiratory muscle fatigue.

Fatigue can be defined, in general, as the inability to maintain an established task (19). If applied to respiratory muscles, fatigue is defined as the inability to maintain an adequate ventilation ($PaCO_2$ less than 40 mmHG).The equation that relates alveolar ventilation to $PaCO_2$ is given by:

$$PaCO_2 = K(VCO_2/VA) \qquad [2]$$

The equation may be arranged and expressed as:

$$PaCO_2 = \frac{KVCO_2}{(1-VD/Vt)(Vt/Ti)(T_I/T_{TOT})}$$

where VD is dead space ventilation, Vt/Ti is mean inspiratory flow, an index of velocity of contraction of the muscular fibers, and T_I/T_{TOT} is called "inspiratory duty cycle", indicating the fraction of total respiratory during which the inspiratory muscle contracts.

The primary site of fatigue is the respiratory muscles and when the muscles perform a fatiguing task the central nervous system, informed by appropriate neurotransmitters, attempts to reduce Vt/Ti in order to preserve the muscles at the expense of hypoventilation. Mean inspiratory flow may be considered to be proportional to the pressure generated and substituting Vt/Ti with PTI the equation on the top becomes:

$$PaCO_2 = KVCO_2/f(PTI-VD) \qquad\qquad [3]$$

PTI is pressure time index and is termed also as "tension time index" per breath which correlates with the energy demands of the inspiratory muscles. If the energy supply is inadequate for respiratory muscles PTI will decrease and this reduction is counterbalanced by an increase in the respiratory rate. Nevertheless this strategy is weak and the frequency is no longer optimal to sustained ventilation: then $PaCO_2$ increases.

COPD patients, during an acute exacerbation of their chronic airway obstruction, present with factors predisposing to respiratory muscle fatigue (19). In fact, in these patients the mechanical workload is markedly increased because of increased respiratory resistances, decreased dynamic respiratory compliance and dynamic hyperinflation, termed also auto PEEP or intrinsic PEEP (PEEPi) (20). Accordingly, the inspiratory muscles are unable to generate the required pressure for adequate alveolar ventilation, and their efficiency is low because of a great increase in oxygen consumption. The ratio between the pressure generated by the inspiratory muscle and their maximal force is elevated, and the greater the F/Fmax ratio the greater is the energy demand. Besides, F/Fmax is inversely related to "limit time" (time interval after which the respiratory muscles express fatigue). Fmax is a function of fiber length and hyperinflation has deleterious effects on the force-length relationship of the respiratory muscles. Then the diaphragm, the principal muscle of respiration, is markedly shortened and flattened (21-26). The radius curvature (r) is increased because of hyperinflation and according to Laplace law the tension developed is much smaller:

$$P = 2T/r$$

Similarly, Fmax may be diminished by other factors found in COPD patients such as malnutrition, weight loss and atrophy.

But in CAO patients the energy supply is decreased. In fact, the energy supply is dependent on the blood flow to the muscles, which is due to the perfusion pressure related to cardiac output (27) and peripheral vascular resistances of the muscles (28). Cardiac output is decreased because of hyperinflation, which determines an increase of intrathoracic pressure causing a reduced venous return to the heart.

Summarizing, COPD patients, during acute exacerbation of airway obstruction, simply develop an imbalance between energy supply and demand of the respiratory muscles that may lead to fatigue requiring the institution of mechanical ventilation (19).

For the vast majority of patient in an intensive care unit who require mechanical ventilation, weaning and extubation is simple and a variety of strategies may be successful (29) (Table 1). According to our experience and to that one of other intensive care units, usually, about 75% of patients mechanically ventilated because of respiratory failure are weaned from the ventilator within 72 hours on the onset of mechanical ventilation. By contrast the remaining 25% of patients present, at different degree of difficulty, problems during weaning. Among these difficult to weaning, COPD patients are, perhaps, the main component (29).

Table 1. Prevalence of patients requiring weaning techniques

Total	Not requiring (%)	Requiring (%)
165	82	18
259	90	10
171	72	28
COPD	20	80

Fatigue of the inspiratory muscles is the cardinal indication to ventilate COPD patients during acute exacerbation of chronic airway obstruction. Two types of fatigue have been recognized from the point of view of EMG analysis: high frequency fatigue, where recovery occurs within a few hours, and low frequency fatigue with recoveries within some days (30, 31). COPD patients with exacerbation are characterized by low frequency fatigue and their inspiratory muscle should be fully supported by mechanical ventilation for a relatively long period of time. During mechanical ventilation the inspiratory muscles are set at rest. It has been shown that the use of ventilatory support reduced or abolished the electrical activity of the diaphragm and also of other inspiratory muscles as the accessory ones. The muscles become unloaded and this approach contributes to the improvement in respiratory muscle strength and ventilatory endurance.

Assessment of respiratory mechanics in mechanically ventilated patients because of respiratory failure is rarely performed routinely in respiratory intensive care units. Nevertheless it is a relatively simple and useful procedure that gives us information about the status and the progress of the disease. Yet, the measurement of respiratory mechanics is important to the problem of weaning (32).

The capability to resume spontaneous ventilation in mechanically ventilated patients (COPD) is dependent upon the balance between the respiratory load and the pressure that the inspiratory muscles are able to generate. This is illustrated by the first degree equation of Rahn which describes the motion of gas into the respiratory system.

$$P = Vt/Crs + Rrs\ (Vt/Ti) \qquad\qquad [4]$$

where P is the pressure that is applied to move the respiratory system and/or the pressure that the inspiratory muscles have to generate to ventilate the lungs, Vt is tidal volume, Crs is the compliance of total respiratory system, Rrs is flow resistance, and Vt/Ti, as we have just seen above, is mean inspiratory flow. Therefore the measurement of the elastic and resistive pressure of respiratory system plus the additional resistance added by the presence of the endotracheal tube and inspiratory line is the main step to evaluate the evolving respiratory workload in COPD patients.

Measurement of respiratory compliance

We can compute respiratory compliance by one of three different methods:

1. The pressure-volume curve obtained during static inflation and deflation of the lung in a stepwise mode, by means of a giant syringe
2. The interrupter technique of expiratory flow during relaxed expiration (33)
3. End inspiratory occlusion maneuver during constant flow inflation of the lungs (34).

We illustrate the third method, which is simple, reproducible and widely used.

Briefly after occlusion of the airway at end inspiration we assist to an immediate drop in airway pressure which gently decreases to an apparent plateau. The plateau pressure value represents the elastic recoil pressure of the respiratory system relative to end inflation tidal volume. Crs is computed by dividing VT by the plateau pressure value minus total elastic recoil pressure at end expiration (i.e., PEEP + PEEPi). If PEEPi is not included in our computation, the value of respiratory compliance can be underestimated up to above 100% in COPD patients (35).

Measurement of respiratory resistance

After having occluded the airways at end tidal inflation, there is an initial drop (P1) in airway pressure followed by a further decrease (plateau pressure). The total drop represents the total amount of dynamic pressure dissipated at end inspiration. The difference in pressure (Pmax-P1) divided by the inspiratory flow preceding the occlusion represents the true "ohmic" resistance of the total respiratory system plus the additional resistance due to viscoelastic properties of the respiratory system and "pendelluft" because of time constant inequalities within the lungs (34).

In normal lung, pendelluft contributes little to additional inspiratory resistance; in contrast, because of time constant inhomogeneities it becomes an important component in COPD patients (35). In fact we have found that the largest Δ Rrs was exhibited by COPD patients (35).

We have used the end inspiratory occlusion technique at constant flow inflation to assess the dose-response and the time course effect of methylxanthines in mechanically ventilated COPD patients (36).

Detection and measurement of dynamic hyperinflation (PEEPi)

Increased airway resistance and an altered breathing pattern (i.e., rapid shallow breathing) prevent complete expiration and dynamic hyperinflation occurs. When the expiratory muscles are relaxed, PEEPi, due to end expiratory elastic recoil, is a corollary of dynamic hyperinflation. In COPD patients, particularly, detection and measurement of PEEPi value is important not only to obtain the "true respiratory compliance", but also to avoid an undesirable drop in cardiac output and in oxygen delivery to the tissue in general and to respiratory muscle in particular. In fact, a moderate value of 8 cmH_2O of PEEPi can determine a significant decrease in cardiac output (0.6 L/min on average) (37).

PEEPi may be easily measured in mechanically ventilated patients by means of the end-expiratory occlusion technique. In contrast during spontaneous breathing and during weaning trials, when the respiratory muscles are not relaxed, measurement of PEEPi requires the use of a nasogastric tube with an esophageal balloon to assess changes in pleural pressure. In those patients, PEEPi is measured on the esophageal pressure tracing as the pressure difference between the point corresponding to the onset of inspiratory effort and the point corresponding to zero flow. Sampling the gastric pressure during that interval is important to assess whether the Δ Pes due to contracting inspiratory muscles rather than to decontracting expiratory muscles (38).

In Table 2 we provide an overview of respiratory mechanics data from 80 consecutive mechanically ventilated patients in our ICU.

We can see that PEEPi is a constant feature of COPD patients, but it is also present, less frequently, in other groups of patients without a history of chronic airway obstruction. Crs is lower in all the patients and the respiratory resistance reaches values as high as 20 $cmH_2O/L/s$ in COPD patients.

It is clear from Table 2 that respiratory workload is determined by an abnormally low compliance, by a marked increase in respiratory resistance and by intrinsic PEEP. This implies that in terms of pressure generated by inspiratory muscles (weaning), the equation of Rahn has to be modified and rewritten as follows:

$$P = (Vt/Crs + PEEPi) + Rtot,rs \ (Vt/Ti) \qquad [5]$$

In conclusion measurements of compliance, resistance and PEEPi provide useful information not only during mechanical ventilation of COPD patients but also for weaning procedures.

Table 2. Respiratory mechanics in mechanically ventilated patients

Diagnosis	Number	PEEPi (cmH$_2$O)	Cst,rs (L/cmH$_2$O)	Rmax,rs (cmH$_2$O/L/s)	Rmin,rs (cmH$_2$O/L/s)
COPD	40	2.8 – 22	0.058 ± 10	20.2 ± 0.5	10 ± 4.7
ARDS	22	1.0 – 8.1	0.035 ± 0.9	11.7 ± 4.5	5.7 ± 2.8
CPE	8	1.0 – 6.0	0.044 ± 0.8	12.0 ± 5.5	8.3 ± 4.1
Others	18	1.0 – 4.1	0.044 ± 20	07.0 ± 3.3	3.5 ± 2.9

COPD, chronic obstructive pulmonary disease; ARDS, adult respiratory distress syndrome; CPE, cardiogenic pulmonary oedema; PEEPi, positive end-expiratory pressure; Cts,rs, respiratory static compliance; Rmax,rs, maximal respiratory resistance; Rmin,rs, minimal respiratory resistance.

The role of PEEPi during weaning procedures in COPD patients

It is well established that the application of an external PEEP may be of benefit in COPD patients during assisted modes of mechanical ventilation and during weaning trials (39). The external PEEP improves respiratory muscle efficiency because PEEPe is not added to intrinsic PEEP but partially substitutes it. In terms of respiratory muscle effort, PEEPi act as an inspiratory threshold load which has to be overcome in order to inflate the lungs. During controlled mechanical ventilation PEEPi is counteracted by the ventilator; by contrast, during patient-machine interaction PEEPi must be overcome by the inspiratory muscles. In this case the muscles contract isometrically without moving air into the lungs but equally consume oxygen (40).

The dynamic hyperinflation that occurs in COPD patients is added to any increase in absolute lung volume due to the loss of elastic recoil pressure. PEEPi provides a significant burden for the inspiratory muscles which can severely impair the ability to resume spontaneous ventilation (40). Obviously reducing PEEPi will be of benefit.

It is well accepted that application of low levels of external PEEP decreases PEEPi and hence the work of breathing during assisted mechanical ventilation and weaning trials (41, 42). Similarly, continuous positive airway pressure (CPAP) is equally effective in reducing inspiratory effort in spontaneously breathing patients being weaned from mechanical ventilation (42). The ability of PEEP to reduce PEEPi is critically dependent upon the presence of flow limitation. In fact, in the presence of flow limitation, any increase in downstream impedance (PEEPe) relative to the site of flow limitation should have little effect on the rate of lung emptying until the applied external PEEP exceeds a critical level that is somewhat lower than the initial PEEPi. In the absence of expiratory flow limitation, the application of PEEPe will decrease driving expiratory pressure and hence expiratory flow with further increase in end-expiratory lung volume (43-45).

Level of PEEP in patients with intrinsic PEEP

There is no exact guideline for the titration of external PEEP in COPD patients. However, pulmonary hyperinflation should not be enhanced by an excessive amount of PEEPe. In fact this tends to negate the beneficial effects of removing PEEPi by further decreasing inspiratory muscle length and force generating capacity. Therefore it is necessary to measure lung volume using respiratory inductance plethysmography (Respitrace) (46). Alternatively PEEPi can be determined from the measurements of the difference between the value in plateau pressure during an end-expiratory occlusion maneuver and the pressure recorded at end expiration without occluding the airways. By this procedure it is possible to evaluate if PEEP replaces or is added to PEEPi.

Pharmacological treatment of pulmonary hyperinflation

The application of an external PEEP lower than the preexisting level of PEEPi supports the inspiratory muscles during weaning in COPD patients. But PEEPi can also be reduced by lengthening the expiratory time. However, this mean is clearly insufficient because of the high value of the time constant of the respiratory system in COPD patients (2-5 s). More efficient is the administration of drugs which affect the smooth bronchial muscle by decreasing airflow resistance (47). Bronchodilators such as methylxanthines and β_2 adrenergic agonists are widely used in the therapy of acute bronchoconstriction.

We have studied nine and seven consecutive mechanically ventilated COPD patients before and after a bolus of 5-6 mg/kg of doxophylline and inhalation of fenoterol (0.4-1.2 mg), respectively. In both instances there was a marked and significant decrease of flow resistance: PEEPi was significantly reduced from 11.7 ($\pm$ 5.4) to 6.1 ($\pm$ 4.9) cmH$_2$O. These data show that both methylxanthines and β_2 agonists are efficient in reducing the ventilatory load and the dynamic hyperinflation in mechanically ventilated COPD patients. In stable COPD patients we have measured changes in maximum transdiaphragmatic pressure (Pdi max, a good index of muscular strength) associated with bronchodilatation induced by inhaled fenoterol. The explanation is a decrease in end-expiratory lung volume paralleling the decrease of PEEPi from 2.5 ($\pm$ 1.5) to 0.9 ($\pm$ 1.3) cmH$_2$O.

The effect of theophylline on respiratory muscle fatigue

In 1981 M. Aubier et al. observed that administration of theophylline reduced respiratory muscle fatigue; in other words this xanthine ameliorated the endurance of inspiratory muscles. Diaphragmatic fatigue decreased transdiaphragmatic pressure and when theophylline was injected, transdiaphragmatic pressure recovered rapidly (36).

Malnutrition and COPD

Recent investigators have recognized that advancing COPD was frequently associated with a progressive loss of body weight (48). Hospitalized COPD patients appear to have a higher incidence of malnutrition and this applies to patients who develop respiratory failure and therefore require mechanical ventilation. A retrospective clinical trial for COPD patients mechanically ventilated has demonstrated that a body weight less than 90% of ideal was associated with an increase in mortality rate. Clinical studies have demonstrated that metabolic adaptation is not present in COPD patients whose resting expenditure energy is 15%-17% above the predicted values. Donahoe et al. have demonstrated that in COPD patients there is a greater energy requirement for respiratory muscle activity than in controls (49). There are many studies but results conflict regarding measurable improvement in muscle strength due to a nutritional repletion. Nevertheless there is general agreement that a biochemical change is the primary mechanism of benefit rather than a significant gain in body weight.

Predictive indexes of weaning from mechanical ventilation

A large number of parameters have been used for predicting a successful weaning trial (Tables 3, 4). We are listing the following:

Oxygenation indexes
Vital capacity
Maximal inspiratory pressure
Total respiratory compliance
Minute ventilation
Maximum minute ventilation
Occlusion airway pressure (P0.1)
Breathing pattern
Work of breathing
Pressure time index
Clinical examination

Table 3. Some predictive weaning indexes

Prediction result index	Weaning failure False positive (%)	Weaning failure False negative (%)
VC	18	50
V_E	11	75
MVV	14	75
Pi max	26	100
WOB	14	14

VC, vital capacity; V_E, minute ventilation; MVV, maximal voluntary ventilation; Pi max, maximal inspiratory pressure; WOB, work of breathing.

Table 4. Weaning indexes

Strength	Endurance
MIP	T_I/T_{TOT}
$P_{0.1}$	PTI
ΔPes	f/Vt
V_E	RR
WOB	

MIP, maximal inspiratory airway pressure; ΔPes, Δ esophageal pressure; V_E, minute ventilation; WOB, work of breathing; T_I/T_{TOT}, inspiratory duty cycle; PTI, pressure time index; RR, respiratory rate; f/Vt, rapid shallow breathing index; $P_{0.1}$, mouth occlusion pressure at 100 ms.

An exhaustive description of all these parameters is beyond the scope of this paper. We specify that conventional standard criteria for weaning from mechanical ventilation include vital capacity, maximal inspiratory force < –20 cmH_2O, minute ventilation < 10 l/min and, finally, VT greater than 5 ml/kg body weight.

Several authors have questioned the accuracy of these mechanical criteria in predicting a successful weaning trial. These parameters failed to predict the outcome during weaning in patients requiring prolonged mechanical ventilation. There is general agreement among the investigators that other parameters such as $P_{0.1}$, pressure time index, work of breathing are better indicators of successful weaning.

Mouth occlusion pressure measured at 100 ms during closure airway maneuver ($P_{0.1}$)

$P_{0.1}$ is a good indicator of inspiratory central drive. In other words $P_{0.1}$ shows how much the patients "want" to breathe. Its normal value in humans is 1-2 cm H_2O but in decompensated COPD patients may reach values as high as 10-12 cm H_2O

with a normal minute ventilation. $P_{0.1}$ is related to the mechanical workload of the inspiratory muscles. The larger the $P_{0.1}$ the greater is the mechanical burden for the inspiratory muscles (50).

M. Aubier et al. (36) have measured $P_{0.1}$ daily changes in COPD patients mechanically ventilated because of respiratory failure. In some of these patients $P_{0.1}$ decreased after some days of mechanical ventilation and pharmacological treatment to 4-5 cmH_2O. This group has been successfully weaned, whereas the others, whose $P_{0.1}$ was substantially unchanged, have not been weaned (50).

Pressure time index (PTI)

Bellemare and Grassino in 1980 (9) demonstrated the relationship between the inspiratory duty cycle (T_I/T_{TOT}) and the critical transdiaphragmatic pressure (Pdi). In their diagram the regression line defines a value of 0.15 for different ratios of Pdi/Pdimax and T_I/T_{TOT}. Above this regression line "the fatigue area" is located, whereas below is "the nonfatigue area". Therefore a PTI more than 0.15 is predictive of unsuccessful weaning: but we must remember that no index used during weaning is 100% predictive and PTI offers a percentage (25%) of false positives and false negatives (51). We can calculate PTI also as the ratio Pes (esophageal pressure)/Pes max multiplying by T_I/T_{TOT}. If an esophageal balloon has not been positioned in the esophagus, it is possible, utilizing Rahn's motion equation, to calculate the workload for the inspiratory muscles. This value is divided by maximal inspiratory pressure and the ratio multiplied by T_I/T_{TOT}.

Mechanical work of breathing

The mechanical work of breathing is an indirect measure of the energy required to breath spontaneously and has been suggested as a weaning parameter. Several studies have demonstrated that there is a level of 1.3-1.8 kgm/min or 0.75 joule/l above which patients cannot sustain ventilation indefinitely. Lung work is a function of V_T, V_E and of mean airway pressure generated by the inspiratory muscles or applied by the ventilator. The work of breathing is reputed to be a good index of the mechanical properties of the respiratory system related to different degree of respiratory failure (52). Actually devices are available which perform in real time some parameters of respiratory mechanics such as PTI, work of breathing, $P_{0.1}$ etc. The following formula gives the respiratory work expressed in joule/l if we measured the mean airway pressure (P) and tidal volume:

$$WOB = P \, V_T(L) \, 98/1000 \qquad [6]$$

Fiastro and coll. have measured work of breathing in 17 mechanically ventilated patients who had to be weaned. WOB less than 1.6 kgm/min or 0.14 kgm/l were both necessary for successful weaning and these threshold values were achieved in all the patients prior to the successful extubation and absent during mechanical ventilation and periods of unsuccessful weaning (52). Fiastro and coll. have found that mechanical support was necessary when total inspiratory work/min was more than 1.8 kgm/min. They found also that WOB/l is the best discriminant. Fiastro and coll. have evaluated 775 measurements of work of breathing and reported a cut-off level of 1.34 kgm/min. The same author found also a 14% rate of both false positives and false negatives (Table 3).

Techniques of discontinuing ventilator support

Weaning techniques include trial of spontaneous breathing through a T-tube circuit, intermittent mandatory ventilation (IMV) and pressure support ventilation (PSV).

There is no fixed rule in timing the initiation of the weaning trial; nevertheless this timing must be carefully selected because if delayed it will increase the risk connected with prolonged mechanical ventilation. By contrast if it is performed prematurely the patient can suffer a cardiorespiratory decompensation with further damage for himself.

When the physician believes that a weaning trial can be successful, the mechanical support is stopped and the patient is allowed to breathe via a T-tube circuit. To date there is no standardized rule for how long the patient should breathe through a T-tube. Obviously the duration of the T-tube weaning trial depends on the ability of the patient to maintain an adequate value of $PaCO_2$. A persistent normal $PaCO_2$ can be predictive of successful extubation. In contrast, a rapid increase in $PaCO_2$ suggests stopping the weaning trial and reinitiating mechanical support. After an unsuccessful weaning trial a further attempt can be made after a 24-h time interval.

IMV involves a gradual reduction in minute ventilation delivered to the patient by the machine and allows the patient to breathe spontaneously between mechanical breaths (53). To date no controlled studies have demonstrated the superiority of either IMV or T piece in patients difficult to wean (54). Concern has developed over the potential risk for increased inspiratory work and expiratory resistances that may be associated with some IMV delivering systems. This is true especially for demand-flow IMV systems. Concern has also centered around the potential increase, during an IMV trial, of dynamic hyperinflation because of the overlapping of expiration of a mechanical tidal breath with an inspiratory breathing effort. This will cause a further deleterious effect on respiratory muscle performance.

Pressure support ventilation differs from assisted-control ventilation and from IMV as the physician sets, on the ventilator, a level of pressure (10-15 cmH$_2$O) in order to augment every spontaneous patient effort (55). Pressure support may be considered as an adjunctive muscle of inspiration that works as we want according to the imbalance between workload and inspiratory muscle strength (56) (Table 5). During pressure support ventilation the patient triggers expiration; in fact the preset airway pressure is maintained until inspiratory flow falls below a certain level that usually is 25% of peak inspiratory flow. The tidal volume can change from breath to breath and is determined by the preset support pressure, from duration of patient inspiratory effort and finally by pulmonary mechanics (compliance, resistance and PEEPi) (57). As the magnitude of the inspiratory pressure support increases this may serve to unload completely the inspiratory muscles. As a preset support pressure decreases the muscles work proportionally more, yet avoiding the development of respiratory muscle fatigue and disuse atrophy. However, the amount of work necessary to prevent respiratory muscle atrophy in patients undergoing prolonged mechanical ventilation is unknown. From this point of view pressure support ventilation may be the key to maximize respiratory rest when muscle fatigue is a major factor (56) and to keep them trained. But further clinical studies will be required to address these issues in patients during mechanical ventilation and weaning trials (58).

Table 5.

	PS 10 cmH$_2$O	PS 5 cmH$_2$O	CPAP 5 cmH$_2$O
Vt (L)	0.55	0.40	0.32
f (b/min)	25	28	32
ΔPes (cmH$_2$O)	14	18	22
PTPes (cmH$_2$O/min)	250	285	390
WOB	0.85	1.25	1.7

Data collected during an unsuccessful weaning trial in a COPD patient. Note the progressive deterioration of all the parameters from pressure support (10 cmH$_2$O) to CPAP mode.

References

1. Macklem PT, Permutt S (1979) Lung biology in health and disease. The lung in transition between health and disease, vol 12. Dekker, New York
2. Mahler DA (ed) (1993) Pulmonary disease in the elderly patient. Dekker, New York, pp 159-188
3. Burrows B (1991) Clinical implications: epidemiologic evidence for different type of chronic airflow obstruction. Am Rev Respir Dis 143:1452-1454
4. Burrows B, Earle RH (1969) Course and prognosis of chronic obstructive lung disease. A prospective study of 200 patients. N Engl J Med 280:397-404
5. Borrows B, Bloom J, Traver JA, Cline MG (1987) The course and prognosis of different forms of chronic airway obstruction in a sample from the general population. N Engl J Med 286: 912-918

6. Greaves IA, Colebatch HJH (1980) Elastic behaviour and structure of normal and emphysematous lung post-mortem. Am Rev Respir Dis 121:127-136
7. Nagels J, Landser FJ, Van Der Linder L et al (1980) Mechanical properties of lungs and chest wall during spontaneous breathing. J Appl Physiol 49:408-416
8. Grimby G, Takashima W, Macklem PT, Mead J (1968) Frequency dependence of flow resistance in patients with chronic obstructive lung disease. J Clin Invest 47:1455-1465
9. Bellamare F, Grassino A (1983) Force reserve of the diaphragm in patients with chronic obstructive lung disease. J Appl Physiol 55:8-15
10. Similowski T, Yan S, Gauthier AP, Macklem PT, Bellemare F (1991) Contractile properties of the human diaphragm during chronic hyperinflation. N Engl J Med 325:917-923
11. Butler J, Caro CG, Alcala R et al (1960) Physiological factors affecting airway resistance in normal subjects and in patients with obstructive respiratory disease. J Clin Invest 39:584-591
12. Leaver DG, Tattersfield AE, Pride NB (1973) Contribution of loss lung recoil and of enhanced airway collapsibility to the airflow obstruction of chronic bronchitis and emphysema. J Clin Invest 52:2117-2128
13. Burrows B, Saksena FB, Diener CF (1966) Carbon dioxide tension and ventilatory mechanics in chronic obstructive lung disease. Ann Intern Med 65:685-700
14. Park SS, Janis M, Shim CS, Williams MH (1970) Relationship of bronchitis and emphysema to altered pulmonary function. Am Rev Respir Dis 102:927-936
15. Byrd RB, Hyatt RE (1968) Maximal respiratory pressure in chronic obstructive lung disease. Am Rev Respir Dis 98:848-856
16. Cherniack RM, Hodson A (1963) Compliance of the chest wall in chronic bronchitis and emphysema. J Appl Physiol 18:707-711
17. O'Connell JM, Campbell AH (1976) Respiratory mechanics in airway obstruction associated with inspiratory dispnoea. Thorax 31:669-677
18. Cherniack RM (1969) The oxygen consumption and efficiency of the respiratory muscles in health and emphysema. J Clin Invest 38:494-499
19. Roussos CH, Macklem PT (1986) Inspiratory muscle fatigue. In: Macklem PT (ed) Mechanics of breathing, part 2. Oxford University Press, New York (The respiratory system, vol III; Handbook of physiology, sect 3)
20. Pepe PE, Marini JJ (1982) Occult positive end expiratory pressure in mechanically ventilated patients with airflow obstruction. Am Rev Respir Dis 126:166-170
21. Oliven A, Supinsky GS, Kelsen SG (1986) Functional adaptation of diaphragm in chronic hyperinflation in emphysematous hamsters. J Appl Physiol 60:225-231
22. Arora NS, Rochester DF (1987) COPD and human diaphragm muscles dimension. Chest 91: 719-724
23. Rochester DF, Braun NM (1985) Determinants of maximal inspiratory pressure in chronic obstructive pulmonary disease. Am Rev Respir Dis 132:42-47
24. Roussos CG, Fixley M, Gross D, Macklem PT (1979) Fatigue of inspiratory muscles and their synergic behaviour. J Appl Physiol 45:897-904
25. Roussos CH, Macklem PT (1977) Diaphragmatic fatigue in man. J Appl Physiol 43:189-197
26. Roussos C, Macklem PT (1982) The respiratory muscles. N Engl J Med 307:786-797
27. Aubier M, Tippenbach T, Roussos C (1981) Respiratory muscle fatigue during cardiogenic shock. J Appl Physiol 51:499-508
28. Schnader J, Juan G, Howel S, Fitzgerald R, Roussos Ch (1985) Arterial CO_2 partial pressure affects diaphragmatic function. J Appl Physiol 58:823-829
29. Tobin MJ, Alex CG (1994) Discontinuation of mechanical ventilation. In: Tobin MJ (ed) Principles and practice of mechanical ventilation. McGraw-Hill, New York, pp 1177-1206
30. Kadefors R, Kaiser E, Petersen I (1968) Dynamic spectrum analysis of myopotentials with special references to muscle fatigue. Electromyogr Clin Neurophysiol 8:39-74
31. Kaiser E, Petersen I (1962) Frequency analysis of action potentials during tetanic contraction. Electroencephalogr Clin Neurophysiol 14:955

32. Milic-Emili J (1986) Is weaning an art or a science? Am Rev Respir Dis 134:1107-1108
33. Gottfried SB, Rossi A, Higgs BD et al (1985) Noninvasive determination of respiratory system mechanics during mechanical ventilation for acute respiratory failure. Am Rev Respir Dis 131:414-420
34. Rossi A, Gottfried SB, Zocchi L et al (1985) Respiratory mechanics in mechanically ventilated patients with respiratory failure. J Appl Physiol 58:1849-1858
35. Broseghini C, Brandolese R, Poggi R et al (1988) Respiratory mechanics during the first day of mechanical ventilation in patients with pulmonary edema and chronic airway obstruction. Am Rev Respir Dis 138:355-361
36. Aubier M, Roussos CH (1981) Pharmacotherapy in the thorax, part B. In: Roussos CH, Macklem PT (ed). Dekker, New York, pp 1373-1405
37. Brandolese R, Broseghini C, Milic-Emini J, Brandi G, Rossi A (1993) Effect of intrinsic PEEP on pulmonary gas exchange in mechanically ventilated patients with pulmonary edema. Eur Respir J 6:358-363
38. Dal Vecchio L, Polese G, Poggi R, Rossi A (1990) Intrinsic positive end expiratory pressure in stable COPD patients with CAO. Eur Respir J 3:74-80
39. Rossi A, Brandolese R, Milic-Emili J, Gottfried SB (1990) The role of PEEP in patients with chronic obstructive disease during assisted ventilation. Eur Respir J 3:818-822
40. Milic-Emili J, Gottfried SB, Rossi A (1987) Dynamic hyperinflation: intrinsic PEEP and its ramifications in patients with respiratory failure. In: Vincent JL (ed) Update in intensive care medicine. Springer, Berlin Heidelberg New York, pp 192-198
41. Smith TC, Marini JJ (1988) Impact of PEEP in lung mechanics and work of breathing in severe airflow obstruction. J Appl Physiol 65:1488-1499
42. Calderini E, Petrof BJ, Gottfried SB (1989) Continuous positive airway pressure improves the efficacy of pressure support ventilation in severe chronic obstructive pulmonary disease (COPD). Am Rev Respir Dis 139:A155
43. Brandolese R, Bernasconi M, Poggi R et al (1988) Effects of PEEP on respiratory mechanics and gas exchange in mechanically ventilated patients with ARDS and acute exacerbation of COPD. Am Rev Respir Dis 137:A470
44. Gay PC, Rodarte JR, Hubmayr RD (1989) The effect of positive end expiratory pressure on isovolume and dynamic hyperinflation in patients receiving mechanical ventilation. Am Rev Respir Dis 139:621-626
45. Simkowitz P, Brown K, Goldberg P et al (1987) Interaction between intrinsic and externally applied PEEP during mechanical ventilation. Am Rev Respir Dis 135:A202
46. Hoffmann RA, Ershowsky P, Krieger BP (1989) Determination of auto PEEP during spontaneous and controlled mechanical ventilation by monitoring changes in end expiratory thoracic gas volume. Chest 3:613-616
47. Brandolese R, Poggi R, Dal Vecchio L, Rossi A (1990) Pharmacological treatment of pulmonary hyperinflation. In: Gullo A (ed) APICE 1990
48. Arora N, Rochester D (1982) Effect of body weight and muscularity on human diaphragm muscle mass, thickness and area. J Appl Physiol 52:64-70
49. Donahoe M, Rogers R, Openbrier D, Wildon D (1989) Effect of calorie intake on muscles strength in malnourished COPD. Am Rev Respir Dis 139:A334
50. Murciano D, Boczkowski J, Milic-Emini J, Pariente R, Aubier M (1988) Tracheal occlusion pressure: a simple index to monitor respiratory muscle fatigue during acute respiratory failure in patients with chronic obstructive pulmonary disease. Ann Intern Med 108:800-805
51. Annat GJ, Viale GP, Dereymez CP et al (1990) Oxygen cost of breathing and diaphragmatic pressure time index. Measurements in patients with COPD during weaning with pressure support ventilation. Chest 98:411-414
52. Fiastro JF, Habib MP, Shon BY, Campbell SC (1988) Comparison of standard weaning parameters and the mechanical work of breathing in mechanically ventilated patients. Chest 94;2:232-238
53. Weisman IH, Rinaldo JE, Rogers RM et al (1983) Intermittent mandatory ventilation. Am Rev Respir Dis 127:641-647

54. Tomlinson JR, Miller KS, Lorch DG et al (1989) A prospective comparison of IMV and T pice weaning from mechanical ventilation. Chest 96:348-352
55. McIntyre NR (1986) Respiratory function during pressure support ventilation. Chest 89: 677-683
56. Brochard L, Harf A, Lorino H, Lemaire F (1989) Inspiratory pressure support prevents diaphragmatic fatigue during weaning from mechanical ventilation. Am Rev Respir Dis 139: 513-521
57. Brochard L, Rua F, Lorino H et al (1991) Inspiratory pressure support compensate for the additional work of breathing caused by endotracheal tube. Anesthesiology 75:739-745
58. Esteban A, Frutos F, Tobin MJ et al (1995) A comparison of four methods of weaning patients from mechanical ventilation. N Engl J Med 332:345-350

Respiratory Support Strategies in AIDS

E. Calderini, I. Salvo, C. Gregoretti, L. Stella

Introduction

The first cases of acquired immunodeficiency syndrome (AIDS) were reported by the Centers for Disease Control (CDC) in 1981 (1). Later on the causative virus was discovered and initially called the human T-lymphotrophic virus type III/lymphadenopathy-associated virus (HTLV III/LAV) by scientists at the Pasteur Institute (2) and the National Institutes of Health (3), respectively, and successively renamed human immunodeficiency virus (HIV). It quickly became evident that the disease was a worldwide problem and that persons outside the originally described risk groups (intravenous drug abusers and male homosexuals) could also be afflicted (4). AIDS consists of a profound immunosuppression, predominantly of cell-mediated immunity, that leads to a variety of opportunistic diseases, particularly certain infections and neoplasms. The main cause of the immune defect in AIDS is a quantitative and qualitative deficiency in the subset of thymus-derived (T) lymphocytes termed the T4 population. These cells are defined phenotypically by the presence of the CD4 surface molecule, which is the cellular receptor for HIV. Virtually any human cell that expresses CD4 receptors can be infected; among them the monocyte-macrophage lineage is of particular importance. Once the T4-lymphocyte count drops to 200 cells/µl or less, the chances of developing an opportunistic infection such as *Pneumocystis carinii* pneumonia are high, and this level of T4 cells is prognostic of a serious clinical complication.

The lung is the principal target organ of the infectious complications of AIDS and why this occurs is not entirely evident. Part of the explanation lies in the fact that lungs are the more frequent portal of entry of many infectious agents. Besides, the lungs may be predisposed to infectious complications because their immunologic capabilities may be even more suppressed than those of other organs. This is probably due to a direct infection of alveolar macrophages with HIV (5) and to a decreased production of soluble factors by lymphocytes (6). The spectrum of pulmonary disorders associated with HIV infection includes both infectious and noninfectious diseases (Table 1).

Table 1. More frequent pulmonary disorders of HIV infection [Modified from Murray and Mills (7)]

Infections
    Viruses
        CMV, EBV, VZV, HSV, HIV
    Bacteria
        Pyogenic organisms
        Mycobacterium tubercolosis, MAC
    Fungi
        Candida species, *Cryptococcus neoformans*, Aspergillus
        Pneumocystis carinii
    Protozoars
        Toxoplasma gondii
Malignancies
    Non-Hodgkin's lymphoma, Kaposi's sarcoma
Interstitial pneumonias

Pneumocystis carinii pneumonia

Pneumocystis carinii pneumonia (PCP) is the most commonly reported serious opportunistic infection in adult patients with AIDS. It is the index diagnosis for 66% of patients and occurs during the course of their illness in more than 80% of patients with AIDS (7). *Pneumocystis carinii* has been classified as both a parasite and a fungus, although the more recent opinion favored its inclusion with fungi (Table 1). *Pneumocystis* is virtually exclusively a pulmonary pathogen and its transmission is predominantly by the airborne route as either small particle aerosols or droplet nuclei. Although most cases of PCP are thought to result from reactivation of latent infection, there are several instances of small outbreaks of infection that could be attributed to airborne transmission of infection (8-11).

The histopathology of *P. carinii* is distinctive. Alveoli are filled with an acellular, eosinophilic, proteinaceous material that contains cysts and trophozoites of the organism with few inflammatory cells within the alveoli. The interstitial spaces contain predominantly mononuclear inflammatory cells.

The pathophysiologic abnormalities are characterized by impaired gas exchange, primarily from ventilation-perfusion mismatching or right-to-left shunts from impaired ventilation of alveoli filled with microorganisms or inflammatory debris. Most patients are hypoxemic and hypocarbic; more severely ill patients may become hypercarbic as respiratory failure worsens, and pulmonary compliance is markedly reduced.

PCP occurs only in immunosuppressed patients with a CD4 lymphocyte count below 200/mm^3 (12).

Diagnosis is usually made by broncho-alveolar lavage with a sensitivity of 86%. Other diagnostic tools are the examination of Gram-stained specimens obtained by sputum induction or, less frequently, the transbronchial biopsy (sensitivity 87%).

In a 3-year period (1991-1994) we admitted in our ICU dedicated to infectious diseases 38 patients with AIDS and respiratory failure due to *P. carinii*. PCP represents in this population more than a half (55%) of the total number of episodes of acute respiratory failure requiring mechanical ventilation. Other causes of respiratory failure were *Staphylococcus a.* (17%), *Pseudomonas a.* (13%) and *Aspergillus f.* (16%). CMV was also detected on 16% of BAL samples, usually associated to other microorganisms.

Patients with a terminal illness who develop respiratory failure are often reluctant to undergo endotracheal intubation and mechanical ventilation, even when respiratory failure is acute, potentially reversible, and not a direct manifestation of the disease. They have an understandable fear of spending their final days attached to a machine that deprives them of autonomy and of the ability to communicate with others. After endotracheal intubation patients are unable to verbalize, and many patients experience pain and discomfort. Not surprisingly, many patients who have been previously intubated often refuse to repeat this experience. Besides, when a patient with AIDS develops acute respiratory failure, the physician may not have a clear understanding of the possible outcome and has the difficult task of assessing the risk vs benefits of an invasive treatment that will affect the patient's quality of life.

Patient and family support in the decision-making may also be difficult to achieve, particularly when ventilatory assistance is urgently needed. Furthermore, patient may become ventilator dependent and the decision to withdraw life support is difficult and has an emotional cost for all those who are involved.

Besides, the high financial cost to the hospital for supporting patients with respiratory failure and mechanical assistance is not fully recovered by the new diagnosis-related regional reimbursment (DRG).

Noninvasive ventilation

The concept of noninvasive mechanical ventilation by full face or nasal mask was initially developed for patients with neuromuscular disease (13) or chronic obstructive lung disease (14) necessitating rest of fatigued respiratory muscles.

More recently several authors applied continuous positive airway pressure (CPAP) to hypoxemic patients with *Pneumocystis carinii* pneumonia. CPAP improves oxygenation by the same mechanism whether delivered by endotracheal tube or mask. Functional residual capacity and lung compliance rise, $\dot{V}/Q$ matching improves, and shunt decreases (15, 16). CPAP reexpands collapsed alveoli by preventing early airway closure and increasing ventilation to areas of low $\dot{V}/Q$.

Gregg et al. (17) applied 5 cmH$_2$O CPAP by face mask to 18 patients with PCP with a mean pre-treatment PaO$_2$/FiO$_2$ = 75. All patients experienced relief of dyspnea, improved PaO$_2$/FiO$_2$ up to 180, and reduced work of breathing within 2 h from the beginning of treatment. Mask CPAP therapy lasted an average of 4.5 days and the authors underlined how all patients were able to speak and cough. Side effects were represented by dry mouth, necrosis of the bridge of the nose (27%) and conjunctivitis (12%). Two patients experienced recurrent gastric distension and one had pneumothorax. ICU mortality in this population was 37% and hospital mortality 55%. The reported mortality for patients with AIDS and PCP requiring intubation and mechanical ventilation in a total of more than 200 patients evaluated in the literature ranges from 84% to 91% (17-23). Gregg et al. concluded that CPAP by mask could identify a less severely ill or more responsive group of patients.

In a study performed in 1991 in conscious and collaborative patients with AIDS and PCP, Miller and Semple (24) demonstrated the efficacy of CPAP ventilation by an improvement of oxygenation and a reduction of respiratory rate and respiratory work. Gachot et al. (25) compared patients with PCP treated with CPAP by mask or with intubation and conventional mechanical ventilation and observed again that CPAP allows identification of a less acutely ill subset of patients, and avoids intubation and mechanical ventilation in many of them (19-25). In 1990 Brochard et al. (26) published a paper in which they demonstrated that pressure support ventilation (PSV) by face mask can obviate the need for conventional mechanical ventilation in patients with acute exacerbations of chronic obstructive pulmonary disease. Inspiratory pressure support is a method of ventilatory assistance designed to deliver a preset level of positive pressure during spontaneous inspiration. The patient's spontaneous inspiratory activity regulates the frequency and duration of inspiratory assistance. During PSV the assistance is cycled according to the inspiratory flow and stops before the flow drops to zero. The authors were able to show that PSV by mask was able to ameliorate gas exchange and to also reduce inspiratory effort evaluated by trans-diaphragmatic pressure time index and diaphragmatic EEG, provided that a tight fitted face mask was used.

The efficacy of this form of ventilation was successively confirmed in both acute and stable COPD patient by others (27-30). A tight mask is a major concern for patients ventilated for several days: facial pressure necrosis at the site of mask contact with ulcers of the bridge of the nose are frequent complications of mask ventilation causing patient discomfort.

We have recently demonstrated (31) that the mask can be loosened to improve comfort without altering the significant respiratory effort reduction and gas exchange improvement usually seen during mask ventilation. This was made possible by using a time-cycled instead of a conventional flow-cycled pressure support ventilation technique. The Siemens Servo Ventilator C permits the modification of the maximum pressurization time during PSV by adjusting the

RR knob. We set RR at 60 to achieve a maximum inspiratory time of 0.8 s corresponding to 80% of a controlled breath. Conventional flow-cycled PSV could not be used in the presence of air leaks because the flow does not drop below the preset expiratory trigger threshold (25% of inspiratory flow with Servo Ventilator). Inspiratory time is prolonged and inspiratory "hang up" and patient-machine asynchronism occur. Table 2 summarizes the results of the study.

Table 2. Data are means ± SE (*$p < .05$ **$p < .01$ vs SB $p < .05$ vs PSVfc)

	ΔPes (cmH$_2$O)	PTPes (cmH$_2$O.s/min)	RR(es-aw) (bpm)	SaO$_2$ (%)	PaO$_2$/FiO$_2$	PaCO$_2$ (mmHg)
SB	16 ± 3	392 ± 63	–	89 ± 3	148 ± 22	30.6 ± 3.4
PSVfc	15 ± 2	342 ± 58	9 ± 2	95 ± 1	–	–
PSVtc	11 ± 2*	230 ± 29**	1 ± 0.6	96 ± 1*	222 ± 39*	30.6 ± 3.3

SB, Spontaneous breathing; PSVfc, flow-cycled PVS; PSVtc, time-cycled PSV; RR(es-aw), difference between respiratory rate calculated on esophageal and airway pressure curve

In conclusion this study demonstrated that respiratory effort reduction and gas exchange improvement can be achieved during mask ventilation with air leaks provided that a time-cycled PSV is used.

Therefore since 1993, mask ventilation represents the first step treatment in the ventilatory management of patients with AIDS and respiratory insufficiency in our department.

In our last (unpublished) trial we considered 11 patients with AIDS and respiratory failure (most PCP) meeting the conventional criteria for intubation and mechanical ventilation (i.e., PaO$_2$/FiO$_2$ = 109 ± 20; RR = 40 bpm; and bilateral diffuse alveolar-interstitial pulmonary infiltrates). In these patients we were able to demonstrate a rapid improvement of oxygenation after mask ventilation with PSV (PaO$_2$/FiO$_2$ = 173 ± 64 at 1 h and 190 ± 70 at 24 h). Three out of 11 patients (27%) avoided tracheal intubation and were successively discharged from the ICU. The remaining eight patients were intubated and five of them died (63%), confirming the high mortality rate of intubated patients with AIDS and severe respiratory insufficiency (more recent reported mortality rate in literature = 89%) (32).

Our results indicate that mask ventilation is safe, well tolerated and able to avoid the need for tracheal intubation in about 30% of treated patients. It can effectively improve gas exchange and possibly prevent respiratory muscle fatigue by decreasing the workload of the respiratory muscles when adequate gas volumes are delivered.

Permissive hypercapnic ventilation

Once mask ventilation has failed and patients have to be intubated because of worsening of respiratory failure, permissive hypercapnic ventilation (PHC) is used as ventilatory treatment of choice in our department.

PHC was first introduced into clinical practice by Hickling et al. in 1990 (33). They suggested that peak inspiratory pressure limitation (PIP < 40 cmH$_2$O) led to a lower hospital mortality rate in 50 patients with ARDS when compared to mortality rate estimated by APACHE II scoring system or by the "ventilator score". Reduction of peak inspiratory pressure was obtained by reducing tidal volume, allowing spontaneous breathing with SIMV and disregarding hypercapnia. They had moved from animal studies which suggested that the use of large tidal volumes and high peak inspiratory pressures during mechanical ventilation resulted in the development of acute lung injury with the production of hyaline membranes and granulocyte infiltration (34, 35).

The following few randomized studies confirmed an improved outcome, even if not with the dramatic reduction described by Hickling (36, 37).

According to Tuxen (38) the ventilatory strategy for PHC can be summarized as follows:

1. PEEP should be titrated to the point of maximal alveolar recruitment as determined by lung mechanics (inflection point on the P-V static curve).
2. After optimal PEEP has been determined, tidal volume should be gradually reduced from 7 ml/kg to as low as 4 ml/kg in order to maintain the plateau pressure (Pplat) < 30 cmH$_2$O.
3. Suggestions about respiratory rate are less clear; some authors recommend mechanical ventilator rates < 30 bpm while Hickling reported intermittent mandatory rates of 14 to 20 bpm.
4. Whichever approach to ventilator rate is chosen, hypercapnia of greater or lesser degree will occur. To counteract hypercapnia one can sedate and cool the patient, reduce CO$_2$ production by paralysis and restriction of glucose intake and give sodium bicarbonate to correct a pH < 7.25.
5. Concerning oxygenation, FiO$_2$ should not exceed 0.6 and mean airway pressures should be elevated accordingly by increasing inspiratory time rather than tidal volume or external PEEP.

Adverse effects of PHC include cerebral vasodilatation, high cardiac output state with maintenance of blood pressure and enhanced hypoxic vasoconstriction with increased pulmonary vascular resistance.

Avoidance of alveolar overdistension through volume or pressure limitation has a significant support based on animal models and deleterious effects of the associated hypercarbia in severe lung injury do not appear to be an important limiting factor in preliminary human clinical trials. At present there are no data on the use of PHC in AIDS patients with PCP or other opportunistic pulmonary infections. However, we believe that the severe prognosis of these patients and the predisposition to develop life-threatening pneumothorax during mechanical ventilation should encourage the use of PHC even without conclusive experimental results.

References

1. Gottlieb MS, Schanker H, Fan P, Saxon A, Weisman JD (1981) Pneumocystis pneumonia-Los Angeles. MMWR 30:250-252
2. Barre-Sinoussi F, Chermann JC, Rey F et al (1983) Isolation of a T-lymphotropic retrovirus from a patient at risk for acquired immune deficiency syndrome (AIDS). Science 220:868-871
3. Popovic M Sarngadharan MD, Read E, Gallo RC (1984) Detection, isolation, and continuous production of cytopatic retroviruses (HTLV-III) from patients with AIDS and pre-AIDS. Science 224:497-500
4. Curran JW, Jaffe HW, Hardy AM, Morgan WM, Selik RM, Dondero TJ (1988) Epidemiology of HIV infection and AIDS in the United States. Science 239:610-616
5. Salahuddin SZ, Rose RM, Groopman JE, Markham PD, Gallo RC (1986) Human T-lymphotrophic virus type III infection of human alveolar macrophages. Blood 68:281-284
6. Beck JM, Shellito J (1989) Effects of human immunodeficiency virus on pulmonary host defenses. Semin Respir Infect 4:75-84
7. Murray JF and Mills J (1990) Pulmonary infectious complications of human immunodeficiency virus infection. Am Rev Respir Dis 141:1356-1372
8. Mills J (1986) Pneumocystis carinii and Toxoplasma gondii infection in patients with AIDS. Rev Infect Dis 8:1001-1010
9. Ruebush TK II, Weinstein RA, Baehner RL et al (1978) An outbreak of Pneumocystis pneumonia in children with acute lymphocytic leukemia. Am J Dis Child 132:143-148
10. Singer C, Armstrong D, Rosen PP, Shottenfeld D (1975) Pneumocystis carinii pneumonia: a cluster of 11 cases. Ann Intern Med 82:772-777
11. Chusid MJ, Heyrman KA (1978) An outbreak of Pneumocystis carinii pneumonia at a pediatric hospital. Pediatrics 62:1031-1035
12. Masur J, Frederick P, Ognibene FP et al (1989) CD4 count as predictors of opportunistic pneumonias in human immunodeficiency virus (HIV) infection. Ann Intern Med 111:223-231
13. Ellis ER, Bye PTP, Bruderer JW, Sullivan CE (1987) Treatment of respiratory failure during sleep in patients with neuromuscolar disease: positive-pressure ventilation through a mask. Am Rev Respir Dis 135:148-152
14. Marino W (1991) Intermittent volume cycled mechanical ventilation via nasal mask in patients with respiratory failure due to COPD. Chest 99:681-684
15. Gregory GA, Kitterman JA, Phibbs RH, Tooley WH, Hamilton WK (1971) Treatment of the idiopathic respiratory distress syndrome with continuous positive airway pressure. N Engl J Med 284:1333-1340
16. Rasanen J, Down JB, DeHaven CB (1987) Titration of continuous positive airway pressure by real time dial oximetry. Chest 92:853-859
17. Gregg RW, Friedman BC, Williams JF, McGrath BJ, Zimmerman JE (1990) Continuous positive airway pressure by face mask in Pneumocystis carinii Pneumonia. Crit Care Med 18:21-24
18. Maxfield RA, Sorkin IB, Fazzini EP, Rapoport DM, Stenson WM (1986) Respiratory failure in patients with acquired immunodeficiency syndrome and Pneumocystis carinii pneumonia. Crit Care Med 14:443-449
19. Wachter RM, Luce JM, Turner J, Volberding P, Hopewell PC (1986) Intensive care of patients with the acquired immunodeficiency syndrome; outcome and changing patterns of utilization. Am Rev Respir Dis 134:891-896
20. Schein RM, Fischl MA, Pitchenik AE, Sprung CL (1986) ICU survival of patients with the acquired immunodeficiency syndrome. Crit Care Med 14:1026-1027

21. Murray JF, Felton CP, Garay SM, Gottlieb MS, Hopewell PC, Stover DE, Tirstein AS (1984) Pulmonary complications of the acquired immunodeficiency syndrome: report of a National Heart, Lung and Blood Institute Workshop. N Engl J Med 310:1682-1688

22. Baumann WR, Jung RC, Koss M et al (1986) Incidence and mortality of adult respiratory distress syndrome: a prospective analysis from a large metropolitan hospital. Crit Care Med 14:1-9

23. Rosen MJ, Cucco RA, Teirstein AS (1986) Outcome of intensive care in patients with the acquired immunodeficiency syndrome. J Intensive Care Med 1:55-60

24. Miller RF and Semple SJG (1991) Continuous positive airway pressure ventilation for respiratory failure associated with Pneumocystis carinii pneumonia. Respir Med 85:133-138

25. Gachot B, Clair B, Wolff M, Regnier B, Vachon F (1992) Continuous positive airway pressure by face mask or mechanical ventilation in patient with human immunodeficiency virus infection and severe Pneumocystis carinii pneumonia. Intensive Care Med 18:155-159

26. Brochard L, Isabey D, Piquet J et al (1990) Reversal of acute exacerbations of chronic obstructive lung disease by inspiratory assistance with a face mask. N Engl J Med 323: 1523-1530

27. Ambrosino N, Nava S, Bertone P, Fracchia C, Rampulla C (1992) Physiologic evaluation of pressure support ventilation by nasal mask in patients with stable COPD. Chest 101:385-391

28. Nava S, Ambrosino N, Rubini F, Fracchia C, Rampulla C, Torri G, Calderini E (1993) Effect of nasal pressure support ventilation and external PEEP on diaphragmatic activity in patients with severe stable COPD. Chest 103:143-150

29. Fernandez R, Blanch LI, Valles J., Baigorri F, Artigas A (1993) Pressure support ventilation via face mask in acute respiratory failure in hypercapnic COPD patients. Intensive Care Med 19:456-461

30. Appendini L, Patessio A, Zanaboni S, Carone M, Gukov B, Donner CF, Rossi A (1994) Physiologic effects of positive end-expiratory pressure and mask pressure support during exacerbations of chronic obstructive pulmonary disease. Am J Respir Crit Care Med 149: 1069-1076

31. Calderini E, Salvo I, Stella L, Puccio PG, Francavilla N, Torri G, Gregoretti C (1995) Flow-cycled vs time-cycled pressure support mask ventilation in AIDS. Am J Respir Crit Care Med 151:A423

32. Hawley PH, Ronco JJ, Guillemi SA et al (1994) Decreasing frequency but worsening mortality of acute respiratory failure secondary to AIDS-related Pneumocystis carinii pneumonia. Chest 106:1456-1459

33. Hickling KG, Henderson SJ, Jackson R (1990) Low mortality associated with low volume pressure limited ventilation with permissive hypercapnia in severe adult respiratory distress syndrome. Intensive Care Med 16:372-377

34. Webb HH, Tiemey DF (1974) Experimental pulmonary edema due to intermittent positive pressure ventilation with high inflation pressures: protection by positive end-expiratory pressure. Am Rev Respir Dis 110:556-565

35. Dreyfuss D, Saumon G (1991) Lung overinflation: physiologic and anatomic alterations leading to pulmonary edema. In: Zapol W, Lemaire F (eds) Adult respiratory distress syndrome, 2nd edn. Dekker, New York (Lung biology in health and disease, vol 50), pp 433-450

36. Amati MBP, Barbas CSV, Medeiros DM, Deheinzelin D, Kalralla R, Carvalho CRR (1993) Improved lung mechanics and oxygenation achieved through a new approach to mechanical ventilation in ARDS: the importance of reducing the "mechanical stress" on the lung. Am Rev Respir Dis 147:A890

37. Lee PC, Helmoortel CM, Cohn SM, Fink MP (1990) Are low tidal volumes safe? Chest 97:425-429

38. Tuxen DV (1994) Permissive hypercapnic ventilation. Am J Respir Crit Care Med 150: 870-874

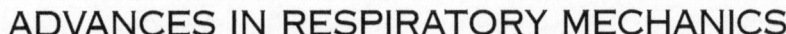

ADVANCES IN RESPIRATORY MECHANICS

Mathematical Models in Respiratory Mechanics

W.A. ZIN, R.F.M. GOMES

The respiratory system, as well as its pulmonary and chest wall components, is comprised of a multitude of elements. The undisputed necessity to interpret the meaning of measurable variables such as volume, airflow, and pressure under both physiological and pathological conditions has imposed the need for relatively simple models that should be able to describe as accurately as possible the mechanical behaviour of the system. The components of such models and their associated parameters should have reasonable physiological counterparts, naturally.

One-compartment model

The simplest model of the respiratory system, which is still the most commonly used, incorporates two lumped elements: one resistance (associated with the pipe) and one elastance (balloon), as depicted in Fig. 1A. The "equation of motion of the respiratory system" describes its behaviour:

$$P(t) = R\dot{V}(t) + EV(t) \qquad [1]$$

where P is the driving pressure, R is the resistance of the pipe to airflow ($\dot{V}$), E is the balloon elastance, V represents the change in volume of the balloon above its relaxed configuration, and t is time. This single-compartment linear model assumes that R and E are independent of $\dot{V}$ and V, respectively, and that inertial forces are negligible. The latter postulate is probably acceptable within the physiological breathing frequencies up to 2 Hz (1).

The electrical analogue of the linear one-compartment model (Fig. 1B) associates an ohmic resistance to a capacitance of magnitude 1/E, which are subjected to the same flow.

From the mechanical point of view (Fig. 1C), the deformation (i.e., volume V) results from the movement of a Voigt body (one dashpot and a spring arranged in parallel constitute a Voigt body).

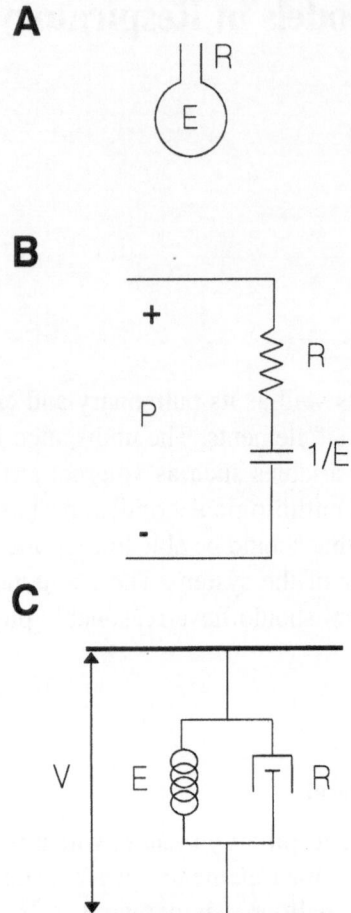

Fig. 1A-C. Linear one-compartment model. **A** anatomic representation. **B** Electrical representation. **C** Rheological representation by a Voigt body

The values for R and E can be determined during continuous breathing by fitting Eq. 1 to P, $\dot{V}$, and V using multiple linear regression (2, 3) or the electrical subtraction method (4). Alternatively, R and E can be obtained during relaxed expiration (5).

Although attractive, the linear single-compartment model cannot explain certain mechanical phenomena presented by the respiratory system, such as: (1) the slow decay in pressure observed after an end-inspiratory occlusion (6-8); (2) the double-exponential profile of expiration sometimes found in animals and humans (9, 10); (3) the frequency dependence of resistance and elastance in the range of 0 to 2 Hz (3, 11-14); and (4) the quasi-static pressure-volume hysteresis in isolated lungs. Therefore, in order to better describe the respiratory system mechanical behaviour more complex models are required.

Two-compartment models

Linear two-compartment models increase the mechanical degrees of freedom of the system, and explain frequency dependence of respiratory parameters, stress adaptation, and the two-exponential decay of expired volume under relaxed conditions. They are divided into two main types: gas redistribution and rheologic models.

Gas redistribution models

These models describe the mechanical properties of the respiratory system based on inhomogeneities of gas distribution within the lungs. In this context, they can be divided into two sub-types: parallel and series redistribution.

The parallel gas redistribution model (15) consists of two alveolar compartments with elastances E_1 and E_2 served by parallel airways with fixed resistances R_1 and R_2 (Fig. 2A). Additionally, a resistance common to the two compartments can be added to the model, to represent central airways resistance (16). Electrically, the model is made up of two serially arranged RC elements organized in parallel (Fig. 2B). Mechanically (Fig. 2C), the model serially associates two Voigt bodies characterized by their respective springs (E_1 and E_2) and dashpots (R_1 and R_2). The total deformation (i.e. volume V) is the sum of each of their respective deformations. This model associates stress adaptation to parallel Pendelluft, which consists of alveolar pressure equilibrium during airflow interruption, and depends on the difference between the two peripheral time constants ($\tau = R/E$), and on volume history.

In the serial gas redistribution model (17), homogeneous lungs (represented by an alveolar compartment with elastance E_2 and distal airways with resistance R_2) are served by central airways with an elastance E_1 and a resistance R_1 (Fig. 3A). The electrical analogue of this model (Fig. 3B) is comprised of a resistance R_1 in series with R_2 and E_2, which, in turn, are in parallel with a capacitance 1/E. This capacitance behaves as a buffer between alveolar and driving pressures. Hence, a given fraction of the inspired volume remains in the central airways, depending on central and peripheral time constants (τ_1 and τ_2, respectively), thus decreasing the volume available for gas exchange. The mechanical representation of the model (Fig. 3C) is obtained by substituting mechanical elements in series for electrical ones in parallel (and those in parallel for electrical ones in series), since mechanical bodies in parallel undergo the same deformation rate and are submitted to an identical pressure when arranged in series. This kind of model is particularly useful in the interpretation of pathological conditions, such as chronic obstructive pulmonary disease. When elastic and resistive data of normal individuals are considered, the serial gas distribution model cannot explain frequency dependence of resistance and elastance in the normal range of breathing frequencies. However, when the peripheral resitance R_2 increases, the model confers a time dependence to R and E compatible with the real behaviour of COPD lungs. Finally, there are alternative anatomical interpretations for E_1, such as that it would be associated with either an alveolar gas compliance or a lung region with negligible resistance (18, 19). However, the original association of E1 with central airways elastance still prevails (18, 20).

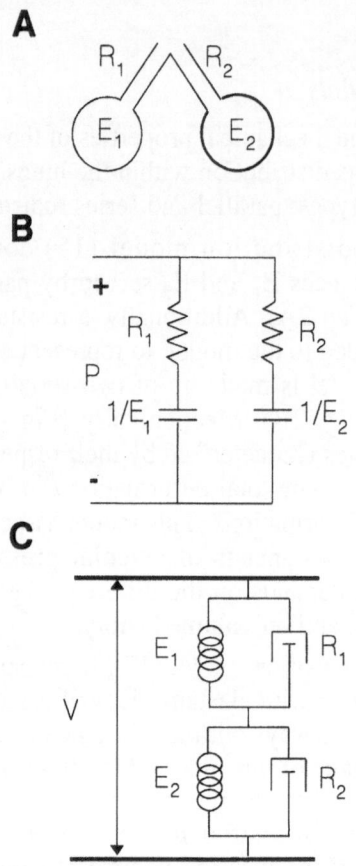

Fig. 2A-C. Linear parallel two-compartment gas redistribution model. **A** Anatomic representation. **B** Electrical representation. **C** Rheological representation by two Voigt bodies (R_1, E_1 and R_2, E_2) associated in series

As also displayed by the parallel two-compartment model, there is gas redistribution between the compartments after flow interruption. In fact, the behaviour of both models may be identical, depending on the values chosen for the four parametres, since they are described by the same differential equation (21):

$$P(t) + a\dot{P}(t) = bV(t) + c\dot{V}(t) + d\ddot{V}(t) \qquad [2]$$

where $\dot{P}(t)$ is the first time derivative of $P(t)$ and $\ddot{V}(t)$ corresponds to second time derivative of $V(t)$.

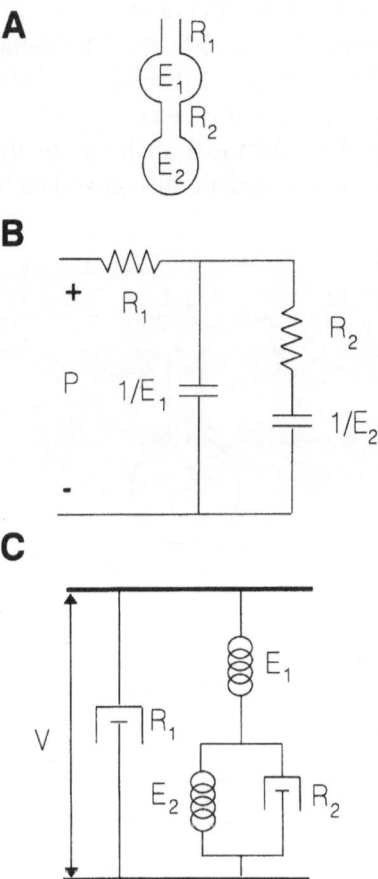

Fig. 3A-C. Linear serial two-compartment gas redistribution model. **A** Anatomic representation. **B** Electrical representation. **C** Rheological representation by a dashpot (R_1) associated in parallel with a spring (E_1) serially coupled with a Voigt body (R_2, E_2)

Rheological models

The rheological models do not assume the existence of an uneven distribution of ventilation. Supporting this notion no inhomogeneity of gas distribution could be detected under normal conditions (22, 23). In fact, the rheological models extend the one-compartment model by incorporating a viscoelastic (24, 25) or plastoelastic (26, 27) element in parallel with the Voigt body depicted in Fig. 1C.

In the viscoelastic model of the respiratory system (24, 25, 28) stress adaptation originates from lung/chest wall tissues and/or surfactant viscoelastic properties (R_2 and E_2, Fig. 4C). A Kelvin body, which is made up of a Maxwell body (R_2, E_2) in parallel with E_1, represents the viscoelasticity in Fig. 4A. The Maxwell body associated in parallel with a Voigt body (R_1, E_1) constitute the mechanical viscoelastic model of the lung. E_1 represents static elastance, and, according to recent experiments involving alveolar capsules, R_1 corresponds to airway resistance in normal animals (22, 23). The deformation of the Maxwell body is the sum of the deformations of its resistive and elastic elements, and its slow time constant ($\tau_2 = R_2/E_2$) might be responsible for the tissue stress adaptation phenomenon. The electrical analogue of the viscoelastic model is depicted in Fig. 4B. Finally, this model is also governed by a differential equation like Eq. 2.

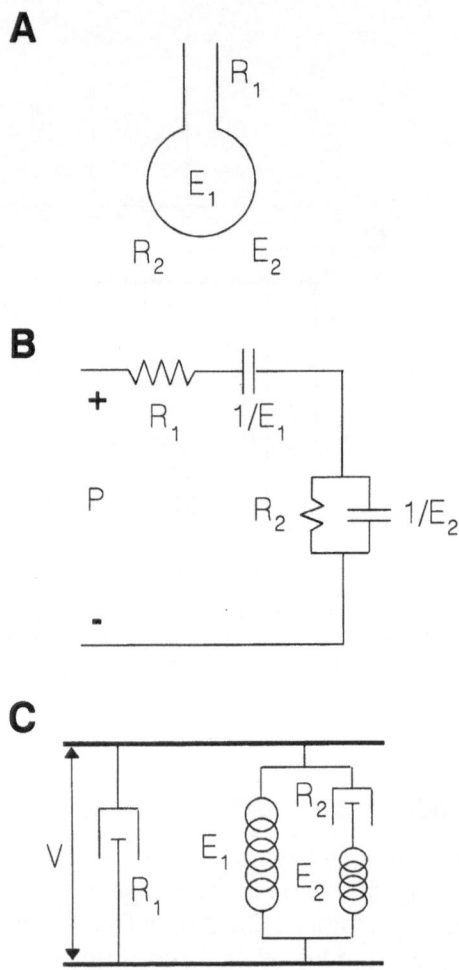

Fig. 4A-C. Linear viscoelastic two-compartment model. **A** Anatomic representation. **B** Electrical representation. **C** Rheological representation by a dashpot (R_1) associated in parallel with a spring (E_1) coupled in parallel with a Maxwell body (R_2, E_2)

The plastoelastic model differs from the viscoelastic one by the substitution of a dry friction (Coulomb) element for the viscous element (R_2) in the Maxwell body, thus forming the Prandtl body (29). The Coulomb element will only start moving after a pressure threshold has been reached. Henceforth, energy is continuously dissipated independently of the rate of displacement. This model could account for the quasi-static pressure volume hysteresis in isolated lungs. However, the plastoelastic model is rarely used in vivo under small volume excursions, where its parameter values have sometimes been found difficult to be interpreted mechanically (30, 31).

Multi-compartment models

An attempt to more accurately describe a set of experimental data can be performed by means of multi-compartment models. Hence, a varying number of Voigt, Kelvin, or Maxwell bodies could be added in parallel to the aforementioned models. In this line, a model has been proposed in which *P(t)* decreases linearly as a function of the logarithm of the time subsequent to a step change in volume (*V*), according to the equation (26, 32, 33):

$$P(t)/V = A - B \times \ln t \qquad [3]$$

Naturally, the existence of a multitude of time constants is implicit in this particular model. Nevertheless, the multi-compartment models yield a great deal of parameters, whose direct assigment to mechanical elements is unwarranted.

Nonlinear models

Another way of increasing the complexity of the mechanical models of the respiratory system is to make the existing elements nonlinear. The simplest one consists in adding a flow-dependent (turbulent) term to the parameter representing airway resistance:

$$P(t) = K_1\dot{V}(t) + K_2\dot{V}(t)^2 + EV(t) \qquad [4]$$

where K_1 and K_2 are Rohrer's constants (34).

A nonlinear viscoelastic model, where both tissue resistance and elastance depend upon squared breathing frequency, is capable of quantitatively accounting for the known amplitude and frequency-dependent properties of lung tissue (35). The nonlinear viscoelastic model can be used instead of a plastoelastic one (26), also able to explain the same phenomena.

Another nonlinear model states that the decay of *P(t)* after the volume increment V can be represented by:

$$P(t)/V = A \times t\text{-}k^{-k} \qquad [5]$$

where *A* and *k* are constants (36, 37). Conversely, it can be concluded that tissue and lung impedances are inversely related to a given power of the breathing frequency.

Studies dealing with nonlinearities have provided interesting conclusions. It has been demonstrated that even an extremely inhomogeneous lung structure can produce virtually homogeneous mechanical behaviour (36). Furthermore, because of nonlinearities, it is feasible to measure respiratory system and pulmonary impedances during conventional mechanical ventilation only at and above normal breathing frequency (38).

Choosing the appropriate model

Naturally, the choice of the model to be used will depend upon the intended physiological or pathophysiological goal. In other words, the most adequate model is that one whose elements closely reproduce the actual system under study (21, 38). Thence, it is virtually impossible to use a "perfect" model. However, the use of simple models that satisfactorily represent the general mechanical behaviour of the respiratory system and its lung and chest wall components is of paramount importance to the respirologist.

The models are to be chosen according to the scientific questioning, techniques and methods to be used, and, of course, the experimental condition. Furthermore, the easy gathering of the parameters of a given model should never thwart the quest for the most appropriate physiological interpretation of the data.

References

1. Sharp JT, Henry JP, Sweany SK, Meadows WR, Pietras RJ (1964) Total respiratory inertance and its gas and tissue components in normal and obese men. J Appl Physiol 43:503-509
2. Hantos Z, Daróczy B, Klebniczki J, Dombos K, Nagy S (1982) Parameter estimation of transpulmonary mechanics by a nonlinear inertive model. J Appl Physiol 52:955-963
3. Bates JHT, Shardonofsky F, Stewart DE (1989) The low-frequency dependence of respiratory system resistance and elastance in normal dogs. Respir Physiol 78:369-382
4. Mead J, Whittenberger JL (1953) Physical properties of human lungs measured during spontaneous respiration. J Appl Physiol 5:779-796
5. Zin WA, Pengelly LD, Milic-Emili J (1982) Single-breath method for measurement of respiratory mechanics in anesthetized animals. J Appl Physiol 52:1266-1271
6. Hughes R, May AJ, Widdicombe JG (1959) Stress relaxation in rabbits' lungs. J Physiol (Lond) 146:85-97

7. Don HF, Robson JG (1965) The mechanics of the respiratory system during anesthesia. Anesthesiol 26:168-178
8. Bates JHT, Rossi A, Milic-Emili J (1985) Analysis of the behavior of the respiratory system with constant inspiratory flow. J Appl Physiol 58:1840-1848
9. Bates JHT, Decramer M, Chartrand D, Zin WA, Böddener A, Milic-Emili J (1985) The volume-time profile during relaxed expiration in the normal dog. J Appl Physiol 59:732-737
10. Chelucci GL, Brunet F, Dall'Ava-Santucci J, Dhainaut JF, Paccaly D, Armaganidis A, Milic-Emili J, Lockhart A (1991) A single-compartment model cannot describe passive expiration in intubated, paralysed humans. Eur Respir J 4:458-464
11. Barnas GM, Yoshino K, Loring SH, Mead J (1987) Impedance and relative displacements of relaxed chest wall up to 4 Hz. J Appl Physiol 62:71-81
12. Brusasco V, Warner DO, Beck KC, Rodarte JR, Rehder K (1989) Partitioning of pulmonary resistance in dogs: effects of tidal volume and frequency. J Appl Physiol 66:1190-1197
13. Hantos Z, Daróczy B, Suki B, Galgoczy G, Csendes T (1986) Forced oscillatory impedance of the respiratory system at low frequencies. J Appl Physiol 60:123-132
14. Hantos Z, Daróczy B, Suki B, Nagy S (1987) Low-frequency respiratory mechanical impedance in the rat. J Appl Physiol 63:36-43
15. Otis AB, McKerrow CB, Bartlett RA, Mead J, McIlroy MB, Selverstone NJ, Radford EP (1956) Mechanical factors in the distribution of pulmonary ventilation. J Appl Physiol 8: 427-444
16. Bates JHT, Baconnier P, Milic-Emili J (1988) A theoretical analysis of interrupter technique for measuring respiratory mechanics. J Appl Physiol 64:2204-2214
17. Mead J (1969) Contribution of compliance of airways to frequency-dependent behavior of lungs. J Appl Physiol 26:670-673
18. Eyles JG, Pimmel RL (1981) Estimating respiratory mechanical parameters in parallel compartment models. IEEE Trans Biomed Eng 28:313-317
19. Peslin R (1986) Methods for measuring total respiratory impedance by forced oscillations. Bull Eur Physiopathol Respir 22:621-631
20. Michaelson ED, Grassman ED, Peters WR (1975) Pulmonary mechanics by spectral analysis of forced random noise. J Clin Invest 56:1210-1230
21. Lorino AM, Lorino H, Harf A (1994) A synthesis of the Otis, Mead, and Mount mechanical respiratory models. Respir Physiol 97:123-133
22. Bates JHT, Ludwig MS, Sly PD, Brown K, Martin JG, Fredberg JJ (1988) Interrupter resistance elucidated by alveolar pressure measurement in open-chest normal dogs. J Appl Physiol 65:408-414
23. Saldiva PHN, Zin WA, Santos RLB, Eidelman DH, Milic-Emili J (1992) Alveolar pressure measurement in open-chest rats. J Appl Physiol 72:302-306
24. Mount LE (1955) The ventilation flow-resistance and compliance of rat lungs. J Physiol (Lond) 127:157-167
25. Bates JHT, Brown KA, Kochi T (1989) Respiratory mechanics in the normal dog determined by expiratory flow interruption. J Appl Physiol 67:2276-2285
26. Hildebrandt J (1970) Pressure-volume data of cat lung interpreted by a plastoelastic, linear viscoelastic model. J Appl Physiol 28:365-372
27. Fredberg JJ, Stamenovic D (1989) On the imperfect elasticity of lung tissue. J Appl Physiol 67:2408-2419
28. Sharp JT, Johnson FN, Goldberg NB, van Lith P (1967) Hysteresis and stress adaptation in the human respiratory system. J Appl Physiol 23:487-497
29. Similowski T, Bates JHT (1991) Two-compartment modelling of respiratory system mechanics at low frequencies: gas redistribution of tissue rheology? Eur Respir J 4:353-358
30. Navajas D, Farré R, Cannet J, Roger M, Sanchis J (1990) Respiratory input impedance in anesthetized paralyzed patients. J Appl Physiol 69:1372-1379
31. Shardonofsky F, Sato J, Bates JHT (1990) Quasi-static pressure-volume hysteresis in the canine respiratory system in vivo. J Appl Physiol 68:2230-2236

32. Hildebrandt J (1969) Dynamic properties of air-filled excised cat lung determined by liquid plethysmography. J Appl Physiol 27:246-250
33. Hildebrandt J (1969) Comparison of mathematical models for cat lung and viscoelastic balloon derived by Laplace transform methods from pressure-volume data. Bull Math Biophys 31:651-667
34. Rohrer F (1915) Der Strömungswiderstand in den menschlichen Atemwegen und der Einfluss der unregelmässigen Verzweigung des Bronchialsystems auf den Atmungsverlauf in verschiedenen Lungenbezirken. Arch Ges Physiol 162:225-300
35. Suki B, Bates JHT (1991) A nonlinear viscoelastic model of lung tissue mechanics. J Appl Physiol 71:826-833
36. Hantos Z, Daróczy B, Suki B, Nagy S, Fredberg JJ (1992) Input impedance and peripheral inhomogeneity of dog lungs. J Appl Physiol 72:168-178
37. Lutchen KR, Suki B, Zhang Q, Peták F, Caróczy B, Hantos Z (1994) Airway and tissue mechanics during physiological breathing and bronchoconstriction in dogs. J Appl Physiol 77:373-385
38. Rotger M, Peslin R, Navajas D, Farré R (1995) Lung and respiratory impedance at low frequency during mechanical ventilation in rabbits. J Appl Physiol 78:2153-2160.

Evolution of Theories and Interpretation of Respiratory Mechanics Data

J. MILIC-EMILI

Single compartment models

The simplest mechanical model of the respiratory system was introduced in 1950 by Otis et al. (1). It consists of a single compartment of constant elastance (E) served by a pathway of constant flow resistance (R). It is based on the assumption that the mechanical properties of the respiratory system are independent of lung volume and flow, and that inertial factors are negligible. These are reasonable assumptions for normal resting breathing, and even the gross overimplification of a single compartment has been useful for making qualitative predictions (2). This mechanical model can be represented by a single first order differential equation:

$$P(t) = EV(t) + R\dot{V}(t) \tag{1}$$

where at any instant t, $P(t)$ is the driving pressure which produces volumes displacement $V(t)$ from the resting end-expiratory level and instantaneous flow $\dot{V}(t)$. However, E and R are not constant but vary with $\dot{V}$ and V.

Volume-dependence of E and R. The S-shaped nature of the static volume-pressure relationship of the relaxed respiratory system was described long ago by Rahn et al. (3). The fact that airway resistance decreases with increasing lung volume was shown by Briscoe and Dubois in 1958 (4).

Flow-dependence of R. Rohrer was the first to estimate Raw (5). Lacking a method for direct measurement of the resistance offered by gas flowing through the airways (Raw) he undertook the formidable task of estimating it by applying the laws governing the flow of gas through tubes to postmortem measurements of the dimension of the airways. Based on these estimates he described the following relationships, which are known as Rohrer's equations:

$$Pres = K_1\dot{V} + K_2\dot{V}^2 \tag{2}$$

and

$$Raw = K_1 + K_2\dot{V} \tag{3}$$

where *Pres* represents the pressure dissipations within the airways owing to gas flow ($\dot{V}$), and K_1 and K_2 are constants. Equation 3 is obtained by dividing both sides of Eq. 2 by $\dot{V}$. Although the specific physical connotations assigned by Rohrer to his constants are no longer accepted, Eqs. 2 and 3 are still used because they provide a close empirical description of experimental results (6). The tissues of the chest wall (w) exhibit ohmic (Newtonian) behaviour, which can be quantified in terms of a fixed resistance (Rint,w) (7). If this is added to Eq. 3, the total resistance of the respiratory system is obtained (*Rrs*):

$$Rrs = Rint,w + K_1 + K_2\dot{V} \tag{4}$$

In this connection it should be noted that the tissues of the lung do not offer any appreciable ohmic resistance (8). Until recently, Eq. 4 was one of the tenets of respiratory mechanics, namely that in normal subjects, at a given lung volume, Rrs should increase with $\dot{V}$. Another basic tenet was that, at a given flow, Rrs should decrease with increasing lung volume because of a decrease in both Raw (4) and Rint,w (9).

The model of Otis et al. (1) also predicted that in normal subjects both E and R should not vary with the frequency of breathing (10). This, however, is not true both in normal subjects and patients with lung disease.

Viscoelastic model

In 1955 Mount measured the dynamic work per breath on the lung (Wdyn,L) in open-chest rats, using sinusoidal variations in lung volume (11). To explain the relatively high values of Wdyn,L at the lower frequencies and the progressive decrease in dynamic pulmonary compliance with increasing frequency, he proposed a four-parameter viscoelastic model of the lung that "confers time dependency of the elastic properties". Until the 1970s, his model was largely ignored. Since then, however, it has been recognized that the viscoelastic properties of the respiratory system play a substantial role in respiratory dynamics.

The lungs and chest wall comprise a large number of elements. This complexity, coupled with the necessity to explain respiratory dynamics under physiological and pathological conditions, has generated the need for relatively simple models that can mimic the mechanical behaviour of the respiratory system. From the pioneering work of Mount (11), Bates and associates (12) have proposed the eight-parameter spring-and-dashpot model of the respiratory system shown in Fig. 1. The model consists of two submodels, the lungs and chest wall, which are arranged mechanically in parallel because they both undergo the same volume changes. The lung submodel consists of a dashpot representing Raw (= Rint,L) arranged in parallel with a Kelvin body, which consists of a spring representing static elastance (Est,L), in parallel with a Maxwell body, that is a spring (E_2,L) and a dashpot (R_2,L) arranged serially. The latter, together with the corresponding time constant (τ_2,L = R_2,L/E_2,L), accounts

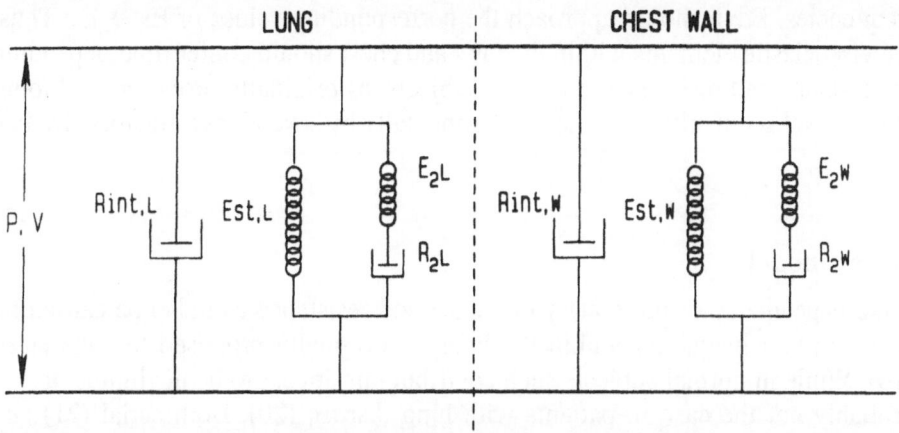

Fig. 1. The eight-parameter spring-and-dashpot viscoelastic model for interpretation of respiratory mechanics. Respiratory system consists of interrupter resistance of lung (*Rint,L*, airway resistance) and chest wall (*Rint,w*) in parallel with (1) *Est,L* and *Est,w* and (2) series spring-and-dashpot bodies (E_2 and R_2, respectively) of lung and chest wall that represent viscoelastic (*stress adaptation*) units. The distance between the *two bars* is analogous to lung volume (*V*), and tension between the bars is analogous to pressure applied to the respiratory system (*P*)

for the viscoelastic properties of the lung. Similarly, the chest wall comprises a resistance (Rint,w) and a Kelvin body consisting of static chest wall elastance (Est,w) and corresponding viscoelastic parameters (E_2,w and R_2,w, τ_2,w). It should be stressed (1) that currently the precise structural basis of the viscoelastic parameters in Fig. 1 is poorly understood, and (13) that the model is clearly too simplistic to be a true representation of the respiratory system.

More complex models have been proposed (14, 15). Nonetheless, the model in Fig. 1 is useful because it mimics and explains several aspects of respiratory dynamics. Also, the viscoelastic units might be functionally important to the extent that they would tend to smooth stress distribution within the thoracic tissues, thereby minimizing local distortions during sudden displacements and reduce regional differences in ventilation distribution caused by time constant inequality.

As a result of viscoelastic pressure dissipations, the effective resistance of the respiratory system (Rrs,eff) is higher than that described by Eq. 4, particularly at low respiratory frequencies (f). By contrast, at high f, Rrs,eff should approximate Rrs in Eq. 4. Indeed, at high respiratory frequencies (f), the springs E_2 in Fig. 1 will oscillate so fast that there will be insufficient time for their tension to be dissipated through the dashpots R_2. By contrast, at low frequencies, the dashpots R_2 are given time to move and dissipate the elastic energy stored in E_2. In the limit, as frequency tends to zero, the springs E_2 should remain at fixed length (i.e., resting length at which tension is zero). This implies that the dynamic lung and chest wall elastances (Edyn) should increase with increasing f. At high frequencies, Edyn should approach the corresponding values of Est + E_2. Thus, the viscoelastic elements within the lung and chest should confer time-depending of elastance and resistance in normal subjects, as originally proposed by Mount (11) and subsequently confirmed experimentally by several investigators (16-19).

Other models

Time dependency of pulmonary elastance and resistance can also be caused by time-constant inequality within the lung, as originally proposed by Otis et al. (10). While in normal subjects such contributions appear to be negligible, this is probably not the case in patients with lung disease (20). Both serial (21) and parallel (10) models of time-constant inequality have been proposed. Until now it has been virtually impossible to separate these effects from those due to viscoelastic behaviour (22).

Implications of viscoelastic behaviour on expiratory flow

Although the dynamic work attributable to airway resistance represents energy that is dissipated as heat, part of the elastic energy stored during inspiration in springs E_2 in Fig. 1 can be recovered during expiration to overcome expiratory airway resistance. Indeed, at f > 0.5 Hz, virtually all of the elastic energy stored in springs E_2 during inspiration should be available as expiratory-driving pressure. Thus, during increased ventilation (e.g., muscular exercise), some of the requirements for increased expiratory flow rates are intrinsically met by the increase in Edyn,L and Edyn,w because of the higher frequencies. Since the elastic energy stored in the lung and chest wall is greater with rapid than with slow inspirations, lung deflation should be faster following rapid inflation. Augmentation of the expiratory-driving pressure through a viscoelastic mechanism was originally described by Mortola et al. (23), who found that passive lung deflation was slower if the expiration was preceded by an end-inspiratory hold. This phenomenon has been confirmed in several subsequent studies (20, 24). Viscoelastic mechanisms have important effects both on relaxed expiration and on forced expiratory maneuvers.

Relaxed expiration. Based on the simple model of Otis et al. (1), Brody (25) theorized that the time course of volume (V) during passive expiration should be described by a single exponential function:

$$V(t) = Vo \cdot e^{-t/\tau_{rs}} \qquad [5]$$

where t is time and Vo is initial volume above the relaxation volume of the respiratory system. Equation 5 is the kernel of various methods for measurement of respiratory mechanics, such as that based on the addition of known expiratory resistances (26) and the "single-breath method" of Zin et al. (27). However, Bates et al. (13) have shown that, in anaesthetized, paralysed dogs, the time course of volume during passive expiration following inflation with a 5-s breathhold can better be described in terms of a double-exponential function:

$$V(t) = A \cdot e^{-t/\tau'} + B \cdot e^{-t/\tau''} \qquad [6]$$

This behaviour, which was attributed to viscoelastic mechanisms, has also been observed in normal, anaesthetized, paralysed humans (28).

Forced expiration. Figure 1 implies that, under dynamic conditions, the effective elastic recoil pressure of the lung can exceed the static elastic pressure as a result of the additional elastic pressure (PL) stored in spring E_2,L. Therefore, the maximal flows during forced expiration should be greater when the manoeuvre is performed following a rapid lung inflation (with a concomitant increase in ΔPL) and without an end-inspiratory pause (to avoid dissipation of this energy into dashpot R_2,L) than after a slow inflation or forced expiration preceded by an end-inspiratory pause. This hypothesis has been recently confirmed in experiments on both normal subjects (29) and COPD patients (30).

References

1. Otis AB, Fenn WO, Rahn H (1950) The mechanics of breathing in man. J Appl Physiol 2: 592-607
2. Mead J (1960) Control of respiratory frequency. J Appl Physiol 15:325-336
3. Rahn H, Otis AB, Chadwick LE, Fenn WO (1946) The pressure-volume diagram of the thorax and lung. Am J Physiol 146:161-178
4. Briscoe WA, DuBois AB (1958) The relationship between airway resistance, airway conductance and lung volume in subjects of different age and body size. J Clin Invest 37: 1279-1285
5. Rohrer F (1915) Der Strömungswiderstand in den menschlichen Atemwegen und der Einfluss der unregelmässigen Verzweigung des Bronchialsystems auf des Atmungsverlauf verschiedenen Lungenbezirken. Arch Gesamte Physiol Mens Tiere 162:225-299
6. Mead J, Agostoni E (1964) Dynamics of breathing. In: Fenn WO, Rahn H (eds) Respiration, vol. 1. Washington, DC, American Physiological Society, pp 411-427. Handbook of physiology, Section 3
7. D'Angelo E, Prandi E, Tavola M, Calderini E, Milic-Emili J (1994) Chest wall interrupter resistance in anesthetized paralyzed subjects. J Appl Physiol 77:883-887
8. Bates JHT, Ludwig MS, Sly PD, Brown K, Martin JG, Fredberg JJ (1988) Interrupter resistance elucidated by alveolar pressure measurement in open-chest normal dogs. J Appl Physiol 65:408-414
9. Grimby G, Takishima T, Graham W, Macklem P, Mead J (1968) Frequency dependence of flow resistance in patients with obstructive lung disease. J Clin Invest 47:1455-1465
10. Otis AB, McKerrow CB, Bartlett RA, Mead J, McIlroy MB, Selverstone NJ, Radford EP (1956) Mechanical factors in distribution of pulmonary ventilation. J Appl Physiol 8:427-443
11. Mount LE (1955) The ventilation flow-resistance and compliance of rat lungs. J Physiol (Lond) 127:157-167

12. Bates JHT, Brown K, Kochi T (1987) Identifying a model of respiratory mechanics using the interrupter technique. In: Proceedings of the Ninth American Conference I.E.E.E. Engineering Medical Biology Society, pp 1802-1803

13. Bates JHT, Decramer M, Chartrand D, Zin WA, Boddener A, Milic-Emili J (1985) Volume-time profile during relaxed expiration in the normal dog. J Appl Physiol 59:732-737

14. Fredberg JJ, Stamenovic D (1989) On the imperfect elasticity of lung tissue. J Appl Physiol 67:2408-2419

15. Hildebrandt J (1970) Pressure-volume data of cat lung interpreted by a plastoelastic linear viscoelastic model. J Appl Physiol 28:365-372

16. Barnas GM, Yoshiro K, Loring STL, Mead J (1987) Impedance and relative displacements of relaxed chest wall up to 4 Hz. J Appl Physiol 62:71-81

17. D'Angelo E, Calderini E, Torri G, Robatto F, Bono D, Milic-Emili J (1989) Respiratory mechanics in anesthetized-paralyzed humans: effects of flow, volume and time. J Appl Physiol 67:2556-2564

18. D'Angelo E, Robatto FM, Calderini E, Tavola M, Bono D, Torri G, Milic-Emili J (1991) Pulmonary and chest wall mechanics in anesthetized paralyzed humans. J Appl Physiol 70: 2602-2610

19. Hantos Z, Daroczy B, Suki B, Galgoczy G, Csendes T (1986) Forced oscillatory impedance of the respiratory system at low frequencies. J Appl Physiol 60:123-132

20. Eissa NT, Ranieri VM, Corbeil C, Chassé M, Robatto FM, Braidy J, Milic-Emili J (1991) Analysis of behavior of the respiratory system in ARDS patients: effects of flow, volume, and time. J Appl Physiol 70:2719-2729

21. Mead J (1969) Contribution of compliance of airways to frequency-dependent behaviour of lung. J Appl Physiol 26:670-673

22. Bates JHT, Baconnier P, Milic-Emili J (1988) A theoretical analysis of interrupter technique for measuring respiratory mechanics. J Appl Physiol 64:2204-2214

23. Mortola JP, Magnante D, Saetta M (1985) Expiratory pattern of newborn mammals. J Appl Physiol 58:528-533

24. Guérin C, Coussa M-L, Eissa NT, Corbeil C, Chassé M, Braidy J, Matar N, Milic-Emili J (1993) Lung and chest wall mechanics in mechanically ventilated COPD patients. J Appl Physiol 74:1570-1580

25. Brody AW (1954) Mechanical compliance and resistance of the lung-thorax calculated from the flow recorded during passive expiration. Am J Physiol 178:189-196

26. McIlroy MB, Tierney DF, Nadel JA (1963) A new method of measurement of compliance and resistance of lungs and thorax. J Appl Physiol 18:424-427

27. Zin WA, Pengelly LD, Milic-Emili J (1982) Single-breath method for measurement of respiratory system mechanics in anesthetized animals. J Appl Physiol 52:1266-1271

28. Chelucci GL, Brunet F, Dall'Ava-Santucci J, Dhainaut JF, Paccaly D, Armaganidis A, Milic-Emili J, Lockhart A (1991) A single-compartment model cannot describe passive expiration in intubated, paralyzed humans. Eur Respir J 4:458-464

29. D'Angelo E, Prandi E, Milic-Emili J (1993) Dependence of maximal flow-volume curves on time-course of preceding inspiration. J Appl Physiol 75:1155-1159

30. D'Angelo E, Prandi E, Marazzini L, Milic-Emili J (1994) Dependence of maximal flow-volume curves on time course of preceding inspiration in patients with chronic obstructive pulmonary disease. Am J Respir Crit Care Med 150:1581-1586

Assessment of the Viscoelastic Constants Using the Rapid Airway Occlusion Technique

V. Antonaglia, F. Beltrame, U. Lucangelo, A. Grop

During mechanical ventilation, the technique of rapid airway occlusion (RAO) during constant flow inflation (1-4) and the "single-breath" method (5-9) are probably the most commonly employed for measuring the respiratory mechanics.

The latter permits to assess the mechanical behaviour of the respiratory system during passive expiration in anaesthetized humans.

RAO permits to assess the static respiratory parameters in response to volume inputs and emphasize the stress relaxation that takes into account the gas redistribution and viscoelasticity during the occluded breath. This method has been used, particularly, to test the linear viscoelastic model proposed by Bates et al. (10) in response to volume inputs (11, 12). The results of most of recent studies on anesthetized subjects (13, 14), animals (15) and patients with adult respiratory distress syndrome (16, 17) and with COPD (18) during mechanical ventilation have been interpreted according to this model.

The viscoelastic model parameters are obtained by performing a series of iso-flow occlusions at different lung volumes, or a series of occlusions at a fixed lung volume achieved with different inflation flows.

The viscoelastic constants of the respiratory system can be assessed by fitting the equation

$$\Delta R_{rs} = R_2 \left(1 - e^{-T_i/\tau_2}\right) \tag{1}$$

to the experimental data, where T_i is the inspiratory time and ΔR_{rs} is the additional resistence that takes into account the viscoelastic behaviour and time constant inequalities of the lung and the chest wall.

Eq. [1] is the final value, at $t = T_i$, of the following function

$$\Delta R_{rs,ins}(t) = R_2 \left(1 - e^{-t/\tau_2}\right) \tag{2}$$

that represents the exponential increase of additional resistance in response to a ramp of applied volume at constant-flow inflation according to Bates analysis (19).

The viscoelastic model

ΔR_{rs} are represented by the viscoelastic branch of the "spring-and-dashpot" rheological model proposed by Bates (10, 19) and based on Mount (20) and Sharp et al. (21) studies.

This model is made up of two parallel compartments: a dashpot representing $R_{int,rs}$, and a Kelvin body (22). The latter is made up of a spring, E_1, representing the static elastance of the respiratory system, $E_{st,rs}$, in parallel with a Maxwell body (22), i.e. a spring, E_2, and a dashpot, R_2, placed in series. E_2 and R_2 represent the viscoelastic properties of the respiratory system. The time constant, τ_2, of the Maxwell body is reflected by the R_2/E_2 ratio. These two compartments are placed in parallel between two equidistant bars. One is fixed and the other is moving at a constant rate. This rate corresponds to constant flow inflation, Φ, and at the end of inflation the distance between them corresponds to the volume that entered the lung. This model is shown in Figure 1.

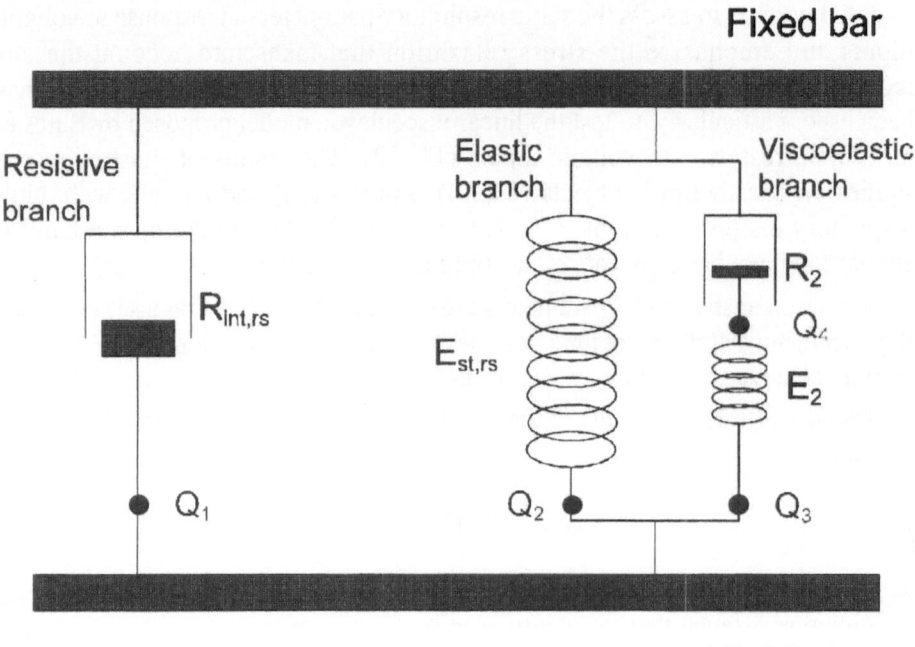

Fig. 1. The "spring-and-dashpot" rheological model during inflation

The model during inspiration

With reference to Fig. 1, if the distance between the two bars increases with Φ, starting from the elastic equilibrium volume, points Q_1, Q_2 and Q_3 move at the same constant speed, Φ. If we remove the bonds due to the springs and dashpots, points Q_1, Q_2 and Q_3 may be seen as the mobile seats of three different forces $F_1(t)$, $F_2(t)$ and $F_3(t)$ corresponding to the pressures of the system, i.e. respectively to the flow-resistive pressure, the elastic pressure and the viscoelastic pressure of the respiratory system. These forces hinder the mobile bar's movement and their total sum, $F(t)$, with opposite sign respect to $F_1(t)$, $F_2(t)$ and $F_3(t)$ corresponds to the total distending pressure of the model. In our analysis this pressure is represented from the tracheal pressure, P_{tr}.

P_{tr} may be used as a substitute of mouth pressure to avoid the resistance caused by the endotracheal tube, tubing and measuring equipment.

In particular, point Q_1 in the resistive branch is dragged at the same Φ and the relevant dashpot reacts with a force $F_1(t)$.

Similarly, the point Q_2 in the elastic branch is dragged at the same Φ and spring $E_{st,rs}$ applies an elastic return force $F_2(t)$ corresponding to $E_{st,rs}$ $V(t)$.

The viscoelastic branch behaves in a different way because of the combined presence of spring E_2 and dashpot R_2. While point Q_3 is dragged at the same Φ, point Q_4 reaches this constant speed only after a period of time ($t > 3$ τ_2). The force diagram of the model at Ti is shown in Fig. 2.

During the inflation, pressure components cannot be selectively distinguished. RAO permits to determine each single component of distending pressure of the model.

The model during occlusion

When the flow is suddenly interrupted and the airway occlusion prolonged, then the bars of the model remain at the same distance because the inflated volume, $V(t)$, is trapped into the lungs and in the airways. In particular, based on its characteristics, dashpot $R_{int,rs}$ completes its work at $t = T_{i+}$ and the related pressure goes down to zero. Spring $E_{st,rs}$ is blocked between the bars and continues to apply the elastic return force F_2 (T_i). On the other hand, in the viscoelastic branch, Q_3 is blocked, while Q_4 is moving in the same direction as before airway occlusion. During the occlusion the spring E_2 may go back to its equilibrium length (which corresponds to resting conditions) whereas dashpot R_2 continues to lengthen until 3 τ_2 are reached.

After occlusion a rapid drop is present in the recorded pressure ($P_{max} - P_1$), which is followed by a gradual decrease in pressure to an apparent plateau value (P_2).

The initial pressure drop corresponds to the resistive pressure related to the airway distal to the measurement point. This value, divided by the immediately preceeding steady flow, Φ, provides the interrupter resistance, $R_{int,rs}$ reflecting airway resistances (11). The force $F_1(t)$ in the resistive branch at the end of inspiration is $F_1(T_i) = R_{int,rs}$ Φ.

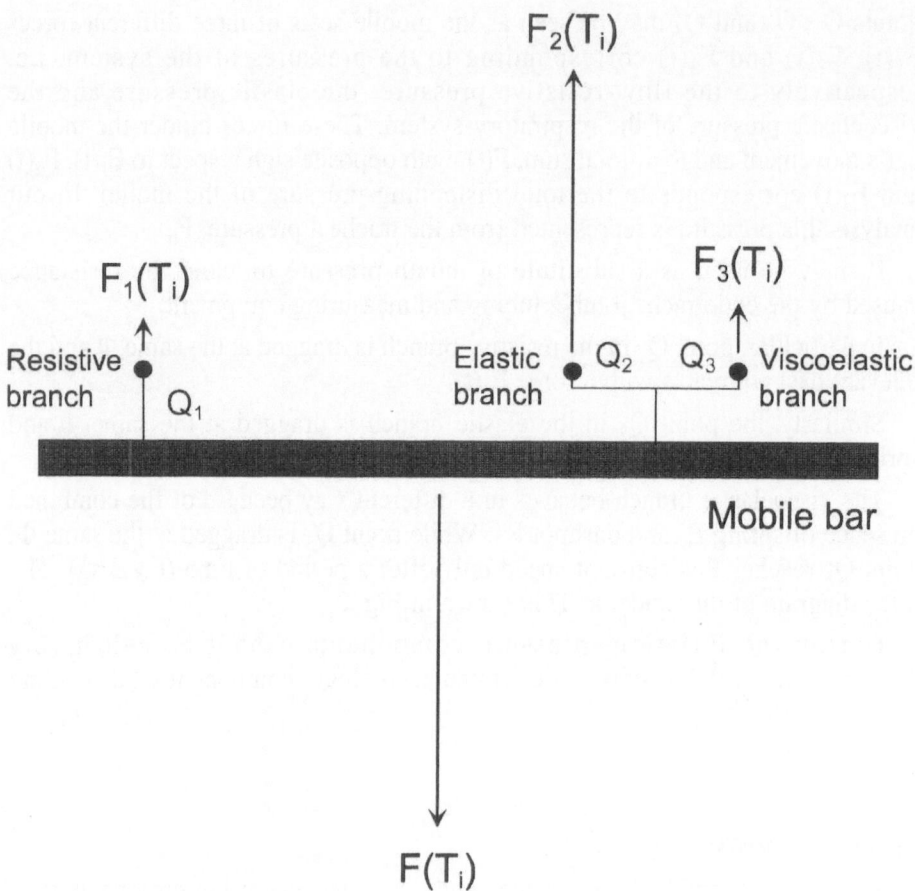

Fig. 2. Force diagram of the "spring-and-dashpot" rheological model at Ti

The slow decay of pressure ($P_{diff} = P_1 - P_2$) represents the stress relaxation that takes into account the viscoelastic behaviour and time constant inequalities of the lung and the chest wall. P_{diff} divided by preceeding occlusion Φ yields the additional resistance ΔR_{rs}.

If the occlusion time is long enough, P_2 is taken to represent the static end-inspiratory elastic recoil pressure of the respiratory system ($P_{st,rs}$).

During airway occlusion, the "spring-and-dashpot" rheological model may be drawn as in Fig. 3. The relevant force diagram is shown in Fig. 4.

In Fig. 4, at time $t = 3\,\tau_2$ after airway occlusion, the additional force $F_4(t)$ applied on point Q_3 in the viscoelastic branch goes down to zero. Summarizing, the distance between the two bars remains the same, but the force applied between

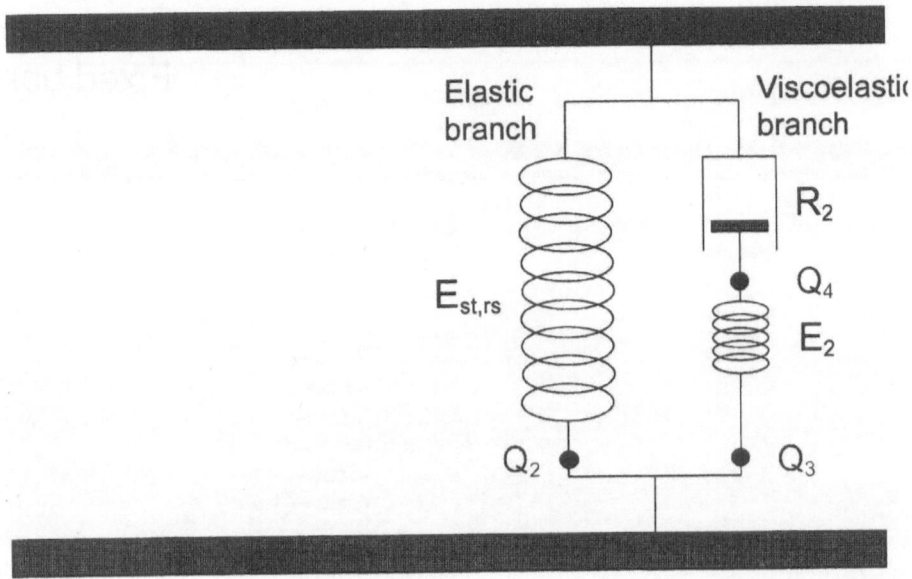

Fig. 3. The "spring-and-dashpot" rheological model during the end-inspiratory occlusion, $t < 3\,\tau_2$ after airway occlusion

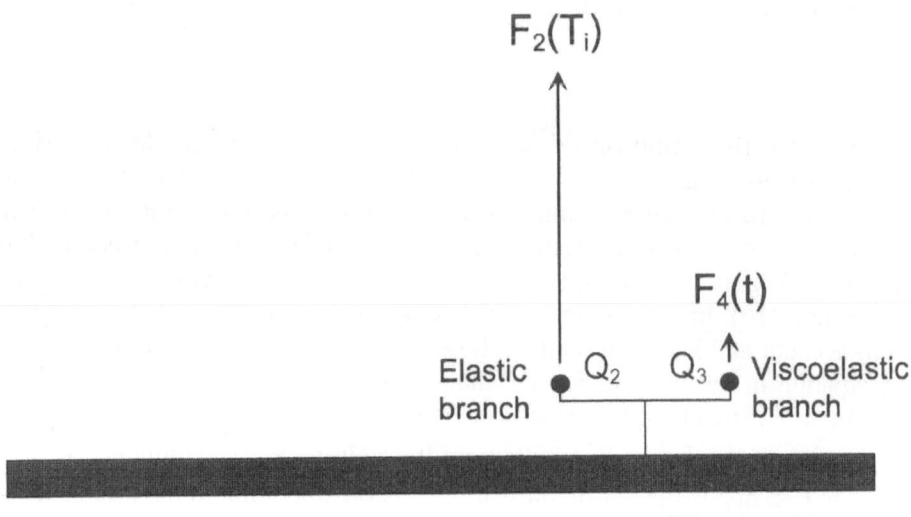

Fig. 4. Force diagram of the "spring-and-dashpot" rheological model shown in Fig. 3

the bars changes until reaching a constant value at $t > 3\,\tau_2$ because of spring $E_{st,rs}$ remaining blocked at a fixed length as shown in Figs. 5 and 6.

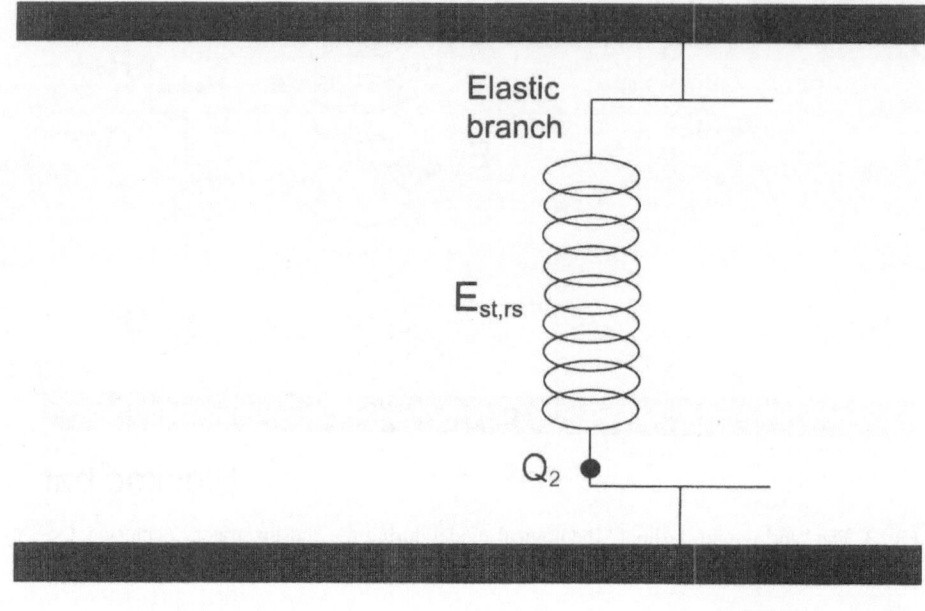

Fig. 5. The "spring-and-dashpot" rheological model during the end-inspiratory occlusion, with $t > 3\,\tau_2$ after airway occlusion

Because the equation of motion of the respiratory model describing inhomogeneous lungs (23) is comparable to that of Bates model (19), it is quite impossible to discern how much stress relaxation is due to inhomogeneities within the lung or to viscoelastic behaviour. In ARDS patients it was found that the inhomogeneities within the lung contributed relatively little to stress relaxation (16). In the present analysis only the viscoelastic behaviour is taken into account and P_{diff} reflects the relaxation of the spring E_2 resulting in energy dissipation in the dashpot R_2, i.e. the viscoelastic pressure. It depends on the degree of E_2 stretch at occlusion time.

During the occlusion P_{tr} results from the addition of two components.

The first one is the elastic pressure, $P_{st,rs}$ corresponding to the product of the volume inspirated above the resting position and elastance $E_{st,rs}$. $P_{st,rs}$ equals the steady-state postocclusion pressure. The second one is the function concerning

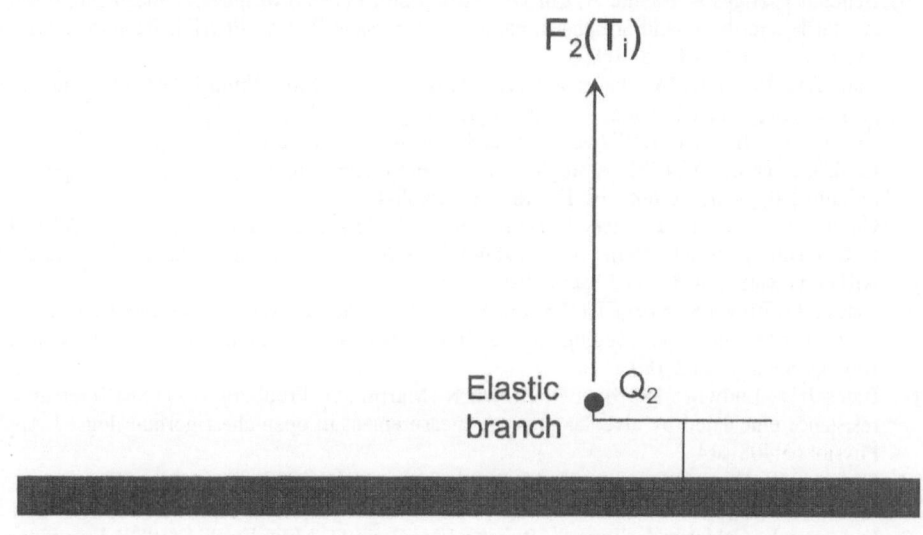

Fig. 6. Force diagram of the "spring-and-dashpot" rheological model shown in Fig. 5

additional pressure which, during the occlusion, takes into account the viscoelastic behaviour.

It has been possible to obtain the viscoelastic constants of the respiratory system by analyzing the decay of P_{tr} curve during the occlusion.

In conclusion, the technique of rapid airway occlusion during constant flow inflation allows an easy assessment of the static mechanical properties of the respiratory system, the airway and chest wall newtonian resistance, and the viscoelastic constants which are the expression of the time-dependent behaviour of normal lung and chest wall.

References

1. Mead J, Whittenberger JL (1954) Evaluation of airway interruption technique as a method for measuring pulmonary airflow resistance. J Appl Physiol 6:408-416
2. Bates JHT, Rossi A, Milic-Emili J (1985) Analysis of the behaviour of the respiratory system with constant inspiratory flow. J Appl Physiol 58:1840-1848
3. Bates JHT, Baconnier P, Milic-Emili J (1988) A theoretical analysis of interrupter technique for measuring respiratory mechanics. J Appl Physiol 64:2204-2214
4. Kochi T, Okubo S, Zin A, Milic-Emili J (1988) Flow and volume dependence of pulmonary mechanics in anaesthetized cats. J Appl Physiol 64:441-450
5. Zin WA, Pengelly L, Milic-Emili J (1982) Single breath method for measurement of respiratory mechanics in anesthetized animals. J Appl Physiol: Respirat Environ Exercise Physiol 52:1266-1277

6. Behrakis P, Higgs B, Baydur A, Zin WA, Milic-Emili J (1983) Respiratory mechanics during halothane anesthesia and anesthesia-paralysis in humans. J Appl Physiol: Respirat Environ Exercise Physiol 55:1085-1092

7. Bates JHT, Decramer M, Chartrand D, Zin W, Boddener A, Milic-Emili J (1985) Volume-time profile during relaxed expiration in the normal dog. J Appl Physiol 59:732-737

8. Chelucci G, Brunet F, Dall'Ava-Santucci J, Dhainaut J, Paccaly D, Armaganidis A, Milic-Emili J, Lockhart A (1991) A single-compartment model cannot describe passive expiration in intubated, paralysed humans. Eur Respir J 4:458-464

9. Guttmann J, Eberhard L, Fabry B, Bertschmann W, Zeravik J, Adolph M, Eckart J, Wolff G (1995) Time constant/volume relationship of passive expiration in mechanically ventilated ARDS patients. Eur Respir J 8:114-120

10. Bates JHT, Brown K, Kochi T (1987) Identifying a model of respiratory mechanics using the interrupter technique. Proceedings of the Ninth American Conference, Engineering Medical Biology Society 1802-1803

11. Bates JHT, Ludwig MS, Sly PD, Brown K, Martin JG, Fredberg JJ (1988) Interrupted resistance elucidated by alveolar pressure measurement in open-chest normal dogs. J Appl Physiol 65:408-414

12. Ludwig MS, Dreshaj I, Solway J, Munoz A, Ingram RH (1987) Partitioning of pulmonary resistance during constriction in the dog: effect of volume history. J Appl Physiol 62:807-815

13. D'Angelo E, Calderini E, Torri G, Robatto FM, Bono D, Milic-Emili J (1989) Respiratory mechanics in anesthetized paralyzed humans: effects of flow, volume, and time. J Appl Physiol 67:2556-2564

14. D'Angelo E, Robatto FM, Calderini E, Tavola M, Bono D, Torri G, Milic-Emili J (1991) Pulmonary and chest wall mechanics in anesthetized paralyzed humans. J Appl Physiol 70: 2602-2610

15. Similovski T, Levy P, Corbeil C, Albala M, Pariente R, Derenne JP, Bates JHT, Jonson B, Milic-Emili J (1989) Viscoelastic behaviour of lung and chest wall in dogs determined by flow interruption. J Appl Physiol 67:2219-2229

16. Eissa NT, Ranieri VM, Corbeil C, Chassé M, Robatto FM, Braidy J, Milic-Emili J (1991) Analysis of behaviour of the respiratory system in ARDS patients: effect of the flow, volume and time. J Appl Physiol 70;6:2719-2729

17. Tantucci C, Corbeil C, Chassé M, et al (1992) Flow and volume dependence of respiratory system flow resistance in ARDS patients. Am Rev Respir Dis 145:355-360

18. Tantucci C, Corbeil C, Chassé M, et al (1991) Flow resistance in COPD patients in acute respiratory failure: effects of flow and volume. Am Rev Respir Dis 144:384-389

19. Bates JHT, Brown K, Kochi T (1989) Respiratory mechanics in the normal dog determined by expiratory flow interruption. J Appl Physiol 67:2276-2285

20. Mount LE (1955) The ventilation flow-resistance and compliance of rat lungs. J Physiol Lond 127:157-167

21. Sharp JT, Johnson N, Goldberg NB, Van Lith P (1967) Hysteresis and stress adaptation in the human respiratory system. J Appl Physiol 23:487-497

22. Reiner M (1958) Rheology. Handbook of Physics. McGraw-Hill, 3:40-49

23. Otis AB, McKerrow CB, Bartlett RA, Mead J, McIlroy MB, Selverstone NJ, Radford EP (1956) Mechanical factors in distribution of pulmonary ventilation. J Appl Physiol 8:427-443

INVASIVE AND NONINVASIVE
HAEMODYNAMIC MONITORING

Technical Aspects of Haemodynamic Monitoring

M. Dei Poli, B. Allaria, A. Trivellato, P. Ferrario

Measurements are frequently made of pulmonary artery pressure (PAP), systemic arterial, central venous (CVP), and pulmonary capillary wedge pressure (WP) in the critically ill patient. In our rapidly evolving technological world, intravascular pressure monitoring is substantially unchanged, in contrast with the fields of imaging or surgery. Despite noteworthy advances in tip transducers catheter technology, fluid filled manometer systems are widely used for clinical cardiovascular monitoring purposes.

Equipment necessary to display and measure a pressure waveform include an appropriate intravascular catheter, fluid-filled noncompliant tubing with stopcocks, mechanoelectrical transducer, a transducer dome, a constant flush device; an electronic monitoring equipment, which usually consist of a connecting cable, monitor with amplifier, oscilloscope display screen, and recorder.

Using this equipment, intravascular pressure changes are transmitted through the hydraulic (fluid filled) elements to the transducer, which converts mechanical displacement into a proportional electrical signal. The signal is amplified, processed by the monitor, and the waveform displayed on the oscilloscope screen, accompanied by a digital readout.

The instrumentation cascade starts with intravascular catheters (arterial, venous or pulmonary artery), for providing access to blood sample withdrawal and connection to the system of measure. A stopcock is placed along the fluid filled tubing: the length of this line varies from a few centimeters to more than 1 m. The quality of signal recording is inversely proportional to the tubing length. A second stopcock is often encountered in a system assembly: it must be remembered that all stopcocks are critical in generating air bubbles.

Perfect priming is strictly required for a good signal transfer.

The continuous flush device is used to fill the pressure monitoring system and helps prevent blood from clotting in the catheter by continuously flushing fluid through the system.

The catheter-transducer system is completed by the pressure transducer, almost universally used in form of disposable device. The transducers are resistive devices that convert the movement of their sensing diaphragm into an electrical signal.

There has been great confusion in the past in matching transducers, cables and monitors of different vendors and brands: the AAMI/ANSI standards have greatly simplified an interchangeable use of transducers with any monitor. Graphic display of the pressure waveform is performed after signal amplification: only recently microprocessor based monitors and dedicated PCs have completely replaced older oscilloscope based monitors.

An optimal anesthesia management and the accuracy of intensive care procedures greatly rely on qualitative cardiovascular monitoring: the precision of pressure measurements has an important role in this scenario.

Many works has been written about problems and inaccuracy of hydraulic pressure monitoring. In 1903 Otto Frank described the criteria for an accurate pressure waves recording. Since 1946 the research in this field extensively covered many topics: as examples the theoretic formulation of catheter-manometer system, the pressure waveform frequency composition and the dynamic response of the system (1).

For a system to be reliable means the generation of a nondistorted signal in response to a physical phenomenon: it depends mainly on the quality of the system components.

The major problems in blood pressure measurements using a catheter system are:
1. Improper zeroing and zero drift
2. Improper transducer/monitor calibration
3. Inadequate dynamic response
4. The improper determination of derived data from the available pressure signals

Careful setup and testing of the complete monitoring system is essential to acquire accurate data. The zeroing is the single most important step in the setting of the catheter-transducer system, since an error in this step could generate large differences in recording all pressures, particularly the weaker ones (CVP, pulmonary artery and wedge pressure).

Zeroing is done by opening the system to the atmosphere after aligning the transducer at the midaxillary line, assuming this as expression of the right heart position in the recumbent body.

The major calibration problems, associated with improper transducer setup or dome application, could be eliminated by the use of the recently introduced disposable pressure transducers.

For accurate pressure recording a catheter transducer system must fulfill three requirements:
1. Static accuracy
2. Physiological reaction
3. Dynamic accuracy

Static accuracy

The static accuracy describes the ability of the system in measuring stationary or very slowly changing events. A fixed ratio is demonstrable between the input signal to the transducers and the output, whichever the physiological range of the measure performed. If the output signal varies with the pressure modifications, the transducer shows some "hysteresis": it is mandatory to exclude this property before using the system.

Physiological reaction

An interaction between the catheter and the vessel that contain it could affect the flow and subsequently an even accurate measure.

Dynamic accuracy

It is difficult to guarantee this property in a measuring system, but is mandatory that the system could record phase and amplitude rapidly changing events. If not recorded in time, phase and amplitude variations could distort the output signal. The response to amplitude and phase variation represents the system dynamic response.

Amplitude response

The physiological pressure and flow are periodic events in which the cardiac rhythm plays a central role. The heart rate is the fundamental frequency and is 1 Hz at a heart rate of 60 beats per minute. If the fundamental frequency is 1 Hz, it means a heart rate of 60 beats per minute, if 2 Hz a rate of 120 beats per minute, and if 3 Hz a rate of 180.

Complex waves may be reduced to their harmonic components by the application of a mathematical principle known as Fourier analysis. Any complex wave could be considered as composed of many simple periodic functions (sine or cosine): the simple function having the same frequency as the original complex wave constitutes the fundamental or first harmonic. Those having twice or thrice this frequency are named second, third, ... harmonics. When the pressure wave harmonics are known (for instance 12 Hz for the sixth harmonic) it is possible to understand if the measuring system is able to correctly record the signal.

It is well known that the aortic pressure has five main harmonics, and that harmonics after the fifth are scarcely significant in amplitude: they are comparable to noise. The major signal contribution is due to the first and second harmonics, but good recording are obtained when six to ten harmonics are considered (12 to 20 Hz for a 120 beats per minute rate).

When considering ventricular pressures the Fourier analysis shows five main harmonics, and that a system able to record at 20 Hz is adequate. For atrial pressures the system needs to consider at least ten harmonics. The resynthesis of 15 harmonics is necessary for dP/dt max recording.

Phase response

The recording of pressure waves will scarcely be accurate if the harmonics are irregularly spread over time, that is, not in phase. There is phase distortion when the pressure wave harmonics are not conducted at a uniform speed from the source to the transducer. The shifting of the harmonic components relative to each other in time may result in alteration of the recorded waves, in shape and in amplitude.

The conventional catheter-manometer systems which employ long fine cannulae almost always induce phase distortions. The phase distortion is frequency dependent and increases at high frequences.

The catheter-transducer systems, as defined by Gardner (2), usually behave as an "underdamped second order dynamic system". The three mechanical parameters that describe a second order system are: *elasticity*, due usually to the transducer diaphragm flexibility; *mass*, of the fluid moving inside the system; and *friction*, due to the movement of the fluid in the pressure tubings under pulsatile forces action.

The elasticity, the mass and the friction produce two measurable parameters: the damped natural frequency (Fn), referred to the frequency of the system oscillation, and the damping factor (ζ), that describes how quickly the system stops. The accurate description of the system Fn and ζ is the most common technique to indicate the dynamic response of a catheter-transducer system. The accuracy of measurements is affected by these two factors.

Low values for Fn and ζ (i.e. underdamped) are undesirable and lead to errors in pressure measurements, especially when the waveform of the pressure contains high-frequency components. The requirements for catheter-manometer systems have been set from values as low as 6 Hz (3) to a minimum of 25 Hz for the Fn (4) and a ζ between + 0.64 (5) and + 0.707.

The required range of dynamic response is termed the bandwidth, where the "useful bandwidth" is defined as the range of spread of frequencies over which the catheter-manometer system can accurately measure the blood pressure – typically from just above zero Hz to two-thirds of the natural frequency.

The effect of underdamping on blood pressure waveforms results in inaccuracies in waveforms recordings and critical significant values derived from those (i.e dP/dt max) (6). Maximum dP/dt and peak systolic values may be distorted by artifact due to an inadequate measuring system.

The catheter, the tubings, the fast flush device and the transducer could distort the pressure signal. The fast flush device test could give assurances about the adequacy of the recorded waveforms and parameters.

Two methods are commonly used to describe the dynamic response of the catheter, the tubings and the transducers. The first method states that the system frequency response remains unchanged up to a specific cutoff frequency. This is strictly related to the number of harmonics of the original pressure wave (usually ten harmonics are specified). The second method uses the specification of the natural frequency (Fn) and the damping coefficient (ζ).

The Fn and ζ are easily measurable on the measuring system in use and could be employed to define the dynamic of the catheter-transducer system. When placed on a two-dimensional diagram Fn and ζ describe five areas, where only two of these refer to an adequate and optimal reproduction of the pressure wave. The remaining three refer to distorted waves.

The majority of the catheter-transducer systems are underdamped. If the Fn is lower than 7.5 Hz the shape of the pressure waveform will be distorted, whichever the dumping factor ζ. When the Fn is increased to 24 Hz, ζ does not distort the waveform in a range between 0.15 and 1.1.

In order to optimize the dynamic response of a measure system, the Fn should be increased as much as possible. A high Fn is obtainable with short tubings, large diameter catheters, low compliance transducers and components.

The fast flush device test has been used extensively for catheter-transducer systems testing since Gardner published his work in 1982. After inducing a square wave flushing the system and evaluating the subsequent oscillations the natural frequency and the damping factor could be measured. This approach could be criticized on a theoretical base (7): the combination of catheter, tubing, transducer and monitor leads to a system of order superior to the second, as proposed by Gardner. Moreover, the dynamic response is only incompletely described by the square wave theory.

Billiet and Colardyn (8) suggested a measuring structure based on an amplitude/phase frequency diagram (the Gabarith system). This may describe the accuracy and the consistency of the intravascular pressure measurement and may evaluate the precision and accuracy of catheter-transducer systems.

The systolic pressure is first influenced by an unsatisfactory system dynamic response; the diastolic pressure can tolerate better scarce performances of the components of the system itself.

Many factors could induce a weak dynamic response of the catheter-transducer system:

- Air bubbles
- Kinking of the tubing, T connections
- Too long tubings
- Too high compliance of tubings
- Too high compliance of pressure transducer or fast flush device
- Clots along the tubing

In the clinical assessment the best method to increase the system dynamic response is to ameliorate the Fn.

This could be obtained through:

1. Air bubble elimination. The fast flush device must be placed after the transducer, so that the air bubbles from the device could be trapped in the transducer dome.
2. System assembly simplification. This could be facilitated by using disposable preassembled packages.
3. Using only short and low compliant tubings.
4. Eliminating blood clots from the catheter.

A Fn of more than 20 Hz could be generated by paying attention to all of these factors. If the system still does not perform adequately, an adjustable damping device (Accudynamic, Abbott; Rose, Resonance OverShoot Eliminator) should be used.

References

1. Anderson HR, Bergsten O (1982) Blood pressure measurements and methods. Albertslund. S & W Mediko Teknic A/S, pp 4-74
2. Gardner RM (1981) Direct blood pressure measurement – dynamic response requirements. Anesthesiology 54:227-236
3. Wood EH (1956) Physical response requirements of pressure transducers for the reproduction of physiological phenomena. Trans Am Inst Electr Eng Commun Electr 75:32-40
4. Bruner JMR, Krenis LJ, Kunsman JM, Sherman AP (1981) Comparison of direct and indirect methods of measuring arterial blood pressure, part 1. Med Instrum 15:11-21
5. Gardner RM (1981) Direct blood pressure measurements – dynamic response requirements. Anesthesiology 54:227-236
6. Boonzaier DA (1978) Resonance artifact in intravascular blood pressure measuring systems: a technique for on line digital computer correction. Afr J Sci 74:250-255
7. Billiet E, Colardyn F (1992) Hazardous information from bedside fast flush device test for fluid filled pressure monitoring systems. J Vasc Dis Angiol 43:988-995
8. Billiet E, Colardyn F (1992) The Gabarith: a new approach in evaluating fluid filled pressure monitoring systems. World Congress of Anesthesiologists, Den Haag, Abstracts 70

Pressure Wave Modifications in Different Cardiac and Respiratory Events

B. Allaria, M. Dei Poli, M. Favaro, G.L. De Filippi

Heart and respiration may affect the morphology and the absolute values of pressure waves to such an extent that we would advise everyone to have a screen or, better, a recorder presenting, at the same time, ECG values, a respiration curve identifying inspiration and expiration, and the pressure wave to be monitored. We would also advise everyone to acquire a thorough knowledge of the normal morphology of pressure waves and their relationships with the cardiac cycle. Unfortunately, neither nursing nor medical students are made aware of the need for an accurate cardiovascular monitoring. Perhaps this is why the reading of pressure waves is generally approximate and difficult tracings are often misinterpreted.

Central venous pressure and wedge pressure tracings are recorded to acquire information about the right ventricular end-diastolic pressure (RVEDP) and the left ventricular end-diastolic pressure (LVEDP).

When ventricular Swan Ganz catheters are available, there is no need to measure the central venous pressure (CVP), since RVEDP data are directly available. Similarly, with a catheter in the left ventricle there is no need to measure the wedge pressure (WP).

If no direct measurements are available, CVP and WP must be analyzed. The analysis of these two pressure waves is often rather complex since they are influenced by respiratory as well as cardiac events. It is therefore mandatory to know exactly their normal morphology, the relationships between specific points characterizing pressure waves, and the cardiac cycle analyzed by means of an ECG.

As may be seen in Fig. 1, both CVP and WP are characterized by an "a" wave, an expression of the atrial contraction, and by a "v" wave, an expression of the atrial filling when the tricuspid or the mitral valve close. On the descending limb of the "a" wave there may be a small wave ("c" wave) which is likely to be related to the closing of the tricuspid or the mitral valve. An important difference between CVP and WP is the time location of "a" and "v" waves.

In CVP the "a" wave starts during the P-Q interval of ECG, and the "v" wave in the subsequent T-P space, generally close to the T wave. In WP, the "a" wave is somewhat delayed and generally starts during QRS or at the end of it. The

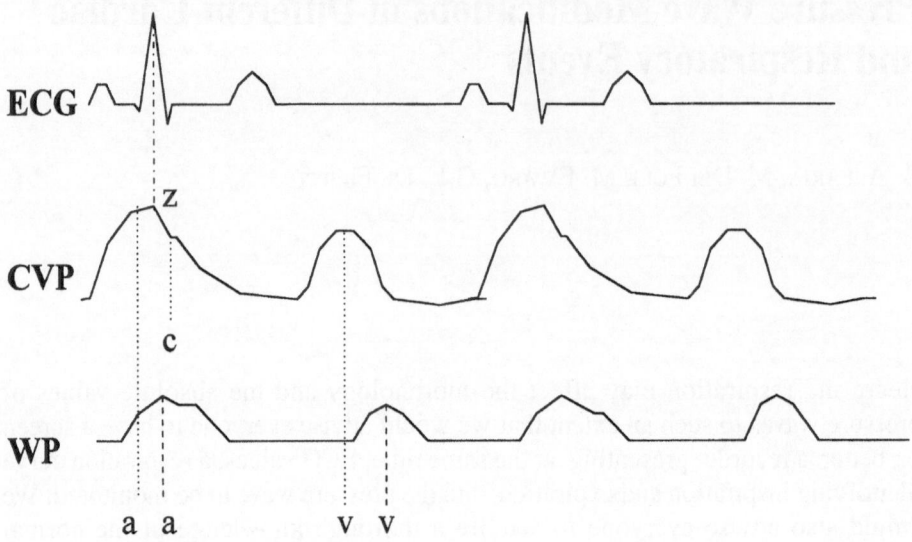

Fig. 1. Relationships between CVP, WP and ECG. The "a" wave of CVP starts in correspondence with the P-Q, and the "v" wave in correspondence with the subsequent T-P interval, immediately after the end of the T wave. In WP "a" and "v" waves are delayed for two reasons:
1) The left atrial contraction is delayed with respect to the right
2) Wp measurement is made at a certain distance from the left atrium, and therefore with a certain delay

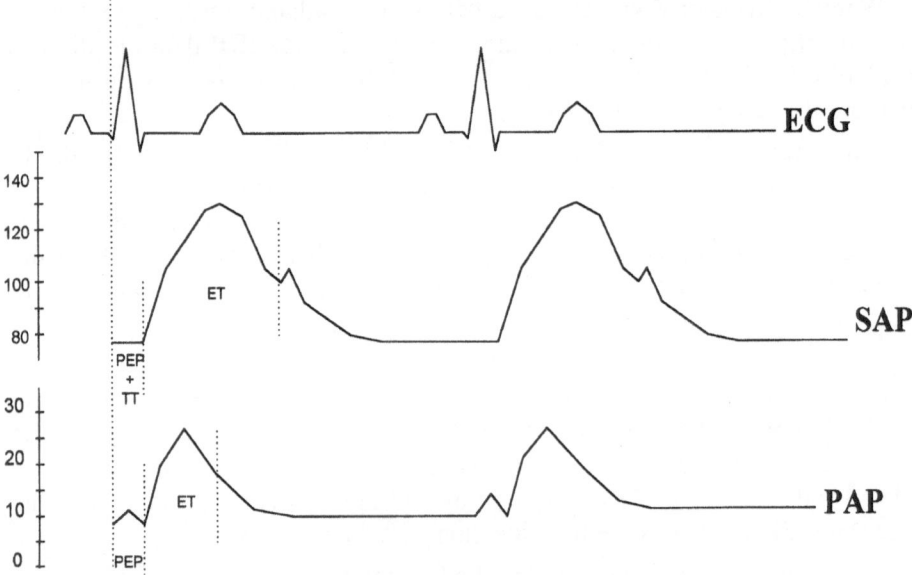

Fig. 2. Systemic arterial pressure and pulmonary artery pressure. To be noted: the presystolic wave, which must be excluded from the measurement of the pulmonary end-diastolic pressure, and the relationships between ECG and pressure waves

beginning of the "v" wave is delayed as well and while appearing in the same T-P space as the "v" wave of CVP it starts close to P.

As will be shown later, knowledge of the time relations between pressure waves and the cardiac cycle is crucial when interpreting complex signs.

Particularly interesting is the "z" point, coinciding with the end of the diastole, when right ventricular and atrial pressures are in equilibrium - monitoring this point means monitoring RVEDP (1).

The most common anomalies of CVP and WP caused by the cardiac activity will now be considered. There are basically three heart-related reasons for the onset of CVP and WP anomalies:

1. Valvular alterations
2. Heart rate alterations
3. Alterations of the haemodynamic status

Tricuspid and mitral stenoses lead to an abnormal elevation of the "a" wave in CVP and WP respectively. Tricuspid or mitral failure leads to giant "v" waves.

The presence of giant "a" or "v" waves may complicate the reading of the tracings, and a tracing with giant waves may sometimes be hastily mistaken for a pulmonary artery pressure tracing. A careful observation of the time relations between these events is the precondition for a correct diagnosis.

It should be kept in mind that in chronic ventricular failure with atrial distention, the presence of a giant "v" wave means that the maximum distention of the atrium has been reached and is thus a sign of pulmonary stasis. A giant "a" wave is often caused by impairment of the ordinary atrio-ventricular contraction sequence, with simultaneous atrial and ventricular systole (junctional rhythm, second- and third-degree atrioventricular blocks).

Clearly, the presence of giant "a" or "v" waves disrupts venous tracings and makes them unsuitable to predict ventricular end-diastolic pressures. For giant "v" waves, though, RVEDP may be predicted by reading CVP during QRS ("z" point, or end-diastole point).

The "a" wave may be absent in patients with atrial fibrillation, and the "v" wave may get smaller and almost disappear in hypovolemic patients with high-compliance atria.

As regards arterial tracings (pulmonary artery and systemic pressure), it is appropriate to present normal situations first. The pulmonary artery pressure wave is characterized by a presystolic wave, which may be absent but is sometimes very large, thus being a misleading factor in the measuring of end-diastolic pressure (Fig. 2). It used to be regarded as secondary to left atrium contraction, but this is not the case - the presystolic wave is present even when the patient has no more atrial contraction.

This wave must be excluded in the measurement of end-diastolic pressure which must be read at the foot of the real, subsequent, pulmonary artery pressure wave. As is known, the interval between the foot and the dicrotic notch of arterial

waves corresponds to the left ventricle ejection time (systemic pressure) or to the right ventricle ejection time (pulmonary pressure); and the time between the ECG Q wave and the foot of the arterial pulses corresponds to the right pre-ejection time (pulmonary artery) and to the left pre-ejection time (systemic pressure).

Actually, the right pre-ejection time (PEP) is real and is about 100 ms, whereas the left PEP, being measured peripherally (the wrist for the radial artery) is increased by the transmission time, which in healthy adults is about 70 ms (personal data).

The left PEP, measured peripherally, in a healthy subject with a normal heart rate, is about 180 ms, i.e., the central PEP (110 ms) plus the transmission time (70 ms).

These aspects have been stressed because PEP monitoring may provide additional information about the ventricular filling, and monitoring of the PEP/ET ratio may be useful in monitoring the contractility of the right and left ventricles.

A good correlation has been recently demonstrated between right PEP/ET and right ventricle ejection fraction (RVEF), whereas the correlation between left ventricle ejection fraction (LVEF) and left PEP/ET has been known for decades.

One of the cardiac factors most frequently leading to modifications of the pressure waves is the loss of the normal atrioventricular contraction sequence. As atrial contraction significantly contributes to ventricular filling (25%), the lack of it leads to a dramatic decrease in the stroke volume (SV) with a subsequent reduction in systemic and pulmonary artery pressure values. Premature ventricular contractions (PVC) cause a loss of the normal atrioventricular contraction sequence and a reduction in the filling time.

PVC thus lead to reduced SV and have obvious repercussions on arterial pressure, which may be very serious in case of PVC sequences or ventricular tachycardia.

As will be shown later, modifications of the respiratory activity may cause alterations of the pulmonary artery pressure values: these modifications are generally artifacts, and the real pressure value must be assessed excluding the respiratory effects. In pressure alterations caused by arrhythmias, there are no artifacts, but pressure values actually reflecting the hemodynamic situations.

Great caution is required when pressure values are assessed in arrhythmic patients (atrial and ventricular extrasystole, atrial fibrillation). When extrasystolic events are more frequent, or when the ventricular frequency of an atrial fibrillation is higher, SV is further reduced and arterial pressure values decrease accordingly.

Average values rather than values at a given point in time should therefore be recorded. Values displayed on a monitor – which are average values calculated over several contractions – are closer to reality than instantaneous recordings.

In normal respiratory activity, inspiration facilitates venous return, increases SV and therefore slightly increases arterial pressure. The opposite is true when there is an increase in pericardial pressure. In such a situation the increased venous return further increases pericardial pressure, which hinders ventricular movement, thus reducing SV and arterial pressure.

This phenomenon, known as "pulsus paradoxus", may be useful when pericarditis is suspected.

Modifications of arterial tracings are present also in case of valvular defects. Aortic failure, for instance, makes it almost impossible to identify the dicrotic notch of the peripheral arterial sphygmogram. Diastolic pressure gradually decreases until the end of the diastole, when the new systole begins. The tracing is such that the automatic reading of the arterial pressure by the monitor is very difficult, and sometimes an extraordinarily low diastolic pressure is recorded (20 mmHg or slightly more).

Ahrens and Taylor (2) rightly suggest disregarding the lowest values and read the diastolic value some 0.20 s after QRS for systemic arterial pressure recorded in the radial artery.

After briefly describing the interference of the cardiac activity on venous and arterial pressure tracings, the interference on pressure waves of the respiratory activity will now be described. We shall not deal with the real hemodynamic effects of spontaneous and artificial respiration as this issue would deserve a paper of its own. Rather we shall concentrate on the artifacts caused by ventilation which often complicate the reading of pressure tracings.

Artifacts almost always concern pressure waves recorded in intrathoracic regions (CVP, WP, PAP, etc.). Respiration-related variations of systemic arterial pressure are real and do not present any particular reading problem.

The difference between intrathoracic pressure waves and systemic arterial pressure waves depend on the fact that while the environment surrounding the most commonly used arteries (radial artery) is at atmospheric pressure, i.e., the pressure used for the transducer zero value, the intrathoracic regions where pressure is recorded are surrounded by a variable-pressure environment, similar to the pleural pressure.

As pleural pressure is not easily measured clinically, esophageal pressure is used instead.

If, for example, CVP is 8 mmHg and the pleural pressure is −2 mmHg, the actual CVP will be:

$$CVP = 8 - (-2) = 10 \text{ mmHg}$$

If CVP is 8, but the pleural pressure is +5 (under artificial ventilation, for example), the actual CVP will be:

$$CVP = 8 - (+5) = 3 \text{ mmHg}$$

Obviously the clinical interpretation of these two apparently equal venous pressure values will be completely different.

However, since esophageal pressure is not easily recorded either, the most common way to record pressure values which are close to actual values is recording them when the intrathoracic pressure is very close to environmental pressure, i.e., at end expiration, both with spontaneous and artificial ventilation.

Clearly these problems would not exist if catheters with distal transducers, i.e. on the site where pressure is recorded, were available. These catheters, however, are too expensive to be commonly used.

Clearly, in spontaneous ventilation, pressure values measured at end expiration correspond to the highest recorded values, whereas in artificial ventilation pressure values measured at end expiration correspond to the lowest values.

Contrary to what is generally believed, spontaneous respiration produces more artifacts than artificial ventilation. Spontaneous ventilation directly causes variations in pleural pressure, whereas artificial ventilation leads to pressure changes in the airways which are only in part transmitted to the pleural space and are very slight in low-compliance lungs. In most spontaneously breathing patients it is easy to identify the end of expiration: expiration is longer than inspiration and is characterized by higher pressure values.

Things are more complex in high-rate spontaneous respiration: in this case it is difficult to identify a point of end expiration with a respiration flow equal to zero. Furthermore, since expiration is active, pleural pressure goes up and recorded pressure values are higher than actual values.

It should be kept in mind that in tachypneic patients, then, venous and pulmonary artery pressure values may be overestimated. This is particularly important in patients for whom acute hypovolemia on a hemorrhagic basis is suspected and in whom, in the early stages, Ht is not indicative and CVP and WP values are important in order to make a diagnosis.

Another condition which may cause important artifacts is the forced expiration of patients with asthma or COPD. In these cases the reading in the highest points of the pressure wave, during expiration, gives higher than real values. In order not to have abnormally high or wrong pressure values, the point of end expiration must be identified.

In artificial ventilation the highest values are recorded during inspiration and it is appropriate to measure pressure values at end inspiration when the flow is close to zero.

The availability of a pressure curve and/or airway flow helps in choosing the time at which pressure values should be recorded. If there are no pressure or airway flow data, it will be enough to make the reading during the lowest pressure part of the pressure tracing (expiration). It is important, however, not to mistake the expiration phase for a low point in the tracing, corresponding to the inspiration effort of a patient under assisted ventilation or a patient who has not adapted to ventilation.

In weaning COPD patients, the transmural systolic pressure of thoracic aorta is important. This value expresses the afterload of the left ventricle and its elevation is one of the causes of the LVEF reduction observed in these patients when being weaned from the respirator. Since systemic systolic pressure (SBP) basically coincides with aortic pressure, the transmural pressure of intrathoracic aorta (TAP) is equal to SBP minus pleural pressure: if the pleural pressure during inspiration is −6 mmHg and SBP is 150 mmHg, the transmural aortic pressure will be:

$$TAP = 150 - (-6) = 156 \text{ mmHg}$$

Work done for weaning may increase SBP. Furthermore, in COPD patients, forced inspiration with important pleural depressions is not infrequent. The afterload may thus increase significantly, leading directly to a decrease in LVEF or, in coronaropathic patients, to left ventricular ischemia with a further LVEF decrease.

An accurate recording of TAP is therefore useful in monitoring COPD patients during weaning (3), in particular patients with coronary disease and/or history of left ventricular failure.

References

1. Allaria B, Dei Poli M, Brunetti B, Trivellato A (1994) Computerized analysis of biologic cardiovascular signals. 9th European Congress of Anesthesiology. Jerusalem, October 2-7;373
2. Ahrens TS, Taylor LA (1992) Haemodynamic waveform analysis. WB saunders Company ED, USA 1992
3. Richard CH, Teboul JL, Archambaud F, Hebert JL, Michaut P, Auzepy P (1994) La funzione ventricolare sinistra durante svezzamento respiratorio in pazienti con COPD. Intensive Care Med (ed. ital.);3:155

Noninvasive Pressure Measurements

D. CATHIGNOL, R. MUCHADA

Introduction

Blood pressure measurement started in the eighteenth century. In 1773, an English theologian and scientist Stephan Hales measured a horse's mean blood pressure directly without anaesthetic. Blood pressure measurement has since improved through a succession of scientific studies. Although the method of reference continues to be intra-arterial catheterisation, clinicians now have noninvasive methods at their disposal, which allow them to measure the mean, diastolic and systolic blood pressures either manually or automatically. More recently, devices have appeared on the market that allow a continuous blood pressure curve to be recorded, which is very close to the actual intra-arterial pressure curve.

Before describing the various methods that allow blood pressure to be measured, we would like to point out that the ideal situation would be a recording which is the same as a pressure curve produced by a catheter in the ascending aorta, just after the sigmoid valves. Such a measurement should be able to produce this curve in the correct shape and size, continuously, in real time, and under any physiological or pathological conditions. The reason that clinicians do not use the method of reference is that it has many associated disadvantages that restrict its use: numerous iatrogenic risks, a high cost and is relatively complex to set up. However, it enables blood pressure to be measured even at extreme values, in particular in hypotension.

All noninvasive measurements have the characteristic of the measurement site (humeral artery, radial artery or the digital artery) being some distance away from the ideal measurement site (ascending aorta). Even in the absence of any pathology, the blood pressure at these sites is noticeably different to measurement at the aortic arch. Figure 1 illustrates these differences clearly. More specifically, the systolic blood pressure is seen to increase and the time curve becomes rounder as the measurement site becomes more distal from the ascending aorta. The different measurement methods can be divided into three main groups: manual methods that produce successive readings of the systolic, diastolic and mean blood pressures; automatic methods that give the same readings but repeatedly; and finally methods that provide a continuous blood pressure recording as a curve.

Unobtrusive manual methods

Auscultation

The commonest noninvasive method for measuring blood pressure used today is auscultation.

A cuff of the right size is wrapped around the arm and inflated to a pressure greater than the occlusion pressure. It is then deflated gradually. When the pressure in the cuff becomes less than the systolic blood pressure, the Korotkoff sounds are heard (Fig. 2). As deflation continues, their sound changes and they then disappear. Even though it is unanimously accepted that the appearance of the Korotkoff sounds corresponds to the systolic pressure, the criteria for measuring the diastolic pressure are more controversial (1). Some feel that it corresponds to when the sounds change, others when they disappear. Accuracy of this method (and of all methods using a pneumatic cuff) depends greatly on the cuff being the right size for the arm. The cuff should be at least as wide as the arm circumference and the inflatable bladder should if possible be circumferential (2). Despite the fact that the stethoscope incorporated into the cuff may be of a different material, it is important to make sure that there is very good skin contact. For better sensitivity, a binaural stethoscope with thick rubber tubing is to be preferred, even if it is less practical for the clinician.

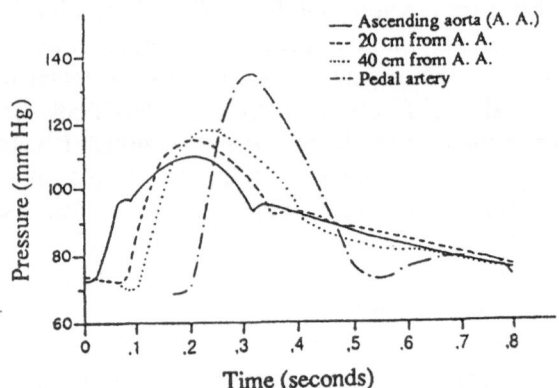

Fig. 1. The time wave form of the blood pressure is dependent on the site

If these rules are not respected, large errors can occur, particularly in obese patients in whom a cuff that is too small causes overestimation of the blood pressure. Hypotension is another cause of failure of this method. If the blood pressure is too low, especially if there is associated arterial vasoconstriction (in shock), the Korotkoff sounds cannot be heard (3).

Oscillometry

Oscillometry is another noninvasive method for monitoring blood pressure in which variations in the pressure of the blood pressure cuff are detected (3, 4). The type of oscillometer commonly used today has a valve which allows either the absolute value of the cuff pressure to be displayed or the amplitude of oscillations in the cuff, irrespective of the pressure (Fig. 2). The cuff is used by inflating it until there are no oscillations. It is then deflated slowly until rapid fluctuations in the cuff pressure are seen on the gauge. The cuff pressure is then read. Numerous studies have shown that this point is at or close to the systolic pressure (3). The cuff is then further deflated until the oscillations reach their maximum and then begin to decrease. This point has been shown to be close to the mean blood pressure, not the diastolic pressure as previously thought. The diastolic pressure cannot be measured with any certainty by oscillometry, although certain authors have shown the rapid decrease in the amplitude of the oscillations inside the cuff to be correlated to the diastolic pressure.

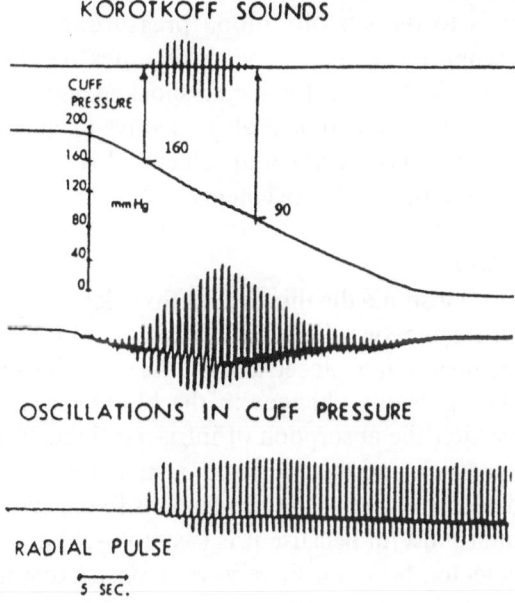

Fig. 2. Comparison between Korotkoff sounds, cuff pressure oscillations and radial pulse

It remains to be shown if very low blood pressures can be measured accurately, especially in situations where intense arterial vasoconstriction is liable to reduce the oscillations (shock).

Blood flow methods

Three methods may be described which detect the reappearance of blood flow as soon as the pressure inside the cuff drops below the systolic pressure.

Palpation

This technique requires a minimum of equipment: an inflatable cuff, and an anaeroid or mercury manometer. The cuff is inflated until the radial pulse can no longer be felt. It is then slowly deflated and the systolic pressure is considered as the point when the pulse can be felt again. The main advantages of this method are its simplicity and the fact that it is not dependent on the hearing of the observer. This method is, however, unsuitable for systolic pressures less than 80 mmHg (5).

Doppler ultrasound

A more sensitive method for measuring blood flow is an ultrasonic blood flow detector that uses the Doppler principle (5, 6). The detector is placed over the distal radial artery and the characteristic swishing sound of the arterial blood flow is listened for as the cuff is deflated. The pressure at which the arterial flow is heard corresponds to the systolic blood pressure. Some users detect the diastolic pressure when the Doppler sound becomes regular. This method is highly sensitive and particularly useful in cold shocked patients whose peripheral pulses are faint or absent. This method is also sensitive to electromagnetic sounds and is therefore of little or no use when the electrical scalpel is being used. It is also very sensitive to the patients' movements.

Photoelectric method

Photoelectric devices constitute the third blood flow detection method which can be used for measuring the systolic blood pressure. This technique measures absorption of light from a source placed against the skin, the most convenient site being the finger. The pulsatile changes in the blood volume associated with pulsatile blood flow alter the absorption of infra-red light. If the cuff is inflated above the systolic pressure and then deflated, a sudden oscillation in the output of the blood flow detector is seen. This corresponds to the systolic pressure. This technique is particularly useful because it is easy to use, but errors can occur by movement of the detector. It fails if there is vasoconstriction in the finger blood vessels due to the cold or a drop in the blood pressure.

Automatic blood pressure measurement methods

Automatic blood pressure devices appeared in the 1960s. As a rule, they use the same principles as their manual counterparts. The function performed by the clinician occurs automatically.

Oscillometric method

The principle of this method is similar to that described in "Oscillometry" and Fig. 2. The cuff is inflated and deflated periodically and characteristic points are detected automatically. The first of these devices to become widespread was the Dinamap (7, 8). The latest generation of these devices shows the diastolic, systolic and mean blood pressures as well as the cardiac rhythm. The oscillometric method is very sensitive to muscle activity. An automatic detection system stops deflation of the cuff when this occurs. These successive periods when the cuff remains inflated are very unpleasant for the patient and in certain cases, skin, vascular or neurological lesions have been described, apparently due to excessive compression. This method works just as well on the forearm, the upper arm or even the legs, which may be useful for obese patients or during operations where the arm is inaccessible.

Auscultatory method

Another approach to automatic blood pressure measurement is by using a device that measures systolic and diastolic pressure by auscultation. Like the Dinamap, the Infrasonde works by automatic inflation of a cuff on the arm (9). Two crystal microphones, positioned over the brachial artery, determine the point at which the Korotkoff sounds first appear. The cuff then deflates at a rate selected by the operator and the systolic, diastolic and mean blood pressures are measured. As may be imagined, the major drawback with this technique is that the sensors must be placed accurately over the artery. If they are moved away from the artery, the signal strength weakens and the blood pressure indicated by the machine is inaccurate. The operator should therefore take great care to ensure that the sensors are correctly positioned and that the cuff is tightly fastened. Unlike Dinamap, Infrasonde does not work over the distal parts of the limbs.

Doppler method (Arteriosonde)

This must surely be the first automatic system on the market. It is based on detection of blood flow appearing by the Doppler effect (10). Just like its manual cousin, this device measures systolic and diastolic pressure. A pump automatically inflates the cuff to a preselected pressure and then gradually deflates the cuff. As soon as the first jet of blood is detected under the cuff, a valve closes, thus stopping the mercury column, that indicates the systolic pressure, from falling any further. The diastolic pressure column continues to fall until the device detects that the arterial walls have stopped moving and that no more turbulence is caused by the cuff. At this point, the machine indicates that the measurement has been made. Correct positioning of the sensors is crucial.

Measurement methods giving pressure curves

Photo-plethysmography

The Finapress (finger arterial pressure) uses a technique based on work done by Penaz (11). The finger cuff includes a photo-plethysmograph and a combined infra-reduction transmitter and receptor. The wavelength of the light emitted is characteristic of the absorption of haemoglobin, this allowing variations in blood volume to be measured. The principle of this method is to maintain the finger blood volume at a constant level by use of a mini-cuff, whose pressure is regulated according to the light signal received by the receptor (Fig. 3).

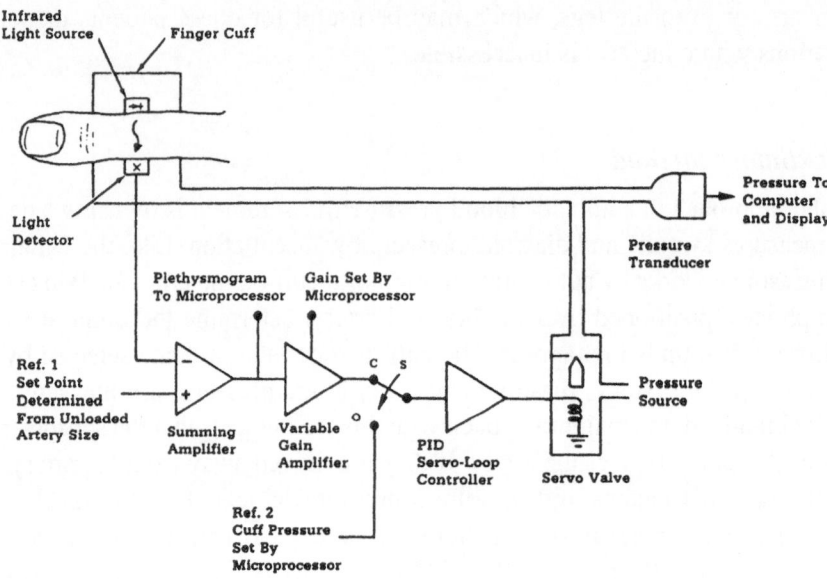

Fig. 3. Block diagram of the servocontrol loop of the Finapress

Initially, the device is set up in an open loop, with the mini-cuff being inflated until the maximum of variations in the recorded light is obtained, this corresponding to the mean blood pressure. Then the device is set up in a closed loop. When the cuff is kept under pressure, this maintains the light signal at a constant value. The maintenance pressure varies according to the digital intra-arterial pressure, this being continuously recorded and indicated. As the pressure of the cuff is equal at all times and opposite to the intra-arterial pressure, the transmural pressure is always zero. In order to take account of any changes in volume that may occur in the finger, the device recalibrates itself regularly about every minute.

The main advantage is that it produces a continuous pressure curve, from which the systolic, diastolic and mean blood pressures and the heart rate can be deduced.

However, there are certain conditions in which the blood pressure measured inexplicably does not correspond with that from traditional methods, particularly under extreme conditions, so many authors consider that this method is not a substitute for traditional methods in all cases.

Cor-medical system

This relatively recent method has not yet been included in many publications. Its principle is as follows: during the heart cycle, the blood pressure varies between a minimum value (diastolic pressure) and a maximum value (systolic pressure) (12). This intra-arterial variation causes the arterial diameter to change and hence the corresponding muscle volume. This device's mode of action rests on two important principles: firstly, the possibility of measuring changes in the muscle volume during the heart cycle and secondly, recognising the relationship linking movement of the arterial wall to the intra-arterial pressure. The volume is measured by a cuff placed over the chosen site for the measurements. Volume changes cause slight differences in the pressure inside the cuff, which are detected by an electropneumatic sensor. The arterial stress/strain relationship is obtained by using the cuff in the same way as in oscillometry with occlusion. It is therefore possible to determine the corresponding variations in arterial volume for the systolic, diastolic and mean blood pressures respectively (Fig. 4). With three points on a curve and the law of variation, it is therefore possible to reconstruct the pressure/movement relationship. The volume variations can therefore be translated into blood pressure variations. The main advantage of this method is that the measurements are made without occluding the blood vessel, under the best possible physiological conditions.

As this is a recent method, it is too soon to be able to comment on whether measurements which are closely linked to the stress/strain curve are valid.

Conclusion

As we have seen, there are many different methods available, which allow not only successive measurements of the systolic, diastolic and mean blood pressures to be made, but also a continuous blood pressure curve with respect to time to be obtained in real time. Research in progress hopes to increase the frequency and reliability of measurements. More sensitive receptors and more powerful software will gradually allow the measurement frequency to be increased. To enhance reliability, some manufacturers consider combining two methods and continually checking which method gives the best concordance between the signal and the sound.

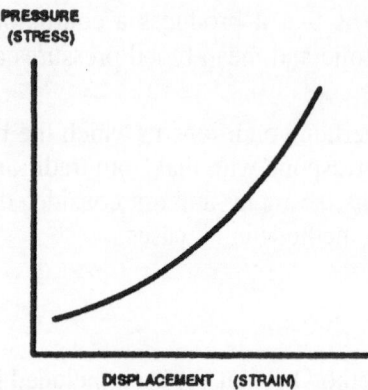

Fig. 4. Artery stress/strain relationship. The curve is determined by the three characteristics points: systolic pressure, mean pressure, and diastolic pressure

Numerous comparisons have been made between the reference method and the different methods described. As a general rule, the correlations are poor, but obviously the measurement conditions are completely different: (i) the sites are distant from each other, (ii) invasive methods measure the pressure inside the artery whereas (iii) noninvasive methods are based on measurements of flow distribution in occluded arteries. Efforts should, in our opinion, particularly be concentrated on making these measurements repeatable under extreme conditions, rather than on correlations which will continue to be open to question for some time to come. Pains have been taken to transfer information from intra-arterial pressure curves to the curves obtained by noninvasive methods.

References

1. Meyer PH (1977) Physiologie humaine. Flammarion, Paris
2. Kirkendall WM, Burton AC et al (1967) Recommendation for human blood pressure determination by sphygmomanometers. Circulation 980
3. Geddes LA (1970) The direct and indirect measurement of blood pressure. Year Book Medical, St. Louis
4. Roy CS, Adami JG (1980) Heartbeat and pulse-wave. Practitioner 45:20
5. Gravenstein JS, Newbower RS et al (1979) Essential non invasive monitoring in anesthesia. Grune and Statton, New York
6. Medasonics Co, 340 Pioneer Way, PO Box M, Mountain View, CA 94042, USA
7. Kimble KJ, Darnall RA et al (1981) An automated oscillometric technique for estimating mean arterial pressure in critically ill newborns. Anesthesiology 54:423-425
8. Francoual M, Himmich H et al (1980) Evaluation d'une méthode oscillométrique de mesure automatique de la pression artérielle. Agressologie 21:157-161

9. Puritan-Bennett Corporation of California, 12655 Beatrice Street, Los Angeles, CA 90086, USA
10. Roche Medical Electronics Division, Hoffman LaRoche, Inc., Cranbury, NJ, USA
11. Penaz J (1973) Photoelectric measurement of blood pressure, volume and flow in the finger. Digest 10th Int Conf Med Biol Eng 104
12. User Manual. COR Medical Catalog Item. 7001-89-80

Noninvasive Cardiac Output Measurements

D. CATHIGNOL, R. MUCHADA, B. LAVANDIER, J. JOSSINET

Doppler ultrasound method

Principle of the measurement

By definition, flow (q) as a function of time, passing through a section of a vessel is written:

$$q(t) = s(t).\bar{v}(t)$$

$s(t)$ is the section of the vessel at time t;
$v(t)$ is the mean velocity of the blood through the whole of the vessel's section (mean spatial velocity), that is the speed which could replace all the different speeds occurring on a section, with the flow remaining the same (Fig. 1).

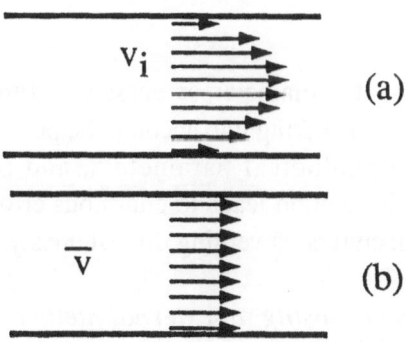

Fig. 1a, b. $\bar{v}$ is defined as the mean velocity which gives the same flow as in **a**

Calculation of the flow q requires measurement of:
- The section at any time
- The mean velocity on the whole of the section at any time

The different techniques on offer differ according to the methods used to measure the section and the velocity and by the measurement site, which can be suprasternal, oesophageal or tracheal.

Measurement of the section

For a circular vessel, the section $s(t)$ is linked to the diameter by:

$$s(t) = \frac{\pi \, d^2(t)}{4}$$

where $d(t)$ is the diameter at time (t).

There are four different possibilities:

Absence of diameter measurement

When this solution is chosen, it is not possible to speak of flow. It has been used for a long time by devices using a suprasternal approach. Light and Cross named it aortovelography (1). If the ascending aorta is the chosen site for measurement of the velocity, it is possible to speak of relative variation in the flow, because the diameter fluctuates little with time. The situation is not the same if the measurement site is the descending aorta, where the aortic diameter varies with time, especially in children.

Use of tables

Tables exist which give the diameter of vessels in function of physiological parameters of an individual. Taking into account the poor correlation between the diameter and the morphological parameters, and the width of standard distributions curves, this solution leads to enormous errors (2). To suggest their use, as do some manufacturers, is verging on dishonesty.

Measurement of diameter using an external method

Measurement of the diameter of a vessel, in which velocity is to be measured is possible either by X-ray or by ultrasound (3, 4). The measured diameter is then taken as constant with time, a fairly accurate assumption for the ascending aorta in adults, but often incorrect for the descending aorta or for children. Measurement of the diameter by X-ray makes the method complicated and measurement by ultrasound on the chosen site can often be tricky. Some authors recommend a compromise, where the diameter of a different artery than the one to be used later is measured, a correction then being made using tables.

Continuous measurement of the diameter

This method becomes a possibility if the ultrasonic transducer is linked to a measuring probe. This method allows both the diameter to be monitored with time and the correct positioning of the probe to be checked. Two methods are available: either directly with the diameter being measured by an ultrasonic time motion system (5), or by measurement of the energy reflected back from the target zone, which varies according to the section of the vessel (6). This last technique is less accurate than the other one, because the variation in the energy reflected back depends on the tissues in between and on the positioning at any one time of the sensor with respect to the different surfaces.

Measurement of blood flow velocity

Measurement of the blood flow velocity is performed using a continuous or pulsed emission Doppler velocimeter.

Doppler effect

Let us consider a vessel and a particle p moving at a speed v. If f_e is the frequency of the ultrasound emitted, it can be shown that the frequency difference between the frequency of the ultrasound emitted and the ultrasound received f_r is called the Doppler frequency, this being written:

$$f_r - f_e = f_d = -\frac{f_e\, v\left(\cos\theta_1 + \cos\theta_2\right)}{c}$$

where c is the speed of the ultrasound which is equal to 1520 m/s in the blood (Fig. 2).

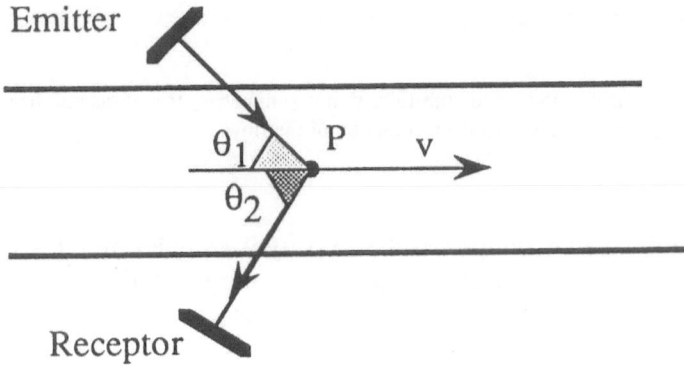

Fig. 2. Principle of the Doppler effect. When the pulsed Doppler system is used, only one transducer is needed. This transducer is used as emitter and receptor

This relationship only allows the velocity to be calculated if the angle θ is known. In the suprasternal method already mentioned, the angle is near 0 degrees and any errors produced by not knowing the exact angle are small. For the oesophageal method, there is a region between the 5th and 6th posterior intercostal space where the oesophagus is practically parallel to the aorta and therefore θ can be known accurately. In the tracheal method, the angle is only known if an X-ray is taken.

Influence of the distribution of the velocity

The speed inside a vessel is not constant over the whole of the section. Using a narrow beam can lead to measurement errors (7). In fact, the operator generally directs the ultrasonic beam in such a way as to obtain the greatest possible deviation. The operating mode inevitably leads to overestimation of the flow at any one moment in time (Fig. 3). In some configurations, the spatial distribution of the flow is not in the axis of symmetry of the vessel, and so the probe is badly positioned.

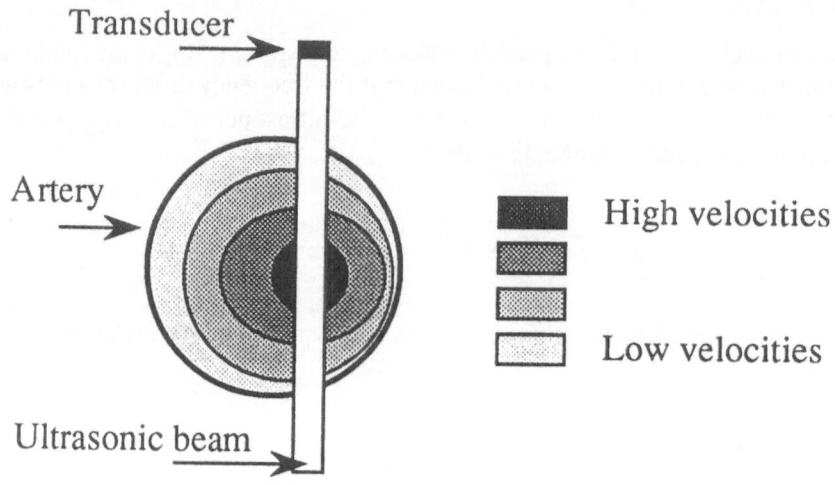

Fig. 3. When the spatial distribution of the flow is not symmetric, the ultrasonic beam is not oriented in the right position, giving an overestimation of the flow

During diastole, the distribution of the velocity is complex and it is possible to have positive, negative and zero velocities at the same time. The surface covered by zero velocity may represent practically the whole of the vessel's area. Nevertheless, if the transducer of the velocimeter is directed towards the red blood cells that are moving, it shows a velocity that unfortunately is multiplied by the total surface of the vessel, greatly overestimating the flow at that moment. This phenomenon is at the origin of highly negative flows at the end of diastole.

Some manufacturers try to solve this by filtering out the low frequencies, but this only masks the problem. A more accurate solution consists of estimating the relationship between the surfaces of the zones in movement with the zones which are still in movement and correcting the measurement according to this relationship (5).

The approach

Suprasternal approach

This technique allows the cardiac blood flow (excluding the coronary arteries) to be measured, because the measurement can be made at the ascending aorta, if the following problems are resolved (1) (Fig. 4).

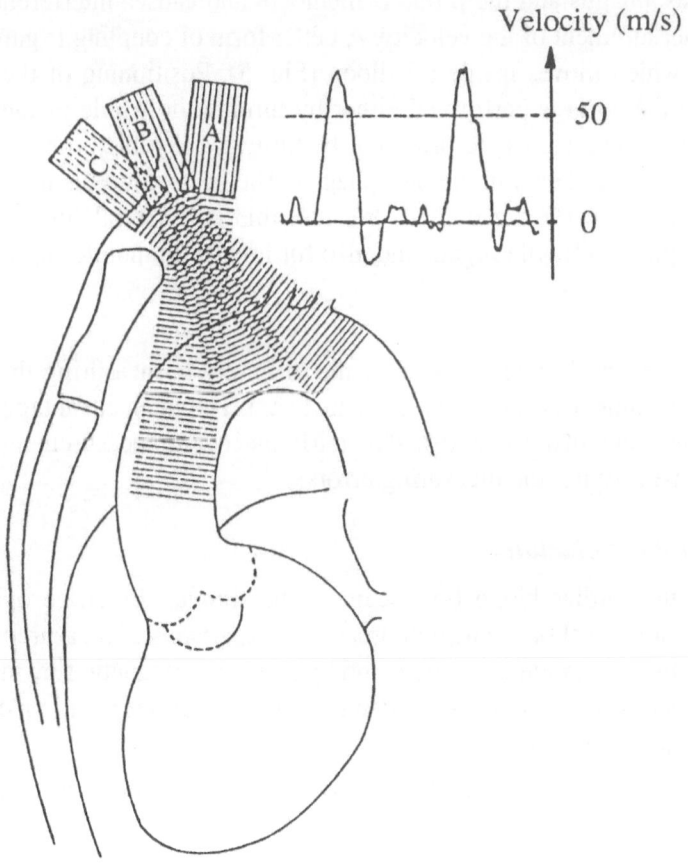

Fig. 4. Using the suprasternal approach, it is theoretically possible to measure the flow in the ascending aorta (transducer position in A), in the descending aorta (C) and to measure the diameter (B)

In general, the problems posed by this method are:

- False estimation of the angle θ because of curving of the aorta
- Poor reproducibility because the velocity is not constant on the whole of the surface of the vessel
- Difficulty in keeping the sensor in place over long periods
- The need to filter out frequencies which correspond to movements of the wall and the valves, especially when a continuous emission velocimeter is used

Oesophageal approach

This was first suggested by J. Reid. The probe is situated facing the descending aorta and the blood flow measured excludes the coronary arteries and the brachiocephalic trunk. As the oesophagus is parallel to the aorta between the 5th and 6th posterior intercostal space, the angle θ is therefore determined by the geometrical position of the probe (5). With an uncovered probe, coupling between the oesophagus and the probe is mediocre and causes interference and errors in the measurement of the velocity. A better form of coupling is gained by using a probe which moves inside a balloon (Fig. 5). Positioning of the probe with respect to the aorta is performed either by turning the whole of the probe inside the oesophagus (uncovered probe) or by turning a flexible probe which is inside a soft immobile sheath in the oesophagus. The last solution is much safer and more comfortable for the patient. We feel this is essential for neonates, whose oesophagus is a fragile organ, and also for long-term monitoring (8).

Tracheal approach

This method is not used much because of the difficulty in measuring the angle between the ascending aorta and the ultrasonic beam. The main advantage is that the probe is cheap and disposable (9). This fairly inaccurate measurement of the diameter increases further the measuring errors.

Discussion and conclusion

Monitoring of the cardiac blood flow seems to be simplest by an oesophageal rather than a suprasternal or tracheal approach. Comparisons of measurement of the blood flow by the oesophageal route and by an electromagnetic flowmeter in the pig, rabbit or dog are excellent provided that the precautions mentioned in the previous paragraphs are taken into account.

Solutions for measurement of the blood flow, which do not include measurement of the diameter or calculate the section from morphological tables, are unsuitable. Association of measurement of the blood flow with other haemodynamic or physiological parameters should allow the clinical condition of the patient to be known more accurately.

Impedance cardiography

Impedance plethysmography has been widely evaluated for monitoring the heart. Efforts have been made to quantify several aspects of cardiac function. The estimation of absolute or relative stroke volume or cardiac output has been studied by many researchers. Measures of left ventricular contractility or vigour have been studied. Techniques used to estimate the severity of mitral or aortic valve regurgitation, monitor changes in thoracic fluid volume, detect patent ductus arteriosus, and aid the management of several clinical conditions have also been evaluated. These applications will be reviewed below after discussing the underlying theory.

Theory

Thoracic impedance measurements are made using a four-electrode technique as illustrated in Fig. 5. A high frequency (> 10 kHz), constant low intensity (< 5 mA) current (i) is injected between circumferential electrodes, one placed high on the neck and another around the abdomen. The voltage difference v(t) produced across the thorax is picked up by two electrodes, one placed around the base of the neck and the other at xyphoid level.

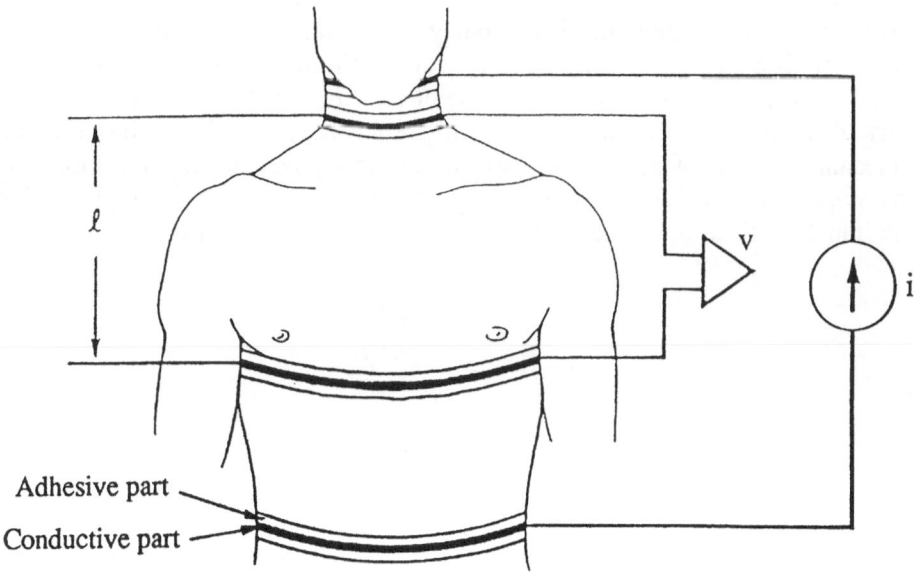

Fig. 5. The circumferential electrode array is generally used for impedance cardiography

The ratio:

$$R(t) = \frac{v(t)}{i}$$

gives the electrical resistance between the two electrodes in function of time.

If we consider a thorax model composed only of two parts: the first one corresponding to the resistance of the chest R_c and the second to the resistance of the aorta approximated as a blood cylinder, we have:

$$R_v(t) = \rho\, l^2\, V(t)$$

Where r is the resistivity of the blood, l the length between the two sensing electrodes and $V(t)$ the time function of the blood volume.

It may be possible to demonstrate, if $V(t)$ is the time volume of blood cylinder that:

$$\Delta V(t) = \frac{-\rho\, l^2\, \Delta R}{R^2(t)} \qquad [1]$$

The time variation of ΔR is given in Fig. 6.

If it can be considered that the velocity stroke wave is constant during the systole and if we consider also that the outflow at the beginning of the systole is not modified by the input flow (equivalent to a perfect compliant artery) then the ratio $\Delta R/\Delta t$ at the beginning of the systole corresponds to the velocity stroke wave, considered as mentioned previously as constant (Fig. 6). To estimate the total variation ΔR that the systolic ejection volume would have given, it is necessary to project the systolic up-slope of the ΔR signal to the end of systole, marked by the dicrotic notch. The difference between this value and the impedance at start of systole corresponds to the equivalent total variation ΔR. The slope of the curve corresponds to the maximal value of the time derivative function $\Delta R/\Delta t$ and the systolic ejection volume is now given by

$$\Delta V = \frac{-\rho\, l^2\, T \left(\dfrac{dR}{dt} \right)_{max}}{R^2} \qquad [2]$$

R is the baseline of the impedance.

The dependence of the stroke volume estimates on the actual flow wave form has been studied. The sensitivity of stroke volume to the rise time and the fall time of the velocity stroke wave form was evaluated. The results show that the wave form can greatly affect the accuracy of stroke volume estimates by Eq. 2.

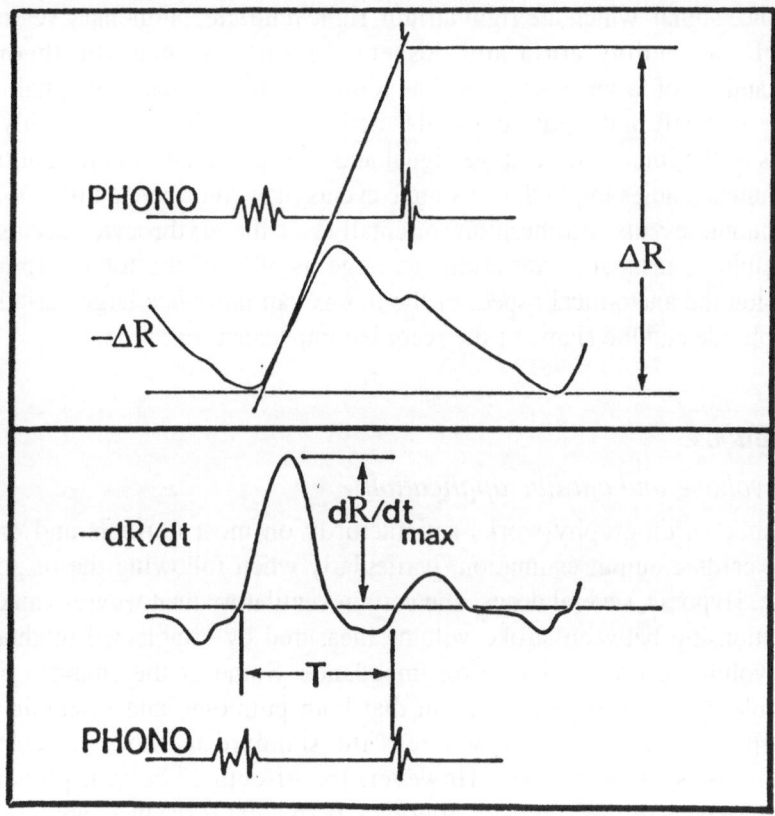

Fig. 6. Time variation and derivative time variation of the electrical impedance during the cardiac cycle

The accuracy of Eq. 2 is also affected by blood resistance or/and fluid collecting in the chest. Stroke volume is particularly sensitive to fluid between the chest wall and the left lung.

What is sampled

Pulsatile blood volume and flow changes are due to every component of the thoracic vasculature from the vena cava to the arteries of the chest wall. How much do the changes in each contribute to the total impedance signal? How variable is the proportion due to each? A number of studies have addressed these questions.

Theoretical, animal, and human studies have been used to define what is sampled and how to predict stroke volume from impedance recordings. The widely used equation for estimating stroke volume from impedance is based on a simple, two-component model, while there are six major contributors to the impedance signal, which are right atrium, right ventricle, pulmonary vessels, left ventricle, ascending aorta and descending aorta. Hence, the theoretical understanding of what is sampled has room for improvement. Animal studies indicate that left and right ventricular activity normally cause roughly equal portions of the impedance change signal and that their relative contribution may vary. Human studies imply that systemic events may contribute a little more than the pulmonic events. Furthermore orientation or the erythrocytes seems to be responsible to resistance variations as large as 50% of the total variation. In conclusion the anatomical aspect of the thorax can introduce large variations of the amplitude and the shape of the recorded impedance variation.

Applications

Stroke volume and cardiac application

Impedance cardiography works satisfactorily on most normals and *only for relative* cardiac output estimation, particularly when following the response to exercise. Hypoxia, several drugs, and certain ventilatory manoeuvres can change the relationship between stroke volume measured by established methods and stroke volume estimates based on impedance. Some of the changes may be explicable based on the observation that both pulmonic and systemic events affect the impedance signal, whereas the standard methods reflect either pulmonic or systemic flows. However, the effects of certain physiologic variables, e.g., inotropy, preload, afterload, peripheral resistance, and/or arterial compliance, appear not to be properly accounted for since physiological changes occasionally lead to low correlation, even within one subject. While good correlation between impedance and reference method cardiac outputs have been reported, enough poor correlations have been reported to cast doubt on the reliability of stroke volume estimates based on impedance. In certain clinically encountered circumstances, this is true even of relative stroke volume estimates by impedance.

Ventricular performance evaluation

For clinical management, it is often desirable to evaluate ventricular performance, particularly during exercise in response to treatment. The appropriate measure of ventricular performance depends on the application. Myocardial contractility can be defined using velocity length-tension diagrammes; however, global measures of performance are often preferred.

A number of indexes for estimating ventricular performances have been derived from the thoracic impedance signal. The height of the impedance derivative and the time between characteristic points have been used, separately and in combination, as indexes of ventricular performances. The indexes generally used are:

$$\left(\frac{dz}{dt}\right)_{max},$$

the time between the R_{wave} to the $\left(\dfrac{dz}{dt}\right)_{max}$,

the Heather index defined by $\dfrac{\left(\dfrac{dR}{dt}\right)_{max}}{\left[R_{wave}-\left(\dfrac{dR}{dt}\right)_{max}\right]\text{interval}}$,

and the STI intervals measured from the impedance curves.

It is important to note that the correlation between the STI measured by the impedance cardiography correlate with those measured using the triple trace method (ECG, phonocardiogram and carotid pulse).

Other uses and methods

Additional uses for thoracic impedance measurements have been investigated, such as thoracic fluid monitoring, aortic and mitral regurgitation, evaluating cardiovascular response, guiding treatment of patent ductus arteriosus, monitoring respiration, and so on.

Conclusion

Thoracic impedance measurements made with band electrodes around the neck and torso have been used by many investigators. Clinical studies have evaluated the utility of impedance recordings in a number of situations. Conflicting results have been reported concerning its accuracy for stroke volume estimation, and this implies that impedance stroke volume estimates will be unreliable in a small percentage of patients. Never may impedance cardiography be considered as a cardiac blood flowmeter. Only relative variations may be recorded. Characteristic points can often be identified in the impedance derivative which reliably correspond to physiologic events, e.g., the start of ejection. The timing of these points and the shape of the impedance derivative should be useful for the early diagnosis of ventricular decompensation and for quantifying mitral or aortic valve regurgitation. The baseline impedance and changes therein are useful for monitoring the thoracic fluid volume. These abilities may make it a valuable addition to stress testing and decision making in critical care patients.

References

1. Cross G, Light LH (1974) Non invasive intra-thoracic blood velocity measurement in the assessment of cardiovascular function. Biomed Eng 464-470
2. Klotz KF et al (1995) Continuous measurement of cardiac output during aortic cross-clamping by oesophageal Doppler monitor O.D.M. 1. Br J Anesth 74:655-660
3. Lang-Jensen T, Berning J, Jacobsen E (1983) Stroke volume measured by pulsed ultrasound Doppler and M. Mode echocardiography. Acta Anaesthesiol Scand 27:454-457
4. Kumar A et al (1989) Non invasive measurement of cardiac output during surgery using a new C.W. Doppler oesophageal probe. Am J Cardiol 64:793-798
5. Lavandier B, Cathignol D et al (1985) Non invasive aortic blood flow measurement using an intraoesophageal probe. Ultrasound Med Biol 11(3):451-460
6. Evans JM, Skidmore R, Luckman NP, Wells PNT (1989) A new approach to the noninvasive measurement of cardiac output using an annular array Doppler technique-I. Theoretical considerations and ultrasonic fields. Ultrasound Med Biol 15(3):169-178
7. Vieli A, Jenni R, Anliker M (1986) Spatial velocity distributions in the ascending aorta of healthy humans and cardiac patients. IEEE Trans Biomed Eng BME-33(1):28
8. Lavandier B, Muchada R et al (1991) Assessment of a potentially non invasive method for monitoring aortic blood flow in children. Ultrasound Med Biol 17(2):107-116
9. Abrams JH, Weber RE et al (1989) Transtracheal Doppler: a new procedure for continuous cardiac output measurement. Anesthesiology 70(1):134-138
10. Penney BC (1986) Theory and cardiac applications of electrical impedance measurements. CRC Crit Rev Biomed Eng 13(3):227-281
11. Lamberts R, Visser KR, Zijlstra WG (1984) Impedance cardiography. Van Gorcum, Assen

Haemodynamic Profile and PetCO$_2$ Monitoring in Patients at Risk

R. MUCHADA

Introduction

Haemodynamic profile

Non-invasive haemodynamic profile monitoring can be performed nowadays thanks to a device recently introduced on the market, the Dynemo 3000 Sometec (1). The combination of a 10 mHz ultrasonic echo scan and a 5 mHz Doppler velocimeter connected to an endo-oesophageal probe allows continuous measurement of the aortic diameter and of the blood flow velocity in the descending aorta. These two parameters not only make measurement of the aortic blood flow (ABF) possible, but also accurate and reproducible (2), avoiding some of the criticism made of this technique (3).

The addition of external devices (electrocardiogram and sphygmomanometer) provides the signals and data necessary for obtaining a non-invasive haemodynamic profile, which includes information on the ABF and factors affecting its regulation (afterload, left ventricular contractility, heart rate, and electrical intracardiac conduction and stimulation) (4).

Preload cannot be assessed directly, but can be calculated indirectly by continual analysis of the evolution of the different parameters or by a filling test under continuous monitoring of the haemodynamic data.

End tidal CO$_2$ pressure (PetCO$_2$)

Although this monitoring allows haemodynamic changes to be seen, no information is obtained on the final function of the cardiovascular system, that is, *tissue perfusion*.

For this reason, by integration of the recorded variations of PetCO$_2$ into the cardiovascular profile, an attempt can be made to provide additional information in order to ascertain if an improvement in the haemodynamic conditions helps to maintain tissue perfusion (5). The following facts justify this integration:

Expired CO$_2$ is produced by metabolism and is the result of O$_2$ consumption in the mitochondria. After several enzymic reactions, the cycle ends with the production of ATP, heat, H$_2$O and CO$_2$. Thanks to its specific characteristics and to a pressure gradient, CO_2 diffuses easily into the interstitial space and into the venous capillaries. If perfusion is sufficient, the CO_2 is transported, to be eliminated by the ventilated lungs. In the absence of perfusion, the remaining intracellular O_2 (PcellularO_2 = 40 mmHg) allows aerobic metabolism to be maintained in the mitochondria (PmitochondrialO_2 = 4 mmHg) for a short period of time. During this time, CO_2 continues to be produced. In the absence of perfusion, the CO_2 produced accumulates in the intracellular interstitial spaces and the venous capillaries, followed by a reduction in the PetCO$_2$ (6).

When normal perfusion is restored after a brief period of hypoperfusion, a wash out phenomenon occurs with an increase in expiratory CO_2 excretion. This then produces an increase in the PetCO$_2$. Variations in the PetCO$_2$ are generally used as a parameter in respiratory monitoring, but when combined with simultaneously recorded ABF variations or changes in other circulatory parameters, they can provide an index of tissue perfusion, as long as certain restricted observation conditions are observed (stable metabolism, stable alveolar ventilation, no large changes in the ventilation-perfusion ratio ($\dot{V}/Q$) as calculated by the arteriolar/PetCO$_2$ gradient [P(a-et) CO$_2$]).

Variation in the P(a-et)CO$_2$ has been described as being the main factor responsible for variations in PetCO$_2$ under stable metabolic and ventilation conditions (7). However, if the measurement of this gradient is to remain reliable, reproducible and useful, a number of fundamental rules need to be adhered to. The sucker of the side stream capnograph should be positioned as close as possible to the patient's respiratory tract, so that artefacts caused by an increase in the dead space (intratubular compression volume and reduced in true alveolar ventilation produced by variations in lung compliance) can be avoided. In addition, the capnograph should be calibrated using the same gas mixture as that used to calibrate the apparatus used by the laboratory to measure the blood gases. Finally, the blood sample for measuring PaCO$_2$, which is needed for calculating the gradient, should be taken using a glass syringe and should be tested less than 5 min after sampling. The blood sample must be taken during a period of stability as regards ventilation, metabolism and circulation.

Variations in the ABF-PetCO$_2$

When the variations in ABF and PetCO$_2$ are observed simultaneously, three main modifications may be detected:

1. A rapid drop in the PetCO$_2$ without change in the ABF. This is due mainly to an alteration in the alveolar ventilation or a problem with the ventilatory device.
2. A slow, gradual drop in both PetCO$_2$ and ABF followed by stabilization. This is often seen under general anaesthesia (GA) and may be the result of a gradual slowing of the cellular metabolism caused by the GA.
3. A rapid simultaneous drop of both the PetCO$_2$ and the ABF. Taking into account the restricted observation conditions described above, this fall should

be interpreted as an alteration in tissue perfusion. These are the most interesting variations for our monitoring of the haemodynamic and PetCO$_2$ profile. These changes should be rapid (occurring in less than 5 min) and in order to be recorded, the drop of the PetCO$_2$ should be at least 10% to 15% from the initial value. Once again, it should be underlined that the changes should be analysed in patients without any variation in the ventilatory status. In our own experience, standard ventilation with a tidal volume (V$_t$) of 8 ml/kg at a frequency of 12 cycles/min, in patients without any respiratory disease, allows the PetCO$_2$ to be maintained between 32 and 36 mmHg. This means that even without any drop in the PetCO$_2$, the observation of a PetCO$_2$ less than 30 mmHg in patients being ventilated according to the constants recommended in the previous paragraph already suggests that there is an alteration in tissue perfusion. This can be confirmed by haemodynamic monitoring of ABF.

General anaesthesia and non-invasive haemodynamic-PetCO$_2$ monitoring

Combined haemodynamic and capnographic monitoring has proved its usefulness during GA to diagnose, treat and observe evolution of cardiovascular changes and alterations in tissue perfusion.

This technique, which is adapted to the monitoring requirements under GA, is especially useful because it is non-invasive, easy to use, measures continuously and produces objective results.

One of the main advantages with this monitoring technique is that it allows a rapid, accurate and early diagnosis of any haemodynamic changes, in particular myocardial failure due to the anaesthetic, thanks to the integration of systolic time intervals (STI) into the haemodynamic profile.

A treatment which is adapted to each clinical situation can therefore be administered and the effects can be monitored by the gradual haemodynamic and PetCO$_2$ changes. This method avoids the use of an empirical treatment, which is sometimes recommended during GA.

It also allows one of the fundamental aims of GA, protection of the patient against the autonomic nervous system reaction (stress), to be met thanks to a sufficient level of anaesthesia being maintained and to extrinsic compensation of the cardiovascular alterations.

Thus, systematic observation between January 1989 and January 1993 of 585 patients aged over 50 years old under GA (382) operated for peripheral arterial disease, 112 on the gastrointestinal tract, 62 orthopaedic operations and 19 gynaecological operations under balanced GA; induction: propofol 2 mg/kg, phenoperidine 0.014 mg/kg, Norcuron 0.7 mg/kg; maintenance isoflurane at 1% (inspired concentration), phenoperidine 0.014 mg/kg/h and recurarization with

0.3 mg/kg Norcuron every 60 min; stable ventilation (12 cycles/min, V_t 8 ml/kg, FiO_2 0.4, FiN_2O 0.6) allowed haemodynamic and capnographic alterations to be detected, so that suitable action could be taken. Out of all of the patients, 281 (48%) had myocardial depression around 20 min after introduction of the isoflurane, with a haemodynamic profile which included a drop in the ABF, in stroke volume (SV) and in the mean arterial blood pressure (MAP) with an increase of the pre-ejection period (PEPi), of the PET/left ventricular ejection time (LVET) ratio and total systemic vascular resistances (TSVR). At the same time, the $PetCO_2$ was reduced by about 15% compared with the level observed after ventilation has been stabilized.

All of the patients received dobutamine (mean dose of 4 mcg/kg/min) after checking that there was no hypovolaemia. The results were positive for all of the patients treated, except for 11 of them (3.9%) who, under dobutamine perfusion, had an increase in heart rate (HR), a slight increase in the ABF and a shortening below the normal level of the PEPi and the PEP/LVET ratio, but without correction of the $PetCO_2$ and without significant change or even a reduction in the SV. These changes were interpreted as the result of a positive beta-1 action acting by stretching the myocardial fibres but without producing adequate shortening during systole. In this small group of 11 patients, the association of enoximone allowed the hoped-for haemodynamic response to be obtained and hypocapnia to be corrected.

This series of 585 patients, who were selected from a total of more than 6500 patients having a GA and monitored by this technique between 1986 and 1995, is presented here just as a specific example of the cardiovascular variations that can be diagnosed and treated by this method.

Non-invasive haemodynamic monitoring-PetCO$_2$ in intensive care

The same system is used in the intensive care unit. Our experience in this setting is much more limited because up until now, it has only been used for a smaller number of patients (about 650).

It is particularly useful because of the detailed characteristics mentioned above and especially for the speed with which the user can diagnose cardiovascular alterations, notably in shock. In patients presenting with clinical haemodynamic alterations, this non-invasive examination allows results to be obtained in less than 10 min that help the diagnosis to be made, to decide on the treatment, and once the treatment has been started, to assess its effect.

This is of course not suitable for continuous long-term monitoring, but allows the changes in parameters to be followed over several hours as long as the ultrasound probe is kept in the right position. Any alteration in the position of the sensors should be corrected manually by turning the handle on the oesophageal probe. This requires there being staff present who are used to operating this noninvasive haemodynamic device. Monitoring can continue without any problem for long periods (8 to 12 h in our experience), but taking into account the ease with which it is set up, it is perfectly possible to monitor for shorter periods and to reinstall the device if there is clinical suspicion or observation of haemodynamic alterations.

It is therefore interesting to comment on non-invasive haemodynamic monitoring of a series of 18 patients in septic shock who were admitted to our intensive care unit. This is summarized in Table 1.

Table 1. The continuous and non-invasive haemodynamic and PetCO2 monitoring determined a radical change on the treatment in those patients with a clinical and biological shock syndrome

Septic and cardiogenic shock- ICU (1991-1994)
non-invasive haemodynamic monitoring

Patients	M	W	Age	Septic shock	Cardiogenic shock
18	13	5	72 ± 8	12	6

Septic shock
N = 12
Etiology

Aortic surgery	Laparoscopy	Acute Pancreatitis	Pneumonia
6	1	1	4

Blood culture = 8 G – / 3 Gram + / 1 Gram + and –

Primary treatment

Dobut	Dopamine	Dobut + Dopamine
1	5	6

Secondary treatment after
non-invasive haemodynamic study

Dobut	Dopamine	Dobut + Dopamine	Norep	Norep + Dobut
0	1	0	2	5

Norep + ß-blockers
4

Hospitalisation: mean = 15 days (max = 62 days, min = 11 days)
Evolution = survivors = 11   Deaths = 1 (ARDS)

Cardiogenic shock
N = 6
Etiology

Myocardial infarction	Cardiac arrest	Cardiac failure
4	1	1

Primary treatment

Dobut	Dopamine	Dobut + dopamine	(+ Trinitrine)
5	0	1	6

Secondary treatment after
non-invasive haemodynamic study

Dobut + trinitrine	Dobut + norep	Dobut + perfane
2	2	2

Hospitalisation: mean = 6 days (max = 8 days, min = 4 days)
Evolution = survivors = 5   Deaths = 1 (cardiac failure)

Dobut, dobutamine; Norep, norepinephrine

The analysis summarized in Table 1 brings up a number of points which are worth commenting on.

1. Non-invasive haemodynamic exploration allows a rapid accurate diagnosis of cardiovascular alterations to be made.

2. Non-invasive haemodynamic monitoring of patients in intensive care led to modification of the treatment in most cases, which produced a rapid correction of the haemodynamic changes and secondary stabilization.

3. The primary choice of treatment (beta-mimetics alone or associated with other drugs) was altered and the use of beta-1 mimetics and/or vasoconstrictors allowed the flow/pressure balance to be restored and good renal function to be recovered (return of diuresis and probably of tissue perfusion, although the changes in $PetCO_2$, which is used like a label of tissue perfusion under GA, need confirmation in intensive care patients).

4. The use of beta-blockers in certain types of shock seems difficult to be admit; however, some of our patients benefited from this treatment.

5. All the patients showed a haemodynamic improvement and a good secondary evolution. In five patients, the length of the hospital stay was over 15 days, as a result of secondary complications. There were unfortunately two deaths on the 6th and 8th day after improvement of haemodynamic parameters; one from end-stage cardiac failure and the other from a pyocyanic bacterial lung infection which caused irreversible acute respiratory failure.

Comments about the patients with septic shock treated with beta-blockers

These four patients had all the clinical characteristics of septic shock syndrome and were under stable mechanical ventilation.

The basic treatment was begun by intravenous fluid replacement and an association of beta-mimetics: dopamine (10 ± 2mcg/kg/min) and dobutamine (8 ± 3 mcg/kg/min). Haemodynamic non-invasive monitoring showed a uniform profile for the four patients with a decreased ABF, a near normal MAP, and a high total systemic vascular resistance (TSVR), but the four patients had tachycardia, over 150 b/min with a low SV and a PEPi and a PEP/LVET ratio below normal.

The tachycardia, reduction of SV and the shortening of the PEPi and PEP/LVET ratio caused by the beta-mimetics suggested stopping them temporarily. This was followed by a noticeable reduction in the TSVR and of the MAP, a slight reduction in the ABF, but a persistently shortened PEPi and PEP/LVET ratio, continued tachycardia and a reduced SV.

These four patients therefore received a noradrenaline infusion at a mean dose of 0.75 ± 0.25 mcg/kg/min which helped to increase the MAP and the TSVR. But tachycardia and a shortened PEPi and PEP/LVET ratio persisted. The SV remained low.

Under these circumstances, an endogenous beta-mimetic stimulation should be evoked. This possibility was based on the fact that there was persistent tachycardia, shortening of PEPi and PEP/LVET ratio and a tendency to vasoplegia when dopamine was stopped.

In this situation, use of a beta-blocker may be considered, to reduce the HR, increase the left ventricular filling time, increase the isometric contraction time, improve systolic emptying (increasing the SV), and reduce the left ventricular parietal tension, allowing an improvement in coronary blood flow and a drop in the MvO$_2$, and finally to improve the ABF and tissue perfusion.

There are of course two risks to take into account:

1. Myocardial depression can occur with beta-blockers, but in our observation, endogenous beta stimulation was sufficient to avoid this.
2. The aggravation of arterial hypotension under beta-blockers actions did not help the blood flow to be evenly distributed. This situation could be counterbalanced by adding noradrenaline.

The beta-blocker used (Esmolol-Brevibloc) has some special characteristics, in particular its very short half-life which gives it a short duration of action. This means that the situation can be reversed quickly in the case of major haemodynamic upset.

In the group of four patients, the dose used was 0.5 mg/kg as a bolus, followed by an infusion at a mean dose of 10 ± 2 mcg/kg/min. The infusion continued for a minimum of 10 h and a maximum of 70 h. The treatment was stopped after gradually reducing the infusion by 2 mcg/h.

Follow-up of the haemodynamic profile showed a favourable response to the treatment used (increase in ABF, stable TSVR, no changes in the MAP, reduction in the HR, and increase in the PEPi and of the PEP/LVET ratio).

This haemodynamic recovery was accompanied by a gradual marked increase in the PetCO$_2$ in those patients whose ventilation remained stable. This increase in the PetCO$_2$ could indicate a recovery of tissue perfusion, this being confirmed at least in the kidney by the return of diuresis.

Figure 1 shows the gradual changes in the haemodynamic parameters and the PetCO$_2$ in one of the patients in this small series.

The treatment used could be proposed because the haemodynamic changes were followed up with the continuous and non-invasive monitoring, allowing suitable cardiovascular and general evolution of the patients to be demonstrated.

However, such a decision should be based only on an objective pathophysiological diagnosis and the good results obtained in this small series of patients need to be confirmed by larger studies in the future.

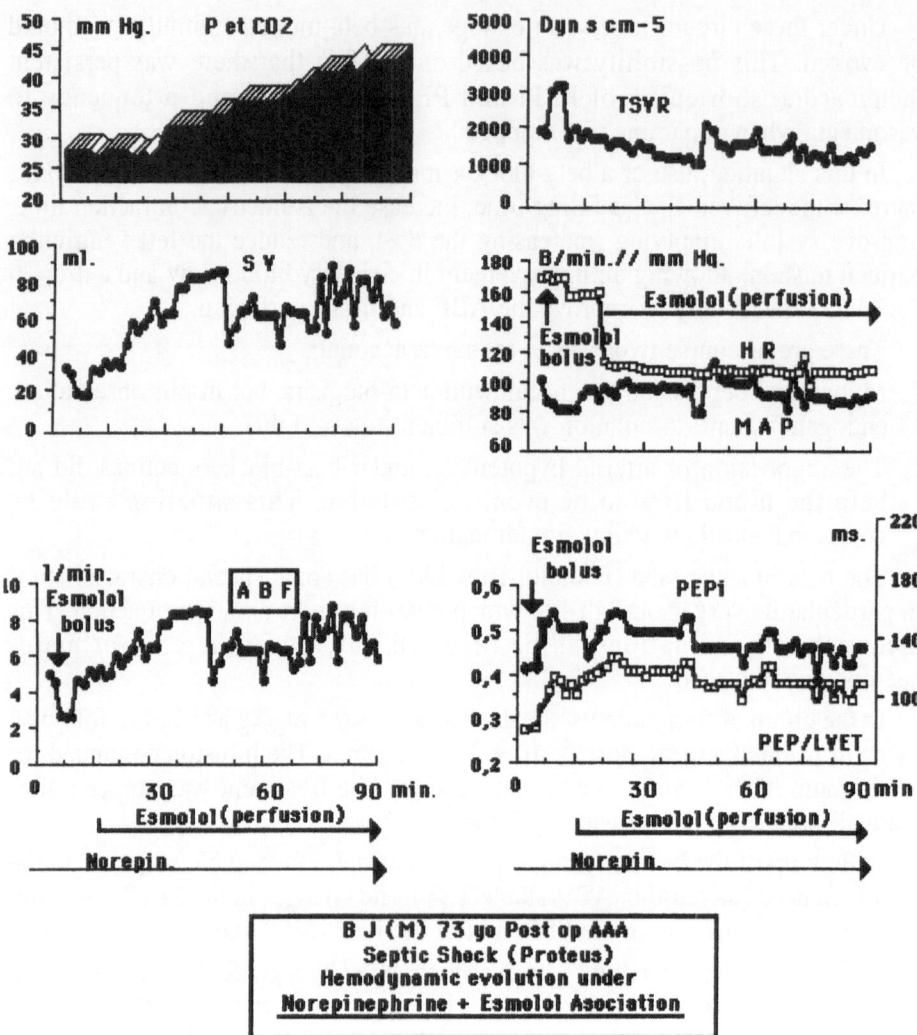

ABF, aortic blood flow; *HR*, heart rate; *SV*, stroke volume; *MAP*, mean arterial pressure; *TSVR*, total systemic vascular resistances; *PEPi*, pre ejection period; *LVET*, left ventricular ejection time; *PEP/LVET*, PEP-LVET ratio; *PetCO₂*, end tidal CO_2 pressure

Fig. 1. Non-invasive haemodynamic profile of a patient with septic shock treated with the association of norepinephrine (*Norepin.*) - esmolol. After stopping the initial treatment (dopamine 10 mcg/kg/min - dobutamine 8 mcg/kg/min), he did not have any modification of the PEPi, PEP/LVET ratio and the HR. The norepinephrine perfusion keeps a correct MAP, but without improvement of the other haemodynamic parameters. The use of a beta-blocker increased the PEPi and the PEP/LVET ratio, but decreased HR. This fact was followed up by an increase of ABF, SV, and of the PetCO₂. This improvement of the cardiovascular and tissue perfusion situation should be determined by the break of an endogenous ß stimulation, allowing a correct left ventricular filling. The recovery of the SV and of the ABF with constant TSVR ensure, thanks to a stable perfusion pressure, an adequate tissue perfusion, seen by the increase of the PetCO₂

Conclusion

The benefit of non-invasive haemodynamic monitoring and of the $PetCO_2$ in patients at risk can be summarized by the following points:

1. Possibility of access to a rapid objective non-invasive diagnosis of haemodynamic and tissue perfusion modifications.

2. Monitoring of the haemodynamic profile including information on the ABF and on the factors involved in its regulation, particularly on left ventricular contractility (STI).

3. Preload cannot be assessed directly but can be evaluated either by analytical deduction from the changes in the various parameters, or by a filling test under haemodynamic non-invasive control.

4. Simultaneous monitoring of the $PetCO_2$ under restricted observation conditions gives clear information on the state of tissue perfusion during GA and would also seem useful in intensive care, but this fact needs to be confirmed by other larger, more thorough comparative studies.

5. The diagnosis, the choice of a treatment and continuous follow-up of cardiovascular and tissue perfusion evolution has gradually and simply become accessible with this new approach to non-invasive monitoring.

References

1. Lavandier B, Muchada R, Chignier E, Fady JF, Birer A, Cathignol D (1991) Assessment of a potentially noninvasive method for monitoring aortic blood flow in children. Ultrasound Med Biol 17:107-112
2. Muchada R, Rinaldi A, Lavandier B, Cathignol D (1992) Echo doppler transesofageo nel bambino: importanza dell'esatta misura del diametro aortico e delle sue variazioni nel tempo per il calcolo della gittata aortica. Minerva Anestesiol 58:347-355
3. Kamel DG, Symreng T, Starr J (1990) Inconsistent oesophageal doppler cardiac output during acute blood loss. Anesthesiology 75:95-103
4. Muchada R, Rinaldi A, Verenier F, Fady JF, Lavandier, Cathignol D (1990) Monitorizzazione emodinamica non invasiva attraverso l'integrazione dei dati ottenuti con l'ECG, con il flusso aortico mediante sonda esofagea Doppler e con pletismografia digitale. Minerva Anestesiol 50:147-156
5. Brunel D, Muchada R (1991) Evaluation de la perfusion tissulaire par surveillance simultanée du débit aortique et de la capnographie. Presse Med 20:1665-1666
6. Gazmuri RJ, von Planta M, Weil MH, Rackow EC (1989) Arterial PCO_2 as an indicator of systemic perfusion during CPR. Crit Care Med 17:237-240
7. Sholomo A. (1991) Can changes in end tidal PCO_2 measure changes in cardiac output? Anesth Analg 73:808-881

TRAUMA OPERATIVE PROCEDURES (T.O.P.)

The Development of the Trauma System: Epidemiological Data

G. Berlot, M. Viviani, M. Soiat

Introduction

In the developed countries, trauma is the main cause of death in people younger than 30 years (1). In Italy alone, more than 8000 people die every year within the first year following a car crash. Many classical retrospective studies demonstrated that the mortality of trauma patients has a trimodal distribution (1): roughly 50% of them die in the first hour after the initial event, due to injuries incompatible with life: thus, it appears that an improved survival of this group of patients is more based on the adoption of preventive measures including speed limits, airbags, helmets etc. than to medical intervention. Another 30% of patients die within few hours after the trauma, due to factors which are, at least partially, preventable, including delays in the rescue, in the triage and in the transportation to referral centers, missed or underevaluated lesions etc. It is likely that the outcome of many of them could be improved by a more comprehensive resuscitative strategy, as well by the improvement of either out-of-hospital and in-hospital management. The remaining deaths are due to delayed and indirect complications of the initial event, generally associated with the development of sepsis and multiple organ dysfunction syndrome (MODS). It is conceivable that in these patients, too, an early and aggressive treatment could reduce the mortality, because the factors responsible for sepsis and its associated cardiorespiratory and metabolic derangements are probably present from the very early posttraumatic phase (see later).

From the data outlined above, it appears that (a) the appropriate treatment of trauma patients should be target-oriented against either the more immediate life-threatening alterations and their delayed consequences and (b) due to heterogeneity of factors which can influence the individual clinical settings and the final outcome, including the age, the presence of coexisting diseases, the assumption of drugs etc., trauma patients should be managed by experienced teams, particularly committed to the care of patients with multiple and severe pathophysiological derangements.

When looking at the epidemiological data deriving from trauma patients, we believe that, besides the rough numbers deriving from a merely statistical analysis (how many patients/year, sex, age etc.), it is necessary to recognize (a) if the existing system is sufficient or needs some implementation(s), and (b) if, where and when potentially harmful management errors occur.

The validation of a trauma system

As it happens in every field of medicine, the simplest way to evaluate the efficacy of an intervention is to compare its effects in a treated and in an untreated group. Dealing with trauma patients, the management of the victims by a skilled team during either the out-of-hospital and in-hospital phase can be considered the intervention whose efficacy is under evaluation. Many factors influence the final outcome, so modifying the epidemiology of trauma. It should be recalled that the prehospital treatment affects the final result of a process, which includes the alert of the emergency system, the dispatch of the trauma team and its arrival on the scene. Every delay in the first phases can influence both the short- and long-term outcome. The early in-hospital treatment is another key moment: the immediate treatment of trauma patients is typically multidisciplinary, involving many specialists, with often conflicting views about the diagnostic and therapeutic priorities. Moreover, experiences deriving from different socioeconomic conditions are not always comparable; a classical example of this latter obstacle is the different rate of penetrating injury among American and European trauma patients.

Thus, we think that the effects of a trauma system should be evaluated on a step-by-step basis, starting with the out-of-hospital phase.

The prehospital phase

The clinical approach to trauma patients has changed during the last 20 years. All over Europe, a number of emergency systems have been implemented, whose main aims were (a) to assess the patients' conditions and to provide the basic, and somewhere, the advanced life support care and (b) to move the injured patients to the more appropriate hospital (2).

Several investigations have been published in Europe and in the USA, which addressed the impact of the improved prehospital trauma care on the survival of injured patients.

To assess the effects of a trauma system, recently Sauaia et al. (3) compared patients included in a previous study (1977) with those treated in 1992, after the implementation of the system. Although the mechanisms of injury, the demographics and the cause of death were not changed, the number of early deaths was reduced and there was an increased number of late deaths related with brain injuries and MODS. Interestingly, the already described, trimodal distribution of death was no more apparent. The authors ascribed these effects to the earlier care and to the improved access to the hospital facilities. Other investigators demonstrated a three-fold increase survival rate in patients after a 50-m fall (with an estimated impact speed of 98 km/h) (4) after the implementation of a prehospital trauma system manned with paramedics. An improved prognosis, which has been attributed to a better trauma care, has been observed even among elderly patients, who are considered more prone to injury-related systemic complications (5).

Also the use of the emergency medical helicopter service (EMHS) provides a good example of the impact of training on trauma-related mortality. A previous American study demonstrated that for injured patients transported by air either from the scene of the accident or from a peripheral hospital to a trauma center the deteminant factor was not constituted by the speed of the transport but by the improved quality of care provided by the EMHS team (6).

More recently, another study compared two different EHMS systems, located in the USA and in Germany, respectively (7). The American team was made up of nurses and paramedics whereas the German team included a trauma surgeon, experienced in airway management and thoracic decompression. The patients were comparable in terms of severity of injuries (assessed with the injury severity score, ISS), mechanisms of injury, age and time of flight. The overall mortality was slightly lesser among German patients (9.5% vs 11.3, p:n.s.); in particular, in this group, there were fewer early deaths, and the authors attributed these results to the better airway and ventilation management provided by the flight surgeon. In a recent study, Nardi et al. (8) assessed the impact of EHMS on survival by comparing three groups of trauma patients, treated by paramedics on a load-and-go basis (Group A), by emergency physicians with basic life support (BLS) (Group B) and by experienced intensive care specialists, with 10 years of experience in the management of critically ill trauma patients (Group C). Patients of the three groups were similar in terms of ISS, mechanisms of injury and age. In-hospital mortality was 38% in group A, 32% in group B and 12% in group C ($p < 0.005$ A vs C and $p < 0.05$ B vs C, respectively). Analyzing the possible causes of these results, the authors observed that the mean rescue time (i.e. the time elapsed from the first emergency call and the arrival at the trauma center) was longest in Group A, shortest in group B and intermediate in group C (162, 28 and 55 min, respectively) and concluded that the speed of rescue did not play a major role in the improved mortality. Instead, in this group there was a higher rate of immediate tracheal intubation, volume resuscitation was more aggressive and pneumothoraces were more frequently recognized and decompressed.

The aggressive prehospital volume resuscitation has been recently questioned by Brickell et al. (9), who observed, after penetrating torso injuries, a better outcome and less postoperative complications in hypotensive patients rushed directly to the emergency ward, compared with those volume-resuscitated in the prehospital phase. Surprisingly, the untreated patients presented a mean increase in their systolic arterial pressure of 41 mmHg (from 72 to 113 mmHg) in the interval from their arrival to the trauma center and the entry into the operating room. The authors hypothesized that the worse prognosis of the treated group could be attributed to the increased blood loss due to the volume resuscitation. Actually, there is some experimental evidence suggesting that attempts to increase the arterial pressure during uncontrolled bleeding is associated with inceased blood loss, hemodilution, with the consequent reduction of the hemoglobin and coagulation factors, and mortality (10).

It is not clear if the same experimental and clinical considerations could be applied for patients with blunt torso injury, much more common in European countries, who are currently treated with volume resuscitation via two or more large-bore peripheral i.v. lines, according to the guidelines established by the American College of Surgeons (AMC) through its Advanced Trauma Life Support (ATLS) course.

The inhospital phase

The hospital treatment of trauma patients include two fundamental, contemporary steps. The first can be considered a temporal extension of the management protocol used in the prehospital phase and includes the definitive management of the airways and the correction of hypovolemia/anemia. The second consists in the thorough research of surgical indications, including possible sources of bleeding, intracranial hematomas and bone and soft tissue injuries. Evaluating the results obtained in seriously injured patients (mean ISS 30.1) treated in a well organized trauma system, van der Sluis et al. (11) reported a mortality rate of 25.7%, which was principally associated with the advanced age and severe head and cervical lesions. Half of the survivors were discharged home and the rest was transferred to rehabilitation units, mainly due to the sequelae of neurologic injuries. In a series of 83 severely traumatic fall patients (mean ISS = 29.1), we observed a mortality of 51%; however, most of deaths occurred immediately after the admission, while the diagnostic investigations were still running or in the first 24 h: in both cases, severe head trauma, in some patients in association with extensive retroperitoneal bleeding (unpublished data), was responsible for the death. Actually, in outpatients, shock at the admission (considered as a systolic arterial pressure < 90 mmHg) was positively correlated with death ($p < 0.05$), probably indicating that the prehospital treatment was inadequate in most of cases. In the above mentioned study Fortner et al. (4) were able to demonstrate that the improvement in survival in a similar population was associated to a more aggressive prehospital treatment. In our patients, like in other series (1, 3, 11), most of late deaths were due to the development of sepsis and MODS. This latter point deserves particular attention, because the occurrence of infection and sepsis has been associated to different factors, which can be at least partially reduced by a better in-hospital management. First, trauma patients are particularly prone to infections, due to contaminated wounds, tracheal aspiration and nonsterile invasive procedures performed on the scene (especially insertion of large-bore intravenous cannulae etc.). Second, a number of immunologic abnormalities have been described following trauma and hemorrhage, probably associated with the release of endogenous immunodepressing substances (12, 13). Third, several investigations demonstrated that in critically ill septic and trauma patients the reduction of the splanchnic perfusion is reduced from the early postinjury phase, as reflected by a low gastric intramucosal pH (pHi) and that persistently low values are associated with a worse prognosis (14-17). This finding has been correlated with the escape of bacteria or bacteria-derived substances from the gut lumen into the bloodstream: Rush et al. (18) observed a high rate of positive blood cultures in 56% of trauma patients in shock within 3 h after admission, in some cases associated with endotoxemia. Reed et al. (19) demonstrated that splanchnic nodes of a high percentage of patients undergoing emergency surgery after abdominal trauma contained relevant amounts of live enteric bacteria; however, this finding was not associated with an increased rate of complications, including sepsis and septic shock, nor with an increased length-of-stay in the hospital. Thus, it is conceivable that, even if the findings from Brickell's group (9) should be borne in mind, particularly in the case of penetrating, bleeding wounds, a more aggressive treatment either in the prehospital and in the in-hospital phase could influence both the short- and the long-term outcome.

The analysis of the results of a trauma system should be largely incomplete without taking into account the errors of management and their possible consequences on the final outcome. However, for partially understandable reasons, relatively few investigations have been published on the issue. By evaluating the outcome of severe head injury (Glasgow Coma Scale -GCS- ≤ 8) of 717 patients admitted to National Traumatic Coma Data Bank, Chestnut et al. (20) demonstrated that hypotension and hypoxia at admission were independently associated with a significant increase in morbidity and mortality. In particular, hypotension was associated with a 150% increase in mortality, when compared with normotensive patients. When both factors coexisted, the consequent mortality or ever residual neurological disabilities (including persistent vegetative state) were 75% and 19%, respectively.

In a recent Italian survey, Stocchetti et al. (21), evaluated the rate of in-hospital preventable deaths in 110 severely injured patients and found that in 11 of them it would have been preventable. The authors attributed this finding to a failure in recognizing and treating hypovolemia and sources of bleeding, despite the availability of adequate diagnostic and therapeutic facilities. In a similar study, which involved 13500 cases, Cayten et al. (22) reported 12% preventable deaths (i.e. death occurring in patients with a probability of survival ≥ 50%, established through the use of different severity scoring systems). Also these authors concluded that the delays in surgery accounted for most of preventable deaths in patients suffering from either penetrating or blunt injuries. Besides the delay of surgery, there are some lesions, including cervical spine and carotid injuries, which can go unrecognized and, if left untreated, can carry a high mortality and severe long-term disabling sequelae (23-25). In our series of 83 traumatic fall patients, using a standard diagnostic protocol, which includes extensive radiologic investigations, we found four treatment-needing injuries which went undetected at the admission: however, only two of them (precisely a subdural hematoma and a posttraumatic pneumothorax which were not evident at the initial examination) were life-threatening and required an immediate intervention.

Conclusions

Trauma can be considered as a multisystem disease, whose outcome (either in terms of mortality or long-term consequences) is dependent on many factors, including the severity of the injuries, the pretraumatic pathophysiologic conditions, the age, and the overall treatment. Several investigations demonstrated that the implementation of a comprehensive trauma system, which includes a fast-response reaction by a trained rescue time, quick transport to trauma center and an appropriate diagnostic and therapeutic work-up, is associated with an improved survival. However, a consistent number (around 10%) of potentially preventable deaths still occur. At the present time, now that the usefulness of a trauma system has been established, it appears that more attention should be devoted to the identifications of weak points and bottlenecks both in the prehospital and in-hospital treatment.

References

1. Trunkey DD (1991) Initial treatment of patients with severe trauma. New Engl J Med 324: 1259-1263
2. Bossaert L (1992) A survey of emergency medical service systems in Europe. In: Vincent JL (ed) Yearbook of intensive care and emergency medicine. Springer, Berlin Heidelberg New York, pp 663-672
3. Sauaia A, Moore FA, Moore EE, Moser Ks, Brennan R, Read RA, Pons PT (1995) Epidemiology of trauma death: a reassessment. J Trauma 38:185-192
4. Fortner GS, Oreskovich MR, Copass MK, Carrico CJ (1983) The effects of prehospital trauma care on survival from a 50 meter fall. J Trauma 23:976-981
5. Riggs JE (1993) Mortality from accidental falls among the elderly in the United States, 1962-1988: demonstrating the impact of improved trauma management. J Trauma 35:212-219
6. Moylan JA (1988) Impact of helicopters on trauma care and clinical results. Ann Surg 208:673-677
7. Schmidt U, Frame SB, Nerlich ML, Rowe DR, Blaine LE, Maull KI, Tscherme H (1992) On-scene helicopter transport of patients with multiple injuries - comparison of a German and an American system. J Trauma 33:548-555
8. Nardi G, Massarutti D, Muzzi R, Kette F, De Monte A, Carnelos GA, Peressutti R, Berlot G, Giordano F, Gullo A (1994) Impact of emergency medical helicopter service on mortality for trauma in north-east Italy. Eur J Emerg Med 1:69-77
9. Brickell H, Wall MJ, Pepe PE et al (1994) Immediate versus delayed fluid resuscitation for hypotensive patients with penetrating torso trauma. New Engl J Med 331:1105-1109

10. Capone AC, Safar P, Stezoski W, Tisherman S, Peitzman AB (1995) Improved outcome with fluid restriction in treatment of uncontrolled hemorrhagic shock. J Am Coll Surg 180:49-56
11. van der Sluis CK, ten Duis HJ, Geertzen JHB (1995) Multiple injuries: an overview of the outcome: injury, infection and critical care. J Trauma 38:681-686
12. Schmand JF, Ayala A, Chaudry IH (1994) Effects of trauma, duration of hypotension, and resuscitation regimen on cellular immunity after hemorrhagic shock. Crit Care Med 22: 1076-1083
13. Abraham E (1989) Host defense abnormalities after hemorrhage, trauma and burns. Crit Care Med 17:934-939
14. Ruomen RMH, Vreugde JPC, Goris JA (1994) Gastric tonometry in multiple trauma patients. J Trauma 36:313-316
15. Chang MC, Cheatham ML, Nelson LD, Rutherford EJ, Morris JA (1994) Gastric tonometry supplements information provided by systemic indicators of oxygen transport. J Trauma 37,3: 488-494
16. Doglio GR, Pusajo JF, Egurrola MA et al (1991) Gastric mucosal pH as a prognostic index of mortality in critically ill patients. Crit Care Med 19:1037-1040
17. Gutierrez G, Palizas F, Doglio G et al (1992) Gastric intramucosal pH as a therapeutic index of tissue oxygenation in critically ill patients. Lancet 339:195-199
18. Rush BF, Sori AJ, Murphy TF, Smith S, Flanagan JJ, Machiedo GW (1987) Endotoxemia and bacteremia during hemorrhagic shock. The link between trauma and sepsis? Ann Surg 207: 549-554
19. Reed L, Martin M, Manglano R, Newson B, Kocka F, Barrettt J (1994) Bacterial translocation following abdominal trauma in humans. Circ Shock 42:1-6
20. Chestnut R, Marshall LF, Klauber MR, Blunt BA, Baldwin N, Eisenberg HM, Jane JA, Marmarou A, Foulkes MA (1993) The role of secondary brain injury in determining outcome from severe head injury. J Trauma 34:216-222
21. Stocchetti N, Pagliarini G, Gennari M et al (1994) Trauma care in Italy: evidence of in-hospital preventable deaths. J Trauma 36:401-405
22. Cayten CG, Stahl WM, Agarwal N, Murphy JG (1991) Analyses of preventable deaths by mechanism of injury in 13500 trauma admissions. Ann Surg 214:510-521
23. Davis JW, Phreaner DL, Hoyt DB, Mackersie RC (1993) The etiology of missed cervical spine injury. J Trauma 34:342-346
24. Berlot G, Viviani M, Gullo A (1992) Traumatic carotideal dissection after blunt cervical injury: an elusive clinical entity. Am J Emerg Med 10:396-398
25. Berlot G, Viviani M, Magnaldi S, Gullo A (1995) Delayed traumatic cervical cord transection: case report. Am J Emerg Med 13:101-103

Evaluation and Triage
Current Use and Utility of the Trauma Scoring Systems

P. CARLI

In the last 25 years many scores have been proposed to evaluate the trauma patients. Many parameters have been introduced to try to assess patient status, describe the injuries and finally predict the outcome. Obviously considering the multiple scores available in the current literature none is perfect. The main scores proposed are listed in Table 1. We will limit our analysis to the scores that have been specifically designed for the patient in emergency or during initial management.

The aim of scoring

Until recently the analysis of trauma patient management and the evaluation of the injury severity were based on anecdotes and non scientifically based opinions. A modern injury scoring system is a more objective method. It can provide accurate information for triage (prehospital or in hospital), to monitor patient care and the response to treatment. It is not surprising that many of these scores have been developed in North America, because they may be also a very efficient tool for quality assessment and an indication of the proper use of the resources.

Physiological scores

They are based on very simple clinical parameters obtained by physical examination. They can determine very simply the physiological derangement provoked by the injuries and consequently the severity of the case. These scores are very important in North America for triaging the trauma patient in the prehospital settings. Their use is mandatory because physicians are not involved in prehospital care on scene. Then, EMT or paramedics need guidelines to decide to which of the available facilities the patient must be admitted. From a practical point of view, these scores decrease over triage: patient is oriented to regional Trauma centers without major injury.

Table 1. Scoring systems used for trauma patients

Year	Abbreviations	Denominations
1969	SYMBOL	SYMBOL Rating and Evaluation System
1971		Trauma Index
1971	AIS	Abbreviated Injury Scale
1972	CRIS	Comprehensive Injury Scale
1974		Prognostic Index for Severe Trauma
1974	GCS	Glasgow Coma Scale
1974		Renal Index
1974	TISS	Therapeutic Intervention Scoring System
1974	ISS	Injury Severity Score
1975	RI	Respiratory Index
1977		CHOP Index
1977	PEBL	Penetrating-blunt Code
1979	IISS	Illness-Injury Severity Score
1980		Triage Index
1980	MISS	Modified Injury Severity Scale
1980	RESP	Revised Estimated Survival Probability
1980	AI	Anatomic Index
1980		Hospital Trauma Index
1981		Global Score
1981	TS	Trauma Score
1981		Penetrating Abdominal Trauma Index
1981	PODS	Probability of Death Score
1982	CRAMS	CRAMS Scale (circulation-respiration-abdomen-motor-speech)
1985	MES	Mangled Extremity Syndrome
1985	APACHE II	Acute Physiology and Chronic-Health Evaluation (revised)
1986		Prehospital Index
1986	RTS	Revised Trauma Score
1987	TRISS	Trauma Score Injury Severity Score
1987	PTS	Pediatric Trauma Score
1988	OPS	Outcome Predictive Score
1989	OIS	Organ Injury Scaling
1989	AP	Anatomic Profile
1990	ASCOT	A Severity Characterization of Trauma

Glasgow Coma Scale

Created by Teasdale and Jennett (13) in the early 1970s for the head trauma patients this score is particularly simple and accurate. It is clearly one of the most frequently used scoring tool that correlates to patient outcome (10). Recently it has been modified for patients endotracheally intubated and for children. GCS may be used alone or as neurologic component in combination with other parameters in more sophisticated scoring system.

Revised Trauma Score

Specifically designed for the prehospital care of multiple trauma patient this score is derived from the Triage Index and the Trauma Score both developed by Champion et al. (7). This score simply assess the respiratory, circulatory, and neurological status of the patient. The relative value of these three parameters as predictor of survival has been calculated by a regression analysis based on a large north American data set. This score is described in Table 2. RTS is currently used and correlates with the probability of survival. However, a score of 4 or less to determine patient admission to a trauma center may be discussed.

Table 2. Revised Trauma Score for Champion et al. (7)

Glasgow Coma Scale (GCS)	Systolic arterial pressure (mmHg)	Respiratory rate (c min⁻¹)	Factor "C"
13-15	> 89	10-29	4
9-12	76-89	> 29	3
6-8	50-75	6-9	2
4-5	1-49	1-51	1
3	0	0	0

$$RTS = 0.9368 \ GCS \ \text{"C"} + 0.7326 \ PAS \ \text{"C"} + 0.2908 \ FR \ \text{"C"}$$

CRAMS

This physiological score is also based on the presence of life threatening problems (9). It also included parameters related to the injury pattern derived from clinical examination of the abdomen and the thorax. CRAMS is also correlated to prognosis but its efficiency as a triage tool as compared to RTS and several other scores may be discussed.

The limits of triage score

An important limitation of triage scores is that they do not take into account information related to the mechanism of the injury and to the patient physiological status prior to the trauma. Baxt and coworkers (3) observed that triage scores are accurate in predicting mortality however the sensitivity and the specificity is barely of 70% to predict survival. Conversely Emerman et al. (8) observe that finally EMT opinion on scene is at least as efficient as any formal score (11). Such a pragmatic approach is the origin of a very simple tool like the "trauma triage rule" (3). A severe trauma mandatory transported to a trauma center is then defined by a systolic arterial pressure less than 85 to or a motor component of the GCS less than five or when a penetrating trauma of the head, neck or torso is observed. A more sophisticated approach, based on a decision tree has been elaborated by the American College of Surgeon's Committee on trauma (1).

Triage tool in Europe

Triage scores are not so routinely used in Europe as in North America. This is probably explained by the sophisticated prehospital care system, involving physicians on scene that exist in several countries (France, Belgium, Italy, Germany,...) (5). However, this is also a consequence of the lack of quality assessment program of prehospital care in many of these countries. Scoring system utilization is limited to scientific evaluation to determine comparable groups of patients in a study.

Anatomical scores

The severity of the trauma is assessed by the ranking of the injuries. Consequently a precise diagnosis is needed and these scores are determined afterwards when the patient is in hospital.

Abbreviated Injury Scale (AIS)

Introduced in 1969 this score provides a ranking of injuries from 1 (minor) to 6 (lethal). After 5 different updating, more than 1200 injuries are since 1990 listed in a dictionary. However, this score is not linearly related to the severity (15).

Injury Severity Score (ISS)

Derived from the AIS this score is specifically designed for patients with multiple injuries. Multiple trauma patients are scored by adding together the squares of the three highest AIS scores in predetermined regions of the body. Only AIS scores of 1-5 are used in the calculation of ISS. By convention a patient with an AIS = 6 in any body region is given an overall ISS of 75. It should be noted that the ISS is non-linear. There is pronounced variation in the frequency of different scores. For example, 9 and 16 are very common, 14 and 22 unusual, and 7 and 15 unattainable. This type of distribution precludes the use of parametric statistics in analysis. The overall ISS of a group of patients should be identified by the median value and the range, not the mean value, and analyses should be undertaken using non-parametric statistics. Considering its calculation may provide the same score for patients with very different pattern of injuries. Only the three major injuries in three different territories are analysed and consequently a second lesion, even severe, in any of these territories is not taken into account. Recently a new anatomical score (the Anatomic Profile) includes these characteristics (15).

Evaluation of quality assurance

Quality assurance according to the diversity of mechanism and type of injury, the delivery of care, and the patient status is particularly difficult in trauma patients. More than 10 years ago data collection on trauma was initiated to develop a statistical analysis of survival based on scoring systems. This Major Trauma Outcome Study (MTOS) (6) has included near 200 000 patients and was extended to England and Australia (15). The aim of this study was to outline patients with unexpected outcome that will be interesting cases for a peer review of their file. MTOS was based on the TRISS methodology.

TRISS index

TRISS is a combination of anatomic and physiological indices to determine a probability of survival (Ps) (6); mathematical calculation of Ps is detailed on Table 3.

Table 3. TRISS methodology

Probability of survival of individual patient

$$Ps = \frac{1}{1+e^{-b}}$$

Where e = natural logarithm and

$$b - b_0 + b_1 (RTS) + b_2 (ISS) + b_3 (A)$$

b_{0-3}, weighted coefficients based on a major trauma outcome study (United States). These differ for blunt and penetrating injuries. RTS, revised trauma score; ISS, injury severity score; A, age (score 0 if < 54, score 1 if ≥ 55)

   Ps is merely a mathematical calculation; it is not an absolute measure of survival but only of the probability of survival. Charts can be compiled to identify patients whose Ps are on the "wrong side" of a line that represents 50% mortality (i.e. unexpected survivors or unexpected deaths). Although such charts may be helpful in identifying some patients who could be usefully discussed at departmental meetings they should be not used as the sole measure of performance.

   The TRISS methodology can also be used to assess the performance of an institution. The "W statistics" measures the difference between the actual and the predicted numbers of deaths or survivors treated by the institution. The "Z statistics" measures the significance of W.

TRISS methodology in Europe

Several attempts have been made to develop a MTOS like study in European countries. In the UK TRISS is now commonly used as a tool of quality assurance by the North Western Injury Research Center in Manchester (15).

This method has also been used in limited series of patients in France and Germany to analyse efficiency of prehospital care (12, 14).

ASCOT

A severe characterization of trauma is a more statistically reliable indicator than TRISS of probability of survival (1). ASCOT attempts to improve TRISS by incorporating the number, the location and the severity of all the injuries. Age of patients is also incorporated more precisely in the index calculation. ASCOT is particularly reliable in penetrating trauma patients.

Conclusion

To evaluate the severity and the outcome of trauma patients scoring based on physiological status and anatomical description of the injuries have been currently used. In addition several of these methods provide accurate information on the quality control of the patient care and the overall efficiency of the trauma care systems.

References

1. ACSCOT (1990) American College of Surgeon's Committee on Trauma. Resources for optimal care of the injured patient. Chicago
2. Baker SP, O'Neil B (1976) The Injury Severity Score: an update. J Trauma 16:882-885
3. Baxt W, Jones J, Fortlage D (1991) The trauma triage rule: a new resource-based approach to the prehospital identification of major trauma victims. Ann Emerg Med 19:1404-1406
4. Boyd CR, Tolson MA, Copes WS (1987) Evaluation of trauma care: the TRISS method. J Trauma 27:370-378
5. Carli P, Riou B, Barriot P (1993) Trauma anesthesia practices throughout the world: France. In: C Grande (ed) Textbook of trauma anesthesia and critical care. Mosby Saint-Louis, pp 199-205
6. Champion HR, Copes WS (1990) The major Trauma Outcome Study: establishing national norms for trauma care. J Trauma 30:1356-1365
7. Champion HR, Sacco WJ, Copes WS, Gann DS, Gennarelli TA (1989) A revision of the trauma score. J Trauma 29:623-629

8. Emerman CL, Shade B, Kubincanek J (1991) A comparison of EMT judgment and pre-hospital trauma triage instruments. J Trauma 31:1369-1375
9. Gormican S (1982) CRAMS scale field triage of trauma victim. Ann Emerg Med 11:132-135
10. Jennett B, Teasdale G, Braakman R (1979) Prognosis of patients with severe head injury. Neurosurgery 4:283-289
11. Ornato J, Mlinek EJ (1985) Ineffectiveness of the Trauma Score and the CRAMS scale for accurately triaging patients to trauma centers. Ann Emerg Med 14:1049-1054
12. Schmidt U, Frame SB, Nerlich ML, Rowe DW, Enderson BL, Maull KI (1992) On-scene helicopter transport of patients with multiple injuries. Comparison of a German and an American system. J Trauma 33:548-555
13. Teasdale G, Jennett B (1974) Assessment of coma and impaired consciousness: a practical scale. Lancet 2:81-84
14. Yates D, Carli P, Woodford M, Soleil C (1994) Towards statistical comparison of French and British systems of initial trauma care. Jeur 2:88-93
15. Yates DW (1990) Scoring systems for trauma. Br Med J 301:1090-1094

What Can We Do During the "Golden Hour"?

H.H. Delooz

Introduction

The golden hour after trauma is spent for about 50% on the site and during transport to the hospital, the other half in the emergency department. Traditionally the focus is on the ABC of emergency care: airway, breathing and circulation, although we have stressed adequate immobilization, staunching and wound care as another priority (1).

Airway, breathing and circulation are the links of the physiological chain of events responsible for two vital functions: ventilation or carbon dioxide elimination and oxygenation or oxygen transport to the tissues. How important are these functions during the early phase after injury in determining mortality, morbidity and disability? How dangerous are hypercapnia and hypoxia of the tissues?

Ventilation or CO_2 elimination

It has been stressed that permissive hypercarbia in patients with severe adult respiratory distress syndrome may improve outcome (2). A recent article by Simon et al. (3) is entitled "Hypercarbia: is there a cause for concern?".

As far back as 1980 we have used in our department a protocol for status asthmaticus which indicated as mode for controlled ventilation:
- "Slow inspiration (ex: 33% of cycle)
- No inflation hold
- Slow expiration
- Low frequency (6-8 min)
- Small tidal volume, limiting inspiratory pressure to < 50 cm H_2O
- Duration of expiration to adapt to the duration of expiratory wheezing, checked by auscultation
- → Voluntary hypercapnia"

We advocated this mode of ventilation because our goal was to maintain adequate oxygenation, while ventilation was considered of little or no importance. Death as a result of status asthmaticus is due to high respiratory work and oxygen consumption in the presence of poor oxygen transport due to the "tamponade" effect of increasing intrathoracic pressure. The combination causes accumulated oxygen deficit or oxygen debt. Controlled ventilation with voluntary or permissive hypercapnia aims at abolishing the respiratory work, while minimizing the tamponade effect and the risk for barotrauma, and assuring oxygen delivery through prolonged contact time at the alveolar-capillary interface and a shift of the oxygen-hemoglobin-dissociation curve to the left as a result of respiratory acidosis.

Only voluntary hypercapnia has allowed us to decrease the in-hospital mortality of status asthmaticus, at a time when this had not been achieved during the previous two decades, although the introduction in medical practice of artificial ventilation and corticosteroids had been witnessed.

In 1992 Potkin et al. (4) published the case report of a 46 year old male who sustained severe accidental hypercapnia during anesthesia in an outpatient surgical center. He was admitted to the emergency department with a pH of 6.60 and a P_aCO_2 of 375 mmHg. The context, however, was clear: the patient's arterial saturation had been continuously monitored and had always been maintained above 90%. The authors conclude that survival is possible in acute severe respiratory acidosis as long as tissue anoxia and ischemia are prevented. They mention that recent studies of the intracellular pH regulation have revealed the ability to regulate intracellular pH to a much greater extent than is observed in the extracellular space, among other mechanisms by active extrusion of protons (5). They rightfully stress the fact that the mechanisms involved are directly or ultimately energy consuming and require that the cells remain well oxygenated and perfused.

Looking back at the previously cited paper of Simon et al. (3), it is clear from the table comparing survivors and nonsurvivors of severe pulmonary dysfunction at the time of the highest P_aCO_2 that the difference in both groups in P_aCO_2 is not significant, while the bicarbonate and lactate concentrations are. We consider this as evidence of the fact that survivors and nonsurvivors are not differentiated by hypercapnia but by the oxygen availability being capable or not of meeting the oxygen requirement.

We conclude that hypercapnia, although not a goal in early trauma care, can be accepted if oxygenation is preserved. Of course we will discuss further in this paper the effect of ventilation on brain perfusion and oxygenation.

Oxygen transport

Oxygen delivery is dependent on the oxygen content of the arterial blood and the cardiac output. Consumable oxygen, however, is limited to the product of the cardiac output and the difference between the arterial oxygen content and the content at a PO_2 of 20 mmHg, for this represents the mixed venous oxygen content at maximal oxygen extraction. Determinant for mortality and morbidity is the occurrence of oxygen deficit (6, 7) as a result of the consumable oxygen not being able to meet the oxygen requirement or oxygen need. Consumable oxygen deficit over time constitutes the incurred oxygen debt.

Oxygen need

Edwards et al. (8) stated in 1988 that the occurrence of an "ebb phase" after injury in man is an attractive hypothesis, but cannot be supported by the evidence available. Cuthbertson's claim (9) for a reduced oxygen consumption after injury for up to a period of 48 h, although it was quoted for four decades, cannot be supported by any evidence, not even by that originally presented by the author. We completely agree with Edwards' statement: "it is the delivery of oxygen to the tissues which determines the metabolic response to injury and the maintenance of this above critical levels that determines outcome".

Oxygen delivery

In our ongoing major trauma outcome study Leuven, a first clinical impression is required from the first physician to see the patient, whether at the scene, during transport or in the emergency department. Five clinical symptoms have to be recorded: agitation, shock, cyanosis, asymmetrical respiratory movements and subcutaneous emphysema.

As shown in Table 1 mortality in the group of patients that was observed with signs of shock was 41% as opposed to 3.4% in the group without signs of shock. Mortality in the group observed with cyanosis was 55% as opposed to 4.3% in the group without cyanosis. Both shock and cyanosis were independent predictors of outcome (Log-Rank test $p < 0.0001$).

Table 1. MTOS Leuven

First clinical impression (prehosp. or ED)		Mortality	
Agitation	yes	23/177	13%
	no	135/2625	5%
Shock	yes	69/167	41%
	no	89/2635	3.4%
Cyanosis	yes	40/73	55%
	no	118/2729	4.3%
Asymm. resp.	yes	32/147	22%
	no	126/2655	4.7%
Subcut. emphys.	yes	9/36	25%
	no	149/2766	5.4%

Hypoxia and multiple organ failure (MOF)

Several experimental studies have been aiming at the identification of the events or cascades responsible for the development of organ failure in general and adult respiratory failure (ARDS) in particular. Duchateau et al. (10) for instance looked at complement activation in patients at risk of developing ARDS. They found C5a-like activity only in patients at risk for ARDS. It was highly associated with clinical conditions that predispose to ARDS, but it could not be considered as a real predictor of ARDS occurrence in these patients. Their observations suggest that other factors such as hypoxia may influence the development of ARDS.

Larsen et al. (11) in experimental work on rabbits conclude that complement activation, as an isolated event, will not cause a significant increase in lung permeability. However, combining complement activation with an episode of hypoxia leads to an increase in lavage albumin.

Nuytinck et al. (12) investigated the effects in New Zealand white rabbits of a 4-h infusion of activated complement and its combination with short hypoxic periodes (20 min) on respiratory function, leukocyte count, platelet count and morphology of lungs, heart, liver, kidney and spleen. The combination of hypoxia and systemic complement infusion appeared to aggravate microvascular injury to the lungs, with the occurrence of protein rich alveolar edema and hemorrhage in the lungs and accumulation of PMN debris, containing macrophages, in the spleen.

The inflammatory reaction found in all other organs examined may represent the early phase of MOF.

Hypoxia, hypotension and secondary brain injury

The Traumatic Coma Data Bank (TCDB) prospectively studied the outcome from severe head injury patients (GCS score ≤ 8) in 717 cases and investigated the impact of hypotension [systolic blood pressure (SBP) < 90 mmHg] and hypoxia ($P_aO_2 \leq 60$ mmHg or apnea or cyanosis in the field) on secondary brain insults, occurring from injury through resuscitation. Miller et al. (13) in 1982 published the first detailed studies of the prevalence and significance of secondary systemic insults in 225 prospectively studied patients at the Medical College of Virginia. These patients, however, were only studied at arrival at the trauma center and do not represent events resolved before the patient reached the hospital. Their categories were also not mutually exclusive (i.e., the category of hypoxia included patients who also incurred a hypotensive period and vice versa).

Chesnut et al. (14) analyzed hypoxia and hypotension as four mutually exclusive categories: neither hypotension nor hypoxia, hypoxia alone, hypotension alone, hypotension and hypoxia combined. Prevalence and effects were evaluated for the expanded time interval from injury through resuscitation.

Analysis of the association of outcome with hypotension controlled for hypoxia, age and severe multiple trauma reveals hypotension to have been extremely significant ($p < 10^{-6}$). Analysis of the independent association of outcome with hypoxia was also significant ($p = 0.013$). The frequency of occurrence was 45.6% for hypoxia and 34.6% for hypotension. In the discussion of the paper Chesnut et al. stress the fact that in the past, the finding of ischemic neuropathological conditions in patients dying as a result of severe head injury (15) mainly served as an impetus to the recognition and treatment of elevated intracranial pressure (ICP) in order to avoid compromised cerebral perfusion pressure and resultant ischemia, whereas the results of Miller (13) and the present study explain another significant cause for the frequency of ischemic damage by elucidating the high incidence and grave consequences of *early* post-traumatic hypotension.

The addition of hypotension with or without hypoxia doubles the mortality and significantly increases the morbidity of severe head injury. The influence of hypoxia may be tempered by the highly developed intubation and ventilation protocols employed by emergency medical services very early in field resuscitation.

The disparity between hypotension and hypoxia as secondary brain insults may lie in the differential sensitivity of the brain to hypoxemia and deficient perfusion. The highly developed ability of the brain to extract oxygen protects it from hypoxia if normal perfusion is maintained. In contrast the disruption of autoregulation that occurs with head injury results in ischemia from systemic hypotension, resulting from systemic hypotension despite adequate oxygenation of the blood. Sensitivity to hypotension of patients with head injury makes them fundamentally different from other patients with multiple injuries. The authors conclude that resuscitation protocols for brain injured patients should assiduously avoid hypovolemic shock on an absolute basis.

Pigula et al. (16) studied the effect of hypotension and hypoxia on children (< 17 years) with severe head injury (GCS < 8). In their study hypoxia alone was not associated with increased mortality in normotensive patients ($p = 0.34$). Hypotension, however, significantly increased mortality even without concomitant hypoxia ($p < 0.00001$). The authors conclude that in pediatric head injury, adequate resuscitation is probably the single most critical factor for optimal survival. The period in the field, during extrication and during transport, may be particularly critical in the development of secondary brain injury through the occurrence of hypotension.

Chesnut et al. (17) in another paper in 1993 conclude that probably the cut off point for CPP should be elevated (to the range of 70 mmHg or more) after brain injury. In this light a SBP of 90 mmHg would generally represent a CPP that is unacceptable even in the absence of intracranial hypertension.

Experimental work by Ishige et al. (18) studying the effect of hypoxia on rats subjected to a standardized traumatic brain injury (fluid percussion impact pressure of 5 to 6 atm for 20 ms) showed that whereas ischemia was not present in rats with either impact injury of hypoxia alone, the perfusion staining of injured cerebral tissue in vivo with 2,3,5-triphenyltetrazolium chloride showed an area of extensive ischemia around the impact site in rats with hypoxic insult. The authors also showed increases in neurologic deficit and brain electrical function, when hypoxia was associated with the traumatic brain injury.

Cruz (19), when continuously monitoring global cerebral oxygenation, perfusion pressure and expired CO_2 in 69 adults with acute severe closed brain injury, found that profound but brief desaturation was not associated with neurological deterioration, while profound and prolonged (> 10 min) desaturation was accompanied by significant decreases in Glasgow Coma Scale score, even though intracranial pressure levels were not significantly different in these two groups of patients. The author concludes that global cerebral hypoxia that does not respond promptly to treatment appears to be independently deleterious to neurological function in severely head injured patients.

On the other hand Schmoker et al. (20) studied a porcine model of traumatic injury receiving a cryogenic lesion plus hemorrhage to a mean arterial pressure of 50 mmHg for 45 min.

Hemorrhagic hypotension following TBI produced a significant and sustained reduction in cerebral oxygen delivery associated with a lower cerebral metabolic rate for oxygen and higher intracranial pressure and cortical water content than seen with the traumatic lesion alone. This occurred despite adequate early restoration of systematic oxygen delivery. M.J. Rosner (Birmingham, Alabama) in the discussion of the paper stresses the fact that hypotension will be much more effective at producing low flow in damaged tissue that it is in normal tissue. He adds that systolic pressures of 90 mmHg or even slightly above are ridiculously low in the phase of brain injury.

The role of CO_2 elimination in secondary brain injury

Fortune et al. (21) have measured internal carotid blood flow and oxygen delivery under normo-, hypo- and hypercapnia conditions and progressive hypoxemia in normal volunteers. Their data suggest that hypoxia and carbon dioxide changes will alter cerebral blood flow simultaneously and additively, with only a slight reduction in oxygen delivery when hypoxia is combined with hypercapnia, while the effect of hypoxia on the cerebral blood flow completely compensates for the effect of diminished saturation under normocapnia and hypocapnia.

Zhuang et al. (22) in the previously mentioned porcine model of focal cryogenic brain injury questioned whether maintenance of CPP prevents cerebral ischemia and secondary brain damage. They found that adequate CPP did not normalize cerebral perfusion after brain injury, since CBF and cerebral oxygen delivery in the experimental group progressively decreased throughout the entire experiment and were significantly lower than controls. These data suggest that maintenance of CPP may not prevent ischemia after focal brain injury, probably as a result of a significant increase in cerebral vascular resistance. The authors conclude that medical interventions to reduce cerebral vascular resistance may be required to improve cerebral blood flow and oxygen delivery and to prevent secondary brain injury.

Bouma and Muizelaer (23) in a review on cerebral blood flow, cerebral blood volume and cerebrovascular reactivity after severe head injury report that recent data indicate that low CBF and ischemia probably occur within the first few hours after injury. The authors also underline the importance of the cerebral blood volume as determinant of cerebral blood flow and stress the fact that CBF is determined by mean arterial blood pressure, intracranial pressure, blood viscosity and the diameter of arteries and arterioles. Cerebral blood volume, however, is a function of vascular diameter alone. They conclude that we can only speculate about the possible causes for early post-traumatic ischemia. One possible explanation is vasospasm of the large conducting arteries. If vasospasm is indeed the cause, this also means that raised arterial blood pressure in these cases will not increase ICP or enhance cerebral edema. Early hyperventilation to prevent raised ICP may likewise not be useful or even be dangerous by provoking ischemia (24).

As a result of all these studies we can conclude that hypoxia has to be avoided by all means, that hypotension has to be controlled but a systemic systolic blood pressure routinely considered acceptable may not be sufficient to assure adequate cerebral perfusion in the brain injured patient and finally since ischemia seems to occur very early after brain injury even under adequate cerebral perfusion pressure, hyperventilation or hypocapnia in the golden hour may be deleterious. Maintenance of normocapnia is indicated in brain injury patients.

Clinical practice

Mateer et al. in 1993 (25) performed continuous pulse oximetry during emergency endotracheal intubation and demonstrated that hypoxemia (sat < 90%) occurred more frequently in nonmonitored than in monitored attempts, while the duration of severe hypoxemia (sat < 85%) was significantly greater for nonmonitored attempts. They conclude that continuous pulse oximetry monitoring reduces the frequency and the duration of hypoxemia associated with emergency endotracheal intubation attempts.

Nardi et al. (26) in a study on the impact of emergency medical helicopter service on mortality for trauma demonstrated very elegantly that decreased mortality (12% versus 38% and 32%) for identical injury severity scores correlated with intubation rates on the scene of 81% versus 0% to 2%, thoracic drainage on scene of 14% versus 0% and an average volume administration of 1400 ml versus 0 ml in the prehospital phase. All these interventions served to maintain adequate oxygen delivery.

Trupka et al. (27) compared in a prospectively studied trauma population a group of patients who were intubated within 2 h after injury with a group of patients with delayed intubation and found that although the injury severity score of the first group was significantly higher (39 versus 29), both groups had comparable incidence of respiratory failure, while the delayed intubation group had an even higher, though not significantly different, multiple organ failure rate and mortality. The authors conclude that emergency prehospital endotracheal intubation is indicated in shock, GCS ≤ 8, and apparent respiratory failure, but they also advocate early intubation in major chest trauma, ISS > 24, and a combination of two or more fractures with crush injury.

Deakin (28) debates the merits of early fluid resuscitation and argues that fluid resuscitation before definitive hemostasis has been achieved may accelerate blood loss, cause hypothermia and result in a dilutional coagulopathy. But identifying ongoing, uncontrolled hemorrhage in the field may be very difficult (29).

Deakin et al. (30) in a critical review of the use of field stabilization state that it is unlikely that all trauma patients are best treated by either field resuscitation or scoop and run approach and that the most effective form of prehospital care may depend upon the type of injuries sustained. The authors also stress the importance of scene time if stabilization has to be attained.

In our opinion these statements support the fact that the best prehospital care will be provided by the team with the broadest experience and the greatest expertise. This of course seems to be obvious for the whole of medical practice, but is still subject to debate when it comes to pre-hospital care in general and trauma care in particular.

The future?

Finally a completely different approach is currently researched with support of the US Army (31). The traditional approach in emergency trauma care, as described above, aims at all cost and unfortunately in the severely traumatized patient often without success to maintain adequate oxygen transport in order to meet the oxygen requirement.

A drastic cut down on the oxygen need through the introduction of a process well known in certain animals as hibernation would bring the patient in a state in which definitive treatment can be postponed until arrival at the proper care facility. The product responsible for hibernation has been identified as a delta morphinoid produced by the corpus pineale and when injected into an animal it promptly produces hibernation.

This process not only lowers very efficiently the oxygen need, but because of the lowering of the oxygen consumption also allows the flux of oxygen from the hemoglobin to the tissues to slow down to such an extent that the gradient between hemoglobin and cells falls and extraction will become almost total.

The future of prehospital resuscitation may be limited to the prompt introduction of hibernation and the transport of the patient to the facility, wherever it is located, where complete repair of the injuries can be achieved, followed by the reversal of the hibernation. Although it has the flavor of science fiction, it may, although probably not in such a simple form, come about in a future which still may be ours to see.

References

1. Delooz H (1991) Organization and implementation of emergency services in the treatment of major trauma. J Neurotrauma 8 [Suppl]:S7-S12
2. Hickling KG, Henderson SJ, Jackson RL (1990) Low mortality associated with low volume pressure limited ventilation with permissive hypercapnia in severe adult respiratory distress syndrome. Intensive Care Med 16:372
3. Simon RJ, Mawilmada S, Ivatury RR (1994) Hypercapnia: is there a cause for concern? J Trauma 37:74-81
4. Potkin RT, Swenson ER (1992) Resuscitation from severe acute hypercapnia. Determinants of tolerance and survival. Chest 102:1742-1745
5. Hoffman EK, Simonsen LO (1989) Membrane mechanisms in volume and pH regulation in vertebrate cells. Physiol Rev 69:315-382
6. Guyton AC, Crowell JW (1961) Dynamics of the heart in shock. Fed Proc 10:51
7. Shoemaker WC, Appel PL, Kram HB (1988) Tissue oxygen debt as a determinant of lethal and non lethal postoperative organ failure. Crit Care Med 16:1117-1120
8. Edwards JD, Redmond AD, Nightingale P, Wilkins RG (1988) Oxygen consumption following trauma: a reappraisal in severely injured patients requiring mechanical ventilation. Br J Surg 75:690-692
9. Cuthbertson DP (1932) Observations on the disturbance of metabolism produced by injury to the limbs. Q J Med 1:233-246
10. Duchateau J, Haas M, Schreyen H, Radoux L, Sprangers I, Noel FX, Braun M, Lamy M (1984) Complement activation in patients at risk of developing the adult respiratory distress syndrome. Am Rev Respir Dis 130:1058-1064
11. Larsen GL, Webster RO, Worthen GS, Gumbay RS, Henson PM (1985) Additive effect of intravascular complement activation and brief episodes of hypoxia in producing increased permeability in the rabbit lung. J Clin Invest 75:902-910
12. Nuytinck JKS, Goris RJA, Weerts JGE, Schillings PHM, Schuurmans Stekhoven JH (1986) Acute generalized microvascular injury by activated complement and hypoxia: the basis of the adult respiratory distress syndrome and multiple organ failure? Br J Exp Pathol 67:537-548
13. Miller JD, Becker DP (1982) Secondary insults to the injured brain. J R Coll Surg Edinb 27:292-298
14. Chesnut RM, Marshall LF, Klauber MR, Blunt BA, Baldwin N, Eisenberg HM, Jane JA, Marmarou A, Foulkes MA (1993) The role of secondary brain injury in determining outcome from severe head injury. J Trauma 34:216-222
15. Graham DI, Adams JH, Doyle D (1978) Ischaemic brain damage in fatal non-missile head injuries. J Neurol Sci 39:213
16. Pigula FA, Wald SL, Shackford SR, Vane DW (1993) The effect of hypotension and hypoxia on children with severe head injuries. J Pediatr Surg 28:310-316

17. Chesnut RM, Marshall SB, Piek J, Blunt BA, Klauber MR, Marshall LF (1993) Early and late systemic hypotension as a frequent and fundamental source of cerebral ischemia following severe brain injury in the traumatic coma data bank. Acta Neurochir 59 [Suppl]:121-125
18. Ishige N, Pitts LH, Hashimoto T, Nishimura MC, Bartkowski HM (1987) Effect of hypoxia on traumatic brain injury in rats: part 1: changes in neurological function, electroencephalograms, and histopathology. Neurosurgery 20:848-853
19. Cruz J (1993) On-line monitoring of global cerebral hypoxia in acute brain injury. Relationship to intracranial hypertension. J Neurosurg 79:228-233
20. Schmoker JD, Zhuang J, Shackford SR (1992) Hemorrhagic hypotension after brain injury causes an early and sustained reduction in cerebral oxygen delivery despite normalization of systemic oxygen delivery. J Trauma 32:714-722
21. Fortune JB, Bock D, Kupinski AM, Stratton HH, Shah DM, Feustel PJ (1992) Human cerebrovascular response to oxygen and carbon dioxide as determined by internal carotid artery duplex scanning. J Trauma 32:618-628
22. Zhuang J, Schmoker JD, Shackford SR, Pietropaoli JA (1992) Focal brain injury results in severe cerebral ischemia despite maintenance of cerebral perfusion pressure. J Trauma 33: 83-88
23. Bouma GJ, Muizelaar P (1992) Cerebral blood flow, cerebral blood volume, and cerebrovascular reactivity after severe head injury. J Neurotrauma 9 [Suppl]:S333-S348
24. Cruz J (1993) Combined continuous monitoring of systemic and cerebral oxygenation in acute brain injury: preliminary observations. Crit Care Med 21:1225-1232
25. Mateer JR, Olson DW, Stueven HA, Aufderheide TP (1993) Continuous pulse oximetry during emergency endotracheal intubation. Ann Emerg Med 22:675-679
26. Nardi G, Massarutti D, Muzzi R, Kette F, De Monte A, Carnelos GA, Peressutti R, Berlot G, Giordano F, Gullo A (1994) Impact of emergency medical helicopter service on mortality for trauma in north-east Italy. A regional prospective audit. Eur J Emerg Med 1:69-77
27. Trupka A, Waydhas C, Nast-Kolb D, Schweiberer (1994) Early intubation in severely injured patients. Eur J Emerg Med 1:1-8
28. Deakin CD (1994) Early fluid resuscitation in haemorrhagic shock. Eur J Emerg Med 1:83-85
29. Lechleuthner A, Lefering R, Bouillon B, Lentke E, Vorweg M, Tiling T (1994) Prehospital detection of uncontrolled haemorrhage in blunt trauma. Eur J Emerg Med 1:13-18
30. Deakin C, Davies G (1994) Defining trauma patients subpopulations for field stabilization. Eur J Emerg Med 1:31-33
31. Personal communication. International Resuscitation Research Conference '94, Pittsburgh, May 5-8, 1994

Care of Trauma Patients: In-hospital Phase

A. DE MONTE, G. NARDI

The chain for survival of trauma patients includes several links: identification, notification, first aid on the scene, safe prehospital transportation, diagnostic procedures, treatment of life-threatening lesions first and definitive stabilisation of trauma injuries later, until hospital discharge. The strength of the chain is given by its weakest link and therefore each single passage of this survival chain has to "run" at its fastest speed but synchronising with the others. For example, all the advantages of an efficient and top level prehospital care might be nullified by a less efficient in-hospital working phase.

During the past years, trauma prevention and prehospital care have received a tremendous impulse by technological advances and their application in general security (seat belts, etc.) and on medical treatment. The benefits of an advanced rescue support on the scene of accident (i.e. golden hour concept) has been debated and supported by international consensus (i.e. ATLS, etc.) and by public and private training programmes (1-3). However, an equivalent consensus has not been reached yet with concern to in-hospital treatment (4-13).

In this chapter we will analyse the organisational aspects of in-hospital assistance to trauma patients.

Organisational planning

The idea of a trauma care system has been developed since the 1960s, when the USA National Research Council (14) identified traumatic events as the leading cause of death in the under forties population. In this report, trauma was defined as "the neglected disease of modern society".

The concept of a trauma care system, supports the philosophy of regionalisation of trauma patients in the effort to improve the quality of care associated with a more rational utilisation of resources (4, 6, 7, 15-18).

In this organisational planning, the trauma centre becomes the cornerstone upon which the system is based on and it has to be interconnected.

The ideal trauma centre is built up to treat specifically all trauma patients and it is provided with all the facilities for diagnosis and therapy. Therefore, all

architectural barriers have to be avoided. Diagnostic procedures should be
centralised and integrated and they have to pivot on the patient to minimise the
loss of time and superfluous displacements of the patient itself (Fig. 1). Adequate
laboratories, operating rooms and intensive care facilities have to be available 24
h a day. Portable and fixed equipment of vital functions has to be available too.

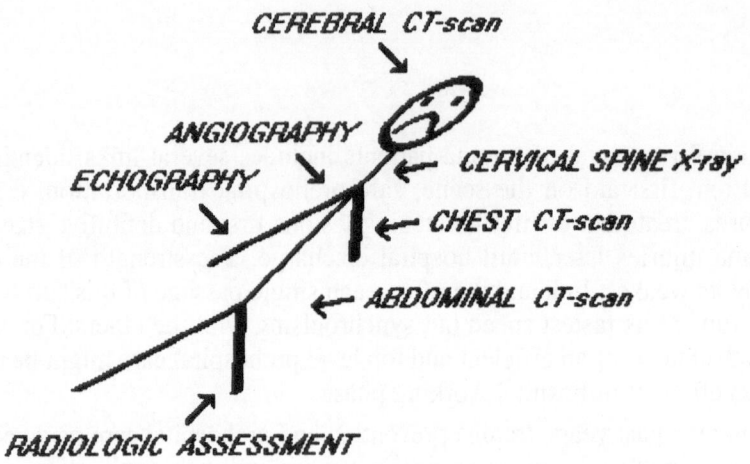

Fig. 1. Diagnostic investigations that should rotate around a trauma patient

The centralisation of trauma patients in level I regional hospitals improves the
capability and the skill of medical and paramedical staff. In fact, only 10% of
trauma patients require specific facilities which are available in a first level
trauma centre (11). Therefore the process of regionalisation of patients has also
the advantage of reducing the time required to complete the learning curve of
junior staff with respect to level II and III centres. The advantages of this
organisational model are reported in Table 1.

Table 1. Main advantages of a dedicated trauma centre

- Good use of time
- Rational employment of medical and nonmedical staff
- Less opportunity of iatrogenic damage due to
  - Changes of surgical bed or decubitus
  - Bone fracture dislocation
  - Dislodgement of tracheal tube
  - Drains malpositioning
  - Accidental change on drug administration rate
- Safer manipulation of instrumental facilities
- Increasing competence of the personnel

Although plenty of scientific reports and economical and political planning agree with such a strategy, reality is far from conforming to this theory. Probably, it is not possible to reach a general agreement on the treatment of trauma patients because of the great number of factors involved in the quality of care and organisation of trauma centres, with respect to local requirements. In 1988 in the USA, only Maryland and Virginia had their trauma care assistance programme completed; 29 states had not even initiated the regional categorisation of trauma centres, whilst the remainders were still at the beginning of planning (11, 12, 18).

We don't have any data to show European reality is any different. It is quite normal for a trauma patient to enter a regional hospital and to be forced in a sort of pilgrimage to reach the different diagnostic and surgical facilities, with consequent loss of precious time. Moreover, accordingly with local organisation, some instrumental examinations (i.e. abdominal echography) can be or cannot be carried out in ICU and the distance between ward and imaging diagnostic units is an "independent variable". As a consequence, the heterogeneity concerning logistic aspects influences the diagnostic and therapeutic approaches which change among different institutions. In Table 2 we report the information we obtained from 40 Italian hospitals concerning the basic facilities available in their centre regarding trauma care. The hospitals we considered include a total of 32,000 beds and among them 486 were ICU beds (general, cardiac or neurosurgical), only 1.5% of the total beds, significantly lower than 3% as recommended by European committees. Among the 17 hospitals classified as level I centres, only nine have a centralised diagnostic department and the opportunity to perform diagnostic procedures in ICU, 12 have round the clock availability of angiography. Five centres have a cerebral CT scan situated between 100 and 500 m away from the ICU, while in two cases the distance is over 500 m; in one hospital thoraco-abdominal CT scan is not available 24 h a day.

Table 2. Facilities available in 17 Italian first level trauma centres

	Centralisation of diagnosis		Angiography 24 h		Echo in ICU		CT-ICU > 100 m	
Availability	Yes	No	Yes	No	Yes	No	Yes	No
Number	9	8	12	5	9	8	7	10

In-hospital treatment protocols

It is not a simple matter to define a uniform in-hospital treatment protocol for trauma patients. Certainly, there are several conditions where methods of approach are obvious and unanimously accepted. For example, no one will argue the fact that an extradural haematoma 5 cm wide has to be drained as soon as possible.

On the other hand, there are a great number of borderline conditions whose treatment is not so obvious. Moreover, other factors such as local habits, organisational and surgical aspects as well as patient condition can support an aggressive or cautious approach. In our institution, we share the rule of ATLS guidelines to consider a trauma patient affected by an acute series of life-threatening lesions until proved otherwise, and previously existing pathologies should not be regarded as the leading cause of the actual patient condition. Of course this attitude can induce one to perform a redundant number of diagnostic investigations but it can produce a tremendous impact in the expectancy and quality of life of a trauma patient. For example, all trauma patients entering our unit have the spine completely evaluated by plain X-ray and if C7-T1 alignment is not correctly visible, CT scan is performed for further evaluation. Following this policy, we established that 27 (18%) patients out of a series of 145 trauma patients admitted to our centre presented with a spine lesion. In 50% of cases, the damage was located in the cervical section and half of them involved the C7-T1 area.

Remarkably, 50% of patients with cervical spine fractures were free from evident neurologic lesions and they underwent successful emergency stabilisation surgery.

Plain chest X-ray has many limitations too. In another group of 52 chest trauma patients we observed that half of them had their chest drained because of pneumothorax. However, diagnosis was correctly performed with chest radiogram in 30% of the cases only, while the remainder was detected by computed tomography of the chest.

These clinical findings raise the problem of indication and quality control of imaging diagnostic procedures and the indications for them. Clear guideline consensus is difficult to reach due to the nothomogeneous attitude in medical practice and in the specific background of operators. As an example of this, we have a questionnaire filled out by specialists of 40 major Italian hospitals; 15 of them claimed to have a good knowledge of ATLS guidelines, in six cases the knowledge was assumed as "sufficient" while in the remaining 17 the level of know-how is thought to be poor. Moreover, various centres supposed to be "level I" have no thoracoabdominal CT scan and angiography available 24 h a day.

Time as a crucial factor

Time is a crucial factor when we deal with trauma patients during the acute phase. Therefore it has to be best utilised. There is a different scale to measure the time during the out or in-hospital treatment. In fact, the out-hospital rescue phase does not lasts more than 60 min, no matter if "scoop and run" or "stay and play" strategy is preferred. On the other hand, the acute phase of in-hospital treatment can be prolonged for many hours. Accordingly with the local organisation, the patient may pass from one specialist's care to another and from a diagnostic section to another one. The clinical consequences can also be noteworthy because the higher the number of passages, the higher will be the possibility of losing clinical information. In our centre for example, a patient rescued by helicopter requiring a cerebral and a thoracic CT scan, undergoing open celioscopy and general ICU admission, changes between six and eight litters or surgical beds (19). It is obvious that each passage may potentially damage the patient status or the instrumentation, as pointed out in Table 1.

Recently, in our centre we analysed the time required for the acute stabilisation of a severe trauma patient, from hospital entrance to ICU admittance. In particular we measured the time spent for primary and secondary survey in the emergency room, which is necessary to perform diagnostic procedures, and the interval elapsed before entering the ICU. The results are reported in Tables 3-5; it is worthwhile to underline that for each patient we required on average more than 4 h (from 2 h to 11 h!) before ICU admittance.

Table 3. Number and type of examination performed in a series of 60 severe trauma patients

Diagnostic investigation	n
Skull X-ray	20
Cervical spine X-ray	49
Thoracolumbar X-ray	40
Pelvic X-ray	13
Other X-ray	21
Abdominal echography	33
Cervical spine CT-scan	13
Cerebral CT-scan	44
Thoracic CT-scan	21
Thoracolumbar CT-scan	18

Table 4. Timing of the acute stabilisation period phase (see text for further information)

Timing	Min (range)
First aid	36 (15-100)
Standard X-ray examination	55 (15-110)
Total time	245 (105-700)

Table 5. Surgical interventions during the acute phase stabilisation

Surgical intervention	n (%)
Neurosurgery	12 (20)
General surgery	10 (16.6)
Orthopaedics	7 (11.6)
Chest drainage	7 (11.6)

Conclusion

In-hospital trauma care guidelines definition is hindered by different logistic and organisational aspects of each single local institution. Regionalisation of the trauma care system can concur to homogenise the approach to this pathology, overcoming structural gaps and addressing the patients towards the most suitable structures. As a result, the work load will be better distributed according to available resources. Of course, this is a long lasting process which includes several phases:

- Census and categorisation of facilities available in each medical centre
- Local and regional consensus according to specific single resources
- Re-planning and adaptation of existing structures, in order to exploit all local existing facilities
- Recurring updating meetings for protocols revising and critical analysis of the results

Of course, the meaning of all topics mentioned in this chapter, loses part of its meaning if the trauma centre is not interconnected with a well-organised hospital emergency system.

References

1. American College of Surgeons Committee on Trauma (1991) Advanced Trauma Life Support Course Student Manual. American College of Surgeons, Chicago
2. Skinner D, Driscoll P, Earlam R (eds) (1991) ABC of major trauma. Br Med J
3. De Monte A, Nardi G (1994) Protocolli ATLS per il trattamento del politrauma. In: Associazione di pubblica assistenza (ed) Testo ufficiale Corso Nazionale di Emergenza VTLS, Signa
4. Clemmer PT, Orme FJ, Thomas OF et al (1985) Outcome of critically injured patients treated at level I trauma centres versus full-service community hospitals. Crit Care Med 13:861-863
5. Shackford RS, Mackersie CR, Hoyt BD et al (1987) Impact of a trauma system on outcome of severely injured patients. Arch Surg 122:523-527
6. Eastman BA, Lewis RF, Champion RH, Mattox LK (1987) Regional trauma system design: critical concepts. Am J Surg 154:79-87
7. West GJ, Williams JM, Trunkey DD, Wolferth CC (1988) Trauma systems. Current status-future challenges. JAMA 259:3597-3600
8. Maull IK, Schwab WC, McHenry DS et al (1986) Trauma center verification. J Trauma 26: 521-524
9. Ornato PJ, Craren JE, Nelson MN, Kimball FK (1985) Impact of improved emergency medical services and emergency trauma care on the reduction in mortality from trauma. J Trauma 25:575-579
10. Gibson G (1978) Categorization of hospital emergency capabilities: some empirical methods to evaluate appropriateness of emergency department utilization. J Trauma 18:94-102
11. Mesnick P (1991) Emergency medical services, trauma care, and disaster planning. In: Capan ML (ed) Trauma: anesthesia and intensive care. Lippincott, Philadelphia, pp 845-859
12. Hurst MJ (1991) Trauma: an overview. In: Rippe MJ (ed) Intensive care medicine. Little, Brown, Boston, pp 1455-1458

13. Wilson FW (1989) Trauma. In: Shoemaker CW (ed) Textbook of critical care. Saunders, Philadelphia, pp 1230-1271
14. National Research Council (1966) Accidental death and disability: the neglected disease of modern society. Washington DC
15. Shackford RS, Hollingworth-Fridlung P, Cooper FG, Eastman BA (1986) The effect of regionalisation upon the quality of trauma care as assessed by concurrent audit before and after institution of a trauma system: a preliminary report. J Trauma 26:812-820
16. Eggold R (1983) Trauma care regionalisation: a necessity. J Trauma 23:260-262
17. Ammons AM, Moore EE, Pons TP et al (1988) The role of a regional trauma system in the management of a mass disaster: an analysis of the Keystone, Colorado chairlift accident. J Trauma 28:1468-1471
18. Trunkey DD, Blaisdell WF (1988) Epidemiology of trauma. In: Wilmore WD (ed) Care of the surgical patient. Scientific Am IV;6:1-7
19. De Monte A, Nardi G, Giordano F et al (1995) Il politraumatizzato dal primo soccorso al ricovero in terapia intensiva. Fase intraospedaliera. In: Pasetto (ed) Le nuove frontiere dell'impegno anestesiologico: il sistema di emergenza, i trapianti e la terapia antalgica domiciliare. Atti del convegno, pp 34-37

Prehospital Care for Severe Trauma Patients: What Do We Mean by ALS?

G. NARDI, A. DE MONTE

Introduction

The reduction of trauma morbidity and mortality is one of the priorities of all health services around the world. In the USA injuries cause the loss of more years of life than do cancer and heart disease combined and the total injury-related costs are higher than the costs of any other disease process (1). Two of the most effective ways of combating this public health problem are prevention and the establishment of a trauma system.

In recent years major effort has been made in many countries to improve the quality of trauma care by means of the implementation of an integrated approach, including the development of trauma centers and the amelioration of prehospital care. A strategy of centralization of severe trauma patients to large institutions specifically organized to care for them (trauma centers) has been shown to decrease both mortality rate and the number of preventable deaths (2, 3). In a recent analysis on the outcome in severely injured patients (Injury Severity Score - ISS - > 15) before the implementation of a dedicated trauma program in California (4) Demetriades observed a 33% reduction of mortality in severe blunt trauma with a trend toward lower permanent disabilities.

However, it should be kept in mind that a large percentage of trauma deaths occur before admission to any hospital. In an epidemiological survey in the South West Thames region in England, Daly and Thomas (5) observed that as many as 53% of all the deaths occur in the prehospital setting and the figure is even higher (58%) in Wales according to Gorman et al. (6).

These data are consistent with the results of a recent audit in a population of 1 million people in northeast Italy (7). Two hundred twenty-two severely injured patients (ISS > 15) who were still alive on arrival of the first EMT were entered into this study. Among the 68 patients (30.8%) who eventually died (Fig. 1), 20 (29%) died on the scene or during transportation and 17 more patients (25%) died on admission to the nearest rural hospital before referral or within 30 min of admission to a trauma center. Only 46% of the total deaths occurred in the ICUs or in the operating rooms during emergency surgery. Therefore, as stated by Daly "... if important reductions in deaths from severe injury are to be made, then prehospital care needs to be improved".

When do the severely injured patients die: analysis of 67 deaths
Data of the Regional audit: 1st august 1992 - 28 february 1993

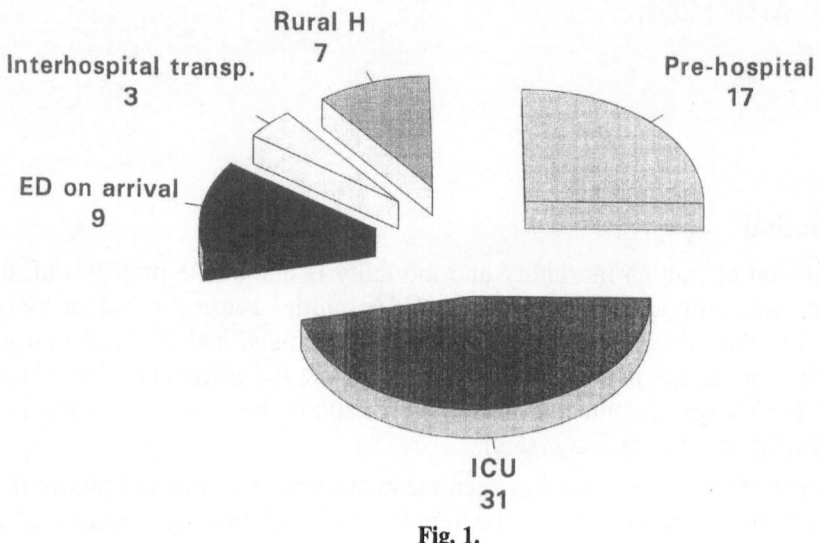

Fig. 1.

To improve the quality of prehospital care in many health services paramedics and physicians are trained to provide advanced supportive therapy (ALS) including tracheal intubation, decompression of tension pneumothorax and the establishment of i.v. lines for fluid resuscitation.

Many different studies have been carried on in the USA to evaluate the advantages of ALS vs. BLS. Most of the time (3) these studies were unable to demonstrate any benefit of ALS at the scene in terms of survival and reduction of hospital stay. In Europe, in contrast, the large majority of the people involved in trauma care strongly believe that prehospital advanced trauma life support (ATLS) could be of paramount importance in reducing mortality and morbidity due to trauma (7).

In a regional audit (8) that took into consideration all the victims of unvoluntary trauma over a period of 7 months, we observed a highly significant reduction in mortality in the group of patients rescued by the EHMS through an ALS strategy, which will be discussed in further detail.

There are several possible explanations for these discrepancies: first, in the USA there is an extremely large number of penetrating injuries while in Europe most of the injured patients sustain a blunt trauma. As clearly demonstrated by Lerer and Knottenbelt (9) the key to improving survival in penetrating injuries lies in rapid transportation by the quickest available means, including private transports. Prehospital stabilization for patients with major injuries involving the heart or the large intrathoracic vessels is probably just a loss of time and ALS offers no advantage (10).

Smidt and coworkers (11) retrospectively evaluated the results of *"on scene helicopter transport"* of patients with multiple injuries. They compared two different systems: one in Germany and the second in the USA. Two groups of patients were considered: 221 in Germany and 186 in the USA. The patients of the two groups were comparable regarding mechanism of injury, age, mean ISS, ISS distribution and number of severe injuries per body region.

Surprisingly the intubation rate in the German group was three times higher (37.1% vs 13.4%), the rate of thoracic decompression on the scene was 10% vs. 0.5% and the amount of fluids infused in the prehospital setting was more than the double (1800 ml vs. 825 ml) as an average. Both groups were said to have been treated by ALS. Thus a second explanation for the inconsistency among data from different authors and different countries lies in major differences in the adopted protocols and therefore in the definition of ALS.

How many trauma patients can benefit of ALS procedures

It has been estimated that 60 million injuries occur in the USA each year (12). Although 5% of them require hospitalization (3 million), the percentage of severe trauma is a minimal fraction of this figure.

There are extremely few data on the epidemiology of severe trauma in Europe. In a study from Gordman and coworkers, where the definition of severe trauma was applied to patients with ISS > 15, the authors reported an incidence of 1088 patients per year on a population of 3.2 millions people: 340 per million per year. In our study in northeast Italy the estimated incidence referred to victims who were found alive was 385 per million, consistent with data from England. In our study, the overall mortality rate (prehospital and hospital) for patients with ISS > 15 was 30.8%. This figure is consistent with data reported by Spaite et al. (13) in Arizona using the same method (32.6%) and with the figures reported by Demetriades et al. in California (4). It seems therefore reasonable that patients with ISS > 15, who have an expected mortality around 30%, might benefit from ALS in the prehospital setting. In this case the target for a trauma team with ALS skills should be estimated in 300-400 patients per million/year. However, in a recent prospective study performed to estimate the potential benefits of ALS, on a population of one million people in Northern Ireland, McNicholl (14) evaluated that the projected annual intubation figures are 30 patients per annum. In this evaluation only apneic patients and comatose patients who eventually aspirated were considered potential candidates for on scene intubation. Not surprisingly, as many as 85% of these patients died.

McNicholl's study raises an extremely important point. To understand which is the best organization of a prehospital emergency service caring for trauma patients, we ought to define at first which interventions are useful in prehospital setting and make clear which is the target population for ALS trained teams. If we agree with McNicholl that no more than 30 patients per million people yearly will require prehospital intubation, then the rationale to train paramedics has to be challenged, as it is difficult to assume that anybody who performs intubation once or twice a year will be able to maintain an adequate level of skills.

Consensus and controversies on ABC

Airway and cervical spine protection

Data from the literature point out that 15%-35% of all patients with severe head injury suffer a secondary brain injury from hypoxia and hypovolemia before hospital admission (15). In a study from the University of Texas it was shown that those unconscious head-injured patients who had endotracheal intubation carried out on the field have a 40% better chance of survival with a good neurologic outcome.

Endotracheal intubation is the definitive procedure for establishing an airway and optimizing ventilation. However, the decision to intubate injured patients at the scene is difficult to make. Intubation in trauma patients may be extremely difficult and unlike cardiac arrest where any intervention is better than none (the outcome being death), an inadequate attempt to intubate a trauma patient may, through complications, worsen the injury. There are no well-defined criteria for intubation in trauma. Oswalt et al. (16) recently showed that a delay in tracheal intubation is associated with a mortality rate higher than predicted by TRISS method in trauma patients with a GCS lower than 13.

The ATLS guidelines (American College of Surgeons) do not include the use of anesthetic induction agents and neuromuscular blockers. Without these agents the airway management of reactive trauma patients might be extremely difficult and not always feasible. This can explain the huge differences in intubation rate among reports from the USA and Europe.

Vilke et al. (17) compared field intubations by the nasotracheal route to rapid sequence induction orotracheal intubation and noninduced orotracheal intubation. In this study rapid sequence orotracheal intubation was associated with a higher success rate, fewer complications and a better patient outcome. However, the prehospital use of neuromuscular agents can be extremely dangerous in unskilled hands.

For these reasons standards of prehospital airway care must not be merely good but have to be excellent.

One of the major concerns of this maneuver is that tracheal intubation might have harmful effects on patients with a traumatic cervical spine injury by inducing further neurological damage. To avoid movement of the cervical spine, previous editions of the ATLS guidelines have recommended nasotracheal intubation. The current guidelines (18) state that the most important determinant of whether to proceed with orotracheal or nasotracheal intubation depends on the experience of the physicians. In experienced hands, rapid sequence induction with neuromuscular blockers with manual in-line stabilization of the head and neck, followed by oral intubation has also proven safe in patients with cervical spine injuries (19).

Breathing

Pneumothorax is one of the most frequent and life threatening complications of severe injuries involving the chest. In a previous study we observed that unrecognized tension pneumothorax was the most important cause of preventable death in trauma patients who died within 30 min of admission to the Emergency Department of the Hospital of Udine, a level 1 trauma center in northeast Italy (20). Moreover in a series of 52 consequent severe chest trauma (AIS ≥ 3) submitted to CT scan soon after admission, 50% had a pneumothorax. There is little doubt that emergency decompression of tension pneumothorax is a potentially life saving procedure and that early detection and treatment of this condition is an important part of ALS strategies. However, once again, there are impressive differences in the percentage of trauma patients who are submitted to thoracic decompression by different ALS teams (11).

Circulation

Another controversial topic is the prehospital administration of fluids to trauma patients. Conventional on the scene treatment includes prompt intravenous infusion of crystalloids or colloids in order to maintain adequate perfusion of cerebral and myocardial tissue with well oxygenated blood. Up to now, the controversy in fluid resuscitation has been over which type of fluids to use. The practice of initiating fluid administration in the prehospital setting has now been challenged.

Kaweski et al. (21) analyzed the effects of prehospital intravenous fluids on survival in 6855 patients. Two groups of patients were compared: one received fluids while the other group did not. The mean prehospital time was 36 min in both groups. Within each group, no difference in mortality rate was recorded when patients who received fluids were compared to those who did not. The authors concluded that mortality rate following trauma is not influenced by the prehospital administration of fluids but is related to the severity of underlying injuries. Smith et al. (22) in Sacramento reviewed 52 cases of trauma patients who had a BP of less than 100 mmHg either on the scene or on arrival to the emergency department. He stated that a percentage of the 14 patients who died had a treatable surgical lesion and with a more rapid access to the hospital they might have been saved. Moreover the fluid volume infused had been proven of little influence on final outcome. Smith therefore concluded that the prehospital stabilization of the critically injured is a failed concept. The majority (65.4%) of the patients in Smith's study were victims of penetrating injuries. Five deaths out of 14 were due to stab wounds or gunshot to the heart or major vessels, which were considered to be surgically treatable.

More recently Bickell et al. (23) conducted a prospective trial comparing immediate resuscitations with fluids versus no fluids over 598 hypotensive patients with penetrating injuries to the torso. Patients who did not receive fluids before surgery had a lower mortality rate (30% vs. 38%) and fewer complications (23% vs. 30%) compared with patients who received fluids before surgery. The authors conclude that aggressive administration of intravenous fluids to patients with penetrating injuries should be delayed: intravenous fluids may promote hemorrhage by diluting coagulation factors and decreasing the resistance to flow around an incomplete thrombus (23).

The statements of these studies need some comments:

1. As clearly stressed by the Houston group (23), their conclusions refer only to hypotensive patients with penetrating injuries requiring immediate surgery. Moreover as many as 176 patients with RTS = 0 (no recordable pressure) were excluded from the analysis. Some experimental data on animals (24) suggest that administration of fluids to ensure a low blood pressure (40 mmHg) may help to ensure a limited tissue perfusion without enhancing blood loss. Whether patients with the most severe penetrating injuries could benefit from fluid resuscitation need therefore to be further investigated. Based on the results of their studies, Smith et al. (22) and Kaweski et al. (21) conclude that prehospital administration of fluids is of no value but they fail to distinguish between patients with blunt and penetrating injuries. While penetrating injuries caused by gunshot or stab wounds are a major problem in the USA with over 24 000 people killed annually (25), in Europe blunt trauma as a consequence of road traffic accidents or work accident are the large majority. The results of studies based on a population where 40% or more of the severe injuries are penetrating cannot be extrapolated to different realities.

2. In Bickell's study the average of Ringer's solution administered in the prehospital setting in the immediate resuscitation group was 870 ml and the volumes administered before surgery at the trauma center was 1608 ml. The same amount of fluids, less than 1 l of crystalloids, were infused in Smith's series, while in Kaweski's study the volume of crystalloids infused in the group of patients with ISS > 50 and BP < 90 was 1245 ml on average, which means an effective volume replacement of less than 250 ml even in the most severely injured patients with hemorragic shock... Such a volume is by far too low to bring to any significant change in hemodynamics.

Moreover according to Smith the time spent by the EMTs to establish an i.v. line ranged between 8.6 and 11.5 min, with a percentage of failed attempts varying from 40% to 11% and being more frequent in patients with more profound hypotension.

It makes no sense to waste 11 min to establish an i.v. line to infuse a few milliliters of saline and again an i.v. line doesn't mean an ALS!

Theses studies demonstrate the limited value of an insufficient prehospital administration of fluids rather than of prehospital infusion of fluids itself, at least in cases of blunt trauma.

The large majority of severely injured patients involved in motor vehicle accidents also have head trauma. Both hypoxia and hypotension have been shown to worsen the outcome in head injury (26). There is little doubt that undertreatment of hypovolemia in the prehospital setting is associated with major risks of brain ischemia. Some authors feel, however, that resuscitation with large volumes of fluids could enhance the development of brain edema and that fluid restriction will help limit any increase in intracranial pressure.

In a recent study Scalea (27) evaluated the hemodynamic responses and the effects of volume resuscitation on intracranial pressure in patients with severe blunt trauma and head injury. The patients in this study required a mean of 5 l of electrolyte solution in the first 24 h and had a positive balance of 3.6 l averaged. Despite volume loading, intracranial pressure did not increase. The only patient who presented a sustained increase in intracranial pressure had a negative balance during the first 24 h. Moreover when invasively monitored, many of the patients with diffuse blunt trauma and close-head injuries, although normotensive, had a low cardiac output and evidence of impaired peripheral perfusion. As many as 80% of the patients in this series were underresuscitated when invasively monitored. Volume loading to these patients was associated to an augmentation of cardiac output but no increase in intracranial pressure. Hypovolemia may increase the dangers related to other treatment, enhancing the risks of brain ischemia in patients submitted to hyperventilation. As hypotension is one of the later manifestations of inadequate perfusion, it is possible that hypoperfusion without hypotension may also affect neurologic outcome.

According to the guidelines of the American College of Surgeons (28), young traumatized patients with hypotension are expected to have a blood loss of at least 30%-40% of the total blood volume (i.e. 2000 ml of blood for an 80-kg man). Very large amounts of fluids are required to restore volemia in these cases if crystalloids are employed. Recently hypertonic saline and hyperoncotic dextran have been suggested for prehospital resuscitation, because of their ability to expand blood volume and elevate systemic blood pressure and cardiac output in a small volume and during a short time (29).

An increasing number of studies report promising results with this technique; however, in the controlled studies hypertonic saline/dextran infusion (HSD) was compared with an equal amount of normal saline or Ringer's solution (30, 31). Again, as no more than 250 ml of HSD were employed to avoid the risk of hypernatriemia, the control group received an insignificant amount of fluids. Mattox et al. reported an improved blood pressure and a better survival in the HSD subgroup requiring surgery and Vassar et al. (31) a tendency toward improving survival in patients with severe head injuries. No study has yet been performed to compare hypertonic saline and HSD to adequate volume of colloids or crystalloids.

One of the major technical problems in order to obtain an adequate volume replacement in the prehospital setting concern the maximum rate of infusion. The use of bags under pressure, although associated with a small risk of air embolism (32), allows a sharp increase in the rate of infusion (Table 1). The same amount of fluids can be infused through bags under pressure, even when the bags are on the stretcher at the patient's level, thus allowing to continue infusions even during field transportation (33).

Table 1. Maximum flow rate through a standard infusion set attached to i.v. catheters for peripheral vein of different calibers

Gauge	22	20	18	17	16	14
Calibre (mm)	0.8	1.0	1.2	1.4	1.7	2.0
Maximum flow rate (ml/min)						
Normal saline (NS) (h 120 cm)	27	43	67	98	109	146
Emagel (h 120 cm)	25	37	48	72	97	130
NS in pressure bag (h 120 cm)	74	137	160	266	332	432
Emagel in pressure bag (h 120 cm)	68	120	152	249	295	322
NS in pressure bag at the patient's level (h = 0)	65	109	147	195	303	352

Data refer to catheters that are not inserted in vein. Measurement conditions are the following: infusion bags kept at 120 cm height and atmospheric pressure (A), pressure bags inflated at a constant pressure of 300 mmHg and kept either at 120 cm above the catheter (B) or at the catheter level (C).
Normal saline is used as a standard colloid and gelatines (Emagel) in 1000 ml bags as standard colloids.
From Nardi et al. (33)

ALS strategy for an emergency helicopter service

In 1991 we carried out an audit on the outcome of the severely injured patients admitted to our hospital. The study highlighted that a high percentage of patients died soon after admission as a consequence of mistreatment in the prehospital phase. Fifty-three percent of the early deaths were considered to be preventable. Unrecognized tension pneumothorax was the most important cause of preventable deaths, followed by undertreated hemorrhagic shock.

The results of the study were widely discussed and great effort was made to improve the quality of trauma care.

In August 1992 an emergency helicopter medical service (EHMS) was set up. The EHMS, based at Udine hospital, cares for the whole area of Friuli, an administrative region in the northeastern part of Italy. The region has a surface of 8600 km^2 with a population of 1.25 million people and is basically a rural area.

In order to ensure a high degree of care in the prehospital phase, the most experienced physicians and paramedics were involved. The EHS team consists of one anesthesiologist with at least 10 years of experience in the ICU, and two ICU nurses with prolonged experience in prehospital care as part of ambulance EMT. Three years later, more than 50% of all severe trauma patients (ISS > 15) in this region are rescued being at the scene by the EHMS. This percentage is much higher (80%) when only accidents that occur during daylight are taken into consideration.

The ALS strategy adopted by the EHMS is shown in Table 2.

Table 2. ABC treatment

ATLS strategy (FVG regional emergency helicopter service)
A   Airways and cervical spine:
On scene orotracheal intubation through rapid sequence induction
if GCS $\leq$ 12 or hypoxia (SaO_2 < 90% and FiO_2 = 0.8)
B   Breathing:
Aggressive treatment of pneumothorax
C   Circulation:
Aggressive fluid resuscitation with colloids and crystalloids through large bore i.v. lines and bags under pressure

A: Airways. According to the adopted guidelines, injured patients with GCS $\leq$ 12 or who present with severe hypoxemia are submitted to orotracheal intubation through a rapid sequence induction with neuromuscular blockers. The cervical spine is kept in-line manually and stabilized with a semi-rigid collar before intubation.

Two hundred ninety-seven trauma patients were intubated at the scene in 30 months by the EHMS. Of the 208 patients with a GCS < 9 rescued during the same period, 202 were submitted to tracheal intubation at the accident scene and only 6 were not. In five cases the guidelines were not applied by decision of the anesthetist. In one case no airway could be established in spite of repeated attempts of orotracheal and nasotracheal intubation: the anesthetized patient was assisted by mask ventilation until admission to the emergency department with no consequences (Fig. 2). Seventy-two injured patients had a GCS $\geq$ 9 and $\leq$ 12: 36 of them were intubated and 26 were not (Fig. 3). Among the patients who were not intubated three vomited and one of them aspirated. Another patient had an epileptic attack with severe hypoxia and subsequent cardiac arrest. After CPR he did well. No complications were reported in the group of patients who underwent tracheal intubation.

B: Breathing. All physicians involved in the EHMS are skilled both in decompression of tension pneumothorax and thoracic drainage. Patients who present with hypoxemia, hypotension and either subcutaneous emphysema or unilateral hypoventilation are submitted to an explorative thoracentesis at the

On the scene intubation
GCS < 9 (208 severely injured patients)

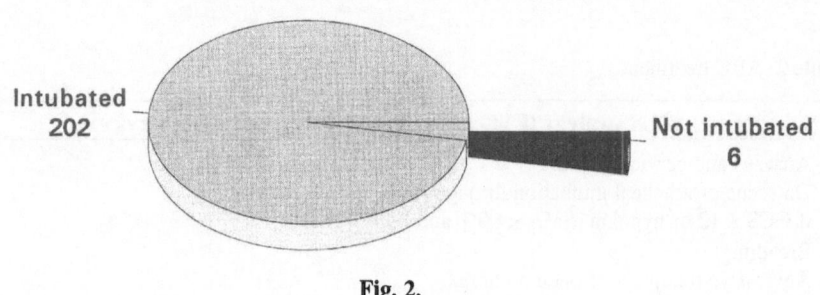

Fig. 2.

On the scene intubation
GCS > = 9 and < = 12   (72 patients)

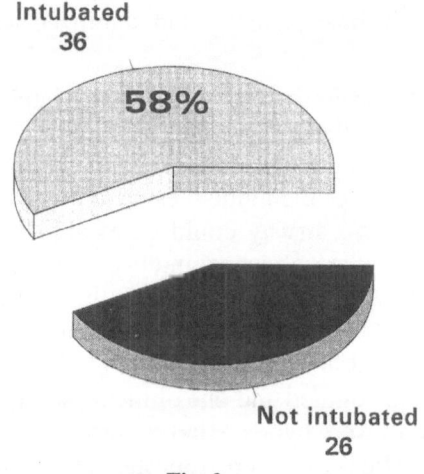

Fig. 3.

scene. If air under tension is recorded thoracic decompression is performed by means of a large 2.2 mm ∅ needle connected to a Heimlich's valve.

From August 1, 1994 to May 31, 1995 (10 months), 17 patients with tension pneumothorax were treated by chest decompression. In three cases a bilateral thoracic drainage was inserted. In spite of all measures taken to identify and treat pneumothorax at the scene, five patients with unrecognized tension pneumothorax brought in by the EHMS required emergency chest decompression soon after admission to the Emergency Department. However, during 30 months, not a single patient treated by the EHMS died because of pneumothorax neither in the prehospital or early hospital phase.

C: Circulation. According to the guidelines all the hypotensive patients with blunt trauma are treated with massive infusions of both colloids and crystalloids using bags under pressure and with the aim to achieve a blood pressure of 100 mmHg. Two large bore i.v. lines are considered to be mandatory.

A prospective study on all the hypotensive blunt trauma patients is now in progress. During the first 6 months of the survey, 36 consecutive patients with BP < 90 were entered into the study. The average time to insert one i.v. line was 1 min for the first line while 55 s more were needed for the second line. In one case no i.v. line could be started on the field. The average fluids infused in the prehospital setting was 1848 (0-5600) with an average of 863 mls of crystalloids (0-3800) and 985 mls of colloids (0-3000). Four patients had no recordable pressure when first seen. Two of them were found in cardiac arrest but successfully resuscitated. One patient died in the prehospital setting. All the others were admitted to the emergency department with a BP of 70 mmHg or higher.

The efficacy of the ALS strategy applied by the regional EHMS has been evaluated by means of a prospective regional audit and of a trauma center intra-hospital survey. Both the overall (8) and hospital (20) mortality rates were significantly lower if compared with patients submitted to BLS by ambulance teams. The rate of preventable mortality decreased threefold.

More than 2500 trauma patients have been rescued by the EHMS during the first 30 months since its implementation. Although the EHMS cares for the most serious injured patients, among patients still alive when first rescued at the scene, only six died before hospital admission. This means a prehospital mortality rate of less than 2% for patients with ISS > 15. The expected prehospital mortality rate for patients with ISS > 15 submitted to BLS according to the results of 1993 regional audit was 12%: six times higher (Fig. 4).

Conclusions

Our data support the importance of ALS at the scene as a cornerstone to increasing survival for trauma patients. Artificial ventilation, spine control, drainage of pneumothorax and aggressive treatment of hypovolemia are all associated with a better survival rate and bring few risks in skilled hands.

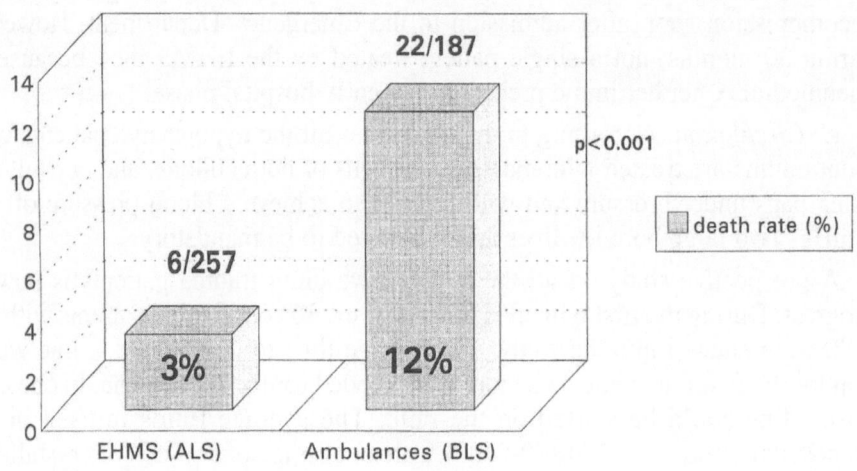

Severe trauma (ISS > 15)
Prehospital mortality

Fig. 4.

However, there is a need for a better definition of "ALS" in trauma care in order to allow comparison of the results of the different studies and to establish a widely accepted strategy.

References

1. Trunkey DD, Blaisdell WF (1988) Epidemiology of trauma. In: Wilmore WD (ed) Care of the surgical patients. Sci Am 6:1-7
2. Cales RH (1984) Trauma mortality in Orange County: the effect of implementation of a regional trauma system. Ann Emerg Med 13:15-23
3. Sampalis JS, Lavoie A, Williams JI et al (1993) Impact of on-site care, prehospital time and level of in-hospital care on survival in severely injured patients. J Trauma 34:(2)256-261
4. Demetriades D, Belzberg H, Asensio J et al (1995) The impact of a dedicated trauma program on outcome in severely injured patients. Arch Surg 130:216-220
5. Daly KE, Thomas PR (1992) Trauma deaths in the South West Thames region. Injury 23(6): 393-396
6. Gorman DF, Teanby DN, Sinha MP et al (1995) The epidemiology of major injuries in Mersey region and North Wales. Injury 26(1):51-54
7. Delooz HH (1991) Organization and implementation of emergency services in the treatment of major trauma. J Neurotrauma 8 [Suppl 1]:S1-S6
8. Nardi G, Massarutti D, Muzzi R et al (1994) Impact of emergency medical helicopter service on mortality for trauma in North-East Italy. A regional prospective audit. Eur J Emerg Med (1):69-77

9. Lerer LB, Knottenbelt JD (1994) Preventable mortality following sharp penetrating chest trauma. J Trauma 37(1):6-12
10. Buckman RF, Badellino MM, Mauro LH et al (1993) Penetrating cardiac wounds: prospective study of factors influencing initial resuscitation. J Trauma 34(5):717-725
11. Schmidt U, Frame SB, Nerlich M et al (1992) On-scene helicopter transport of patients with multiple injuries-comparison of a German and an American system. J Trauma 33:4(548-553)
12. Spaite Dw, Tse DJ, Valenzuela TD et al (1991) The impact of injury severity and prehospital procedures on scene time in victims of major trauma. Ann Emerg Med 20(12):1299-1305
13. National Safety Council (1986) Accident facts. Chicago, Illinois
14. McNicholl BP (1994) The golden hour and prehospital trauma care. Injury 25:251-254
15. Champion RH, Sacco W (1991) Triage of trauma victims. In: Trunkey D, Lewis F (eds) Current therapy of trauma. Lewitt, Philadelphia, pp 97-103
16. Oswalt JL, Hedges JR, Soifer BE (1992) Analysis of trauma intubations AM. J Emerg Med 10(6):(511-514)
17. Vilke GM, Hoyt DB, Epperson M et al (1994) Intubation techniques in the helicopter. J Emerg Med 12(2):217-224
18. The American College of Surgeons Committee on Trauma Advanced Trauma Life Support program for Physicians (1993) Instructor manual. Chicago
19. Criswell JC, Parr MJA (1994) Emergency airway management in patients with cervical spine injuries. Anaesthesia 49:900-903
20. Nardi G, Massarutti D, Giordano F et al (1994) Interhospital transport for severe trauma patients. Mutz NJ, Koller W, Benzer H (eds) Proceeding of the European Congress on Intensive Care Medicine. Monduzzi, Bologna, pp 631-639
21. Kaweski SM, Sise MJ, Virgilio RW (1990) The effect of prehospital fluids on survival in trauma patients. J Trauma 30:1215-1218
22. Smith JP, Boday BI, Hill AS et al (1985) Prehospital stabilization of critically injured patients: a failed concept. J Trauma 25:65-68
23. Bickell WH, Wall MJ, Pepe PE (1994) Immediate versus delayed fluid resuscitation for hypotensive patients with penetrating torso injuries. N Engl J Med 331:1105-1109
24. Stern SA, Dronen SC, Birren P (1993) Effect of blood pressure on hemorrhage, volume and survival in a near-fatal hemorrhage model incorporating a vascular injury. Ann Emerg Med 22:155-163
25. Schwab CW (1993) Violence: America's uncivil war-presidential address. Sixth scientific assembly of the eastern association for the surgery of trauma. J Trauma 35:657-665
26. Chestnut RM, Marshall LF, Klauber MR (1992) The role of secondary brain injury in determining outcome from severe head injury. J Trauma 34:216-222
27. Scalea TM, Maltz S, Yelon J et al (1994) Resuscitation of multiple trauma and head injury: role of crystalloid fluids and inotropes. Crit Care Med 22:1610-1615
28. American College of Surgeons (1988) Traumatic shock. Adv Trauma Life Support 125-130
29. Krausz MM (1995) Controversies in shock research: hypertonic resuscitation. Pros and Cons. Shock 3:69-72
30. Mattox KL, Maningas PA, Moore EE et al (1991) Prehospital hypertonic saline/dextran infusion for post-traumatic hypotension. The USA multicenter Trial. Ann Surg 213(5):482-491
31. Vassar MJ, Perry CA, Holcroft JW (1993) Prehospital resuscitation of hypotensive trauma patients with 7.5% NaCl with added dextran: a controlled trial. J Trauma 34(5):622-632
32. Pitera R, Hershman Z, Cardoso R et al (1994) The potential for venous air embolism from one liter crystalloids bags. Crit Care Med 22:1(A21)
33. Nardi G, Di Silvestre A, Peressutti R et al (1995) Il trauma vertebro midollare: strategia e rischi delle manovre di estrinsecazione. In: L'emergenza sanitaria in Italia. Peris A (ed). Signa, pp 97-108

Multivariable Physiologic Monitoring as a Guide to the Severity and Appropriate Therapy of Posttrauma ICU Patients

J.H. SIEGEL, D. RIXEN

Clinical care and therapeutic decision making in the severely injured patient whose course is complicated by shock, sepsis or one of the various organ failure syndromes has been complicated by a lack of a precise methodology of *classification* of the nature of these disease processes and stratification of their severity. One important additional consequence of the lack of an effective methodology for *stratification* of critically ill patients with posttraumatic and/or septic syndromes into groups of homogeneous severity has been the paucity of significant advances in basic science mechanisms linking the production of various shock mediators to the different categories of the human host defense response. As a therapeutic consequence, the results of recent human clinical trials where a variety of antiendotoxin or anticytokine mediators have been tested in the therapy of sepsis have been either disappointing or equivocal in their outcome.

Several systems of disease classification have been utilized as an approach to the problem of quantifying or qualifying the host defense response in man. The Sepsis Syndrome: SIRS (1, 2) definitions of the host defense response, with or without the delineation of bacterial septicemia, have proven ambiguous and have blurred the distinctions which they attempted to define. The APACHE methodology (3, 4) which is based on a quantitative grouping of physiologic variables using a heuristic methodology, while representing a distinct improvement over more qualitative systems, has not been shown to have sufficient precision to enable bedside decision making, especially with regard to the posttrauma patient (5, 6).

Recently, a *Physiologic State Severity Classification* (PSSC) methodology developed from 17 cardiorespiratory and metabolic variables which can be obtained dynamically in an intensive care setting has been shown to permit the *classification* of the human host defense response into a data dependent grouping of physiologically similar states (7). The PSSC method also permits the *stratification* of an individual patient at a specific moment in time with regard to the severity of his host defense adaptive response within a given physiologic state classification. This Physiologic State Severity Classification (PSSC) methodology has been used to examine and quantify the human response to severe sepsis, the evolution of the adult respiratory distress syndrome and the prediction of outcome in critically injured trauma patients (8, 9). This methodology has been compared in posttrauma patients to the system of *classification* into sepsis syndrome and systemic inflammatory response (SIRS) (1), to the criteria of the HA-1A Sepsis Study (8) and to that of the Veterans Administration Systemic Sepsis Co-operative Study (9). With regard to severity *stratification*, it has been compared with regard to specificity, sensitivity and accuracy with the APACHE II derived risk of hospital death (ARDEATH) computed from the weighted coefficients developed by Knaus for use in the posttrauma patient (3, 4).

Classification of the physiologic host defense response by the physiologic state classification methodology

The classification methodology used in this study for qualification of the nature of the host defense response is the Physiologic State Classification (7). This methodology was originally developed from 1120 multivariable data sets of 17 physiologic variables obtained from 338 critically ill or surgical patients, including critically injured trauma patients. The physiologic state classification methodology was then validated on a separate group of 205 trauma patients not in the original study and shown to permit meaningful and significant groupings into consistent host defense response patterns which could be validated in new patient groups not in the original development set (10). The variables used in this methodology are the cardiac index (CI); the heart rate (HR); the mean arterial blood pressure (MAP); the oxygen consumption index $\dot{V}O_2/M^2$; the mixed venous pH (pHv); the arterial base excess computed as the extra cellular component (BEA); the mixed venous CO_2 (PvCO_2); the total peripheral resistance (TPR); the cardiac mixing time (Tm), which reflects the left ventricular ejection fraction; the pulmonary vascular dispersive mean transit time (Td), which used together with the cardiac output can develop an estimated pulmonary blood volume; the systolic ejection time (ET); the right atrial pressure (RAP); the respiratory index (RI); the pulmonary shunt (QS/QT); the arterial CO_2 tension (PaCO_2); the arteriovenous O_2 content difference (Ca-vO_2D) and the mixed venous oxygen tension PvO_2. In developing this methodology, each of the variables in a given patient data set was normalized by the mean and standard deviation of the same variable in a data set obtained from a group of recovering trauma patients (the reference-R STATE). The resulting normalized 17 variable sets were then clustered to delineate data-dependent physiologic patterns which represented prototypic physiologic states. The critical point is that with this normalization all of the states are delineated with respect to the prototype of the R State and are scaled in dimensions of standard deviations ("distance") from R State.

Seven state clusters (STATES) resulted, the reference R State of normal trauma recovery, the A State of normal stress response, the B State of metabolic insufficiency, the C_1 State of moderate and C_2 State of severe respiratory sufficiency, the D State of cardiogenic decompensation and the H State of hypovolemia without shock. Figure 1 shows the prototypic patterns of the mean values for the R, A, B, C_2 and D STATES.

Each State prototype can be considered as a grid point in a physiologic space which can be considered to be analogous to a physical space. At any given moment in time, the multivariable physiologic pattern (the State of a new patient) can be classified by measuring that patient's specific "distance" from each of the prototypic state centers and the closest "distance" to any prototype cluster center defines the State classification of that patient. This is shown in Fig. 2. However, as shown in this figure, each patient has a quantifiable "distance" from every State. Consequently, the patient's movement over time within this physiologic space, as the patient recovers or becomes more severe, can be related to the patient's changing physiologic patterns and his other State "distances" and can be monitored at each time point. Moreover, as the relationship of the physiologic State to patient outcomes was examined it became clear that certain regions within this State space, reflecting patient similarities to the various prototype States, were associated with better outcomes and other regions had a greater likelihood of death.

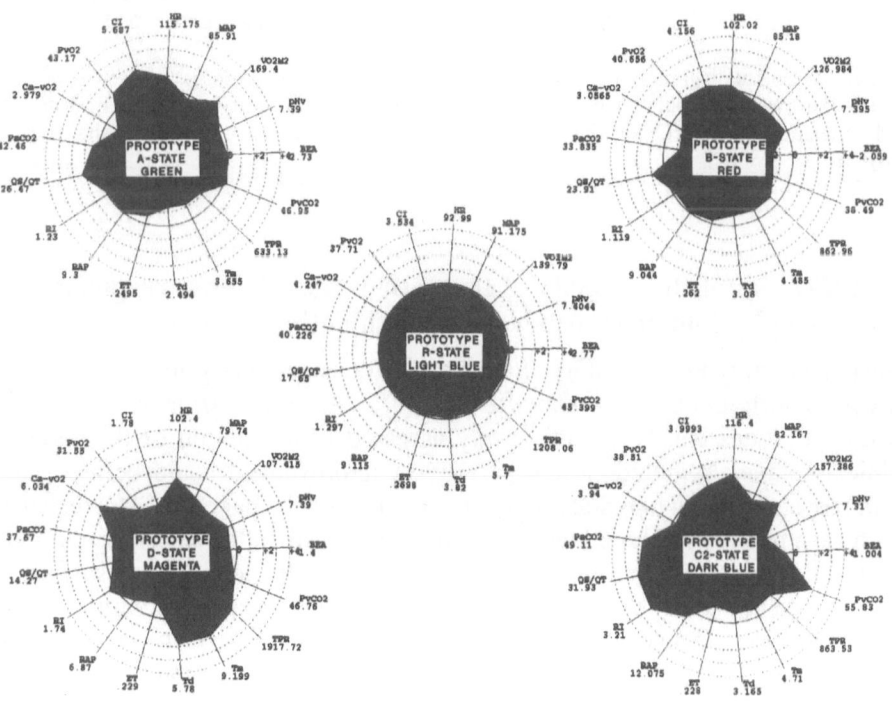

Fig. 1. Five examples of prototypes of physiologic States (R State, A State, B State, C_2 and D State)

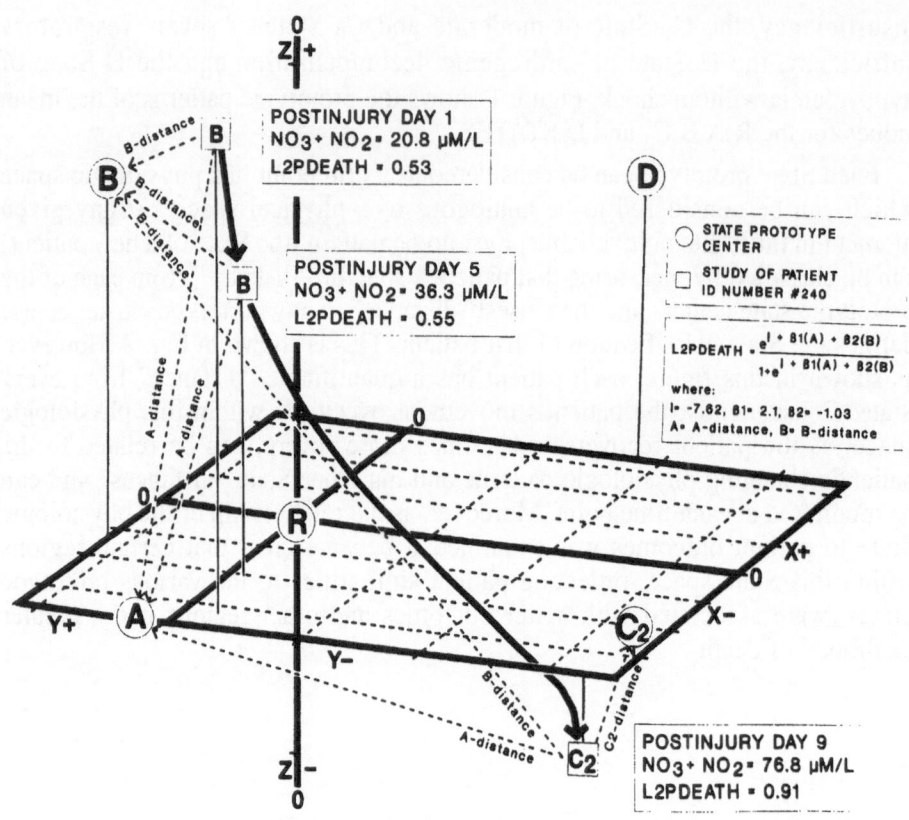

Fig. 2. Conceptual diagram of the "multidimensional physiologic hyperspace" with State protocol centers illustrated. Computation of a specific patient's L2PDEATH from A and B State "distances" and its relation to Nitric Oxide shock mediator levels as clinical course worsens is shown. From (14)

Stratification of the severity of the patient host defense response using the physiologic state severity classification system

Since the prototypic physiologic States can be considered as grid points within a physiologic hyperspace, a specific patient's "distance" from each of these prototype States can be quantitatively assessed as a function of the patient's clinical course. As noted earlier, severity or improvement could be associated with movement from one State region to another and the patient's State distances from each of the prototype States related to improvement or deterioration in his clinical course. As a result, using the Physiologic State Classification system, an index for severity stratification was developed which was approximated by a linear logistic model (L2PDEATH) (7, 11). In this model *severity* was shown to be related to movement away from the normal expected posttrauma physiologic host defense response (A STATE) toward a State of either metabolic insufficiency B STATE or respiratory insufficiency C_2 STATE. In the posttrauma patients the movement from the A STATE appears to be highly correlated with movement toward the C_2 STATE with an independent component added by the B STATE direction movement. This linear logistic model uses the equation:

$$L2PDEATH = \frac{e^{\,I + \beta 1(A) + \beta 2(B)}}{1 + e^{\,I + \beta 1(A) + \beta 2(B)}}$$

Where I = –7.62, β_1 = 2.1, A = A-distance β_2 = –1.03, B = B-distance

L2PDEATH has been shown to produce a highly accurate prediction of the likelihood of death which can be used as an index of severity (7). The sensitivity, specificity and correctness of the prediction are shown in Table 1 and compared to the predicted power of the APACHE derived ARDEATH for the same group of patients (7, 11). These data show that the APACHE derived index of the probability of death (ARDEATH) and the L2PDEATH stratification of severity equally predict (% = % correct) the outcome amongst survivors, but the ARDEATH index substantially *underpredicts* the risk of death. This has significant implications, since it might lead a trauma surgeon or critical care physician to underestimate the patient's severity and therefore undertreat a potentially correctable life threatening event.

Table 1.

	APACHE II (ARDEATH)		L2PDEATH		Total
	n	*%*	*n*	*%*	*n*
Survivors (S)	34	97.1	34	97.1	35
Deaths (D)	12	48.0	20	80.0	25
Total (S + D)	46	76.6	54	90.0	60

From (7).

With regard to the delineation of sepsis syndrome, SIRS and the stratification of the severity of the septic state. When the Physiologic State Severity Classification system is applied to the delineation of the presence and the severity of the septic condition, it can be shown to be more specific than any of the current definitions of sepsis, including the sepsis criteria of American College of Chest Physicians/Society of Critical Care Medicine Consensus Conference (1), the sepsis criteria of the HA-1A sepsis study (8), the criteria of the Veterans Administration Systemic Sepsis Cooperative Study (9) and the Systemic Inflammatory Response Syndrome, SIRS criteria of the members of the American College of Chest Physicians Society of Critical Care Medicine (2).

Within each definition, comparing 416 studies from 60 patients with the physiologic scoring provided by the APACHE II methodology shows substantial overlap between APACHE scores of patients with bacterial septicemia with the score ranges of the other categorizations of the septic process (Fig. 3).

In contrast, the Physiologic State Classification tends to group patients with sepsis primarily in the B and C STATES of physiologic response, with patients having demonstrated bacterial septicemia having a higher incidence of being in the C_2 STATE of combined metabolic and respiratory insufficiency (Fig. 4).

However, when the quantitative State "distance" relationships are used for severity stratification of Sepsis Syndrome: SIRS patients there is a meaningful separation of sepsis severities in post injury patients. Figure 5 shows a three dimensional projection of the A,B,C_2 State space with regions of overlapping ranges for studies from patients who were in the systemic inflammatory response syndrome (SIRS), or the sepsis syndrome as defined by the Bone group (1, 2) and

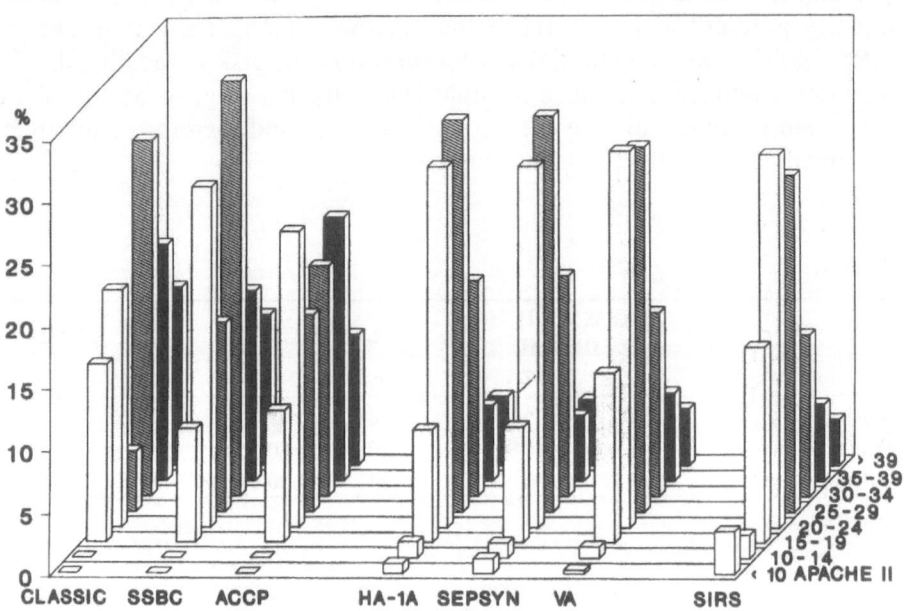

Fig. 3. Distribution of different definitions of "sepsis" and "systemic inflammatory response" with regard to the range of APACHE II score points in each definition. Application of current definitions of "sepsis" and "systemic inflammatory response" to 416 studies (100%) in 60 multiple trauma patients. Criteria of sepsis; sepsis syndrome with (CLASSIC, SSBC or ACCP), or without (HA-1A, SEPSYN, VA) confirmed positive culture from blood or an intraperitoneal source; sepsis criteria (SEPSYN) of the Members of the American College of Chest Physicians/Society of Critical Care Medicine Consensus Conference, SEPSYN, with the systemic response to infection proven by positive cultures from blood or an intraperitoneal source (ACCP); (VA) sepsis criteria of Veterans Administration Systemic Sepsis Cooperative Study; (SIRS) Systemic Inflammatory Response Syndrome criteria of the Members of the American College of Chest Physicians/Society of Critical Care Medicine Consensus Conference. From (7)

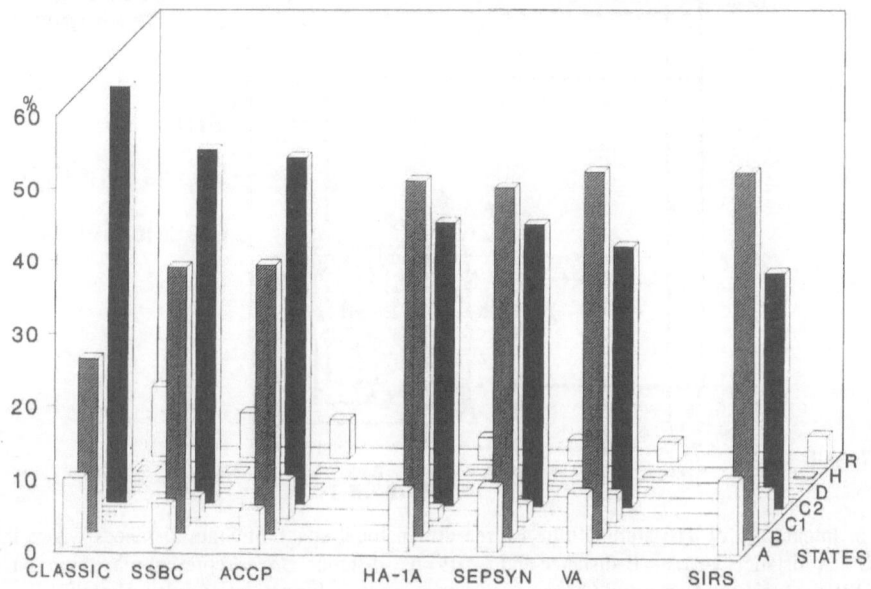

Fig. 4. Distribution of different definitions of "sepsis" and "systemic inflammatory response" within various physiologic States of the Physiologic State Severity Classification. For abbreviations see caption to Fig. 3. From (7)

for patients with Classic sepsis, indicating those with sepsis syndrome who also had demonstrated bacteremia. When the individual studies from 416 observations of 60 patients were plotted within the State space defined by the patient's physiologic "distance" to the A,B and C_2 States, it can be seen that the distribution of patients with regard to sepsis severity (as defined by their outcome of survival or death) is not homogeneous within any clinical definition. Therefore, in the selection of patients with sepsis syndrome for a randomized prospective trial, it is clear that if one reached into the State space box to pluck out a patient who at a given time in his or her clinical course fell within the overall area of occupancy of sepsis syndrome patients, depending on whether one reached shallow or deep into the State space box, or to the right or to the left into the State space box, one might pull out a different nonrandom distribution of patient severities. This clearly demonstrates that using sepsis syndrome: SIRS criteria one cannot select two homogeneous randomized groups for a prospective clinical trial.

However, as shown in Fig. 6, within the same State space box, when the regions defined by the L2PDEATH severity index as a vector within the A,B,C_2 STATE space are used, it can be seen that more homogeneous distributions of severity can be defined. Patients whose physiologic severity would predict a higher *probability of death* are found to be in a region of the State space marked

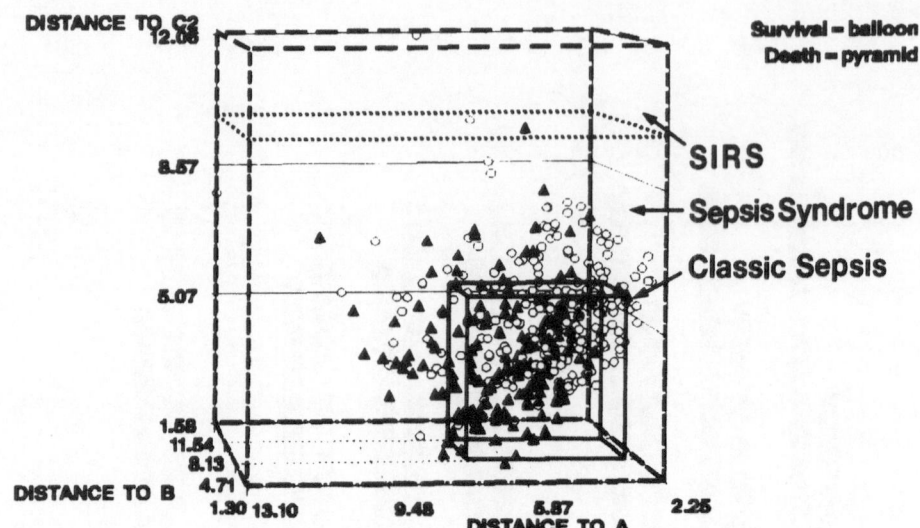

Fig. 5. Integration of 416 studies into a three dimensional space of State distances where the *x-axis* = A-distance, *y-axis* = B-distance and *z-axis* = C$_2$-distance. *Boxes* represent maximum range % of SIRS, sepsis syndrome and Classic or bacteremic sepsis for patient samples. From (7)

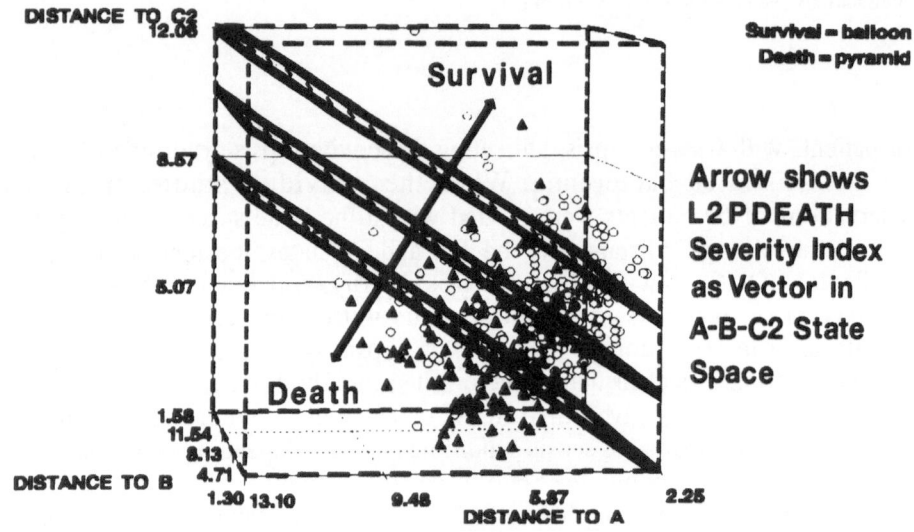

Fig. 6. Integration of 416 studies into a three dimensional space of State distances where the *x-axis* = A-distance, *y-axis* = B-distance and *z-axis* = C$_2$-distance. *PLANES* delineate regions of increasing *probability of death* (from *right* to *left*) based on patient sample State "distances" according to *L2PDEATH* logistic model. From (7)

off by the L2PDEATH criteria as being distinctly different from that occupied by patients with lesser degrees of severity secondary to sepsis. Thus, it is suggested that this transformation of the primary physiologic data from physiologic monitoring into an information based approach may allow better prospective randomized clinical trials and also can be used to quantify significant changes in an individual patient's status from a more to a less severe State in response to therapy.

Relationship of mediators of shock process to physiologic STATE

When the pattern of cytokine mediators (TNF, IL-1, IL-6, IL-8), histamine and nitric oxide was examined in the light of their Physiologic State Classification, it became clear that patients in the A State of normal stress response not only had the lowest incidence of death (no patients primarily in the A State died), but they also had the lowest incidence of the circulating cytokine mediators TNF, IL-1 and IL-6 (12), and also had the lowest incidence of elevated histamine or nitric oxide levels (13, 14). Conversely, as the patient's Physiologic State Severity Classification worsened from the A State normal stress response to the B State of metabolic insufficiency, or to the C_2 State of combined metabolic and respiratory insufficiency, the incidence of circulating levels of the inflammatory cytokines increased (12), as did the incidence and quantity of histamine (13) and the incidence of increased circulating levels of nitric oxide (measured as $NO_3 + NO_2$) (14). Moreover within the physiologic state space the patient's "distance" ratio between the various States describes the severity of that patient's condition and also allows one to delineate regions of greater *probability of death* which also have the highest level of these shock mediators. Movement into these State space regions is associated with the evolution from nonseptic injury to sepsis and with the development of the various postinjury failure syndromes, such as ARDS. Thus movement within the Physiologic State space would appear to be a manifestation of the nature and severity of underlying shock mediator host defense response.

These data strongly suggest that from bedside physiologic monitoring methodologies similar to those used in present day in intensive care units, a quantitative index for evaluation of patient severity can be developed which delineates the specific patient's physiologic metabolic pattern of response and the likelihood of shock mediator elaboration. This Physiologic State pattern provides information relative to the application of specific modalities of therapy. A use of this methodology to obtain a more quantitative method of patient monitoring which provides information rather than data is being developed to interface with patient monitoring systems amenable to continuous monitoring using standard clinical physiologic sensors. The Physiologic State Severity Classification stratification system described here can be used as a basis for randomization in prospective clinical trials of new agents or for the evaluation of the effects of a standard modality of therapy on an individual patient.

References

1. Bone RC, Fisher CJ, Clemmer TP et al (1989) Sepsis syndrome: a valid clinical entity. Crit Care Med 17:389-392
2. Bone RC and Members of the American College of Chest Physicians/Society of Critical Care Medicine Consensus Conference Committee: American College of Chest Physicians/Society of Critical Care Medicine Consensus Conference (1992) Definitions for sepsis and organ failure and guidelines for the use of innovative therapies in sepsis. Crit Care Med 20:864-874
3. Knaus WA, Draper EA, Wagner DP, Zimmerman JE (1985) APACHE II: a severity of disease classification system. Crit Care Med 13:818-829
4. Knaus WA, Draper EA, Wagner DP, Zimmerman JE (1986) An evaluation of outcome from intensive care in major medical centers. Ann Intern Med 104:410-418
5. Giangiuliani G, Mancini A, Gui D (1989) Validation of a severity of illness score (APACHE II) in a surgical intensive care unit. Intensive Care Med 15:519-522
6. Cerra FB, Negro F, Abrams J (1990) APACHE II score does not predict multiple organ failure or mortality in post operative surgical patients. Ann Surg 125:519-522
7. Siegel JH, Rixen D, Friedman H (1995) Physiologic classification and stratification of illness severity of posttrauma "sepsis" patients as a basis for randomization of clinical trials. J Endotoxin Res 2:177-188
8. Ziegler EJ, Fisher CH, Sprung CL et al (1991) Treatment of gram-negative bacteremia and septic shock with HA-1A human monoclonal antibody against endotoxin - a randomized, double blind, placebo-controlled trial. N Engl J Med 324:429-436
9. Hinshaw L and The Veterans Administration Systemic Sepsis Cooperative Study Group (1987) Effect of high-dose glucocorticoid therapy on mortality in patients with clinical signs of systemic sepsis. N Engl J Med 317:659-665
10. Siegel JH, Goodzari S, Coleman WP et al (1993) Quantifying the severity of the human response to injury and sepsis as a guide to the interpretation of pathophysiologic cytokine effects. In: Schlag G, Redl H, Traber D (eds) Third Wiggers Bernard Conference on Shock, Sepsis and Organ Failure. Springer, Berlin Heidelberg New York, pp 163-204
11. Rixen D, Siegel JH, Friedman HP (1995) "Sepsis/SIRS", physiologic classification, severity stratification, relation to cytokine elaboration and outcome prediction in posttrauma critical illness. J Trauma (submitted for publication)
12. Rixen D, Siegel JH, Friedman H (1995) Physiologic state severity classification as an indicator of posttrauma cytokine response. Shock 4:27-38
13. Rixen D, Siegel JH, Bertolini M, Espina N (1995) Histamine, cytokine and metabolic relationships in posttrauma critical illness. Surgery (submitted for publication)
14. Rixen D, Siegel JH, Espina N, Bertolini M, Friedman HP (1995) Nitric oxide production as a correlate of sepsis and the severity of the physiologic state of the host defense in posttrauma critical illness (1995). J Trauma (submitted for publication)

Optimisation of Oxygen Transport in Polytraumatised Patients

B. Kremžar, A. Špec-Marn

Introduction

The number of polytraumatised patients in Slovenia as in the rest of the world is constantly increasing. The leading causes of death are primary brain trauma, failure of one vital organ or multiple organ failure (MOF).

However, close haemodynamic monitoring at an early stage, as well as measurements of oxygen transport and tissue oxygenation, coupled with optimisation of oxygen transport may greatly improve the prognosis in polytraumatised patients.

Definition of polytrauma

In the literature, several definitions of polytrauma have been proposed (1).

At the Ljubljana Central Intensive Care Unit, the term polytrauma refers to trauma affecting at least three organs or organ systems (in various parts of the body), of which at least one organ injury represents an immediate threat to the patient's life.

The Modified Injury Severity Scale (MISS) is used for evaluation of the severity of polytrauma (2). According to our definition, severe injuries with a MISS score of 25 or more are defined as polytrauma and have to be treated in the intensive care unit.

The response of the organism to trauma

In polytraumatised patients, the local and systemic effects of trauma trigger mechanisms involved in the maintenance of homeostasis. The most important pathophysiological mechanism is the activation of the neuroendocrine system, responsible for various metabolic disorders, electrolyte and fluid imbalance. Even though traumatic haemorrhagic shock is known to be the leading inducing event, some other equally significant factors have recently been implicated, such as endotoxins and humoral degradation products released from the injured tissues. Recently, the role of inflammatory cytokines released from macrophages, and lymphocytes has been emphasised. These cytokines act synergistically with the endocrine mediators involved in the metabolic response to trauma (3).

The management of trauma patients has been based on the principle of "ebb" and "flow" phases of metabolic response to injury as described by Cuthbertson. However, this concept of "ebb" phase has been questioned lately (4). The "ebb" phase probably reflects acute systemic underperfusion; with appropriate resuscitation and stabilisation the "ebb" phase rapidly evolves into the hypermetabolic "flow" phase, suggesting that the response of the organism to trauma is in fact hypermetabolic (5).

A better understanding of the pathophysiology of polytrauma and recent technological developments have allowed faster restoration of normal blood flow, ventilation and oxygenation. However, severely traumatised patients are still at risk of developing acute respiratory distress syndrome (ARDS), failure of other organs and sepsis. These complications are most likely to develop in patients with shock and with resulting tissue hypoxia.

Therefore close monitoring of oxygen transport and tissue oxygenation is of utmost importance in early detection and prevention of tissue hypoxia in polytraumatised patients.

Monitoring of oxygen transport

The maintenance of oxygen balance depends on the interaction of the following variables: oxygen uptake in the lungs, oxygen transport and oxygen extraction in the tissue. Disturbances of any of these processes may lead to tissue hypoxia, with the clinical manifestations of disturbed consciousness, oliguria, tachycardia, cutaneous underperfusion and hypotension. Since these clinical signs occur too late and are not specific, we prefer to monitor oxygen transport variables, including cardiac output (CO), arterial oxygen saturation (SaO_2), mixed venous oxygen saturation (SvO_2), oxygen delivery (DO_2) and oxygen consumption ($\dot{V}O_2$). The above mentioned parameters are indirect measures of tissue oxygenation. Direct measurement of tissue oxygenation has unfortunately not been introduced into clinical practice yet.

Theoretically partial mixed venous oxygen pressure (pvO_2) or SvO_2 indicate global tissue oxygenation and the ratio between tissue oxygen delivery and tissue oxygen consumption.

SvO_2 is calculated by the following equation derived from Fick's equation

$$\dot{V}O_2 = CO \times (CaO_2 - CvO_2)$$
$$\dot{V}O_2 = CO \times Hb\ (SaO_2 - SvO_2) \times 1.36 \times 10$$
$$SvO_2 = SaO_2 - (\dot{V}O_2/(CO \times Hb \times 1.36 \times 10))$$

As indicated by the equation, SvO_2 increases with the increase of the following DO_2 variables: arterial oxygen saturation, cardiac output and haemoglobin levels. SvO_2 decreases in parallel with the increase in oxygen consumption. Because of that, SvO_2 is an useful index of respiratory, cardio-vascular and metabolic functions of the organism.

Under normal physiologic conditions, SvO_2 levels range from 70% to 75% (6). These values suggest a normal relationship between oxygen delivery and oxygen requirements, provided that normal compensatory mechanisms and normal blood flow distribution have been preserved (7).

In addition to continuous monitoring of SvO_2, it is equally important to measure blood lactate levels, which represent an important index of tissue hypoxia and anaerobic glycolysis.

Pulse oximetry is a simple, reliable and noninvasive technique for continuous monitoring of arterial oxygenation, a valuable parameter in a variety of clinical situations (8).

The main goals of invasive haemodynamic monitoring of oxygen transport, used alone or in combination with noninvasive methods, are the assessment of patient's stability, to alert the ICU personnel of the patient's instability, and to evaluate the efficacy of the employed therapeutic procedures (9).

Optimisation of oxygen transport

The majority of our polytraumatised patients are in shock, need massive blood transfusion, and their average MISS score is 40. All polytraumatised patients with a MISS score higher than 25 have continuous invasive SvO_2 monitoring by means of fibreoptic Swan-Ganz catheter and simultaneous continuous SaO_2 measurements by a pulse oximeter.

It is well known that polytraumatised patients with associated hypovolemic and haemorrhagic shock maintain stable tissue oxygen consumption despite reduced oxygen delivery, by increased oxygen extraction (O_2ER) leading to decreased SvO_2 if the microcirculation is intact (10). Our main therapeutic goal is to maintain normal SvO_2 levels by providing adequate DO_2, including SaO_2, haemoglobin and CO, on the one hand, and by elimination of the factors that increase $\dot{V}O_2$ (pain, temperature, anxiety etc.), on the other hand.

Once hypovolaemia and hypoxia have been controlled, the patient's needs for inotropic support have to be assessed. This is done by the dobutamine test. The dobutamine test is based on the principle that low-dose dobutamine (5 μg/kg/min) increases CO and DO_2 without increasing $\dot{V}O_2$, except in the presence of lactic acidosis. Therefore, infusion of low dose dobutamine is used to assess the dependency of $\dot{V}O_2$ on DO_2 (11). DO_2 and $\dot{V}O_2$ levels are measured prior to and 30 min after the administration of dobutamine under the same condi-tions. The test is positive when the increase in DO_2 is associated with a simultaneous increase in $\dot{V}O_2$ by more than 10%. The test is repeated when necessary. The dobutamine therapy given in larger doses augments $\dot{V}O_2$ by enhancing metabolism through catecholamine-induced thermogenesis (12). However, the dobutamine administration has to be titrated. Evaluation of SvO_2 only is not an accurate measure of tissue oxygenation. The levels of the arterial blood lactate have to be monitored synchronously. Increased lactate concentration is the marker of tissue hypoxia and has an important negative prognostic value (13, 14). Markedly elevated blood lactate levels may occur immediately upon admission to the ICU as the result of lactate washout from underperfused hypoxic tissue and follows immediately the initiation of perfusion (5). Early after trauma the overall lactate trend rather than individual lactate measurement should be considered in the prognosis (15).

In 1993, Pinsky proposed that an excessive increase of DO_2 is not beneficial for critically injured patients; on the contrary, he stated that it may have adverse effects on the patient. Blood volume replacement may increase the risk of pulmonary and peripheral oedema. In addition, dobutamine increases $\dot{V}O_2$ in the myocardium resulting in cardiac arrhythmias and elevation of overall tissue $\dot{V}O_2$ (16). Therefore precautious replacement of the lost blood with fluids, stored blood products, and precautious usage of vasoactive substances is recommended.

There is not a general consensus concerning optimal haemoglobin and haematocrit levels. Some authors recommend moderate haemodilution to a haematocrit level of 20%-30%; this produces a significant increase in tissue oxygen extraction capabilities due to decreased blood viscosity. Other authors claim that in traumatised patients who have received massive transfusion and are at risk of developing recurrent haemorrhage or coagulation disorders, haematocrit levels should be increased to a level greater than 35% (5). We use this last approach.

We attempt to attain optimal CO in polytraumatised patients primarily by resuscitation of the lost circulating volume, thus enhancing pulmonary capillary wedge pressure (PCWP) to 18 mmHg. When these therapeutic measures fail to provide the desired DO_2, inotropic support with dobutamine is initiated. In the majority of polytraumatised patients with normal myocardial function, adequate CO levels are usually obtained by circulating blood volume resuscitation. This is, however, not the case in polytraumatised patients with cardiac contusion.

Another important task involved in optimisation of oxygen transport is the maintenance of SaO_2 levels greater than 90%. In patients with severe multiple injuries, the development of ARDS may be precipitated by several risk factors (17).

Positive end expiratory pressure (PEEP) is applied when nontoxic oxygen concentrations fail to maintain SaO_2 at a level greater than 90%. However, PEEP has not only beneficial effects. It may also act adversely by causing the reduction in venous blood flow and subsequent decrease in CO (18). ARDS patients on

PEEP need close monitoring to determine the effects of PEEP on pulmonary and cardiac function, as well as on DO_2 and $\dot{V}O_2$.

Conclusion

The primary goal in the management of polytraumatised patients is to manipulate oxygen transport variables until stable $\dot{V}O_2$ levels are reached. This must be achieved without a decrease in SvO_2 and without the elevation of O_2ER, with blood lactate levels remaining within normal limits. At that point optimal DO_2 is achieved, providing for optimal $\dot{V}O_2$ and aerobic metabolism. Optimal DO_2 should be determined for each patient individually.

References

1. Olerud S, Allgower M (1985) Evaluation and management of the polytraumatised patient in various centres. World J Surg 143-148
2. Mayer T, Maltak ME, Johenson DG, Walker MI (1980) The modified injury severity scale in paediatric multiple trauma patients. J Pediatr 15:719-26
3. Arnold J, Little RA (1991) Stress and metabolic response to trauma in critical illness. Curr Anaesth Crit Care 2:139-148
4. Edwards JD (1991) Hemodynamic monitoring in trauma. In: Dhainaut JF, Payen D (eds) Strategy in bedside hemodynamic monitoring. Springer, Berlin, Heidelberg, New York, pp 197-209 (Update in intensive care and emergency medicine)
5. Morre FA, Haenel JB, Moore EE, Whitehill TA (1992) Incommensurate oxygen consumption in response to maximal oxygen availability predicts postinjury multiple organ failure. Trauma 33:58-67
6. Gullo A, Giordano F, Toš L (1989) Monitoring of SvO_2 in critically ill. 4th Post graduate course A.P.I.C.E. Physiology and pathophysiology of oxygen transport. In: Gullo A (ed) Series in critical care and emergency medicine. Club A.P.I.C.E. Trieste, 10-17
7. Nelson LD (1988) Application of venous saturation monitoring. In: Civetta JM, Taylor RW, Kirby RR (eds) Critical care. Lippincott, London, 327-334
8. Lamiell JM (1991) Pulse oximetry. In: Ducer JP, Kirby RR, Taylor RW (eds) Problems in critical care. Oxygen monitoring. Lippincott, Philadelphia, pp 44-54
9. Johnston KS (1991) Clinical application of oxygen monitoring. In: Ducey JP, Kirby RR, Taylor RW (eds) Problems in critical care. Oxygen monitoring. Lippincott, Philadelphia, pp 110-125
10. Edwards JD, Redmand AD, Nightingale P, Wilkins RG (1988) Oxygen consumption following trauma: a reappraisal in severely injured patients requiring mechanical ventilation. Br J Surg 75:690-692
11. Vincent LJ, Roman A, Backerb DL et al (1990) Oxygen uptake, supply dependency. Effects of short-term dobutamine infusion. ARRD 2:142
12. Krachman SL, Lodato RF, Morice R, Guitierrer G, Dantzker DR (1994) Effect of dobutamine on oxygen transport and consumption in the adult respiratory distress syndrome. Intensive Care Med 20:130-137
13. Hayes MA ,Yau EHS, Timmins AC, Hlinds CJ, Watson D (1993) Response of critically ill patients to treatment aimed at achieving supranormal oxygen delivery and consumption. Relationship to outcome. Chest 103:886-895

14. Bakker J, Coffernils M, Leon M, Gris F, Vincent JL (1991) Blood lactate levels are superior to oxygen-derived variables in predicting outcome in human septic shock. Chest 99:956-962
15. Ronco JJ, Fenwick JC, Wiggs BR, Phang PT, Russel JA, Tweeddale MG (1993) Oxygen consumption is independent of increases in oxygen delivery by dobutamine in septic patients who have normal or increased plasma lactate. ARRD 147:25-31
16. Pinsky MR (1993) Oxygen delivery and uptake in septic patients. In: Vincent JL (ed) Yearbook of intensive care and emergency medicine. Springer, Berlin Heidelberg New York, pp 357-383
17. Ralph DD, Robertson HT, Weaver LJ (1985) Distribution of ventilation and perfusion during positive end-expiratory pressure in the adult respiratory distress syndrome. ARRD 131:54-60
18. Hyers TM (1994) Risk factors and outcome in ARDS. In: Vincent LJ (ed) Yearbook of intensive care and emergency medicine. Springer, Berlin Heidelberg New York, pp 463-473

The Role of the Anesthesiologist During Nonconventional War

A. PEREL, H. BERKENSTADT

Background

Chemical warfare was used extensively during World War I and was part of the weapon arsenal of many countries during World War II and the years afterwards (1). During the last two decades chemical weapons have become the "nuclear weapons of the poor countries", since they are easily produced from ordinary chemicals and because of their potential lethality (2). In the 1980s Iraq used chemical warfare against Iran (3) and recently, chemical gases were used against the civilian population by terrorists in Japan.

During the Gulf War the Israeli civilian population suffered from daily missile attacks. Although only conventional weapons were used there was a constant fear of the use of nonconventional warfare. This fear led to the situation that all the population was equipped with a special protecting kit which included gas masks that were used during the attacks until the presence of nerve gases was ruled out. Each house had a sealed room to minimize gas exposure.

This situation led the Israeli health services to increase their preparedness to treat a large number of chemical weapon casualties, mainly by "nerve agents", since these materials are the most adaptable to long range attacks upon the civilian population (4). This medical system is also appropriate for the treatment of toxicological disasters, like the one in India in 1984, when thousands of people were injured after an explosion in an insecticide factory (5). In this chapter we will attempt to describe the most important factors in the organization of such medical services, concentrating on the important role of the anesthesiologist.

The intoxication

The nerve agents owe their activity to their ability to irreversibly inhibit the enzyme cholinesterase, with a resultant cholinergic crisis. Increased muscarinic activity produces excessive bronchial, salivary, ocular and intestinal secretions, sweating, miosis, bronchospasm, and bradycardia. Nicotinic effects include muscle fasciculations, twitching, weakness and paralysis. Central nervous system injury includes loss of consciousness, convulsions and depression of respiratory drive. These signs, their time of onset, and the rapidity of propagation depend on the dose of the nerve gas and the route of exposure. Inhalation of a large dose of nerve agent may cause very fast clinical deterioration with respiratory arrest within 5 min. Cutaneous exposure to toxic drops will generally be followed by a longer period before onset of signs (6, 7).

The treatment

The first principle in the treatment of nerve gas poisoning is the minimizing of exposure. These protective measures include a gas mask, adequate protective cover, and the ingestion of pyridostigmine tablets, a reversible inhibitor of the enzyme acetylcholine esterase. The pharmacological treatment of nerve gas poisoning is mostly empirical and is based upon the experience in the treatment of organophosphate pesticide intoxication, on animal experimental data and on the few accidental human exposure data (6-9). The postexposure treatment includes respiratory support in the form of oxygen, suction, and artificial airway and mechanical ventilation after tracheal intubation. Specific antidotal treatment includes mainly atropine in order to treat the cholinergic muscarinic effect of intoxication. Centrally acting cholinolytic drugs such as scopolamine are used to treat the central nervous system signs of intoxication in combination with anticonvulsive therapy by benzodiazepines. Oximes, such as toxogonin, are used in order to disconnect the toxic agent from the target enzyme before they bind irreversibly (10).

Hospital logistics

A nerve gas attack will have all the characteristics of a mass casualty event. Thousands of injured people will seek medical aid in a short period of time, including children and the elderly, some of them suffering from previous illnesses that may influence the severity of the intoxication. In order to prevent nerve gas exposure the population is instructed to wear gas masks and to enter closed sealed rooms after any missile or airplane attack. Further instructions are given by the media. In the case of intoxication the population is encouraged to open their personal kits, use atropine autoinjectors and perform self-decontamination. Medical units of the civilian defense forces are responsible for further treatment, evacuation and decontamination. Patients who need further medical interventions are evacuated to hospitals especially organized for this task (11).

In order to prevent the uncontrolled arrival of worried family members, and in order to prevent the spread of toxic materials from the contaminated casualties, the entrance to the hospital is restricted to one gate. After entering the hospital a triage of the casualties is done. Walking casualties are considered to be mildly injured, while patients who cannot walk are considered moderately or severely injured according to their respiratory status. Casualties with combined traumatic and toxicological injury are considered as a separate group.

After life-saving treatments, given by hospital staff wearing full protective gear, casualties are decontaminated by water and soap. Only after decontamination are the casualties moved to the clean hospital area and are approached by unprotected medical personnel.

In order to make this complex system work hospitals have to make the following preparations:

1. The logistics of traffic control, crowd control and patients traffic, within the hospital, have to be established and implemented within short notice.
2. Large numbers of stretcher bearers, workers for the contamination area and security personnel have to be trained.
3. A large decontamination area with warm water supply has to be built. This area has to be equipped with many metal stretchers on wheels.
4. Medical personnel have to be trained to recognize the intoxication signs and symptoms, to give antidotal treatment and to ventilate the patients.
5. Antidotal drugs, respirators, oxygen supply and suction units have to be available in sufficient quantities.

The role of the anesthesiologist

From our experience the anesthesiologist has a major role in the preparedness of the hospital for such a nerve gas attack. Due to their intimate acquaintance with resuscitation, emergency airway management, trauma, mechanical ventilation and intensive care, the anesthesiologists automatically become key physicians in the organization and operation of the hospital. Resuscitation and manual skills are needed in the decontamination area, the various emergency rooms (general pediatric, combined injuries and the one for ventilated patients) and in the operating room.

During the Gulf War we realized that aggressive resuscitation should start in the decontamination area, where a secure airway should be established before the decontamination process (5-8 min) is complete. We have therefore examined the ability of anesthesiologists to intubate while wearing full protective gear. The basic components of the individual protective system consist of a gas mask, a suit, gloves and boots. These items impose a physiological and psychological burden which may compromise performance: the common gas mask may increase the respiratory effort and restrict the visual fields; the gloves interfere with normal dexterity; the multilayered overgarment often causes subjective discomfort and may precipitate excessive heat load (12). However, in a study done by our department it was shown that anesthesiologists can perform tracheal intubation in adults and children while working in full protective gear, although the time needed to perform the intubation was somewhat longer compared to "conventional" conditions. These results are limited by the fact that the study was done on mannequins without hypersecretions, convulsions, etc. In another study done by the Medical Corps, emergency medical technicians were asked to perform a series of tasks relevant to a toxicological disaster situation. Protective clothing induced a 30% prolongation of task performance. The quality of performance was, however, unchanged, and a prolonged stay of 8 h in full protective gear (including a gas mask) did not affect performance (13).

Combined injuries

Treatment of patients with combined (chemical and conventional) injuries is another challenge for the anesthesiologist in this situation. These patients can be severely intoxicated since open wounds are a port of entry for the toxic agent, and since their conventional injury was probably caused due to their proximity to the explosion (14).

Anesthesia for these patients may be complicated by the characteristic bronchospasm and bronchial hypersecretions, the hypovolemia due to sweating, vomiting and diarrhea, possible arrhythmias and some behavioral deficits and disturbances in the subacute stage of intoxication. Another major factor is the hemodynamic status due to the conventional injury itself.

Anesthetic considerations

Selection of anesthetic drugs in this situation is based on theoretical considerations since almost no data exist regarding this problem.

Hypnotics: The use of barbiturates as hypnotics and anticonvulsants is limited by the patient's hemodynamic status. Benzodiazepines seem to be the drug of choice since their use is followed by minor hemodynamic changes.

Analgesics: Fentanyl seems to be the opiate of choice in this situation, since morphine can induce bradycardia, part of which is mediated by a vagolytic effect, and meperidine may induce hypotension by a decrease in myocardial contractility. It has to be remembered that fentanyl can induce bradycardia as well. Although ketamine is the drug of choice in the anesthesia of many trauma cases, and although NMDA receptor antagonists were shown to protect the brain from nerve gas induced convulsions in animal studies (15), the use of this drug seems to be unwarranted because it may worsen the patient's respiratory status due to hypersecretions and enhance the behavioral and psychiatric changes induced by the intoxication.

Muscle relaxants: Pancuronium bromide seems to be the muscle relaxant of choice because of its vagolytic induced tachycardia. Other common nondepolarizing muscle relaxants (*d*-tubocurarine, vecuronium bromide, atracurium) have no muscarinic effect on the heart, and the histamine release induced by some of them may worsen hemodynamics and respiration. The use of succinyl choline may be dangerous because of the hyperkalemia that may be induced by convulsions, and because of the bradycardia that may occur in patients with high sympathetic tone. The use of a nerve stimulator in this situation is mandatory since the pharmacodynamics of muscle relaxants may be altered because of the intoxication and because of pyridostigmine pretreatment.

Volatile anesthetics: The bronchodilatatory effect of halothane makes it a suitable agent for the anesthesia of these patients. Its use is, however, limited by the hemodynamic effects of this drug.

In conclusion, anesthesia to patients intoxicated by nerve agents should include the use of specific antidotes, respiratory therapy as in conventional patients with severe bronchospasm, and anesthetic drugs that include a benzodiazepine, fentanyl as an opiate, pancuronium bromide as a muscle relaxant, and volatile anesthetics depending on the patient's hemodynamic status.

The postoperative period

The postoperative period presents unique problems such as the necessity to put a gas mask on a patient fresh out of surgery. We have found that the drinking straw of the mask can serve as a route for oxygen supplementation, and that gas masks as a rule increase the work of breathing in a limited manner only. These considerations, in addition to the degree of intoxication, will affect the timing of extubation. Last but not least one has to deal with excessive anxiety, of patients and medical personnel alike, who often tend to demonize nonconventional weapons and attribute to them unrealistic powers of destruction. Cool headedness is an essential part of optimal professional performance in this situation.

References

1. Robinson JP (1971) The problem of chemical and biological warfare. Stockholm International Peace Research Institute (SIPRI). Humanities Press, New York
2. Sidel VW (1989) Weapons of mass destruction: the greatest threat to public health. JAMA 262:680-682
3. Hu H, Cook-Deagan R, Shukri A (1989) The use of chemical weapons: conducting an investigation using survey epidemiology. JAMA 262:640-643
4. Karni A, Shemer J, Revach M (1985) Hospital deployment for the management of chemical warfare casualties. Harefua 108:560-563 (in Hebrew)
5. Lorin HG, Kulling PE (1986) The Bophal tragedy - what has the Swedish medicine planning learned from it? J Emerg Med 4:311-316
6. Grob D (1956) The manifestation and treatment of poisoning due to nerve gas and other organic phosphate anticholinesterase compounds. Arch Intern Med 98:221-239

7. Sidell FR (1974) Soman and sarin: clinical manifestation and treatment of accidental poisoning by organophosphates. Clin Toxicol 7:1-17
8. Grob D, Harvey AM (1953) The effects and treatment of nerve gas poisoning. Am J Med 14:52-63
9. Grob D, Harvey JC (1958) Effects in man of the anticholinesterase compound sarin. J Clin Invest 37:350-368
10. Dunn MA, Sidell FR (1989) Progress in medical defense against nerve agents. JAMA 262: 649-652
11. Shapira Y, Bar Y, Berkenstadt H, Atsmon J, Danon YL (1991) Outline of hospital organization for a chemical warfare attack. Isr J Med Sci 27:616-622
12. Caeter BJ, Cammermeyer M (1985) Biopsychological responses of medical unit personnel wearing chemical defense ensemble in a simulated chemical warfare environment. Milit Med 150:239-249
13. Arad M, Berkenstadt H, Zelingher J, Laor A, Shemer J, Atsmon J (1993) The effects of continuous operation in chemical protective ensemble on performance of medical tasks. J Trauma 35:800-804
14. Berkenstadt H, Marganitt B, Atsmon J (1991) Combined chemical and conventional injuries-pathophysiological, diagnostic and therapeutic aspects. Isr J Med Sci 27:623-626
15. Braitman DJ, Jaax NK, Sparenborg S (1988) MK-801 protects against seizures and brain damage induced by the cholinesterase inhibitor soman. Soc Neurosci Abstr 14:240

CEREBRAL AND SPINAL DYSFUNCTION

Coma, Persistent Vegetative State, and Death

E. FACCO

Coma and its worse consequences, persistent vegetative state (PVS) and brain death (BD), are a very complex and intriguing problem, involving not only medical knowledge, but also philosophical, psychological, cultural, ethical as well as economical aspects. The sum of these different conditions can be considered as a major health problem, owing to its increasing frequency, social and economical costs, and problems related to the diagnosis of BD and organ transplantation.

In epidemiological studies on head injury an incidence of 9-24 deaths/10^5 population/year (1) has been reported. The estimated incidence of subarachnoidal hemorrhage is about 4-10/10^5 population/year, with an overall mortality of about 50% and more than half of survivors with major neurological deficits (2, 3); stroke is the third cause of mortality in the USA, with some 85,000 deaths and 10^6 neurological disabilities/year (4). Furthermore, the overall rate of coma, severe disability, PVS and death becomes much higher, when untreatable mass lesions (e.g. brain tumor), anoxia, dementia and congenital diseases are included.

Many years ago, it was estimated that as many as 3% of admissions to the emergency ward were comatose patients (see 4). Since then the development of neurological intensive care has allowed a progressive decrease in mortality, but the rate of prolonged unconsciousness and PVS is increasing more and more. Up to 30%-40% of severely head injured patients undergo such an evolution (5): this causes an annual incidence of 600 new PVS patients in the UK with a prevalence of 1,500 (6), and an estimated presence of 1,000 cases in France (7); in the USA an estimated presence of 5,000-10,000 cases has been reported in 1991 (8), and of 10,000-25,000 adults plus 4,000-10,000 children in 1994 (9). The progressive increase in patients with PVS yields crucial ethical, social and economical dilemmas regarding the definition of the "appropriate" management.

Though a substantial clarification of the concepts of coma, PVS and BD has been achieved in the past two decades, considerable confusion between different neurological conditions with different prognosis still persists in the population, mass media and even doctors, leading to harmful as well as unfounded controversies. The confusion depends also on the wide range of terms used, where often diagnosis and prognosis are unduly mixed up: *unconsciousness, coma, deep coma, prolonged coma, irreversible coma, vegetative state, PVS, akinetic mutism, apallic coma, mute responsiveness, coma depassé, cerebral death, neocortical death, brain death.* Some of them are sometimes wrongly used synonomously, while others are inappropriate and should be withdrawn.

This persistent confusion yields three main consequences: a), wrong diagnosis [37% rate of misdiagnosis has been reported in a study on patients admitted to a rehabilitation center (10)]; b) inappropriate treatment; c) false hopes in patients' relatives; d), polemics on the certainty of BD and organ donation. Thus, the concepts of coma, PVS, BD and related conditions are to be clearly defined and distinct in clinical practice in order to avoid misunderstandings and misleading conclusions.

Coma

The definition of coma implies the definition of consciousness, a word with so many different meanings and implications: the Oxford dictionary defines consciousness as "being conscious" and "all the ideas, thoughts, feelings, wishes, intentions, recollections of a person" (11). Most of the aspects of consciousness are not merely medical, but philosophical, ethical, moral, literary, religious and psychologic: nevertheless, both their quantitative (different levels of arousal) and qualitative changes (mood, emotion, intellect, behaviour, language) are often a matter of medical evaluation and diagnosis, making hard, if possible, an absolute division between the medical and nonmedical aspect of consciousness. As far as the word "unconscious" is concerned, it has again many different meanings, since it can be attributed both to a sleeping, stuporous or comatose person, or to unrecalled impulses and memories of a wakeful one (when this term is used in a psychoanalytic context). The lack of awareness observed in both comatose and PVS patients gave rise in the past years to the mentioned confusion.

Trying to fix the boundaries of consciousness in the context of definition of coma, we can consider the former characterized by three essential aspects: a) arousal; b) awareness of self and environment; c) environmental interaction. The arousal depends upon reticular formation and allows one to be awake; the awareness refers to the content of cognitive processes and depends upon hemispheres and the interaction between their different regions; the environmental interaction requires the whole brain to perceive both external and internal environment and to elaborate proper responses. Awareness requires wakefulness, but wakefulness does not imply awareness, and interaction requires both of them.

It is worth noting that in medical practice we can only evaluate the awareness from the interaction, but absolutely cannot explore it directly. This is very crucial in the definition and evaluation of PVS, which can only be behavioural and phenomenological, since it is impossible to check with certainty whether a residual glimpse of awareness, of intrapsychic elaboration or the capability of suffering at some level are preserved in a condition of extreme disability: this is the link between different clinical conditions like vegetative state, catatonia, apatia and abulia. The ticklishness of this matter requires much wisdom in the problem of choosing the appropriate management (from intensive management to withdrawal of treatment, including nutrition and hydration) of PVS patients.

Granted the mentioned features of consciousness, the definition of coma in terms of their loss becomes easier: coma is a condition of unarousability, loss of awareness and environmental interaction (with the already mentioned limits of a neurobehavioural evaluation). In other (and more practical) words, the comatose patients has the eyes closed, does not obey commands and does not utter words (1). It is to emphasize that closed eyes are an essential feature in the diagnosis of coma: they mean the absence of arousal, which discriminates coma from other conditions of decreased consciousness, such as PVS.

Unawareness and loss of environmental interaction must be better defined in order to avoid the confusion already yielded in the past with the term "unresponsiveness" (12). The environmental interaction (likewise responsiveness) is referred to meaningful behaviours (13): the comatose patient shows neither intentional movements, nor sustains visual pursuit movements of the eyes through a 45° arc in any direction when the eyes are held open manually; reflex movements such as posturing, withdrawal from pain can of course be preserved. The sustained visual pursuit movements, although unlikely to be observed in the early stage, can be a relevant sign of meaningful behaviour in the subacute or chronic phase, when the patient is going to come out of coma.

As far as the clinical course of coma is concerned, it lasts from hours to several weeks, with most survivors beginning to open eyes and breathe spontaneously within 1 month: therefore, the term *irreversible coma*, sometimes used in the past to define PVS as well as BD, is absolutely wrong for two reasons: a) irreversible coma does not exists as a clinical entity, since opening the eyes implies recovery from coma, by definition; b) BD is simply the death of the patient, which is, by definition, beyond coma (the former regards corpses, the latter alive patients). The only acceptable meaning of such a term might perhaps be prognostic, namely the exact prediction that a given comatose patient will die before opening eyes, but it does not seem to be so relevant. Likewise, the archaic term *apallic coma*, already used as synonymous with PVS, should also be abandoned for two reasons: a) if it means vegetative state, it is no longer coma; b) the word apallic refers to a neuropathological feature (the loss of neocortex), while many different brain lesions yield a PVS, thus the latter term is much more suitable to describe this clinical condition. Finally, the *coma depassé,* described by Mollaret and Goulon in 1959 (14), has nowadays mainly a historical meaning, being replaced by the concept of BD: what is worth noting is that the adjective *depassé* used by the authors properly meant that the patient had gone *beyond* coma.

Coma scales

The common use of words such as light and deep coma show the need of staging the loss of consciousness into different levels, in order to better define its severity and prognosis: this aspect is of paramount importance, since only an effective and well standardized grading of coma can assure a reliable evaluation, information exchange between doctors and comparison between series. More than 20 coma scales have been published in the literature in the past two decades (15, 16): their considerable number clearly shows the difficulty of achieving the ideal result (namely, effectiveness and simplicity). Furthermore, their relevant number yielded in the past confusion rather than a proper information exchange in clinical practice: for example, classifying a patient as coma of grade four tells nothing unless the coma scale used is not specified.

Generally speaking, coma scales classify the severity of coma in two ways, giving stepwise gradings (which define "levels" of coma) or numerical scores: in the former, each level is defined by the coexistence of groups of signs in a hierarchical scale; in the latter all signs are checked independently of each other and the coma score is the sum of the values arbitrarily given to each sign. The most important scales of each type are the one proposed by Plum and Posner (17) and the Glasgow Coma Scale (GCS) (18), respectively. Some criticism can be addressed to both scales: according to Jennett and Teasdale (1), the scale by Plum and Posner would not adequately describe brain dysfunction in the comatose patient, since motor responses, ocular reflexes, breathing patterns etc. may reflect focal damage rather than brain dysfunction as a whole, thus the correlation between them and the depth of coma may not be close. On the other hand, the GCS in comatose, intubated patients mainly reflects the best motor response: comatose patients have the eyes closed, while the verbal response cannot be checked. Although the motor response in GCS is not a sign of focal damage (being the *best*), again, it gives an estimate of the depth of coma reflecting essentially the posture (e.g. decorticate or decerebrated), namely the level of rostrocaudal evolution: since brain areas involved in the regulation of consciousness are not those controlling motor function, the GCS seems to have conceptually the same limits in grading the depth of coma as the scale by Plum and Posner (when GCS < 8). Once again, the major problem in defining the severity of consciousness impairment in coma depends on the absence of meaningful responses: not being able to explore directly the content of consciousness, we can only assess the overall severity of brain dysfunction, where the severity of rostrocaudal evolution is generally assumed to define the depth of coma. In this regard, the inclusion of brain stem reflexes can add substantial information on the severity of neurological deterioration and on the likely outcome: in 1986 we reported that oculocephalic and light reflexes showed a closer correlation to the outcome than the GCS (19), while in the paediatric versions of GCS (20) the need for including brain stem reflexes has been emphasized, in order to improve the assessment of brain injury.

Although the GCS is absolutely the most widely used coma scale and is nowadays a standard routinely used in all centres, due to its simplicity, the scale by Plum and Posner retains all its value; in comatose patients it can provide more detailed information on the level and severity of brain stem dysfunction and, thus, on prognosis. The best protocol in clinical practice is, obviously, to record a careful neurological examination: then any scale can be built up *a posteriori* without losing information.

As far as the cause of coma is concerned, it is worth recalling that the GCS was created to assess head injured patients, but in the past two decades it has been more and more used to evaluate coma of any origin. In a series of more than 15,000 nontraumatic patients admitted to the ICU it has been reported that the inclusion of GCS in the APACHE III Prognostic Scoring System improved the prognostic evaluation (21), but a lack of sensitivity was found in the intermediate range of GCS. Likewise, in our experience on subarachnoidal hemorrhage (in preparation) the GCS is significantly related both to the outcome and to evoked potentials. However, a GCS = −4 can predict poor outcome more accurately than a GCS = 5-8 can predict a good one, with a rate of falsely optimistic predictions close to 50%. This low sensitivity of GCS has been reported in severe head injury as well (19), leading to overrating the likelihood of recovery.

Two other aspects of the GCS are worth being mentioned: a) in patients with GCS > 4 a given value may be the result of the sum of different E,V,M responses: thus, different clinical situations are joined in the same score (perhaps this is one of the possible causes of low GCS sensitivity); b) the score assigned to each sign is arbitrary and probably a better estimation of its relative weight would improve the accuracy of the GCS. Recently, in a mathematical analysis of the GCS (22) it has been argued that only 15 out of the 120 possible mathematical combinations of E,V,M responses are clinically valid (e.g. a combination of normal verbal response with decerebrate posturing does not seem to be possible) and that the motor responses are generally dominant, suggesting that weighted numerical values might improve precision.

Duration of coma

Once coma has been defined and graded, the recovery of consciousness can be assessed, but the mechanisms of recovery remain greatly unknown.

Different signs can mark the reappearance of consciousness: a) stimulated eye opening; b) spontaneous eye opening; c) capability of visual tracking; d) localized pain responses; e) recovery of speech; f) capability of obeying commands.

Some of these functions often return in close succession, but in many cases substantial discrepancies may occur regarding the order of reappearance, the time elapsed from the insult as well as the time required from the first sign of arousal to the full recovery of consciousness. The most frequent sequence of recovery, as defined by the GCS, seems to be E2 → M5 → E4 → M6 (23). As far as speech is concerned, patients can speak before obeying commands or *vice versa*, but this sequence cannot always be checked due to tracheal intubation.

The stimulated eye opening suggests that arousal is going to recover, while the spontaneous eye opening means the full recovery of wakefulness, but, as mentioned before, it does not necessarily imply the recovery of awareness: therefore, spontaneous eye opening (E4) shows that the patients has come out of coma, but this sign gives no information on the quality of survival (recovery of consciousness or PVS). The visual tracking (i.e. the capability of sustaining visual pursuit movements) may be an early sign of meaningful behaviour and is, by definition, absent in coma as well as in PVS (9).

A correlation appears to exist between the duration of coma, mechanisms of recovery and final outcome. When recovery occurs within a few days, the cause of coma is probably a reversible neural dysfunction. When coma is more prolonged, the recovery time is also longer: this suggests that structural rather than functional damage has occurred and, different mechanisms of recovery, including some amount of compensation by alternative routes, may be required. A significant correlation between coma lasting more than 2 weeks and poor outcome has been found by us in children but not in adults (19), while the time between the onset of stimulated eye opening and the appearance of localized pain response seems to depend upon the duration of coma (23).

Persistent vegetative state

The term persistent vegetative state, introduced by Jennett and Plum in 1972 (24), defines a chronic state of wakefulness with no behavioural signs of meaningful environmental interaction (and, therefore, no apparent awareness), in which respiration, blood pressure, and generally all life sustaining functions are preserved. This chronic condition, which has been also defined "a fate worse than death" (25), can be the result of three main groups of causes: a) coma due to anoxia, brain injuries (traumatic or nontraumatic) or untreatable mass lesions (such as brain tumors); b) the end stage of degenerative brain diseases, such as Alzheimer's or Jacob-Creutzfeld disease, multi-infarct dementia; c) anencephaly and other congenital diseases. Therefore, two different subpopulations with PVS can be recognized: an elderly group, mainly with dementia and cerebrovascular disorders, and a younger group (including children), mainly in PVS due to anoxia, head injury, brain tumors, and congenital diseases. The development of neurological intensive care has progressively decreased mortality in the past three decades and improved the quality of survival, by decreasing secondary brain damage. On the other hand, the number of PVS patients has increased more and more, due to, a) increased incidence of brain injuries, and b) stabilization and survival of severe cases, who in the past would have died. Thus, PVS is the victory of neurological ICU and represents the cost for assuring the highest probability of recovery, but this "by-product" is now raising crucial ethical, medical and economical dilemmas.

Likewise coma, the wide range of terms used to indicate PVS, gave rise in the past to some confusion. Furthermore, some additional problems have been caused by terms such as *persistent:* in fact, a prognostic value is generally attributed to this adjective, leading to harmful conclusion about the ultimate fate of the patient when unproperly used. The mentioned confusion and high rate of misdiagnosis (10) calls for reassessing PVS and clearly defining the proper terms, their exact meaning and diagnostic criteria.

The already mentioned terms, such as *apallic syndrome, prolonged coma, neocortical death* etc. are to be abandoned; according to the ANA Committee on Ethical Affairs, only the word *vegetative state* should be used (26). The adjective *persistent* should be intended as a diagnosis of the actual neurological conditions and not as a prognostic judgement on the patient's future: it refers only to the past, namely the observation that this condition has steadily kept over time (24). Only the term *permanent* has a strong prognostic value, indicating that this condition is irreversible, thus referring to the future. Misunderstanding the proper meaning of the word persistent may lead to a negative therapeutic approach, due to the belief that the patient will not benefit from the treatment; this is why the American Congress of Rehabilitation Medicine has suggested withdrawing it and advocated only specifying the time elapsed from the onset of vegetative state (13). In contrast, once the proper meaning of the term persistent is clarified and accepted, there is no reason for concern, but this is a matter of consensus yet to be reached.

Definition and diagnosis of PVS

In their original description, Jennett and Plum (24) described PVS as a condition in which there is no evidence of "any adaptive response to the external environment, the absence of any evidence of a functioning mind which is either receiving or projecting information, in a patient who has long periods of wakefulness". A common consent on this definition can be drawn by the reports of the Multisociety Task Force on PVS (19), the American Congress of Rehabilitation Medicine (13), the ANA Committee on Ethical Affairs (26), the AMA Council on Scientific Affairs (27) and the Child Neurology Society Ethic Committee (28). The main discrepancies only regard the use of the term persistent, as already discussed (29), and the lower importance attributed to absent visual tracking in the diagnosis by the members of the Child Neurology Society (28).

The essential clinical criteria for the diagnosis of PVS are (13):

a) The patient opens the eyes spontaneously and has sleep-wake cycles.

b) Breathes spontaneously.

c) Does not obey commands.

d) Does not utter recognizable words.

e) Does not show intentional movements.

f) Does not show any evidence of awareness, meaningful or learned behaviour.

g) Does not sustain visual pursuit movements of the eyes through a 45° arc in any direction, but may show spontaneous eye movements.

h) Does not withdraw from threatening gestures.

i) Bowel and bladder incontinence is present.

j) Brain stem, spinal and primitive reflexes (e.g., sucking, rooting, chewing, swallowing) may be preserved.

k) The diagnosis cannot be made during concomitant acute systemic complications (such as high fever, infections, cardiorespiratory failure, etc.) or sedative administration (29).

l) Investigative techniques, such as EEG, multimodality evoked potentials, CT scan, MRI, SPECT and/or PET can confirm the presence of severe brain damage.

The absence of intentional movement does not exclude the presence of meaningless movements, including unintentional mimic reflexive reactions (e.g. crying, smiling), the origin of which is pseudobulbar. The latter often leads the relatives, and sometimes the attending doctor, to false beliefs and hopes on the actual status and prognosis of the patient, looking like signs of awareness. Likewise, the absence of visual tracking does not exclude possible reflexive reactions, such as turning the eyes towards peripheral stimuli. Since a reproducible sustained visual pursuit is often one of the earliest signs of reappearing consciousness, its correct assessment is very important both for diagnosis, prognosis and the evaluation of the need for suitable rehabilitation programs; however, remember that a few PVS patients may show some degree of visual tracking without further improvement in their conditions.

Investigative techniques, such as CT scan, MRI, EEG, multimodality evoked potentials, SPECT, PET, can add substantial information in the assessment of PVS: much caution is required in formulating a diagnosis and predicting a poor prognosis in a clinically vegetative patient with completely normal tests. Conversely, even if some investigations are powerful prognostic indicators (e.g. multimodality evoked potentials), much care and caution are always needed when correct prognostic formulations are to be made.

The importance of proper diagnosis is emphasized by the papers of Tresh et al. (8) and Childs et al. (10), who reported an overall rate of misdiagnosis of 17% and 37%, respectively: the probability of inaccurate diagnosis was higher when it was performed more than 3 months post-injury and/or the cause of coma was trauma (10). This high probability of diagnosing PVS in patients who are aware of themselves and/or environment depends on the already discussed terminological problems as well as on superficiality of diagnosis: a clear definition of PVS and qualified physicians are essential to decrease errors to a minimum. Since the reappearance of consciousness may be a slow process, especially in patients with severe brain lesions and prolonged coma, also its behavioural signs may not be strictly reproducible in the early stage of recovery. Thus, an extended observation, together with criticism and inclination to listen to the reports of relatives and nurses, is required.

The diagnosis of PVS also requires this clinical picture be kept over time before it can be defined as persistent. There is a substantial agreement that PVS can be diagnosed when lasting more than 1 month (9, 26), excluding use of the term persistent before this time has gone by. The prognostic aspect of PVS, which is implicit in the definition of permanent VS, is much more ticklish: in fact, the need for absolute certainty of diagnosis and exact prognosis is required by the ethical, social and economic consequences. In this regard, the diagnosis of PVS has the same implications as the diagnosis of BD and requires the same attention devoted to it in the past two decades. Worth mentioning is the wise position of the ANA Committee on Ethical Affairs (26): "Defining PVS has as much practical importance as developing standards for diagnosis of brain death... whenever possible it becomes the physician's responsibility to determine when, with overwhelming probability, a patient's higher brain function, including his or her self-awareness is permanently lost... The public must be assured that the PVS can be diagnosed with a high degree of certainty by well-defined clinical criteria. The medical definition... is not influenced by ethical, legal or other matters. All subsequent decisions making regarding management of this condition must start from its accurate diagnosis".

Prognosis of PVS

The assessment of prognosis (namely, the definition of permanent VS), requires the knowledge of the causes of PVS, its duration and the age of the patient. The latter must be taken into account, since young patients and children have usually a slightly better prognosis of both coma and PVS than older people. It has been suggested that the diagnosis of irreversibility can be made with reasonable certainty after 3 months from nontraumatic insults and after 12 months from severe head injury (9, 29). Walshe and Leonard (30) observed 29 PVS patients over a period of 3 years: not one of them recovered consciousness, justifying the conclusion that these patients should be treated without undue intervention to preserve a mindless life; likewise, Sazbon et al. (31) reported that patients with nontraumatic PVS, if they recovered consciousness, did so within 5 months in all cases, and continued to suffer from severe disability. In contrast, a similar study on 650 head injured patients (32) has shown that a few cases (about 6%) can regain consciousness during the second year from the trauma; similar results have been reported by Higashi (33) in a 5-year follow-up of 110 PVS patients: only 10% of them recovered partially from the PVS, most showing only a minimal reactivity, but one of them becoming alert and well oriented following 3 years in postanoxic PVS. Of course, PVS patients cannot be considered as terminally ill, since they can potentially survive for a long time, once nutrition and hydration are continued.

The prognostic criteria of PVS in adults cannot be directly applied to children, due to their higher chances of recovery; however, the likelihood of regaining consciousness in children appears to be only slightly higher than in adults. In a long-term follow-up study only a minimal reactivity was at best observed after an average of 4.5 years from the onset of PVS (34).

As a general rule, a permanent VS in children can be diagnosed with reasonable certainty, granted a longer period of observation than the one required for adults: a substantial agreement exists among the members of the Child Neurological Society that PVS can be diagnosed after no less than 6 months from the insult in children younger than 2 years, while in older ones only 3-4 months are required for anoxic and ischemic injuries and 6 for head trauma (28). Some reluctance to diagnose PVS in the first few months of life is understandably present, due to the limitations of neurological examination and the effects of development in the potential for recovery: the use of investigative techniques is strongly recommended to improve the assessment of brain damage, but this is a good practice in adults too. In this regard, multimodality evoked potentials (MEPs) are worth being used: MEPs are powerful prognostic indicators in the acute phase of coma, being able to assess the likelihood of recoverying consciousness in most cases (see 35, 36 as reviews). For example, in postanoxic coma a steady absence of cortical N20 in somatosensory evoked potentials and preserved auditory brainstem responses is closely related to a final outcome in PVS. The usefulness of MEPs has been studied less in the chronic phase, but there is some evidence that they may be helpful in the evaluation of both prognosis of PVS and the presence of remaining cognitive abilities (37).

In summary, a clear and safe diagnosis of PVS can be obtained in clinical practice, once all the criteria and recommendations are met. When prognosis is concerned, the evaluation of irreversibility of PVS can be achieved with a high degree of certainty, once aetiology, age, duration of PVS and neurodiagnostic tests are taken into account. It has been estimated that only patients younger than 40 years with carefully diagnosed PVS have small chances of recovery: when PVS duration is more than 3 months, they have less than $1/10^3$ likelihood of recovery (38). Probably we cannot perform an unerring prediction of irreversibility in all cases, but we can do it in most cases, critically analysing the whole of the clinical and laboratory data. At the moment this looks to be the best way to avoid misdiagnosis.

Once permanent VS has been diagnosed, new problems face both physicians and patient's relatives, regarding what is the "appropriate" management, a dilemma with ethical and economic facets. In this cases the attending doctor has a very hard job, very well described by Celesia (39): "...physicians must gather their communication skills; rely on their humanity, kindness, and understanding; and rise above the artisan and scientist to become at the same time the friend and the adviser. It is not easy; it never will be".

Ethical and economic problems

A detailed analysis of this topic is beyond the aim of this contribution; nevertheless, a few essential remarks must be outlined, since they are relevant in decision making.

Ethics and economics are clearly distinct matters, and the former cannot be dependent upon the latter; nevertheless, a wise evaluation of economic problems can help evaluating what is really meaningful in the management of hopeless conditions, allowing better definition of the cost/benefits ratio.

PVS patients can survive for many years: the length of survival depends on the occurrence and severity of systemic complications and, hence, on the level of medical care and routine sustenance. The management requires artificial feeding and hydration plus considerable efforts to prevent or treat decubiti, infections, ankylosis, and respiratory failure; in other words, a long survival can be obtained only with aggressive medical treatment. In fact, most PVS patients routinely require one or a combination of the following procedures most of the time: a) intravenous line; b) nasogastric or gastrostomy tube (about 20%-60% of cases); c) tracheostomy (more than 30% of cases); and d) indwelling urinary catheters (up to 75% of cases) (8, 33, 40). Furthermore, they periodically need aggressive in-hospital treatment of acute complications or intercurrent diseases: 1/3 to 2/3 of patients develop pneumonia, urinary tract infections, decubiti, or, less frequently, more severe complications, such as gastric bleeding. The costs of such sustained medical efforts range from about $250 and $1,000/day, depending on the level of treatment required and its place (home or hospital) (34, 40).

The need for aggressive management (including surgical procedures), its high cost and the poor prognosis, together with the ethical implications, are the essential factors for the definition of the appropriate management and of the right behaviour of both physicians and relatives.

The problem of withholding or withdrawing treatment in PVS, including nutrition and hydration, is still controversial and definitive answers are not available. Some inclination to consider morally justified withdrawal of artificial nutrition and hydration is prevailing (6, 26-29, 38, 41-43), but different legal positions and rulings exist in different countries, including the value and recognition of living wills; the latter is better defined in the USA, less in the UK and much less in Italy.

The justification for withdrawal derives from considering artificial nutrition and hydration as medical treatments requiring surgical procedures (e.g. gastrostomy) and/or medical monitoring (29), and not simple ordinary care. In contrast, this position has given rise to some concern and criticism: it has been argued that surgical procedures and nasogastric tube are medical treatment, but certainly food and water are not (44). Whatever the position, withdrawal of nutrition causes, as a matter of fact, starvation to death. Also the assumption that withdrawing treatment is justified to avoid further suffering seems to be contradictory to the statement that PVS patients have no capacity to experience pain or suffering (29); again, the patient's presumptive will is not so easily evaluable if not declared before the insult, while a mindless patient simply has no will.

The Church is also opposed to overtreatment of hopeless conditions, when it does not preserve the best interests of the patients. Formerly, Pope Pius XII in 1957 (45) answered questions on resuscitation before a congress of anaesthetists, as follows: "life, health, all temporal activities are subordinate to spiritual aims... it is the physician's duty, and specially of the anesthetist, to define dying and the moment of death of a person, who dies in a state of unconsciousness... Physicians' duties and rights depend upon those of the patient... family rights generally depend upon the presumptive will of the patient... Duties oblige only to use ordinary care... in hopeless conditions and when one cannot honestly impose the burden of extraordinary means of treatment, the family can insist in order that physicians stop resuscitation and they can comply with it... In this case there is no euthanasia, which never will be allowed". According to Pius XII, recently the US Bishop Pro-life Committee has stated that even in permanent VS the withdrawal of nutrition and hydration (being "ordinary" means) is not justified (46).

As a general rule, we must be aware that any position, even if philophically and ethically correct in a medical environment, may lead as well to harmful conclusions when used in a different context, for example to state general rules in politics, when ethical and economic implications might wrongly be intermingled. Even if today we can morally accept feeding withdrawal in individual cases following the patient's or surrogates' will and court judgement, a rash extension of this position to the whole PVS population would be dangerous: economic interests being a strong incentive for human behaviour, euthanasia could be easily justified for a useless and expensive population, whose costs can be on the order of several thousand million dollars/year in countries like the USA (given the quoted incidence and costs). It might lead to, or be the expression of, a harmful inclination to eugenics like in ancient Sparta or, much worse, in the Third Reich... This is the reason for thinking with much care and prudence about proper PVS management, a very narrow and uneven track between euthanasia and a ruthless therapeutic obstinacy, where the meaning and value of a patient's life is not so easy to judge. It does not depend only on the patient himself, but also on the feeling of the relatives tending to him, especially when the vegetative patient is their beloved son.

Minimal responsiveness

The Glasgow Outcome Scale, which nowadays is universally used, classifies the outcome into five well known grades: death, PVS, severe disability, moderate disability and good recovery (47). Although this section does not deal with disability of conscious patients, it is worth outlining the concept of minimal responsiveness (MR), which is the link between PVS and severe disability. The need for defining one more outcome level comes from the wide range of conditions included in severe disability, from nearly vegetative patients to those dependent only for certain activities.

MR includes patients with inconsistent responses, but showing some meaningful interaction with the environment (13): it can be observed in patients coming out from VS and represents the tail-light of severe disability. Such patients are no longer in PVS but cannot properly be defined as severely disabled.

The essential clinical criteria for the diagnosis of MR are (13):

1. Presence of meaningful response following a specific command, question, or environmental prompt.
2. When the meaning is doubtful, the response should at least occur significantly more often during the above mentioned stimuli and should have been observed at least once during formal testing.

The term akinetic mutism is a further cause of confusion, since it has been used for both PVS and MR patients. The need for consensus on terminology is again pressing, since the ANA Committee on Ethical Affairs has suggested withdrawing it (being synonymous with PVS) (26), while the American Congress of Rehabilitation Medicine has defined akinetic mutism as a condition of severe decrease in neurologic drive or intention, in patients with fully intact visual tracking (13): according to this definition they are not in a PVS, but rather they would belong to the MR group. Since the use of the term akinetic mutism causes confusion anyway it is better to avoid it at the moment.

Death

The death of a patient is by definition the worst defeat of medical treatment. Although physicians face death routinely, it is generally beyond the clinical interest of the attending doctors (once occurred), while in coroners the object of interest is the cause of death and not the biological process and the pathophysiology of dying.

For many centuries death was defined as the arrest of breathing; from seventeenth century the moment of death could be defined by cardiac arrest, following the discovery of the systemic and pulmonary circulation by William Harvey. In the recent past the development of medical technology has yielded a new picture of death, formerly called coma depassé (14), a macabre waste-product of modern intensive care.

The diagnosis of BD is an intriguing problem, involving not only biological and medical knowledge of dying, but also substantial philosophical, religious, cultural, ethical and psychological aspects. Cultures and religions can give different meanings to the death of the body, leading more or less to the inclination to accept this unavoidable event. Just mentioning the three most widespread doctrines, in Judeo-Christian culture death means the departure of the soul from the body, where the spiritual aspect is the only important thing. As to the diagnosis, Pope Pius XII (45) stated that "on the practical level one needs to be mindful of the connotation of the terms 'body' and 'separation'... As to the pronouncement of death... the answer cannot be inferred from religious and moral principles, and consequently it is an aspect lying outside the competence of the Church". In a materialistic view, the death of the body is the end, *tout court*. In Buddhism a more complex belief is present, where the concept of karma (moral behaviour and its consequences) and reincarnation are the way of allowing one to leave the Samsara (life on the earth) and reach Nirvana (spiritual illumination); but it is said as well that Nirvana is in the Samsara and the latter is part of Nirvana, while the theory of Anatta (in Theravada doctrine) denies the existence of the soul, looking often as poser to a superficial western reader (48). A beautiful review of the biological, philosophical, religious and cultural aspects of death and their implication on its diagnosis (with much attention to BD) has been published in 1986 by Christopher Pallis in the Encyclopaedia Britannica (49).

In the context of diagnosis of BD, many controversies have been raised in the past two decades in the population, media, and even among physicians, bewildered at the prospect of declaring dead a corpse with the heart still beating. Thus, a clear definition of death is required, while the criteria for diagnosis are a direct consequence of definition.

Definition of death and ethical implications

Turning once again to the Oxford Dictionary (11), death can be defined as "dying; ending of life", but it is only a tautology.

A few points must be analysed to get a clear definition of death:

1. The first aspect to be clarified is whether death is an event or a process. The former probably can happen only during a nuclear explosion, while in all other instances death is a process requiring time. It is well known that heart, liver and kidney may still be kept viable for the short time required between donation and transplant, while the drawing of a viable cornea can be performed several hours after terminal cardiac arrest. According to the 22nd World Medical Assembly held in Sydney in 1968 death can be considered as "a gradual process at the cellular level, with tissues varying in their ability to withstand deprivation of oxygen. But the clinical interest lies not in the state of preservation of isolated cells, but in the fate of the person. Here the point of death of the different cells and organs is not so important as the certainty that the process has become irreversible, whatever techniques of resuscitation may be employed" (50).

2. It is essential to define what is essential to the nature of man, the loss of which implies death: considering the brain as the centre and source of the integral

functions of the body and of psychic life, the death of man can be identified with the death of the brain in all instances, with two components: a) brain stem, as the site of *breathing, wakefulness* and *vegetative life*; b) the cerebrum, as the site of higher functions, including *awareness*. The loss of the former yields the loss of the latter, but not the opposite. The loss of both is the death of the patient; the loss of higher functions only is the most severe loss a man can suffer, but it is not death. If death could be defined simply, as considered in the past, by the arrest of breathing or heart, cardiopulmonary resuscitation could not exist. Conversely, any resuscitation manoevre fails and/or can honestly be stopped when the brain stem is dead.

3. If death is defined in all instances by the death of the brain, BD is only a particular clinical form of death yielded by artificial ventilation (namely, a macabre artefact): in other words, death is always the same, while only the clinical forms may change and, as a consequence, the criteria of diagnosis. The term "diagnosis of death with neurological criteria" would be much more correct than "brain death": the latter leads one understand that only one organ, the brain, is dead, but not necessarily the patient, while it must be clear, especially for a patient's relatives, that the only difference between natural and BD is in the procedure for diagnosis.

4. The main aim of the diagnosis of BD is not letting a terminal patient die (like in euthanasia), but withdrawing ventilation in a corpse. This has some useful and ethically valuable consequences: a) preserving the dignity of death (the BD patient is similar to a heart-lung preparation); b) avoiding useless waste of resources; c) assuring proper treatment to patients who really need it; d) allowing organ transplant. As far as the latter is concerned, it is worth emphasizing that the diagnosis of death is only the *condicio sine qua non* for organ transplant, but the two have nothing else in common.

The very concept of BD has undergone a substantial evolution in the past three decades. Formerly, the concept of BD implied in the Harvard Criteria (51) was the *death of the whole central nervous system*, since in the criteria spinal reflexes were included. Later on, the concept of *brain stem death* has been more focused as the kernel of death (52-55). A dead brain stem undoubtedly means that the patient is dead, having lost forever consciousness, breathing and vegetative life: there are no chances of residual survival, even in PVS. Thus, any concept of BD cannot help including in the criteria for diagnosis death of the brain stem, but two different concepts are accepted in different countries today: the already described brain stem death, and the *death of the whole brain*, including the brain stem. The former has been adopted in the UK, while the latter is preferred in the USA and other European countries, including Italy. The essential difference is that brain stem death considers the death of the brain stem enough to pronounce death, while the death of the whole brain requires checking also the absence of cortical function. The clinical criteria are the same in both cases (since a clinical evaluation of the cortex in a deeply comatose patient is nonsense), while the main difference is the use of neurodiagnostic investigations as ancillary tests, which have also the advantage of giving an "objective" confirmation of the diagnosis.

A third concept of brain death has been suggested, fortunately with no wide consensus and no practical consequences so far, which is centred upon cognitive aspects of the human being: this is *cortical death*, where death is defined as the loss of an ethically relevant life, of environmental interaction and of expression of individuality (56). Indeed, cortical death is only one of the terms to be abandoned, as mentioned at the beginning of this chapter, since it is a bad synonym for PVS. The concept of cortical death cannot be absolutely accepted for many reasons:

a) Individual expression is of course one of the most important aspects of human beings, but the life itself also has some value. In the Judeo-Christian view, human life is of infinite worth; as a consequence, also a reduced life has infinite value as well, and euthanasia is not justifiable. But understanding this concept requires a good deal of feeling and *pietas*; this position is probably also shared by Buddhism, since compassion was one of the most important virtues of Siddharta Gotama.

b) The evaluation of brain stem death can be absolutely certain and objective. In contrast, psychic life can be evaluated only behaviourally, and probably we never will be able to explore directly the mazes of intrapsychic life. Thus, the concept of cortical death yields at best uncertainty, discretion and negligence in a diagnostic procedure which must be absolutely certain; at worst, it means active euthanasia, or even murder.

c) According to Pallis (52), cortical death is the "first step along a slippery slope. If one starts equating the loss of higher functions with death, then, which higher functions? Damage to one hemisphere, or both? If to one hemisphere, to the 'verbalising' dominant one, or to the 'attentive' non-dominant one? One soon starts arguing frontal versus parietal lobes". The slippery slope includes PVS patients today, may add psychiatric ones tomorrow, then severely disabled and so on in a range where a corpse is at one extremity and a depressed patient at the other. All socially unuseful and possibly expensive people can be arbitrarily included in this view. Ancient Sparta gets closer and closer...

d) The prospect of declaring PVS patients dead leads one to propose organ donation in human beings still breathing. This introduces an ethically unjustifiable practice, incompatible with the only true aim of any medical act, that is to say patient's benefit: PVS patients could become a sort of organ tank, and therefore be the instruments and not the aims of medical activity (organ banks or concentration camps?).

e) Such a position is not compatible with common sense: if a PVS patient is considered dead, he should be buried, but it is not acceptable to bury still breathing beings, neither human nor animal. Should we simply bury them or should we do something before in order to stop breathing (such as suffocate them)? This position does not require further comments, but only a veil of silence.

The last important aspect is not directly related to the diagnosis of death, but is joined to organ transplant and is causing unacceptable ethical violations. There is increasing evidence that executed prisoners are the main source of organs for transplant in China (57); this, in turn, leads authorities to an extensive use of the death penalty, including political offenders and other nonviolent criminals. Among other despicable consequences worth mentioning are possible wrongful executions, violation of medical ethics, errors in BD diagnosis, economic interests promoting an "organ market" for highpaying foreign patients. Again, this is a clear example of how single ethically meaningful matters, like brain death and organ transplantation, can lead to unacceptable distortions when unduly intermingled with politics and economics. Here the slippery slope leads from medicine to torture.

References

1. Jennett B, Teasdale G (1981) Management of head injuries. Davis, Philadelphia
2. Pakarinen S (1967) Incidence, etiology and prognosis of primary subarachnoidal hemorrhage. Acta Neurol Scand 43:1-127
3. Phillips LH, Whishnant JP, O'Fallon WM et al (1980) The unchanging pattern of subarachnoid hemorrhage in a community. Neurology 30:1034-1046
4. Adams RD, Vitors M (1989) Principles of Neurology. Mc Graw-Hill, New York
5. Marshall LF, Becked DP, Bowers SA, Cayard C, Eisenberg H, Gross CR et al (1983) The National Traumatic Coma Data Bank. J Neurosurg 59:276-284
6. Institute of Medical Ethics Working Party on the Ethics of Prolonging Life and Assisting Death (1991) Withdrawal of life-support from patients in a persistent vegetative state. Lancet 337:96-98
7. Blin F (1991) L'état végétatif chronique, une question toujours d'actualité. Agressologie 32:213
8. Tresh DD, Sims FH, Duthie EH, Goldstein MD, Lane PS (1991) Clinical characteristics of patients in persistent vegetative state. Arch Intern Med 151:930-932
9. The multi-Society Task Force on PVS (1994) Medical aspects of the persistent vegetative state. N Engl J Med 330:1499-1508
10. Childs NL, Mercer WN, Childs HW (1993) Accuracy of diagnosis of persistent vegetative state. Neurology 43:1465-1467
11. Hornby AS, Cowie AP, Gimson AC (1974) Oxford Advanced Learner's Dictionary of Current English. Oxford University Press, Oxford
12. Frowein RA (1976) Classification of coma. Acta Neurochir 34:5-10
13. American Congress of Rehabilitation Medicine (1995) Recommendations for use of uniform nomenclature pertinent to patients with severe alterations in consciousness. Arch Phys Med Rehabil 76:205-209
14. Mollaret P, Goulon M (1959) Le coma depassé. Rev Neurol 101:3-15
15. Giron GP, Facco E (1987) Stato di coma. Acta Anest Ital 38:539-553
16. Spittler JF, Langenstein H, Calabrese P (1993) Die Quantifizierung krankhafter Bewusstseinsstorungen. Gutekriterien, Zwecke, Handlichkeit. Anasthesiol Intensivmed Notfallmed Schmerzther 28(4):213-221
17. Plum F, Posner JB (1983) The diagnosis of stupor and coma. Davis, Philadelphia

18. Teasdale G, Jennett B (1974) Assessment of coma and impaired consciousness. Lancet ii:81-84
19. Facco E, Zuccarello M, Pittoni G, Zanardi L, Chiaranda M, Davià G, Giron GP (1986) Early outcome prediction in severe head injury: comparison between children and adults. Childs Nerv Syst 2:67-71
20. Simpson DA, Cockington RA, Hanieh A, Raftos J, Reilly PL (1991) Head injuries in infants and young children: the value of the Paediatric Coma Scale. Review of literature and report on a study. Childs Nerv Syst 7(4):183-190
21. Bastos PG, Sun X, Wagner DP, Wu AW, Knaus WA (1993) Glasgow Coma Scale score in the evaluation of outcome in the intensive care unit: findings from the Acute Physiology and Chronic Health Evaluation III study. Crit Care Med 21:1459-1465
22. Bhatty GB, Kapoor N (1993) The Glasgow coma scale: a mathematical critique. Acta Neurochir (Wien) 120:132-135
23. Van de Kelft E, Segnarbieux F, Candon E, Couchet P, Frerebeau P, Daures JP (1994) Clinical recovery of consciousness after traumatic coma. Crit Care Med 22:1108-1113
24. Jennett B, Plum F (1972) Persistent vegetative state after brain damage: a syndrome in search of name. Lancet 1:734-737
25. Feinberg WM, Ferry PC (1984) A fate worse than death. The persistent vegetative state in childhood. Am J Dis Child 138:128-130
26. ANA Committee on Ethical Affairs (1993) Persistent vegetative state: report of the American Neurological Association Committee on Ethical Affairs. Ann Neurol 33:386-390
27. American Medical Association Council on Scientific Affairs (1990) Persistent vegetative state and the decision to withdraw support. JAMA 263:426-430
28. Ashwal S, Bale JF Jr, Coulter DL, Eiben R, Garg BP, Hill A, Myer EC, Nordgren RE, Shewmon DA, Sunder TR et al (1992) The persistent vegetative state in children: report of the Child Neurology Society Ethics Committee. Ann Neurol 32:570-576
29. Position of the American Academy of Neurology on certain aspects of the care and management of the persistent vegetative state patient (1989). Neurology 39:125-126
30. Walshe TM, Leonard C (1985) Persistent vegetative state. Extension of the syndrome to include chronic disorders. Arch Neurol 42:1045-1047
31. Sazbon L, Zagreba F, Ronen J, Solzi P, Costeff H (1993) Course and outcome of patients in vegetative state of nontraumatic aetiology. J Neurol Neurosurg Psychiatry 56:407-409
32. Levin HS, Saydjari C, Eisenberg HM, Foulkes M, Marshall LF, Ruff RM, Jane JA, Marmarou A (1991) Vegetative state after closed head injury. A traumatic coma data bank report. Arch Neurol 48:580-585
33. Higashi K, Hatano M, Abiko S, Ihara K, Katayama S, Wakuta Y, Okamura T, Yamashita T (1981) Five-year follow-up study of patients with persistent vegetative state. J Neurol Neurosurg Psychiatry 44:552-554
34. Fields AI, Coble DH, Pollack MM, Cuerdon TT, Kaufman J (1993) Outcomes of children in a persistent vegetative state. Crit Care Med 21:1890-1894
35. Facco E, Munari M, Baratto F, Behr AU, Giron GP (1994) Long term monitoring in intensive care patients: Electroencephalogram, evoked responses and brain mapping. In: Shulte am Esch J, Kochs E (eds) Central nervous system monitoring in anesthesia and intensive care. Springer, Berlin Heidelberg New York, pp 257-279
36. Facco E, Munari M, Baratto F, Behr AU, Giron GP (1993) Multimodality evoked potentials (auditory, somatosensory and motor) in coma. Neurophysiol Clin 23:237-258
37. Guerit JM (1994) The interest of multimodality evoked potentials in the evaluation of chronic coma. Acta Neurol Belg 94:174-182
38. Council on Scientific Affairs and Council on Ethical and Judicial Affairs (1990) Persistent vegetative state and the decision to withdraw or withhold life support. JAMA 263:426-430
39. Celesia G (1993) Persistent vegetative state. Neurology 43:1457-1458
40. Kaufman DM, Lipton RB (1992) The persistent vegetative state: an analysis of clinical correlates and costs. N Y State J Med 92(9):381-384

41. Weir RF, Gostin L (1990) Decisions to abate life-sustaining treatment for nonautonomous patients. JAMA 264:1846-1853
42. Gerber P (1994) Withdrawing treatment from patients in a persistent vegetative state. Med J Aust 19,161:715-717
43. Guidelines on the vegetative state: commentary on the American Academy of Neurology statement (1989). Neurology 39:123-124
44. Spencer SJG (1993) Inconsistency and confusion cloud the debate. BMJ 307:202 (letter)
45. Pio XII (1958) Risposte ad importanti quesiti sulla rianimazione. In: Discorsi e radiomessaggi di Sua Santità Pio XII, XIX anno di Pontificato 2.3.1957-1.3.1958, Tipografia Poliglotta Vaticana, Città del Vaticano, pp 613-621
46. US Bishops' Pro-life Committee (1992) Nutrition and hydration: moral and pastoral reflections. Origins 21:705-712
47. Jennett B, Bond M (1975) Assessment of outcome after severe brain damage. Lancet i:480-484
48. Humphreis C (1962) Buddhism. Penguin Books Ltd
49. Pallis C (1986) Death. Encyclopaedia Britannica 1986, Edition, pp 1030-1042
50. Gilder SSB (1968) Twenty Second World Medical Assembly. BMJ 3:493-494
51. Harvard Medical School Ad Hoc Committee to Examine the Definition of Brain Death (1968) A definition of irreversible coma. JAMA 205:337-340
52. Pallis C (1982) ABC of brain stem death. Reapparaising death. BMJ 285:1409-1412
53. Pallis C (1982) ABC of brain stem death. From brain death to brain stem death. BMJ 285:1487-1490
54. Pallis C (1982) ABC of brain stem death. Diagnosis of brain stem death I. BMJ 285:1558-1560
55. Pallis C (1982) ABC of brain stem death. Diagnosis of brain stem death II. BMJ 285:1641-164
56. Beresford HR (1978) Cognitive death: differential problems and legal overtones. Ann N Y Acad Sci 315:339-348
57. China. Organ procurement and judicial execution in China (1994). Human Rights Watch Asia 6:1-42

Pathophysiology and Monitoring of Cerebral Edema

F. Della Corte, O. Piazza, A. Clemente, M.A. Pennisi

After primary neurologic damage due to a traumatic, ischemic, hypoxic or metabolic event, a secondary lesion may arise, worsening it and becoming a vicious circle. Locally, the initial energetic breakdown or the tissue mechanical disruption set off a number of biochemical chain reactions leading to a derangement of molecular structures and liberating toxic mediators. Globally, these reactions are responsible for brain edema and disorders of microcirculation (1).

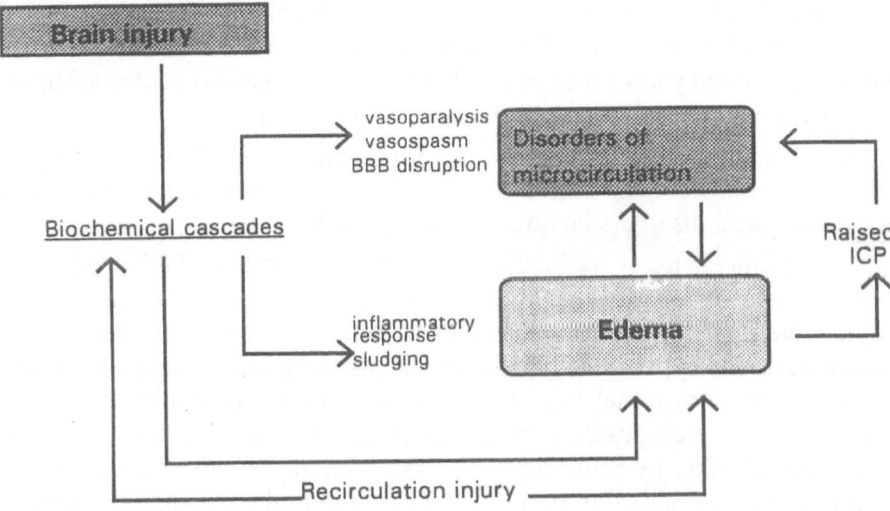

Fig. 1. Some mechanisms involved in the pathophysiology of brain edema

Brain edema defines an increase of the brain water and sodium contents that, when severe, may be responsible for major focal or diffuse signs of brain dysfunction due to the focal encroachment on blood vessels and regional flow impairment. The rise in tissue and in intracranial pressures (ICP) is surely the most threatening consequence of brain edema for the reduction of global perfusion and finally for compression and herniation of brain tissue.

Klatzo (2) classified cerebral edema into two major categories: vasogenic and cytotoxic edema. A third category, defined as interstitial edema, is related to the the increase in brain water in case of hydrocephalus (Table 1).

Vasogenic edema, the most frequent kind of edema, associated with brain neoplasms, head injury and ischemia, is characterized by the increased permeability of brain capillary endothelial cells and extravasation of protein-rich fluid from the intravascular to the interstitial space following injury of the vascular endothelium and blood brain barrier. Factors leading to cerebrovascular dilation and hyperperfusion (hypercapnia, hypoxia, hyperpirexia and systemic hypertension) increase vasogenic edema formation. The cerebral white matter is particularly vulnerable to vasogenic edema because of the lesser amount of cells than in the gray matter and a different disposition of the cellular channels, so that it offers less resistance to edema spreading.

Cytotoxic edema is characterized by the swelling of all brain components with a concomitant reduction of the brain extracellular space. It is caused by ischemia, hypoxia, reduced osmolality, meningitis and toxins that impair cell membrane pump mechanisms. Every pathologic event which damages Na^+/K^+ ATPase membrane pump causes an increase of intracellular Na^+: water moves from the blood into the cerebral tissue to balance the ionic equilibrium. When endothelial cells are particularly affected, the capillar lumen is encroached upon, giving rise to an increased resistance to arterial perfusion.

Notwithstanding these differences, it is very difficult to define how much the pathogenesis of a secondary lesion is to ascribe to vasogenic or cytotoxic edema since biochemical disorders involve the brain globally.

Even if brain edema is well defined as an increase in brain bulk attributable to an increase of its water and sodium content, the term edema is often inappropriately used to define other causes of increased brain volume which may induce intracranial hypertension. In many patients, the predominant pathogenetic mechanism for intracranial hypertension is an increase of the blood volume contained in the cerebrovascular bed. This is called *"brain engorgement"* and may be caused either by active arterial vasodilation or by passive distension of the vascular tree secondary to raised blood pressure in the presence of impaired autoregulation, or obstruction to cerebral venous outflow (3). In the latter case, an increased blood volume but not an increased blood flow is observed. In these patients, with reduced intracranial compliance, small increases in cerebral blood volume lead to considerable increases in ICP, reduction in cerebral perfusion pressure (CPP) and, at last, to brain edema.

Differential diagnosis of classical models of cerebral edema (cytotoxic, vasogenic and interstitial) is easier when the primary cause of cerebral damage is well known. In this case, the diagnosis is achieved by traditional facilities (computerized tomography, magnetic resonance, echography in hypoxic children) but it is much more difficult to follow edema along its development and to prevent its consequences.

Table 1. Features of the different types of brain edema

	Vasogenic	Cytotoxic	Interstitial
Pathogenesis	Increased capillary permeability	Cellular swelling, glial, neuronal, and endothelial	Increased brain fluid due to block of cerebrospinal fluid absorption
Location of edema	Chiefly white matter	Grey and white matter	Chiefly periventricular white matter in hydrocephalus
Edema fluid composition	Plasma filtrate, including plasma proteins	Increased extracellular water and Na^+	Cerebrospinal fluid
Extracellular fluid volume	Increased	Decreased	Increased
Capillary permeability to large molecules	Increased	Normal	Normal
Associated syndromes	Brain tumor, abscesses, infarction, trauma, hemorrage, lead encephalopathy, purulent meningitis	Hypoxia or hypo-osmolality (water intoxication), purulent meningitis	Obstructive hydrocephalus, pseudotumor, purulent meningitis
Electroencephalographic changes	Focal slowing	Generalized slowing	Tracing often normal

Since it is impossible, up to now, to monitor directly the development of brain edema, one must detect it through an impending condition of raised ICP and inadequate CPP. The mismatch between cerebral metabolic rate in O_2 ($CMRO_2$) and cerebral blood flow (CBF) is the first cause of cerebral deterioration and then of brain edema. On this basis, especially to correct inadequate CPP that leads to cytotoxic edema, continuous ICP, arterial pressure and cerebral perfusion pressure (CPP) monitoring are the fundamental means for the detection and treatment of different types of cerebral edema. Moreover, quantitative and qualitative analysis of the ICP pulse waveform and dynamic studies of the intracranial system may add further information about the monitoring of edema.

Finally, other helpful means for cerebral monitoring, directly available at the patient's bedside, are at the disposal of the clinician such as: transcranial Doppler sonography, jugular venous oxygen saturation (SjO_2) and near infrared spectroscopy (NIRS).

Transcranial Doppler (TCD) sonography provides a noninvasive means for the identification of cerebral ischemia monitoring blood flow velocities (systolic, diastolic and mean flow velocity) at the level of the basal intracranial vessels (most commonly the middle cerebral artery) through the temporal bone (temporal window). The pulsatility index (PI) is derived from systolic (SV) minus diastolic (DV) divided by mean velocity (MV) (PI = SV − DV/MV). Normal MV is 60 cm/s; normal value for PI is below 1. Increased MV (more than 100 cm/s) indicates an increased flow. Blood flow velocity is proportional to the regional CBF and to the caliber of the vessel being examined but the interpretation of blood flow velocity values as an index of CBF requires caution for the diameter of intracranial vessels may vary. Thus, TCD cannot measure absolute values of CBF but can evaluate velocity changes, gives some useful pieces of information about autoregulation (CO_2 vasal reactivity, responsivity to barbiturate and to carotid compression) and could help to evaluate the degree of impairment of the intracranial system and to recognize causes of vasogenic and cytotoxic edema. The TCD waveform is different if the increase of blood flow velocity is due to hyperemia or instead to nonhyperemic causes, the latter being characterized by a diastolic notch. Finally, blood flow velocity values and their waveform shapes may be associated with arterojugular difference in O_2 ($AJDO_2$) values to define patients at higher risk of ischemia (4).

As far as the *jugular bulb venous oxygen saturation* (SjO_2) is concerned, it is now considered a useful tool for the evaluation of the adequacy of cerebral blood flow to the metabolic needs and for the identification of global cerebral hyperemia, hypoperfusion and ischemia, especially after head injury.

Rearranging the Fick's equation ($CjvO_2 = CaO_2 - CMRO_2/CBF$, where $CjvO_2$ is the jugular oxygen content drawn at the jugular bulb and CaO_2 the arterial oxygen content and where $CjvO_2$ is directly dependent from SjO_2), the continuous monitoring using fiber optic technology or intermittent measurements of SjO_2 may represent a potential means to evaluate cerebral circulation.

Despite many limitations of this technique either for continuous monitoring (linked to frequent repositioning and recalibration) and for intermittent measurements (significant episodes of abnormal saturation may not be detected), SjO_2 has confirmed its utility in the management of acutely ill neurological patients, especially when evaluated in combination with other parameters. A prognostic role of SjO_2 has been recently demonstrated by Gopinath (5) who observed that severe head injured patients with multiple episodes of jugular venous desaturations had a poorer outcome.

Normal adult SjO_2 is 50%-75%. Global hypoperfusion occurs when SjO_2 goes below 50% without a change in cerebral metabolic rate for oxygen ($CMRO_2$) or increase in arterojugular lactate concentration (AJDL) and global ischemia develops when $SjO_2 < 50\%$, $AjDO_2 > 9$ ml/dl, $CMRO_2 < -0.06$ mmol/g/min and LOI (lactate oxygen index = $-AJDL/AJDO_2$) exceeds 0.08 (6).

Near infrared spectroscopy (NIRS) has been proposed as a new technique for analyzing changes in tissue oxygenation. Since the pioneering work of Jobsis (7), several authors have attempted to monitor the oxygenation state of hemoglobin and the redox state of cytochrome oxidase in living tissue by NIRS. Infrared light between 650 and 1100 nm penetrates human tissue quite well: this light can pass through extracranial tissue into the brain and return to a sensor with valuable information concerning intracerebral attenuation of light. This attenuation is attributed to chromophores including oxyhemoglobin, deoxyhemoglobin, and oxidized cytochrome c oxidase.

Spectrophotometry for hemodynamics is based on the dual wavelength of reflected light from a tissue. One wavelength is used to measure a change in the oxygenation state of hemoglobin and the other to compensate for a possible change in the total hemoglobin concentration. The latter wavelength is most conveniently an isosbestic point of hemoglobin and the absorbance difference between these wavelengths is recorded as a change of the oxygenation state. For NIRS, several investigators used 805 nm as an isosbestic point. Cytochrome oxidase possesses a broad absorption band in this region. Thus the quantitative analysis has been hampered by the redox change of this enzyme. Cytochrome aa3, also known as cytochrome c oxidase, is the terminal member in the mitochondrial electron transport chain. This enzyme serves as the ultimate indicator of mitochondrial oxygen sufficiency within brain tissue.

Simultaneous monitoring of oxygenated hemoglobin (O_2 Hb) and deoxygenated hemoglobin (HHb), within the tissue under observation, provides information on oxygen delivery: total hemoglobin indicates relative tissue blood volume. In Hazeki's study (8), the addition of 5% CO_2 to the inspired gas in rat increased the absorbance at 805 nm. This can be explained by the increase of total hemoglobin in the rat head, probably reflecting the dilatation of cerebral blood vessels. Hoshi et al. (9) have confirmed that NIRS has the potential for real time functional brain imaging: in healty voluntears they confirmed the reability of NIRS by PET study. McCormick et al. (10) have suggested two clinical applications of NIRS: for the study of cerebral hemodynamics and for cerebral oximetry. According to McCormick, NIRS allows evaluation of cerebral blood flow through the measure of transit time of an indocyanine green bolus. The indocyanine green is a tracer which absorbs in the infrared spectrum. The tracer injected via a central venous catheter is detected at the cerebral level by NIRS. The mathematical analysis of time activity curves is identical to that for nondiffusible radioisotope tracers and assumes a monoexponential washout of a single compartment. Transit time is not the golden hemodynamic measure, but frequently collected, it could be an index of changes in CBF. In fact, the transit time is the blood volume (CBV) divided by volumetric CBF (t = CBV/CBF and then CBF = CBV/t). The problem is measuring or estimating CBV, introducing an additional error in evaluating CBF.

The infrared technology is suited for providing an index of adequacy of cerebral oxygen delivering (DO_2) for a given level of oxygen consumption. The infrared light encounters both arterial and venous vascular beds and in the brain venous predominates (70%-80%). Thus cerebral oximetry represents primarily the venous compartment and the cerebral venous saturation (SvO_2). One can obtain, through a mathematical elaboration of data to clinical variables, the measurement of cerebral oxygenation in the form of a more familiar variable: saturation. Similarly to pulse oximetry, in concept, the measurement is non-invasive and continuous and its potential implications in diagnosis and therapy is evident.

The limitation of this technique is primarily related to the lack of information concerning the behavior of infrared light in a complex medium such as the head. Up to now preliminary data seem to demonstrate a good correlation between regional saturation obtained by NIRS and SjO_2, in absence of hematoma or ischemia below the sensor.

References

1. Siesjo B (1992) Pathophysiology and treatment of focal cerebral ischemia. Part I. J Neurosurg 77:169-184
2. Klatzo I, Seitelberger F (1967) Brain edema. Springer, New York
3. Miller JD, Staneck A et al (1972) Concepts of cerebral perfusion pressure and vascular compression during intracranial hypertension. Elsevier, Amsterdam, pp 411-432 (Progress in brain research, vol 35)
4. Chan KH, Miller JD, Dearden NM, Andrews PJD, Midgley S (1992) The effect of changes in cerebral perfusion pressure upon middle cerebral artery blood flow velocity and jugular bulb venous oxygen saturation after severe brain injury. J Neurosurg 77:55-61
5. Gopinath SP, Robertson CS, Contant CF, Hayes C, Feldman Z, Narayan RK, Grossman RG (1994) Jugular venous desaturation and outcome after head injury. J Neurol Neurosurg Psychiatry 57:717-723
6. Dearden NM (1991) Jugular bulb venous oxygen saturation in the management of severe head injury. Curr Opin Anesth 4:279-286
7. Jobsis F (1977) Non invasive, infrared monitoring of cerebral and myocardial oxygen sufficiency and circulatory parameters. Science 189:1264-67
8. Hazeki O, Tamura M (1988) Quantitative analysis of hemoglobin oxygenation state of rat brain in situ by near infrared spectrophotometry. J Appl Physiol 64:796-802
9. Hoshi Y, Onoe H et al (1994) Non-synchronous behavior of neuronal activity, oxidative metabolism and blood supply during mental task in man. Neurosci Lett 172:129-133
10. McCormick P, Stewart M et al (1991) Noninvasive cerebral optical spectroscopy for monitoring cerebral oxygen delivery and hemodynamics. Crit Care Med 19:89-97

Monitoring of Cerebral Dysfunction: Treatment of Post-traumatic Cerebral Injury

N. Stocchetti, F. Buzzi, P. Ceccarelli, M. Cormio, S. Rossi

Introduction

Treatment of post-traumatic cerebral injury is a challenging task. It is based on the meticulous detection of cerebral disturbances, on their aggressive therapy and, sometimes, on their prevention. In this review we will shortly underline the pathophysiologic mechanisms of cerebral damage, mostly for identifying the possible targets of therapeutic intervention. It is impossible to cover here the broad spectrum of therapies indicated for head injury. Instead we will focus on some simple points which are well accepted theoretically, but not applied everywhere in daily practice.

Secondary damage

Treatment of post-traumatic brain injury is aimed at reducing damage, since a complete restoration of the pre-traumatic cerebral condition is beyond our capabilities. Damage usually results not only by the initial mechanical insult but also by a complex chain of events called "secondary brain damage" (1).

This concept, originally restricted to the occurrence of ischemic damage, can be appropriately extended to traumatic brain injuries for many reasons. In fact the main mechanisms of damage are basically the same in ischemic and in traumatic injuries. Moreover, ischemia is widely recognized as the main cause of secondary aggravation of all types of severe head injuries (2). Global ischemia-hypoxia are very often observed in trauma due to associated systemic injuries and/or respiratory disorders inherent to comatose states. Accordingly, global cerebral ischemia can also result from elevated intracranial pressure. Focal ischemia is common around expansive lesions, creating local tissue pressure gradients. Penumbra conditions in ischemia and in focal trauma are similar.

In ischemia the failure of energy triggers biochemical reactions that produce, around the central core, edema formation and alteration of the microcirculation which secondarily extends the lesion. In trauma the disruption of tissue directly produces biochemical disorders resulting in similar edema and similar microcirculatory disturbances, leading to secondary perifocal ischemia and further enlargement of the lesion.

Finally, at the molecular level, the mechanisms of destruction are basically the same even though they may operate in different sequences and with a different time course and intensity in various situations of ischemia and/or trauma.

The central nervous system has very little endogenous fuel and essentially no reserve of oxygen. Since the brain extracts approximately one third of the total blood oxygen content, with cessation of blood flow the brain depletes its supplies of oxygen within seconds. The glycogen content of the brain is also low (2-3 mmol/g), and therefore the total amount of glucose and glycogen is thus only sufficient to sustain the normal rate of oxygen consumption for approximately 5 min.

For all these reasons the brain is very vulnerable to insults that compromise its oxygen or substrate supply, such as hypoxia and ischemia.

It is possible to identify two distinct thresholds of ischemia: one for functional impairment and the other for the initiation of structural damage. The critical CBF threshold for electrical failure in the cerebral cortex is fairly constant in all studied species (3) and in man around 16-18 ml/100g/min. At this level the ATP concentration remains close to normal. With further reduction of flow, energy stores are progressively decreased. At a threshold of around 8-12 ml/100g/min, ion pumping is stopped, cells are depolarized and the destructive reactions leading to structural alteration are triggered.

Together with the absolute level of flow the duration of low flow also determines the irreversibility of damage (4, 5). Heiss and Rosner (3) established in cats that critical for the survival of neurons is residual flow below 5 ml/100g/min for more than 20 min, or below 8 ml/100g/min for more than 30 min, or below 14 ml/100g/min for more than 45 min. A flow around 18 ml/100g/min would be tolerated indefinitely, provided there is a low level of consumption.

Strategies for treatment

Strategies for treatment have been developed, and some are still in the process of being developed, considering the different phases of treatment.

Generally speaking, strategies for reducing secondary damage are based on three lines of action:

1. Hemodynamic and respiratory handling to avoid ischemia and, therefore, to guarantee an adequate delivery of substrates, after exclusion of surgical masses. When ischemia is caused by an expanding lesion, such as a subdural hematoma, the only reasonable approach is prompt surgical evacuation.
2. Various pharmacological or physical methods intended to reduce the cerebral metabolic demand if ischemia is in some measure inevitable.

3. When specific mediators of secondary damage can be identified, they can be counteracted, and some promising compounds are under development.

Early phase

In the immediate phase after trauma specific goals should be pursued. The fundamental goal of resuscitation is restoration of circulating volume, blood pressure, oxygenation and ventilation. In fact, the deleterious impact of secondary insults such as arterial hypotension and hypoxia have been documented (6). A level of arterial oxygen saturation close to 100% has to be obtained, avoiding any unnecessary reduction of $PaCO_2$. In practice, comatose patients require tracheal intubation and controlled ventilation. Recently the widespread use of myorelaxant for head injured patients has been questioned (7). By definition any unnecessary drug has to be avoided, but during the rescue phase a smooth intubation and ventilation can often be achieved only after sedation and paralysis.

Accordingly, arterial pressure has to be measured as soon as possible and corrected if lower than 110-120 mmHg systolic. Correction requires volemic restoration, both stopping bleeding and infusing isotonic fluid, and sometimes infusion of vasopressors.

Since early detection and removal of intracranial surgical masses is of paramount importance, appropriate delivery of patients to a hospital where a CT scan and surgery can be performed on emergency basis is crucial.

Intensive care

The main objectives of intensive care have been to maintain adequate cerebral perfusion and oxygenation and to avoid medical and surgical complications. Uncontrollable intracranial hypertension remains the most frequent cause of death in aggressively managed head injured patients. The poor prognosis accompanying sustained elevations of intracranial pressure (ICP) has been well established. A large scale study of ICP involving 1030 patients was conducted as part of the Traumatic Coma Data Bank (8). Of this group, ICP data were studied from 428 patients who met monitoring criteria. As expected, age, admission motor score and abnormal pupils were highly significant in explaining outcome. Beyond these factors, the percentage time that ICP was above 20 mmHg was highly significant ($p < 0.0001$).

The first issue in neuro-oriented critical care is that ICP must be measured, together with arterial pressure, allowing monitoring and management of cerebral perfusion pressure (CPP).

Much more emphasis has been placed on CPP in the last decade and in most centres the overall management is more focused on CPP preservation than in ICP control "per se". It has been reported that CPP should be kept above 60 mmHg, but greater levels have also been suggested (1, 9).

Relationship between cerebral blood flow and cerebral oxygen consumption may probably be estimated by measuring arteriovenous differences of oxygen ($AVDO_2$) or cerebral extraction of oxygen (10). Patients with inadequate oxygen supply to the brain can be identified regardless of the occurrence of intracranial hypertension and before any clinical deterioration is detectable. That is expected to minimize brain damage and to improve both survival and quality of survival. Since $AVDO_2$ = hemoglobin concentration x 1.34 x arteriojugular venous oxygen saturation percentage, when arterial oxyhemoglobin saturation, Hb concentration and the position of the Hb dissociation curve remain constant, the ratio of global cerebral blood flow over oxygen consumption is proportional to the venous oxygen saturation at the jugular bulb.

Episodes of venous desaturation (< 50%) have been reported (11) in nearly 40% of patients with a Glasgow coma score less than 8 after severe head injury using continuous monitoring. Most of the episodes were less than 1 h in duration, and it is likely that many of them would not have been detected without continuous measurement of $SjvO_2$. Episodes of desaturation were most common on day 1 after injury and twice as common in patients with a reduced cerebral blood flow as compared to patients with a normal or elevated cerebral blood flow. The most common causes of reduced $SjvO_2$ include systemic hypotension, increased ICP and hypocarbia.

Hypothermia may limit secondary brain injury by reducing cerebral metabolism (12), stabilizing cell membranes and suppressing the high levels of extracellular excitotoxic amino acids present after head injury (13).

As a general rule, hypothermia reduces $CMRO_2$ by an approximately 5% °C reduction in body temperature (14). In patients with head injury, hypothermia to 32-33 °C reduced $CMRO_2$ approximately 11%.

Clinical investigations have only recently attempted to record human brain temperature (15). Intracranial temperature varied from 0.5 to 2.0 °C higher than body temperature in severely head injury patients. A randomized trial in a consecutive series of 40 patients with severe head injury established that lowering the brain temperature to 32-33 °C with cooling blankets and cold saline gastric perfusion is feasible and safe. This study demonstrated that such a small difference in brain temperature produced a 26% reduction of CBF with a 40% drop in ICP. A trend is observed toward better outcome in the treated group.

Hypothermia may have a future in brain protection. But the impact of brain temperature on $CMRO_2$ should always be kept in mind today in clinical practice. Since hyperthermia aggravates metabolic stress and is additive to ischemic injury, metabolic protection begins with solid measures against hyperthermia.

Pharmacological intervention

Promising compounds, capable of acting at different levels of the biochemical cascade causing cellular and vascular damage after head injury, have been developed in the experimental setting. Among them are calcium entry blockers, excitatory amino acid antagonists, and drugs active against free radicals, such as superoxide dismutase (SOD). Some of them, as SOD and tirilazad mesylate, are supported by impressive experimental evidence. In different models, for example, the 21-aminosteroid, U74006F, tirilazad mesylate, appears to be 100 times more potent than methylprednisolone in the inhibition of lipid peroxidation (16).

Despite the amount of data suggesting benefits, introduction of new drugs in the therapeutic regimen must be very cautious. Only well planned and conducted clinical trials may provide a solid answer to our expectations.

Rehabilitation

All the efforts spent on the scene of accident, in the operating room, and in intensive care are just the premise for a complete recovery. This final goal cannot be achieved unless a scientific and comprehensive program of rehabilitation is started early and continued as long as necessary.

Conclusions

Secondary damage is associated with higher mortality, lower recovery rate and poorer outcome. It is therefore necessary to identify and to treat vigorously every additional insult to the CNS after trauma. New strategies, and old principles, are available but incompletely applied. Final outcome can only be viewed as the sum of the best efforts devoted during several phases of treatment, starting in the field and finishing years after trauma, with the financial and psychological support that the social environment can provide.

References

1. Miller JD (1982) Physiology of trauma. Clin Neurosurg 29:103-130
2. Graham DI, Ford I, Adams JH, Doyle D, Teasdale GM, Lawrence AE, McLellan DR (1989) Ischemic brain damage is still common in fatal non-missile head injury. J Neurosurg Psychiatry 52:346-350
3. Astrup J, Siesjo BK, Symon L (1981) Threshold in cerebral ischemia. The ischemic penumbra. Stroke 12:723-725
4. Heiss WD, Rosner G (1983) Functional recovery of cortical neurons as related to degree and duration of ischemia. Ann Neurol 14:294-301

5. Kaplan B, Brint S, Tanabe J, Jacewiz M, Wang XJ, Pulsinelli W (1991) Temporal thresholds for neocortical infarction in rats subjected to reversible focal cerebral ischemia. Stroke 22:1032-1039
6. Chesnut RM, Marshall LF, Klauber MR, Blunt BA, Baldwin N, Eisenberg HM, Jane JA, Marmarou A, Foulkes MA (1993) The role of secondary brain injury in determining outcome from severe head injury. J Trauma 34:216-222
7. Hsiang JK, Chesnut RM, Crisp CB, Klauber MR, Blunt BA, Marshall LF (1994) Early, routine paralysis for intracranial pressure control in severe head injury: is it necessary? Crit Care Med 22:1471-1476
8. Eisenberg HM, Gary HE, Aldrich EF, Saydjary C, Turner B, Foulkes MA, Jane JA, Marmarou A, Marshall LP, Young HF (1990) Initial CT findings in 753 patients with severe head injury. J Neurosurg 73:688-698
9. Pickard JD, Czosnyka M (1993) Management of raised intracranial pressure. J Neurol Neurosurg Psychiatry 56:845-858
10. Cruz J, Miner ME, Allen SJ, Alves WM, Gennarelli TA (1991) Continuous monitoring of cerebral oxygenation in acute brain injury: assessment of cerebral hemodynamic reserve. Neurosurgery 29:743-749
11. Gopinath SP, Robertson CS, Contant CF, Hayes C, Feldman Z, Narayan RK, Grossman RG (1994) Jugular venous desaturation and outcome after head injury. J Neurol Neurosurg Psychiatry 57:717-723
12. Astrup J (1982) Energy requiring cell functions in the ischemic brain. Their critical supply and possible inhibition in protective therapy. J Neurosurg 56:482-497
13. Busto R, Globus MYT, Dietrich WD, Martinez E, Valdes I, Ginsberg MD (1989) Effect of mild hypothermia on ischemia-induced release of neurotransmitters and free fatty acids in rat brain. Stroke 20:904-910
14. Michenfelder JD, Milde JH (1991) The relationship among canine brain temperature, metabolism, and function during hypothermia. Anesthesiology 75:130-136
15. Mellergard P, Nordstrom C (1991) Intracerebral temperature in neurosurgical patients. Neurosurgery 28:09-713
16. Hall ED (1989) Free radicals and CNS injury. Crit Care Clin 5:793-805

The Glasgow Coma Scale After 20 Years

J.D. MILLER

Introduction

In 1974, just over 20 years ago, Teasdale and Jennett published a paper in the *Lancet*, "Assessment of Coma and Impaired Consciousness. A Practical Scale" that has become one of the most widely cited papers in the neurological literature (1). Twenty years on, what is the status of the Glasgow Coma Scale today? The purpose of this brief review is to try to answer this question.

The introduction of the Glasgow Coma Scale (Table 1) was a response to a need to introduce simplicity and objectivity into the grading of loss of consciousness. At that time, a number of coma scales were in existence that were unidimensional but depended upon the use of terms such as stuporose, semicomatose and comatose, that were not defined in objective terms. Teasdale and Jennett proposed that consciousness could be resolved into three components - arousal that was manifested by eye-opening, awareness of and responsiveness to changes in the environment that were manifest in the verbal and motor responses. For each of these components they described a series of response levels related to the stimuli required to elicit the response which was described in objective terms. For example, motor responses at the lower end of the scale were referred to as abnormal flexor referring to flexion at the elbow and an abnormal component that consisted of pronation and wrist flexion, and extensor referring to extension at the elbow, rather than using the terms decorticate and decerebrate which themselves required definition. Before publishing their paper, considerable effort was expended in Glasgow in testing the new scale for inter-observer variability by having numbers of observers examine the same patient or watch a video of examination of the patient (2). The scale was also compared for reliability between different user groups, including senior and junior doctors, nurses, allied health personnel, and medical students. Comparison studies were also made between native English speakers and non-native English speakers. The value of these latter studies was later confirmed when the Glasgow Coma Scale was adopted in a number of other countries and translated into several different languages, including most European languages, Japanese and Chinese.

One of the points emphasised by Teasdale and Jennett was the value of the scale in enabling realistic comparisons to be made between groups of head injured patients studied in different centres. The Glasgow Group set up a collaboration in collection of head injury data with two centres in Holland (Groningen and Rotterdam) and with a centre in the United States (University of Southern California at Los Angeles) (3).

Table 1. Glasgow Coma Scale

Eye opening	4	Spontaneous
	3	To command
	2	To pain
	1	Nil
Verbal response	5	Oriented speech
	4	Confused speech
	3	Words only
	2	Sounds only
	1	Nil
Best motor response	6	Obey command
	5	Localise pain
	4	Flexor withdrawal
	3	Abnormal flexion
	2	Extension
	1	Nil

At this stage, the Glasgow Coma Scale was attracting a number of critics, some of whom criticised the scale for being too complex, while others claimed that the scale was too simple. A pragmatic interpretation of these criticisms would be that the scale was probably pitched at the correct level of complexity to combine adequate description of the state of the patient, yet to allow statistical analyses of adequate sized groups. In an editorial article in the Journal of Neurosurgery, Langfitt made a strong plea for widespread adoption of the Glasgow Coma Scale to allow comparison of different series of head injured patients and critical examination of claims that one or other mode of management of head injury did or did not produce improvements in head injury outcome (4). Langfitt's recommendations bore fruit. A detailed comparison was made between the Glasgow/Rotterdam/Los Angeles databank and a group of more than 200 severely head injured patients treated in Richmond, Virginia, and a similar sized group of patients treated in San Diego (5, 6). The Glasgow Coma Scale was incorporated into the American Traumatic Coma Data Bank that was set up as a joint venture between the Office of Biometry of the National Institutes of Health and four neurosurgical centres in the US, later expanded to five centres (7, 8).

The applications of the Glasgow Coma Scale have also been extended beyond head injury to description of the level of consciousness in patients with subarachnoid haemorrhage and patients with many forms of medical coma including craniospinal infection and hepatic coma. In the case of subarachnoid haemorrhage, most investigators had used the Hunt and Hess Scale which was in turn a modification of the Botterell Scale that graded patients into one of five categories depending upon the level of consciousness and the presence of signs of meningism and abnormal neurological signs. A further modification was introduced by a Sub-committee of the World Federation of Neurosurgical Societies to incorporate Glasgow Coma Score values into the Scale which was then renamed the WFNS Scale (Table 2). This is now the most widespread system for describing patients with subarachnoid haemorrhage (9).

Table 2. WFNS scale for subarachnoid haemorrhage

Grade	Criteria	
1	GCS 15, neurologically intact or isolated cranial nerve palsy	
2	GCS 15, neurologically intact, but with headache and vomiting	
3	GCS 13-14,	
	a	without neurological deficit
	b	with focal neurological deficit
4	GCS 8-12, with or without neurological deficit	
5	GCS 3-7, in coma with or without abnormal motor positioning	

Comparison with other coma scales

While a number of other scales have been proposed and used over the years, very few have been subjected to the detailed studies of inter-observer error, reliability and value for prognosis that has been applied to the Glasgow Coma Scale. Exceptions are the Glasgow Liege Coma Scale and the Swedish Reaction Level Scale.

The Glasgow Liege Scale was an attempt to incorporate brain stem responses into the scoring system as a fourth scale, additional to the eye-opening, motor response and verbal response scores used in the Glasgow Coma Scale (10). Implicit in this system was the belief that with progressive impairment of brain function there was a hierarchical loss of brain stem reflexes starting with the vertical oculofistibular response and ending with the oculocardiac reflex. It is by no means certain that such a hierarchical loss is the rule and the scale has not found widespread acceptance. Impairment or loss of brain stem reflexes does, in any case, form part of the head injury prognostic algorithm that has been developed in Glasgow for use alongside the coma scale and incorporating additional prognostic factors such as age.

The Swedish Reaction Level Scale (RLS 85) (Table 3) was introduced as an improvement on a unidimensional coma scale that was in widespread use in the

Scandinavian countries (11). In the Swedish Scale the distinction between consciousness and unconsciousness is determined by one or more of a series of possible responses that include the uttering of recognisable words, orienting eye movements, obeying commands or warding off painful stimuli. The purpose of using this form of differentiation was to allow assessments to be made in patients in whom eye-opening was not possible because of swelling or speech was impossible because of intubation or aphasia. The Swedish Scale has been subjected to detailed comparison with the Glasgow Coma Scale and to studies of repeatability and reliability (12).

Table 3. Swedish Reaction Level Scale (RLS - 85)

1. Alert - no delay in response
2. Drowsy or confused - responds to light stimulus
3. Drowsy or confused - responds only to strong stimulus
YES
MENTAL RESPONSE: at least one of - utters words; orienting eye movement; obeys commands; wards off pain
NO
4. Unconscious - localises but does not ward off pain
5. Unconscious - withdraws from pain
6. Unconscious - stereotyped (abnormal) flexion to pain
7. Unconscious - stereotyped extension to pain
8. Unconscious - no response to pain

A comparison study of these two scales has been carried out in Edinburgh, which may be regarded as a neutral centre without a vested interest in the promotion or development of either scale. The study was carried out in 239 head injured patients in whom the level of consciousness ranged from fully awake to deeply comatose. A group of nine doctors were trained in the use of both the Glasgow Coma Scale and the Swedish Reaction Level Scale. They evaluated patients and scored each patient on both of the scales (13).

Using each of the two assessment scales, patients were allocated into categories of minor head injury (GCS 13-15; RLS 85 1-2), moderate head injury (GCS 9-12 and 7 or 8 with eye opening; RLS 85 3), and severe head injury (GCS 3-8 with no eye opening; RLS 85 4-8). Percentage agreement levels between GCS and RLS 85 were obtained and the weighted kappa coefficient was calculated.

There was a good overall agreement level between GCS and RLS 85 in terms of allocating patients to the three categories of head injury severity (Table 4). The percentage agreement was 88% and the weighted kappa coefficient 0.87. This overall level of reliability, however, was not reflected in allocating all three of the degrees of severity of head injury. The percentage agreement levels were 95% for minor head injury and 91% for severe head injury, but for patients classified as having a moderate head injury there was only 45% agreement. From another viewpoint, only 41% of the total number of patients allocated by either method to the category of moderate head injury were common to both groups. In the remaining 59% of cases where one or other scoring method allocated the patient to a category other than moderate head injury, neither scale systematically allocated patients to a better or a worse category.

Table 4. Comparison of GCS and RLS 85

RLS 85	Glasgow Coma Scale			Total
	Severe (3-8.E1)	Moderate (9-12)	Minor (13-15)	
Severe (4-8)	31 (91%)	4 (14%)	0	35
Moderate (3)	1 (3%)	13 (45%)	9 (5%)	23
Minor (1,2)	2 (6%)	12 (41%)	167 (95%)	181
TOTALS	34 (100%)	29 (100%)	176 (100%)	239

In practice, the use of the RLS 85 scale was at times advantageous when patients were unable to be scored for eye opening or verbal response but this number of cases was relatively small and the use of the RLS 85 scale was found not to be any more accurate than the more widely adopted Glasgow Coma Scale. It was therefore concluded that in Edinburgh, where the Glasgow Coma Scale was already in use, there were insufficient grounds to warrant changing the type of coma scale used for assessment of head injured patients.

Glasgow Coma Scale and prognosis

Soon after it had been shown that the Glasgow Coma Scale was a reliable means of describing the level of consciousness in head injured patients, it became clear that it was also a powerful prognostic tool (14). Although it was never intended that the three component scores of the Glasgow Coma Scale would be summated, because it is an ordinal and not a cardinal scale, nevertheless, the Glasgow Coma Sum Score was closely related to head injury mortality (15). In a series of 1919 head injured patients reported from Edinburgh, the mortality was approximately 40% for those scoring 8 or less on the coma scale, for those scoring 9-12 points on the GCS sum score the mortality was 4% and, for those scoring 13, 14 or 15 points on the GCS, the mortality was 0.4% (16).

The Glasgow Coma Scale was incorporated into an outcome prediction algorithm in Glasgow, together with other important prediction factors including age, pupil light responses and reflex eye movements and the presence of an intracranial haematoma on CT. The Glasgow Prediction Algorithm was based on Bayesian Statistics which allow prediction to proceed even when some data are missing. A similar exercise was carried out by Stablein and his associates using a logistic regression model (17). This allowed ranking of the prognostic factors in their order of importance for prognosis. This exercise confirmed the major importance of the motor score element of the Glasgow Coma Scale as being one of the most important single prognostic factors in head injury (18-20).

In nearly all series described, the prognostic algorithm, once developed, is tested upon a further series of patients treated in the same institution. We have recently completed an independent assessment of the Glasgow Prognostic Algorithm involving 426 predictions in 325 patients with head injuries treated in Edinburgh. The prediction algorithm provides the percentage probability of outcome in each of three possible outcome groups, dead or vegetative, severely disabled and moderately disabled or good recovery as defined on the Glasgow Outcome Scale of Jennett and Bond. In appropriate patients predictions would be calculated on admission after resuscitation, prior to evacuation of an intracranial haematoma for those patients who had such a lesion, and at 24 h, 3 days or 7 days after the onset of coma lasting at least 6 h. Our aim was to assess how often clinically useful predictions could be calculated in head injured patients presenting acutely and to compare the predicted with the actual outcome of the patients as assessed at 6 to 24 months after injury using the latest available true outcome assessment (21).

By far the most frequent reason for predictions to be impossible was that the patients were intubated, paralysed and artificially ventilated. This was the case in 15% of patients already upon admission to the neurosurgical unit and in 76, 59 and 35% of patients in whom prediction was attempted at 24 h, 3 days and 7 days after onset of traumatic coma (Table 5).

When predicted outcome was compared with actual outcome, overall, 76% of predictions were correct, 15% were pessimistic, that is the outcome was better in truth than the predicted outcome and 10% of predictions were optimistic, where the patients actually had a poorer outcome than was predicted. The prediction algorithm was correct in 84% of patients whose true outcome was good or moderate. The prediction algorithm was also correct in 84% of predictions of death or vegetative survival. In contrast, of those predictions that forecast survival with severe disability, only 12% were correct (Table 6).

It could be concluded from this independent assessment that although the Glasgow Prediction Algorithm accurately forecast outcome in three quarters of head injured patients, there are nevertheless predictions that are quite wrong despite being made at a high level of confidence, that is at 95% or greater probability of a particular expected outcome. It would therefore be inappropriate to use it as a reason to limit or withdraw care from patients. The prediction algorithm is least accurate in forecasting survival with severe disability. This is unfortunate because this is the very group of patients in whom it would be helpful to have an early identification of need and early application of intensive rehabilitative measures. Finally, largely because a number of patients are already intubated, paralysed and ventilated when seen by the neurosurgical team, assessment of the Glasgow Coma Score and calculation of a prediction is not possible in a number of cases.

Table 5. Feasibility of prediction of outcome using Glasgow algorithm

Time of admission	No of cases	Prediction possible n (%)	Not possible n (%)
Admission	183	139 (76)	44 (24)
Pre-operative for haematoma	141	137 (97)	4 (3)
24 h after coma lasting 6 h or more	180	35 (19)	145 (81)
3 days after coma	145	49 (34)	96 (66)
7 days after coma	124	66 (53)	58 (47)

Table 6. Predicted vs actual outcome for all predictions made

Predicted outcome	Actual outcome		
	Good/moderate	Severe disability	Dead/vegetative
Good/moderate	225 (84%)	23 (47%)	15 (13%)
Severe disability	14 (5%)	6 (12%)	3 (3%)
Dead/vegetative	28 (11%)	20 (41%)	92 (84%)
Total	267 (100%)	49 (100%)	110 (100%)

The Glasgow Coma Scale today

The GCS has been widely accepted on a world-wide basis, largely because it is simple, objective and reliable and this in turn means that it is a useful medium for communication between doctors, nurses and hospitals, allowing everyone who discusses the patient to have a clear idea of the level of responsiveness in that individual. The increased use of early intubation and artificial ventilation in head injured patients does pose a problem for the doctor in the hospital, who may have to rely upon the assessment of a non-medical individual made at a time when the patient has not been resuscitated. This may pose major problems in clinical trials of specific therapy where the severity of the patient's head injury may be over estimated or under estimated at the early roadside assessment. This is one area in which the simplicity and objectivity of the Glasgow Coma Scale becomes of paramount important in enabling an accurate assessment of the level of response to be possible at the scene of the accident by any trained personnel, provided that the patient's airway, circulation and oxygenation are adequate at the time and the patient is not under the influence of a sedative or depressant drugs. Alcohol presents a common and a difficult problem because of its analgesic as well as sedative properties in patients who have consumed large quantities of alcohol. The amount of pain stimulation may be insufficient to elicit a response on the Glasgow Coma Scale. Despite these problems the Glasgow Coma Scale remains in 1995, the bench mark, world wide, for assessment of the level of consciousness of patients who have suffered head injury, subarachnoid haemorrhage or who have become comatose following any one of a number of severe medical disorders.

References

1. Teasdale G, Jennett B (1974) Assessment of coma and impaired consciousness: a practical scale. Lancet 2:81-83
2. Tesdale G, Knill-Jones R, Van der Sande J (1978) Observer variability in assessing impaired consciousness and coma. J Neurol Neurosurg Psychiatry 41:603-610
3. Jennett B, Tesadale G, Galbraith S, Pickard J, Grant H, Brackman R, Vezaat C, Maas A, Minderhoud J, Vecht CJ, Heiden J, Small R, Caton W, Kurze T (1977) Severe head injuries in 3 countries. J Neurol Neurosurg Psychiatry 40:291-298
4. Langfitt TW (1978) Measuring the outcome from head injuries. J Neurosurg 48:673-678
5. Miller JD, Butterworth JF, Gudeman SK, Faulkner JE, Choi SC, Selhorst JB, Harbison JW, Lutz H, Young HF, Becker DP (1981) Further experience in the management of severe head injury. J Neurosurg 54:289-299
6. Bowers SA, Marshall, LF (1980) Outcome in 200 consecutive cases of severe head injury treated in San Diego County; a prospective analysis. Neurosurgery 6:237-242
7. Foulkes MA, Eisenberg HM, Jane JA, Marmarou A, Marshall LF and the Traumatic Coma Data Bank Research Group (1991) The Traumatic Coma Data Bank: design, methods and baseline characteristics. J Neurosurg 75 [Suppl]:S8-S13
8. Marshall LF, Gauteille T, Klauber MR, Eisenberg HM, Jane JA, Luerssen TG, Marmarou A, Foulkes MA (1991) The outcome of severe closed head injury. J Neurosurg 75 [Suppl]: S28-S36
9. Drake CD, Hunt WE, Sano K (1988) Report of World Federation of Neurological Surgeons Committee on a universal subarachnoid haemorrhage grading scale. J Neurosurg 68:985-986
10. Born JD, Albert A, Hans P, Bonnal J (1985) Relative prognostic value of best motor response and brain stem reflexes in patients with severe head injury. Neurosurgery 16:595-601
11. Starmark JE, Stalhammar D, Holmgren E (1988) The Reaction Level Scale (RLS 85): Manual and Guidelines. Acta Neurochir 91:12-20
12. Starmark JE, Stalhammar D, Holmgren E, Rosander B (1986) A comparison of the Glasgow Coma Scale and the Reaction Level Scale (RLS 85). J Neurosurg 69:699-706
13. Johnstone AJ, Lohlun JC, Miller JD, McIntosh CA, Gregori A, Brown R, Jones PA, Anderson SI, Tocher JL (1993) A comparison of the Glasgow Coma Scale and the Swedish Reaction Level Scale. Brain Injury 7:5-1-506
14. Teasdale G, Jennett B (1976) Assessment and prognosis of coma after head injury. Acta Neurochir 34:45-55
15. Teasdale G, Jennett B, Murray L, Murray G (1983) The Glasgow Coma Scale: to sum or not to sum. Lancet 2:678
16. Miller JD, Jones PA (1985) The work of a regional head injury unit. Lancet 1:1141-1144
17. Stablein DM, Miller JD, Choi SC, Becker DP (1980) Statistical methods for determining prognosis in severe head injury. Neurosurgery 6:243-248
18. Jennett B, Teasdale G, Brackman R, Minderhoud J, Knill-Jones R (1976) Predicting outcome in individual patients after severe head injury. Lancet 1:1031-1034

19. Barlow P, Teasdale G (1986) Prediction of outcome in the management of severe head injuries: the attitudes of neurosurgeons. Neurosurgery 19:989-991
20. Murray LS, Teasdale GM, Murray GD, Jennett B, Miller JD, Pickard JD, Shaw MDM, Achilles J, Bailey S, Jones P, Kelly D, Lacey J (1993) Does prediction of outcome alter patients management? Lancet 351:1487-1491
21. Nissen JJ, Jones PA, Signorini DF, Miller JD Assessment of the Glasgow Head Injury Outcome Prediction Programme. (Submitted)

Clinical Trials in Acute CNS Injuries

F. SERVADEI, G. GIULIANI, M.T. NASI, A. ARISTA

Introduction

Acute central nervous system injuries include head injury, spinal cord injury, focal and global cerebral ischemia and subarachnoid hemorrhage (SAH). Our paper focuses on brain injury and on SAH. Trauma is the first cause of death below the age of 45 in many countries all over the world (1); head injury contributes in the vast majority of cases. An average of 200 patients per 100.000 population per year are admitted to the hospital following a head injury. About 20 per 100.000 population per year are the deaths related to the brain injury (1). Many cases among the survivors present neurological sequelae leading to severe disability. SAH is less frequent (11 cases per 100.000 inhabitants per year); mortality and morbidity in this disease are mainly related to the occurrence of vasospasm (40% to 60% of patients) (2). Both in brain injury and in SAH patients there is primary brain damage due to mechanical factors in head injuries and to hemorrhagic stroke in SAH. This primary damage is followed by secondary damage due to biochemical processes in the tissue surrounding the primary injury. Secondary ischemia, which is present both following brain injury and during vasospasm, leads to loss or reduction of blood flow and oxygen supply. With the improvement in our knowledge concerning this biochemically induced damage, a new set of drugs has been tested in animal models. A few of these drugs reached a phase II - III clinical trial both in SAH and in brain injured patients.

Results of the clinical trials

SAH

Calcium antagonist have been proved to reduce brain damage in experimental models of cerebral ischemia and hemorrhage. The *calcium antagonist nimodipine* does not reduce the incidence of vasospasm detected by angiography in humans or primates but it reduces the size of cerebral infarcts in animals only when given before occlusion of a cerebral artery (3). The role of nimodipine in the prevention or treatment of delayed ischemic dysfunctions after SAH has been studied (4) in seven prospective randomized, double blind clinical placebo-controlled clinical trials using either oral nimodipine (five studies) or intravenous nimodipine (two studies). The largest trial was a British multicenter study which included 554 patients who were treated with oral administration of 60 mg nimodipine for 21 days versus placebo (5). Poor outcomes were reduced by 40% in the treated group ($p = 0.001$). Furthermore, a reduction (34%, $p = 0.003$) in the incidence of cerebral infarction was found in the nimodipine patients. The second largest trial included 215 patients enrolled in one institution (6) who received either intravenous nimodipine followed by oral nimodipine or placebo. One patient of the nimodipine group (1%) and nine patients (8%) of the placebo group died as a result of ischemic deterioration. A further consideration was that the combination of early aneurysm surgery and nimodipine treatment resulted in the best neurological outcome (6).

The efficacy of *tirilazad, a nonglucocorticoid 21 amino steroid* to avoid focal brain ischemia and to act against the opening of the blood brain barrier (7) has been studied in animal models. Further studies demonstrated that the drug can prevent the occurrence of vasospasm (8). These favorable preclinical data led to clinical studies.

A safety study to test a range of doses in patients with aneurysmal SAH and to develop pilot information for trials of efficacy was conducted in 12 Canadian neurosurgical centers (9). From July 1990 to May 1992, 245 patients were entered in the study. Three tirilazad doses were tested: 0.6 mg/kg, 2 mg/kg and 6 mg/kg. No serious side effects were observed at any of the three dosages despite close monitoring of hepatic and cardiac toxicity. A trend toward improvement in the overall 3 month outcome was seen in the 2 mg/kg per day compared to vehicle treated groups. The conclusion is that tirilazad is safe at doses up to 6 mg/kg and is a promising drug in the treatment of aneurysmal SAH patients.

A large clinical trial was then conducted in Europe and Australia enrolling 1015 patients with aneurysmal SAH: 253 were treated with placebo, 257 with tirilazad 0.6 mg/kg, 249 with tirilazad 2 mg/kg and 256 with tirilazad 6 mg/kg (10). All the patients received nimodipine as concomitant therapy. The treatment was started on average 32 h after bleeding and mean Glasgow Coma Score was 12 in every subgroup of patients. In each group the surgical rate was 90%. Adverse events were present in about 2% of the patients with no difference concerning the various subgroups. The highest incidence of good recovery (64%) and the lowest mortality rate (12%) were observed in the 6 mg/kg group whereas in the placebo group good recovery was 53% and mortality 21% ($p = 0.007$ and 0.006, respectively). Symptomatic vasospasm was 18% in the 6 mg/kg group and 26% in the placebo group ($p = 0.04$). In spite of the above-mentioned clinical results, the narrowing of cerebral vessels seen at angiography was not modified by the treatment. In conclusion, it appears that tirilazad associated to nimodipine at the dosage of 6 mg/kg is more effective than nimodipine alone in reducing morbidity and mortality related to aneurysmal SAH. If we consider the results separately, according to gender, mortality was, at the dosage of 6 mg/kg, 3% in males and 17% in females. To verify these data, a multicenter trial only in females at the dosage of 15 mg/kg was started a few months ago.

Head injury

The possibility of calcium antagonists to reduce brain damage in experimental models of ischemia (3), which is a typical form of secondary brain damage following severe head injury, led to clinical trials with *nimodipine* in head injured patients. The first trial, British and Finnish, (HIT 1) (11) had as an endpoint the effect of nimodipine (or placebo) administration on outcome in 350 severely head injured patients. Only "a modest but clinically valuable benefit was shown". HIT 2, European multicenter study (12), enrolled 852 severely head injured patients. No effects of nimodipine were demonstrated concerning overall outcome. In a subset of patients showing signs of SAH on CT scanning a statistically significant ($p = 0.05$) difference was shown concerning unfavorable outcomes in favor of the nimodipine treated group. A third multicenter study (German) is still ongoing.

The initial release or formation of highly reactive free radicals following CNS injury is thought to induce a cascade of secondary or delayed tissue damage due primarily to lipid peroxidation (13).

The radical scavenger *PEG-SOD* has been shown to have beneficial effects on intracranial pressure after experimental cold injury and a clinically significant effect in experimental brain injury (14). This compound has been tested in two large American multicenter clinical trials. The first of these trials randomized 463 patients. Results show 46% favorable outcomes in the placebo group versus 55% in the treated group. However, this difference was not statistically significant (15).

Tirilazad mesilate (U-74006F) is the first member of a new class of synthetic 21 aminosteroids and it has been shown to be a potent inhibitor of lipid peroxidation. This compound was extensively tested in animal models of brain injury and it was shown to improve neurological outcome in spite of not reducing edema formation (16), to reduce mortality (17) and to increase survival rate (18). These results were really the most promising ones and led to two large clinical trials in moderately and severely head injured patients, at the dosage of 10 mg/kg.

The first study, American and Canadian, stopped enrollment at 1191 patients due to a significant interaction between treatment and one factor, presence of hypotension. Since the mortality in vehicle treated patients is markedly lower than would be expected from previous studies, an ongoing investigation is due to explain these differences.

The second study, European and Australian, completed the enrollment at 1132 patients. Overall mortality was 27.5% but data elaboration is not yet available. Among the inclusion criteria for this study, the most important one was a very short therapeutic window. The drug (or placebo) should be administered within 4 h from injury. According to experimental studies (13), the earliest drug administration should ensure the best clinical outcome.

There is evidence from several animal studies that excitotoxic damage to neurons and glia also develops as a consequence of excessive release of excitatory amino acids after primary impact injury, ischemic events and hematoma (19). Therefore a clinical benefit can be expected from the use of excitatory amino acid antagonists such as NMDA antagonists. Only two competitive NMDA antagonists, *GCS 19755* and *D-CPP-end* had completed safety assessments in humans in 1992 (19), whereas another promising one, *MK801*, was withdrawn from clinical use. Selfotel, GCS 19755, is now being tested in two large multicenter studies (American and European-Canadian-Australian), also with a short therapeutic window (8 h from injury). Other non-NMDA antagonist drugs together with blockade of presynaptic glutamate release and kappa opiate antagonist are of interest for the future.

Conclusions

In SAH patients who recover from the initial effect of bleeding often deteriorate a few days later because of arterial narrowing associated with delayed ischemic dysfunction (4). The incidence of angiographic vasospasm has been reported to be as high as 50%-70% with 20%-30% of these patients developing clinical symptoms (2). Nimodipine, a calcium antagonist, is capable of reducing morbidity and mortality in aneurysmal SAH patients. Tirilazad, a new non-glucocorticoid 21-amino steroid, has been shown in two clinical studies to be more effective than nimodipine alone. Both drugs ameliorate clinical outcomes in spite of not reducing the incidence and severity of angiographic vasospasm; therefore the exact mechanism of action is still to be explained.

There is clear evidence from clinical and neuropathological studies that a substantial proportion (30%-40%) of those patients who die after severe head injury have spoken at some stage after impact (19). This suggests that secondary processes are involved at least in a part of the brain damage. This provides opportunity for drug treatment (19). The new concept which developed according to the experimental studies was delivery of the drug within a few hours (4 to 8) from injury. This treatment requires a good network of patients' transportation in order to be able to assess the patient before drug delivery within such a short time frame. Nimodipine was tested in severely head injured patients but it only showed an effect in a small subset of patients with post-traumatic SAH. Free radical scavengers such as PEG-SOD have not been shown to date to present a significant effect on outcome. Large clinical studies conducted with tirilazad (one of the most promising drugs on experimental bases) are over but substantially the results are not yet available. Clinical trials with excitatory amino acid antagonists are now ongoing.

References

1. Kraus JF (1991) Epidemiologic features of injuries to the central nervous system. In: Anderson W, Schoenberg D (eds) Neuroepidemiology: a tribute to Bruce Schoenberg. CRC, Boca Raton
2. Wier B, Rothenberg CH, Grace M, Davis F (1975) Relative prognostic significance of vasospasm following subarachnoid hemorrhage. Can J Neurol Sci 2:109-114
3. Gotoh O, Mohamed AA, McCullogh J et al (1986) Nimodipine and the hemodynamic and histopathological consequences of middle cerebral artery occlusion in the rat. J Cerebr Blood Flow Metab 6:321-331
4. Tettenborn D, Dycka J (1990) Prevention and treatment of delayed ischemic dysfunction in aneurysmal subarachnoid hemorrhage. Stroke 21 [Suppl IV]:85-89
5. Pickard JD, Murray GD, Illingworth L et al (1989) Effect of oral nimodipine on cerebral infarction and outcome after subarachnoid hemorrhage. Br Med J 298:636-642
6. Ohman J, Heiskanen O (1988) Effect of nimodipine on outcome of patients after aneurysmal subarachnoid hemorrhage and surgery. J Neurosurg 6:683-686
7. Zuccarello M (1989) Protective effects of 21 aminosteroid on the blood brain barrier following subarachnoid hemorrhage in the rat. Stroke 20:367-371
8. Steinke DE, Wier BKA, Findlay JM et al (1989) A trial of 21 aminosteroid U74006F in a primate model of chronic cerebral vasospasm. Neurosurgery 24:179-186
9. Haley Clarke E, Kassel NF, Wayne M et al (1995) Phase II trial of tirilazad in aneurysmal subarachnoid hemorrhage. J Neurosurg 82:786-790
10. Kassel NF (1995) Unpublished data presented at the World Congress of Neurosurgery. Acapulco, Mexico, 1993
11. Teasdale G on behalf of the cooperative study (1992) Randomized trial of nimodipine in severe head injury: Hit 1. J Neurotrauma 9 [Suppl 2]:S545-S550
12. The European Study Group on Nimodipine in Severe Head Injury (1994) A multicenter trial of the efficacy of nimodipine on outcome after severe head injury. J Neurosurg 80:797-804
13. Smith DH, Gennarelli TA, McIntosh T (1995) The potential of 21 aminosteroids as neuroprotective therapies in CNS injury. CNS Drugs 3(3):159-164
14. Muizelar JP, Marmarou A, Young HF et al (1993) Improving the outcome of severe head injury with oxygen radical scavenger polyethylene glycol conjugate superoxide dismutase: a phase II trial. J Neurosurg 80:797-804
15. Muizelar JP (1995) Unpublished data presented at the First World Congress on Brain Injury, Copenhagen
16. Sanada, Nakamura T, Nishimura MC et al (1993) Effect of U74006F on neurologic functions and brain oedema after fluid percussion injury in rats. J Neurotrauma 10:65-71
17. McIntosh TK, Thomas M, Smith DH et al (1992) The novel 21 aminosteroid U74006F attenuates cerebral oedema and improves survival after brain injury in the rat. J Neurotrauma 9:33-40
18. Hall ED, Yonkers PA, McCall JM et al (1988) Effects of the 21 aminosteroid U74006F on experimental head injury in mice. J Neurosurg 68:456-461
19. Bullock R, Fujisawa H (1992) The role of glutamate antagonists for treatment of CNS injury. J Neurotrauma 9 [Suppl 2]:S443-S461

Biochemical Mechanisms of Neuronal Degeneration and Plasticity

G. SAVETTIERI, I. DI LIEGRO, A. CESTELLI

The signs and symptoms of neurologic disorders, often bewildering in their clinical manifestations, present extreme diagnostic and therapeutic challenges to physicians. It is necessary to have a good knowledge of the biochemical processes involved in the damage in order to select therapeutic strategies aimed to re-establish, at least in part, the injured physiological functions.

The symptomatology of some well studied chronic diseases results from damage of specific cell populations. This specificity is known as "selective vulnerability". For example, the weakness and muscle atrophy which characterize both poliomyelitis and amyotrophic lateral sclerosis are caused by the destruction of lower motor neurons, whereas the varied symptoms which afflict patients with multiple sclerosis derive from localized foci of degeneration of the myelin sheath and oligodendroglia. On the other hand, in most acute pathologies, such as ischemia or trauma, the initial insult induces a series of secondary events which cause even more damage than the original insult itself: among these secondary events, cytotoxicity and microvascular damage are being studied with an ever increasing detail.

Clinical neurochemistry has always focused on the aetiology and the molecular mechanisms that lead to dysfunction/degeneration of neural cells. In the last decade, in addition, molecular neurobiology has begun proposing a wide spectrum of therapeutic approaches aimed to influence, restore or replace components of neural circuits afflicted by a particular pathology. A further substantial progress in understanding the genetic and epigenetic basis of a number of neurologic diseases has been made thanks to the use of cell cultures, which offer the unique opportunity to probe cause-effect relationships simply by testing the action of a given compound on metabolism and behaviour of specific cell types (1).

Trophic factors and brain insults

In the nervous system repair mechanisms involve two main categories of trophic factors. The first one comprehends neurotrophic molecules secreted by glial as well as other cell types: these molecules act on receptor-bearing neurons to influence their survival and the expression of genes involved in maintenance and repair. The second one comprehends gliotrophic molecules secreted mainly by neurons that regulate glial proliferation, myelination, and the synthesis of neurotrophic molecules by the glial cells. In this section we will refer mainly to neurotrophic factors which are relevant to the survival of injured neurons and the regeneration of damaged axons: these molecules are members of the families of neurotrophins (NTs), fibroblast growth factors (FGFs), epidermal growth factors (EGFs), insulin-like growth factors (IGFs), transforming growth factors ß (TGF ß) and ciliary neurotrophic factor (CNTF) (2-5). That NT expression in brain is regulated by the afferent activity was suggested for the first time by the finding that NGF mRNA levels increased after recurrent limbic seizures (6). Axonal severing in the CNS of adult mammals often causes neurons to die. This catastrophic event is probably due to loss of the trophic support provided both by the targets and the glial cells that surround the axonal processes. A strict dependency of axotomized CNS neurons on the exogenous supply of specific neurotrophic factors has been thoroughly studied by several laboratories. It has been shown that axotomized neurons are temporarily rescued when neurotrophic factors are infused into the site of insult; this beneficial effect is, however, suddenly reverted if the administration of the neurotrophic molecule is discontinued (7). Recent experiments involving infusions of one or more growth factors into the CNS of animals with traumatic chemical or ischemic damage indicate further that these molecules are able to rescue a wide range of cell functions (8-11).

A number of conditions have to be met, however, for the safe and effective use of neurotrophic factors in the treatment of neurologic recovery after injury. These include the development of noninvasive techniques of administration and the maintenance of therapeutic levels of neurotrophic factors in the area of injury. Although repeated injections by osmotic micropumps can be beneficial, the penetration of the compound into the injured area is only limited to a narrow rim around the infused site and long-term steady levels are difficult to maintain (12). The recent development of new biodegradable implantable receptacles might provide a release device of therapeutic relevance (13). The implantation of cells genetically engineered into selected regions of the nervous system is another promising strategy for the long-term administration of proteins: fibroblasts engineered to express NT have been successfully grafted to the brain of laboratory animals to facilitate neuronal survival and regeneration after lesion (14). A problem encountered in some of these experiments is that engineered immortalized cells may continue to grow and form tumors at the site of implantation. A tentative solution seems to include the cells into selectively permeable polymer capsules (15). Recent progress in molecular neurobiology has contributed new and ingenious ways for introducing genes or gene products into mature brain. Herpesvirus and adenovirus vector systems are being developed for gene targeting in neurons, but much remains to be done before these techniques can be considered safe and useful tools for gene therapy (16, 17). In the PNS, where fewer neurons die after axotomy, it is believed that a local supply of growth factors by Schwann cells and other nonneuronal cells residing in the neural stump mitigates the effects of the insult (18).

Neural recognition molecules and extracellular matrix in disease and regeneration

Neuronal migration, axonal extension and synaptic connectivity are basic mechanisms both in development and regeneration of the nervous system. All these phenomena depend on the availability of adequate recognition molecules, which play their role through three different molecular mechanisms:

1. Specific lock-and-key interactions between either homophilic or heterophilic molecules located alternatively on opposing membranes or on a plasma membrane and the extracellular matrix.
2. Differences in the mode of distribution of recognition molecules, as clusters or single molecules, that influence the strength of the interactions between the molecules.
3. The transduction to the cell interior of signals triggered by binding events at the cell surface. Recognition molecules include an extraordinarily large number of structurally related molecules of the immunoglobulin superfamily (19), as well as cadherins (20), integrins (21), and lectins (22).

A significant amount of information has been obtained in vitro for some of these molecules. More recently, experiments with transgenic animals, null for specific genes, not only confirmed the importance of these molecules in the nervous system, but deserved in addition unexpected surprises. Of importance was the realization that the spatial and temporal context in which these molecules are presented can lead to the subtle differences that are observed in different cell types. A fine tuning of cell interactions that goes beyond the simple "stop and go" signals for neurite outgrowth can now, at least in part, be attributed to particular carbohydrate moieties carried by the recognition molecules (23).

Characterization of the phenotype of the mutant mouse deficient in the gene encoding P0, the major glycoprotein of PNS myelin, led to the conclusion that this molecule is involved in the formation and maintenance of PNS myelin (24). The homophilic and heterophilic adhesive properties of P0 reside in its extracellular immunoglobulin-like domain carrying the HNK-1 (human natural killer-1) carbohydrate structure, itself serving as a ligand for cell adhesion molecules. Several point mutations in the human P0 gene have been recognized and classified as Charcot-Marie-Tooth disease type 1B (25, 26) or Déjérine-Sottas disease (27), respectively , depending on the nucleotide sequence mutated. The peripheral myelin protein -22 (PMP-22), whose mutations are responsible for Charcot-Marie-Tooth disease type 1A, has now been identified as a recognition molecule, as it carries the HNK-1 glycan (28). Thus, two genes encoding two PNS-myelin-specific recognition molecules, P0 and PMP-22, produce abnormalities with very similar clinical pictures: distal muscle weakness and atrophy, reduced nerve conduction velocity, and de- and remyelination with onion bulb formation occurring with varying degrees of severity and time of onset.

Mutations in the human gene for the L1 neural adhesion molecule have been related to X-linked hydrocephalus (HSAS: hydrocephalus resulting in the stenosis of the aqueduct of Sylvius). This appears to be secondary to deficits in homophilic and heterophilic L1-related functions in neuronal cell migration, axonal outgrowth and fasciculation and synaptic activity (29): disturbances of neuronal migration and proliferation may lead to cytoarchitectural abnormalities, resulting in stenosis with obstructions of the drainage of the cerebrospinal fluid and, as a consequence, hydrocephalus.

The simple concept that extracellular matrix glycoproteins of the nervous system, such as laminin, fibronectin, tenascin-C, tenascin-R, thrombospondin, vitronectin and agrin either inhibit or promote axonal outgrowth is no longer tenable. Especially for laminin, tenascin-C and tenascin-R, the dual actions of inhibition or promotion are found in the same molecule (30). For example, tenascin-C has distinct domains involved in vitro in adhesion, promotion of neurite outgrowth, neuronal migration, repulsion of neuronal cell bodies and growth cones, and polarization of neuronal morphology.

The distinction between adhesion/repulsion and contact/diffusible ligands for the growth cone are probably somewhat artificial: one ligand (whether diffusing or cell bound) could, via distinct domains, elicit a particular directional response, depending on the nature of the receptors on the growth cone. Thus one molecule can well exert different functions and the question arises over which of these functions is predominant at a particular time and at a particular location for a responding neuron. Evidence is emerging that the association of tenascin-C and tenascin-R with other extracellular molecules, such as fibronectin or proteoglycans, might modify the accessibility of the different domains to their neuronal receptors (31).

Yet another exciting step in understanding the molecular mechanisms governing axonal growth was the recent finding of a growth-cone collapsing molecule, termed collapsin, that is structurally related to molecules that promote axonal growth, such as fasciclin IV. These molecules are part of an emerging family known as semaphorins, phylogenetically conserved from flies to chickens and humans (32).

The existence of axon growth-inhibitory molecules associated with oligodendrocyte membranes and CNS myelin was established some years ago and has important implications for functional CNS regeneration. Antibodies against these proteins, if delivered to the lesion site together with specific NT, enhances the local sprouting of injured axons and prevents retrograde neuronal degeneration (33). Combined effects from several molecules are thus requested to induce axonal outgrowth, particularly because of the ability of NT and cytokines to modulate the expression of adhesion molecules (34, 35).

Mitochondrial neurological diseases

Each mitochondrion contains two to ten copies of supercoiled double stranded circular DNA molecules (mtDNA), only 16.5 kilobases (kb) long. mtDNA exhibits a mutation rate of approximately 1 per 7000 bases leading to two to three mismatched nucleotides per cycle of replication. The half life of mtDNA (6-10 days), relatively short as compared to that of nuclear DNA, ensures a high evolutionary rate. This high mutation rate is related, at least in part, to the location of mtDNA within the mitochondrial matrix, and thus to its exposure to the high concentrations of superoxide ions (O_2^-) generated by the respiratory chain during aerobic respiration. The lack of a histone coat and adequate repair systems are responsible for the vulnerability of mtDNA to free radical induced injury (36, 37).

Chronic progressive external ophthalmoplegia (CPEO) is characterized by bilateral ophthalmoplegia and ptosis with retinal pigmentation. Kearns-Sayre syndrome (KSS) is defined by the onset of CPEO and retinal degeneration before 20 years of age, together with ataxia, hearth-block and high levels of cerebrospinal fluid proteins. Deletions of the mtDNA are found in 40% of CPEO patients and in 90% of those with KSS. Deletions in these disorders are usually single and may vary in size up to 11 kb (38).

Ciafaloni et al. (39) have recently reviewed the clinical and biochemical features of 23 patients with the myopathy, encephalopathy, lactic acidosis and stroke-like episodes (MELAS) phenotype. The heteroplasmic mutation involving an A to G transition at position 3243 in tRNA$^{Leu(UUR)}$ gene has been identified in 21 over 23 MELAS patients (39).

Myoclonic epilepsy with ragged red fibres (MERRF) is characterized by the onset in adolescence or early adulthood of myoclonus, ataxia and myoclonic or generalized seizures. An A to G transition at position 8344 in the mtDNA tRNA^{Lys} gene has been identified in several MERRF families (40).

Susceptibility to deafness induced by the antibiotic aminoglycoside is maternally inherited in a significant proportion of cases. These antibiotics affect bacterial rRNA: given the similarity among bacteria and mitochondria, it has been hypothesized that some antibiotics might also affect some mitochondrial function. A homoplastic point mutation at position 1555 in a highly conserved region of the mtDNA 12S rRNA has been in fact found in families with aminoglycoside-induced deafness as well as in an Arab-Israeli family with maternally inherited deafness (41). A specific deficiency in mitochondrial complex I activity was first identified in Parkinson's disease (PD) in 1989 (42).

This particular defect seems to be confined to the substantia nigra in the CNS, is specific for PD and not related to L-DOPA therapy (38).

Amyloidogenesis in Alzheimer's disease

Alzheimer's disease (AD), the most prevalent cause of dementia in the elderly, is characterized by memory loss and impairment of cognition, language, visual-spatial skills, judgement and behaviour. The disease is classically characterized by two types of brain abnormalities:

1. Neurofibrillary tangles (NFTs), composed of highly phosphorylated forms of the microtubule-associated protein tau in neurons of the cortex, hippocampus and amygdala (compacted plaques)
2. Extracellular deposits (diffuse plaques) of the 40-42 residue amyloid ß-protein (Aß), in cerebral parenchyma and around blood vessels (43)

The fact that some subjects with Down's syndrome who die in their teens show amorphous deposits of Aß (diffuse plaques) in the absence of other cytological lesions of AD has supported the concept that Aß deposition can occur prior to detectable neuronal alteration. It is difficult to establish rigorously such a temporal sequence in AD, because brains are only examined at the end of the disease. However, the presence of a large number of diffuse plaques, always outnumbering compacted plaques, in Alzheimer's brains, and the fact that the amyloid lesions of Down's syndrome are indistinguishable from those of AD suggest that diffuse plaques might represent the earliest distinguishable lesions also in AD.

Although the aetiology of this disease is complex, at least three different genetic loci that confer inherited susceptibility to this disease have been identified:

1. The ε4 (112 Cys to Arg) allele of the apolipoprotein E *(ApoE)* gene is associated with AD in a significant proportion of cases with late onset (> 60 years) (44).
2. Mutations in the gene for the ß-amyloid precursor protein *(ßAPP)* have been found in a small number of families (< 3% of cases) with disease onset before 65 years of age (45).
3. A third mutation, associated with susceptibility to a very aggressive form of AD, has been recently identified in a gene whose product (designated *S182*) is predicted to contain multiple transmembrane domains (46).

The only known protein that shares substantial homology with S182 is SPE-4, an integral membrane protein of 465 amino acids, expressed in the sperm of the nematode *Caenorabditis elegans*. On the basis of phenotype analysis of sterile *spe-4* mutant worms, the protein appears to be a constituent of the Golgi-derived membranous organelles of primary spermatocytes and is required for proper attachment of the organelles to the so-called fibrous bodies of these spermatid precursors (47). Formation of such complexes is essential for correct intracellular transport and distribution of various proteins during meiotic cell divisions in *C. elegans* sperm.

Families with this genetic form of AD develop typical AD almost a decade earlier, on average, than families bearing mutations in ßAPP itself. The Aß peptide, which is the main component of the amyloid plaques in AD, is constitutively expressed by ßAPP-expressing cells (such as neurons, microglia and endothelial cells) and is released by proteolysis of ßAPP in mildly acidic environments, including endosomes and late-Golgi secretory compartments. Mutations in S182, by interfering with the normal membrane trafficking pathways, might cause ßAPP to stay for a longer time in an amyloidogenic organelle.

Triplet repeat mutations in neurological diseases

In the last few years a new mechanism of genetic disease has been identified that underlies severe neurological disorders and seems very likely to be the cause of many others. Since 1991, when the mutation responsible for the fragile X (FraX) syndrome was evidenced as an outstanding expansion of an exonic CGG-repeat, other human genetic diseases have been similarly demonstrated to be due to such mutations. Each of these diseases shows the phenomenon of *genetic anticipation*, characterized by a tendency for a worsening in disease severity in successive generations and for a decrease in the age of onset of the disorder. This phenomenon, once thought to be due to an imprecise clinical diagnosis, has now clearly been shown to have a direct genetic basis (48). The genetic mechanism involved is an abnormal expansion of trinucleotide repeats (triplets), usually localized in a coding region or, less frequently, in a noncoding region of genomic DNA. This expansion, increasing through generations, appears to account for the observed phenotypic feature of anticipation.

FraX syndrome is an X-linked dominant disorder with reduced penetrance. The syndrome is the main cause of inherited mental retardation in humans and is associated with a chromosomal fragile site at Xq 27.3. The reduced penetrance is variable within families where the mutation becomes penetrant only when maternally transmitted; the chance of penetrance increases in successive generations. The *FMR1* (*fragile X mental retardation 1*) gene normally bears in the first exon polymorphic CGG-repeats formed by 6-52 (with an average of 29) copies of the triplet. In the mutant FMR 1 gene, the repeat length increases dramatically up to 600 or more copies of the triplet. Concomitant with this large expansion, referred to as the full mutation, an abnormal methylation of restriction sites within a CG-rich region (CpG island) occurs immediately upstream of the gene (49, 50). This condition inhibits *FMR1* transcription from "full mutation" alleles (51).

Huntington disease (HD) is characterized by choreic movements, changes of personality and progressive dementia which usually begins to appear in midlife. HD is genetically transmitted by an autosomal dominant gene (52). In 1993 the Huntington Disease Collaborative Research Group reported the identification of the HD gene (53). Near the 5′ of the coding sequence, a repeat of 21 CAG trinucleotides has been evidenced, encoding a putative polyglutamine stretch in the protein. This trinucleotide repeat is normally polymorphic with lengths ranging from 11 to 36 CAG repeats (98% of normal subjects have ≤ 24 triplets). Among HD patients, this module expands to sizes between 42 and approximately 100 triplets. The length of the repeat appears to be correlated with the severity of the disease, such that juvenile cases fall within the high end of the abnormal allele lengths. The change in the CAG trinucleotide repeat would predict a variable number of glutamines within the HD protein (called huntigtin). Since normal mRNA levels were observed in cell lines derived from both hetero- and homozygous patients, the increase of glutamines beyond 44 residues likely results in a gain-of-function.

Neuropathology of virus infections

Viruses are being increasingly implicated in causing CNS damage. How they gain access in the first place is far from being straightforward. It is clear that there is not a single mechanism, so that each virus gains access to neurons and affects the immune system in a variety of ways; furthermore, different species of host animals can respond quite differently when infected by the same virus. The studies on specific viral infections are beginning to develop strategies that may be applied to contain a variety of viral diseases.

Neurological diseases occurring in the setting of human immunodeficiency virus (HIV) infection exhibit a remarkable spectrum. The most devastating clinical expression is dementia. The brains of these individuals show alterations in neurons, changes in the glial cells and evidence for increased microglial and macrophage activity (54). Although HIV infects both neural and glial cells in vitro, these cells do not exhibit high levels of infections in vivo. There are evidences in favour of the existence of specific neurotropic strains: it has been recognized that viruses isolated from the brain infect cultures of macrophages more readily than cultures of T cells, while viruses isolated from blood and spinal fluid will readily infect cultures of stimulated T cells. Even within the same patient, sequences obtained directly from viral DNA from brain and spleen or from cerebrospinal fluid and blood show differences, suggesting that there may be brain-specific sequences.

Prion diseases

Prion diseases are neurodegenerative disorders identified both in animals and humans (55, 56). Four different diseases are known to be due to prions in humans: kuru, Creutzfeldt-Jacob disease (CJD), Gerstmann-Straussler-Scheinker disease (GSS) and fatal familial insomnia (FFI); among these, kuru has been known for a long time as an infectious disease transmitted through the ritualistic cannibalism of brains from dead relatives in New Guinea; FFI is an inherited disorder, while CJD and GSS can be sporadic, inherited or infectious. In animals, at least six encephalopathies can be recognized as prion diseases; among these the most common is scrapie, in sheep. All of these diseases are frequently transmissible to laboratory animals and in the past were attributed to unknown infectious pathogens such as bacteria or viruses. Although the unusual biochemical properties of the scrapie agent were first recognized in the late 1940s, only in the 1980s did the large number of experimental data collected indicate convincingly that the scrapie infectious particles were devoid of nucleic acids and composed instead largely, if not entirely, by PrP^{Sc} protein (57, 56). The term "prion" was then introduced to indicate the peculiarity of the agent and to distinguish it from other kinds of infectious particles.

PrP^{Sc} is an abnormal isoform of a cellular protein, PrP^C, that is synthesized in the endoplasmic reticulum, modified in the Golgi apparatus and transported to the plasma membrane where it is inserted through an anchor of glycosylphosphatidyl inositol (GPI). The PrP^C protein seems to reenter the cell through caveolae, like other GPI-proteins, and is protease-sensitive. The abnormal protein, PrP^{Sc}, is, in contrast, protease-insensitive and much evidence suggests that it differs from the normal counterpart only for conformation; the normal protein folds into four conserved α-helical segments that constitute its central core; three of these segments have also the potentiality to form ß-structures, probably the kinds of folds present in PrP^{Sc} (55). Studies with transgenic animals have demonstrated that the infectious process depends on transformation of the endogenous, normal isoform into the abnormal form through a biochemical mechanism that is likely to involve a direct interaction between PrP^{Sc} and PrP^C (58). That the propagation of the prion is to be ascribed to the conversion of PrP^C into PrP^{Sc} under the influence of PrP^{Sc} has been recently confirmed by the finding that no propagation of prions is possible in PrP null mice (59). In the case of inherited prion diseases, mutations have been identified in the sequence encoding the α-helical core of PrP; this finding suggests that mutant PrP molecules might undergo spontaneous conversion into PrP^{Sc}; the accumulation of an excess of this latter form should eventually cause CNS degeneration (56). What is the function of PrP in the brain? Although this protein is highly conserved among mammals and widely expressed during development, homozygous null mice do not show any apparent defect; very recently, however, these mice have been reported to have weakened $GABA_A$ (γ-aminobutyric acid type A) receptor-mediated fast inhibition and impaired long-term potentiation (60). A similar impaired synaptic inhibition might be also the basis for the epileptiform activity found in CJD and for the early synaptic loss and neuronal degeneration that characterize prion diseases in humans (60).

From a more general point of view, nobody really knows how PrP propagation causes cell damage. The scrapie proteins accumulate in the lysosomes of cultured neurons and it is possible that in the brain the lysosomes, swollen to abnormal sizes, might eventually burst, pouring their contents into the cytoplasm. This event might lead to cell death and to further propagation of prions from dead cell lysates to neighbouring cells. Moreover, prion-infected brains contain rod-shaped particles which are ultrastructurally indistinguishable from many amyloids; these amyloid plaques contain extracellular deposits of polymerized protease-resistant PrP (56). One of the most challenging features of prion diseases is the existence of distinct "strains", each able to induce a different pathological syndrome; these different strains possess some sort of cell-specific tropism and induce the PrP^C to PrP^{Sc} conversion only in a limited population of cells. These phenomena have been difficult to explain by the "protein-only hypothesis". However, it has been recently suggested that self-propagation of PrP^{Sc} polymers with distinct three-dimensional structures could be the biochemical basis of scrapie (and possibly other) prion strains (61). According to this hypothesis, prion strains would be alternative conformations or packing arrangements of PrP^{Sc} polymers. Since the chemical environment can strongly affect both PrP^C to PrP^{Sc} conversion and the polymerization kinetics, it is possible that diversity in intracellular conditions determine the "strain-specific" appearance of these diseases and the rate of formation of abnormal proteins (61).

An unexpected help to the understanding of the biochemical basis of prion origins came recently from the finding that some determinants in yeast that were considered extrachromosomally inherited are instead nuclear-encoded proteins which exist in alternative conformations much like the brain prions (62). It appears therefore that prion-like proteins may be much more frequent in nature than expected. Moreover, it is possible that what we have been learning from the study of prion functions could be also useful to the understanding of the causes of other, more common, neurodegenerative diseases, including PD and AD.

Neuronal cell grafting in restorative neurology

Grafting neuronal cells into a patient brain poses ethical problems to be kept in mind well before any attempt to do it. The specific developmental history of every human brain is, from many points of view, unique, in that genetic and environmental factors have sculptured that CNS through a series of hierarchical choices. From this history arise not only a mature brain, but also a mind and a unique personality. How extensive might the manipulations be on brain without affecting personality? On the other hand, would it be correct to restrain from trying an ameliorating intervention if the patient's personality has been already severely impaired by a degenerative disorder?

The ethical principles relating to the rights of human subjects involved in all types of clinical research must be of the utmost importance, especially when remembering the cases of abuse, such as the war crime trials at Nuremberg, the Tuskegee syphilis study, and the Willowbrook Hospital hepatitis study (63).

Starting with Thompson's preliminary work with intracerebral grafting in 1890, the difficulties to achieve good survival of the tissue implanted became immediately clear (64, 65). Because mature, end-differentiated neurons do not, under normal circumstances, divide either in the brain or in culture, the key appears to derive normal neurons from normal neural precursors.

Fetal tissue can be an appealing source of suitable cells since it has been known for a very long time that immature CNS retains a plasticity not usually seen in the adult. The cells from fetal tissue show, indeed, a lively cell cycle (that may enable efficient ex vivo gene modification via retrovirus vectors), pluripotency (allowing for a wide range of phenotypic and regional fates), facile engraftability (particularly into germinal zones), and are often capable of expedited movement through the migratory germinal zones, present in the CS throughout the life span, from development to adulthood. The engrafting of these cells into the germinal zone, where they are able to settle as integral members, could provide a mean for a diffused delivery and integration of gene products throughout the CS.

However, progenitors removed from the brain do not normally remain in a constant proliferative state in vitro: after a finite number of mitoses, they cease dividing and differentiate. An intervention is necessary to maintain them in a proliferative state. The generation of cell lines from progenitors using immortalizing genes transduced by replication-incompetent retroviral vectors or by chronic exposure to mitogenic growth factors circumvents these limitations (66). Whether such progenitors are representative of the majority of progenitors within mammalian CNS or are merely a minor subtype is uncertain: this uncertainty represents one of the limitations in the use of immortalized neuronal cell lines. It has been shown, in fact, that immortalized progenitors derived from the external germinal layer (EGL) of mouse cerebellum could, upon transplantation, give rise to a wide range of interneurons and glia in the adult cerebellum; cultures of primary EGL cells similarly implanted were instead unipotent, giving rise exclusively to granule cells (67).

In spite of these limitations, the attempts to approach brain degenerative diseases through transplantation strategies are very promising, especially because of the fact that, as already discussed, the limitations of the other therapies are much more serious. Pharmacologic agents administered systematically, for example, not only may have erratic effects and transient efficacy, possibly due to restrictions imposed by the brain-blood barrier, but frequently produce undesirable side effects. A direct targeting of genetic material to the host neural tissue may be achieved, on the other hand, by gene therapy. However, the presently available vectors are difficult to be delivered specifically to the right districts and are often unable to enter the cells: retroviral vectors, for example, infect only cells in the S phase of their cell cycle, and most neurons in an adult nervous system are definitively postmitotic; moreover, the safety and efficacy of herpes and adenovirus vectors for adult nervous system is, at most, questionable (17). Therefore, the recent demonstration that transplanted immortalized neural progenitors could integrate into the CNS in a nontumorigenic, anatomically, and perhaps, functionally correct fashion, and that they stably express a retrovirally transduced gene makes this strategy an attractive alternative for gene therapy and repair of the CNS (68, 69).

So far, more than 100 PD patients have received human embryonic mesencephalic grafts in their caudate nucleus and/or putamen (5). The only partial functional recovery observed in most cases could result from an insufficient volume and density of reinnervation or, alternatively, a poor integration of the graft within the host neural circuitries. In the rat PD model, an extensive dopaminergic reinnervation of the striatum has been recently demonstrated by multiple grafting intervenctions (70): this has also led significant improvements of complex sensorimotor integration, such as the recovery of skilled forelimb use and disengage behaviour, that are not ameliorated by standard transplantation procedures. These findings suggest that optimal symptomatic relief in PD patients requires complete engraftment in the striatum. In the patients operated so far, the graft-derived reinnervation has probably reached only part of the caudate or putamen.

Concluding remarks

Over the past two decades, dramatic advances have been made in identifying the genetic and biochemical mechanisms that control neuronal plasticity. The impressive progresses made in the understanding of some of the clues to the normal developmental control devices, together with the identification of genetic mutations responsible for many neurodegenerative disorders, make us confident that neurobiology is no more in its infancy and that it will be able to face successfully the difficult issue of recovering a damaged nervous system in the very near future.

References

1. Cestelli A, Savettieri G, Salemi G, Di Liegro I (1992) Neuronal cell cultures: a tool for investigations in developmental neurobiology. Neurochem Res 17:1163-1180
2. Isackson PJ (1995) Trophic factor response to neuronal stimuli or injury. Curr Op Neurobiol 5:350-357
3. Lindsay RM (1995) Neuron saving schemes. Nature 373:289-290
4. Lindvall O, Kokaia Z, Bengzon J, Elmér E, Kokaia M (1994) Neurotrophins and brain insults. Trends Neurosci 17:490-496
5. Lindvall O, Odin P (1994) Clinical applications of cell transplantation and neurotrophic factors in CNS disorders. Curr Op Neurobiol 4:752-757
6. Gall CM, Isackson PJ (1989) Limbic seizures increase neuronal production of mRNA for nerve growth factor. Science 245:758-761

7. Jelsma TN, Aguayo AJ (1994) Trophic factors. Curr Op Neurobiol 4:717-725
8. Chiu AY, Chen EW, Loera S (1994) Distinct neurotrophic responses of axotomized motor neurons to BDNF and CTNF in adult rats. Neuroreports 5:693-696
9. Skaper SD, Negro A, Facci L, Dal Toso R (1993) Brain derived neurotrophic factor selectively rescues mesencephalic dopaminergic neurons from 2,4,5-Trihydroxyphenylalanine-induced injury. J Neurosci Res 34:478-487
10. Koliatsos VE, Clatterbuck RE, Winslow JW, Cayouette MH, Price DL (1993) Evidence that brain derived neurotrophic factor is a factor for motor neurons *in vivo*. Neuron 10:359-367
11. Mitsumoto H, Ikeda K, Klinkosz B, Cedarbaum JM, Wong V, Lindsay RM (1994) Arrest of motor neuron disease in wobler mice cotreated with CNTF and BDNF. Science 265: 1107-1110.
12. Morse JK, Wiegand SJ, Anderson K, You Y, Cai N, Carnahan J, Miller J, Di Stefano PS, Altar CA, Lindsay RM, Alderson RF (1993) Brain-derived neurotrophic factor (BDNF) prevents the degeneration of medial septal cholinergic neurons following fimbria transection. J Neurosci 13:4146-4156
13. Maysinger D, Jalssenjack I, Cuello AC (1992) Microencapsulated nerve growth factor: effects on the forebrain neurons following devascularizing cortical lesions. Neurosci Lett 140:71-74
14. Frim DM, Uhler TA, Galpern WA, Beal MF, Breakefield XO, Isackson O (1994) Implanted fibroblasts genetically engineered to produce brain-derived neurotrophic factor prevent 1-methyl-4-phenylpyridinium toxicity to dopaminergic neurons in the rat. Proc Natl Acad Sci USA 91: 5104-5108
15. Hoffman D, Breakefield XO, Short MP, Aebischer P (1993) Transplantation of polymer-encapsulated cell line genetically engineered to release NGF. Exp Neurol 122:100-106
16. Wolff JA (1993) Postnatal gene transfer into the central nervous system. Curr Op Neurobiol 3:743-748
17. Fisher LJ, Ray J (1994) *In vivo* and *ex vivo* gene transfer to the brain. Curr Op Neurobiol 4:735-741
18. Bunge RP (1993) Expanding role for the Schwann cell: ensheatment, myelination, trophism and regeneration. Curr Op Neurobiol 3:805-809
19. Buck CA (1992) Immunoglobulin superfamily: structure, function and relationship to other molecules. Seminars Cell Biol 3:79-188
20. Ranscht B (1994) Cadherins and catenins: interactions and functions in embryonic development. Curr Op Cell Biol 6:740-746
21. Haas TA, Plow EF (1994) Integrin-ligand interaction: a year in review. Curr Op Cell Biol 6:656-662
22. Feizi T (1993) Oligosaccharides that mediate mammalian cell-cell adhesion. Curr Op Struct Biol 3:701-710
23. Varki A (1993) Biological roles of oligosaccharides: all the theories are correct. Glycobiology 3:97-130
24. Schachner M (1994) Neural recognition molecules in disease and regeneration. Curr Op Cell Biol 4:726-734
25. Kulkens T, Bolhuis PA, Wolterman RA, Kemp S, Te Nijenhuis S, Valentjin LJ, Hensels GW, Jennekens FGI, De Visser M, Hoogendijk J, Baas F (1993) Deletion of the serine 34 codon from the major peripheral myelin protein P0 gene in Charcot-Marie-Tooth disease type 1B. Nature Genet 5:35-39
26. Su Y, Brooks DG, Li L, Lepercq J, Trofatter JA, Ravetch JV, Lebo RV (1993) Myelin protein zero gene mutated in Charcot-Marie-Tooth patients. Proc Natl Acad Sci USA 90:10856-10860
27. Hayasaka K, Himoro M, Sawaishi Y, Nanao K, Takahashi T, Takada G, Nicholson GA, Ouvrier RA, Tachi N (1993) De novo mutation of the myelin P0 gene in Déjérine-Sottas disease (hereditary motor and sensory neuropathy type III) Nature Genet 5:266-268
28. Snipes GJ, Suter U, Shooter EM (1993) The genetics of myelin. Curr Op Neurobiol 3:694-702
29. Jouet M, Rosenthal A, McFarlane J, Donnai D, Kenwrick SA (1993) Missense mutation confirms the L1 defect in X-linked hydrocephalus (HSAS). Nature Genet 4:331

30. Letourneau PC, Condic ML, Snow DM (1994) Interaction of developing neurons with the extracellular matrix. J Neurosci 14:915-928
31. Schachner M, Taylor J, Bartsch U, Pesheva P (1994) The perplexing multifunctionality of janusin, a tenascin-related molecule. Perspect Develop Neurobiol 2:33-41
32. Schwab ME, Kapfhammer JP, Bandtlow CE (1994) Inhibitors of neurite growth. Annu Rev Neurosci 16:565-595
33. Keynes RJ, Cook GMW (1995) Repulsive and inhibitory signals.Curr Op Neurobiol 5:75-82
34. Hopkins SJ, Rothwell NJ (1995) Cytokines and the nervous system II: actions and mechanisms of action. Trends Neurosci 18:130-136
35. Rothwell NJ, Hopkins SJ (1995) Cytokines and the nervous system I: expression and recognition. Trends Neurosci 18:83-88
36. Wallace DC (1992) Diseases of the mitochondrial DNA. Ann Rev Biochem 61:1175-1212.
37. Holt IJ, Jacobs HT (1994) The structure and expression of normal and mutant mitochondrial genomes. In: Darley-Usmar V, Schapira AHV (eds). Mitochondria: DNA, proteins and disease. Portland Press Res Monograph, London and Chapel Hill, pp 27-54
38. Schapira AHV (1993) Mitochondrial cytopathies. Curr Op Neurobiol 3:760-767
39. Ciofaloni E, Ricci E, Shanske S, Moraes CT, Silvestri G, Hirano M, Simonetti S, Angelini C, Donati MA, Garcia C et al (1992) MELAS clinical features, biochemistry and molecular genetics. Ann Neurol 31:391-398
40. Hammans SR, Sweeney MG, Brockington M, Lennox GG, Lawton MF, Kennedy CR, Morgan-Hughes JA, Harding AE (1993) The mitochondrial DNA transfer RNA^{Lys} A → G (8344) mutation and the syndrome of myoclonic epilepsy with ragged red fibers (MERRF). Brain 116:617-632
41. Prezant TR, Agapian JV, Bohlman MC, Bu X, Otzas S, Qiu W-Q, Arnos KS, Cortopassi GA, Jaber I, Rotter JI et al (1993) Mitochondrial ribosomal RNA mutation associated with both antibiotic-induced and non-syndromic deafness. Nature Genet 4:289-294
42. Schapira AHV (1994) Evidence for mitochondrial dysfunction in Parkinson's disease - a critical appraisal. Mov Disrd 9:125-138
43. Selkoe DJ (1994) Cell biology of the amyloid ß-protein precursor and the mechanism of Alzheimer's disease. Annu Rev Cell Biol 10:373-403
44. Strittmater WJ, Saunders AM, Schmechel D, Perciak-Vance M, Enghild J, Salvesen GS, Roses AD (1993) Apolipoprotein E: high avidity binding to ß-amyloid and increased frequency of type 4 allele and the risk of Alzheimer's disease in late onset families. Proc Natl Acad Sci USA 90:1977-1981
45. Goate A, Chartier-Harlin MC, Mullan M, Brown J, Crawford F, Fidani L, Giuffra L et al (1991) Segregation of a missense mutation in the amyloid precursor protein gene with familial Alzheimer's disease. Nature 349:704-706
46. Sherrington R, Rogaev EI, Liang Y, Rogaeva EA, Levesque G, Ikeda M, Chi H, Lin C, Holman K et al (1995) Cloning of a gene bearing missense mutations in early-onset familial Alzheimer's disease. Nature 375:754-760
47. L'Hernault SW, Arduengo PM (1992) Mutation of a putative sperm membrane protein in Caenorabditis elegans prevents sperm differentiation but not its associated meiotic divisions. J Cell Biol 119:55-68
48. Caskey CT, Pizzuti A, Fu YH, Fenwick RG, Nelson DL (1992) Triplet repeat mutations in human disease. Science 256:784-789
49. Bell MV, Hirst MC, Nakahori Y, McKinnon MR, Roche A, Flint TJ, Jacobs PA, Tommerup N et al (1991) Physical mapping accross the fragile X hypermethylation and clinical expression of fragile X syndrome. Cell 64:861-866
50. Vincent A, Hezitz D, Petit C, Kretz C, Oberlè I, Mandel JL (1991) Abnormal pattern detected in Fragile X patients by pulsed-field gel electrophoresis. Nature 349:624-626
51. Warren ST, Nelson DL (1993) Trinucleotide repeat expansion in neurological disease. Curr Op Neurobiol 3:752-759
52. Dunnett SB, Svendsen CN (1993) Huntington's disease: animal models and transplantation repair. Curr Op Neurobiol 3:790-796

53. Huntington Disease Collaborative Research Group (1993) A novel gene containing a trinucleotide repeat that is expanded and unstable on Huntington disease chromosomes. Cell 72:971-983
54. Johnson RT (1992) Retroviruses and nervous system disease. Curr Op Neurobiol 2:663-670
55. Cohen FE, Pan KM, Huang Z, Baldwin M, Fletterick RJ, Prusiner SB (1994) Structural clues to prion replication. Science 264:530-531
56. Prusiner SM, De Armond SJ (1994) Prion disease and neurodegeneration. Annu Rev Neurosci 17:311-339
57. Prusiner SM (1991) Molecular biology of prion diseases. Science 252:1515-1522
58. Prusiner SM, Scott M, Foster D, Pan K-M, Groth D, Mirenda C, Torchia M, Yang S-H, Serban D, Carlson GA, Hoppe PC, Westaway D, DeArmond SJ (1990) Transgenic studies implicate interactions between homologous PrP isoforms in Scrapie prion duplication. Cell 63:673-686
59. Sailer A, Bueler H, Fischer M, Aguzzi A, Weissmann C (1994) No propagation of prions in mice devoid of PrP. Cell 77:967-968
60. Collinge J, Whittington MA, Sidle KCL, Smith CJ, Palmer MS, Clarke AR, Jefferys GR (1994) Prion protein is necessary for normal synaptic function. Nature 370:295-297
61. Bessen RA, Kocisko DA, Raymond GJ, Nandan S, Lansbury PT, Caughey B (1995) Non-genetic propagation of strain-specific properties of scrapie prion protein. Nature 375:698-700
62. Cox B (1994) Prion-like factors in yeast. Curr Biol 4:744-748
63. Hoffer BJ, Olson L (1991) Ethical issues in brain-cell transplantation. Trends Neurosci 14:384-388
64. Bjorkglund A (1991) Neural transplantation - an experimental tool with clinical possibilities. Trends Neurosci 14:319-322
65. Fisher LJ, Gage FH (1993) Grafting in the mammalian central nervous system. Physiol Rev 73:583-616
66. Snyder EY (1994) Grafting immortalized neurons to the CNS. Curr Op Neurobiol 4:742-751
67. Gao WQ, Hatten ME (1994) Immortalizing oncogenes subvert the establishment of granule cell identity in developing cerebellum. Development 120:1059-1070
68. Renfranz PJ, Cunnigham MG, McKay RDG (1991) Region-specific differentiation of the hippocampal stem cell line HiB5 upon implantation into the developing mammalian brain. Cell 66:713-719
69. Snyder EY, Deitcherb DL, Walsh C, Arnold-Aldea S, Hartwieg EA, Cepko CL (1992) Multipotent neural cell lines can engraft and participate in development of mouse cerebellum. Cell 68:33-51
70. Nikkhah G, Duan W-M, Knappe U, Jodicke A, Bjorklund A (1993) Restoration of complex sensorimotor behavior and skilled forelimb use by a modified nigral cell suspension transplantation approach in the rat Parkinson model. Neuroscience 56:33-43

Oxidative Stress in the Early Phase of Traumatic Central Nervous System Injury: Clinical Data

A. Paolin, E. Bosco, B. Bonivento, L. Nardin, L. Rehak, C. Torri, F. Marzatico

Introduction

Cerebrovascular and metabolic changes associated with traumatic injury to the CNS may be related, in part, with pathological alterations in the intracellular neurochemical system. These events may include alterations in neurotransmitter synthesis and release or changes in pre/or postsynaptic receptor activity. Other changes may include alterations in the synthesis and activity of endogenous neuroprotective compounds (e.g. enzymatic and non-enzymatic antioxidant) or pathological expression and release of endogenous "autodestructive" compounds associated with inflammation and/or with altered oxidative metabolism (e.g. free radicals). Although the timing of the precise cascade of neurochemical events following traumatic brain injury is poorly understood, there is now extensive experimental support for early occurrence and pathological importance of oxygen radical species (ROS) formation and cell membrane lipid peroxidation (LP) (1-4). The potential sources of oxygen radicals within the brain after trauma insult include the arachidonic acid cascade, catecholamine oxidation, electron "leakage" from the mitochondrial electron transfer chain, oxidation of extravasated hemoglobin and later infiltrating neutrophils (Figs. 1, 2). The radical dependent lipid peroxidation of nervous and vascular cell membranes and myelin is catalyzed by free iron released from hemoglobin, transferrin and ferritin by either lowered tissue pH or oxygen radicals. The LP is a geometrically progressing process that spreads over the surface of the cell membrane causing impairment to phospholipid-dependent enzymes, disruption of ionic gradients, membrane lysis and cell death. Criteria for the establishment of the pathophysiological significance of oxygen radical reactions include: a) the demonstration of increased post-traumatic levels of oxygen radicals and lipid peroxides after CNS trauma; b) the spatial and temporal correlation between oxygen radical formation and physiological and pathological alterations (e.g. decrease of oxygen consumption, energy failure, loss of microvasculature regulation, edema and progressive post-traumatic ischemia development); and c) a striking similarity between post-traumatic CNS pathology and experimental chemical peroxidative insult (e.g. ironmicroinjection).

A. Paolin, E. Bosco, B. Bonivento et al.

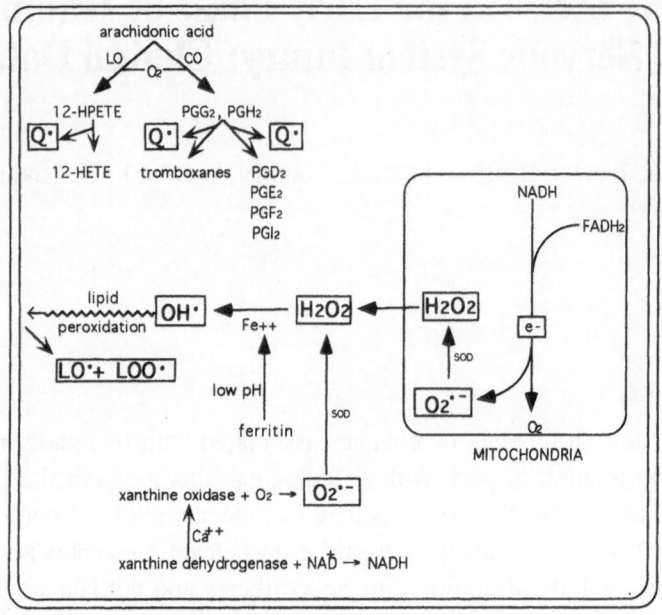

Fig. 1. Possible mechanisms of free radical production. *LO*, lipoxygenase; *CO*, ciclooxygenase; *12-HPETE*, 12-hydroperoxy-eicosatetraenoic acid; *12-HETE*, 12-hydroxyeicosatetraenoic acid; *PGG₂*, *PGH₂*, prostaglandins endoperoxides; *Q*, free radicals; *SOD*, superoxide dismutase; *LO*, *LOO*, lipid radicals

Role of lipid peroxidation in secondary injury processes after a traumatic event

LP is the free radical-mediated cell and tissue injury that forms lipid peroxides within cell membranes and organelles. LP is proportional to the polyunsaturated fatty acid content and inversely proportional to the chain breaking antioxidants. The initiation and propagation phases of the LP chain reaction are depicted in Fig. 3. The chain reaction, affecting the side chains of polyunsaturated fatty acids, begins with the abstraction of an atom of hydrogen by initiating radicals (Fig. 3). Reduction of oxygen to water is a normal process that proceeds through superoxide anion to hydrogen peroxide and finally to water (Fig. 4). During the periods of post-traumatic metabolism, superoxide anion is produced by mitochondrial dysfunction, as a by-product of various enzyme substrate reactions (xanthine/xanthine oxidase, prostaglandin synthase, 5-lipoxygenase) (Fig. 1). Electron transfer chains in the mitochondria and endoplasmic reticulum are major sources of superoxides. When mitochondrial function is altered, some of the electrons which leak from the electron transfer chain react with oxygen, forming superoxide anions. Superoxide anion is not itself particularly reactive and it does not cross the cell membrane very well. However, it can become more dangerous by either accepting a proton or by dismutating to hydrogen peroxide.

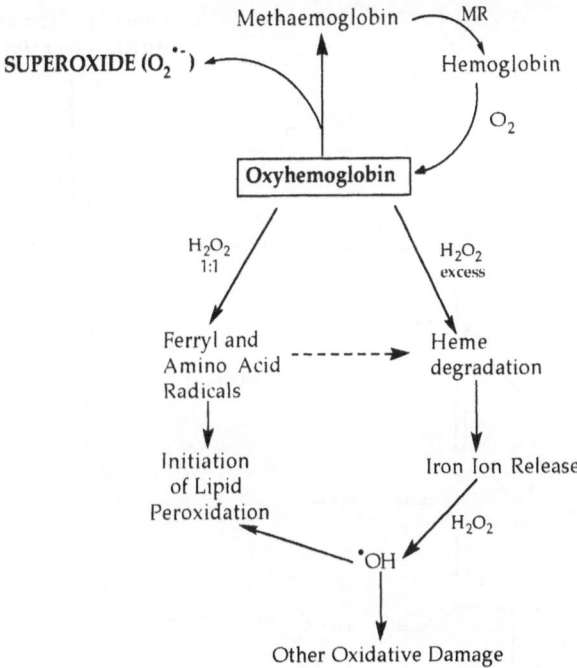

Fig. 2. Free radical production mechanisms associated with extravasated hemoglobin. After the breakdown of the cells, hemoglobin outside of the erythrocyte potentially is highly dangerous because it can be degraded and liberate iron. *MR*, Methaemoglobin reductase

Protonated superoxide anion can better penetrate the membrane where it can initiate LP. Hydrogen peroxide can be produced directly by inflammatory cells, by monoamino oxidase, or by chemical or enzymatic (superoxide dismutase, SOD) conversion of superoxide anion. Mitochondria are rich in SOD: so the superoxides that they produce become hydrogen peroxide. Hydrogen peroxide reactivity is low, but it crosses cell membranes easily, thereby making itself available for radical reaction in the presence of transition metals at sites distant from where it was formed, causing significant injury to the lipid bilayer. It does this by reacting with Fe^{2+} to yield the highly reactive hydroxyl radical. Hydrogen peroxide can be detoxified by two enzymes: glutathione peroxidase (GSH Px), which utilized the reduced glutathione as reducer and catalase (CAT). In normal conditions the reaction from oxygen to water is well controlled by SOD, GSH Px, CAT and endogenous antioxidants. Vitamin E is the most important membrane-bound antioxidant. However, following traumatic insult, the cellular antioxidant control could be overwhelming and reactive free radicals invade the membranes and LP begins. Nitric oxide (NO) is an important molecule that regulates several functions such as the immune system and relaxation of blood vessels; moreover it plays a neurotransmitter role. However, NO could be potentially pathologic; the NO-synthase is easily activated and widespread in

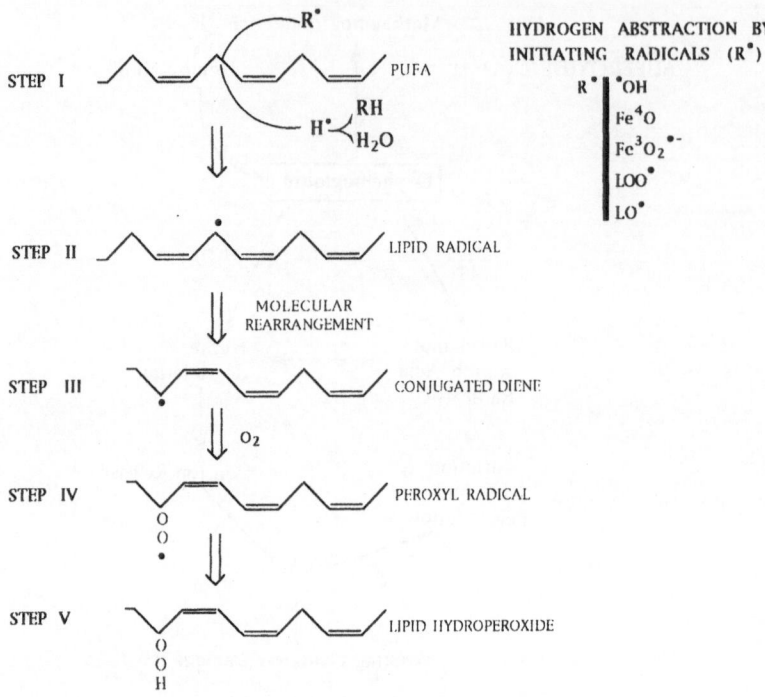

Fig. 3. Lipid (PUFA, polyunsatured fatty acid) peroxidation can be extensive after a single initiating event because resultant radicals, via the chain reaction described, can reinitiate lipid peroxidation, so the process is self-propagating

brain (5). NO is itself a reactive radical and can react with superoxide anion to form peroxynitrite anion ($ONOO^-$) that is readily protonated to form HOONO, particularly if the pH is low. The HOONO is dangerous; it can move across membranes and later decompose to form hydroxyl radical and nitrogen dioxide. Thus, peroxynitrite may deliver hydroxyl radicals (6) and have a vasoconstrictor effect, too (7). As illustrated in Fig. 3, iron plays a crucial role in the LP cascade. The iron is included by the cells in iron-containing proteins or stored in the ferritin. Superoxide anion or lipid hydroperoxides react with ferritin and release the reactive Fe^{2+} (8). Free iron is also released by hydrogen peroxide degradation of hemoglobin (Fig. 2) (9). Fe^{2+} can convert hydrogen peroxide to hydroxyl radical and it is oxidized to Fe^{3+} (Fenton reaction) (10); Fe^{3+} can be reduced to Fe^{2+} by superoxide anion. Lipid hydroperoxides (LOOH) can react with Fe^{2+} to form lipid alkoxides (LO$^\bullet$). Iron/oxygen complexes are probably the most important initiators of LP. The damage during ischemic injury from excess hydrogen peroxide and superoxide anions will be affected by the location and amount of iron and other catalyst ions (e.g. copper). Damage will be limited if metal ions are not available (11). Unfortunately, during CNS traumatic injury, transition metals become available because reactive oxygen frees iron from

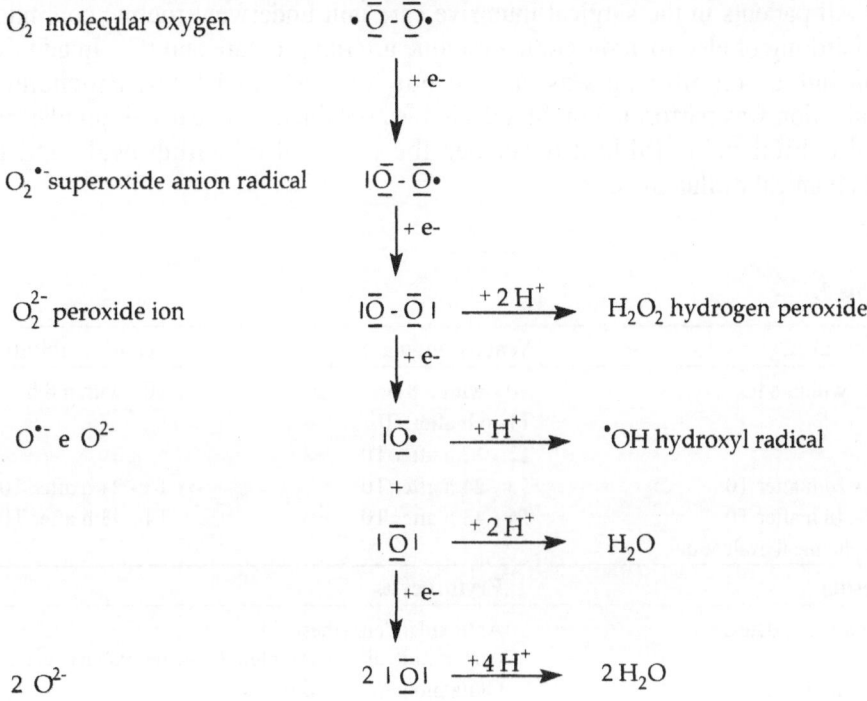

O$_2$ molecular oxygen

O$_2$$^{\bullet-}$ superoxide anion radical

O$_2^{2-}$ peroxide ion $\xrightarrow{+2H^+}$ H$_2$O$_2$ hydrogen peroxide

O$^{\bullet-}$ e O^{2-} $\xrightarrow{+H^+}$ $^{\bullet}$OH hydroxyl radical

                                                             $\xrightarrow{+2H^+}$ H$_2$O

2 O^{2-} $\xrightarrow{+4H^+}$ 2 H$_2$O

Fig. 4. Univalent reduction of molecular oxygen to water

transport and storage proteins, and because the extravasated erythrocytes release hemoglobin at the damage site.

Materials and methods

Twenty-five patients with acute brain traumatic injury were selected for the study. The clinical protocol with inclusion and exclusion criteria is shown in Table 1.

Table 1.

Inclusion criteria	Exclusion criteria
Closed brain injury	Areflexic coma
Admission within 8 h	Diffuse and severe trauma
Age (15-65 years)	Post-traumatic severe hypotension (systolic pressure < 90 mmHg) and/or hypoxic condition (PaO$_2$ < 70 mmHg)
Glasgow Coma Scale (4-8)	

All patients in the surgical intensive care unit underwent routine continuous monitoring of electrocardiogram, systemic arterial pressure and ICP. In addition, continuous monitoring was carried out for SaO_2 and SjO_2. Biochemical evaluation was performed on blood samples obtained from carotid, jugular bulb and cubital vein. Table 2 describes the protocol of withdrawals and the biochemical evaluations.

Table 2.

Arterial	Venous (jugular)	Venous (cubital)
T0 - within 8 h	T0 - within 8 h	T0 - within 8 h
	T1- 6 h after T0	
	T2 - 12 h after T0	
T3 - 24 h after T0	T3 - 24 h after T0	T3 - 24 h after T0
T4 - 48 h after T0	T4 - 48 h after T0	T4 - 48 h after T0
Biochemical evaluations		

Plasma	Erythrocytes
Lipid peroxidates	Antioxidant enzymes
	(superoxide dismutase, glutathione peroxidase, catalase)
Vitamin E	Glutathione (reduced form)

At the set times the blood samples were immediately centrifuged; plasma and erythrocytes were refrigerated at $-70°$ C until analysis. The lipid peroxides such as malonyldialdehyde (MDA) were evaluated using the LPO-586 Bioxytech kit. Vitamin E was determined with HPLC according to Bieri et al. (12). The SOD, GSHPx and CAT activities were performed by spectrophotometric assays (13-15) on lysed erythrocytes. Reduced glutathione (GSH) was determined using the GSH-400 Bioxytech kit. One-way analysis of variance (ANOVA) followed by Fisher's test for multiple comparisons was used and the significance was accepted for $p < 0.05$.

Results

The mean age of the patients was 44 years (15-65 years), the mean admission GCS value was 5, and the mean SjO_2 value was 61.85 mmHg and increased significantly at T2, T3 and T4 as shown in Fig. 5. At T0 all biochemical parameters evaluated in jugular blood (central samples) showed different levels with respect to normal plasmatic and erythrocytic patterns (data not shown). The traumatic events cause biochemical changes that are linked with cerebral oxidative stress and a lipoperoxidative insult as shown in Table 3. The same parameters evaluated in the peripheral blood (cubital vein) showed different patterns without significant differences during the time of the study (data not shown).

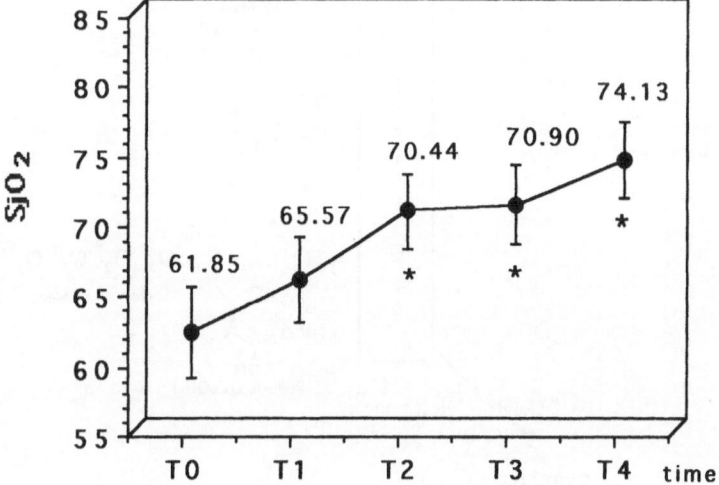

Fig. 5. Oxyhemoglobin saturation of the jugular bulb blood at admission (T0), 6 (T1), 12 (T2), 24 (T3) and 48 (T4) h in patients after CNS traumatic injury. Statistical analysis, see Table 3

Table 3.

	SjO_2	SOD	Vitamin E	MDA
T0	61.85	0.90	9.24	5.99
	+ 3.19	± 0.12v	± 1.02	± 0.90
T1	65.67	0.89	5.21 •	12.59 •
	± 3.11	± 0.12	± 0.96	± 1.72
T2	70.44 •	1.59 •	6.08 •	13.60 •
	± 2.66	± 0.15	± 0.88	± 1.12
T3	70.90 •	1.21	7.43	8,63 •
	± 2.83	± 0.18	± 0.99	± 0.94
T4	74.13 •	1.15	7.69	10.04 •
	± 2.72	± 0.18	± 1.01	± 0.65

The SjO_2 are expressed as mmHg, SOD activity as µg/mgHb, vitamin E as µg/mL and MDA as µmol/L of plasma. The results are expressed as means ± standard error. Statistical significance: T0 vs. T1, T2, T3, T4 • $p < 0.05$.

The SjO_2 increase suggested a progressive reduction of the cerebral oxidative capacity. After 12 h, the SOD activity showed a significant increase, probably

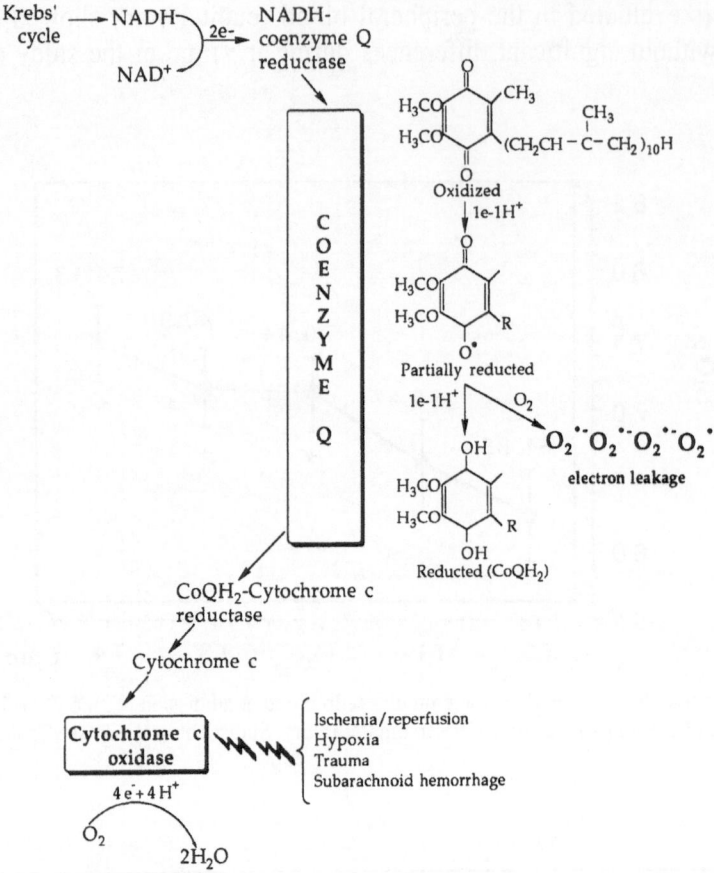

Fig. 6. Mitochondria electron leakage. Fully active cytochrome oxidase keeps all the partial reduced O_2 intermediates tightly bound to its specific sites, preventing other components from leaking electrons directly onto O_2 (coenzyme Q). Partially active cytochrome oxidase keeps only few partial reduced O_2 intermediates tightly bound to its specific sites, permitting other components to leak electrons directly onto O_2 (coenzyme Q)

due to an enhanced superoxide production. The vitamin E decreased significantly after 6 and 12 h, probably due to its enhanced consumption as a lipoperoxidative chain-breaking antioxidant. The increased free radical reactions after brain injury provoke marked increment of lipid peroxides (MDA) at T1, T2, T3 and T4. Furthermore, the MDA level at T0 was three times the normal plasma value.

Discussion

Head injury is one of the most serious problems facing medicine today. Trauma is the most common cause of mortality in people younger than 45 years of age and head injury is most highly associated with mortality in the trauma population (16, 17). Despite continuous advances in our understanding of head injury, its treatment remains somewhat nebulous. Over the past decade, an impressive number of studies have suggested the importance of oxygen radical formation and cell LP in the sequela of neurochemical events that induced the secondary damage in CNS injury. The formation of destructive oxygen free radicals has been associated with a wide variety of CNS damage, including brain edema (18, 19), cerebral ischemia (20-23), spinal cord trauma (24-27) and brain trauma (1, 28, 29). Recently endogenous antioxidants such as vitamin E, vitamin A, vitamin C and coenzyme Q have been shown to be markedly depleted following experimental spinal cord trauma (30), suggesting that a loss of this type of endogenous protective mechanism following traumatic CNS injury may allow the uncontrolled progression of peroxidative damage to cell membranes. Despite several experimental studies that support the central role of free radical reactions in brain post-traumatic events, very few clinical data are available to describe the correlation between post-traumatic physiological parameters and biochemical evaluations that make clear the time course and the intensity of the brain lipoperoxidative events. The purpose of this work was to tentatively establish: a) the role of free radicals and lipoperoxidative events in clinical situations; b) if the blood samples obtained from jugular bulb could represent a tool to study the district (cerebral) post-traumatic phenomena; c) if biochemical changes evaluated in jugular blood samples could be a mirror of the free radical reactions of the microvascular system in post-traumatic patients; d) the time course of cerebral changes of the antioxidant defenses and lipid peroxidative events; and e) if physiological and biochemical parameters could support the hypothesis of the role of free radicals in secondary damage in CNS injury.

The significant increase of SjO_2 suggests an impairment of the cerebral oxidative machinery due to molecular changes in the mitochondrial respiratory chain which then influence oxygen reduction. For example, any alteration in the functionality of cytochrome oxidase can lead to the release of the partially reduced oxygen intermediates (superoxide and hydroxyl radicals), since only cytochrome oxidase is able to retain all the partially reduced oxygen intermediates in the active sites before their complete reduction to water. If, instead, cytochrome oxidase is damaged by the hypoxic or ischemic process, it cannot "drain off" the partially reduced form of oxygen (Fig. 6). Since oxygen accepts one electron at a time, other elements in the respiratory chain give rise to these partially reduced forms, without, however, being able to retain them until they have been completely reduced to water (31, 32). In our patients the amount of oxygen available was much higher than the amount really utilized by the CNS injured. This oxygen could be partially reduced to superoxide, inducing an "oxidative stress". In fact at T2 when the SjO_2 begins to increase significantly the SOD reaches a significant peak (Table 3). There is still insufficient knowledge about both the kinetics and molecular regulation of the antioxidant enzymes (e.g. SOD) in mammalian tissues. Activation by either allosteric or covalent modification of the enzyme molecules is possible by partial occupancy of the enzyme molecules by their substrates and is known to increase their catalytic activity (33). Furthermore, there was a marked correlation between consumption of plasma vitamin E and increase in lipid peroxide production (MDA) in the early phase (8-20 h) of CNS injury (Fig. 7). Our clinical data support the role of free

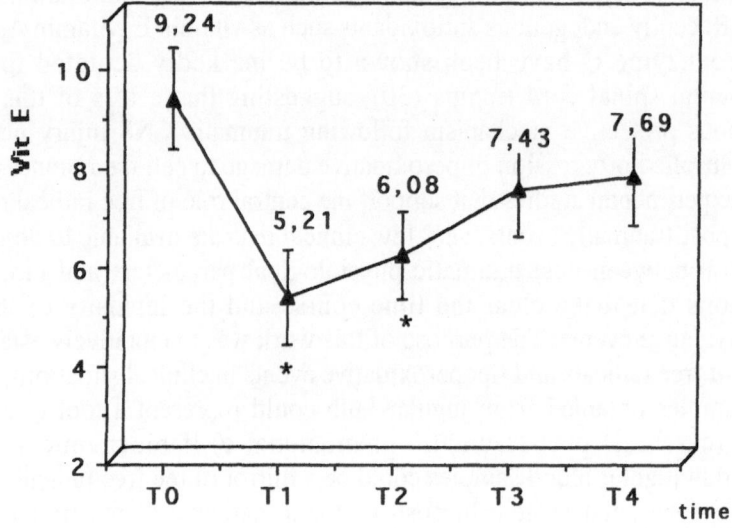

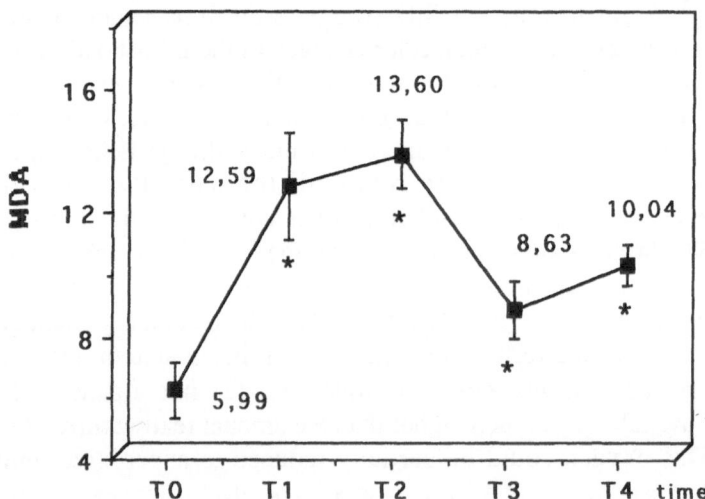

Fig. 7. Vitamin E and malonyldialdehyde (MDA) in blood samples obtained from jugular bulb at admission (T0), 6 (T1), 12 (T2), 24 (T3) and 48 (T4) h in patients after traumatic CNS injury. Statistical analysis, see Table 3

radicals and lipoperoxidative events after CNS trauma injury and suggest the potential beneficial effects of post-traumatic administration of free radical scavengers and antioxidants.

References

1. Kontos HA, Povlishock JT (1986) Oxygen radicals in brain injury. CNS Trauma 3:257-263
2. Braughler JM, Hall ED (1989) Central nervous system trauma and stroke. I. Biochemical consideration for oxygen radicals formation and lipid peroxidation. Free Radic Biol Med 6: 289-301
3. Hall ED, Braughler JM (1989) Central nervous system trauma and stroke. II. Physiological and pharmacological evidence for the involvement of oxygen radicals and lipid peroxidation. Free Radic Biol Med 6:303-313
4. Hall ED, Braughler JM (1993) Free radicals in CNS injury. In: Waxman SG (ed) Molecular and cellular approaches of the treatment of neurological disease. Raven, New York, pp 81-105
5. Hope BT, Michael GJ, Knigge KM, Vincent SR (1991) Neuronal NADPH diaphorase is a nitric oxide synthetase. Proc Natl Acad Sci USA 88:2811-2814
6. Beckman JS, Beckman TW, Chen J, Marshall PA, Freeman BA (1990) Apparent hydroxyl radical production by peroxynitrite: implication for endothelial injury from nitric oxide and superoxide. Proc Natl Acad Sci USA 87:1620-1624
7. Laurindo FRM, da Luz PL, Uint L, Rocha TF, Jaeger RG, Lopes EA (1991) Evidence for superoxide radical dependent coronary vasospasm after angioplasty in intact dogs. Circulation 83:1705-1715
8. Bolan BJ, Ulvik RJ (1990) On the limited ability of superoxide to release iron from ferritin. Eur J Biochem 193:899-904
9. Puppo A, Hallywell B (1988) Formation of hydroxyl radicals from hydrogen peroxide in the presence of iron: is haemoglobin a biological Fenton catalyst? Biochem J 249:185-190
10. Hallywell B, Gutteridge JMC (1990) Role of free radicals and catalytic metal ions in human disease: an overview. In: Packer L, Glazer AN (eds) Methods in enzymology. Academic, San Diego, vol 186, pp 1-85
11. Hallywell B (1992) Reactive oxygen species in the central nervous system. J Neurochem 59: 1609-1623
12. Bieri JG, Tolliver TJ, Catignani JL (1979) Simultaneous determination of alpha-tocopherol and retinol in plasma or red cells by HPLC. Am J Clin Nutr 32:2143-2149
13. Flohè L, Otting F (1984) Superoxide dismutase assay. Methods Enzymol 105:93-104
14. Flohè L, Gunzler WA (1984) Assay glutathione peroxidase. Methods Enzymol 105:114-121
15. Aebi H (1984) Catalase in vitro. Methods Enzymol 105:121-126
16. Backer CC, Hoppenheimer L, Stephens B, Lewis FR, Trunkey DD (1980) Epidemiology of trauma deaths. Am J Surg 140:144-150
17. Trunkey DD, Lim RC (1974) Analysis of 425 consecutive trauma fatalities: an autopsy study. JACEP 3:368-381
18. Chan P, Fishman R (1980) Transient formation of superoxide radicals in polyunsaturated fatty acid induced brain swelling. J Neurochem 35:1004-1007
19. Chan P, Fishman R (1985) Oxygen free radicals: potential edema mediators in brain injury. Springer, Berlin Heidelberg New York
20. Demopoulos HB, Flamm ES, Seligman ML, Pietronigro DD (1982) Oxygen free radicals in central nervous system ischemia and trauma. In: Arfors KE (ed) Pathobiology of CNS injury. Academic, London, pp 127-155
21. Gingsberg M, Watson BD, Busto R (1988) Peroxidative damage to cell membranes following cerebral ischemia. A cause of ischemic brain injury? Neurochem Pathol 9:171-193

22. Lundgren J, Zhang H, Agardh CD, Smith ML, Ivans PJ, Hallywell B, Siesjo BK (1991) Acidosis-induced ischemic brain damage: are free radicals involved? J Cereb Blood Flow Metab 11:587-596
23. Traystman RJ, Kirsch JR, Koehler RC (1991) Oxygen radicals mechanism of brain injury following ischemia and riperfusion. J Appl Physiol 71:1175-1195
24. Anderson DK, Saunders R, Demediuk P, Means E (1992) Lipid hydrolysis and peroxidation in injured spinal cord: partial protection with vitamin E or selenium. J Neurotrauma 2:257-268
25. Hsu C, Halushka P, Hogan E, Banik N, Lee W, Perot P (1985) Alteration of thromboxane and prostacycline levels in experimental spinal cord injury. Neurology 35:1003-1009
26. Pietronigro DD, Hovsepian M, Demopoulos HB, Flamm E (1983) Loss of ascorbic acid from injured feline spinal cord. J Neurochem 41:1072-1076
27. Xu J, Beckman JS, Hogan EL, Hsu CY (1991) Xantine oxidase in experimental spinal cord injury. J Neurotrauma 8:11-19
28. Kontos HA (1989) Oxygen radicals in central nervous system damage. Chem Biol Interact 72:229-255
29. Siesjo BK, Wielock T (1985) Brain injury: neurochemical aspects. In: Becker DP, Povlishock J (eds) Central nervous system trauma status reports. National Institutes of Health, Bethesda, pp 513-532
30. Lemke M, Frei B, Ames BN, Faden AI (1990) Decrease in tissue levels of ubiquino-9 and -10, ascorbate and alpha-tocopherol following spinal cord impact trauma in rats. Neurosci Lett 108:201-206
31. Benzi G, Pastoris O, Marzatico F, Villa RF, Dagani F, Curti D (1992) The mitochondrial electron transfer alteration as a factor involved in the brain aging. Neurobiol Aging 13: 361-368
32. Rehncrona S, Westenberg E, Akesson B, Siesjo BK (1982) Brain cortical fatty acids and phospholipids during and following complete and severe incomplete ischemia. J Neurochem 38:84-93
33. Chance B, Sies H, Boveris A (1979) Hydroperoxide metabolism in mammalian organs. Physiol Rev 59:527-605

Monitoring and Management of Patients with Cerebral and Spinal Dysfunction in Postintensive Care

L. Saltuari, M. Marosi, K. Berek, P. Bramanti

Brain trauma is the most disabling disease of young adults in the twentieth century. About 10% of global mortality is due to trauma, and 68% of these deaths are related to brain trauma (USA) (1, 2). Similar figures were recorded in1991 in the countries of the European Union, with more than 600 000 craniocervical injuries (3). Head injury is a major cause of death and disability, especially in young adults, and peaks between the ages of 15 and 24 years. Over 50% of head injuries are caused by traffic accidents and about 25% by accidents at work.

The increasing severity of a trauma heightens the probability of concomitant brain injury, which in more than 50% of cases will become the main injury.

After drug overdose and severe trauma, cardiac arrest is the third most common cause of coma and/or death. Advances in resuscitation, life support and intensive care medicine have improved the survival and neurologic outcome of patients suffering severe brain damage due to various causes (4-6). About 80% of successfully resuscitated patients remain in coma for variable lengths of time (4, 5).

The annual incidence of spinal cord injury is estimated at 30 to 40/1 000 000 cases per year, with 65% of these patients aged below 35 years (7).

Neurorehabilitation comprises the activation of partially damaged brain areas or parts of the spinal cord, reducing the initial diaschisis and leading to a functional induction of new pathways by bypassing irreversible lesions. The basis for a successful neurorehabilitation is an exact evaluation of the acute condition of a patient and a global summary of the actual functional state.

The therapeutic community is a team of physicians, nurses, physiotherapists, ergotherapists and close relatives, who will care for the specific defects of the patient. Close relatives are important partners of rehabilitation during the subacute phase and take on the most importance for the patient in the reintegration phase, when the patient is trained by the therapeutic community to become independent from the support. Step by step, the patient is reintegrated in his family and the daily life of his community.

Prognosis

The necessity of securing vital functions such as respiration and circulation as well as prophylaxis and treatment of cerebral edema mostly call for rapid intubation, sedation, relaxation and artificial respiration. During this acute phase the patient's clinical neurological evaluation is hampered by these interventions, restricting diagnosis to neuroimaging and electrophysiological methods.

Uncertainty in assessing the outcome of comatose patients combined with the possibility of prolonging a patient's suffering or leaving him with an unacceptable quality of life poses humanitarian and ethical problems for the attending physician. Therefore, early prognosis is considered a major factor in the physician's decision on therapy management.

In clinical research various attempts have been made at early prediction of outcome of the critically ill. Various systems as well as laboratory findings have been used to predict brain injury severity and/or probability of death.

All scientific studies on this topic aim to define a reliable parameter of prognosis within the first 3-7 days after brain damage. According to the current state of the art, it is not possible to predict the outcome of a comatose, brain damaged patient with absolute certainty by using coma scales, electrophysiological techniques, neuroimaging methods, biochemical parameters or combinations of these (8-15).

After severe damage of the brain and/or the spinal cord secondary to traumatic injury, ischemia or anoxia, the first medical activities focus on management of vital functions. Prognostic evaluation is restricted to technical methods.

In the subacute phase clinical neurological evaluation dramatically enlarges the prognostic possibilities. It is of utmost importance to gain information about the patient's remaining neurological capabilities in order to predict his probable outcome and plan the rehabilitation program.

An exact neurological examination reveals the deficiencies of each patient and enables a specific rehabilitation program to be developed for each individual. Several factors require a scientifically accurate prognosis to be established during the subacute phase:

- Clinical decision-making concerning the energy and resources put into the treatment
- Evaluation of the treatment program
- Setting a rehabilitation goal
- Necessary information for close relatives

Clinical evaluation

Increasing intracranial pressure due to edema or acute intracerebral masses caused by traumatic (epidural, subdural, intraparenchymal hemorrhage), ischemic, hypoxic, infectious or neoplastic lesions may result in a downward displacement of the brainstem structures (uncal or central transtentorial herniation), presenting the different stages of midbrain syndrome (16).

With increasing intracranial pressure a progressive deterioration of brainstem functions in the sense of a rostrocaudal descending functional disintegration occurs, manifesting itself in various spontaneously occurring or provokable motor signs, which can be assessed by clinical neurological investigation.

These clinical signs can be arranged in a systematic order by using the classification of midbrain syndrome stages.

Midbrain syndrome stage I: somnolent patient, spontaneous body and limb movements, finalized motor responses to avoid nociceptive stimuli.

Midbrain syndrome stage II: sopor (with reduced spontaneous motor responses) or coma, nonfinalized movements to painful stimuli, divergent bulbus position, slightly increased muscle tone.

Midbrain syndrome stage III: typical decortication pattern with flexed upper and extended lower limbs provoked by external stimuli or spontaneously, the latter indicating a progression, increasing muscle tone, hyperreflexia and pyramidal signs, machine-like breathing.

Midbrain syndrome stage IV: typical decerebration pattern with increased extensor muscle tone of upper and lower limbs occurring spontaneously or by external stimuli, spontaneous pyramidal signs may occur.

Ongoing deterioration leads to bulbar brain syndromes I and II with reduced muscle tone, areflexia and slow deterioration toward brain death.

Patients with the clinical signs and symptoms of midbrain syndromes 1 and 2 mostly recover directly or via a prolonged midbrain syndrome in a relatively short time. All other patients, namely, those with a midbrain syndrome 3 or 4, develop a prolonged midbrain syndrome or an apallic syndrome (AS). About 30% of trauma-induced (17) and nearly 40% of hypoxia-induced severe brain injuries (5) result in AS, more or less a synonym for persistent vegetative state. The development toward AS is characterized by systematic progress (18), and independent of its etiology AS is remarkably uniform, representing a restriction of brain functions at the mesodiencephalic level (19).

Clinically, AS is characterized by the reappearance of day- and night-independent sleep/wake rhythm, blank staring eyes, missing blink reflex, mastication patterns, reflectory primitive motoricity and a vegetative dysfunction in the sense of an enhanced sympathicotonia. This vegetative dysfunction is still present in the initial stages of remission.

Although AS is generally regarded as having a very poor prognosis, remission of AS (19-22) is observed in a relatively high percentage of patients previously documented in a study where 35% of patients with improving AS were classified as rehabilitated (independent) and some of them back at work (18).

The term persistent vegetative state was suggested by Plum and Jennet in 1972 (23, 24), who proposed the following characterization:

These patients may open their eyes (with sleep and wake rhythms), may be able to follow an object with their eyes, but not speak, do not obey commands and do not show a response that is psychologically meaningful to the objective observer.

Several descriptions of AS (16, 21, 22, 25) existed prior to this redescription by Jennet and Plum. Probably, redefinition seemed to be necessary in order to have an international classification.

Two recent consensus statements (1993 American Neurological Association and 1994 Multisociety Task Force) redefine the persistent vegetative state (PVS). The Task Force definition requires no evidence of awareness or of interaction with others; no evidence of sustained, reproducible, purposeful or voluntary behavior or responses to visual, auditory, tactile or noxious stimuli; no evidence of language comprehension or expression; intermittent wakefulness with preserved cranial nerve and spinal reflexes, and preserved hypothalamic and brainstem autonomic functions.

According to these descriptions, some differences exist between our definition of AS and that of PVS.

Jennet et al. describe roving movements of the eyes in PVS patients which, according to our definition, represent the stage of a prolonged midbrain syndrome (23, 24).

Reaction to acoustic or visual stimuli with the eyes and head are defined by us as the sign of early remission stage I; following a moving object with the eyes is remission stage I to II. Thus, PVS represents a mixture of the clinical signs and symptoms of a full-blown AS and those of remission stages I and II.

An important aspect of the clinical signs and symptoms of a full-blown AS is an enhanced sympathicotonia with signs of chronic stress reaction. This vegetative dysfunction can still be observed during the initial phases of remission, however, with a slowly progressing normalization as of stage V.

Clinically speaking, remission of AS is a developing process, manifesting itself in several stages (RES I-VIII). Nevertheless, in many patients recovery stops at an early stage and they remain severely disabled.

First signs of remission are emotional reactions to the patient's surroundings, optical staring at and turning toward persons (phase I). Following with the eyes, purposeful movement and the obeying of instructions are related to phases II and III. Phases IV and V of AS remission are characterized by symptoms of the so-called Klüver-Bucy syndrome (26). Coherent verbalization as well as a slowly increasing improvement in the highest cortical performance characterize remission stages VI-VIII.

Neurological examination of a cooperative patient suspected of having a traumatic transection of the spinal cord involves no methodological difficulties, because it is possible to segmentally localize and abjectivize the myotome paralysis. On the other hand, it can be very difficult to clinically assess a non-cooperative patient for spinal cord function. For reasons of biodynamics, the combination of cerebral and spinal cord injuries is not infrequent. In 1993 the Department of Traumatology of Innsbruck University Hospital treated 38 000 emergency cases, of which 1410 (3.7%) involved spinal trauma, with 316 cases considered serious. The combination of a serious cerebral injury and a serious spinal trauma was diagnosed in 21 patients.

Imaging techniques provide valuable information on the morphology of structural changes, so that morphological structural changes along with the ensuing spinal cord injury can even be shown in comatose patients.

Gerrelts et al., Gerrelts bd., Petersen eu., Marby J., Petersen Sr., Journal/ Trauma 1991 Dec. 31 (12:16 22/6) examined over a period of 32 months 1331 victims of a blunt polytrauma for whom an X-ray of the cervical vertebral column was taken in the acute phase. In 61 of these patients the cervical vertebral column was seen to be injured. In five patients (4%) the diagnosis was overlooked during acute assessment and was only clinically established in the subsequent period (2-21 days). Reid et al. showed 38 (19.3%) late diagnoses in a further study of 274 cervical vertebral injuries.

These findings go to show that it is not infrequent for cervical vertebral injuries to be overlooked or not diagnosed in the acute phase. This is above all the case for combined craniocerebral traumas, where a classic neurological examination of uncooperative patients is not possible. Despite this problem, it should be possible to perform a clinical neurological assessment of a patient in the acute phase. Early detection of spinal injuries prevents incorrect positioning, incorrect transport, and subsequent dislocations caused by intubation and permits better early radiological evalution.

Clinical neurological assessment depends on a precise anamnesis of how the accident occurred. Thorough examination with verification of any possible contusion marks is also necessary.

The patient's respiration can provide important information with regard to a transection of the spinal cord: a high-level lesion (above C4) is accompanied by respiratory insufficiency and marked innervation of the scalene muscles, a lesion from C4 to C6 affects so-called diaphragmatic respiration, and lower lesions influence so called shallow respiration.

In craniocerebral trauma patients with reduced wakefulness motoricity can provide information on spinal cord function. While a patient with midbrain syndromes I or II responds to nociceptive stimuli with finalized and nonfinalized motor responses, we have observed in midbrain syndromes III and IV the so-called decortication or decerebration patterns with marked increase in muscle tone. Injuries of the spinal cord produce pseudo flaccid paralysis below the level of the lesion, which is caused by spinal shock.

The tendon reflexes also serve to localize spinal lesions, because in the case of acute midbrain syndrome the enhanced reflexes below the level of the lesion during spinal shock cannot be triggered.

In patients with midbrain syndrome the level of sensation can be verified by means of nociceptive stimuli. Special attention must be paid to assessing the level of sensation at the transition from cervical to thoracic vertebrae, where the supraclavicular nerves (C4) border directly on D2, so that the lesion can be presumed to be too low if the extremities are not examined precisely.

In the case of prolonged midbrain syndrome and remission of spinal shock, the various manifestations of the spastic hypertonia in the remission phases can provide additional clinical information on concomitant spinal lesions. Examination of the bulbocavernosus reflex is an additional neurological means of detecting functional disturbances in the spinal cord.

Clinical suspicion of a concomitant spinal cord injury naturally demands a new, precise, radiological reevalution or electrophysiological diagnosis by means of tibialis SSEP and motor-evoked potentials. From the standpoint of rehabilitation management, it is important for patients with spinal cord transection to be positioned regularly (turned every 2 h) in order to prevent typical flexor spasms, which must be interpreted as complex shortening reactions as part of deafferentation.

Vertical positioning on an upright table is sometimes difficult for these patients and often can only be performed in the framework of an antispastic therapy with oral or intrathecal baclofen.

Electrophysiological investigations

Supplementary electrophysiological examinations such as electroencephalography and evoked potential measurements are aids for determining clinical prognosis.

The reliability of electrophysiological examination differs strongly, depending on the etiology of the cerebral injury. In patients with craniocerebral trauma the brainstem auditory evoked potentials are seen to be extremely sensitive in terms of a negative outcome prognosis. Of patients with a very abnormal bilateral BAEP (massive prolonged I-III or III-V interpeak latency), 90% have a poor outcome. The exception here are patients with direct brainstem trauma. Somatosensory evoked potentials tend to predict a good outcome, provided early cortical response is normal, while unilateral prolonged or lacking potentials do not permit a reliable prognosis, because the multifocal lesions can cause a selective influence on the lemniscis medialis or the thalamocortical pathways and thus no conclusions can be drawn on the patient's remission tendency.

Motor-evoked potentials are unreliable because patients who remain in full-blown AS can show normal motor-evoked potentials, although they present clinically massive decortication patterns. This can be explained by the fact that the motor-evoked potentials reflect only 10% of the corticospinal tract, and extrapyramidal motoricity cannot be assessed from this examination.

In the case of hypoxic injuries, somatosensory-evoked potentials are seen to be highly sensitive. A definite prognosis can be made within the first 4 days, because at this time a bilateral or unilateral lack of cortical response can clearly predict a poor outcome. The presence of an early response, even with minor latency delay can predict a positive outcome with 96% certainty already on day 3. BAEP and MEP are only suitable for assessing outcome development and overall with the somatosensory-evoked potentials.

Event-related potentials (ERP) are an additional method for establishing a prognosis by means of electrophysiological parameters.

ERP are an electrophysiological method to evaluate attentiveness or cognitive processing, applied by the classic "oddball paradigm".

A low-frequency acoustic stimulus is repeated at 1-s intervals, while randomly added high-frequency acoustic stimuli (rare stimulus) must be recognized by the proband. After approx. 200 ms a negative potential, so-called mismatch negativity (N 200), is produced that is interpreted as the expression of a more complex automatic processing function of the brain without primary cognitive activity. Repeated occurrence of this potential is very possibly the expression of an increase in the functional activity of the brain, but gives no indication of cognitive processing mechanisms. In contrast, P 300 (300 ms) is a parameter for attentiveness or the expression of cognitive processing.

The classic oddball paradigm cannot be applied in apallic patients, because they do not meet the prerequisites for active cooperation in recognizing the rare stimulus. For this reason we have modified this method so that the patient's name is used as the rare stimulus in order to give it an emotional component commanding the patient's attention. This modification permits uncooperative patients to be examined without prior instruction. By changing the oddball paradigm we attempted to employ a significant stimulus as the rare stimulus.

Patients in AS show different electrophysiological reactions. In several patients with full-blown AS or in the initial remission stages of AS, a P300-like wave was determined as the expression of cognitive processing. We found that even clinically identical patients can be on various cognitive levels of development. The method represents a parameter for AS remission capability in order to give further information about possible rehabilitation programs.

The value of biochemical variables has been studied recently but at present such measures are not routinely used to determine prognosis.

Clinical findings during remission

Remission of AS is characterized, as mentioned above, by several signs and symptoms representing both the reintegration of caudorostral neurological functions and the inner cerebral trauma. These signs and symptoms must be diagnosed in a very early stage to enable a carefully directed neurological and neuropharmacological intervention.

Frequent pathologies during remission

1. Posttraumatic Parkinson - like symptomatology (PTP)
2. Posttraumatic cerebellar dysfunction (PTCD)
3. Posttraumatic mutism (PM)
4. Communicating hydrocephalus
5. Increasing spasticity
6. Joint calcifications
7. Contractures
8. Polyneuropathy (bed rest, critical illness polyneuropathy)

In 1929 Crouzon reported on a patient presenting the symptoms of Parkinson's disease secondary to brain trauma. According to his observation traumatic Parkinson's disease should be characterized by:

* Severe brain trauma
* Obvious latency between trauma and onset of extrapyramidal symptoms
* Clear progression

Adams and Victor as well as several other authors refused to accept trauma as a trigger of Parkinson's disease. A posttraumatic symptomatology was discussed in the sense of rostrocaudal reintegration.

Gerstenbrand et al. (16) observed the close similarity between posttraumatic and postencephalitic Parkinson's. They proposed L-Dopa treatment for these patients.

According to our observations a Parkinson-like symptomatology does exist, and about 40% of our patients benefit from L-Dopa treatment. Nevertheless, we did not perform a double-blind randomized study with L-Dopa.

The main symptoms of PTP are:

* Amimia
* Rigidity
* Bradykinesis

Tremor is hardly observed and vegetative symptoms improve.

All patients are treated with L-Dopa in an average dosage of 375-750 mg per day. No central induced side effects such as dyskinesia occurred. Peripheral side effects such as hypotonia probably due to forced dosage were observed in some cases.

The rigid akinetic variant of PTP resembles the symptoms seen in patients suffering from so-called arteriosclerotic Parkinson's, also based on multilocal lesions. According to Anjulie and Rugerie central side effects also rarely occur in these patients.

The posttraumatic Parkinson symptomatology with rigid muscle tone and akinesis is partially reversible and represents the neurophysiological consequence of the neuropathological patterns of the innercerebral trauma.

The signs and symptoms of posttraumatic cerebellar dysfunction occur in 25%-30% of severely brain injured with a peak in young patients.

Symptoms are characterized by static and dynamic ataxia, dysarthria, dysmetria, wing-beating tremor together with cranial nerve palsy and disturbed oculomotion. First signs occur during the initial stages of remission.

According to Rundino, posttraumatic cerebellar malfunction correlates with the duration of coma, which agrees well with our observations when cerebellar dysfunction mostly was observed in patients with a coma duration of more than 30 days.

Pathophysiologically, this symptom is based on a torsion of the brachii ad pontem secondary to a mechanism described previously by Lindenberg, lesioning cerebellorubral and cerebellovestibular fibers.

Physiotherapeutic treatment consists of walking, training in water or leadcuff charging of the extremities, based on the theory of agonist/antagonist coordination.

Posttraumatic cerebellar dysfunction is secondary to the strain of the cerebellar peduncles and induces a physicotherapy-resistant dysmetria as well as trunk ataxia.

INH was reported to have a positive influence on cerebellar malfunction symptoms in patients suffering from encephalitis disseminata. We investigated the INH therapy with a dosage of 600 mg per day and 150 mg B6 substitution. Comparing this treatment with a propanolol dosage of 60 mg per day we found a 25% improvement of fine motor functions and of dysarthria. In contrast to propanolol, INH therapy was stressed with increasing liver enzymes and increasing ataxia. Nevertheless, traumatic cerebellar malfunction improves within years and especially in younger patients.

Posttraumatic mutism (PM) represents a partial remission with improving consciousness and cognitive functions but retarded improvement of speech. It is characterized by a lack of phonation and verbal communication but preserved ability for gesticulative and written communication, without clinical signs and symptoms of aphasia, dysarthria or laryngeal malfunction.

Neurophysiologically, Cramon (34) explains this symptomatology as a trauma-induced transitory dysfunction of the periaqueductal gray matter, tegmentum and fibers to the Ncl. ambiguus, structures essential for species-specific phonation in primates.

Lindval et al. report on dopaminergic neurons in this region projecting to frontal and endorhinal brain structures.

We observed a partial or complete remission in all our patients suffering from PM within 3-25 weeks. According to our observations, three stages of PM remission can be differentiated:

* Full-blown PM with lack of phonation and verbalization and lack of voluntary expiration
* Dysphonic vocalization and verbalization, decreased voluntary expiration
* Dysphonic verbalization but ability to execute normophonic verbalization by voluntary effort, normal voluntary expiration

L-Dopa administration in a range of 375-750 mg per day seems to force remission, probably secondary to a stimulation of dopaminergic neurons of the mesolimbic system, as mentioned above.

PM mostly occurs after the third or fourth stage of remission. It is the consequence of temporary dysfunction of the periaqueductal gray matter or of the mesolimbic system and responds very well to oral L-Dopa administration.

The definition of spasticity proposed by Lance describes a velocity-dependent increase in tonic stretch reflexes and increased tendon jerks resulting from disinhibition of the stretch reflex as one component of an upper motor neuron lesion. From the clinical viewpoint, spasticity presents with phasic or tonic clinical features or a mixture of both. Phasic spasticity is characterized by exaggerated phasic stretch reflexes, tendon jerks, clonus, short-lasting plantar flexion withdrawal reflexes and occasionally occurring spontaneous phasic spasms. Tonic spasticity, in contrast, presents with exaggerated tonic stretch reflexes and a typical antigravity pattern of the upper and lower limbs.

Complete spinal cord injury presents with phasic spasticity as opposed to the incomplete spinal cord injury characterized by a more pronounced spasticity with additional tonic reflex activity, which represents supraspinal influence upon segmental neurons.

Supraspinal tonic spasticity is the result of a mismatch of descending facilitation and inhibition secondary to damaged or disconnected cerebral structures. The spinal cord is disinhibited as a consequence of interrupted cortical excitatory inputs to the medullary reticular formation, the output of which via the lateral reticulospinal tract inhibits spinal reflexes and promotes voluntary movements. Facilitated promotion of extensor reflexes via facilitatory reticulospinal and vestibulospinal pathways is less affected by cortical lesions, as they are not under direct cortical control.

Despite the very sophisticated diagnostic tools at our disposal, we are not able to cure every patient. Spasticity as one symptom of upper motor neuron lesion is, in fact, pharmacologically susceptible. Spinal spasticity responds in only about 75%, supraspinal spasticity in far less than 50% satisfactorily to oral antispastic treatment. A new and more effective means of treatment seems to be intrathecal application of baclofen via an implanted drug delivery system. Intrathecal application of baclofen is considered the treatment of choice in patients suffering from spinal spasticity, who insufficiently respond to conventional oral antispastic medication. This approach has also been used successfully in cases with spasticity of supraspinal origin.

To achieve a good therapeutic response in supraspinal spasticity the amount of intrathecal baclofen must be approximately twice the dosage required for spinal spasticity.

Supraspinal spasticity is characterized by a reduction of inhibitory influences while facilitatory influences are preserved (27).

The spinal cord is disinhibited secondarily to interruption of the normal excitatory inputs to the medullary reticular formation, which normally inhibits antigravity (extensor) reflexes and promotes voluntary (flexor) movements. Facilitation of extensor reflexes via pontine reticulospinal and vestibulospinal pathways is less affected by cortical lesions in humans since they lack direct cortical control (28-30). Baclofen (β-[4-chlorophenyl]-GABA), Lioresal, is a slightly lipophilic GABA-analogon that selectively acts on GABA - B receptors (31). It is not antagonized by bicuculline. The muscle-relaxing effect is mediated by presynaptic and at high concentrations also by postsynaptic actions (32). Activation of GABA - B receptors causes a reduction of CA^{++} influx into presynaptic terminals, thus resulting in less transmitter release. L-Glutamate- and L-Aspartate-dependent primary afferences seem to be under presynaptic GABA-ergic control (33).

Baclofen is effective in supraspinal spasticity, having more influence on mono- than on polysynaptic reflexes, which is probably due to the drug's presynaptic activity.

Side effects rarely occur, such as epileptic seizures (rare) or catheter displacement. Meningitis or local infections are avoidable if absolute sterility is maintained, particularly when refilling the pump. None of our patients suffered such complications. The risk of intoxication is inherent, especially with baclofen bolus injections. Therefore, close observation following bolus administration or dose adjustments is necessary.

A not infrequent complication is hydrocephalus absorptivus, whose symptoms are mainly seen in craniocerebral trauma patients who suffered traumatic subarachnoid hemorrhaging in the acute phase. Partial obstruction of the arachnoid granulations disturbs absorption of the bloody fluid, which manifests itself in enlargement of the lateral and third ventricles. Increase of pressure on the brain in followed by secondary enlargement of the Virchow-Robin space, which is tomographically seen from its periventricular high lucency. The clinical symptoms are often difficult to recognize, because the occurrence of hydrocephalus delays the patient's remission without a marked deterioration in clinical condition. The symptoms seldom present as the typical clinical symptoms of progressive akinesis and amimia or an increase in primitive oral patterns.

Diagnosis is established as follows:

1. Clinical observations: stagnant clinical progress
2. Computed tomography: increasing enlargement of the waist of the lateral an third ventricles as well as periventricular high lucency
3. Isotope cysternography: demonstration of isotopes in the lateral ventricle 24 h after administration is definite proof of disturbed absorption

For normal-pressure hydrocephalus, implantation of an atrioventricular or atrioperitoneal shunt with an adjustable valve system is recommended. An improvement in hydrocephalic symptoms should be seen within 10 days or 1 month. Persistence of symptoms means that the valve system urgently needs checking.

Periarticular calcification occurs in approximately 15% of adolescent craniocerebral trauma patients. Prediction points are the hip and elbow joints. Periarticular calcification can have a very negative affect on rehabilitation because local pain symptoms increase tone, while inhibition of flexion, extension and internal rotation of the hip prevent early verticalization of the patients. For this reason periarticular calcification is surgically removed early in remission; surgery is also performed when the bone scan is positive or there is elevated alkali phosphatase.

A prospective study conducted from 1989 to 1994 showed that in 67 surgically treated joints in 52 patients recalcification with renewed functional impairment of the joints occurred in only two cases. These findings show that recalcification, formerly considered a frequent occurrence, is a very seldom complication following surgery.

In conclusion it can be said that precise diagnosis and a neurorehabilitation program tailored to the situation can promote early detection and treatment of tertiary injuries with good rehabilitation outcome, even for severe cerebral lesions.

In a catamnestic study of 376 patients treated at our clinic following severe craniocerebral trauma, 34% of patients who presented with full-blown AS in the course of remission were able to be reintegrated into their social surroundings or were able to return to work (35).

These figures demonstrate the efficacy and necessity of early, intensive and skilled rehabilitation in patients following severe, acute damage of the central nervous system.

References

1. Cooper PR (1993) Head injury, 3rd edn. Baltimore, Williams and Wilkins.
2. Frankowski RF, Annegers JF Whitman S (1985) Epidemiological and descriptive studies. Part 1. The descriptive epidemiology of head trauma in the US. In: Becker DP, Povlishock JT (eds) Central nervous system trauma status report. National Institutes of Health NINCDS, Bethesda, pp 33-43

3. WHO Statistics Annual (1993)
4. Brain resuscitation clinical trials II study group (1991) A randomized clinical study of calcium entry blocker (Lidoflazine) in the treatment of comatous survivors of cardiac arrest. N Engl J Med 324:1225-1231
5. Longstreth WT, Diehr P, Inui TS (1988) Prediction of awakening after out hospital cardiac arrest. N Engl J Med 308:1378-1382
6. Bell JA, Hodgson HJF (1974) Coma after cardiac arrest. Brain 97:361-372
7. De Vivo MJ, Fine PR, Maetz HM et al (1980) Prevalence of spinal cord injury: a re-estimation employing life table techniques. Arch Neurol 37:707-708
8. Lancet prediction IBK - GCS
9. Benzer A, Traweger C, Öfner D, Marosi M, Luef G, Schmutzhard E (1955) Statistical modelling in analysis of outcome after trauma - Glasgow Coma Scale and Innsbruck Coma Scale. Anasthesiol Intensivmed Notfallmed Schmerzther
10. Mullie A, Buylart W et al (1988) Predictive value of Glasgow Coma Score for awakening after out of hospital cardiac arrest. Lancet i:137-140
11. Marosi M, Gerstenbrand F, Luef G, Zimmermann S et al (1991) Scoring of coma. Lancet 337:1043
12. Lechleitner P, Felber S et al (1993) Is early determination of neurological outcome after prehospital resuscitation possible in patients after cardiocirculatory arrest? Circulation [Suppl] 88:1
13. Madl C, Grimm G et al (1993) Early prediction of individual outcome after cardiopulmonary resuscitation. Lancet 341:855-858
14. Martin GB, Paradis MA et al (1992) Nuclear magnetic resonance spectroscopy study of human brain after cardiac resuscitation. Stroke 22:462-468
15. Karkela J, Pasanen M et al (1992) Evaluation of hypoxic brain injury with spinal fluid enzymes, lactate and pyruvate. Crit Care Med 20:378-386
16. Gerstenbrand F et al (1967) Das traumatisch apallische Syndrom. Springer, Vienna New York
17. Dalle Ore G, Gerstenbrand F, Lücking CH et al (1977) The apallic syndrome. Springer, Berlin Heidelberg New York
18. Berek K, Luef G, Marosi M, Saltuari L (1993) Apallic syndrome - to treat or not to treat. Lancet 341:899
19. Rosenblath W (1989) Über einen bemerkenswerten Fall von Hirnerschütterung. Dtsch Arch Klin Med 64:406-424
20. Strich SJ (1956) Diffuse degeneration of the cerebral white matter in severe dementia following head injury. J Neurol Neurosurg Psychiatry 19:163-185
21. Ule G, Döhner W, Bues E (1961) Ausgedehnte Hemissphärenmarkschädigung nach gedecktem Hirntrauma mit apallischem Syndrom und partieller Spätrehabilitation. Arch Psychiat 155-176
22. Vigouroux R, Naquet R, Baurand C, Choux M, Salomon G, Khalil R (1964) Evoulution electro radio clinique de comas graves prolonges post traumatiques. Rev Neurol 110:72-81
23. Jennet B, Plum F (1972) Persistent vegetative state after brain damage. Lancet 1:734-737
24. Braakman R, Jennet WB, Minderhound M (1988) Prognosis of the posttraumatic vegetative state. Acta Neurochir 95:49-52
25. Kretschmer E (1940) Das apallische Syndrom. Z gesamte Neurol Psychiatr 169:576-579
26. Gerstenbrand F, Poewe W, Aichner F, Saltuari L (1983) Klüver Bucy Syndrome in man: experiences with posttraumatic cases. Neurosci Biobehav Res 7:413-417
27. Brooks VB (1986) The neural basis of motor control. Oxford, New York
28. Howe JR, Ziegelgänsberger W et al (1986) D-baclofen does not antagonize the actions of L-baclofen on rat neocortical neurons in vitro. Neurosci Lett 72:99
29. Kroin JS, Penn RD et al (1984) Reduced spinal reflexes following intrathecal Baclofen in the rabbit. Exp Brain Res 54:191
30. Lance JW (1980) Symposium synopsis. In: Feldman, Young, Koella (eds) Spasticity: disordered motor control, Year Book, Chicago, pp 485-494

31. Bowery NG, Doble A et al (1981) Bicuculline-insensitive GABA receptors on peripheral autonomic nerve terminals. Eur J Pharmacol 71:53
32. Davidoff RA (1985) Antispastic drugs: mechanisms of actions. Ann Neurol 17:107
33. Zieglgänsberger W, Howe JR et al (1988) The neuropharmacology of baclofen. In: Müller H (eds) Local spinal therapy of spasticity, Springer, Berlin Heidelberg New York, pp 37-49

CSF Filtration: Scientific and Clinical Update

R. Heusslein, S. Rother, C. Trömel, K.-H. Wollinsky, E. Schmutzhard,
D. Pöhlau

Introduction

The filtration of cerebrospinal fluid (CSF) was first used by Wollinsky and
coworkers in severely affected GBS patients who did not respond to other
therapies (1). Recently published data describing in vitro studies, animal
experiments and clinical experience in Ulm, Germany (2-6) encouraged other
centres to use this technique. We are actually facing an increase in clinical data
on CSF filtration (1, 6-18) with enlargement of the range of indications as well
as an understanding of the possible mechanism of CSF filtration in various
neurological diseases (3-5, 18-22). Even though it is still an experimental
approach more than 40 hospitals – predominantly situated in the German
speaking countries – are presently using CSF filtration. Clinical experiences are
based on the treatment of more than 250 patients. This increased usage is partly
based on the fact that the technique is easy to perform and associated with a low
incidence of side effects. The main reason for the growing acceptance of CSF
filtration, however, is the increasing number of publications indicating that CSF
filtration offers the opportunity to intervene in the course of diseases even in late
chronic stages.

The aim of CSF filtration is to remove cellular and soluble components from
the CSF known to be involved in the pathologic and inflammatory processes. In
order to perform CSF filtration an 18G catheter is placed intrathecally in the
lumbar region under sterile conditions (6). CSF is automatically sucked (pressure
and flow being controlled by a special pump; Infors Flofors) via the bypass of a
prefilled filter system (Pall, CSF1) into a syringe and then is reinjected through
the filter. Filtration is repeated several times during one session in order to reach
a total volume of 200-250 ml. The catheter usually remains in place for 5 days
and the treatment is repeated daily (6).

The materials of the filter housing and the membrane are biocompatible and
suited for implantation. The affinity of the surface modified 0.2 μm membrane to
certain molecules allows efficient retention of proteins or peptides much smaller
than the pore size (23, 24; Fig. 1).

The in vitro validation of the filter system revealed that inflammatory
cytokines or complement, for example, are significantly reduced while albumin

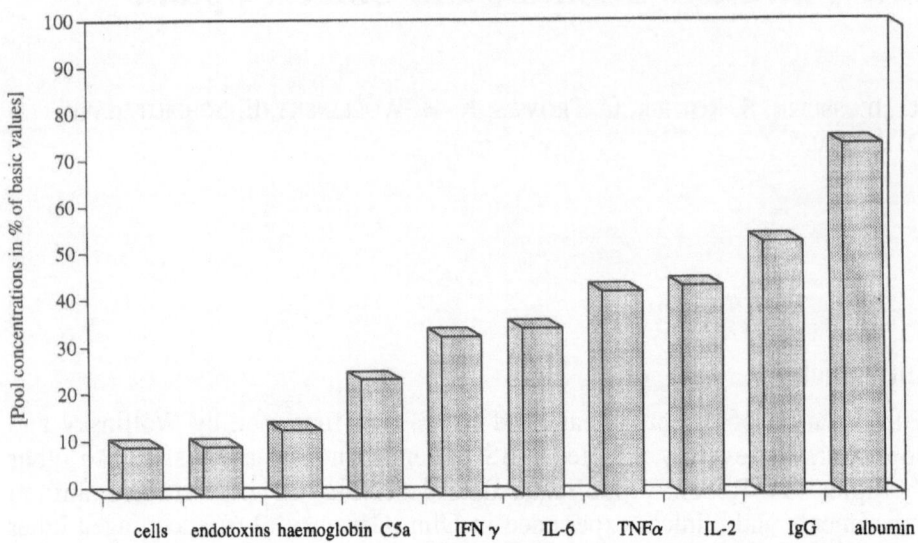

Fig. 1. Residual concentrations of various cellular and soluble CSF components in 100 ml artificial CSF after filtration of 150 ml (3 x 50 ml). Cells and endotoxins had been measured with *Escherichia coli* under conditions representing cell concentrations in bacterial meningitis. Glucose and electrolytes are not retained by the filter (data not shown). Initial concentrations of inflammatory mediators immunoglobulins were comparable to clinical values described for various autoimmune neuropathies. *IFN*, interferon; *IL-6*, interleukin 6; *TNFα*, tumour necrosis factor α; *IgG*, immuno-globulin G

almost completely passes the membrane (23, 24). The free passage of albumin through the filter membrane must be regarded as desirable since high albumin concentrations are described as "proexcitatory" with respect to the conductance of sodium channels (5). Cells or bacteria are mechanically retained by the filter membrane, thus giving a sterile filtrate. The efficiency of adsorptive filtration is a function of the affinity of the molecule to the membrane and the capacity (inner surface) of the membrane. For example, initial concentrations of 1.06 and 2.8 mg/dl haemoglobin (representing values which normally occur on the fifth to seventh day after a subarachnoidal bleeding) (25) were reduced by 50%-86% (to 0.15 and 1.41 mg/dl, respectively; see Fig. 1) after filtration of 150 ml volume. It should be noted that all data on filtration efficacy were obtained under worst case conditions with respect to concentration and total amount of proteins and cells.

In addition to those substances known to be involved in degenerative inflammatory processes, CSF filtration also efficiently retains small-sized molecules which are not yet fully characterized but described by their cytotoxic or electrophysiological activity. One example is the presence of a sodium channel blocking factor, detected in the CSF but not the serum of GBS patients, which can be effectively reduced by CSF filtration (3, 5). Other conduction blocking factors are further discussed (for review see 26).

Acute and chronic inflammatory demyelinating polyneuropathies

The theoretical background for introducing the technique in GBS was the intrathecal occurrence of potentially pathogenic factors, such as autoantibodies and complement proteins throughout the course of the disease (27-29). Since it is well known that plasma exchange is effective by removing humoral components from the blood it also appeared useful to remove those factors from the CSF. The hypothesis that blood derived humoral factors are also of pathogenic relevance in the CSF was supported, for example, by animal experiments revealing that anti-ganglioside antibodies cause severe demyelination at the spinal roots of rabbits when administered intrathecally (30). In this context it has to be considered that plasma exchange alone is not suited to reduce humoral factors efficiently from the CSF (31). This presumably also applies to specific conduction blocking factors detected in the CSF but not in the blood of GBS patients with acute or long-term neurological deficits (3, 5).

Several authors have already described that GBS patients in early and even later stages of disease, not responding to plasma exchange and/or high dose intravenous immunoglobulins, draw benefit from CSF filtration (1, 6, 8, 11, 12, 13, 15). Wollinsky et al. (8) recently presented clinical data on nine GBS patients suffering from long-term deficits (disease duration on average 20.1 months). In these patients 4-21 CSF filtrations (on average 9.5 filtrations) were performed over an average period of 2.6 months. Three patients did not respond to CSF filtration (remained on score of 4) whereas six patients improved by scores of 1-2, resulting in a median improvement from a score of 4 to 3. This result is particularly promising when disease latency before CSF filtration (on average 20.1 months) and the treatment period under CSF filtration (on average 2.6 months) are compared.

Up to now more than 40 GBS cases treated with CSF filtration have been published (there are unpublished data on more than 80 GBS patients). A multicentre randomized crossover study is currently comparing the clinical effects of CSF filtration and plasma exchange in acute GBS. Intermediate results will be published in 1996. Positive clinical effects after CSF filtration were also observed in chronic demyelinating polyneuropathy (Wollinsky, in preparation; Dachsel, personal communication) and the CNS variant Miller-Fisher syndrome (14).

A summary of case reports on acute GBS ($n = 24$; 6, 8) already indicates that CSF filtration accelerates the recovery rate when compared with conservative, non-GBS specific therapies (literature data 6, 8). Furthermore the clinical effects of CSF filtration even seem to be comparable with literature data on other GBS-specific therapies such as plasma exchange and high dose intravenous immunoglobulins. As a result of the experiences of various users CSF filtration is regarded to be beneficial with respect to side effects, handling and costs when compared with other GBS-specific treatments.

Multiple sclerosis (MS)

Myelin destruction in MS is a consequence of a multi-component autoimmune reaction involving cells (32), inflammatory cytokines (33-37), complement factors (28, 38) and autoantibodies (39, 40). Recent investigations confirmed the occurrence of further factors of proteineic nature (17 kD) in the CSF, which are specifically toxic for astrocytes but not primarily toxic for oligodendroglial cells (20, 21). Dobransky et al. described high gliotoxic activity in the CSF of MS patients during acute exacerbations but not in remission. After clinical CSF filtration this cytotoxicity was clearly reduced (20). Eluates from the filters revealed that this factor was highly retained. Since astrocytes incubated with the gliotoxic factor in vitro produce high amounts of inflammatory cytokines, a secondary cytotoxic effect on oligodendrocytes cannot be excluded and offers a new pathway in the pathophysiology of MS (21).

Furthermore Brinkmeier et al. demonstrated in vitro using patch clamp recordings that CSF from MS patients interferes with voltage dependent sodium channels (4). After contact with CSF from MS patients, the sodium inward current through those channels was markedly reduced. Therefore, it can be considered that the clinical symptoms are not only caused by demyelination but also by a direct physiological impact on neurons (26).

Clinical results using CSF filtration were first presented by Wollinsky et al. (7). They reported on ten severely affected acute or chronic progressive patients. In all patients rapid objective or at least subjective improvements were described. Additionally, in order to stabilize the clinical improvements Wollinsky et al. applied an immunosuppressive treatment 2 weeks after CSF filtration. Further case reports (8, 11) and a first pilot trial including patients with severe chronic progressive MS (9, 10; see also Haas, this volume) confirmed the beneficial clinical results. The design of further clinical studies is presently discussed.

Amyotrophic lateral sclerosis (ALS)

ALS is characterized by a progressive and specific destruction of lower and upper motor neurons, but the underlying pathophysiological mechanism in sporadic ALS is controversially discussed (autoimmune process? apoptosis?). Increased titres of antiganglioside or anti-Ca^{++}-channel antibodies (41, 42) as well as the presence of immune complexes, IgGs and complement C4 (43, 44), indicate an involvement of the immune system. Furthermore, an abnormal glutamate metabolism in the brain of ALS patients has been described, presumably resulting in an increased intracellular Ca^{++} influx, destabilization of the cytoskeleton and neuronal cell death (45, 46).

This hypothesis is supported by recent work from Couratier et al. (47). Couratier et al. describe that CSF from ALS patients has a cytotoxic effect on rat neurons in culture. As the neurotoxicity can be blocked by CNQX – an antagonist to the AMPA/kainate receptor but not by NMDA antagonists – a specific interaction with a glutamate receptor must be considered. Further evidence was given by Nagaraja et al. (46) showing that ALS-CSF but not serum induces aberrant phosphorylation of neurofilaments, which might finally lead to the degeneration of neurons.

Tests on isolated nerves incubated with CSF from ALS patients indicate that measurable effects can occur within a few hours: a reduction of the sum action potential amplitude (Fig. 2) and induction of degenerative changes (Fig. 3; 19, 22). These paranodal demyelinations could be caused by destabilization of neurofilaments, finally resulting in a detachment of terminal myelin loops. This phenomenon specifically occurred in large myelinated fibres whereas small myelinated fibres remained intact in the same spinal nerve. The observed physiological and morphological effects were reduced by CSF filtration under in vitro conditions (19, 22).

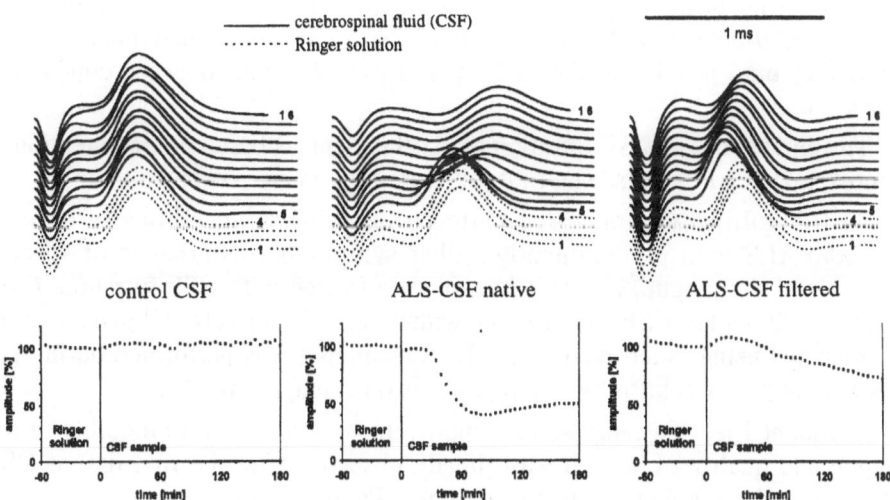

Fig. 2. Electrophysiological changes on bovine spinal roots after incubation with CSF. *Upper row,* Compound nerve action potentials. Time interval between subsequent records 15 min. After 1 h incubation in Ringer solution as reference (1-4, dotted lines), the nerve was in contact with CSF (5-16) for 3 h. *Lower row,* Long term diagram showing maximum amplitude of the compound action potential. The *vertical bar* at time = 0 indicates the change from Ringer solution to CSF. *Left side,* control CSF (normal values, no neuropathy); *middle,* ALS-CSF; *right side,* Same ALS-CSF after in vitro filtration

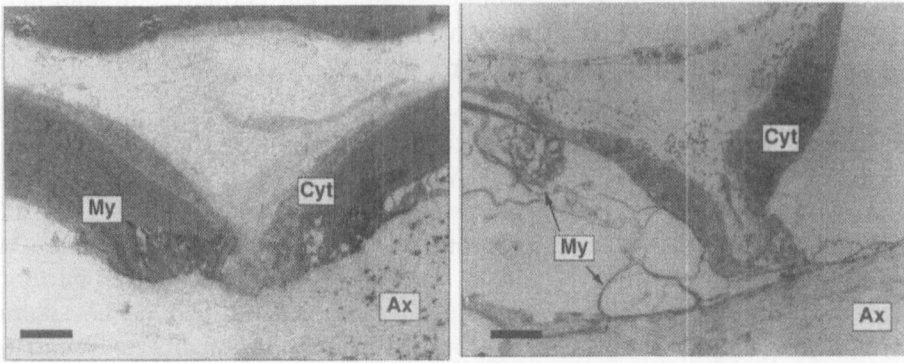

Fig. 3. Morphological changes on ventral bovine spinal roots after 180 min of incubation with Ringer (*left*) or ALS-CSF (*right*). Transmission electron microscope pictures show a longitudinal section of the node of Ranvier from axons with a diameter of ca. 4 μm (nodal) to 10 μm (internodal). Ax, axon; Cyt, cytoplasm of schwann cells; My, Myelin intact on the left but detached from the axon membrane and retracted from node of Ranvier on the right. *Bar*, 1 μm.

ALS is not described as a demyelinating disease. However, anti-GM1-antibodies are frequently detected (57%; 48) in the serum of ALS patients and elevated levels of complement protein C4d were described in CSF (44). Since anti-GM1 antibodies and complement factors are known to be involved in demyelinating processes, their presence could at least partially explain the occurrence of the paranodal destruction. Moreover, it is described that anti-GM1 antibodies bind in ALS to the node of Ranvier (49) and induce a conduction block (50, 51).

The clinical use of CSF filtration on ALS patients is based on the intention to remove toxic CSF factors. The first four case reports are presented here:

K.-H. Wollinsky/Ulm: three patients suffering from clinically defined sporadic ALS with predominantly bulbar symptoms (disturbance of speech, paralysis of the tongue) and atactic gait were treated with CSF filtration. Over 5 days 5 x 200 ml of CSF were filtered without any side effects. All patients were documented using video recordings. Documentation was performed during the whole treatment week; follow-up phase was on average 2 weeks.

In patient 1 (f, 67 years) distinct improvement with regard to mobility of the tongue and quality of speech was already observed after the first day of CSF filtration and remained stable for 2 weeks. Patient 2 (m, 17 years) improved slightly in speech and improved considerably with regard to walking. Patient 3 (m, 74 years) suffered from severe dysfunction of the hands and paretic gait. During the filtration week we observed significant improvement in mobility of the upper limbs. Before CSF filtration he could lift his right arm only several centimetres; after treatment elevation of the arm to the head was possible. Additionally opponing of the fingers and finger stretching was possible after CSF filtration. These improvements remained stable over 2 weeks. The data have to be regarded as preliminary, as no long-term data are currently available.

D. Pöhlau/Bochum: A patient (m, 49 years) suffered from nonfamilial ALS for 2 years. He continuously deteriorated. His disability reached 25 points on Limb Norris scale. CSF filtration (8 x 30 ml CSF daily) was performed for 7 days.

He was scored with the Limb Norris Scale (see Fig. 4). Two days after the last filtration he was able to walk and climb 40 steps compared to four steps before the treatment; also fine motor skills and coordination were clearly improved. The weakness was substantially reduced. This improvement was short lasting (2 weeks). No side effects from CSF filtration were observed.

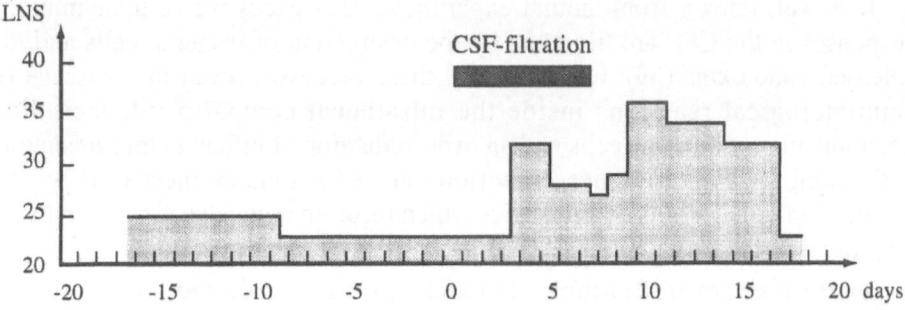

Fig. 4. ALS patient scored with Limb Norris Scale (LNS). The improvement after CSF filtration (*bar*) lasted for ca. 2 weeks

These first case reports indicate that the classical understanding of ALS as a degenerative motoneuron disease obviously does not fully describe the pathology. Slight but relatively quick improvements of motor function after CSF filtration can only be explained by functional impairment of neurons probably by toxic or blocking factors in CSF which are removed by filtration but reproduced within a certain time period. These first case reports must be regarded as encouraging since up to now no comparable effect had been observed using other therapies. If there is an effect in slowing the disease progression further investigation by a controlled study over a longer period of time with repeated treatments is necessary.

Bacterial meningitis

Despite the development of new antibiotics the mortality rate in certain forms of bacterial meningitis, such as pneumococcal meningitis, is still nearly 30% (52).

Another 20%-30% of patients survive only with incomplete remission (52-54). Brain damage, especially brain oedema, is the most important complication in bacterial meningitis, leading to mental retardation, learning disabilities, and focal neurological deficits (54-56).

Inflammatory mediators such as TNF-α are suggested to play an important role in the development of brain oedema and neuronal injuries. This hypothesis is supported by the observation that intrathecal injection of cytokines results in profound effects in the brain and induces *brain oedema in animals* (57). Täuber et al. (56) have demonstrated in vitro that CSF from rabbits infected with bacterial meningitis (pneumococcal or *Escherichia coli* meningitis) is highly neurotoxic and that the neurotoxicity is mainly based on the presence of TNF-α. High intrathecal levels of TNF-α were also reported for patients with bacterial meningitis (34, 58).

It is well known from animal experiments that excessive cellular immune responses in the CSF are triggered by the destruction of bacterial cells and the released endotoxins (59). Once induced these processes result in a cascade of immunological reactions inside the intrathecal compartment, including accumulation of immune cells and an overproduction of inflammatory mediators (60; compare Fig. 5). These reactions are additionally increased by the application of bacteriolytic antibiotics which result in rapid elevation of cell wall fragments in the CSF (59, 61).

Therefore, several authors demand innovative adjuvant strategies in combination with antibiotics for the management of bacterial meningitis and for the reduction of complications (54, 62, 63). As recently described CSF filtration

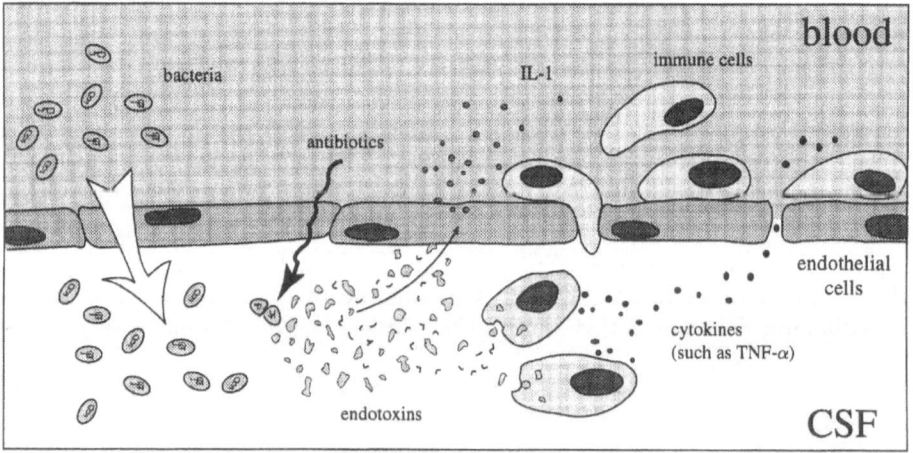

Fig. 5. Bacterial meningitis. The presence of bacteria and the release of endotoxins can initiate a cascade of immune reactions in CSF resulting in the accumulation of cells and the production of inflammatory mediators such as tumour necrosis factor (*TNF*); *IL-1*, interleukin

might represent such a strategy (16, 18). In vitro experiments have revealed that the CSF filter membrane (CSF1, PALL, Dreieich/Germany) efficiently reduces bacteria and endotoxins as well as inflammatory mediators such as TNF-α (23, 24). Based on these findings CSF filtration (9 x 25 ml cycles) was simultaneously applied with intravenous penicillin G in a patient suffering from pneumococcal meningitis (16). CSF was purulent and contained 6700 polymorphonuclear cells per mm^3. CSF-TNF-α was strongly elevated (813 pg/ml). Within 2.5 h CSF filtration resulted in a drop of cell number to 240 cells/mm^3 and the TNF-α level decreased significantly to 39 pg/ml. CSF filtration was only performed one time (directly after lumbar puncture for diagnosis) and antibiotics were administered over 12 days. Clinically, the initial cerebellar syndrome (phase I) improved within 2 days and the patient was mobilized on day 3. He left the hospital fully recovered without sequelae and with normal CSF findings on day 13.

This first case report on the combined therapy antibiotics plus CSF filtration seems to confirm the theoretical considerations. In particular the pronounced positive effect on CSF parameters is promising since antibiotics alone initially increase the intrathecal immune response. Despite this first positive case report the clinical value of this combined therapy must be proven in controlled studies.

Conclusion

Reviewing the actual literature data, increasing evidence is provided that CSF modifications play a role in the pathogenesis of various neurological diseases. CSF filtration here presented as a new therapeutic approach in neurology may provide the necessary tool to influence the CSF content in a relatively mild and acceptable way. The case reports cited indeed show clinical benefit even under extreme negative selection - CSF filtration is still being used as an additive treatment when other strategies failed. Further clinical work is needed to prove this promising trend.

References

1. Wollinsky KH, Weindler M, Hülser PJ, Geiger P, Matzek N, Mehrkens H-H, Kornhuber HH (1991) Liquorpheresis (CSF filtration): an effective treatment in acute and chronic severe autoimmune polyradiculoneuritis (Guillain-Barré syndrome). Eur Arch Psych Clin Neurosci 241:73-76
2. Hülser PJ, Wiethölter H, Wollinsky, KH (1991) Liquorpheresis eliminates blocking factors from cerebrospinal fluid in polyradiculoneuritis (Guillain-Barré syndrome). Eur Arch Psychiatry Clin Neurosci 241:69-72
3. Brinkmeier H, Wollinsky KH, Hülser PJ, Seewald MJ, Mehrkens H-H, Kornhuber HH, Rüdel R (1992) The acute paralysis in Guillain-Barré syndrome is related to a Na$^+$ channel blocking factor in the cerebrospinal fluid. Pflugers Arch 421:552-557
4. Brinkmeier H, Wollinsky KH, Seewald MJ, Hülser P-J, Mehrkens H-H, Kornhuber HH, Rüdel R (1993) Factors in the cerebrospinal fluid of multiple sclerosis patients interfering with voltage-dependent sodium channels. Neurosci Lett 156:172-175

5. Würz A, Brinkmeier H, Wollinsky KH, Mehrkens HH, Kornhuber HH, Rüdel R (1995)
    Cerebrospinal fluid and serum from patients with inflammatory polyradiculoneuropathy have
    opposite effects on sodium channels. Muscle Nerve 18:772-781
6. Wollinsky KH, Hülser PJ, Brinkmeier H, Mehrkens HH, Kornhuber HH, Rüdel R (1994)
    Filtration of cerebrospinal fluid in acute inflammatory polyneuropathy (Guillain-Barré
    syndrome). Ann Med Interne 145:451-458
7. Wollinsky KH, Hülser PJ, Mauch E, Mehrkens HH, Kornhuber HH (1992) Liquorpherese bei
    10 Patienten mit Multipler Sklerose. Verh Dtsch Gesellsch Neurol 7:444-445
8. Wollinsky KH, Hülser PJ, Brinkmeier H, Mehrkens HH, Kornhuber HH, Rüdel R (1995)
    Klinische Erfahrungen mit der CSF filtration. Neuropsychiatrie 9 (in press)
9. Haas J, Düzel E, Tendolkar L, Sailer M, Wurster U, Rieger A, Heinze HJ (1995) Cerebrospinal
    fluid filtration: an experimental therapeutic approach to multiple sclerosis. J Neurol 242
    [Suppl]:S118
10. Haas J, Sailer M, Düzel E, Tendolkar I, Wurster U (1995) Liquorfiltration bei multipler
    Sklerose: eine experimentelle Therapie. Neuropsychiatrie 9 (in press)
11. Allen C, Kepplinger B, Papst H (1995) CSF filtration (cerebrospinal fluid filtration) bei
    demyelinisierenden Erkrankungen. Neuropsychiatrie 9 (in press)
12. Gruber F, Pfausler B, Laich E, Vollert H, Brucker B, Schmutzhard E, Deisenhammer E (1995)
    Einsatz der Liquorfiltration bei Guillain-Barré Syndrom. In: Harms L, Schielke E, Weber JR
    (eds) 12. Tagung Arbeitsgem Neurol Intensivmed Deutsch Gesellsch Neurol, ANIM, Berlin,
    pp 194
13. Gruber F, Laich E, Brucker B, Deisenhammer E (1995) Kombinationstherapie Cerebrospinal-
    flüssigkeits-Filtration/i.v. Immunglobuline bei Guillain-Barré Syndrom. Neuropsychiatrie 9
    (in press)
14. Pfausler B, Auckenthaler A, Grubwieser G, Vollert-Rogenhofer H, Schmutzhard E (1994)
    Miller-Fisher-Syndrom – erfolgreiche Therapie mit Liquorfiltration – ein Fallbericht.
    Neuropsych 8:41
15. Pfausler B, Schmutzhard E (1995) CSF filtration bei neuroimmunologischen Erkrankungen
    (GBS, Miller-Fisher Syndrom, zerebraler Lupus erythematodes). Neuropsychiatrie 9 (in press)
16. Pfausler B, Grubwieser G, Bösch S, Vollert H, Herold M, Schmutzhard E (1995)
    Cerebrospinal fluid-filtration reduces TNF in bacterial meningitis-CSF. Eur J Neurol (in press)
17. Pfausler B, Bösch S, Grubwieser G, Vollert H, Greil R, Hagn C, Schmutzhard E (1995)
    Multimodal therapy in life-threatening cerebral lupus erythematosus: the benefit of
    cerebrospinal fluid pheresis. Int Arch Allergy Immunol 563 (in press)
18. Schmutzhard E, Grubwieser G, Pfausler B (1995) Liquorfiltration - eine adjuvante
    therapeutische Strategie bei der bakteriellen Meningitis. Neuropsychiatrie 9 (in press)
19. Trömel C, Gnatzy W (1995) Elektrophysiologische und morphologische Veränderungen an
    isolierten Spinalwurzeln nach Applikation von GBS-, MS- und ALS-Liquor. Neuro-
    psychiatrie 9 (in press)
20. Dobransky T, Amouri R, Wollinsky KH, Westarp ME, Rieger F (1995) Influence of filtration
    on a new gliotoxic activity in cerebrospinal fluid from multiple sclerosis patients.
    Neuropsychiatrie 9 (in press)
21. Amouri R, Dobransky T, Benjelloun N, Rieger F (1995) A new gliotoxic activity and its
    implications for the immunopathogenesis of multiple sclerosis. Neuropsychiatrie 9 (in press)
22. Trömel C, Gnatzy W (1995) Extracellular records of bovine spinal root bundles incubated
    with cerebrospinal fluid of patients as an animal model for blocking effects in neurological
    diseases. In: Elsner N, Menzel R (eds) Proceedings of the 23rd Göttingen Neurobiology
    Conference: Learning and Memory. Thieme, Stuttgart, New York 2:855
23. Rother S, Knoblauch KD, Kirschfink M (1995) Filtration von Liquor cerebrospinalis (CSF
    filtration): Technisches Konzept und Filtrationseffizienz unter in vitro Bedingungen.
    Neuropsychiatrie 9 (in press)
24. Rother S, Kirschfink M (1994) CSF filtration: a new therapeutical concept - technique and
    scientific background. In: Gullo (ed) APICE 1994. Fogliazza editore, Milano vol 9, pp
    577-586

25. Foley PL, Takenaka K, Kasselli NF, Lee KS (1994) Cytotoxic effects of bloody cerebrospinal fluid on cerebral endothelial cells in culture. J Neurosurg 81:87-92
26. Waxman SG (1995) Sodium channel blockade by antibodies: a new mechanism of neurological disease? Ann Neurol 37:421-423
27. Hartung HP, Schwenke C, Bitter-Suermann D, Toyka KV (1987) Guillain-Barré syndrome: activated complement components C3a and C5a in CSF. Neurology 37:1006-1009
28. Sanders ME, Koski CL, Robbins D, Shin ML, Frank MM, Joiner KA (1986) Activated terminal complement in cerebrospinal fluid in Guillain-Barré syndrome and multiple sclerosis. J Immunol 136:4456-4459
29. Simone IL, Annunziata P, Maimone D, Liguori M, Leante R, Livrea P (1993) Serum and CSF anti-GM 1 antibodies in patients with Guillain-Barré syndrome and chronic inflammatory demyelinating polyneuropathy. J Neurol Sci 114:49-55
30. Schwerer B, Lassmann H, Kitz K, Bernheimer H (1986) Ganglioside GM1, a molecular target for immunological and toxic attacks: similarity of neuropathological lesions induced by ganglioside-antiserum and cholera toxin. Acta Neuropathol (Berl) 72:55-61
31. Graus F, Abos J, Mazzara R, Pereira A (1990) Effect of plasmapheresis on serum and CSF autoantibody levels in CNS paraneoplastic syndrome. Neurology 40:1621-1623
32. Söderström M, Link H, Sun JB, Fredrikson S, Wang ZY, Huang WX (1994) Autoimmune T-cell repertoire in optic neuritis and multiple sclerosis: T-cells recognising multiple myelin proteins are accumulated in cerebrospinal fluid. J Neurol Neurosurg Psychiatry 57:544-551
33. Hartung HP, Jung S, Stoll G et al (1992) Inflammatory mediators in demyelinating disorders of the CNS and PNS. J Neuroimmunol 40:197-210
34. Weller M, Stevens A, Sommer N, Melms A, Dichgans J, Wiethölter H (1991) Comparative analysis of cytokine patterns in immunological, infectious, and oncological neurological disorders. J Neurol Sci 104:215-221
35. Hauser SL, Doolittle TH, Lincoln R, Brown RH, Dinarello CA (1990) Cytokine accumulations in CSF of multiple sclerosis patients: frequent detection of interleukin-1 and tumor necrosis factor but not interleukin-6. Neurology 40:1735-1739
36. Benvenuto R, Paroli M, Buttinelli C et al (1991) Tumor necrosis factor-alpha synthesis by cerebrospinal fluid-derived T cell clones from patients with multiple sclerosis. Clin Exp Immunol 84:97-102
37. Sharief MK, Hentges R (1991) Association between tumor necrosis factor-alpha and disease progression in patients with multiple sclerosis. N Engl J Med 325:467-472
38. Linington C, Morgan BP, Scolding NJ, Wilkins P, Piddlestone S, Compston DAS (1989) The role of complement in the pathogenesis of experimental allergic encephalomyelitis. Brain 112:895-911
39. Catz I, Warren KG (1986) Intrathecal synthesis of autoantibodies to myelin basic protein in multiple sclerosis. Can J Neurol Sci 13:21-24
40. Warren KG, Catz I (1994) Relative frequency of autoantibodies to myelin basic protein and proteolipid protein in optic neuritis and multiple sclerosis cerebrospinal fluid. J Neurol Sci 121:66-73
41. Kimura F, Smith RG, Delbono O, Nyermoi O, Schneider T, Nastainczyk W, Hoffmann F, Stefani E, Appel SH (1994) Amyotrophic lateral sclerosis patient antibodies label Ca^{++} channel alpha 2 subunit. Ann Neurol 35:164-171
42. Apostolski S, Lator N (1993) Clinical syndromes associated with anti-GM1 antibodies. Semin Neurol 13:264-268
43. Apostolski S, Nikolic, Bugarski-Prokoplievic C, Miletic V, Pavlovic S (1991) Serum and CSF immunological findings in ALS. Acta Neurol Scand 83:96-98
44. Tsuboi Y, Yamada Y (1994) Increased concentration of C4d complement protein in CSF in amyotrophic lateral sclerosis. J Neurol Neurosurg Psychiatry 157:859-861
45. Rothstein JD, Tsai G, Kuncl RW et al (1990) Abnormal excitatory aminoacid metabolism in amyotrophic lateral sclerosis. Ann Neurol 28:18-25

46. Nagaraja TN, Gourie-Devi M, Nalini A, Raju TR (1994) Neurofilament phosphorylation is enhanced in cultured chick spinal cord neurons exposed to cerebrospinal fluid from amyotrophic lateral sclerosis patients. Acta Neuropathol 88:349-352

47. Couratier P, Hugon J, Sindou P, Vallat JM, Dumas M (1993) Cell culture evidence for neuronal degeneration in amyotrophic lateral sclerosis being linked to glutamate AMPA/kainate receptors. Lancet 341:265-268

48. Pestronk A, Adams RN, Clawson L, Cornblatz D, Kuncl RW, Griffin D, Drachman DB (1988) Serum antibodies to GM1 gangliosides in amyotrophic lateral sclerosis. Neurology 38: 1457-1461

49. Santoro M, Thomas FP, Fink ME, Lange DJ, Uncini A, Wadia NH, Latov N, Hays AP (1990) IgM deposits at nodes of Ranvier in a patient with amyotrophic lateral sclerosis, anti-GM1 antibodies and multifocal motor conduction block. Ann Neurol 28:373-377

50. Santoro M, Uncini A, Corbo M, Staugaitis SM, Thomas FP, Hays AP, Latov N (1992) Experimental conduction block induced by serum from a patient with anti-GM1 antibodies. Ann Neurol 31:385-390

51. Arasaki K, Kusunoki S, Kudo N, Kanazawa I (1993) Acute conduction block in vitro following exposure to antiganglioside sera. Muscle Nerve 16:587-593

52. Durand ML, Calderwood SB, Weber DJ, Miller SI, Southwick FS, Caviness VS, Swartz MN (1993) Acute bacterial meningitis in adults. A review of 493 episodes. N Engl J Med 328: 21-28

53. Pfister HW (1993) Akut-entzündliche Erkrankungen des Zentralnervensystems. Akt Neurol 20:83-88

54. Pfister HW, Feiden W, Einhäupl KM (1993) Spectrum of complications during bacterial meningitis in adults. Arch Neurol 50

55. Klein JO, Feigin RD, McCracken GHJ (1986) Report of the task force on diagnosis and management of meningitis. Pediatrics 78:959-982

56. Täuber MG, Sachdeva M, Kennedy SL, Loetscher H, Lesslauer W (1992) Toxicity in neuronal cells caused by cerebrospinal fluid from pneumococcal and gram-negative meningitis. J Infect Dis 166:1045-1050

57. Saukkonen K, Sande S, Cioffe C (1990) The role of cytokines in the generation of inflammation and tissue damage in experimental gram-positive meningitis. J Exp Med 171: 439-448

58. Leist TP, Frei K, Kam-Hansen S, Zinkernagel RM, Fontana A (1988) Tumor necrosis factor alpha in cerebrospinal fluid during bacterial, but not viral meningitis. J Exp Med 167: 1743-1748

59. Tuomanen E, Liu H, Hengstler B, Zak O, Tomasz A (1985) The induction of meningeal inflammation by components of the pneumococcal cell wall. J Infect Dis 151:859-868

60. Tuomanen E (1993) Bakterielle Meningitis und die Blut-Hirn-Schranke. Spektr Wissensch 4:86-90

61. Arditi M, Ables L, Yogev R (1989) Cerebrospinal fluid endotoxin levels in children with H. influenzae meningitis before and after administration of intravenous ceftriaxone. J Infect Dis 160:1005-1111

62. Tunkel AR, Wispelwey B, Scheld M (1990) Bacterial meningitis: recent advances in pathophysiology and treatment. Ann Intern Med 112:610-623

63. Quagliarello V, Scheld M (1992) Bacterial meningitis: pathogenesis, pathophysiology and progress. N Engl J Med 327:864-872

SCORING SYSTEMS '95

Acubase: Fundamentals and Perspectives

G. TULLI, G. BOCCONI, R. OGGIONI, E. MESSERI, V. MANGANI, A. VENEZIANI, R. IAMELLO

Introduction

Acubase, a product developed by two young intensive care specialists: Mark Palazzo and John Vogel and realized by Clinical Information System Inc. (CIS) in Seattle (USA), is a clinical data management, research and decision system for health care professionals in the adult and pediatric intensive care units.

Acubase is written in 4th Dimension and is compiled with 4D Runtime, a fully functional version of the 4th Dimension Software, making it unnecessary for the user to purchase 4th Dimension separately. The international version requires that the user have the 4th Dimension Runtime Diskette for occasional insertion as a "key disk".

4th Dimension (4D) is a relational database and 4D Runtime serves as the compiler for the database. 4th Dimension allows Acubase to use all the Macintosh computer interface features including menus, windows, buttons, pop-up menus, scrollable areas, radio buttons, and check buttons.

Acubase is supplied with the appropriate filters for export of data for analysis in other programs and other computer systems, including mainframes, PC's and others. Hardware requirements arc: any Macintosh computer with a 68020 processor or higher, including a Power Macintosh or a Macintosh Power-book, a minimum monitor display of 13" or 14" displaying 640 x 480 pixels (640 x 400 on PowerBook 170, 180), color desirable, operating system 6.05 or higher with system 7.1 or 7.5 strongly recommended, memory DRam-8Mb, hard disk with a minimum of 80 Mb.

Acubase fills a gap in typical hospital information systems by providing an easy to use but comprehensive way to apply complex patient-acuity scoring systems to the management of staffing and treatment protocols. It simplifies the maintenance and analysis of patient data for the ICU. It provides an easily accessible way to continuously monitor both the quality and cost of patient care.

Acubase is useful both for the clinician who requires very simple data collection and for the research worker who wants to record and retrieve complex data for later analysis. The program offers extensive capabilities for audits of unit performance and generates reports which can be either automatic or user-customized. It allows the user to record simple or complex data with equal ease.

In addition to providing for more routine needs, such as automatic generation of entry and discharge letters, Acubase automatically calculates the most commonly used severity of illness scores for purposes of assessment of quality of care and permits analysis and transfer of data.

Acubase in adult and pediatric intensive care units

Acubase provides a wide range of data management services including: calculating critical illness severity scores, retrieving and graphing data and statistics, performing prognostic calculations, and tracking demographic, trauma, hemodynamic, diagnostic, follow-up, daily discharge, nonsurvivor, and organ donation data.

The following is a more detailed description of these services and their function.

General and demographic data

The general data sheet is the starting point for all patient data entry. This sheet consists of six different pages which cover: admission details, diagnostic details, history and examination, past medical history, trauma data, and MPM admission data.

A. Admission details: this page contains demographic data including: ICU number, hospital number, name and first name, date of admission, sex, date of birth, race, address and telephone, contact information, date of hospital admission, date of ICU admission, ICU consulting physician, referring physician, primary care physician and from where the patient was admitted or transferred.

B. Diagnostic details: this page allows the user to enter details concerning the reason for admission, return admissions, diagnosis, patient group, problems and operations. Diagnoses, problems and operations. Fields each have their own modifiable pop-up lists providing options to choose from to document the state of the patients, to ensure consistency in data entry.

C. History and exam: this free-text section enables the user to record the current medical history leading to the patient's admission and physical examination.

D. Past medical history: the past medical history page also allows the user to enter information on medical history, treatment history and allergies.

E. Trauma: the trauma page applies only to those patients who have suffered injuries. Acubase provides a modifiable pop-up list of injuries to choose from, and based on selections, including the complete AIS-90 listing. When an injury is selected, Acubase will automatically calculate the Injury Severity Score (ISS), the Revised Trauma Score (RTS) and the subsequent calculation of the TRISS index with prediction of chance of survival (1-3).

F. MPM 2°: the user may choose to calculate the MPM 2° score and response to a series of physiologic and diagnosis/condition related questions. Coronary, burn, cardiac surgery, pediatric, and readmitted patients are excluded from MPM 2° (4-6).

Daily data sheet

The daily data sheet contains information essential for the calculation of acuity scores and prognoses. Once daily data is entered, a summary report for the day may be printed.

A. Daily data: the daily data page records basic patient information. In addition, senior physicians may enter an evaluation that includes orders for future treatment and a prognosis. Daily data fields are: temperature, systolic blood pressure, diastolic blood pressure, mean blood pressure°, heart rate, ventricular tachycardia or fibrillation, ventilated/CPAP, respiratory rate, %O_2, PaO_2, PaO_2/FIO_2°, history of chronic renal failure, sodium, potassium, creatinine, urea, HCO_3, glucose, urine output, fluid balance°, Hct(%), platelets, albumin, WBC, bilirubin, prothrombin time, systemic anticoagulation (° = automatically calculated value).

B. Daily data page 2: chronic health and Glasgow Coma Scores, entered here, combine with previously entered daily data to provide the basis for APACHE 2°, APS (acute physiology score), SAPS, and OFS (organ failure) scores (7-10).

C. APACHE 3°/SAPS 2°: Acubase calculates an APACHE 3° score based on data entered regarding eye, verbal and motor response. The presence of comorbidity conditions is also entered to generate both APACHE 3° and SAPS 2°. Acubase does not provide for calculation of APACHE 3° prognoses (11, 12). The methodology for these calculations is (at this date) still proprietary information and is unavailable for inclusion in Acubase.

D. Infections and problems: infections and problems may be entered, traced and reported from user modifiable lists. Site of infection, organism involved, problems and evolution are all recorded.

E. Monitoring and treatment: all treatments given, and monitors used, by the patient are recorded daily from lists with default options. Entering monitor and treatment data automatically calculates TISS (therapeutic intervention scoring system) (13). Costs are automatically calculated based on hospital-specific treatment and monitor costs in order to generate a patient's daily cost of care. The monitoring and treatment page also includes a field for documenting a nursing dependency score. The score is based on the guidelines suggested by the British Intensive Care Society and is a useful general descriptor of patient acuity.

F. Daily notes: the user may enter free text about the patient that may be searched or printed at a late date.

G. Other investigations: the investigation page allows the user to enter details of
   any number of additional tests along with their results. This information may
   be searched or analyzed at any time.

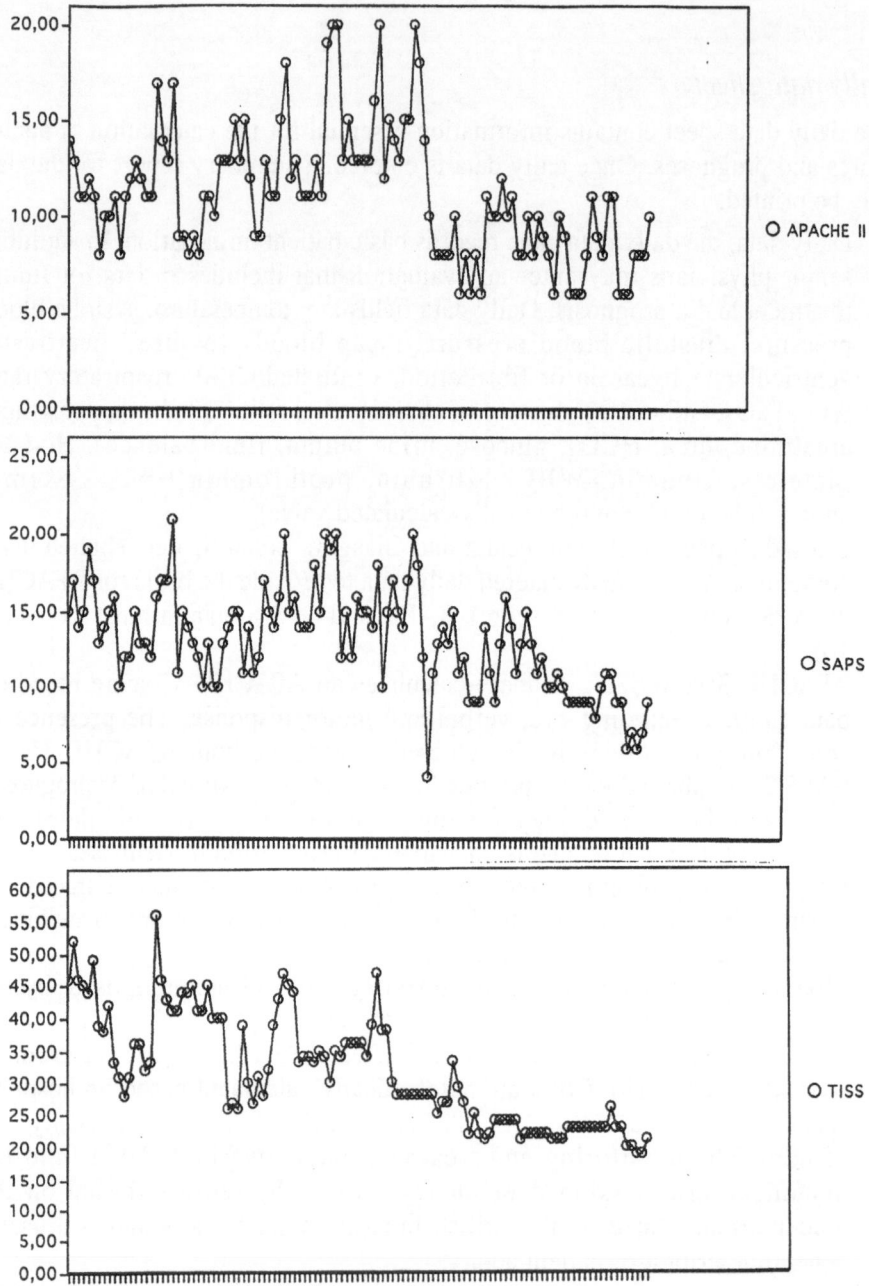

Fig. 1. Day in unit

Other data

Acubase provides for the collection of hemodinamic data at a frequency of 1 h or less, a discharge sheet, the calculation of TISS on discharge, and the calculation of Apache 2° prognosis.

A. Hemodynamic sheet: the hemodynamic sheet provides for recording as many hemodynamic measurements per day as are necessary. The fields included are: time of test, hours post admission, drug used, weight, height, BSA, lactate, Hb, heart rate, mean heart pressure°, cardiac output°, CVP°, meanPAP°, PCWP, systemic vascular resistance°, SVR index°, stroke volume°, LVSWI°, pulmonary vascular resistance°, PVR°, stroke index°, RVSW°, cardiac index°, arterial blood values°, venous blood values° (° = automatically calculated values).

B. Discharge sheet: the discharge sheet allows the user to summarize the patient's progress and record final outcomes. The information on this sheet includes: basic patient information, date of discharge, discharged to, survivor/nonsurvivor, details of death, details of stay, summary of ICU stay, treatment on discharge, points to survey, follow-up data.

C. Calculation of TISS on discharge: some authorities consider that a TISS calculation for the last 24 h in the ICU is a useful monitor of whether a patient has been appropriately discharged to a step down or ward facility. Acubase automatically calculates this score for the last 24 h prior to discharge.

D. Calculation of prognosis/APACHE 2°: on completion of sufficient daily data entry, Acubase calculates six prognostic indices.

Accessed through senior medical in the discharge data sheet, Acubase will first present graphs indicating the change in APACHE 2° and TISS scores with time, and organ system failures (OSF) during the patient's stay. The second page provides a tabulation of prognostic indices based on entered data as follows: the doctor's estimate of prognosis, the risk of death based on the reason for admission coefficient and the worst APACHE 2° score in the first 24 h, the APACHE 2° risk of death based on response to treatment by day 4, the SAPS 2° risk of death on day 1, the OFS and trend analysis, the TRISS chance of survival score, and the MPM 2° prognosis on admission, at 24 h, at 48 h and at 72 h.

Extracting data from Acubase

Data can be extracted from Acubase through several mechanisms including standard reports, user-designed reports, general searchs, and an export data function.

A. Reports and stats menu: the reports and stats menu permits both quick surveys of data and examination of specific data on more detail.
   1° Standard reports and summaries
      Admission report - a summary of patients admitted to the unit.

Unit report - a list of patients in the unit during a user specified time interval.

Diagnosis report - a list of patients by their diagnosis.

Infection report - a list of patients by tipe of infection and/or micro-organism.

Trauma report - a list of patients by injury.

Referring doctor report - a list of patients by referring consultant.

A daily data summary report is also available. This summary is printed directly from the daily data section.

2° General search: the general search allows one to obtain a list of patients with certain search criteria, from simple one level searches to complex searches with multiple variables and search criteria. The results of the search may be printed in user-designed reports or exported for further analysis.

3° Exporting data: exporting commonly required data to a statistics package or spreadsheet is most easily accomplished through the general search quick report function. It may also be exported through the export data function by choosing from lists containing data on entry or data related to ICU stay.

B. Graphs menu: the graphs menu includes options for illustrating occupancy, type of patients, actual versus predicted mortality, and outcomes. Standard graphs include: ISS vs mortality/annum, SAPS 2° vs mortality/annum, SAPS 2° predicted vs actual mortality, APACHE 2° vs mortality/annum, APACHE 2° predicted vs actual mortality, TRISS predicted vs actual mortality, occupancy by unit, patient type, and patient outcome.

Individual patient parameters may be graphed directly from the daily data section to illustrate trends and daily progress.

C. Complex reports: an ICU nonsurvivors report and a prognostic report may be printed based on user specified search parameters. Follow-up letters to send to patients or referring physicians may also be customized through this function.

D. Quick reports: quick reports provides a way to: produce lists of records with summary calculations from all data or user-defined searches.

– Design tabular reports with titles, column headings, and subcategory headings with lists
– Use different fonts, styles, and numerical formats in the report
– Produce unique reports or save standard reports to be run each week, month or quarter
– Export data in ASCII file format for additional analysis

Nursing data

Adequacy of nursing staff for the patient workload may be assessed using information in the nursing audit section. There are four menu choices: enter nursing data, view nursing data, nursing graphs and reports, and search nursing data.

A. Enter nursing data: enter nursing data allows one to enter data on the total beds full per shift, the number of beds closed per shift, the number of nurses per shift, the number of nurses absent per shift and the total nursing dependency score.

Table 1. Acubase server

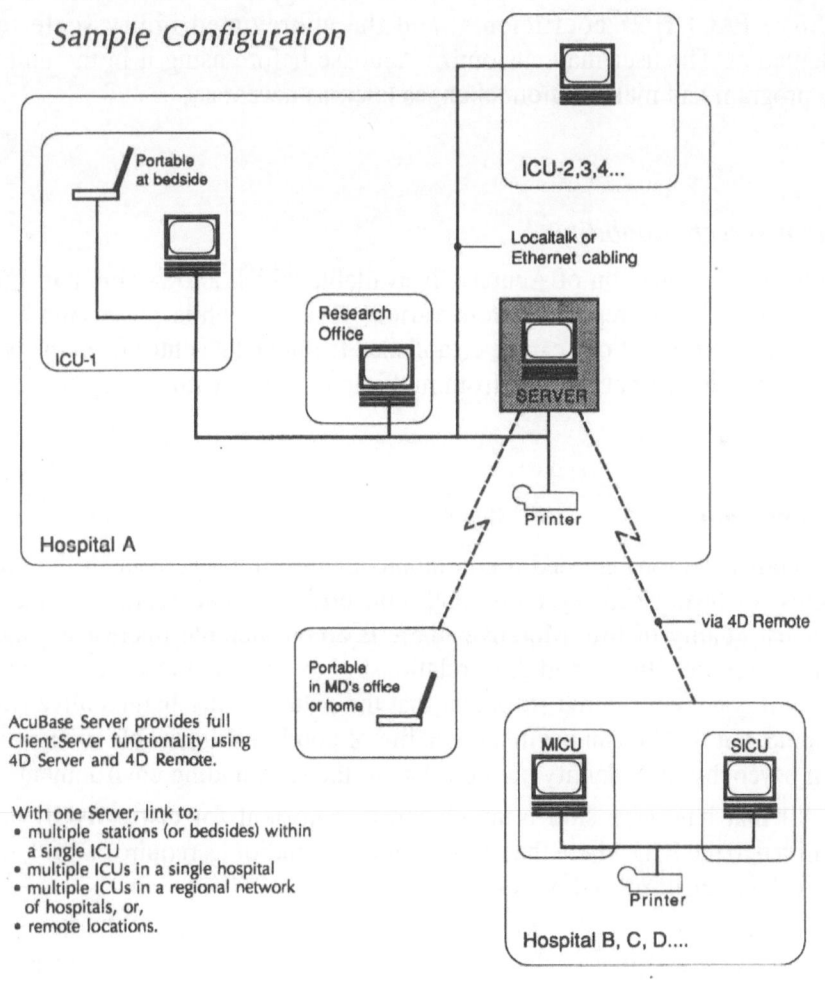

Sample Configuration

Portable at bedside

ICU-2,3,4...

Localtalk or Ethernet cabling

Research Office

ICU-1

SERVER

Printer

Hospital A

via 4D Remote

Portable in MD's office or home

AcuBase Server provides full Client-Server functionality using 4D Server and 4D Remote.

MICU

SICU

With one Server, link to:
- multiple stations (or bedsides) within a single ICU
- multiple ICUs in a single hospital
- multiple ICUs in a regional network of hospitals, or,
- remote locations.

Printer

Hospital B, C, D....

AcuBase Server available now for Apple Macintosh™.
PC (Windows) version available Summer '95.

Clinical Information Systems, Inc.
83 South King Street, Suite 617
Seattle, WA 98104 USA 206/583-0338

B. View nursing data: data entered under enter nursing data may be viewed between the dates requested.
C. Nursing graphs and reports: nursing data may be graphed and reported by date and shift.

Customizing Acubase

Acubase can be customized by the user to meet the needs and circumstances of the hospital, ICUs, physicians and communities.

By customizing, the user can add particular treatments, costs, injuries, diagnoses, and other items to pop-up lists that appear in the program as well as TISS, APACHE 2° coefficients, and the abbreviated injury scale for ISS calculation. The user may customize Acubase before using it in the unit or use the program and make custom changes later, as necessary.

Client-server capability

A client-server version of Acubase is available which allows simultaneous data entry, analysis and reporting from various locations while preserving a central database. Configurations can be established to allow data entry from the bedside, from multiple distinct units or from multiple hospitals within a region (Table 1).

Conclusions

Hospitals have long needed a continuous quality improvement in the complex context of health care systems, both concerning actual treatments and future patients' quality of life. Moreover there is a considerable interest in quality of care, severity of illness and their relationship to costs and resources in the ICU. Today it is not considered sufficient that the patient is discharged alive from the hospital, but that he can begin again a life of good quality, is able to maintain his own psycophysical identity and to relate to the surrounding environment.

All that has been said is much more important for critically ill patients admitted to the ICU where the life-threatening conditions require careful, reliable clinical and instrumental monitoring.

For this reason many severity of illness scorings (severity disease indexes) have been created that enable stratification of patients into different groups of severity, elaborations of statistical probability models of death based on linear uni- or multivariate regression equations, evaluations of staff workloads, costs, and complications (14).

A single severity score, by itself, is not enough to give all these data. Different systems have been created and developed and implemented that have the main advantage of deriving a death probability from a set of data, chosen as the worse ones, recorded in the first 24 h after admission. These data do not reckon complications developing during this time, such as MOFS iatrogenic injuries, emergency surgical interventions etc.

Dynamic systems have been developed that have a better predictive value in comparison to static systems and they are more reliable even if burdensome in recording data and in calculating death probability (15, 16). Following the patient day by day in the evaluation of the initial pathologies, therapeutic effects, monitoring and nursing/medical staffing demonstrate the complexity of the case mix; a single score is not enough to avoid what was previously said, manual elaboration of data, on line recording is a utopia still today in most Italian hospitals. To respond to all these needs many software packages have been developed, among them Acubase totally devoted to ICU.

Acubase provides user help in clinical decision making management and research. Acubase is an easy, user friendly program, it allows one to quantify quality of care with standard international criteria, to apply therapeutic protocol management, to evaluate the use of health care personnel, to simplify continuous patient analysis procedures, monitoring, quality and critical care costs. Demographic data, diagnostic data, hemodynamic data, discharge and follow-up data, and data related to organ procurements are recorded. Automatically daily APACHE 2° and 3°, SAPS 1°, SAPS 2°, MPM 2°, TRISS, ISS, RTS, OFS, TISS are calculated. It is possible to recall data from different categories, matching data and linking them to elaboration and evolution statistical programs, to have prognoses on the final outcome, to evaluate bed occupancy rates, nursing dependency score, daily costs and total costs. All these data can be graphically represented on monitors and printers.

Our experience

From 1/1/1993 Acubase was used in the ICU in Florence, version 3.3M initially and then the new version 3.4M on an Apple Macintosh computer with a Motorola 68030 (Power PC Macintosh) processor. The first record of physiological variables and infections and treatments is done on an appropriately developed flow chart; this happens every day for every admitted patient. A group of intensive care specialists (specifically trained and dedicated part time to Acubase) introduces data in the program and elaborates data, also on request by some ICU doctor.

The annual general review of our ICU is an example of Acubase clinical management (Table 2).

Actually (from July 1995) we are working on a new version 3.5 Acubase.

G. Tulli, G. Bocconi, R. Oggioni et al.

Table 2. Acubase program

	1993	1994
General data		
Admitted	159	193 (+21.38%)
Enrolled	138	182 (+30.43%)
Men	88	124 (+40.91%)
Women	50	58 (+12.00%)
Mean age (men)	66.04	65.03 (−1.53%)
Mean age (women)	65.04	58.50 (−10.05%)
Admission pathology mortality		
Mortality (men)	36 (40.9%)	45 (−4.61%)
Mortality (women)	20 (40%)	18 (−7.86%)
Surgical	64	81 (+20,99%)
Nonsurvivors	22 (34.37%)	91 (+28.57%)
Medical	65	42 (−4.62%)
Nonsurvivors	33 (50.77%)	9
Trauma	9	1
Nonsurvivors	1 (11.11%)	
Mean severity scoring		
Apache 2° 23 SD 8.188		
APACHE 2°	23 ± 8.188	
APACHE 3°	82 ± 28.352	68.22
SAPS 1°	21 ± 5.309	
SAPS 2°		41.36
Medical pathology		
APACHE 2° nonsurvivors	26.46	
Cut-off point 0.5	28	
APACHE 3° nonsurvivors	103.23	90.68
Cut-off point 0.5	82	82
SAPS 1° nonsurvivors	23.42	
Cut-off point 0.5	26	
SAPS 2° nonsurvivors		58.54
Cut-off point 0.5		47
Surgical pathology		
APACHE 2° nonsurvivors	26.46	
Cut-off point 0.5	31	
APACHE 3° nonsurvivors	82.35	
Cut-off point 0.5	83	83
SAPS 1° nonsurvivors	22.41	
Cut-off point 0.5	26	
SAPS 2° nonsurvivors		41.36
Cut-off point 0.5		
Costs and length of stay		
Cost survivors (Italian Lire)	19,370,000 ± 26,080,000	18,429,600 (−4.85%)
Cost nonsurvivors	20,633,000 ± 27,081,041	26,213,302 (+27.02%)
Effective cost survivors	35,777,777	32,646,000 (−8.75%)
LOS		
LOS survivors (day)	12,91 ± 55.159	12.29
LOS nonsurvivors	13.75 ± 19.069	13.60
Global		12.74

Acubase is available worldwide from Clinical Information System (CIS) 83 South King Street, Suite 617 - Seattle, WA 98104 USA - telephone 206/583-0338 - fax 206/583-0349.

References

References on which the Scoring Calculation in Acubase are derived include the following:

1. American Association for Automotive Medicine. The Abbreviated Injury Scale, 1990 Revision, Arlington Heights, IL 60005 (1990)
2. Baker S, O'Neill B (1976) The injury severity score: an update. J Trauma 882-885
3. Body C, Tolson M, Copes W (1987) Evaluating trauma care: the TRISS method. J Trauma 27:370-78
4. Lemeshow S, Teres D, Klar J, Spitz Avrunin J, Gehlbach SH, Rapoport J (1993) Mortality probability models (MPM2°) based on an international cohort of intensive care unit patients. JAMA 270:2478-2486
5. Lemeshow S, Le Gal JR (1994) Modelling the severity of illness of ICU patients: a systems update. JAMA 274:1049-1055
6. Lemeshow S, Klar J, Teres D, Avrunin JS, Gelbach SH, Rapoport J, Rué M (1994) Mortality probability models for patients in intensive care unit for 48-72 hours: a prospective multicenter study. Crit Care Med 22:1351-1358
7. Knaus WA, Draper EA, Wagner DP, Zimmerman JE (1985) APACHE II: a severity of disease classification system. Crit Care Med 818-829
8. Le Gall J, Loirat P, Albertovich A et al (1984) A simplified acute physiology score for ICU patients. Crit Care Clin 231-232
9. Knaus W, Draper E, Wagner D, Zimmerman J (1985) Prognosis in acute organ system failure. Ann Surg 685-693
10. Knaus WA, Wagner D (1989) Multiple system organ failure: epidemiology and prognosis. Crit Care Clin 231-232
11. Knaus W, Wagner D, Draper E, Zimmerman j, Bergner M Bastos P, Sirio C, Murphy D, Lotring T, Damiano A, Harrel F (1991) The APACHE III prognostic system. Chest 1619-1636
12. Le Gall JR, Lemeshow S, Saulnier T (1993) A new simplified acute physiology score (SAPS 2°) based on an European/North America multicenter study. JAMA 270:2957-2963
13. Keene A, Cullen D (1993) Therapeutic intervention scoring system: update 1993. Crit Care Med 1-3
14. Armaganidis A, Beaufils F, Bonfils X, Burchardi H, Cook D, Fagot-Largeault A, Suter P, Thijs L, Vesconi S, Williams A (1994) Predicting outcome in ICU patients. Reanim Urgences 3:141-152
15. Bion JF, Aitchison TC, Edlin SA, Ledingham IM (1988) Sickness scoring and response to treatment as predictors of outcome from critical illness. Intensive Care Med 167-172
16. Chang RW, Jacobs S, Lee B (1988) Predicting outcome among intensive care patients using computerised trend analysis of daily APACHE II scores corrected for organ system failure. Intensive Care Med 558-566

PERIOPERATIVE PROBLEMS
IN OBESE PATIENTS

Obesity and Coexisting Diseases: Anesthesiological Point of View

L. SOLLAZZI, V. PERILLI, P. BOZZA, R. RANIERI, R. TACCHINO, M. CASTAGNETO, M. CROCI, P. PELOSI

Introduction

Obesity is a metabolic disease in which adipose tissue represents a proportion of body tissue greater than normal (more than 30% of body weight). Up to 33% of the population in North America and 20% in Italy can be considered obese, exceeding by 10% or more their ideal body weight. Recently, great improvement has been made in developing new surgical techniques for the treatment of obesity such as ileojejunal bypass and/or gastric binding (1). However, since these patients are characterized by several systemic physiopathological alterations, the anesthesiological management in the perioperative period may present several problems, mainly related to their body habitus, respiratory and cardiovascular derangements (2). In this review, we will briefly discuss the anesthesiological management of obese patients in the perioperative period.

Definition of obesity

In clinical practice the anesthetist may use several methods to assess excess body weight (2): 1) height/weight tables; 2) calculation of the ratio between actual and ideal weight (relative weight) – for calculation of ideal weight in kg, one can substract 100 (men) and 105 (women) from the patient's height in cm; 3) calculation of body mass index (BMI). BMI is simply calculated as weight/height (kg/m²). People are considered obese if the relative weight exceeds 1.1 or BMI > 30 kg/m², while morbid obesity is defined as a relative weight exceeding 2 and BMI > 40 kg/m².

Physiology

Respiratory disorders

Obese patients are characterized by marked disorders in respiratory mechanics, increased respiratory work load and high metabolic demands.

These alterations may be more pronounced during the intra- and postoperative period, particularly in patients with pre-existing respiratory disorders.

Respiratory mechanics

Severe alterations in respiratory system mechanics have been reported both in awake and in anesthetized-paralyzed morbidly obese patients (3-5). However, the individual relative role of the lung and chest wall has not been completely clarified. In fact Naimark and Cherniak (3) supported the idea that the main reason for the reduction in respiratory compliance was the decrease in chest wall compliance, while other authors did not find alterations in the chest wall (6). Recently, Pelosi et al. (4) reported that, at least during anesthesia and paralysis, both chest wall and lung compliance are reduced and lung resistance increased, as a result of increased adiposity (in and around the ribs, diaphragm and abdomen) and smaller functional residual capacity (FRC) (4, 7). The severe reduction in FRC is probably due to the developing of extensive atelectatic areas, as generally occurs in normal people, during anesthesia (8).

Respiratory work

Respiratory work is increased and the efficiency of breathing is decreased in obese patients as a result of decreased respiratory compliance and increased resistance. In normal subjects, respiratory work is divided evenly between lung and chest wall inflation. In contrast, in obese patients, respiratory work is increased mainly as a result of low pulmonary compliance (55%), being the contribution of low chest wall compliance and high pulmonary resistance 30% and 15%, respectively (4).

Metabolic demands and oxygenation

Alterations of respiratory mechanics and increased respiratory work impose high metabolic demands in obese patients (2). These demands are reflected by an increased oxygen consumption ($\dot{V}O_2$) and carbon dioxide production. Moreover, as mentioned above, in obese patients, FRC is markedly reduced, and during anesthesia may decline to less than closing capacity, leading to airway closure, V/Q mismatch and hypoxemia. Several authors found an intrapulmonary shunt of 10%-15% in obese compared with 2%-5% in normal subjects (9). Dead space is usually increased (up to 61% of tidal volume), although normal dead space has been found in both awake and anesthetized obese subjects (4, 10).

Cardiovascular disorders

The cardiac pathology in obese patients is mainly an adaptation of the cardiovascular system to the overweight and increased metabolic demand (11-14). Moreover, obesity itself, may produce anatomic alterations in cardiac structure. The fat excess, in fact, may be localized in the heart structures, inducing severe impairment of the mechanical and electric performance. Generally, extreme obesity is associated with several hemodynamic alterations.

Cardiac output and heart rate

Total blood volume and cardiac output (CO) increase in direct proportion to the amount of the patient's overweight and to the increased $\dot{V}O_2$. High CO is mainly caused by the increased blood flow to the fatty tissue; in fact the total distribution of CO is similar in obese and in normal subjects. Since the increase in CO and $\dot{V}O_2$ are proportional, the arterovenous oxygen difference is normal or slightly increased.

The heart rate being roughly normal, the increase in CO is mainly due to an increase in stroke volume (SV).

Pulmonary artery and systemic hypertension

In the obese, pulmonary artery pressure is increased for several reasons:
1. High CO, independent of the pulmonary vascular resistance
2. Progressive hypoxia and hypercapnia (obesity hypoventilation syndrome) inducing pulmonary artery vasoconstriction with pulmonary artery hypertension

Moreover, there is a frequent association between obesity and systemic hypertension due to increased activity of the renin-angiotensin-aldosterone system, increased total blood volume, increased sympathetic activity and hyperinsulinism. Mortality in hypertensive obese patients is reported to be higher than in nonhypertensive individuals.

Left and right ventricular dysfunction

The consequent elevation of filling pressures, due to the abnormalities in diastolic function, may easily induce congestive heart failure. A larger SV induces an elevation in left and right ventricle work with a consequent increase in cavity size, in accordance with Laplace's law. This predisposes to eccentric ventricular hypertrophy, and consequently, to ventricular dysfunction. However, only exceptionally right heart pathology is predominant in obese patients (Pickwickian syndrome).

Cardiac arrhythmias

Many rhythm disturbances may be present in obesity caused by myocardial hypertrophy and ischemic heart disease. Some authors described a relationship between fatty infiltration, arrhythmias and sudden death.

Ischemic heart disease

Several studies (13, 14) suggest a close relationship between obesity and ischemic heart disease. Recently it has been demonstrated that cardiovascular disease risk factors are related to body fat distribution rather than to total body weight: visceral fat deposition, particularly intraabdominal, constitutes the principal risk factor. Several anthropometric parameters are used to estimate the fat distribution in connection with the cardiovascular risk. The best parameter is the "waist-to-hip" ratio, that is the ratio between the intraabdominal and the subcutaneous fat. Nevertheless the pathogenesis of coronary disease in obesity is again substantially uncertain.

Gastrointestinal disorders

The obese population is characterized by a high incidence of gastroesophageal reflux, a gastric juice volume greater than 25 ml and pH less than 2.5, increasing the risk of gastric content aspiration and subsequent pneumonitis (2).

Pharmacological considerations

Several factors, related both to obesity and the drug used, may modify pharmacokinetics in the obese compared to normal subjects: change in volume distribution and protein binding properties, increased renal clearance and changes in liver clearance (2, 15).

Volume distribution

The etiology of the changes in drug distribution in the obese includes a smaller fraction of total body water, greater adipose tissue content, increased lean body mass and changed tissue protein binding, increased blood volume and modifications in its constituents. Many drugs are administered on the basis of dose per unit body weight, assuming a proportionality between clearance and body weight, however; this assumption is not valid in obesity because of changes in body composition and volume distribution.

Plasma protein binding

Although plasma protein binding is not modified by obesity, altered blood composition (increased lipid concentration) may affect protein binding, thus reducing free drug concentration.

Drug clearance

Renal clearance is increased in obesity, while hepatic clearance is roughly normal.

Anesthetic management

Preoperative care

Preoperative care assessment includes: preoperative physical examination, premedication and preparation for surgery.

Preoperative physical examination

The physician should review the medical history, perform a careful physical examination, detailed assessment of the upper airway and baseline laboratory screening. In particular, the anesthetist should be aware of the problems related to mask ventilation and tracheal intubation in this kind of patient. In fact obese patients are characterized by a fat face, short and fat neck and limited movement of the jaw, neck and head. The cardiovascular and respiratory performance should also be carefully evaluated, especially in patients with a positive history of cardiopulmonary disease.

Premedication

There are no specific guidelines on this subject; however, we may suggest: 1) to not widely use opioids as preanesthetic medication and prescribe small doses of sedatives; 2) to administer histamine H_2 receptor blocking agents; 3) to avoid i.m. premedication because of unpredictability of absorption.

Preparation for surgery

An i.v. peripheral cannulation is mandatory and when possible a central venous cannulation, preferably performed the night before surgery.

Routine monitoring should include inspiratory airway pressure, ECG, pulse oximeter, urinary catheter, and carbon dioxide analysis. Moreover, the use of a nasogastric tube is mandatory. Patients should not lie supine because of possible impairment of ventilation, and possibly, in reverse Trendelenburg's position. A prophylactic anticoagulant therapy should be considered in all obese patients to reduce the risk of pulmonary embolism.

Intraoperative care

Intraoperative care includes the induction and maintenance of anesthesia.

Induction of anesthesia

It has been suggested that more than one anesthetist should be involved in the induction of anesthesia for expected difficult tracheal intubation.

Preoxygenation is mandatory for at least 10-20 min. An awake intubation, with or without a fiberoptic bronchoscope, is suggested, although it is not performed by all anesthetists.

Maintenance of anesthesia

No single anesthetic regimen has been shown to be superior to others; nevertheless balanced anesthesia is preferable to general anesthesia alone.

Large tidal volume (15-20 ml/kg ideal body weight), large manually performed lung inflations and high inspiratory oxygen fraction have been recommended. In contrast, the application of a positive end-expiratory pressure (PEEP) has been discouraged (16), although Pelosi et al. (17) recently demonstrated that low levels of PEEP (5-10 cm H_2O) together with moderate tidal volume (6-8 ml/kg ideal body weight) may improve respiratory mechanics and oxygenation.

Postoperative care

Mortality and respiratory complications, in the postoperative period, are more common in obese than in normal patients (18). Moreover obese patients who suffer from coexisting respiratory diseases more frequently develop postoperative complications than obese patients free of these diseases. In the postoperative period respiratory mechanics and lung volumes are particularly affected, thus causing a marked increase in work of breathing and prolonged hypoxemia (4). However, the need for postoperative ventilatory support is rare. Several measures may decrease the frequency of pulmonary complications, in the postoperative period, among them 1) maintenance of a semirecumbent position, 2) intensive chest physiotherapy and 3) nocturnal nasal continuous positive airway pressure.

Personal experience

Here we report the clinical experience in the Catholic University Hospital of Sacred Heart from April 1990 to April 1995, in 160 patients (127 women and 33 men, age 41 ± 8 years, 1.2 ± 0.4 overweight) who underwent biliopancreatic diversion. Sixty of 160 patients had positive anamnesis for cardiovascular disease (58 hypertension, one ischemic heart disease and one mitral valvular disease). Patients were premedicated with diazepam 0.01 mg/kg p.o.; induction was performed after 5 min denitrogenation with O_2 100%, with penthotal 2-3 mg/kg and fentanyl 3 mcg/kg. Maintenance of anesthesia was conducted with isofluorane 0.5-1.5% and N_2O; neuromuscular blockade was obtained with vecuronium or atracurium. Patients were mechanically ventilated with tidal volume 8 ml/kg and respiratory rate of 10 bpm, aiming to $ETCO_2$ of 30 mmHg.

During surgical procedure blood gases and hemodynamic determinations were collected at the following times (Table 1): 1) after endotracheal intubation; 2) after laparotomy; 3) after positioning of distractors; 4) in reverse Trendelenburg's position; and 5) at the end of surgery (in the recovery room, in spontaneous ventilation, $FiO_2 = 40\%$).

Table 1. Blood gases and hemodynamic determinations

	I	II	III	IV	V
PaO$_2$ (mmHg)	142 ± 52	171 ± 81	176 ± 56	156 ± 73	140 ± 31
PaCO$_2$ (mmHg)	38 ± 4	35 ± 6	32 ± 5	33 ± 5	37 ± 4
P(A-a)O$_2$ (mmHg)	197 ± 122	194 ± 80	211 ± 188	200 ± 118	161 ± 89
PAS (mmHg)	140 ± 19	143 ± 18	142 ± 15	130 ± 21	142 ± 28
PAD (mmHg)	71 ± 17	73 ± 11	76 ± 15	69 ± 12	75 ± 15
HR (bpm)	83 ± 14	85 ± 17	84 ± 13	83 ± 18	80 ± 14

Legend of the table: Data are expressed as mean ± SD. P(A-a)O$_2$, alveolar arterial oxygen pressure; PAS, systolic artery pressure; PAD, diastolic artery pressure, HR, heart rate.
Determinations were obtained at the following times: I, after endotracheal intubation; II, after laparotomy; III, after positioning of distractors; IV, in reverse Trendelenburg's position; V, at the end of surgery (in the recovery room, in spontaneous ventilation, FiO$_2$ = 40%).

References

1. Pace WG, Martin EW, Tetirick T, Fabri PJ, Carey LC (1979) Gastric partitioning for morbid obesity. Ann Surg 190:392-400
2. Shenkman Z, Shir Y, Brodsky JB (1993) Perioperative management of the obese patient. Br J Anaesth 70:349-359
3. Naimark A, Cherniack RM (1960) Compliance of the respiratory system and its components in health and obesity. J Appl Physiol 15:377-382
4. Pelosi P, Croci M, Ravagnan I, Vicardi P, Gattinoni L (1995) Total respiratory system, lung and chest wall mechanics in sedated-paralyzed postoperative morbidly obese patients. Chest (in press)
5. Pelosi P, Croci M, Ravagnan I, Cerisara M, Vicardi P, Lissoni A, Gattinoni L (1995) Analysis of behavior of the respiratory system in sedated-paralyzed morbidly obese patients: effects of flow, volume and time. J Appl Physiol (submitted)
6. Suratt PM, Wilhoit SC, Atkinson RL, Rochester DF (1984) Compliance of chest wall in obese patients. J Appl Physiol 57:403-407
7. Damia G, Mascheroni D, Croci M, Tarenzi L (1988) Perioperative changes in the functional residual capacity in morbidly obese patients. Br J Anaesth 60:574-578
8. Tokics L, Hedenstierna G, Strandberg A, Brismar B, Lundquist H (1987) Lung collapse and gas-exchange during anesthesia: effect of spontaneous breathing, muscle paralysis and positive end-expiratory pressure. Anesthesiology 66:157-167
9. Sodeberg J, Thomson D, White T (1977) Respiration, circulation and anesthetic management in obesity. Investigation before and after jejunoileal bypass. Acta Anesthesiol Scand 21:55-61
10. Hedenstierna G, Santesson J (1976) Breathing mechanics, dead space and gas-exchange in the extremely obese, breathing spontaneously and during anesthesia with intermittent positive pressure ventilation. Acta Anesthesiol Scand 20:248-254
11. DeDivitiis O, Fazio S, Petitto M, Maddalena G, Contaldo F, Mancini M (1981) Obesity and cardiac function. Circulation 64:477-482
12. Kaltman AJ, Goldring RM (1976) Role of circulatory congestion in the cardiorespiratory failure of obesity. Am J Med 60:645-655
13. Manson J, Colditz GA, Stampfer MJ, Willett WC, Rosner B, Monson RR, Speizer FE, Hennekens CH (1990) A prospective study of obesity and risk of coronary heart disease in women. N Engl J Med 332:882-889
14. Rabkin SW, Mathewson FAL, Hsu PH (1977) Relation of body weight to development of ischemic heart disease in a cohort of young North American men after 26-year observation period: the Mannitoba study. Am J Cardiology 39:452-458

15. Blouin RA, Kolpek JH, Mann HJ (1987) Influence of obesity on drug disposition. Clin Pharmacy 6:706-714
16. Salem MR, Dalal FY, Zygmunt MP, Mathrubhutham M, Jacobs HK (1978) Does PEEP improve intraoperative arterial oxygenation in grossly obese patients? Anesthesiology 48: 280-281
17. Pelosi P, Norsa A, Croci M, Vicardi P, Cerisara M, Gattinoni L (1995) Physiologic effects of positive end-expiratory pressure (PEEP) in postoperative sedated-paralyzed morbidly obese patients. Intensive Care Med (in press)
18. Pemberton LB, Manax WG (1971) Relationship of obesity to postoperative complications after cholecystectomy. Am J Surg 121:87-90

Intubation by Fibroscopy in Morbidly Obese Patients

M. Croci, P. Pelosi, A. Pedoto, G. Ferrari, C. Fochi, L. Tarenzi

Visualization of the vocal cords by direct laryngoscopic view during general anaesthesia and muscles paralysis probably is the most popular technique to perform orotracheal or nasotracheal intubation, at least in Italy. However, this manoeuvre shows a variable incidence of difficulty and failure in the general surgical population.

Usually a high degree of difficulty, requiring multiple attempts to obtain endotracheal intubation, is observed in a small number of patients: an overall incidence of 1%-4% of subjects has been reported with impossible exposition of vocal cords (grade III-IV of laryngoscopic view) (1, 2). Obviously the percentage of failed intubation is still less and ranges from 0.05% to 0.35% (1-3), the high end of this range being associated with obstetric patients.

However, also in morbidly obese patients, Lee and coworkers reported an increased difficulty in endotracheal intubation, with a positive correlation between body weight and numbers of failed attempts (4).

Since difficult or failed intubation is associated with higher mortality and morbidity attributable to anaesthesia, it is important to identify in advance those patients in whom this problem could be present. Many factors can indicate difficulty of endotracheal intubation such as dental configuration, extension of atlanto-occipital joint, maxillary length and height, limited mandible movements. Nevertheless, in morbidly obese patients soft tissues rather than bone structures are altered.

Tongue size and mobility are important factors in determining difficulty in airway control (5) and actually morbidly obese patients present alterations of the soft structures of the upper airways, leading to increased resistance, at least in the subset suffering from obstructive sleep apnea syndrome (6). Also large breasts may increase the difficulty of a direct laryngoscopy because there is little room between the breasts and the mouth for the handle of a conventional laryngoscope (7). Moreover, Wilson and coworkers, in a prospective study (8), identified body weight as one of five factors contributing to difficult laryngoscopy; in the same study neck circumference was significantly higher ($p < 0.01$) in patients with laryngoscopic difficulty when compared to subjects with no laryngoscopic difficulty.

Despite the higher probability of difficult endotracheal intubation in morbidly obese patients, one can tell us that "a patient does not die from failure of tracheal intubation but from failure of oxygenation".

Unfortunately this kind of patient presents an increased difficulty in oxygenation, too, associated with difficulties in mask ventilation. Several factors could explain this: a sharp decrease in functional residual capacity is probably the most significant abnormality described during general anaesthesia in morbidly obese patients (9) and could explain the need for a higher inspired oxygen fraction to maintain an adequate arterial oxygen pressure (10); moreover, reduction in compliance and increase in resistance of the respiratory system (11), together with difficulties in maintaining a patent upper airway (12) can jeopardize the patient during face mask ventilation in anaesthetized-paralysed morbidly obese subjects.

Moreover, the increased volume of gastric content in morbidly obese patients, even after an overnight fasting, should be considered when choosing anaesthetic technique (13).

On the basis of these considerations, we believe that an endotracheal tube should be positioned while the patient is awake. Even if this is a rather unpleasant experience for the patient, there are several reasons to choose this option. First of all, patients maintain patency of the natural airway, spontaneously breathing. Moreover, muscle tone maintains the upper airway structures in the usual position so that they are much easier to identify. In contrast, anaesthesia induction and muscle paralysis are associated with changes of the anatomy which make conventional intubation more difficult (14). Furthermore the intubation of the trachea in awake patients was proposed as a method for preventing aspiration in high risk subjects (15).

Several techniques are available to perform an awake endotracheal intubation, the most important are the following: 1) blind oral, 2) blind nasal and 3) fibreoptic tracheal intubation. One of the most popular methods of intubating the trachea of an awake patient is probably the blind nasotracheal route: it has the advantage of being independent from visualization of the glottis and it has a good chance of success in a wide series of patients of different age and body size (16); unfortunately it may cause, in about 20% of patients (16, 17), an upper airway bleeding that could compromise subsequent fibreoptic efforts. Similarly, techniques are described to perform a blind orotracheal intubation (18, 19): under local anaesthesia a laryngeal mask airway is positioned and then a tracheal tube can be advanced, possibly with the support of a gum elastic bougie. Of all these intubation techniques, conventional direct laryngoscopy is perhaps the most stimulating one and requires a very cooperative patient.

The first report of the use of a fibreoptic device to intubate the trachea was by Murphy (20); subsequently fibreoptic intubation has increased in popularity since the introduction of dedicated devices (21). Fibreoptic intubation can be performed using either the oral or the nasal route and the only major impediment is the presence of a significant amount of blood and/or secretions that can interfere with the vocal cord visualization, even if this technique is used in emergency situations, too (22, 23).

Briefly, this technique needs a well lubrificated flexible fibreoptic laryngoscope to be inserted into an endotracheal tube (ETT) and then advanced through the nose or the mouth. Once the fibreoptic laryngoscope has been passed into the trachea, the ETT can be railroaded over the fibrescope and properly positioned, under direct vision, with the tip above the tracheal carina. Then the fibreoptic laryngoscope can be withdrawn, the ETT connected to the breathing circuit and general anaesthesia induced. Numerous devices were proposed to aid fibreoptic intubation through the mouth (24): all of them are designed to bring the tip of the instrument close to the laryngeal aperture without requiring much skill. When using the nasal route, this aim can be reached by advancing the ETT about 15 cm from the nostril in an average adult; in this condition the tip of the ETT will be positioned 1-2 cm proximal to the epiglottis (25).

The awake fibreoptic tracheal intubation technique has also been documented as a feasible and safe tool in subjects considered at high risk of aspiration of gastric content both in elective and emergency surgery (26).

Our experience

We have been using awake orotracheal intubation in morbidly obese patients for many years; about 150 subjects receiving general anaesthesia for elective surgery (gastroplasty or jejunoileal by-pass) were intubated using either a flexible fibreoptic laryngoscope (LF 1, Olympus) and a bite block or conventional direct laryngoscopy; the choice between the two techniques was made on the basis of the personal skill of the anaesthetist present in the operative room. No major complications (such as hypoxia, hypotension or aspiration of gastric content) or failed intubations were reported when the fibreoptic laryngoscope was used; in few poorly cooperative patients conventional laryngoscopy was unsuccessful and fibreoptic laryngoscope was used to perform orotracheal intubation from an anaesthetist skilled in this technique.

One of the major technical problems in fibreoptic orotracheal intubation is the passage of a standard, preformed polyvinyl chloride ETT through the glottic opening because the tube may catch on the epiglottis, arytenoids or aryepiglottic folds (27). To avoid this problem we use rather small ETTs (7-mm ID in female and 7.5-mm ID in male patients) and only in one woman did the ETT not pass through the glottic opening; with a smaller tube (6.5-mm ID) we were able to complete the orotracheal intubation without complications. Alternatively, if the anaesthetist wishes to position an ETT with a larger ID, it is possible to use a flexible, spiral-wound ETT. This is less likely to be impeded by glottic structures, allowing the introduction of a larger ETT into the trachea (28).

As previously stated this technique is rather unpleasant for the patient; however, it should be remembered that awake fibreoptic intubation attenuates (29) or abolishes (30) the hypertensive response usually observed during general anaesthesia and muscle paralysis when conventional laryngoscopy and endotracheal intubation are performed. We perform all these manoeuvres for getting control of the airway under local anaesthesia while the patient is only slightly sedated. In this way we avoided respiratory depression since awake fibreoptic intubation requires a longer time than endotracheal intubation with conventional laryngoscopy under general anaesthesia and muscle paralysis (31). With this approach we never observed desaturation during intubation manoeuvres; in contrast when fibreoptic intubation is performed under general anaesthesia major complications, such as desaturation and cardiac depression, are reported (32).

We conclude that awake fibreoptic tracheal intubation is a safe and useful technique in morbidly obese patients receiving general anaesthesia since this can avoid difficulties that anaesthesiologists could encounter both with conventional tracheal intubation and/or mask ventilation.

References

1. Cormack RS, Lehane J (1984) Difficult tracheal intubation in obstetrics. Anaesthesia 1105-1111
2. Samsoon GLT, Young JRB (1987) Difficult tracheal intubation: a retrospective study. Anaesthesia 42:487-490
3. Lyons G (1985) Failed intubation. Anaesthesia 40:759-762
4. Lee JJ, Larson RH, Buckley JJ, Roberts RB (1980) Airway maintenance in the morbidly obese. Anesthesiol Rev 7:33-36
5. Boliston TA (1985) Difficult tracheal intubation in obstetrics. Anaesthesia 40:389
6. Stauffer JL, Zwillich CW, Cadieux RJ, Bixler EO, Kales A, Varano LA, White DP (1987) Pharyngeal size and resistance in obstructive sleep apnea. Am Rev Respir Dis 136:623-627
7. Kay NH (1982) Mammomegaly and intubation. Anaesthesia 37:221
8. Wilson ME, Spiegelhalter D, Robertson JA, Lesser P (1988) Predicting difficult intubation. Br J Anaesth 61:211-216
9. Damia G, Mascheroni D, Croci M, Tarenzi L (1988) Perioperative changes in functional residual capacity in morbidly obese patients. Br J Anaesth 60:574-578
10. Fox GS, Whalley DG, Bevan DR (1981) Anaesthesia for the morbidly obese. Br J Anaesth 53:811-816
11. Croci M, Pelosi P, Solca M, Vicardi P, Tubiolo D, Valenza F (1994) Respiratory mechanics during anesthesia in morbidly obese patients. Anest Analg 78:S74
12. Teeple E, Ghia JN (1983) An elevated pulmonary wedge pressure resulting from upper respiratory obstruction in an obese patient. Anesthesiology 59:66-68
13. Vaughan RW, Bauer S, Wise L (1975) Volume and pH of gastric juice in obese patients. Anesthesiology 43:686-689
14. Sivarajan M, Fink RB (1990) The position and the state of the larynx during general anesthesia and muscle paralysis. Anesthesiology 79:439-442
15. Thomas JL (1969) Awake intubation. Indications, technique and a review of 25 patients. Anaesthesia 24:28-35

16. Williamson R (1989) Blind nasal intubation and (or) fibreoptic guided intubation? Anaesthesia 44:176-177
17. Coe PA, King A, Towey RM (1988) Teaching guided fibreoptic nasotracheal intubation. An assessment of an anaesthetic technique to aid training. Anaesthesia 43:410-413
18. McCrirrick A, Pracilio JA (1991) Awake intubation: a new technique. Anaesthesia 46:661-663
19. Brain AIJ (1989) Further development of the laryngeal mask. Anaesthesia 44:530
20. Murphy PA (1967) A fibreoptic endoscope used for nasal intubation. Anaesthesia 22:489-491
21. Vaughan RS (1989) Airways revisited. Br J Anaesth 62:1-3
22. Bullingham A, Hampson-Evans D, Palazzo M (1994) An impaled neck. Anaesthesia 49: 866-869
23. Shearer VE, Giesecke AH (1993) Airway management for patients with penetrating neck trauma: a retrospective study. Anest Analg 77:1135-1138
24. Patil V, Stehling LC, Zauder HL, Koch JP (1982) Mechanical aids for fiberoptic endoscopy. Anesthesiology 57:69-70
25. Roger S, Benumof JL (1983) New and easy fiberoptic endoscopy-aided tracheal intubation. Anesthesiology 59:569-572
26. Ovassapian A, Krejcie TC, Yelich SJ, Dykes MHM (1989) Awake fibreoptic intubation in the patient at high risk of aspiration. Br J Anaesth 62:13-16
27. Ovassapian A, Yelich S, Dykes M, Brunner E (1983) Fiberoptic nasotracheal intubation: incidence of failure. Anest Analg 62:692-695
28. Bull SJ, Wiklund R, Ferris C, Connelly NR, Ehrenwerth J, Silverman DG (1994) Facilitation of fiberoptic orotracheal intubation with a flexible tracheal tube. Anesth Analg 78:746-748
29. Ovassapian A, Yelich SJ, Dykes MHM, Brunner EE (1983) Blood pressure and heart changes during awake fibreoptic nasotracheal intubation. Anesth Analg 62:951-954
30. Hawkyard SJ, Morrison A, Doyle LA, Croton RS, WAke PN (1992) Attenuating the hypertensive response to laryngoscopy and endotracheal intubation using awake fibreoptic intubation. Acta Anaesthesiol Scand 36:1-4
31. Shaeffer HG, Marsch SCU (1991) Comparison of orthodox with fibreoptic orotracheal intubation under total IV anaesthesia. Br J Anaesth 66:608-610
32. Smith M, Calder I, Crockard A, Isert P, Nicol ME (1992) Oxygen saturation and cardiovascular changes during fibreoptic intubation under general anaesthesia. Anaesthesia 47:158-161

Total Respiratory System, Lung and Chest Wall Mechanics, Lung Volumes and Gas-Exchange in Morbidly Obese Patients During General Anesthesia

P. Pelosi, M. Croci, P. Vicardi, A. Lissoni, M. Cerisara

Introduction

Morbidly obese patients present an increased risk of developing anesthetic problems during surgery (1, 2). Among them, respiratory complications should be carefully considered since these patients are particularly prone to developing severe hypoxemia, even in the absence of previously demonstrable intrinsic pulmonary disease (3). Respiratory complications may be caused not only by the surgical procedure itself, but also by the severe respiratory mechanical changes occurring during anesthesia and paralysis. Although the mechanical properties of the total respiratory system, the lung and the chest wall have been extensively investigated in spontaneously breathing patients (4-8), little attention has been given to the modifications occurring during anesthesia and paralysis.

In this brief chapter, we will discuss the alterations in respiratory mechanics, lung volumes and gas-exchange induced by anesthesia and paralysis and possible therapeutic interventions to minimize them.

Modeling of respiratory mechanics

Our understanding of the mechanical behavior of the respiratory system is substantially based on theoretical models that should mimic that of the real system and whose parameters should have a physiological meaning.

A few years ago, D'Angelo et al. (9), using the technique of rapid airway occlusion during constant flow ($\dot{V}$) inflation, demonstrated that the respiratory system of normal anesthetized-paralyzed subjects could be explained in terms of a spring and dashpot model incorporating: 1) the airway resistance (Rint,rs) and respiratory elastance (Est,rs) and 2) a spring and dashpot body (Maxwell body) in parallel with Est,rs, reflecting the stress adaptation units within the thoracic tissues (DRrs). The Maxwell body consists in a spring (E2) and a dashpot (R2) arranged serially. The sum of Rint,rs and DR,rs gives the total respiratory system resistance (Rrs). This four-element model predicts that during constant $\dot{V}$ inflation DRrs should increase with inspiratory time (Ti) according to the following function (9, 10):

$$DRrs = R_2 (1 - e^{-Ti/J_2}) \qquad [1]$$

where J_2 is the time constant of the Maxwell body ($= R_2/E_2$). Because during constant flow inflation $Ti = V_T/\dot{V}$, eq. 1 can be rewritten as:

$$DRrs = R_2 (1 - e^{-V_T/\dot{V}J_2})$$ [2]

where V_T is tidal volume.

This equation implies that, at fixed inspiratory $\dot{V}$, *DRrs* will increase exponentially with V_T, whereas at constant inflation V_T, *DRrs* will decrease with increasing $\dot{V}$.

We recently investigated the adaptability of this mechanical model and the volume and flow dependence of Est,rs, Rrs, Rint,rs and DRrs in anesthetized-paralyzed morbidly obese patients (11). Our results were compared with those obtained by D'Angelo et al. in normal anesthetized-paralyzed subjects (9). We found that the spring and dashpot model accurately described respiratory system in morbidly obese patients, too; in fact DRrs strictly followed Ti according to Eq. 1.

Rint,rs. In these patients, Rint,rs was three to four times higher than in normal subjects at each level of flow and increased with flow according to Rohrer's equation (Rint,rs = $K_1 + K_2$ x $\dot{V}$), where K_1 and K_2 are constants. While K_1 was similar to normal (1.1 ± 3.2 cm H_2O x l^{-1} x s and 1.94 ± 0.51 cm H_2O x l^{-1} x s, respectively), K_2 was markedly increased (8.1 ± 6.3 cm H_2O x l^{-2} x s^2 and 0.52 ± 0.08 cm H_2O x l^{-2} x s^2, respectively). In contrast, Rint,rs decreased with increasing V_T, while inspiratory $\dot{V}$ was kept constant. At each level of V_T, Rint,rs was higher in obese patients compared to normal.

DRrs. DR,rs was higher in morbidly obese patients compared to normal at each level of flow (8.2 ± 1.0 cm H_2O x l^{-1} x s and 4.1 ± 0.4 cm H_2O x l^{-1} x s, respectively). Both in normal subjects and in obese patients DRrs decreased progressively with increasing $\dot{V}$ and increased with V_T, accordingly to Eq. 2. Because the changes of DRrs with $\dot{V}$ and V_T were paralleled to the concomitant changes in Rint,rs, their sum (Rrs) was substantially independent, in contrast to normal, from $\dot{V}$ and V_T.

Est,rs. Est,rs was higher than that reported in normal subjects (29.3 ± 5.04 cm H_2O x l^{-1} vs 14.5 ± 2.1 cm H_2O x l^{-1}, respectively). Since Rint,rs was increased, the standard time constant (Rint,rs x Est,rs) was similar to normal (0.14 ± 0.17 s vs 0.21 ± 0.9 s, respectively) and Est,rs was independent of flow. Under iso-V conditions, the behavior of Est,rs with increasing V_T was different from normal subjects. In obese patients the decline in Est,rs with increasing V_T was more pronounced than in normal subjects, particularly up to 0.70 l. This indicated that the volume-pressure curve of obese patients was much more curvilinear (convexity towards the pressure axis more evident) and characterized by an inflection point.

In conclusion the respiratory system of anesthetized-paralyzed morbidly obese patients may be described with a spring and dashpot model as for normal subjects. However, these patients are characterized by a marked increase in static elastance and total resistance of the respiratory system. The increase in the total resistance of the respiratory system is caused by an increase both in airway resistance and in the viscoelastic mechanical properties of the respiratory tissues.

Lung and chest wall mechanics

The relative role of the lung and chest wall in determining alterations in respiratory system mechanics in morbidly obese patients has not been completely clarified. In fact, at least in awake subjects, some authors found an alteration in chest wall but not in lung mechanics (5), while others found a normal behavior of the chest wall (6). In a group of morbidly obese patients, under anesthesia and paralysis, we partitioned respiratory system mechanics into its lung and chest wall components, using the technique of rapid airway occlusion during constant flow (12). We found that: 1) the increased respiratory system elastance was caused by an increase both in lung (Est,L) and chest wall (Est,w) elastance, although the former was prevalent; 2) the increase in respiratory resistance was mainly due to an increase in lung resistance (R,L), chest wall resistance being similar to normal; 3) the increase in Est,L and R,L could be explained by the marked reduction in functional residual capacity (FRC) and not to intrinsic mechanical alterations of the lung tissues and/or airways.

Est,L. Different explanations may be proposed for the altered Est,L in morbidly obese patients. Increased Est,L may be caused by a collapse of alveolar units, intrinsic alterations of the elastic characteristics of lung tissues with surface lining film modifications or to be the result of pulmonary vascular engorgement. Standardizing Est,L for lung volume, we obtained "specific" lung elastance, an index of intrinsic elastic properties of the lung, and we found that it was not different from normal. Consequently, it seems unlikely that increased Est,L was caused by intrinsic mechanical alterations of lung tissues. More probably it may be a consequence of an alteration in the number and/or size of terminal lung units (a terminal lung unit being thought to consist of a small airway airspace, alveolar walls and capillaries), participating in expansion and ventilation, as shown by the marked decrease in lung volume, i.e., in FRC (13).

Est,w. Not only Est,L but also Est,w was increased in morbidly obese patients. An increase in Est,w may be caused by increased adiposity around the ribs, diaphragm and abdomen, limited movements of the ribs caused by thoracic kyphosis and lumbar hyperlordosis from excessive abdominal fat content. Another possible cause is that decreased total thoracic and pulmonary volume may pull the chest wall below its resting level and therefore to a flatter portion of its pressure-volume curve. In a classical clinical study, Sharp et al. (14) found that both explanations, as mentioned above, may be applied in obese patients for the increase in Est,w.

P. Pelosi, M. Croci, P. Vicardi et al.

Resistance. We found that the increase in Rrs was mainly due to lung resistance, on average 83%, chest wall resistance being approximately normal. The increase in lung resistance was due both to airway resistance (Rint,rs) and to "additional" lung resistance (DR,L), which represents the viscoelastic properties and/or inhomogeneities within the lung units ("pendelluft"). In this study (12), Rint,rs averaged 1.9 ± 1.0 cm H_2O x l^{-1} x s^{-1} in normal patients and 4.7 ± 3.1 cm H_2O x l^{-1} x s^{-1} in obese patients. Similar values of airway resistance (5.0 ± 0.05 cm H_2O x l^{-1} x s^{-1}) were obtained in awake obese patients using body plethysmography (8). The increase in Rint,rs in obese patients may be attributed to the airway hyperactivity, vagal reflexes, or reduced lung volume. When Rint,rs was related to FRC, thus obtaining "specific" airway conductance (sGaw), we found that sGaw was not different between normal and obese patients. This indicated that the increase in airway resistance in obese patients is probably caused not by an anatomical narrowing but simply by a reduced lung volume as previously reported in awake obese patients (9).

DR,L in our obese patients could reflect a longer amount of time constant inequalities within the lung or altered stress adaptation properties of the lung tissues. However, the end-inspiratory occlusion method does not allow differentiation between stress adaptation phenomena and time constant inhomogeneities. When DR,L was related to FRC, thus obtaining "specific" additional lung resistance (sDR,L), no significant differences were found in sDR,L between normal and obese patients. Since in these patients FRC was markedly reduced, while V_T delivered was similar to normal, V_T/FRC ratio was higher in obese patients than in normal subjects (115% vs 32%, respectively). Therefore the degree of tissue stress or "pendelluft" measured by DR,L could be higher in obese patients only because of an increase of V_T/FRC ratio.

In conclusion, in morbidly obese patients not only the chest wall but also lung mechanics are altered. In fact, both lung elastance and resistance are increased. The marked reduction in FRC occurring in these patients during anesthesia and paralysis may explain for these severe modifications in lung mechanics.

Gas-exchange

In line with data reported by other authors during spontaneous breathing (4, 15), we found that morbidly obese patients during anesthesia and paralysis are severely hypoxemic compared to normal (12). Hypoxemia may be caused by the developing of collapsing of alveolar units and formation of subsequent atelectasis leading to a ventilation-perfusion (V/Q) mismatch (4) and to a large intrapulmonary blood shunt (16-18).

In our morbidly obese patients, we found not only a marked reduction in PaO_2/PAO_2 ratio (19), but also a significant correlation between PaO_2/PAO_2 ratio and Est,rs, Est,L and FRC (12). This indicated that modifications in respiratory mechanics correlate well with the derangements in pulmonary gas-exchange and, as a consequence, are of great importance in determining hypoxemia. We also found a significant correlation between PaO_2/PAO_2 ratio and lung resistance (Rint,rs and DR,L), indicating that both airway resistance and time constant inhomogeneities within the lung could also play a role in determining hypoxemia in morbidly obese patients.

Thus, increasing lung volume, we should expect a significant improvement in respiratory mechanics and oxygenation. Several methods have been suggested to increase lung volume in morbidly obese patients during anesthesia and paralysis (3): 1) ventilation using tidal volumes as great as 15-20 ml/kg ideal body weight; 2) large, manually performed lung inflations; and 3) application of positive end expiratory pressure (PEEP), although Salem et al. (20) reported that PEEP might actually decrease oxygenation. Recently, we found (21) that, in morbidly obese patients, application of moderate levels of PEEP (5-10 cm H_2O) together with moderate tidal volumes (8-10 ml/kg ideal body weight) during anesthesia and paralysis may increase FRC, improving lung and chest wall mechanics and oxygenation without modifying $PaCO_2$. Thus we suggest the use of moderate levels of PEEP in this kind of patient during anesthesia and paralysis, when it is mandatory to improve oxygenation.

Conclusion

In conclusion, during anesthesia and paralysis morbidly obese patients are characterized by marked derangements in respiratory system, lung and chest wall mechanics caused by the considerable reduction in FRC. These alterations may account for severe hypoxemia frequently occurring in these kinds of patients. Application of low levels of PEEP, increasing FRC, may partially reduce the negative effects on respiratory mechanics and oxygenation induced by anesthesia and paralysis.

References

1. Fox GS, Whalley DG, Bevan OR (1981) Anesthesia for the morbidly obese: experience with 110 patients. Br J Anaesth 53:811-816
2. Vaughan RW (1974) Anesthetic considerations in jejunoileal small bowel bypass for morbid obesity. Anesth Analg 53:421-429
3. Shenkman Z, Shir Y, Brodsky JB (1993) Perioperative management of the obese patient. Br J Anaesth 70:349-359
4. Holley HS, Milic-Emili J, Becklake MR, Bates DV (1967) Regional distribution of pulmonary ventilation and perfusion in obesity. J Clin Invest 46:475-481
5. Naimark A, Cherniack RM (1960) Compliance of the respiratory system and its components in health and obesity. J Appl Physiol 15:377-382
6. Suratt PM, Wilhoit SC, Hsiao HS, Atkinson RL, Rochester DF (1984) Compliance of chest wall in obese subjects. J Appl Physiol 57:403-407
7. Sharp JT, Henry JP, Sweany SK, Meadows WR, Pietras RJ (1964) The total work of breathing in normal and obese men. J Clin Invest 43:728-739

8. Zerah F, Harf A, Perlemuter L, Lorino H, Lorino AM, Atlan G (1993) Effects of obesity on respiratory resistance. Chest 103:1470-1476
9. D'Angelo E, Robatto FM, Calderini E, Tavola M, Bono D, Torri G, Milic-Emili J (1991) Pulmonary and chest wall mechanics in anesthetized paralyzed humans. J Appl Physiol 70: 2602-2610
10. Bates JHT, Rossi A, Milic-Emili J (1985) Analysis of the behaviour of the respiratory system with constant inspiratory flow. J Appl Physiol 58:1840-1848
11. Pelosi P, Croci M, Ravagnan I, Cerisara M, Vicardi P, Lissoni A, Gattinoni L (1995) Analysis of behavior of the respiratory system in sedated-paralyzed morbidly obese patients: effects of flow, volume and time. J Appl Physiol (submitted)
12. Pelosi P, Croci M, Ravagnan I, Vicardi P, Gattinoni L (1995) Total respiratory system, lung and chest wall mechanics in sedated-paralyzed postoperative morbidly obese patients. Chest (in press)
13. Damia G, Mascheroni D, Croci M, Tarenzi L (1988) Perioperative changes in the functional residual capacity in morbidly obese patients. Br J Anaesth 60:574-578
14. Sharp JT, Henry JP, Sweany SK, Meadows WR, Pietras RJ (1964) Effects of mass loading the respiratory system in man. J Appl Physiol 19:959-966
15. Said SI (1960) Abnormalities of pulmonary gas-exchange in obesity. Ann Intern Med 53: 1121-1129
16. Vaughan RW, Wise L (1976) Intraoperative arterial oxygenation in obese patients. Ann Surg 1184:35-42
17. Luce JM (1980) Respiratory complications of obesity. Chest 78:626-631
18. Fisher A, Waterhouse TD, Adams AP (1975) Obesity: its relation to anesthesia. Anesthesia 130:633-647
19. Gilbert R, Auchincloss JH, Kuppinger M, Thomas M (1979) Stability of the arterial/alveolar oxygen partial pressure ratio. Crit Care Med 7:267-272
20. Salem MR, Dalal FY, Zygmunt MP, Mathrubhutham M, Jacobs HK (1978) Does PEEP improve intraoperative arterial oxygenation in grossly obese patients? Anesthesiology 48: 280-281
21. Pelosi P, Norsa A, Croci M, Vicardi P, Cerisara M, Gattinoni L (1995) Physiologic effects of positive end-expiratory pressure (PEEP) in postoperative sedated-paralyzed morbidly obese patients. Intensive Care Med (in press)

Bariatric Surgery: Indications and Complications

S.B. DOLDI, G. MICHELETTO, A. RESTELLI, A. FAVARA

Introduction

The surgical treatment of morbid obesity began in the USA in 1954 to provide an effective treatment to decrease weight for patients 80%-100% overweight where diet, drugs or psychotherapy had failed. Bariatric surgery progress during the last 40 years has been amazing, looking for a safe, effective and low morbidity procedure. Since the 1970s clinical research has been working on two different pathways at the same time:

– Procedures based on intestinal malabsorption
– Procedures based on gastric restriction to reduce the food intake

Jejuno-ileal bypass (JIBP)

After introduction into surgical practice in the 1960's, JIBP has been revised and modified by J.H. Payne and L.T. De Wind (end-to-side JIBP), H. Scott (end-to-end JIBP) and S.B. Doldi and W. Montorsi (1) (side-to-side JIBP). This procedure is easily and completely reversible. Our personal experience up to may 1995 includes 302 patients (Table 1).

Table 1. Jejuno-ileal bypass: personal experience

Patients	302
Male/female	75/227
Age (years)	33.4 ± 9
Preoperative weight (kg)	138.8 ± 25.3
BMI (kg/m^2)	50.7 ± 7.2
Follow-up	10 years

Results

The average weight loss is 37.2%, corresponding to an overweight decrease of 80% after 2 years of follow-up and then remains stable. As a consequence other diseases related to obesity (diabetes, dyslipidemias, hypertension, osteoarticular diseases, dysmenorrhea, Pickwick syndrome) markedly improve and some of them resolve completely. Some 9% of patients have a poor weight loss defined as less than 25% of the preoperative weight at 2 years of follow-up. A reintervention in these patients with a shortening of JIBP gave good results in half of them.

Side effects

Diarrhea is the most common side effect: it is usually severe in the first postoperative period (six to seven evacuations per day) and then improves to two to three evacuations per day of solid stool.

Early complications

Severe diarrhea (more then 15-20 daily evacuations) can occur in 9% of patients, commonly associated with electrolyte imbalance (4.5%). Surgical wound infections are rare (2.2%).

Late complications

Dietary or behavioral mistakes can lead to severe diarrhea (5.9%), electrolyte disorders (6.7%), trace element depletion (8.4%), vitamins depletion (2.2%), usually treated with specific oral therapy or parenteral feedings. Gas bloat syndrome (20%) can be cured with specific antibiotic therapy and dietary treatment (2). Some refractory patients underwent conversion of JIBP to biliointestinal bypass (2.1%). Incisional hernia (16.9%) is usually a mechanical problem. Gallstones (12.8%) are treated following usual indications. Kidney stones (7.5%) can be prevented with daily oral calcium supplementation. Persistent intestinal malabsorption (2.9%) caused by a poor hypertrophic adaptation of the working loop, severe liver failure (1.3%) and interstitial ossalic nephritis (0.8%) are the most dangerous complications requiring reconversion of JIBP. Mortality related to the surgical procedure is 1.2%.

Biliointestinal bypass (BIBP)

Hallberg and Ericksson in the late 1970s introduced the BIBP into bariatric surgery (Fig. 1); as a consequence stool bile salts concentration is decreased (50% less then JIBP), reducing liver damage, diarrhea and blind loop syndrome. BIBP induces a weight loss and advantages as JIBP; considering the side effects and complications, there is a minor number of stool evacuations (three per day), a minor occurrence of blind loop bacterial overgrowth (6%) and an absence of severe liver failure in our 53 patients. BIBP is reversible.

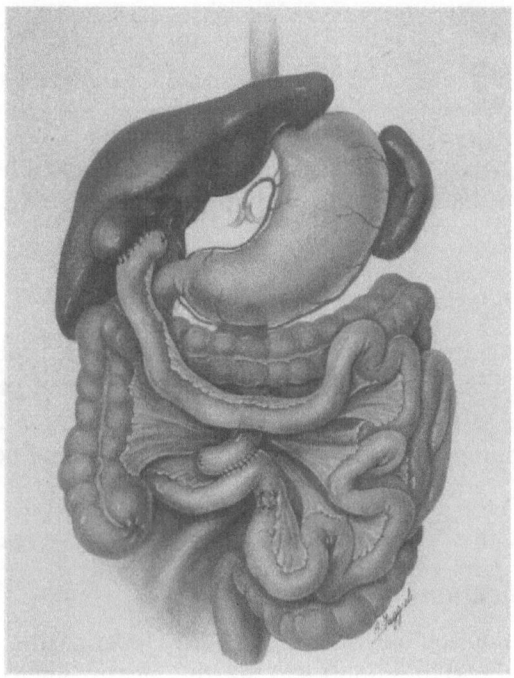

Fig. 1. Biliointestinal bypass

Horizontal gastroplasty (HGP)

Gomez created the HGP in the 1979 using a horizontal gastric partition. The upper pouch volume should not exceed 40-60 ml. The procedure is easy and completely reversible. Our experience (3) with HGP is shown in Table 2.

Table 2. Horizontal gastroplasty: personal experience

Patients	102
Male/female	17/85
Age (years)	39.3 ± 8.2
Preoperative weight (kg)	120.8 ± 19.6
BMI (kg/m^2)	46.4 ± 6.3
Follow-up	5 years

Results

A 72% average decrease of overweight was obtained in 78% of our 102 patients. Poor weight loss occurred in 18%. It can be caused by technical complications (outlet enlargement, staple line disruption) or by incorrect indication (sweet-eaters).

Side effects

Nausea, vomiting, epigastric pain, and gastric distension can occur if the alimentary habits of the patient are not correct.

Metabolic complications

Recurrent vomiting (6.8%) can be associated with electrolyte imbalance or vitamin depletion (4%). Gallstones can occur in 6.8% of patients. Peripheral neuropathy (3.4%) is caused by B group vitamin depletion and it is the most severe metabolic complication, potentially lethal for central neural syndrome of Wernicke's type.

Technical complications

Splenectomy (4%) during our first 30 patients. Upper gastric pouch perforation or dehiscence of the staple line (2%) are the most dangerous complications; ischemia is the common cause. They cause diffuse peritonitis mimicking acute respiratory failure. Their surgical emergency treatment is always complex. Staple line disruption (2.2%) and outlet dilation (10.2%) require appropriate surgical treatment. Outlet stenosis (3.4%) can be treated with endoscopic dilation. The mortality rate is 2.3%.

Silastic ring vertical gastroplasty (SRVGP)

We performed Willbanks-Eckhout's SRVGP in the early 1990s for 4 years. The outlet, after calibration, is reenforced using a silastic ring. The surgical procedure is easily and completely reversible.

Results

A 33.1% weight loss was obtained in 90.7% of our 44 cases after 3 years average follow-up. BMI decrease was 33.2%.

Metabolic complications

Recurrent vomiting (11.3%), gallstones (8.1%) and peripheral neuropathy (2.2%) can occur.

Technical complications

Splenectomy (4.5%) is common at the beginnings. Delayed emptying of the upper pouch (4.4%) without outlet stenosis presents with occasional vomiting episodes. Staple line disruption (2.2%) requires relaparotomy and revision. Intraluminal dislocation of the silastic ring (2.2%) 3 months after the procedure did not require any particular treatment. Abnormal upper gastric pouch dilation (2.2%) requires surgical removal of the silastic ring. Mortality was 0%.

Adjustable silicone gastric banding (ASGB)

The most recent news in bariatric surgery is the ASGB (4). Since November 1993 we have been performing the Kuzmak's (5) ASGB (Fig. 2). It is possible to perform the procedure with laparoscopic technique. Indications and contraindications are similar to those for gastroplasty with a few modifications:

– Second degree obesity (BMI > 30)
– Patients older then 60 years

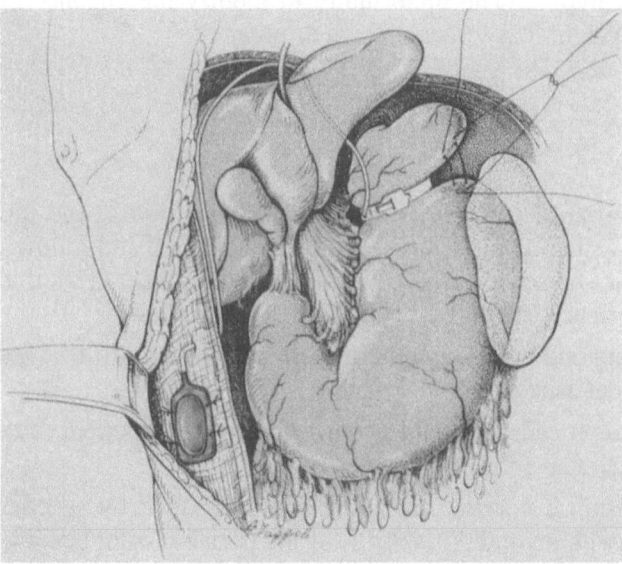

Fig. 2. Adjustable silicone gastric banding

Our surgical experience includes 20 patients, four of them via a laparoscopic approach (Table 3). Twelve patients have had 6 months of follow-up.

Table 3. Adjustable silicone gastric banding: personal experience

Patients	20
Male/female	7/13
Age (years)	39 ± 6.1
Preoperative weight (kg)	135.3 ± 20.9
BMI (kg/m^2)	46.5 ± 5.4
Follow-up	6 months

Results

A 21.7% average weight loss is obtained after 6 months of follow-up. Mortality was 0%.

Complications

Oral overfeeding was the cause of persistent vomiting, requiring recalibration of the channel in one patient. A huge dilation of the upper pouch was caused by a compliance deficit in one patient who underwent conversion of ASGB in biliointestinal bypass. The opportunity to modify the channel's diameter was useful when weight loss was excessive or poor.

Conclusions

Since 1950 bariatric surgery has made sensible progress and today is routine surgery. New technical procedures and better selection and follow-up of patients define bariatric surgery as an effective and safe treatment of morbid obesity. Our personal experience (6) suggests three conclusions:

– Patient selection is of paramount importance and it must evaluate clinical and psychological aspects.
– The surgical procedure should be performed by an experienced team, choosing the best treatment for every single patient.
– The follow-up is imperative, endless and managed by a dedicated team of physicians with enough knowledge of the possible complications.

If these criteria are strictly followed results are good and complications are few and acceptable.

References

1. Doldi BS, Vita PM, Restelli A, Micheletto G, Longoni F, Caspani P, Montorsi W (1990) Y a-t-il encore une place pour le court-circuit jejuno-ileal dans le traitement chirurgical de l'obesite morbide? Ann Chir 44:362-367
2. Venturi M, Zuccato E, Restelli A, Mazzoleni L, Mussini E, Doldi BS (1994) Utility of hydrogen and methane breath-test in combination with X-ray examination after barium meal in diagnosis of small bacterial overgrowth after jejuno-ileal bypass for morbid obesity. Obesity Surgery 4: 144-148
3. Doldi BS, Vita PM, Lattuada E, Restelli A, Micheletto G, Longoni F, Montorsi W (1990) Gastroplastie horizontale dans la chirurgie de l'obesite morbide: une condamnation injiustifiee? Ann Chir 44:356-361
4. Favretti F et al (1994) Bendaggio gastrico regolabile: nostra esperienza su 111 casi consecutivi. Chirurgia Triveneta 1:6-9
5. Kuzmak L (1989) Gastric banding. In: Deitel M (ed) Surgery for morbid obesity. Lea and Febiger, Philadelphia
6. Vita PM, Restelli A, Caspani P, Longoni F, Doldi BS (1992) L'esperienza mondiale attuale nel trattamento chirurgico della grande obesità. Minerva Chir 47:77-88

ANAESTHESIOLOGICAL AND SURGICAL PROBLEMS IN LUNG TRANSPLANTATION

Lung Transplantation: Aspects of Anaesthetic and Early Postoperative Management

J.P. LITTLE, R.D. LATIMER

Introduction

The first isolated lung transplant occurred in 1963. Between then and 1980 some 40 procedures were carried out but the longest survivor lived only ten months after the transplant (1). Technically, the major obstacle to success was impaired healing of the bronchial anastomosis due to a poor post-implantation blood supply. Problems of infection and rejection hampered lung transplantation in common with that of other organs (2).

Improved surgical techniques produced the first long-term survivor in Toronto in 1983 (3). Since the late 1980s there has been a rapid increase in the numbers of lung transplants such that since 1989 they have been more common than heart-lung transplants in the United States (4). The annual number of lung transplants increased from 40 in 1988 to over 400 in 1991 (5). Survival figures have progressively improved to a situation where one year survival for single lung transplant now stands at 73% and three year survival at 63% (6).

Expanding indications for lung transplantation are leading to a greater need for anaesthetists to be familiar with this procedure and the particular demands of single and double lung transplantation.

Recipient selection and assessment

To be considered for lung transplantation patients generally must have progressive pulmonary disease with a life expectancy of less than 18 months (7). Single lung transplantation (SLT) exceeds the numbers of double lung procedures (6) and over 40% of single lung transplants are performed for chronic obstructive pulmonary disease. The commonest current indication for double lung transplantation (DLT) is cystic fibrosis with numbers likely to increase as DLT supersedes heart lung transplantation in these patients (8). Table 1 lists the indications for lung transplantation.

Table 1. Indications for lung transplantation [from (36)]

Single lung
  Parenchymal lung disease without pulmonary infection [e.g. idiopathic pulmonary fibrosis,
  emphysema, chronic obstructive pulmonary disease (COPD)]
  Correctable congenital heart disease with secondary pulmonary hypertension
  (e.g. atrial septal defect)
  Pulmonary vascular disease without severe cardiac failure
Double lung
  Septic lung disease (e.g. cystic fibrosis)
  Severe bullous emphysema
  Correctable congenital heart disease with secondary pulmonary hypertension
  (e.g. atrial septal defect)
  Pulmonary vascular disease without severe cardiac failure

It can be seen that there is considerable overlap between the indications for single and double lung transplantation and there has been a move towards the use of single lung transplantation (SLT) unless there is a specific indication for double lung transplantation (DLT) such as sepsis (2). Even in the setting of pulmonary vascular disease satisfactory results can be obtained from SLT since it has been shown that a marked improvement in right ventricular function can occur postoperatively (9) in patients who in the past would have received a heart-lung transplant in the belief that the right ventricular dysfunction was irreversible. In COPD although DLT provides greater improvement in objective measures of pulmonary function (10), the increase in exercise tolerance is as great with SLT (11). Potential recipients must satisfy a number of criteria related and unrelated to their pulmonary disease (Table 2).

Table 2. Criteria for transplantation [from (2)]

Medical criteria
  Life expectancy from progressive pulmonary disease < 18 months
  Age < 60 years
  Absence of systemic disease with significant end-organ damage
  (especially liver and kidney damage)
  Absence of significant coronary artery disease (on angiogram)
  No previous extensive mediastinal irradiation
  Not on high dose corticosteroids
  Adequate nutrition
  Ambulatory
  Psychosocial criteria
  Compliant with medical treatment
  Psychologically stable

Lung transplantation is now being applied in some centres to conditions previously considered unsuitable such as thromboembolic pulmonary hypertension, respiratory failure associated with connective tissue diseases, ARDS and broncho-alveolar cell carcinoma (12).

Assessment of recipients involves clinical assessment of their pulmonary disease including its likely progression and objective tests of lung function. Such tests may help to decide on referral for transplantation, an FEV_1 of less than 30% predicted being considered a threshold in cystic fibrosis or emphysema (13). Because pulmonary fibrosis may progress rapidly earlier referral is warranted particularly if FVC is less than 65% of predicted (6). Cardiac assessment includes coronary angiography to diagnose the presence of coronary artery disease and right heart catheterisation to measure pulmonary artery pressures and cardiac output. Assessment of right ventricular function is important to predict the response to clamping of one pulmonary artery perioperatively. Failure to maintain an adequate cardiac output at this stage may require the institution of cardiopulmonary bypass (CPB).

Donor organ procurement

Although there has been a report of lung transplantation from a living donor (14), donor lungs are usually obtained from a brain stem dead individual. Of necessity such patients are intubated and ventilated and the lungs are at risk from colonisation and infection by micro-organisms, the incidence of frank pulmonary infection increasing with the amount of time intubated particularly after 48 hours (15). Further lung damage may occur from neurogenic mechanisms (16) or overenthusiastic use of crystalloid fluid resuscitation. In patients with head injury the original trauma may have caused lung damage. Estimates suggest that only 5-15% of available organ donors have suitable lungs (7, 17). Added to this are the scarcity of donors and the large number of potential donors whose organs are not utilised. Donor criteria are summarised in Table 3.

Table 3. Lung donor criteria

Age < 55 years
Normal chest radiograph
PaO_2 > 40 kPa (FiO_2 = 1.0)
Normal bronchoscopic examination
No purulent secretions (Gram stain of aspirate)
No prior chest surgery
No significant chest trauma

Donor lung management aims to avoid lung damage by keeping FiO_2 less than 0.6 to avoid oxygen toxicity and tailoring ventilation to minimise barotrauma and volutrauma (ventilator induced lung injury). Poor oxygenation due to atelectasis will often respond to bronchoscopic clearing of secretions and vigorous expansion of the lungs by hand ventilation (18-20).

Preservation of the donor lung relies on cooling and the infusion into the pulmonary arteries (vasodilated by prior infusion of prostacyclin) of a "pneumoplegia" solution based on a mixture of crystalloid, human albumin solution and donor autologous blood. Research on preservation techniques aims to reduce lung dysfunction secondary to ischaemia and reperfusion ("pulmonary reimplantation response") which is more common when ischaemic time is longer (21). Ischaemic times of 6-8 h are presently considered acceptable (22). Various drugs have been added to the preservative solution to try to reduce the degree of ischaemia/reperfusion injury including glutathione, free radical scavengers and calcium-channel blockers (23, 24). The degree of lung inflation during storage also seems important and it is routine to inflate the lungs with air prior to stapling the trachea.

Anaesthetic management

Conacher has described lung transplantation as "a pneumonectomy in a patient who, under normal circumstances would be adjudged unfit for such an operation" (25).

Preoperative assessment

Time is often at a premium in these patients and a full assessment may not always be possible. Review of the notes and a brief clinical evaluation is usually all that is possible. It is important to be aware of the degree of pulmonary hypertension and cardiac dysfunction if present. Whether CPB is planned should be ascertained. In general these patients have little or no respiratory reserve and as such may be easily compromised.

There is really no role for sedative premedication in these patients in whom drug induced hypercarbia may have deleterious effects on the pulmonary vasculature with subsequent decompensation. Patients with limited respiratory reserve may also become hypoxic if sedated.

Monitoring

Comprehensive monitoring (Table 4) is easily justified in these patients both on the basis of their underlying disease and the nature of the planned procedure.

Table 4. Monitoring requirements

Mandatory
    Electrocardiograph[a]
    Pulse oximeter[a]
    Capnograph
    Arterial line for pressure monitoring and sampling[a]
    Central venous catheter for pressure monitoring and drug infusions
    Temperature probe
    Urinary catheter for urine output
    Monitors of airway pressure and tidal volume
Optional
    Pulmonary artery flotation catheter (PAFC)
    Transoesophageal echocardiography (TOE)
    Gastric tonometer

---

[a] Sited before induction of anaesthesia.

This represents routine practice at our institution, other centres prefer to site central venous lines prior to induction (26) although this is often difficult due to problems in positioning the patient optimally for rapid performance of the procedure. It may, for example, compromise the patient if they are other than sitting upright. Siting central venous lines after induction of anaesthesia improves patient comfort with little compromise in terms of one's ability to detect important changes during anaesthetic induction and institution of positive pressure ventilation. Monitoring of pulmonary artery pressure via a pulmonary artery flotation catheter (PAFC) is considered mandatory in many centres (26) although spurious data may be produced during pneumonectomy (27). Despite such caveats, the potential benefits of measuring pulmonary artery pressure in these patients are manifest and postoperatively the ability to measure pulmonary artery occlusion pressure and cardiac output aids logical fluid management (28). Some centres are using transoesophageal echocardiography for a qualitative assessment of cardiac function (29).

Monitoring of ventilation is vital in these patients where achieving optimal ventilation may be difficult due to varying compliance and the risk of air trapping particularly in emphysematous patients (25, 30) (see below). Monitoring airway pressure, inspired and expired volumes are all important. Adequacy of gas exchange is monitored by continuous pulse oximetry and capnography with intermittent measurement of arterial blood gases. The capnograph trace may exhibit two peaks for each breath due to greatly varying time constants between lungs after donor lung implantation in SLT.

The measurement of gastric intramucosal pH (pHi) using a gastric tonometer may be a useful adjunct to the data provided by more traditional monitoring particularly in the postoperative period. A low pHi may provide evidence of inadequate tissue oxygen delivery earlier than other measures (e.g. lactate) allowing intervention before irreversible changes occur (31-33).

Need for cardiopulmonary bypass

The rise of isolated lung transplantation often makes it possible to avoid the use of CPB. In one series (excluding patients with pulmonary hypertension), only one of 59 SLT patients required CPB whilst 18 of 68 DLT (bilateral sequential technique) did so (34); in another series 6 of 36 patients for SLT required CPB (35). Predicting such patients has proved problematical (34, 35). Patients receiving a donor lung or lungs for pulmonary hypertension nearly always require CPB to maintain haemodynamic stability.

During SLT, a test clamping of the pulmonary artery is made and CPB is used if there is haemodynamic instability or gas exchange deteriorates (36). If DLT is performed en bloc with a tracheal anastomosis then CPB is mandatory (2). It is usual now, however, to perform DLT as a sequential technique with bronchial anastomoses (bilateral sequential lung transplantation) and CPB can often be avoided (37). Additionally, the sequential technique has advantages over the en bloc technique in terms of anastomotic healing.

Avoidance of CPB has the potential advantages of reduced ischaemic time, less pulmonary injury and less postoperative bleeding (36). De Hoyos et al. showed that CPB was associated with a greater incidence of acute lung injury and prolonged intubation (38).

Choice of anaesthetic drugs and conduct of anaesthesia

Drug induced changes in cardiac output, systemic and pulmonary vascular resistance and pulmonary vascular responsiveness must all be reduced to the minimum. Where such effects are unavoidable then they must be recognised quickly and prompt steps taken to restore equilibrium. It can be argued that an awareness of the effects of anaesthetic drugs and an ability to counter them before deleterious consequences occur is more important than the choice of drug per se.

Anaesthetic induction is a period of major cardiorespiratory changes where prudent drug choice can reduce the degree of changes that occur. A technique based on a cardiostable induction agent such as etomidate together with a synthetic opioid such as fentanyl is well proven (25, 39). The dose of opioid may have to be tailored to the planned strategy for postoperative extubation. Moderate to high dose fentanyl (30-50 µg/kg or more) necessitates a period of post-operative mechanical ventilation (39). If this is to be avoided then lower doses (e.g. 10-15 µg/kg) are used which may be at the cost of reduced cardiac stability.

There has been recent interest in the role of propofol in cardiac anaesthesia both for induction and maintenance (40). A study of patients with low cardiac output preoperatively showed the combination of propofol and fentanyl (15 µg/kg) to be no less stable than high dose fentanyl (60 µg/kg) in terms of changes in blood pressure, cardiac output and myocardial contractility but to have distinct advantages in respect to shorter times to wakening and extubation (41). This appears an attractive combination of drugs. The muscle relaxant chosen should optimally cause little change in blood pressure or heart rate and vecuronium fulfils most requirements. Some will prefer a longer acting drug and whilst pancuronium is a traditional choice newer drugs such as doxacurium or pipecuronium can fill the same role without the tendency to cause tachycardia.

In the maintenance phase of anaesthesia there is controversy about the use of volatile anaesthetic agents. There are theoretical objections to their use on the basis of cardiovascular side effects and diminution of hypoxic pulmonary vasoconstriction. In clinical practice, however, low doses of isoflurane or halothane as an adjunct to opioid anaesthesia appears to have little deleterious effect (25). Isoflurane may have a useful role due to its vasodilator action systemically and in reducing the dose of opioid required to suppress the pressor response to noxious stimuli. Whilst nitrous oxide has been shown to increase pulmonary vascular resistance it has been used without adverse effects in lung transplantation (25).

Flexibility is required in the approach to intraoperative ventilation. The recipients native lungs may be non-compliant requiring high inflation pressures. The ability to vary flow rates, inspiratory time, tidal volume and PEEP will be advantageous in many cases.

Airway management

In SLT it is usual to employ a double lumen endobronchial tube with intubation of the main bronchus of the non-operated side. This facilitates ventilation of the intubated lung facilitating surgery on the non-ventilated, collapsed side. Problems may occur with right or left sided tubes. With right sided tubes the variable origin of the right upper lobe bronchus may cause problems as its orifice may be obstructed (42). Left sided tubes may occasionally be difficult to place, the endobronchial portion tending to advance into the right main bronchus. Checking of tube position may be clinically using cuff inflation, clamping and auscultation or using fibreoptic bronchoscopy. Recently a new method of checking position using flow/volume loops has been proposed (43). Whatever method is used, checks must be repeated after changes in patient position as migration has been shown to occur in 33% of tubes after moving from the supine to the lateral position (43). Polyvinyl chloride tubes may have advantages over red rubber tubes as cuff inflation pressures are lower reducing the risk of mucosal ischaemia. Additionally, the cuff shape of right sided PVC tubes makes blocking of the right upper lobe bronchus less likely (44). Airway management for DLT without CPB poses a particular challenge. A simple approach is to use an endobronchial tube and intubate the main bronchus of the lung to be removed second. Removal of the first lung proceeds as for SLT with one lung ventilation. Both lungs are then ventilated after implantation of the first donor lung. The second side is then mobilised whilst still being ventilated with the endobronchial lumen being withdrawn from the main bronchus to enable it to be clamped. The tube remains in a partially withdrawn position after implantation of the second donor lung avoiding intubation near the bronchial suture line (Oduro A., personal communication). A technique using blockers guided into each main bronchus in turn under fibreoptic guidance is also possible but more difficult to manage smoothly. If CPB is to be used then airway management is much simplified for SLT or DLT as a standard single lumen endotracheal tube may be used.

Intraoperative problems

The significant areas that present problems during the operation include ventilation of the native lungs, institution of one lung ventilation, clamping of the pulmonary artery and the time during which the donor lung is perfused but not ventilated. In DLT it may be added the time when the first donor lung is ventilated alone. Additional dissection is often difficult and prolonged, particularly in the presence of previous infection, and blood loss may be considerable.

Ventilation may produce problems very early, particularly in patients with emphysema, in whom air trapping may readily occur if normal tidal volumes and respiratory rates are used and has been described as causing severe hypotension due to tamponade and impaired venous return (25, 30). A high index of suspicion is required and diagnosis is aided if inspired and expired tidal volumes are monitored and care taken not to over inflate the lungs. The possibility of tension pneumothorax producing the same clinical picture must not be forgotten. A period of apnoea allowing expiration to occur will provide relief of air trapping with haemodynamic improvement. A strategy of deliberate hypoventilation with permissive hypercapnia has been described in a patient prone to air trapping (30). A new approach to this problem has been proposed by Conacher - prolonged interval jet ventilation involving the delivery of a "breath" consisting of 3-9 jet pulses followed by a pause of 10-50 s (45). This technique was found to provide adequate oxygenation without air trapping or cardiovascular instability at the cost of a raised $PaCO_2$. Problems may continue into the postoperative period after a SLT procedure for emphysema.

Institution of one lung ventilation may lead to hypoxaemia due to shunt through the non-ventilated lung, and manoeuvres that are used in thoracic anaesthesia are also appropriate in lung transplantation with certain provisos (25). Increasing the inspired fraction of oxygen may be all that is required.

Further approaches include the application of PEEP to the ventilated lung which may cause more problems than it solves by limiting expiration and reducing cardiac output (25). Oxygenation via the operated lung has been attempted by insufflation of oxygen or the application of CPAP (25). Recently it has been suggested that inhaled nitric oxide may improve oxygenation during one lung ventilation (J.V. Booth, personal communication) although the mechanism remains to be elucidated. If all attempts fail to achieve adequate oxygenation then it may be necessary to institute CPB.

Clamping of the pulmonary artery provides a major test during lung transplantation. The ability of the right ventricle to maintain cardiac output in the face of increased afterload is a major determinant in avoiding CPB. Pharmacological support for the right ventricle may be required at this time including inotropes and pulmonary vasodilators to reduce vascular resistance in the ventilated lung. Dopamine or adrenaline may be useful to improve cardiac output but may further increase pulmonary vascular resistance. Concomitant or sole use of a pulmonary vasodilator to off load the right ventricle is a logical approach to this problem (25). Possible drugs include isoprenaline, prostacyclin and inhaled nitric oxide. Isoprenaline and prostacyclin dilate systemic as well as pulmonary vessels and may necessitate the addition of a vasoconstrictor such as noradrenaline or phenylephrine. Failure of these methods will require CPB to be used.

Completion of the vascular anastomoses to the donor lung before the bronchial anastomosis may create a large shunt with consequent hypoxaemia which, whilst often short-lived, may be a significant problem. The best management is probably to avoid the problem by anastomosing the airway first, although this may be technically more difficult (25). Temporary clamping of the pulmonary artery may be required or separate ventilation of the two lungs using a catheter technique with jet ventilation to enable ventilation whilst the airway anastomosis is performed.

Early postoperative care

The early postoperative period may be complicated by problems with pulmonary function, bleeding, and renal and cardiovascular function. Blood loss must be monitored closely and coagulopathy and thrombocytopenia corrected in the face of excessive blood loss. Bleeding is more commonly a problem when CPB is used. Pulmonary, renal and cardiovascular care are considered further below. Meticulous attention is required to the prevention of infection with an agreed policy on changing central venous catheters and the use of antibiotics.

Timing of extubation

This decision will impact on many other areas of postoperative care. Opinion differs with some centres extubating within a few hours of the end of the operation and others ventilating routinely for up to seven days. Early extubation (within six hours postoperatively) has several potential advantages (46). Removal of positive pressure ventilation reduces the chances of ventilator induced lung injury with potential exacerbation of acute lung injury. A further advantage is gained from avoiding a continuing need for sedative drugs which may cause or exacerbate postoperative hypotension. Studies have also shown an improvement in myocardial performance following extubation after cardiac surgery which may be extrapolated to this situation (47). The removal of the tracheal tube restores a natural barrier to bacterial colonisation of the lungs and early extubation may thus reduce the risk of infection in these immunosuppressed patients, a major threat to life after transplant surgery.

The opposite view advocates late extubation and argues that continued ventilation has advantages during the early postoperative period which may be marked by cardiovascular instability and acute lung injury. Oxygen demands can be reduced by sedation and ventilation and oxygenation ensured. It can be argued that continued ventilation is wise whilst there is a risk of the pulmonary reimplantation response, although positive pressure ventilation may exacerbate lung injury. Continued ventilation may pose the problem after SLT of two lungs with very different mechanics and gas exchanging characteristics. The remaining native lung, for example, may be prone to air trapping. Some centres routinely institute differential lung ventilation postoperatively to allow the different requirements of the two lungs to be met.

In general early extubation seems to have more advantages than disadvantages and should be applied in patients who are warm, cardiovascularly stable and have good gas exchange.

The pulmonary reimplantation response

This example of acute lung injury appears to be a result of ischaemia and reperfusion. In common with other examples of acute lung injury the primary site of pathology is in the alveolar capillaries which allow accumulation of interstitial lung water (21, 48). The response is more severe as ischaemia time for the donor lung increases. It seems likely that there is a degree of lung injury in all patients. It presents usually over the first 4 h postoperatively and is at its worst on days 2-4. The radiographic appearances are those of diffuse pulmonary infiltrates and the differential diagnosis includes infection and cardiogenic pulmonary oedema.

The response to ischaemia and reperfusion involves a systemic inflammatory response involving the activation of complement and the migration and sequestration of neutrophils in the lung (49). Activated neutrophils appear to have an important role in the development of the acute lung injury. The presence of oxygen and the development of reactive oxygen species is crucial to the reperfusion injury.

Neutrophil depletion using leucocyte filters has been shown to reduce acute lung injury in animals (49) but potential adverse effects such as increased infection rates may reduce the attraction of this manoeuvre. The phosphodiesterase inhibitor pentoxifylline inhibits neutrophil chemotaxis and activation in animals. It appears safe in man (50).

Perhaps more inviting are steps to reduce the degree of reperfusion injury by actively scavenging oxygen free radicals. A number of drugs have this property including mannitol, allopurinol and acetylcysteine. Currently their role is unclear but may turn out to be a prophylactic one (51).

Reperfusion injury appears potentially easier to prevent than treat. Once established, manipulations of neutrophils and inflammatory mediators have not been shown to have a useful effect on outcome. Treatment of the established syndrome is generally supportive intensive care whilst avoiding ventilator induced lung injury by care to limit peak airway pressure (to less than 45 cmH$_2$O) and over inflation. These aims may be best achieved by alternative ventilation strategies such as pressure limited ventilation although their ability to improve outcome is unclear (51).

Fluid and cardiovascular management

The maintenance of adequate oxygen delivery to vital organs is the goal as it is in any critically ill patient (52). Ensuring this occurs against a background of a patient with a lung or lungs with abnormal capillaries. Protection of the lungs from harm may alter the way in which oxygen delivery is maintained. The maintenance of an adequate cardiac output requires optimal fluid filling but over hydration must be avoided to limit the increase in lung water. The use of a pulmonary artery catheter enabling the measurement of cardiac output may have advantages in guiding therapy but carries an infection risk which may be greater. Monitoring of central venous pressure and urine output is certainly vital in all patients. A relatively non-invasive monitor of adequate oxygen delivery is gastric tonometry with measurement of gastric intramucosal pH (pHi) although it is unproven in this situation. It can, however, provide a useful guide to fluid and inotropic management and a low pHi may be an earlier indicator of problems than more traditional data (31). In the event of a low pHi, dopexamine which is a splanchnic vasodilator appears to have a role in therapy (33). Inotropes, pressors and/or pulmonary vasodilators may all be required in the early postoperative period to optimise cardiac particularly right ventricular function. Support of the right ventricle may require identical measures to those considered above. If renal function is poor and urine output low despite adequate cardiac output then the need for exact fluid balance to protect the lungs will necessitate early recourse to renal support such as haemofiltration.

Pain relief

Analgesia is a particularly important issue if a strategy of early extubation is to be adopted. Only with good analgesia will the patient be able to deep breathe and cough adequately after extubation. Compliance with physiotherapy is also facilitated guarding against sputum retention and the development of infection.

Essentially the problem is that of pain relief after a thoracotomy which has been widely addressed in the past (53).

Available options include parenteral opiates intermittently or by infusion or patient controlled analgesia (PCA). Whilst continuous infusion or PCA can provide adequate analgesia the incidence of sedation, respiratory depression and nausea is often intolerably high in these high risk patients. Interest has focused on the use of the epidural route which is best able to provide the quality of analgesia required. An intense block is possible with local anaesthetic alone but the concentration required may lead to a high incidence of hypotension and a combination of dilute local anaesthetic (e.g. 0.1%-0.125% bupivacaine) with an opioid provides the best ratio of efficacy to safety (54). The most commonly used opioids are fentanyl and morphine. Fentanyl is more lipid soluble than morphine and rostral spread may be less, resulting in a lower incidence of late respiratory depression (55). However, it has been questioned whether fentanyl acts locally in the spinal cord or is merely absorbed systemically from the epidural space (56). Comparisons of intravenous and epidural fentanyl alone have shown similar analgesia by either route but with less side effects when given epidurally (56). The exact site of administration in the epidural space seems unimportant for opioids (56, 57) but is important for local anaesthetics requiring the siting of the catheter close to the dermatomal level of the incision.

The provision of adequate analgesia is possibly the anaesthetists most important contribution to a smooth postoperative course for these patients if early extubation is the chosen plan.

Summary

Lung transplantation is a procedure with increasing application and is likely to become more and more common. The main impediment to its growth is the scarcity of suitable donor organs. The recipients pose particular anaesthetic problems which are added to by the ability to avoid the use of CPB. Ventilation in particular may pose problems not encountered even in the thoracic surgical population and their solution may involve unusual strategies. A policy of good pain relief and early extubation enables the avoidance of the problems of prolonged ventilation at the possible cost of a need for reintubation should lung injury show itself only after extubation.

References

1. Raffin TA (1988) Double lung transplantation for COPD: reversing the irreversible. Am Rev Respir Dis 139:301-302
2. Judson MA (1993) Clinical aspects of lung transplantation. Clin Chest Med 14:335-357
3. Cooper JD, Ginsberg RJ, Goldberg M et al (1986) Unilateral lung transplantation for pulmonary fibrosis. N Engl J Med 314:1140-1145
4. US Scientific Registry of Organ Transplantation and the Organ Procurement and Transplantation Network: Annual Report, 1990
5. Breen TJ, Keck B, Hosenpud JD et al (1992) Thoracic organ transplants in the United States from October 1987 through December 1991: a report from the UNOS Scientific Registry for Organ Transplants. Clin Transplants 33-43
6. Rothfield KP, Firestone S, Firestone LL (1994) Patient selection and outcomes for lung transplantation. Curr Opin Anaesthesiol 7:299-304
7. Egan TM, Kaiser LE, Cooper JD (1989) Lung transplantation. Curr Probl Surg 26:681-751
8. Patterson GA, Cooper JD, Dark JH et al (1988) Experimental and clinical double lung transplantation. J Thorac Cardiovasc Surg 95:70-74
9. Pasque MK, Trulock EP, Kaiser LR, Cooper JD (1991) Single-lung transplantation for pulmonary hypertension. Circulation 84:2275-2279
10. Patterson GA, Maurer JR, Williams TJ et al (1991) Comparison of outcomes of double and single lung transplantation for obstructive lung disease. J Thorac Cardiovasc Surg 101: 623-632
11. Williams TJ, Patterson GA, McClean PA et al (1992) Maximal exercise testing in single and double lung transplant recipients. Am Rev Respir Dis 145:101-105
12. Dark JH (1994) Lung transplantation. Transpl Proc 26:1708-1709
13. Paradis I, Manzetti J, Foust D et al (1993) When to refer for lung transplantation? Characteristics of candidates who die prior vs. those who survive to receive a transplant. Am Rev Respir Dis 147:A597
14. Goldsmith MF (1990) Mother to child: first living donor lung transplant. JAMA 264:2724
15. Egan TM, Boychuk JE, Rosato K et al (1992) Whence the lungs? A study to assess suitability of donor lungs for transplantation. Transplantation 53:420-422
16. Colice GL, Matthay MA, Bass E et al (1984) Neurogenic pulmonary edema. Am Rev Respir Dis 130:941-948
17. Harjula A, Starnes VA, Oyer PE et al (1987) Proper donor selection for heart-lung transplantation: the Stanford experience. J Thorac Cardiovasc Surg 94:874-880
18. Pickett JA, Wheeldon D, Oduro A (1994) Multi-organ transplantation donor management. Curr Opin Anaesthesiol 7:80-83
19. Freeman JW (1993) Donor selection and maintenance prior to multiorgan retrieval. In: Vincent JL (ed) Yearbook of intensive care and emergency medicine. Springer, Berlin Heidelberg New York, pp 671-683
20. Mackersie RC, Bronsther OL, Shackford SR (1991) Organ procurement in patients with fatal head injuries. Ann Surg 213:143-150
21. Sleiman C, Mal H, Dubois F et al (1992) Pulmonary reimplantation response in single lung transplantation. Am Rev Respir Dis 145:A305
22. Kaiser LR, Pasque MK, Trulock EP et al (1991) Bilateral sequential lung transplantation: the procedure of choice for double-lung replacement. Ann Thorac Surg 52:438-446

23. Kirk AJ, Colquhoun IW, Dark JH (1993) Lung preservation: a review of current practice and future directions. Ann Thorac Surg 56:990-1000
24. Novick RJ, Menkis A, McKenzie FN (1992) New trends in lung preservation: a collective review. J Heart Lung Transplant 11:377-392
25. Conacher ID (1988) Isolated lung transplantation: a review of problems and guide to anaesthesia. Br J Anaesth 61:468-474
26. Trintafillou AN, Heerdt PM (1991) Lung transplantation. Int Anesthesiol Clin 29:87-109
27. Wittnich C, Trudel J, Zidulka A, Chu-Jeng Chiu R (1986) Misleading "pulmonary wedge pressure" after pneumonectomy: its importance in postoperative fluid therapy. Ann Thorac Surg 41:192-196
28. Jardin F, Bourdarias JP (1995) Right heart catheterisation at bedside: a critical view. Intensive Care Med 21:291-295
29. Thomas BJ, Siegel LC (1991) Anesthetic and postoperative management of single-lung transplantation. J Cardiovasc Vasc Anesth 5:266-267
30. Quinlan JJ, Buffington CW (1993) Deliberate hypoventilation in a patient with air trapping during lung transplantation. Anesthesiology 78:1177-1181
31. Gutierrez G, Palizas F, Doglio G et al (1992) Gastric intramucosal pH as a therapeutic index of tissue oxygenation in critically ill patients. Lancet 339:196-199
32. Fiddian-Green RG, Baker S (1987) Predictive value of the stomach wall pH for complications after cardiac operations: comparison with other monitoring. Crit Care Med 15:153-156
33. Maynard N, Bihari D, Beale R et al (1993) Assessment of splanchnic oxygenation by gastric tonometry in patients with acute circulatory failure. JAMA 270:1203-1210
34. Triantafillou AN, Pond CG, Cerza RF et al (1993) Cardiopulmonary bypass requirements in lung transplant patients: the Washington University experience. Anesthesiology 79:A47
35. Firestone L, Carrera J, Firestone S, Rothfield K (1993) Single lung transplants: who needs bypass? Anesthesiology 79:A46
36. Rossi J, Bierman MI, Griffith BP (1995) Recent progress in lung transplantation. Curr Opin Crit Care 1:77-83
37. Patterson GA (1990) Double lung transplantation. Clin Chest Med 11:227-233
38. de Hoyos, Demajo W, Snell G et al (1993) Preoperative prediction for the use of cardiopulmonary bypass in lung transplantation. J Thorac Cardiovasc Surg 106:787-796
39. Tinker JH, Roberts SL (1989) Anaesthesia for cardiac surgery. In: Nunn JF, Utting JE, Brown BR (eds) General anaesthesia, 5th edn. Butterworths, London, pp 864-910
40. Sherry KM, Massey NJA, Moore NA, Blackburn A, Peacock JE (1991) Infusion induction and maintenance of hypnosis with propofol in patients presenting for cardiac surgery. In: Prys-Roberts C (ed). Focus on infusion. Current Medical Literature Ltd, London, pp 24-29
41. Bell J, Sartain J, Wilkinson GAL, Sherry KM (1994) Propofol and fentanyl anaesthesia for patients with low cardiac output state undergoing cardiac surgery: comparison with high-dose fentanyl anaesthesia. Br J Anaesth 73:162-166
42. Vaughan RS (1993) Double-lumen tubes. Br J Anaesth 70:497-498
43. Bardoczky GI, Levarlet M, Engelman E, Defrancquen P (1993) Continuous spirometry for detection of double-lumen endobronchial tube displacement. Br J Anaesth 70:499-502
44. Clapham MC, Vaughan RS (1985) Endobronchial intubation. A comparison between polyvinylchloride and red rubber double lumen tubes. Anaesthesia 1111-1114
45. Conacher ID (1995) Prolonged interval jet ventilation. An alternative technique for patients with problematic cardiopulmonary pathophysiology. Anaesthesia 50:518-522
46. Higgins TL (1992) Pro: early extubation is preferable to late extubation in patients following coronary artery surgery. J Cardiothor Vasc Anesth 6:488-493
47. Gall SA, Olsen CO, Reves JG et al (1988) Beneficial effects of endotracheal extubation on ventricular performance. J Thorac Cardiovasc Surg 95:819-827
48. Kirklin JK (1991) Prospects for understanding and eliminating the deleterious effects of cardiopulmonary bypass. Ann Thorac Surg 51:529-531
49. Johnson D, Thomson D, Hurst T et al (1994) Neutrophil-mediated acute lung injury after extracorporeal perfusion. J Thorac Cardiovasc Surg 107:1193-1202

50. Montravers P, Fagon JY, Gilbert C et al (1993) Pilot study of cardiopulmonary risk from pentoxifylline in adult respiratory distress syndrome. Chest 103:1017-1022
51. Kollef MH, Schuster DP (1995) The acute respiratory distress syndrome. N Engl J Med 322: 27-37
52. Shoemaker WC (1995) Invasive and noninvasive cardiopulmonary monitoring of acute circulatory dysfunction and shock. Curr Opin Crit Care 1:189-190
53. Conacher ID (1990) Pain relief after thoracotomy. Br J Anaesth 65:806-812
54. George KA, Wright PMC, Chisakuta A (1991) Continuous thoracic epidural fentanyl for post-thoracotomy pain relief: with or without bupivacaine? Anaesthesia 46:732-736
55. Morgan M (1989) The rational use of intrathecal and extradural opioids. Br J Anaesth 63: 165-188
56. Guinard J-P, Mavrocordatos P, Chiolero R, Carpenter RL (1992) A randomized comparison of intravenous versus lumbar and thoracic epidural fentanyl for analgesia after thoracotomy. Anesthesiology 77:1108-1115
57. Wotherspoon HA, Kenny GNC, McArdle CS (1991) Pain following thoracotomy. A randomised, double-blind comparison of lumbar versus thoracic epidural fentanyl. Anaesthesia 46:915-917

Progress in Lung Transplantation

M. CASTAGNETO, G. NANNI, N. PANOCCHIA

The pioneer era

The first report of lung transplantation dates back to 1906 and is due to A. Carrel and C. Guthrie who performed a heterotopic heart-lung transplant in the cat. However, it was not until 1950 that Iuvenelles and Metras proved in an autotransplantation model in the dog that lung transplantation was technically feasible. It is noteworthy that these authors employed atrial instead of single pulmonary vein anastomosis as well as bronchial artery revascularization.

In 1963, after extensive animal work, Hardy et al. (1) of Jackson-Mississippi University performed the first single lung transplant in a patient with lung cancer and severe chronic obstructive pulmonary disease (COPD). The grafted lung was retrieved after cardiac arrest in a patient who had sustained a massive myocardial infarction. The recipient, treated with steroid and azathioprine based immunosuppression, survived 18 days and, apparently, no histologic evidence of rejection was found on post-mortem examination.

After Hardy's breakthrough 38 more lung transplant operations were performed world wide over a 15-year period; however, no long-term successes could be reported due to technical, physiopathologic, immunological or septic complications. Only one patient, transplanted in Gand (Belgium) by Derom (2), survived as long as 10 months.

It was therefore necessary to go back to the laboratory and delve more deeply into the technical and physiologic problems of lung transplantation. The turning point came when a group of thoracic surgeons, working at Toronto University, resolved to make a careful retrospective analysis of all the clinical experience of lung transplantation available at that point. They noted that out of 20 patients who survived the transplant operation for more than a week, 16 went on to die for complications related to failure of the bronchial anastomosis, which was therefore termed the Achille's heel of lung transplantation (3). Experimental work further demonstrated that poor bronchial healing was due to ischemia secondary to inappropriate harvesting and preservation of the lung as well as to the steroid effect (4). In this regard it must also be noted that cyclosporine, which had just become available at that time, making rejection control more effective, also improved bronchial stump vascularization. In an effort to fast bronchial flow restoration, omentopexy, namely, wrapping the bronchial anastomosis with a pedicle of omentum, proved to be of further advantage.

The new era

With this encouraging experimental background, in 1983 the Toronto group, headed by Dr. Joel Cooper, started a new clinical lung transplant program whose final success has been fundamental for establishing this as an accepted procedure and the sole therapy for many end-stage pulmonary diseases.

We can therefore set 1983 (5) as the starting date of the modern era of lung transplantation: most recent clinical series show that major complications range around 10%-15% with a decreasing trend due to the rapid expansion of knowledge in this new field, whose most relevant aspects can be summarized as follows:

Organ preservation. It is a widely shared contention that the quality of transplanted lung is of paramount importance in determining the fate of the whole procedure. To this end utmost attention should be paid to the appropriate maintenance of the donor, to the correct harvesting technique and to the lung preservation conditions; containment of ischemic damage means a more rapid resumption of gas exchange function, less pulmonary edema, better blood flow and better healing of the bronchial anastomosis and in the end a more rapid patient recovery.

At the present time harvesting of the donor lung is performed after flushing the organ through the pulmonary artery with a cold intracellular perfusion fluid, called modified Collins solution (6). In order to decrease the pulmonary vascular resistance 500 mcg of PGE_1 are injected directly into the pulmonary artery. Recently the Belzer solution (University of Wisconsin solution) was used instead with good results (7).

Surgical technique. While it remains to be established whether a truly telescopic bronchial anastomosis is superior to the common figure 8 stitch techniques, progress in preservation procedures have made the omentopexy optional and in general less popular.

Immunosuppressive therapy. Advances in immunosuppressive therapy made possible by cyclosporine have been beneficial, as already mentioned, also in the healing of bronchial anastomosis through reduction of rejection mediated inflammatory response which in turn causes impairment of microvasculature blood flow. This is why steroids, which were withheld in the first few weeks after grafting because of the adverse effect on wound healing, were more recently employed again after operation (8).

Heart-lung and double lung transplantation. In 1981 B.A. Reitz (9) performed the first few successful heart-lung transplants in patients with pulmonary hypertension and heart failure due to Eisenmenger's syndrome.

Although other centers used this option to treat cystic fibrosis and emphysema it soon became clear that transplanting the heart in this clinical situation in most cases was unnecessary and unwarranted.

In 1986, the Toronto Lung Transplant Group (10) showed that it was possible to graft both lungs without the heart. Over the following years the operation was perfected and simplified and instead of transplanting both lungs en bloc sequential, bilateral lung transplantation became the standard procedure. This operation (11), which is carried out through a transverse thoracotomy, is essentially very much alike the technique of single lung transplantation performed on both sides. It carries a much lower postoperative morbidity and mortality risk and does not require, in most instances, the use of cardiopulmonary by-pass (12).

Indications for lung transplantation

As experience and results of lung transplantation improve, indications also evolve. In general and with few exceptions, we can say that the indications for lung transplantation are progressive, irreversible disabling end stage nontumor pulmonary disease. Table 1 shows which transplant procedure is indicated for what pulmonary disease.

Table 1. Which procedure for what disease

Single lung Tx
Restrictive lung disease
Chronic obstructive pulmonary disease
Pulmonary vascular disease
Infectious lung disease (selected patients)
Bilateral lung Tx
Infectious end-stage disease
Cystic fibrosis
Bronchiectasis
Obstructive and restrictive lung disease with infection
Giant bilateral bullous disease
Pulmonary vascular disease
Heart-lung Tx
Pulmonary hypertension with severe congenite heart disease
End stage pulmonary disease and severe heart defects in young patients

It must be stated, however, that bilateral lung operation, being much harder on the patient, should be reserved for people under 50 years of age.

Timing of transplantation is another crucial point which needs careful consideration (13). There is not a simple parameter, either clinical or physiopathologic, to guide in this difficult decision. In general a life expectancy of 12 to 18 months is considered the reference point. Table 2 shows the severity indices compatible with this criterium.

Table 2. Severity indices of chronic lung disease and timing of transplantation

Chronic obstructive pulmonary disease (COPD) and alpha-1-antitrypsin deficiency emphysema (EMP-A1)

      FEV_1 after bronchodilatators: < 30% of predicted

      Hypoxia at rest (PaO_2 < 55-60 mmHg)

      Hypercapnia

Secondary pulmonary hypertension

      Deteriorating clinical course

      Episodes of lung disease exacerbation

Cystic fibrosis

      FEV_1 after bronchodilatators: < 30% of predicted

      Hypoxia at rest (PaO_2 < 55-60 mmHg)

      Hypercapnia

      Deteriorating clinical course

      Airway colonization with antibiotic-resistant organism (*Pseudomonas, Aspergillus*)

Idiopathic pulmonary fibrosis (IPF)

      VC and TLC < 60% of predicted

      Hypoxia at rest

      Secondary pulmonary hypertension

Primary pulmonary hypertension

      NYHA class III and IV

      Mean atrial pressure > 10 mmHg

      Mean pulmonary artery pressure > 50 mmHg

      Cardiac index < 2,5 $L/m/m^2$

      Unresponsive to Ca channel blockers and PGI_2

In addition the quality of life of the patient must be taken into account and his nutritional status.

Lastly it should be mentioned that when a simple lung transplant is indicated the side should be selected where the most severely diseased lung resides. When both sides are equal it is preferable to graft the left lung for fibrosis and the right for COPD (14). This is done in order to keep the more expanded lung on the left side to lessening the chance of mediastinal shift during mechanical ventilation.

The pulmonary donor

The guidelines for acceptance of donor lungs are showed in Table 3. Moreover it is necessary to provide the prospective recipient with an organ that would best match his or her size. This is done on the basis of anthropometric parameters (15), such as height and submammillary diameter, chest X-ray measurements (horizontal and vertical diameters) and spirometric data such as predictive TLC and VC. A 10% discrepancy between donor and recipient can be tolerated without untoward effects. It is estimated that only 10% of available donors are currently considered acceptable for lung harvesting.

Table 3. Lung donor criteria

ABO compatibility
Age < 45 years
Normal chest X-ray
$PaO_2 > 300$ mmHg on $FiO_2 = 1.0$ and PEEP 5 cm for 5'
Bronchoscopy: clear
No significant pulmonary contusion
No previous thoracic surgery

Technique of lung transplantation

Description of the surgical technique (16, 17) of lung transplantation is beyond the scope of this review. The operation is relatively straightforward and entails a pneumonectomy carried out through a posterolateral thoracotomy on the fifth intercostal space for a single lung or through a transverse thoracotomy for bilateral lung transplantation. The new lung is then sewn in, making an end to end anastomosis of the bronchus first, then of the pulmonary artery, and lastly of the atrial cuff encompassing the two veins.

Postoperative course and complications

Table 4 summarizes the main events occurring after lung transplantation. It must be pointed out that during the first two postoperative weeks pulmonary dysfunction due to the so-called "reperfusion syndrome" (18), rejection reaction or infection are most common. Although reperfusion syndrome appears in the first 2 days while rejection occurs after the first week and infection comes usually later, all three conditions have similar clinical and physiopathological features and often coexist. Hence the difficulty in making a differential diagnosis and employing the appropriate treatment.

Table 4. Postoperative events and complications after lung transplantation

Reperfusion syndrome
Rejection reaction
Infections (Bacteria, viruses, fungi)
Bronchial anastomosis breakdown
Pneumothorax
Other complications: cardiac, neurological, abdominal, hematological, renal

Clinical results of lung transplantation

Overall clinical results of lung transplantation are regularly made available by the St. Louis International Lung Registry. Data came from 142 institutions although there are 77 presently active centers worldwide, 44 of which are within the United States. Prior to 31 December 1994 there are 3836 transplants reported to the registry (19); of these 2346 were singles, 1252 were bilateral sequentials, and 230 were en bloc double lung transplants. The number of transplants performed yearly seems to be levelling off at around 900. The main indications for lung grafting remain, in decreasing order of frequency, COPD, IPF, CF, EMP.A-1, PPH. The largest number of transplants are performed in the 40 to 60 age group. Actuarial patient survival of the total registry experience since 1983 at 1, 2 and 5 years is respectively 71%, 64% and 48%. However, survival rates of 2529 patients transplanted between 1992 and 1994 are at 1 and 2 years respectively 74% and 68%.

As lung transplantation become more and more successful, an increasing number of centers have started new programs in recent years. The Division of Organ Transplantation, to which the authors belong, is one of them. Having been deeply involved in transplantation surgery for the last 25 years with special reference to kidney and liver, the acquired experience was easily applied to the lung transplantation program (20, 21). Although we have done only three single lung and one bilateral lung transplant (22), they are all currently alive and well from 10 to 23 months postoperatively. Clinical courses did not show any surgical complications while immunosuppressive therapy was managed very much like that for our kidney and liver transplant patients; namely, cyclosporine blood levels were kept at 400 ng/ml, steroids rapidly tapered down to 12 mg/day by the end of the first week, while antilymphocytes antibodies were given only for resistant rejection. It is our feeling that the promising results we have so far obtained are based on three factors:

− Previous extensive experience with management of transplant patients
− Thorough preparation of the patient for the surgical procedure, especially from the nutritional and rehabilitative point of view
− Meticulous attention to the details in postoperative care

Conclusion

At last lung transplantation has also become an established therapy for many patients with end-stage pulmonary disease. Unfortunately this convention is not always shared by all people involved in the care of these patients, and all too often transplantation comes as a very last resort and too late. On the other hand, the supply of donor organs remains extremely limited and new strategies must be devised to increase its number if we are to make pulmonary transplantation a realistic option for all the patients who are in need of it.

References

1. Hardy JD, Webb WR, Dalton ML (1963) Lung homotransplantation in man. JAMA 186: 1065-1074
2. Derom F, Barbier F, Ringoir S (1971) Ten month survival after lung homotransplantation in man. J Thorac Cardiovasc Surg 61:835-846
3. Eagan TM, Kaiser LR, Cooper JD (1989) Lung transplantation. Curr Prob Surg 26:10
4. Goldberg M, Lima O, Morgan E (1983) A comparison between cyclosporin a and methylprednisolone plus azathioprine on bronchial healing following canine lung autotransplantation. J Thorac Cardiovasc Surg 85:821-826
5. Cooper JD (1989) Lung transplantation. Ann Thorac Surg 47:28-44
6. Colquhoun IW, Kirk AJB, Au J, Conacher ID, Corris PA, Hilton CJ, Dark JH (1992) Single - flush perfusion with modified Euro-Collins solution experience in clinical lung preservation. J Heart Lung Transplant 11:S209-S214
7. Hardesty HL, Aeba R, Armitage JM, Kormos LR, Griffith BP (1993) A clinical trial of University of Wisconsin solution for pulmonary preservation. J Thorac Cardiovasc Surg, 105: 660-666
8. Inui K, Schaefers HJ, Aoki M, Wada H, Becker V, Ongsiek B, Haverich A (1993) Effect of methylprednisolone and prostacyclin on bronchial perfusion in lung transplantation. Ann Thorac Surg 55:464-469
9. Reitz S, Wallwork JL, Hunt SA (1982) Heart-lung transplantation successful therapy for patients with pulmonary vascular disease. N Engl J Med 306:557-564
10. Toronto lung transplantation group (1986) Unilateral lung transplantation for pulmonary fibrosis. N Engl J Med 314(18):1140-1145
11. Pasque MK, Cooper JD, Kaiser LR, Haydock DA, Triantafillou A, Trulock EP (1990) Improved technique for bilateral lung transplantation rationale and initial clinical experience. Ann Thorac Surg 49(5):785-91
12. Patterson GA, Maurer JR, Williams TJ, Cardoso PG, Scavuzzo M, Todd TR and The Toronto Lung Transplant Group (1991) Comparison of outcomes of double and single lung transplantation for obstructive lung disease. J Thorac Cardiovasc Surg 101:623-632
13. Trulock EP (1993) Recipient selection. 3th International Lung Transplant Symposium, Zurich 1993, June 24-25
14. Mal H, Andreassian B, Pamela P, Duchatelle JP, Rondeau E, Dubois F, Baldeyrou P, Kitzis M, Sleiman C, Pariente R (1989) Unilateral lung transplantation in end-stage pulmonary emphysema. Am Rev Resp Dis 140:797-802
15. Noirclerc M, Shennib H, Giudicelli R, Latter D, Metras D, Colt HG, Mulder D (1992) Size matching for lung transplantation. J Heart Lung Transplant 11:S203-208
16. Cooper JD, Pearson FG, Patterson GA, Todd TR, Ginsberg RJ, Goldberg M, Demajo WAP (1987) Technique of successful lung transplantation in humans. J Thorac Cardiovasc Surg 93: 173-181

17. Patterson GA (1993) Technique for single and bilateral transplantation. 3th International Lung Transplant Symposium, Zurich, June 24-25
18. Alican F, Cayrli M, Isin E, Hardy JD (1971) Left lung reimplantation with immediate right pulmonary artery ligation. Ann Surg 174:34-43
19. St. Louis International Lung Registry: April 1995 report
20. Nanni G, Scotti A, Sganga G, Panocchia N, Caricato A, Modesti C, Perrotta D, Castagneto M, Crucitti F (1991) Single lung transplant in pig beneficial effects of PGI_2 and gluthatione on early lung function. J R Coll Edinb 36:346
21. Panocchia M, Nanni G, Chiarello M, Azzaretto M, Procopio A, Caricato A, Marinelli R, Castagneto M (1994) Comparison of Euro-Collins (EC), low potassium dextrane (LPD) and University of Wisconsin (UW) solutions in preventing formation of oxygen free radicals (OFR) in pig lung transplantation. J R Coll Edinb 39:382-383
22. Nanni G, Castagneto M, Panocchia N, Agnes S, Avolio A, Foco M, Magalini S, Crucitti F, Sollazzi L, Perilli W, Pennisi M, Proietti G, Pirronti T, Marano P, Salvatori M, Valente S, Pagliari G, Ciappi G, Pennestrì F, Morelli P, Possati G (1994) Il trapianto di polmone all'Università Cattolica di Roma: successo dei primi tre casi. Società Italiana di Chirurgia, 96° Congresso Nazionale, Roma 16-19 ottobre 1994, Edizioni Minerva Medica, Roma

Nitric Oxide in Pulmonary Hypertension

J.O.C. AULER Jr.

Introduction

Nitric oxide (NO) has mainly been seen as a toxic agent associated with air pollution. Recently it has been recognized as a primary endogenous mediator of important physiologic processes. Both artery and vein are able to release endothelium-derived relaxing factor (EDRF) in response to different vasodilators (1, 2). Among several functions, the vascular endothelium, which encircles the blood, contributes to the control of vascular tone by releasing compounds that mediate contraction or relaxation of the underlying vascular smooth muscle (3, 4). The endothelium synthesizes vasodilator substances such as prostacyclin, endothelium-derived relaxing factor or nitric oxide (NO) (5, 6) as well as endothelin(s) and endothelium-derived contracting factor which promotes vasoconstriction (3). In response to several stimuli or mediators, the endothelial L-arginine NO pathway is activated by contact with the blood, in addition to receptor utilized mechanisms activated by shear stress, acetylcholine, ADP, bradykinin, substance P, histamine, and platelet-derived products (7). NO diffuses into the smooth muscle cells where it activates the soluble guanylate cyclase to generate cyclic GMP, the second messenger mediating relaxation (6, 8, 9). Endogenous NO seems to be continuously released for accurate regulation of vascular tone. Substances such as acetylcholine or bradykinin are considered as endothelium-dependent dilators and therapeutic nitrates which directly activate soluble guanylate cyclase by releasing NO from their molecules are considered as endothelium-independent dilators. NO is also considered an inhibitor of platelet aggregation, contributing to the vasodilator properties of prostacyclin (7, 10). Vascular smooth muscle relaxation and cyclic GMP accumulation due to the action of several chemical substances on the endothelium are attributed to the release of NO (11, 12). The central role of the endothelium in mediating vessel tone has become of paramount importance since knowing of acetylcholine dependence on EDRF release. Endothelial dysfunction in a number of vascular diseases may be related to an attenuated acetylcholine response and decreased NO release, which may contribute to pulmonary hypertension (13, 14).

Several kinds of injuries to the pulmonary vascular endothelium have been related to the development or exacerbation of pulmonary hypertension. It is important to consider whether the inhibition of the basal release of NO would be followed by some untoward side effects. Several studies have shown that inhibition of NO synthesis could exacerbate vasoconstriction and ischemia (15). In this regard, it is interesting to note that in some conditions where endothelial lesions may occur, such as during organ preservation for transplant and cardiopulmonary bypass, this may be associated with impaired endothelium NO formation (16-18). These observations emphasize the concept that the circulatory system is in a constant state of vasodilation and that the inhibition of that vasodilator tone system results in noticeable vasoconstriction. Endothelial dysfunction as observed in many diseases reflecting altered L-arginine-NO pathway activity can be demonstrated by a decreased cyclic GMP content in the vascular wall or by a reduced response to endothelium-dependent vasodilators such as acetylcholine (19). It has been described that the vasodilatory properties of inhaled NO are mainly restricted to the pulmonary circulation which makes NO an attractive agent to be utilized in several clinical conditions associated with pulmonary hypertension (20). Additionally, inhaled NO seems to selectively dilate vessels of ventilated areas of the lung, causing a decrease in intrapulmonary shunt and improving the oxygenation (21). Pulmonary vascular resistance and pulmonary artery pressure in ARDS patients (22, 23), persistent pulmonary hypertension of the newborn (24-26) and severe pulmonary hypertension (27) have been reduced during NO inhalation. These same effects can also be seen in cardiac surgical patients including children with congenital cardiopathy during hemodynamic diagnostic investigation (28), after pediatric (27) and adult surgical correction (29-31) as well as during heart and lung transplantation. Selective pulmonary vasodilation is a desirable effect after heart (32) and lung transplantation (33) to control severe pulmonary hypertension that may result in right ventricular failure (32). Although inhaled NO seems to counteract hypoxic pulmonary vasoconstriction in volunteers inhaling hypoxic mixtures (34), the reduction in pulmonary artery pressure, and oxygenation improvement are dependent on and related to the degree of the previous levels of pulmonary vascular resistance (35). Current intravenous vasodilators employed to relax the pulmonary vasculature often result in systemic hypotension, an effect not commonly described with inhaled NO because of its rapid inactivation by the hemoglobin (36, 37). Since the time NO was reported to be an EDRF (2), a growing interest in its clinical use has been observed, making the possibility to use an agent that can be circumscribed to a delimited territory very attractive and putting this agent in a possible advantage over the traditional vasodilators for treatment of acute pulmonary hypertension (38) as could be observed in heart transplant patients. As previously described, it has been indicated that inhaled NO is a potent pulmonary vasodilator (39). In this abstract, the hemodynamic effects of 20 ppm of NO in eight adult patients (mean age 40 ± 14 years) submitted to heart transplantation were investigated. Two hours after the surgical procedure, NO was administered together with mechanical ventilation. Conventional hemodynamic data was collected at 30 and 60 min before and after NO inhalation. As can be seen in Table 1, inhaled NO promoted a significant

Table 1. Inhaled nitric oxide hemodynamic effects

	Baseline	30' NO	60' NO	30' after	60' after
HR	113 ± 13	114 ± 14	111 ± 16	115 ± 15	112 ± 14
MAP	77 ± 12	87 ± 11	78 ± 12	78 ± 14	82 ± 9
MPAP	28 ± 7	26 ± 6	26 ± 7	26 ± 6	28 ± 5
CWP	17 ± 7	18 ± 6	19 ± 7	17 ± 5	18 ± 5
CI	4.8 ± 1.1	5.2 ± 1.1	5.4 ± 1.3*	5.1 ± 1.3	4.9 ± 1.3
SVR	693 ± 280	717 ± 224	624 ± 285	675 ± 266	720 ± 279
PVR	108 ± 30	73 ± 25*	59 ± 24*	88 ± 36	93 ± 29

HR, heart rate (beats/min); MAP, mean artery pressure (mmHg); MPAP, mean pulmonary artery pressure (mmHg); CWP, capillary wedge pressure (mmHg); CI, cardiac index ($l/min/m^2$); SVR, systemic vascular resistance (dynes/s/cm^5); PVR, pulmonary vascular resistance (dynes/s/cm^5)

* $p < 0.05$ compared with values before NO inhalation

increase in cardiac index as well as a significant decrease in pulmonary vascular resistance, more evident 60 min after NO inhalation. The elevated vascular resistance in end stage cardiac patients can be a limiting factor in the indication of the transplantation and/or in the postoperative period (40). Kieler-Jensen et al. (41), in heart transplant candidates, compared intravenous vasodilators with NO and observed that NO was more effective as a selective pulmonary vasodilator. In addition, following cardiopulmonary bypass, it is common to observe pulmonary vascular resistance (PVR) exacerbation that can cause right ventricular dysfunction. Intravenous vasodilators are commonly employed to control the PVR; however, they may also cause reduction in systemic blood pressure as well which may additionally require vasopressors (42). Girard et al. (32) described severe right ventricular failure after transplant which responded favorably to NO. Contrary to ARDS patients, it is interesting to note that NO has not significantly modified pulmonary oxygenation when this parameter was previously considered normal. Transpulmonary gradient (mean pulmonary artery pressure minus wedge pressure) seems to be a more accurate index to reflect the real pulmonary resistance than the traditional PVR. Some studies have revealed that TPG is one of the most important predictors of survival after heart transplant; if this gradient exceeds 20 mmHg there is a stepwise increase in early mortality (43). In unpublished data, we have observed a significant decrease in TPG in heart transplant patients during the period in which patients inhaled NO. It may also be beneficial after lung transplantation. The inhaled gas could lower pulmonary artery pressure and pulmonary vascular resistance in addition to improving intrapulmonary shunt fraction by correcting ventilatory/perfusion abnormalities after lung transplantation. Theoretically, the eventual improvement in gas exchange and pulmonary hemodynamics could be maintained with continued NO therapy. Transplanted lungs may be further damaged during reperfusion, resulting in alveolar capillary edema, altered lung compliance and elevation in PVR, factors that could compromise the graft function. As previously mentioned, PVR exacerbation after lung transplantation may be explained by ischemic endothelial damage and impaired endogenous NO production. It is attractive to consider that inhaled NO may temporarily substitute the role of endogenous NO as a vasodilator mediator in the pulmonary vasculature. Adatia et al. (33) demonstrated in a group of five patients with pulmonary hypertension submitted to lung transplantation a significant decrease in mean pulmonary artery pressure, pulmonary vascular resistance as well as in intrapulmonary shunting fraction. According to this study, the necessary doses of NO to be administered after lung transplantation still remains controversial. Even though the effects of inhaled NO on the pulmonary circulation are well demonstrated, its effects on the respiratory system mechanics and gas exchange remain controversial. Although endogenous NO seems to exert an important role on bronchomotor tonus modulation (44, 45), the results of several investigations employing inhaled NO in this area are often contradictory (35). Hypothetically, owing to the fact that they are extremely lipophilic, inhaled NO molecules diffuse through the bronchial epithelium and act upon airway smooth muscle, leading to bronchodilation (44). The relaxation of the terminal bronchioles could be mediated by cyclic-AMP and cyclic-GMP described as the principal intracellular messenger involved with airway smooth muscle relaxation (46). Several investigations have showed the importance of NO in modulating bronchomotor tonus, such as inhibition of endogenous NO synthesis, increasing bronchoconstriction to allergen (47), inhaled NO counteracting methacholine induced bronchoconstriction in guinea pigs (48) and rabbits (49), in addition to a discrete bronchodilating effect observed in asthmatic patients inhaling NO (35, 50). Concomitant to an intraoperative pulmonary vasodilator effect (39), a consistent bronchodilator action of inhaled NO could be very interesting to counteract the increased airway resistance that may occur after lung transplantation. We investigated (51) the effects of 20 ppm of inhaled NO on respiratory mechanics and hemodynamics in twelve postoperative patients (mean age 48.9 ± 14.3 years) submitted to cardiac surgery, including heart transplantation (six patients). During the study all patients remained anesthetized under controlled mechanical ventilation and respiratory mechanics (resistive and elastic properties) were analyzed by the end inflation occlusion method. As can be seen in Figs. 1, 2, the data submitted to a repeated measures analysis of variance (ANOVA) showed a nonsignificant variation on elastic and resistive properties but a significant decrease in pulmonary vascular resistance ($p < 0.05$). Utilizing the same method Puybasset et al. (50) did not demonstrate a bronchodilating effect of NO in ARDS patients. The inconsistency among different studies concerning bronchomotor tonus modulation of exogenous NO may be explained by possible bronchoconstrictive effects induced by byproducts, such as NO_2, generated during administration of the agent.

In conclusion NO may represent a useful and powerful mediator to be used to control pulmonary hypertension after lung and heart transplantation. Some points still need to be clarified, mainly involving doses and side effects related to long-term usage. The role of this agent on respiratory mechanics as well as the gas exchange in relatively normal lungs also requires further studies (52).

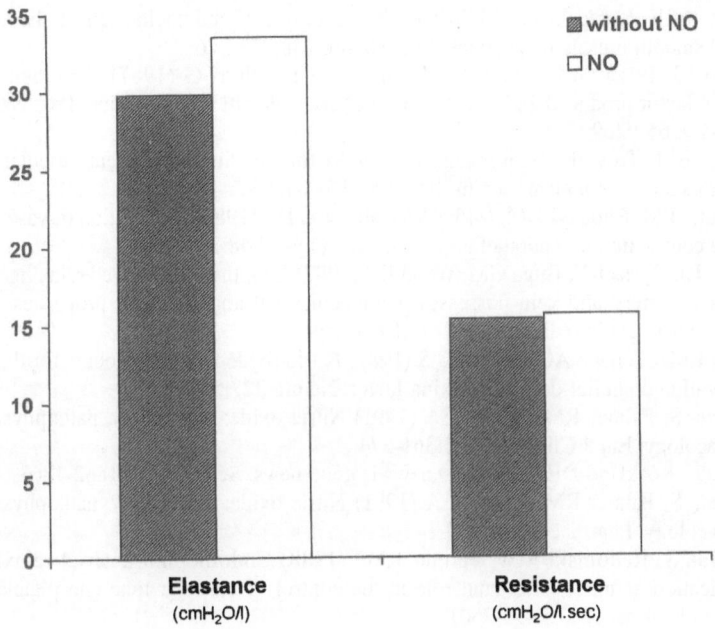

Fig. 1. Values of elastance and resistance of total respiratory system. There is no significant variation before and after nitric oxide (NO) inhalation (20 ppm)

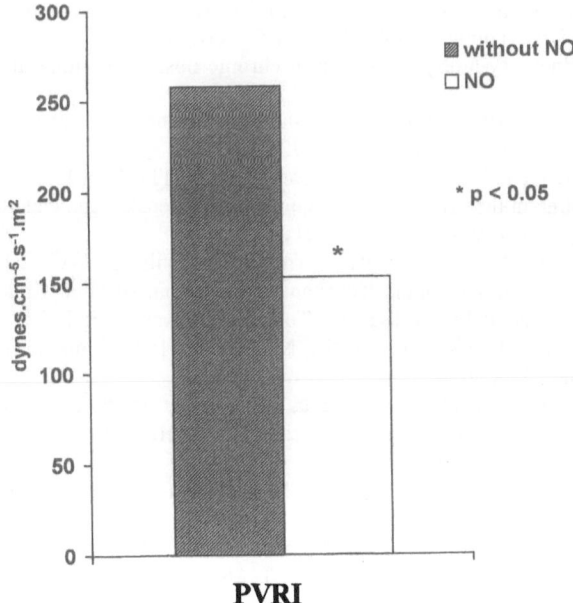

Fig. 2. Impressive and significant decrease in pulmonary vascular resistance after nitric oxide inhalation (20 ppm) $p < 0.05$

References

1. Furchgott RF, Zawadzki JV (1980) The obligatory role of endothelial cells in the relaxation of arterial smooth muscle by acetylcholine. Nature 288:373-376
2. Ignarro LJ, Buga GM, Wood KS, Byrns RE, Chaudhuri G (1987) Endothelium-derived relaxing factor produced and released from artery and vein is nitric oxide. Proc Natl Acad Sci USA 84:9265-9269
3. Brenner BM, Troy JL, Ballermann, BJ (1989) Endothelium-dependent vascular responses. Mediators and mechanisms. J Clin Invest 84:1373-1378
4. Vanhoutte PM, Rubanyi GM, Miller VM, Houston DS (1986) Modulation of vascular smooth muscle contraction by endothelium. Annu Rev Physiol 48:307-320
5. Ignarro LJ, Byrns RE, Buga GM, Wood KS (1987) Endothelium-derived relaxing factor from pulmonary artery and vein possesses pharmacological and chemical properties identical to those of nitric oxide radical. Circ Res 61:866-879
6. Palmer RMJ, Ferrige AG, Moncada S (1987) Nitric oxide release accounts for the biological activity of endothelial-derived relaxing factor. Nature 327:524-526.
7. Moncada S, Palmer RMJ, Higgs EA (1991) Nitric oxide: physiology, pathophysiology, and pharmacology. Eur J Clin Invest 21:361-374
8. Culotta E, Koskland DE (1992) NO news is good news. Science 258:1862-1863
9. Moncada S, Palmer RMJ, Higgs EA (1991) Nitric oxide: physiology, pathophysiology, and pharmacology. Pharmacol Rev 109-142
10. Moncada S, Radomski MW, Palmer RMJ (1988) Endothelium-derived relaxing factor: identification as nitric oxide and role in the control of vascular tone and platelet function. Biochem Pharmacol 37:2495-2501
11. Gruetter CA, Barry BK, McNamara DB, Gruetter DY, Kadowitz PJ, Ignarro LJ (1979) J Cyclic Nucleotide Res 5:211-224
12. Ignarro LJ, Lippton H, Edwards JC, Baricos WH, Hyman AL, Kadowitz PJ, Gruetter CA (1981) J Pharmacol Exp Ther 218:739-749
13. Adnot S, Kouyoumdjian C, Defouilloy C (1993) Hemodynamic and gas exchange responses to infusion of acetylcholine and inhalation of nitric oxide in patients with chronic obstructive lung disease and pulmonary hypertension. Am Rev Respir Dis 148:310-316
14. Dinh-Xuan AT, Higenbottam TW, Clelland CA et al (1991) Impairment of endothelium-dependent pulmonary-artery relaxation in chronic obstructive lung disease. N Engl Med 324:1539-1547
15. Parker JL, Adams HR (1993) Selective inhibition of endothelium-dependent vasodilator capacity by E coli endotoxemia. Circ Res 72:539-551
16. Wessel DL, Adatia T, Giglia TM, Thompson JE, Kulik TJ (1993) Use of inhaled nitric oxide and acetylcholine in the evaluation of pulmonary hypertension and endothelial function after cardiopulmonary bypass. Circulation 88:2118-38
17. Turner-Gomes SO, Andrew M, Coles J, Trusler GA, Williams WG, Rabinovitch M (1992) Abnormalities in von Willebrand factor and antithrombin III after cardiopulmonary bypass operations for congenital heart disease. J Thorac Cardiovasc Surg 103:87-97
18. Toledo-Pereyra LH, Hau T, Simmons RL, Najarian JS (1977) Lung preservation techniques. Ann Thorac Surg 23:487-94
19. Leeman M (1994) Effects of endogenous nitric oxide on the pulmonary circulation. In: Vincent JL (ed) Yearbook of intensive care and emergency medicine. Springer, Berlin Heidelberg New York, pp 101-107
20. Zapol WM, Rimar S, Gillis N, Marletta M, Bosken CH (1994) Nitric oxide and the lung. Am J Respir Crit Care Med 149:1375-80
21. Frostell CG, Fratacci MD, Wain JC, Jones R, Zapol WM (1991) Inhaled nitric oxide: a selective pulmonary vasodilator reversing hypoxic pulmonary vasoconstriction. Circulation 83:2038-2047
22. Rossaint R, Falke KJ, Lopez F, Slama K, Pison U, Zapol WM (1993) Inhaled nitric oxide in adult respiratory distress syndrome. N Engl J Med 328:399-405

23. Gerlach H, Pappert D, Lewandowski K, Rossaint R, Falke KJ (1993) Long-term inhalation with evaluated low doses of nitric oxide for selective improvement of oxygenation in patients with adult respiratory distress syndrome. Intensive Care Med 19:443-449

24. Roberts JD, Polaner DM, Lang P, Zapol WM (1992) Inhaled nitric oxide in persistent pulmonary hypertension of the newborn. Lancet 340:818-819

25. Kinsella J, Neish SR, Shaffer E, Abman SH (1992) Low-dose inhalation nitric oxide in persistent pulmonary hypertension of the newborn. Lancet 340:819-820

26. Pepke-Zaba J, Hogenbottam TW, Dihn-Xuan AT, Stone D, Wallwork J (1991) Inhaled nitric oxide as a cause of selective pulmonary vasodilation in pulmonary hypertension. Lancet 338: 1173-1174

27. Journois D, Pouard P, Mauriat P, Malhere T, Vouhe P, Safran D (1994) Inhaled nitric oxide as a therapy for pulmonary hypertension after operations for congenital heart defects. J Thorac Cardiovasc Surg 107:1129-35

28. Roberts JD, Lang P, Bigatello LM, Vlahakas GJ, Zapol WM (1993) Inhaled nitric oxide in congenital heart disease. Circulation 87:447-453

29. Snow DJ, Gray SJ, Ghosh S et al (1994) Inhaled nitric oxide in patients with normal and increased pulmonary vascular resistance after cardiac surgery. Br J Anaesth 72:185-189

30. Rich GF, Murphy GD Jr, Ross CM, Johns RA (1993) Inhaled nitric oxide: selective pulmonary vasodilatation in cardiac surgical patients. Anaesthesiology 78:1028-1035

31. Girard C, Lehot JJ, Pannetier JC, Filley S, French P, Estanove S (1992) Inhaled nitric oxide after mitral valve replacement in patients with chronic pulmonary artery hypertension. Anesthesiology 77:880-883

32. Girard C, Durand PG, Vedrinne C et al (1993) Inhaled nitric oxide for right ventricular failure after heart transplantation. J Cardiothorac Vasc Anesth 7:481-485

33. Adatia I, Lillehei C, Arnold JH, Thompson JE, Palazzo R, Fackler JC, Wessel DL (1994) Inhaled nitric oxide in the treatment of postoperative graft dysfunction after lung transplantation. Ann Thorac Surg 57:1311-8

34. Frostell C, Blomqvist H, Lundberg J, Hedenstierna G, Zapol WM (1991) Inhaled nitric oxide dilates human hypoxic pulmonary vasoconstriction without causing systemic vasodilation. Anesthesiology 75:989 (abstr)

35. Puybasset L, Rouby JJ (1995) Inhaled nitric oxide in acute respiratory failure. In: Vincent JL (ed) Yearbook of intensive care and emergency medicine. Springer, Berlin Heidelberg New York, pp 331-357

36. Gibson QH, Roughton FJW (1957) The kinetics of equilibria of the reactions of nitric oxide with sheep hemoglobin. J Physiol (Lond) 136:507-526

37. Wennmaln A, Benthin G, Edlund A et al (1993) Metabolism and excretion of nitric oxide in humans. Circ Res 73:1121-1127

38. Kieler-Jensen N, Milocco I, Ricksten SE (1993) Pulmonary vasodilatation after heart transplantation: a comparison among prostacyclin, sodium nitroprusside, and nitroglycerin on right ventricular function and pulmonary selectivity. J Heart Lung Transplant 12:179-184

39. Carmona MJC, Bocchi EA, Auler Jr JOC, Bacal F, Fiorelli AI, Stolf NAG, Amaral RVG, Jatene A (1994) Inhaled nitric oxide in patients submitted to heart transplantation. Circulation 90:I-419 (abstr)

40. Sarris GE, Moore KA, Schroeder JS et al (1994) Cardiac transplantation: the Stanford experience in the cyclosporine era. J Thorac Cardiovasc Surg 108:240-252

41. Kieler-Jansen N, Sven-Erik R, Stenvqvist O et al (1994) Inhaled nitric oxide in the evaluation of heart transplant candidates with elevated pulmonary vascular resistance. J Heart Lung Transplant 13:366-375

42. Vincent JL, Carlier E, Pinsky MR et al (1992) Prostaglandin E1 infusion for right ventricular failure after cardiac transplantation. J Thorac Cardiovasc Surg 103:33-39

43. Kormos RL, Thompson M, Hardesty RL et al (1986) Utility of preoperative right heart catheterization data as a predictor of survival after heart transplantation. J Heart Lung Transpl 5:391 (abstr)

44. Hogman M, Frostell CG, Hedenstrom H, Hedenstierna G (1993) Inhalation of nitric oxide modulates adult bronchial tone. Am Rev Respir Dis 148:1474-1478
45. Miller OI, James J, Elliott MJ (1993) Intraoperative use of inhaled low-dose nitric oxide. J Thorac Cardiovasc Surg 105-550-1
46. Jorens PG, Vermeire PA, Herman AG (1993) L-arginine-dependent nitric oxide synthase: a new metabolic pathway in the lung and airways. Eur Respir J 6:258-66
47. Persson MG, Friberg SG, Hedqvist P, Gustafsson LE (1993) Endogenous nitric oxide counteracts antigen-induced bronchoconstriction. Eur J Pharmacol 249:7-8
48. Dupuy PM, Shore SA, Drazen JM, Frostell C, Hill WA, Zapol Wm (1992) Bronchodilator action of inhaled nitric oxide in guinea pigs. J Clin Invest 90:421-428
49. Hogman M, Frostell C, Arnberg H, Hedenstierna G (1993) Inhalation of nitric oxide modulates methacholine-induced bronchoconstriction in the rabbit. Eur Respir J 6:177-80
50. Puybasset L, Mourgeons E, Segal E, Bodin L, Rouby JJ, Viars P (1993) Effects of inhaled nitric oxide on respiratory resistance in patients with ARDS. Anesthesiology 79:299 (abstr)
51. Auler Jr JOC, Carmona MJC, Saldiva PHN, Gomide do Amaral RV (1994) Effects of inhaled nitric oxide on respiratory mechanics and hemodynamics in patients submitted to cardiac surgery. Clin Intensive Care 5:104 (abstr)
52. Rossaint R, Gerlach H, Pappert D (1994) Inhalation of nitric oxide on severe ARDS. In: Vincent JL (ed) Yearbook of intensive care and emergency medicine. Springer, Berlin Heidelberg New York, pp 108-118

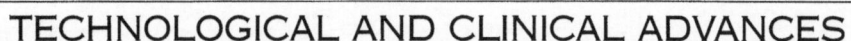

TECHNOLOGICAL AND CLINICAL ADVANCES

Difficult Tracheal Intubation and Airway Management

G. MARTINELLI, C. MELLONI, F. PETRINI, M. VOLPINI

The fundamental responsibility of the anesthesiologist is to maintain adequate gas exchange and particularly oxygenation, while the elimination of CO_2 can be considered a secondary goal, at least for a few minutes.

Studies concerning incidents and accidents, including closed claims analysis, reveal that the leading cause of death and serious damage, particularly cerebral damage, in anesthesia could be attributed to difficulties encountered during attempts at intubation or even difficulties with mask ventilation; it has been very difficult to gather numbers concerning this topic in the past; for instance, Marx et al. (1) collected 2 deaths from failed intubation in 30 000 general anesthetics, excluding obstetrics, but the total number of intubation or the number of successfully managed failed intubation were not given. Recently, a few data became available and those will be discussed at some length because they are very informative: a summary of data gathered from the ASA closed claim study (2) will be presented in Table 1.

Table 1. ASA closed claim study (1990)

- Adverse respiratory events: 34% of total (522/1541)
- Inadequate ventilation 196: 38% of previous cases
- Oesophageal intubation 94: 18%
- Difficult tracheal intubation 87: 17%
- Other mechanisms: airway obstruction, bronchospasm, aspiration, premature unintentional extubation, inadequate O_2 delivery, endobronchial intubation
- Respiratory equipment failures (breathing circuit disconnection or misconnection): 1% of the overall database
- Care judged substandard in 76% of cases
- Better monitoring could probably have prevented the adverse outcome in 72% of cases 85% of respiratory claims gave death or permanent brain damage
- Median payment 240.000 $ for inadequate ventilation, 76.000 $ for difficult tracheal intubation
- Median cost: 200.000 $

The basic limitation of this and similar researches include the inability to generate general estimates of risk, due to lack of denominator data, the absence of a rigorous control group, a probable bias toward adverse outcomes and partial reliance on data from direct participants rather than objective observers.

In order to study the incidence of the problem, unbiased reports or studies of critical accidents or incident monitoring studies are particularly helpful. The AISM (Australian incident monitoring study) (3) included 2000 cases; 4% reported problems with endotracheal intubation; no death was reported albeit one patient suffering from a cardiac arrest was successfully resuscitated. From an analysis of this large body of experience, the following tables help to reveal some points useful for discussion and thought.

Table 2. An analysis of the first 2000 incidents reported to the AISM concerning difficult, including unsuccessful, endotracheal intubation

85 cases (4%)
26 presenting for emergency surgery (31% of total)
19 "out of hours"
27 not predicted (32%)
22 predicted, but serious difficulty reported
17 not intubated (impossible); 20%: roughly 17/85 *4% = %
IPPV by mask presented serious difficulties in 13 (15%); in 2 degree of difficulty increased over time

Table 3. Complications associated with difficult intubations

Oesophageal intubation:	18
Arterial desaturation:	15
Central cyanosis:	7
Oesophageal reflux:	7
Bronchospasm:	5
Laryngospasm:	4
Intubation right main bronchus:	2
Loosed tooth:	2
Epistaxis:	1
Ruptured ETT cuff:	1
ECG ischemic signs:	1
Oesophageal tear:	1
Lacerated tongue:	1
Cardiac arrest:	1

Table 4. Level of training of anesthetists involved in 85 difficult intubations

Consultant specialist:	49%
Trainee:	34%
Trainee non specialist:	10%
Non trainees:	4
Two trainees:	1

Table 5. Factors contributing in difficulty with intubation

See list of obvious causes
Equipment deficiencies:
– failure of scope light
– failure to check: • no suxamethonium available, swap of drugs (pancuronium instead of SCC)
                 • improper ETT tube choice
                 • obstructed mount or tube
                 • no lubrication or softening of the ETT
                 • failure to inject SCC
                 • inexpert assistance; head improperly positioned, excessive cricoid pressure
Lack of supervision

These data show that almost one third of DI were not predicted and that 15% showed simultaneous difficulties with mask ventilation; clearly not all difficult intubations are predictable by any present means and even when they are anticipated prediction of simultaneous difficulty with facemask ventilation is not. It seem therefore extraordinary that the anesthetic literature focuses on getting the tube into the trachea and not on the associated frequently unpredicted but potentially even more deadly situation of the non breathing patient who cannot be intubated or even adequately ventilated; this is illustrated by the present absence of data relating to difficulty with ventilation by facemask alone. Every anesthetist should know, or at least not forget, that patients will succumb not from failure to be intubated, but from failure to be ventilated, as has been the repeated suggestion of The Confidential Enquiry into maternal deaths (4).

The largest number of attempts to intubate with a standard laryngoscope recorded in the closed claims series was 5, in 1 case successful on the 5th; persistent attempts at intubation have been indicated as causes of major complications. An attempt to redirect these priorities has been recently published (6): since these recommendations are illustrated by a great algorithm, that will be presented at the meeting. Another algorithm proposed by Williamson et al. (3) shows that, again, the total number of DI is not known, unless a prospective study on a very large number of patients is examined: Deller et al. (6) reported these data on all patients (8284) admitted in their hospital and presenting for anaesthesia, finding 101 DI (1.2%) out of 254 (3.1%) known (examined according to a protocol); should we conclude that DI oscillate around 1%-3%?

These percentages are confirmed in a more recent prospective study of Rose and Cohen (7).

Since failure to maintain a patent airway for more than a few minutes results in brain damage and death, it is of paramount importance to recognize the difficulties in advance, if possible, and to adopt a protocol for the difficulties in airways management following a series of logical steps.

Since the definition of unable to intubate derives from inexperience and that force and dexterity will make very often the difference, there are situations where the incidence of airway problems are recognized and must be known.

Table 6. Airways difficulties

The case for:
– experience
– force
– skills
– equipment
– trained help

While the application of force has been mainly anecdotic, deriving from personal experience, recently forces applied during laryngoscopy have been measured and related at least to height, weight and presence of maxillary incisors (8); it is interesting to note that forces around 4 kg are developed and that the integral of the forces over time approaches 16 kg in normal patients.

It is known that in obstetrics failed or difficult intubation is the leading cause of anesthetic related maternal mortality, the incidence being much greater than in surgical patients (9, 10). Postulated reasons include the presence of full dentition, increased incidence of laryngeal and pharyngeal edema, obstruction to laryngoscope placement by large breasts, ease of regurgitation and vomiting leading to the dangerous aspiration pneumonia.

Table 7. Casistics of St. James University Hospital, Maternity Unit, Leeds

Year	Number of general anaesthesias	Number of failed intubations
1978	256	1
1979	324	1
1980	362	2
1981	358	1
1982	455	1
1983	576	2
1984 (6 months)	186	1

Table 8. Recognition of the difficult airway

1) Clinical history:
   - the scheduled procedure may indicate a likelihood of airway difficulty
   - any disease or trauma that exists in the vicinity of the path to be followed by the ETT
   - airway history, from patient, previous anesthetic records, medical alert
2) Examination:
   - viewing the patient in the lateral and antero-lateral position, lateral (chin)
   - viewing and palpating the neck anteriorly and laterally
   - extending the neck maximally
   - flexing the neck maximally
   - examining mouth opening, teeth, interdental gap
   - determining patency of the nostrils
   - determining jaw movement (TMJ)
   - determining position and size of tongue

Table 9. Obvious causes of difficult intubation

Congenital:	Pierre Robin syndrome
	Cleft lip and/or palate
	Floppy epiglottis
	Large teeth to larynx distance
	Cockayne syndrome
	(mandibular hypoplasia, large teeth and restricted mouth opening)
	Familiar osseous dysplasia (cherubism);
	Mandibular enlargement with or without maxillary
Involvement	
	Fetal alcohol syndrome
	Mucopolysaccharidoses
	Treacher Collins syndrome (mandibular hypoplasia, macroglossia, glossoptosis, prominent maxilla or maxillary incisors...)
	Tracheal agenesis
	Tracheobronchopatia/osteochondroplastica
	Cystic hygroma
Pharyngeal diverticula	
Inflammatory:	Epiglottis
	Ludwig's angina
	Retropharyngeal abscess
Arthritis of temporomandibular joint or cervical spine	
Ankilosing spondylitis of the cervical spine	
Rheumatoid arthritis	
Still's disease	
Burn contractures	
Fractures involving mandible and/or maxilla or cervical spine	
Endocrine:	Goitre
	Acromegaly
	Diabetes (insulin resist.)
Neoplasia:	Pharyngeal and/or laryngeal tumors
	Pseudoxanthoma protein
Scars, facial or cervical	
Down's syndrome	
Cranio-facial dysmorphias	

When an obvious condition is present, potential difficulties with a conventional approach are recognized and therefore these conditions have not been responsible for many catastrophes (brain damage, death): the majority of problems arose when recognition of possible difficulties with the airways management has been a most subtle issue; i.e. when difficulties arose in patients who were not expected to present any airway problem. From the data presented above it is clear that those unexpected cases occur commonly and call therefore for the adoption of criteria of evaluation of easy versus difficult airways.

In the past, evaluation of airways has been a very difficult task, including a long series of measurements, X-rays and so on (11); some of the most often cited and useful diagrams will be presented.

In order to have great appeal as routine preoperative airway evaluation tools, tests need to be simple and quick to perform, be able to be accomplished at very low cost and highly predictive.

Table 10. Characteristics useful for an ideal test

- Simple
- Quick
- Low cost
- At the bedside
- Predictive

The problem is complicated by the fact that normal anatomical variation is very large, as suggested recently by Janvier et al. (12); they found that it is not possible to define a unique standard model of the upper laryngeal airway; as a matter of fact, this part of the airway consists of two very different regions: one has a morphology that varies little (larynx) and the other has a morphology with random variation (hypopharynx), further complicated by structural changes in the head as a function of body position: the changes found by these authors imply significant deformation in the pharyngolaryngeal structures.

Predictability could be assessed in many ways, but the most informative is founded on the basis of positive and negative criteria, each determining according to various combination sensitivity and specificity.

Table 11.

	FACT	
	+	−
TEST +	A: true pos	B: false pos
−	C: false neg	D: true neg

$a/a + b$ = positive predictive value
$d/c + d$ = negative predictive value
$a/a + c$ = sensitivity, i.e. true +
$d/b + d$ = specificity, i.e. true negative

Moreover, as difficult intubation occurs infrequently and is not easy to define, research has been directed at predicting difficult laryngoscopy (difficult intubation-difficult laryngoscopy).

One of the first scientific approaches to the problem has been the establishment of four grades of laryngoscopic view, defined by Samsoon and Young (13) and Cormack and Lehane (10) as follows:

Grade I: visualization of the entire laryngeal aperture;
Grade II: visualization of the anterior part only of the laryngeal aperture;
Grade III: visualization of the epiglottis only;
Grade IV: visualization of the soft palate only.

However, the preceding classification starts a little too late, while it is possible that even the visualization of the epiglottis cannot be obtained: in other words it cannot exclude problems arising in the upper part of the airways. Moreover, difficult laryngoscopy cannot be accepted as a synonym of DI, because even grade III and IV laryngoscopic views could be transformed into easy intubations with small adjustments like external laryngeal pressure, lifting the epiglottis instead of having the blade in the vallecula and so on.

It is a fortune that we have today at least three predictors that can be used in the preoperative examination, at zero cost and easy to perform, and with a remarkable accuracy in the prediction of subtle ETT intubation difficulties.

Less obvious causes: predictive criteria.

Size of the tongue in relation to the size of the oral cavity can be simply and visually graded by how much the pharynx is obscured by the tongue; the patient sits upright with the head in a neutral position and is asked to open the mouth as widely as possible, protruding the tongue to a maximum; then the airways are classified according to the pharyngeal structures seen, according to Mallampati (14).

	Soft palate fauces		Uvula	Ant. and post tonsillar pillars
Class I	yes	yes	yes	yes
Class II	yes	yes	yes	no
Class III	yes	yes	base only	no
Class IV	yes	yes	no	no

A significant correlation has been found between the ability to visualize the aforementioned structures and the ease of laringoscopy: in patients of class I the laryngoscopic view is grade I in 99-100% of patients, in those of class IV airway the laryngoscopic view is grade III or IV 100% of time. However, patients with intermediate classifications (II and III groups) were found to have a relatively uniform distribution of all grades of laryngoscopic views (15).

Because of that and because of interobserver variability, this test alone has significant false negative and false positive findings and consequently cannot be used alone as an all-or-none predictor, basically since it does not consider other significant factors in the difficult airway, like the mobility of the neck and the size of the mandibular space; however, it does serve in the clinical practice, being able to assess the relative risks in obstetrics for instance, where Rocke et al. (16) quantified the relative risk of DI as being 7.58 times greater for class II patients as compared to class I, while class IV had a 11.2 times greater risk than class I; short neck, receding mandible and protruding maxillary incisors were also significant factors.

Because the low sensitivity (0.42), moderate specificity (0.84) and very low positive predictive value (4.4%) of the Mallampati's test, the test has been criticized; however, it cannot be forgotten that another way of using the oropharyngeal assessment would be to predict the patients in whom there will be no intubation difficulty; of those patients assessed as class I in 96.4% intubation proved to be easy and in a further 3.1% intubation was achieved with only some difficulty; (class II) and no additional risk to the patient; difficulty with intubation was reported only 2/478 class I assessment, but 1/240 poses an additional risk, not being anticipated at all in only 6.6% of class IV assessment subsequently proved to be very difficult.

A slight modification of the Mallampati's classification is the hypopharynx test (17), where hypopharynx examination corresponds well to glottis visualization (667 pts).

Tham et al. (18) showed that the Mallampati's grading observed with the patient in the vertical position did not change when the patient was horizontal; thus the test is still useful when the anesthesiologist is presented with a patient unable to sit up or already on the operating table.

The evaluation for sensitivity, specificity and positive predictability is reported in Table 12.

Table 12.

Author	Patients n.	Difficult intub. %	Sensitivity	Specificity	PPV
Mallampati (14)	210	13	1	0.85	0.51
Cohen (17)	665	7	0.90	0.48	0.12
Pottecher (19)	663	6	0.80	0.66	0.14

Therefore, we are forced to take into account other potential risk factors, like:
1) *Mobility of the neck*: contributes heavily in the laryngoscopic visualization, because when the neck is moderately flexed on the chest and the atlanto-occipital joint is well extended, the axis of the oral, pharyngeal and laryngeal

cavities are best brought in line, universally appreciated as "sniffing" position. In case the neck cannot be extended, as might happen in cases of small occipital-C1 gap, attempts at extending the neck cause the convexity of the cervical spine to bulge anteriorly, pushing anteriorly the larynx and impairing a conventional laryngoscopic view (11, 20-22).

2) *Limited movement of the mandible*: is a recognized cause of DI; this may be related to temporo-mandibular joint dysfunction or trismus, but, in addition, a relatively large mandible and a short thick neck or a mandible with short descending rami may contribute to the problem. Classic teaching is the assessment of the interdental gap: however, two aspects of jaw movement are important in this context, i.e. the aforementioned interdental gap and subluxation of the jaw (maximal forward protrusion of the lower incisors beyond the upper incisors) (23); while mouth opening permits adequate insertion of the laryngoscope, good forward luxation of the mandible provides additional space for forward displacement of the tongue.

3) *The mandibular space* constitutes the space anterior to the larynx and has been expressed as the inside of the mandible to the hyoid bone distance or as the thyromental distance or as the horizontal length of the mandible. The importance of this space and its related measures derives from the fact that the space anterior to the larynx determines how easily the laryngeal axis will fall in line with the pharyngeal axis when the atlanto-occipital joint is extended; if the thyromental distance is short, the laryngeal axis will make a more acute angle with the pharyngeal axis and it will be more difficult for atlanto-occipital extension to bring these two axes in line and viceversa. If there is a large mandibular space, larynx is relatively posterior and the tongue is easily compressed into a large compartment and does not have to be pulled maximally forward in order to reveal the larynx; when there is a very small mandibular space, larynx is relatively anterior and the tongue has to be compressed into a much smaller compartment and must be pulled maximally forward in order to view the larynx.

The thyromental distance and the horizontal length of the mandible have been found to correlate well inversely with the class of pharynx described above (15): a thyromental distance > 6 cm and a horizontal length of the mandible > 9 cm are tightly associated with low tongue-pharyngeal size classification and suggest that direct laryngoscopy will be relatively easy.

It is probable that this measurement is influenced by several factors, namely head extension, position of the larynx, depth and length of the mandible and this is in keeping with the notion that a short, muscular neck causes DI.

A variant of the previous work has been studied by Chou and Wu (24); in 11 patients with documented intubation problems they obtained lateral cervical radiographs with the head in neutral position and the mouth closed and measured the mandibulo-hyoid distance, the vertical distance between the upper margin of the hyoid bone and the lower margin of the mandible. This and other measures were compared with 100 normal patients; patients with difficult intubations had longer mandibulo-hyoid distances, with mandibular angles (angle determined by the intersection of two tangents of lower border of mandible and posterior ramus) tended to position more rostrally and hyoid bone more caudally. The relevance of this work is probably not great and may even be confusing, compared to others who described the high or anterior larynx (20) or the mento-hyoid distance shorter in patients difficult for laryngoscopy and/or intubation (19).

So far, we have discussed the value of a single test as a predictor of difficulties with laringoscopy and/or intubation; would the evaluation be helped by combining several predictive factors together? While common sense would suggest an affirmative answer, and a few reports agree well (23), other workers (25) negate any superiority, finding that both Wilson and Mallampati's tests fail to predict as many as 58% of difficult laryngoscopies; combining Wilson and Mallampati gave no advantage, most probably because no weight was done in the two tests to the atlas-axial gap, so that we are left with impression that using a combination of tests can be useful, but has not been shown, as emerged from two recent studies, unfortunately abstracted (26). A mixture between clinical and anatomical signs seems most promising (27), but the abstract is too concise to explain everything, while it seems that the authors established a score, assigning points depending on the degree of each of seven factors:

– Presence or not of a pathology known to be associated with DI
– Interincisive gap
– Mandible luxation
– Thyromental distance
– Normal or short and broad neck
– Head and neck movement
– Mallampati's test.

If a criticism is allowed, Wilson's score (23) at least presented a lesser degree of interobserver variability.

The search for improved predictive tests continues, but with many difficulties, basically deriving from the need to study prospectively very large number of patients excluding those who originated the study for the predictive evaluation, since a test will inherently perform better on the data used to create it; moreover, even some of the quite large studies performed usually do not contain enough difficult patients to provide acceptable estimates (95% confidence limits) of predictive ability.

The problem could, and has been, approached from its opposite; i.e., you could investigate cases of difficult intubation and analyse the factors involved under well controlled situations; Horton et al. (28) used an X-ray laryngoscopic technique, grading patient on the basis of epiglottic visibility and analyzing airways from the point of views of different angles; the angle between midpoint of the inner surface of the mandibular symphisis, tip of upper incisors and most anterior inferior position of the airway behind the thyroid cartilage and above the vocal cords, this angle appeared to be a sensitive index of degree of difficulty. In all the four cases of greatest difficulty a mechanism was apparent which suggests that airway obstruction during laryngoscopy is almost inevitable in such patients; a phenomenon called "peardrop" and apparently facilitated by a curved blade. This phenomenon is caused by compression of the tongue and postero-inferior displacement results in airway obstruction on insertion of the laryngoscope. While practical implications exist (awake intubation to be preferred, maximum allowable is local analgesia) the "ease of intubation angle" described seems to be a sensitive index of difficulty and is comparable to similar measurement in Bellhouse and Dorè (29) paper. Fahy et al. (30) transferred the angular measure of jaw protrusion from a line joining the upper incisors and a point just above and anterior to the vocal cords to the midpoint of the inner surface of the mandible to previously pregnant patients; the lower angle of this triangle was as important as the angle at the incisors.

Horton et al. (31) suggested a combination index for assessment; XS/JS *XT/IT* sin beta, where I is the tip of upper incisors, T is the anterior airway above the cords, S is a midpoint of inside the jaw, lower border of mandible to incisor tip, J is the condilar midpoint, and X is the intersection of lines IT and JS and beta the angle SXT.

That the epiglottis could be the site of airway obstruction has been known since a long time: that it is one of the most important factors in airway obstruction under anesthesia, contrary to the common belief that attributes all problems to the fall of the tongue, has been suggested by Drummond (32) and Hotchiss (33).

The case of the "floppy epiglottis" has been made when the angle between the epiglottis and the base of the tongue reaches 90°; as a matter of fact with the curved Macintosh blade the optimal position is immediately behind or below the body of the hyoid bone; therefore, the basic mechanism of epiglottic elevation is related to forward traction on the hyoid by the blade tip, so that the hyoid is moved forward and downward. Failure to control the hyoid is cited as a common mechanism in DI with the Macintosh blade, other than calcification of the stylohyoid ligaments. The floppy epiglottis can be elevated by a straight blade laryngoscope, but the blade may impact against the upper teeth and possibly against a cervical vertebra in patients with tight oropharyngeal corners.

According to the already quoted article (29) instead of single measurements, the ratio between the mandibular space to the total length of the tongue is a good predictor of DI, thus introducing the important concept that bony structures should be considered in conjunction with the soft tissues with which they are closely associated.

White and Kander (11) found that the most important factor in determining the ease of direct laryngoscopy is the *posterior depth of the mandible*, i.e. the distance between the alveolus immediately behind third molar tooth and the lower border of the mandible. An increase of this measurement was thought to hinder displacement of the soft tissues by the laryngoscope blade.

Nichol and Zuck (20) suggested that the *atlanto-occipital distance* is a major anatomical factor that determines the ability to extend the head on the neck and exposure of larynx; Bannister and Macbeth (34) stressed the importance of the position of the head and neck in direct laryngoscopy in order to achieve proper alignment of the axes of mouth, pharynx and larynx. The ideal position for axes alignment and intubation can be achieved by raising the head at the atlanto-occipital joint; failure to correctly position the head and neck and bring about alignment of oral, pharyngeal and laryngeal axes is one of the common errors in orotracheal intubation. The amount of extension that can be achieved at this joint is limited by the abutment of the occiput against the posterior tubercle of the atlas; the greater the atlanto-occipital distance, the greater the degree of extension possible: in cases where the posterior tubercle of the atlas is already in contact with the occiput in the neutral position, attempts to extend the head result in anterior bowing of the cervical spine and forward displacement of the larynx. The atlanto-occipital gap may be assessed by lateral radiography of the cervical spine in the neutral position, measuring the distance from the occiput to the spine of the atlas and numerous reports have confirmed its importance (11, 20), stressing the importance of function against distance; raising the occiput above the shoulders helps to eliminate errors in assessment from anterior bowing of the cervical spine. It is important to realize that limitations in head extension are secundary to diseases, like rheumatoid arthritis, but may also occur secondary to anatomical variations at the atlanto-occipital gap in people regarded as normal and those are the cases of unexpected failure of intubation. A recent work (35) has demonstrated that in healthy volunteers undergoing laryngoscopy a mean extension of 25° occurs at C1-C2 and to consider movement between C0-C1 and C1-C2 as separate may be inappropriate.

The anterior larynx has been implicated as a causative factor in DI: distance from upper teeth to thyroid membrane has been repeatedly associated with DI (21 -23).

It is worth noting that in a large prospective study 8 factors tested as predictors failed to reveal any relationship with DI, with discriminant analysis and categorical regression analysis. The 8 factors were visualization of tonsillar pillars, mentum-suprahyoid distance, mentum-sternal notch distance, oral opening distance, range of neck motion, body habitus, receding mandible and buck teeth (26).

Upper teeth have been considered causes of DI; not only teeth and state of the dentition are to be blamed, but also the effective maxillary length and height, even if many authors do not agree (11, 29, 36). Protruding upper incisors have been quoted as relative overgrowth of the premaxilla (37) and Wilson and his colleagues (23) found "buck teeth" to be a risk factor in predicting DI.

A long high-arched palate associated with a long mouth has been indicated as a possible cause of DI, by reducing the space between the posterior angle of the mandible (37): however, case controlled cases have not substantiated these observations.

Concluding this rather long series of signs and measurements, it is time to start a multicenter, large, prospective study on the value of at least a large number of these signs, combined: Pottecher et al. (19) have to be commended for their efforts striving at this demonstration, i.e.:

Table 13.

Sign	Sensitivity	Specificity	Pos. Predictive value
Mouth opening > 4 cm	0.27	0.91	0.21
Mallampati > 1	0.84	0.66	0.14
Chin-hyoid bone	0.52	0.56	0.10
Chin-cart thyroid	0.22	0.97	0.11

However, only PPV improved in their series compared to Wilson (23), while both Wilson > 1 and Mallampati > 1 (14) gave more or less the same numbers; i.e.:

Table 14.

Sign	Sensitivity	Specificity	Pos. Predictive value
Mallampati > 1 (14)	0.40	0.95	0.13
Wilson > 1 (23)	0.50	0.92	0.10

In conclusion, since difficult intubation evaluation ranges widely, Mallampati's (14) scores seem to offer a simple way to evaluate the airways, with a good sensitivity; but, because the positive predictive value remains low, routine use of his classification may result in overestimation of the incidence of DIs. The above mentioned study of Rose and Cohen (7) included 29145 patients over 27 months assisted by an anesthesiologist in the OR. Data were collected on special tick forms prospectively and patients assessed at the preop. visit in a standardized approach aimed at identification of DIs. Overall difficulties in tracheal intubation resulted in 1.8% and awkward in 2.5% (obstetric cases excluded), failure representing 0.3% of cases and postponement of surgery was done in 0.05%: 353 patients were approached with an alternative method instead of direct laryngoscopy under GA. Risk factors resulted: male sex, age between 40-59 years, obesity, while the most important anatomical factors identified included mouth opening, shortened thyromental distance, poor visualization of the hypopharynx and limited neck extension. The combination of 2 or > of these factors increased the risk. This is an example of a jolly good work, suggesting that further studies are necessary to determine if other criteria associations or new signs could enhance detection of problematic intubations. We suggest to try to collect all cases of difficult intubations and propose a leaflet adopted in our Department for this specific purpose (Fig. 1).

Approach to the patient with recognized airways difficulties (obvious or non obvious); awake intubation

Is indirect laryngoscopy useful in prediction? Because there is no predictive study, the answer at the present time would be "no": however, this examination will reveal anatomical abnormalities including obstruction, which would not necessarily indicate a difficult intubation.

Is radiological investigation useful? Yes, as has been reported previously by (11) and (20); however, the problem with any X-ray investigation (or even Magnetic Resonance Imaging) is that they are seldom used unless there is a positive indication; therefore, they give considerable assistance in evaluating the known difficult case, but cannot contribute to prediction in standard clinical practice.

Having recognized since a long time that endotracheal intubation (ETT) is the only way to secure and guarantee the airways, why we stress the term "awake"? Even if this means more time spent by the anesthesiologist, reassuring the patient psychologically, doing a good topical anesthesia, choosing the right drugs in the right dosages for sedation, awake is a prerequisite for the manoeuvre because gas exchange is better maintained thanks to the good muscular tone, that keeps the upper airways structures separated each other and better identifiable with the more restricted view obtainable with the fiberscope.

Anatomo-physiological reasons for awake intubation have recently been pointed out by various authors; Sivarajan (38) demonstrated during general anesthesia (tps) and muscle paralysis (SCC) an anterior displacement of the larynx; along with this displacement the larynx was also stretched longitudinally resulting in separation between vestibular and vocal folds.

Nandi et al. (39) showed with conventional lateral radiography in elderly male patients under general anesthesia (tps/N_2O/O_2/enflurane), spontaneously breathing that there were significant approximations to the posterior pharyngeal wall of the soft palate, tongue base and epiglottis. Apparent radiographic occlusion of the airway occurred most consistently at the level of the soft palate, more rarely at the epiglottis, while the base of the tongue did not touch the posterior pharyngeal wall in any patient and traction on the tongue failed to clear the nasopharyngeal obstruction. Attempted inspiration under anesthesia caused major secondary collapse of the pharynx, with multiple sites of obstruction

DIFFICULT INTUBATION FILE

Date ....../....../...........

First name................................ Family name .... Age...................
Indications for intubation: ···
···
Hospitalized ☐ ....
Ambulant ☐

	Unrecognized difficulty	☐
	Recognized	☐
	Previously reported	☐

Weight...... Height ·········· Soma type..
Neck: Mobile ☐ Hypomobile ☐
Dentition: Complete ☐ Incomplete ☐ ....
Edentulous ☐
TM joint .... Mento-hyoid distance: ....
Frontal oropharyngeal examination:

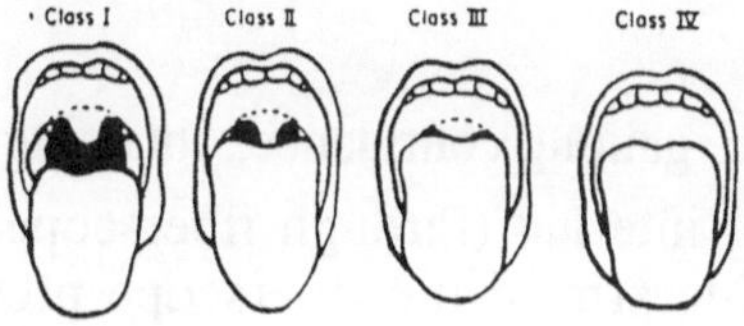

Class I   Class II   Class III   Class IV

MANOEUVRE PERFORMANCE:

Anaesthesiologic technique:
Sedation ☐ No ☐ Yes...
Local anaesthesia ☐ No ☐ Yes...
General anaesthesia ☐ No ☐ Yes ....

Direct laryngoscopy: ....

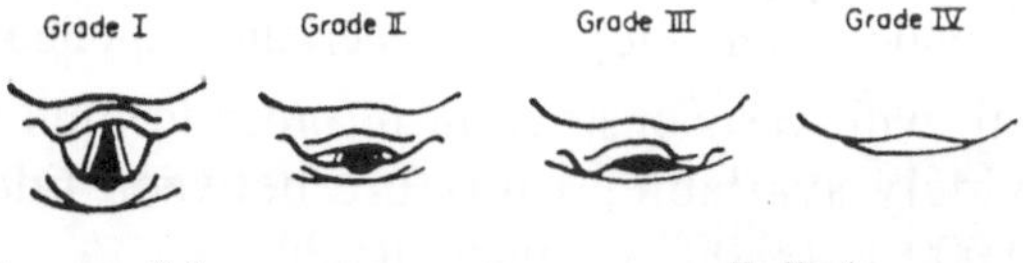

Grade I   Grade II   Grade III   Grade IV

Successful manoeuvre ☐   Failed manoeuvre ☐

Fibrescopy:..
Successful manoeuvre ☐   Failed manoeuvre ☐

Used tube: Type.............. Calibre.....................

Ventilation: ☐ Spontaneous ☐ Assisted ☐ Controlled   Mixture......................
Examination after extubation: ···
···
···
Remarks:···
···

Fig. 1.

similar to that found in obstructive sleep apnea. The reason behind these findings resides most probably in the tone reduction of the muscles of both the tongue and soft palate.

While the first of these two studies was limited in number (9 subjects) and scope and his findings contrast with those of the second study, both investigations stress the fact that the frequent clinical pratice of ascertaining the ease of direct laryngoscopy under awake conditions in patients in whom we suspect difficulties and then inducing general anesthesia to perform tracheal intubation may be fraught with surprise and frustration; in those situations it is best to perform tracheal intubation using topical anesthesia while the patient is awake; while not certainly a pleasant experience for the patient and a little distressing for the anesthesiologist too, it seems safer according to the above mentioned findings.

Proper preparation of the patient with a difficult airway

"PODAS"
– Psychology: explanation, gaining confidence, obtaining cooperation
– Oxygenation; external, internal (through fiberscope); the insufflation of oxygen through the side arm of the fiberscope prevents fogging of the fiberscope and blows the secretion away from the tip of the scope.
  Augmentation of FiO_2 through the cricothyroid membrane has been described, either with an i.v. catheter or with a TTJV (40, 41)
– Dry the mucosa; antisialogogues, better a few minutes before, in order to limit the unpleasant sensations. While widely applied in other fields, precautions against aspiration or vomiting have not been appreciated in these patients, mainly deriving from their alertness. If sedation constitutes an hazard, it is likely that measures to empty the stomach or at least to neutralize gastric acid contents should be undertaken, a topic to be certainly applied in obstetrics
– Anesthesia; topical, with vasoconstriction in order to limit bleeding. Since cocaine is not widely available, a mixture between lidocaine 2% and epinephrine 1:200 000-1:400 000 seems preferable
– Sedation

The intubating attempt

It is of the outmost importance a good start, with the proper positioning of the head and neck of the patient, with the objective to have the oral cavity, larynx, oropharynx and trachea in a as straight line as possible. If the result of the initial laryngoscopy is unsuccessful, the position of the blade should be checked to insure that it is placed as far as possible to the right corner of the mouth, thus reducing the distance to the vocal cords and altering the angle of approach. The tongue is pushed out of the way and any space between upper right molar teeth is utilised. External pressure on the thyroid cartilage by an assistant may be helpful.

Further flexion of the cervical spine could cause persistent difficulty, while the manoeuvre could be useful during the advancement of the tube below the vocal cords, so that they are less likely to impinge on the anterior wall of the trachea. Extension of the cervical spine can bow it forward, lifting the larynx of some patients anteriorly and out of the line of view.

It is wise to remember always that a change of blades could make the intubation possible, depending from the distance of the vocal cords, the need to compress the tongue and soft tissues into the mandibular space, the need to improve blade manoeuvrability in a small mouth; accordingly, the next blade selected should be on the basis of its length, degree and character of curvature, depth of step and width. While a wide choice of blades is recommended, what is probably more important is a rational approach, as atraumatic as possible.

Awake intubation is safe even in cervical injuried patients (42).

Choice of blades and aids: intubation assist devices

Laryngoscope design (43) could be categorized according to problems presented by patients, with reference to their design.

Many other devices have been described and used with variable success: a list would be certainly short of completeness, but a few tricks of low cost are represented by tubes or stylets incorporating a mobile or flexible tip, forceps to be used to advance the tube (Magill) or to grasp the tongue and increase the size of the oral cavity and so on.

Table 15. Laryngoscope design

Problems:	Solutions offered:
– Protruding sternal region increase the angle between blade and handle	Offsetting the blade from the handle
	Decrease the length of the handle
– Narrow space between fully parted incisors teeth	
	Flattening of the flange
	Reduction of the step
– Reduced intra oral cavity	
	Increase flange
	Increase step
	Reversal of flange
	Left handed versions of blades
– The anterior larynx	
	Straight blades
	Wide blade with anterior curve tip
	Raising the middle third of blade + decrease of the curvature radius + extension of tip (44)

Intubating position

For patients presenting DIs standard intubating positions have been suggested (35, 45).

Basic points are reminded in the following scheme:

Recommendations for basic preparation for difficult airway management: the ASA practice guidelines (5):

1) Portable storage unit for difficult airway management:
   - Rigid laryngoscope blades of alternate design and size from those routinely used
   - Endotracheal tubes of assorted sizes
   - Endotracheal tube guides: stylets, lightwand, forceps...
   - Fiberoptic intubation equipment
   - Retrograde intubation equipment
   - At least one device suitable for emergency nonsurgical airway ventilation: transtracheal jet ventilator, hollow jet ventilator stylet, laryngeal mask, oesophageal-tracheal combitube...
   - Equipment for emergency surgical airway access: cricothyrotomy
   - Exhaled CO_2 detector

2) If a difficult airway is known or suspected, the anesthesiologist should:
   - Inform the patient or a responsible person of the special risks and procedures pertaining to management of the difficult airway
   - Ascertain that there is at least one additional individual immediately available to serve as an assistant
   - Consider supplemental oxygen
   - Adoption of specific strategies

It is wise to remember that fiberoptic naso-orotracheal intubation might not always succeed: an analysis of failures was reported by a great expert (46): 1.2% of cases (5/413) were unsuccessful, with 3 not being intubated after successful visualization of the trachea: tricks to slide the tube over the scope have been described by Ovassapian et al. (46) and Katsnelson et al. (47).

Blind nasal intubation (BNI)

BNI involves placing the head and neck of the patient in the best position and passing a well lubricated tube into the nasopharynx with a thorough topical anesthesia; the operator listens at the proximal end of the advancing tube as it approaches and then enters the larynx, at the same time looking at the flow of gases and feeling the ventilation, as well as inspecting a capnogram attached to the proximal end of the nasal tube. The main disadvantage of the manoeuvre resides in the trauma it may produce in the nasal, pharynx, larynx and oesophageal passages. Bleeding and secretions may hinder subsequent fiberoptic visualization of the structures.

Use of a gum elastic bougie or stylet

This method requires prior insertion of a laryngoscope; although the anesthesiologist may see only part of the glottis or indeed none at all, it is often possible to pass a bougie blindly into the trachea; a hollow type may allow visualization of the capnogram with ventilation. The bougie or stylet will then serve as a guide for sliding a tube into the trachea.

Use of fiberoptic instrumentation

The main use of the fiberoptic instrumentation lies in the possibility to railroad the ETT over it into the trachea; the greatest advantages reside in flexibility, ability to pass either the nasal or oral routes, clear visualization of all the structures, normal and abnormal, with the simultaneous possibility of diagnosis. "Tracheal" scopes have become recently more available and have much to be commended thanks to their less delicate structure. Problems reside in the need of familiarization with the equipment, the difficulty of handling secretions, especially in the smaller models, the high cost of the equipment, either for purchasing than for maintenance, including disinfection, sterilization, and considering an inherent delicacy of the instrument, that has to be carefully protected from bites, fall, disinfectants, etc. This list of problems explains its scarce success for emergencies and its absolute superiority on all other methods under elective conditions, with patients awake under topical anesthesia.

Use of a rigid scope has been almost abandoned and it will not be described further.

Use of the light wand

Its principal indications lie in the difficulties associated with restricted mouth opening and cervical rigidity; however, the technique remains relatively blind, since it is based on the visualization of transillumination in darkened surroundings. Continuous inspection of the cricothyroid area allows appreciation of the appearance of the wand behind these membranes; at this point the ETT is advanced and the wand withdrawn. In absence of transillumination the wand is considered to be in the oesophagus.

Use of a LMA

The laryngeal mask has been found of great help even in cases of difficult airways or difficult intubation (48, 49); when it is properly positioned, a guide wire or a tube could be passed trough it.

Laryngeal mask should not be considered an alternative to endotracheal intubation, since it does not offer protection against aspiration and cannot assure a full control on ventilation; however, it is easy to use and is certainly advantageous with respect to the facial mask and has been used as an alternative in cases of DI, even if the ASA did not consider it in its algorithm.

Retrograde intubation

With this approach a catheter or a guidewire is inserted through the cricothyroid membrane and passed in retrograde fashion through the larynx so that it can be attached to the tip of an ETT, pushed and guided down through the larynx. While the technique is technically relatively simple, it cannot be forgotten that the tube may become dislodged during removal of the translaryngeal guidewire and that it is basically a blind technique.

Percutaneous transtracheal jet ventilation

Avoidance of tracheostomy by bypassing the larynx with a needle or a catheter has been studied for many years, the reason being the fear of surgeons and anesthetists to be confronted with a hypoxic patient who cannot be intubated. Initially transtracheal oxygenation was used in patients extremely difficult to intubate, allowing more time for tracheostomy or intubation to be performed. In such situations only a supply of intratracheal oxygen was assured and carbon dioxide could not be eliminated with the rapid development of respiratory acidosis; a 18 g catheter supports an O_2 flow around 4 l/min.

Sanders had the merit to introduce jet ventilation through the narrow lumen of a bronchoscope using oxygen at high pressure and since then air/oxygen mixtures have been injected through small lumen needles or scopes thanks to high pressures. Later on, Spoerel (50) combined jet ventilation with the transtracheal approach and/or high frequency ventilation, with further refinements being represented by the replacement of the metal needle with plastic cannulas and the extension of the principle of mere oxygenation to full ventilation of the patient, either with normal or with high frequencies, thanks to Luer lock connection. Since then many modifications have been proposed, some of them very simple and composed of materials readily available in every OR; e.g., a Teflon (radioopaque) catheter is mounted on a stainless steel needle for attachment to a conventional breathing system via its 15 mm diameter standard male connector or a high source gas such as a high frequency jet ventilation system or a jet device operating at a frequence of 15 to 30/min via a Luer lock female connector. Percutaneous transtracheal ventilation could be applied in the patient difficult or impossible to intubate and/or ventilate, allows the application of oxygenation alone instead of ventilation, allows time to consider elective approaches and could be used during resuscitation even as a method of emergency drugs administration (adrenaline). TTV is useful in microlaryngeal surgery and circumvents the need to use special tubes during laser surgery. In presence of a large tumor at the level of the pharynx or larynx, TTV is an elegant method alternative to tracheostomy.

TTV can be used prophylactically and temporarily, during attempts at DIs, in presence of obvious anatomical difficulties, etc. etc.

From the technical point of view, TTV is safest at the level of the cricothyroid membrane or 5 cm below; air should always be aspirated freely beforehand with a syringe connected to the Luer lock connector and its correct placement should be confirmed endoscopically as soon as technically possible. The catheter in place should be secured firmly and there should always be left an escape route for the insufflated gases, unless the TT catheter is used for oxygenation only. Multiple punctures of the tracheal wall should be avoided and there should be an alarm failsafe control that interrupts the jet inflow automatically when intratracheal pressure rises above a preset value: the development of dangerously high intrapulmonary pressures should be detected at once in order to avoid barotrauma.

Systems available have been reviewed (40, 51); few items will be described here in cases where a jet ventilator is not immediately available, as it happens in the vast majority of ORs the first acceptable TTJV system consists of a jet injector (blow gun) powered by regulated or unregulated central wall oxygen pressure. This tightly jointed system is immediately available, preassembled and reliably could be connected to the transtracheal catheter. The second TTJV system utilizes the anesthesia machine flush valve as the jet injector; this valve will generate a pressure that approaches line pressure. This gas fresh outlet of the anesthesia machine is now standard at 15 mm male outlet and is connected to noncompliant O_2 supply tubing by a standard 15 mm ETT adapter which fits a 4 mm ID ETT. The O_2 supply tubing is connected to the TTJV catheter with either a bonded Luer lock/hose barb connector or through a barrel of a 1 ml syringe.

The mechanism of efficacy is by mass movement of gas from the jet itself as well as by air entrainment by the Venturi principle. Because there are a number of serious TTJV complications these procedures should be undertaken only in desperate emergencies or in carefully thought out elective situations. Since desperate cannot ventilate/cannot intubate emergencies will continue to occur in association with anesthesia, it is highly recommended that every anesthetizing (or resuscitative location) should have immediate availability of TTJV.

Other devices

Many other devices have been proposed in the recent years; among them, the Augustine guide has been widely used in USA, but it is a blind method relying upon the positioning in the glosso-epiglottic space of a blade, used as a guide for a special introductor. It is basically indicated in the problems deriving from rigidity or immobility of the cervical spine.

Instruments like the oesophageal gastric tube airway (OGTA), the oesophageal obturator airway (EOA), the pharyngotracheal lumen airway (PTLA), cannot be accepted in difficult intubation unless in the out-of-hospital emergencies: only the Combitube has been successfully used in DIs, but suffers, like the other devices, from the limitation of the need of a wide mouth opening.

Many investigations have tried to compare the efficacy of a technique against another, on the basis of possible objective indicators, like number of attempts, time elapsed, failure vs successes, % of success, either in the mannikin or in the simulated environment (52); quite few could be considered really objective and comparable, based on a peer review or based on the need of simplicity, ease of teaching and learning, low cost, ready availability in all OR at all times. All techniques requiring long and costly equipment require long learning times, are not always successful and are not available in every OR or ICU. In view of these observations, the multeplicity of the solutions offered is only apparent.

Outcomes of attempted intubation

In case the patient is or has been rendered apneic and is impossible to intubate, there are various courses of action, presented in the ASA, AISM, Obstetric algorithms.

Schematically, assuming that surgery will be short and anesthesia can be safely conducted without intubation, artificial ventilation is continued with the use of an oropharyngeal airway and spontaneous breathing is ultimately restored. If believed necessary, regurgitation can be prevented by inserting a cuffed ETT into the oesophagus top third and inflating the balloon or by having cricothyroid pressure maintained by an assistant. If surgery is to be protracted and not started at once, the wisest course is to artificially ventilate the patient until spontaneous respiration has been restored and elective intubation can be done when consciousness has been regained. If there is the need to continue surgery or it is urgent, another plan of action is at follows:

1. Maintain cricoid pressure
2. Put patient head down or on left side
3. Oxygenate by IPPV; if difficult try with different positions and sizes of airways; aspirate pharynx as required
4. If obstruction persists, try to release cricoid pressure

5a. If oxygenation and ventilation are easy, ventilate with inhalation agents and oxygen and N_2O establishing surgical anesthesia with spontaneous ventilation using a face mask or any other OPA

6a. Empty the stomach with a wide bore NG tube and remove it after having instilled sodium citrate into it

7a. Maintain position of safety, if possible, and (or) maintain anesthesia with RS for the procedure

5b. If oxygenation and/or ventilation are difficult, let the patient wake up

6b. Empty stomach as described in 6a

7b. Use local or regional anesthesia or continue, inducing GA with RS under inhalation anesthesia and deepening as required by the surgical procedure always under RS.

In cases of acute airway obstruction, when repeated attempts at intubation have failed and a failure to ventilate coexist, it is necessary to recourse to mechanical measures, described later.

Unrecognized oesophageal intubation

It is a consequence of failed intubation and has been demonstrated to occur frequently in the etiology of complications of failed intubation, leading to cerebral damage and death. It is therefore necessary to ascertain that the tube is in the trachea beyond every reasonable doubt. This can be accomplished:

Table 16.

Detecting oesophageal intubation
– Measure the $ETCO_2$ and carefully inspect its curve for a few breaths; this is necessary because the stomach could contain some CO_2 following forced mask or OPA ventilation and CO_2 could result from alkalinization of the acid gastric content...
– Check for reservoir balloon movement synchronous with the chest of the patient, either under spontaneous or assisted ventilation
– Check for bilateral equal breath sounds, symmetrically, starting at the axillary left apex
– Check for bilateral symmetrical hemithorax elevation
– Check for epigastric auscultation and elevation
– Check the reservoir bag compliance, refilling
– Check for the presence of tidal volumes with respiration
– Check for unusual noises and/or gurgling sounds
– Palpate ETT cuff trough the neck
– Confirm the persistence and stability of vital signs for two-three minutes following the intubation
– Radiography (non useful in acute situations)

Other complications associated, even if not limited to DIs, consist of oral and nasal hemorrhages. While intraoral hemorrhages are rare, nasal bleeding secondary to repeated transnasal attempts are particularly dangerous, other than rendering a subsequent fibroscopy very difficult if not impossible. It is recommended that nasal passage of a tube should always be attempted gently, with soft tubes and following topical anesthesia with a suitable vasoconstrictor, like cocaine alone or the addition of epinephrine to the local anesthetic in dilution of at least 1:400.000. Materials for immediate control of such hemorrhage include small bore catheters with inflatable balloons and packing.

Extubating a DI

The more difficult an ETT has been to insert, the more reluctant the anesthesiologist, or other personnel, should be to remove the tube, until it is absolutely safe for the patient to have it removed.

Final suggestions and proposals

In closing this long and at some time extenuating review, a few suggestions seem necessary.

From the few reports dealing with DI, it could be excerpted that there are a few points deserving discussion.

Among intubation aids the gum elastic bougie met with the highest success rate, followed by the fiberoptic endoscope, while additional assistance ("trained help") was the most desired aid. It would seem that the use of Magill forceps and of the rigid bronchoscope in difficult intubation is nowadays infrequent. It appears also that "blind" nasal intubation, with the patient awake is a vanishing skill and there is a lack of familiarity and/or availability with the full range of intubating laryngoscopes, blades, attachments presently available. Very rarely, if ever, has a difficult intubation trolley be mentioned.

We propose therefore that in every place where anesthesia is administered a full range of DI aids must be present, starting from bougies, all kind of blades, fiberscope, prisms and ending with a large array of different sizes and forms of face masks and oral/nasal airways, including the LMA and similar devices. Since everything cannot be purchased and even the skills necessary in handling all these items cannot be acquired by all and require time, we suggest to concentrate on a few alternative items, where experience has to be mastered using them routinely in simple normal intubation cases.

The DI trolley seems a highly desirable item; every department has to configure it according to the skills and resources available, but a fiberscope, a series of blades, masks, airways, bougies and a device for a transtracheal jet ventilation seem a minimum list...

From the tables of factors associated with DI, equipment failures cannot be neglected; it is therefore imperative that the anesthesiologist checks all the equipment before embarking on the list of the day, at least once before beginning; all items should be checked, starting from the anesthesia machine, gases and vapors and ending with scopes, blades and so on.

Second, expert supervision should be always available, since we cannot forget that (AISM) in a third of cases the anesthetist was a trainee and in 10% of cases assistance was deeemed inadequate.

The practice of working alone is a danger from this point of view; assuming an incidence of DI around 1%, the occurrence of at least 5-6 cases every year per anesthesiologist seems appropriate; while this number is absolutely insufficient to generate any special skill, it is however leading to a very large number of patients at risk, since, for instance, there are 15 000 practicing anesthesiologists on duty today in our country, cumulating 75 000 cases of DI; applying the same frequencies derived from the literature totalizes 15 000 patients at risk per year, of whom at least 150 will suffer severe damage or death.

It is therefore mandatory to improve our skills, to diffuse the ability to ventilate among the professionals and lay people and for these aims a more detailed knowledge derived from questionnaires and critical incidents or accidents studies will be necessary, in order to be able to:

1) Predict the cases of difficult intubation or ventilation, concentrating them electively in places where equipment and experience are adequate
2) Find the right solution for every case, i.e. where local-regional anesthesia could be appropriately employed instead of general, like in obstetric practice
3) Training for DI.

Special review courses should be organized for anesthesiologists and/or other specialists (otorhinolaryngologists? thoracic surgeons?) and in order to gain the maximum exposure, they should be organized "hands on"; while it is impossible to practice on patients, specially designed mannikins (52) could solve the problem or, alternatively, normal patients could be rendered artificially "more difficult" with various tricks (53). Moreover, at least prospectively, every practitioner of anaesthesia should master at least a few elective techniques, like fiberoptic endoscopy of the upper airways, practicing on normal anatomy, consenting patients. If these proposals sound unethical, the only possibility resides in the field of mannikin simulation.

References

1 Marx GF, Mateo CV, Orkin LR (1973) Computer analysis of postanesthetic deaths. Anesthesiology 39:54-58
2. Caplan RA, Poren KL, Ward RJ, Cheney FW (1990) Adverse respiratory events in anesthesia: a closed claim analysis. Anesthesiology 72:828-833
3. Williamson JA, Webb RK, Szekely S, Gillies ERN, Dreosti AV (1993) Difficult intubation: an analysis of 2000 incident reports. Anaesth Intensive Care 21:602-607

4. Department of Health and Social Services. Report on health and social subjects: report on confidential enquiry into maternal deaths in England and Wales 1982-84, London, Her Majesty's Stationery Office, 1985
5. A report by the American Society of Anesthesiologists Task Force on management of the difficult airway (1993) Practice guidelines for management of the difficult airway. Anesthesiology 78:97-602
6. Deller A, Schreiber MN, Gramer J, Ahnefeld FW (1990) Difficult intubation: incidence and predictability. A prospective study of 8284 adult patients. Anesthesiology 73:A1054
7. Rose DK, Cohen M (1994) The airway: problems and predictions in 18500 patients. Can Anaesth Soc J 41:372-383
8. Bucx MJL, Van Geel RTM, Scheck PAE, Stijnen T, Erdmann W (1992) Forces applied during laryngoscopy and their relationship with patient characteristics. Anaesthesia 47:601-603
9. Lyons G, MacDonald R (1985) Difficult intubation in obstetrics. Anaesthesia 40:1016
10. Cormack RS, Lehane J (1984) Difficult tracheal intubation in obstetrics. Anaesthesia 39: 1105-1111
11. White A, Kander PL (1975) Anatomical factors in difficult direct laryngoscopy. Br J Anaest 47:468-474
12. Janvier G, Bordenaye L, Revel P, Ellison W, Cros AM, Winnock S (1993) Mathematical analysis of the upper respiratory tract from an anthropometric study. Br J Anaest 70: 186-191
13. Samsoon GLT, Young JRB (1987) Difficult tracheal intubation: a retrospective study. Anaesthesia 42:487-490
14. Mallampati SR, Gatt SP, Gugino LD, Desai SP, Waraksa B, Freiberger D, Liu PL (1985) A clinical sign to predict difficult tracheal intubation. Can Anaesth Soc J 32(4):429-434
15. Mathew M, Hanna LS, Aldrete JA (1989) Pre-operative indices to anticipate difficult tracheal intubation. Anesth Analg 68:S187
16. Rocke DA, Murray WB, Rout CC, Gouws E (1992) Relative risk analysis of factors associated with difficult intubation in obstetric anesthesia. Anesthesiology 77:67-73
17. Cohen SM, Laurito, CE, Segil, LJ (1989) Oral exam to predict difficult intubations: a large prospective study. Anesthesiology 71:A936-937
18. Tham EJ, Gildersleve CD, Sanders LD, Mapleson WW, Vaughan RS (1992) Effects of posture, phonation and observer on Mallampati classification. Br J Anaest 68:32-38
19. Pottecher T, Velten M, Galani M, Forrler M (1991) Valeur comparee des signes cliniques d'intubation difficile chez la femme. Ann Fr Anesth Reanim 10:430-435
20. Nichol HC, Zuck D (1983) Difficult laryngoscopy: the anterior larynx and the atlanto-occipital gap. Br J Anaest 55:141-144
21. Roberts JT, Ali HH, Shorten GD (1990) Using the laryngeal indices caliper to predict difficult intubations. Anesthesiology 73:A1011
22. Roberts JT, Ali HH, Shorten GD, Gorback MS (1990) Why cervical flexion facilitates laringoscopy with a Macintosh laryngoscope, but hinders it with a flexible fiberscope. Anesthesiology 73:A1012
23. Wilson ME, Spiegelhalter D, Robertson JA, Lesser P (1988) Predicting difficult intubation. Br J Anaest 61:211-216
24. Chou HC, Wu TL (1991) Mandibuloyoid distance in difficult laryngoscopy. Br J Anaest 71: 335-339
25. Oates JDL, Oates PD, Pearsall FJ, MacLeod AD, Howie JC, Murray GD (1991) Comparison of two methods for predicting difficult intubation. Br J Anaest 66:305-309
26. McDonald JS, Grupta B, Cook RI (1992) Proposed methods for predicting difficult intubation: prospective evaluation of 1501 patients. Anesthesiology 77:A1125
27. Arnè J, Descoins P, Bresard D, Aries J, Fusciardi J (1993) A new clinical score to predict difficult intubation. Br J Anaest 70(Suppl 1):1
28. Horton, WA, Fahy, L, Charters, P (1990) Factor analysis in difficult tracheal intubation: laryngoscopy induced airway obstruction. Br J Anaest 65:801-805
29. Bellhouse CP, Dorè C (1988) Criteria for estimating likelihood of difficulty of endotracheal intubation with the McIntosh laryngoscope. Anaesth Intensive Care 16:329-337

30. Fahy L, Horton WA, Charters P (1990) Factor analysis in patients with a history of failed tracheal intubation during pregnancy. Br J Anaest 65:813-815
31. Horton WA, Fahy L, Charters P (1990) Towards a single index for quantifying osseus factors in difficult laryngoscopy. Br J Anaest 65:583-584P
32. Drummond GB (1989) Site of airway obstruction in anaesthetized patients. Br J Anaest 63:625P
33. Hotchiss RS, Hall JR, Braun IF, Schisler JQ (1988) An abnormal epiglottis as a cause of difficult intubation-airway assessment using magnetic resonance imaging. Anesthesiology 68: 140-142
34. Bannister FB, MacBeth RG (1944) Direct laryngoscopy and tracheal intubation. Lancet 2: 651-654
35. Horton WA, Fahy L, Charters P (1989) Defining a standard intubating position using angle finder. Br J Anaest 62:6-12
36. Van der Linde JC, Roelofse JA, Steenkamp EC (1983) Anatomical factors relating to difficult intubation. African Medical Journal 63:976-977
37. Cass NM, James NR, Lines V (1956) Difficult direct laringoscopy complicating intubation for anaesthesia. Br Med J 1:488-489
38. Sivarajan M, Fink R (1990) The position and state of the larynx during general anesthesia and muscle paralysis. Anesthesiology 72:439-442
39. Nandi PR, Charlesworth CH, Taylor SJ, Nunn JF, Dorè CJ (1991) Effect of general anaesthesia on the pharynx. Br J Anaest 66:157-162
40. Benumof JL, Scheller MS (1989) The importance of transtracheal jet ventilation in the management of the difficult airway. Anesthesiology 71:769-778
41. Baraka A (1986) Transtracheal jet ventilation during fiberoptic intubation under general anesthesia. Anesth Analg 65:1091-1092
42. Meschino MD (1992) The safety of awake tracheal intubation in cervical spine injury. Can Anaesth Soc J 39(2):1114-1118
43. McIntyre JWR (1989) Laryngoscope design and the difficult adult tracheal intubation. Can Anaesth Soc J 36(1):94-98
44. Bellhouse CP (1988) An angulated laryngoscope for routine and difficult tracheal intubation. Anesthesiology 69:126-129
45. Tweedie I, Singh PJ, Williams DR, Charters P. (1990) Is there an "optimum" intubating position? Br J Anaest 64:383P
46. Ovassapian A, Yelich SJ, Dykes MHM, Brunner EE (1982) Fiberoptic nasotracheal intubation-incidence and causes of failure. Anesth Analg 62:692-695
47. Katsnelson T, Frost EAM, Farcon E, Goldiner PL (1992) When the endotracheal tube will not pass over the flexible fiberoptic bronchoscope. Anesthesiology 76:151-152
48. Brain AIJ (1983) The laryngeal mask. A new concept in airway management. Br J Anaesth 55:801-805
49. Brain AIJ (1985) Three cases of difficult intubation overcome by the laryngeal mask airway. Anaesthesia 40:353-355
50. Spoerel WE, Narayanan PS, Singh, NP (1971) Transtracheal ventilation. Br J Anaesth 43: 932-939
51. Patel R (1983) Systems for transtracheal ventilation. Anesthesiology 59:165
52. Hodges UM, O'Flaherty D, Adams AP (1993) Tracheal intubation in a mannikin: comparison of the Bellscope with the Macintosh laryngoscope. Br J Anaest 71:905-907
53. Cobley M, Vaughan RS (1992) Recognition and management of difficult airway problems. Br J Anaest 68:90-97

Airway Management

A. Fantoni

Introduction

The vast majority of the patients admitted in the general ICU present with respiratory problems as primary pathology and thus skilful management of the airways is indispensable for medical staff.

In the normal airway, the first aim is to avoid anatomical damage by applying every measure to make intubation or tracheostomy as harmless as possible. In contrast, in pathological airway conditions a global mastery of the up-to-date techniques is mandatory to impede deterioration of the whole respiratory function.

The airway management subject is wide and includes many conditions that deserve large, separate discussions.

For the sake of brevity, we will restrict our discussion to the more remarkable pathologies and corresponding techniques of treatment, and also to congenital defects such as tracheal stenosis, whose management requires all the combined know-how and technical nuances we apply in the care of the various types of difficult airways.

Retrograde intubation (RI)

In addition to various procedures to facilitate difficult tracheal intubations, RI can hold an important position in the management of airway control.

RI is a manoeuvre that requires a certain skill and good knowledge of anatomical structures of the neck, as it is halfway between simple tracheal intubation and non-surgical tracheostomy.

Methods. After skin disinfection, local anaesthesia of the cricothyroid membrane is performed. Then, the larynx is steadied with two fingers and a 16 gauge needle is inserted into the larynx through the membrane. A guidewire is advanced in cephalad direction until it reaches the oral cavity. The wire, drawn out the mouth, is then introduced into a tracheal tube. Firmly securing the two ends of the guidewire, the tube is pushed towards the glottis until the tip has been completely wedged. At this point the guidewire is removed and the tube is further advanced 5-6 cm into the trachea.

There are many variations in methodology. The use of an extradural catheter with a Tuoy needle has been suggested, with the insertion point in the subcricoid space, between the cricoid cartilage and first tracheal ring (1). The advantages of this method are: less frequent bleeding since, unlike the cricothyroid membrane, which is crossed by an important arterial vessel, the cricotracheal space is devoid of blood vessels; reduction of oedema and risk of stenosis of the glottis on account of the greater distance of the hole from the glottis; and less impinging of the tube against the larynx structures.

The main indications of RI are patients with narrow opening of the mouth, cervical spine lesions or tumour of the mouth.

Thanks to its ease and safety, this technique has been recommended for trauma patients as well. Efficacy and no serious complications of RI were observed during a trial, performed in a prehospital mobile emergency care unit. In this trial, the RI was used first, in cases of failure of conventional techniques of tracheal intubation and then, during a second period, as initial method of choice when failure of conventional methods were anticipated (2).

As a personal comment, it is advisable to acquire a thorough knowledge of the technique and to be able to apply it whenever it would be useful.

The possibility of ventilation by mask is essential: if difficulties occur during the procedure the operator has to stop the RI and start artificial respiration. RI manoeuvres, as well as the conventional intubation attempts, must not exceed 1 min, in order to avoid marked decrease of saturation and subsequent risks. If mask ventilation isn't feasible, there is a clear-cut indication for a tracheostomy.

Tracheostomy

For more than a century, the surgical tracheostomy (ST) reigned supreme without alternatives. With the exception of a few proposal of some sort of nonsurgical methods which were rapidly abandoned, we had to wait until 1985 for the publication of a particular technique of percutaneous tracheostomy adjusted by Ciaglia (3). Small stoma, small wound and fewer inflammatory phenomena are the main advantages of the method. However, there are some drawbacks that reduce its approval and acceptance.

First of all there is danger of injuring the trachea and peritracheal structures and, secondly, the difficulty of introduction of the tracheal tube caused by the larger diameter of the tube compared with that of the introducing probe. To minimize resistances it is necessary to make a larger stoma and utilize rotatory manoeuvres, which can be rather harmful and traumatic.

A new technique has recently been published by us, overturning traditional concepts (4). It is based on the concept of making the stoma by using a particular device composed of flexible plastic cone firmly joined to an armoured tracheal tube. The device is pulled from the mouth to the neck, passing through vocal cords, hence the definition of translaryngeal tracheostomy (TLT). The dilation is made from inside the trachea towards the outside of the neck, thus eliminating the danger of false pathways. In addition, the tracheal cannula has the same diameter as the cone and therefore difficulties can't arise during its passage as it follows the cone.

Other advantages of this technique are the need for only one dilator and, exclusive to this procedure, the tight adherence of the tissues around the cannula that must be considered the most effective factor of prevention against infections of tracheostomy channel.

Lastly, TLT is the only nonsurgical tracheostomy that does not require additional dilation by means of various kinds of forceps, which always involves considerable risk of tracheal damage.

Tracheostomy timing. In one of the most exhaustive studies of this topic (5), the authors affirmed that ST must be performed after 10 days of intubation for the following reasons, some of which are advocated by nurses:

– The tracheostomy is more comfortable for the patient and therefore requires less sedation and restraint.
– The patient can comunicate more effectively.
– Airway care is simplified.

Compared with ST, the dilational, nonsurgical tracheostomy should reduce even more the intubation period as the incidence of complications is lower and the scar generally appears like a remarkably unimpressive dot.

The direct consequence is a marked widening of the indications to include short-term tracheostomies and those in which the length of cannulation cannot be foreseen at the beginning of the respiratory assistance.

With regard to our experience with TLT, its very low trauma and risk, unimaginable until now, justify even earlier tracheostomy that, among other considerations, is supported by our nurses since it simplifies the airway care and control.

Endoscopy

Until 30 years ago, the endoscopy of the tracheobronchial tree remained the exclusive domain of the bronchologist, a specialist coming from pneumology and otorhinolaryngology. The rigid bronchoscope, the only tool available in the past, is difficult to handle and not devoid of risk: for this reason, it is not hard to guess why the anaesthetist tended to delegate the responsibility for endoscopic manoeuvres.

This trend changed with the introduction in clinical practice of the flexible fibreoptic bronchoscope (FFB), which started to be used by other specialists as well. Anaesthetists soon realized the FFB was a valuable tool in airway management in the operating theatre and ICU. The most frequent indications include intubation, changing of endotracheal tubes, extubation and reintroduction of cannula in tracheostomized patients, periodic inspections of the airways during prolonged mechanical ventilation and bronchial secretion sampling to determine the aetiologic diagnosis of pneumonia.

However, one of the main factors of endoscopy's spreading among intensive care specialists was the increasing diffusion of the new techniques of nonsurgical tracheostomies, born as procedures rapidly feasible at the bedside without requiring the anaesthetist's presence.

While testing this method, we became aware of the various risks that a too careless approach could entail. At present, we agree with the majority of authors who judge endoscopic control mandatory during dilational manoeuvres. It has been shown that endoscopic guidance appears to increase the safety of dilational tracheostomies, preventing such complications as pneumothorax, subcutaneous emphysema and paratracheal false passages, previously reported with blinded percutaneous methods (6).

Central airway obstruction

The discussion of this subject is forcedly limited to that kind of pathology in which the intensive care specialist is particularly interested. A list of more frequent causes and an outline on corresponding treatments will be made on the basis of cases treated in the regional centre of our hospital, which for 20 years has admitted patients affected by airway obstruction, with particular focus on the paediatric field (7).

Supraglottitis. In the past it has been improperly named oedema of the glottis. The vocal cords are generally not involved. The preferred method to treat these lesions today is by intubation maintained for 2-3 days with a noncuffed tracheal tube, with a diameter smaller than that normally used for anaesthesia. The oedema of supraglottic structures, epiglottis and ariepiglotticplicae generally disappears in a short time and the patient can be extubated without sequelae. More than corticosteroid therapy, the use of fully saturated and heated gases supplied in a circuit with continuous positive pressure of 5-6 cm of H_2O is absolutely necessary.

In this way, it is possible to promote a return air flow that maintains a constant lubrication of the contact zone between tube and larynx in order to avoid abrasive lesions on already inflamed tissues.

Subglottic stenosis due to intubation. The treatment is exactly like that of supraglottitis but the recovery takes more time. Indeed a therapeutic intubation prolonged for at least 20 days is required.

In the case of unsuccessful extubation, it is advisable to perform a TLT, the only method applicable in children that has a certain safety, and to insert a T-stent for some months.

It is important to remember that use of traditional tracheal cannulae, particularly for children, should be abandoned for two reasons: first, the cannula is not apt to preserve the suprastomal tract from obstruction caused by cicatricial retraction or malacia, which are considered the most frequent factors of decannulation failure. Secondly, the respiration of nonconditioned air through the stoma inevitably leads to a lung deterioration.

T-stent, in contrast, permits respiration through the nose and therefore assures physiological patterns of inhaled gases.

Foreign bodies. Unless there are emergency situations and an undelayable need for intervention, it is sensible to transfer the patient to a specialized centre, as one can never foresee what kind of situation may occur. An unadvised manoeuvre could cause serious airway tree damages. In children, Fogarty balloon catheterization is now considered a well validated method to extract soft and friable foreign bodies, such as peanuts.

The need to treat this kind of patient in only a few efficient centres is sustained by large amount of tools for endoscopy required for this activity and great skill in handling delicate but dangerous instruments.

Congenital obstructions. Treatment of congenital obstrucions of the tracheobronchial tree may be one of the most challenging problems in paediatric care.

We have had a great interest in this field for many years because we sometimes happen to encounter this pathology. We have registered excellent results with conservative methods, essentially based on dilation of the stricture followed by placement of prolonged T-stenting. In our view, surgery has limited indications, only in well selected cases, and is burdened with too many complications.

A review will be made of the most important anomalies in order to obtain satisfactory knowledge of these diseases and their treatment.

Laryngeal malacia. This type of obstruction can depend on an overlong epiglottis or very mobile arytenoids which, continuously or only in certain positions of the head, can provoke an increase of resistance to air flow. Larynx malacia is suspected when stridor, positional indrawing (much more evident in early age with its more pliable rib cage), or sleep and positional apnoea exist. However, only an endoscopic inspection, made during full curarization and during recovery from paralysis can settle diagnostic doubts as well as discover some possible functional obstruction.

Tracheal and bronchial congenital stricture. Deformation of the central airway caused by vascular abnormalities are not exceptional. In some cases the compression on the lumen is the result of surgical correction of congenital cardiovascular disease that requires a neoformation of by-pass or therapeutic channel which hinder the free flow of air. Carina and left main bronchus are more frequently involved.

In these cases, reintervention and shunt elimination are necessary.

Another factor of obstruction, which is also of interest to the anaesthetist, is the stricture of trachea subsequent to a surgical repair of tracheoesophageal fistula, when the suture unduly narrows the lumen.

In addition, an inaccurate ablation of the fistula duct, leaving a long infundibulum, creates a pouch inside the trachea that represents great danger. Indeed the tracheal tube could become wedged in the pouch, leading to asphyxia. These sudden blocks of ventilation are always misinterpreted and attribute to an asthma attack or some other unknown factors, until endoscopic control is made.

Among the strictures of the airway, congenital stenoses of the trachea must be considered. They can be limited to a short tract or involve the whole length of this structure, sometimes extending to the main bronchi. The diameter of stenosis ranges markedly with the corresponding degree of influence on the symptoms.

With the longest and narrowest strictures, the prognosis is ominous, because there is not a practicable therapy.

Some years ago we attempted the use of our conservative method in a case of total tracheal stenosis of 2 mm in diameter. The treatment succeeded because after 3 weeks of gradual dilation with homemade probes, we obtained a lumen normal for the patient's age. A T-stent was then inserted with the aim to stabilize the results and permit spontaneous respiration. After 3 months of treatment, when the infant was near to full recovery, he suddenly died as a consequence of an unrestrainable bleeding, caused by fistula between an unnoticed vascular sling and the trachea.

A second case of stenosis, similar to the first, was transferred to our centre some months ago. Thanks to the previous experience the conservative treatment has run more rapidly, even if it was very strenuous and full of difficulties, especially in the early phases. Today, after 5 months of care, the patient is doing well, breathing spontaneously through a T-stent, made with two extensions for the main bronchi (Y-shaped-stent) to obviate a residual malacia of the carina.

Up to now these two cases are the sole examples of conservative treatment of the worst tracheal stenosis. The results are very promising and are waiting to be made widely known. Many children would benefit.

References

1. Barriot P, Riou B (1988) Retrograde technique for tracheal intubation in trauma patients. Crit Care Med 16:712-713
2. Shantha TR (1992) Retrograde intubation using subcricoid region. Br J Anaesth 68:109-112
3. Ciaglia P, Firsching R, Syniec C (1985) Elective percutaneous dilatational tracheostomy. A new simple bedside procedure: preliminary report. Chest 87:715-719
4. Fantoni A (1993) The translaryngeal tracheostomy. In: Gullo A (ed) Proceedings of APICE, pp 459-465
5. Astrachan DI, Kirchner JC, Goodwin WJ (1988) Prolonged intubation vs. tracheostomy: complications, practical and psychological considerations. Laryngoscope 98:1165-69
6. Paul A, Marelli D et al (1989) Percutaneous endoscopic tracheostomy. Ann Thorac Surg 47: 314-315
7. Fantoni A, Ripamonti D, Favero A (1989) Central airway obstruction in children. In: Vincent JL (ed) Update in intensive care and emergency medicine. Springer, Berlin Heidelberg New York, pp 606-617

Electrolyte Emergencies (Mg,K)

F. Schiraldi, F. Paladino

G.M. Berlyne once defined magnesium as the Cinderella of the divalent ions. Nevertheless an increasing amount of interest is growing on Mg-related problems in the ICU. Magnesium and potassium share a lot of physiological actions and interplay with each other in neuromuscular and cardiovascular functions, which are very likely to be deranged in the critically ill. So theoretical knowledge and practical attention of both of them is required of the intensive care specialist.

Magnesium

Normal values for serum Mg concentration are 1,3-2 mEq/l or 1,8-2,5 mg/dl. Hypomagnesemia has been suggested to probably be "the most underdiagnosed electrolyte deficiency in current medical practice" (1). Besides, as symptomatic Mg depletion is often associated with multiple biochemical abnormalities, such as hypokalemia, alkalosis and hypocalcemia, it may be difficult to define specific manifestations as due to hypomagnesemia (2). The main causes of hypomagnesemia can be related to a) redistribution, b) gastrointestinal losses, and c) renal losses.

a) *Redistribution:* as for calcium, the physiologically active part of Mg is the ion, while the protein-bound and the chelated fractions can be considered inactive; as outlined in Table 1 the relative distribution among the three is closely related to the blood pH. Alkalemic states or the iatrogenic alkalinization of the patient reduce the biologically active fraction of Mg (3).

Table 1. Relationship between Mg^{++} and pH

		Normal pH	↑ pH
Mg^{++}	Ionized	50%	30%
	Protein bound	35%	50%
	Chelated	15%	20%

Other causes of redistribution are the refeeding after starvation and the chelation complicating acute pancreatitis or massive citrated transfusions.

b) *Gastrointestinal losses:* steatorrhea, bowel resection, biliary fistulas and, more frequently, prolonged naso-gastric suction (NGS) may all reduce Mg absorption and, particularly in NGS, induce renal losses due to enhanced renal tubular exchange (↑ ALDO).

c) *Renal losses:* renal Mg wasting, as defined by continued urinary Mg excretion in the face of hypomagnesemia, can be due to renal or extrarenal causes (loop diuretics, aminoglycosides, cyclosporine, Bartter's syndrome, alcohol ingestion, DKA). It is noteworthy that Mg losses in diabetic ketoacidosis are multifactorial, depending on Mg coupling with ketoaciduria, osmotic diuresis and extra-intracellular shifting after insulin.

It is also useful to remember that the renal handling of Mg is finely regulated in normal subjects, urinary elimination being usually less than 15 mEq/day; so that in Mg-depleted patients no more than 1-2 mEq/day should be found, otherwise a renal cause should be suspected (4).

Consequences of Mg depletion

Some of the major effects of low $[Mg]_p$ are related to a multiple ion channel modulation, mainly affecting the Ca channel current and the outward K current (see below). Nevertheless, serum Mg levels of 1 mEq/l or less warrant immediate therapy to prevent important clinical implications (5). Increased neuromuscular excitability up to tetany, anxiety, delirium, psychosis, and hallucinations may all be part of the neurotoxic effects. The most important clinical disturbance is the frequent association of hypomagnesemia with ventricular arrhythmias, particularly during myocardial ischemia (6).

Moreover, Mg deficiency, like K deficiency, sensitizes the patient to digitalis toxicity. Mg administration prolongs the effective refractory period, depresses conduction, increases the membrane potential (makes it more negative) and can control ventricular tachyarrhythmias: in the ICU setting this could be very useful when conventional antiarrhythmic drugs do not succeed. In those patients it could be better to aim for a serum Mg concentration of 2.8-3.5 mEq/l, infusing Mg salts as suggested in Table 2 (7).

Table 2. Emergency administration of Mg

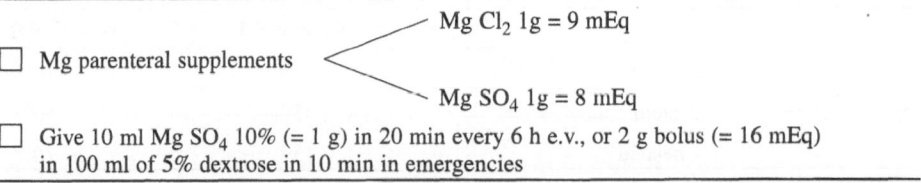

Mg parenteral supplements
- $Mg\ Cl_2$ 1g = 9 mEq
- $Mg\ SO_4$ 1g = 8 mEq

☐ Give 10 ml $Mg\ SO_4$ 10% (= 1 g) in 20 min every 6 h e.v., or 2 g bolus (= 16 mEq) in 100 ml of 5% dextrose in 10 min in emergencies

Moreover there are several reports on the improved efficacy of digoxin combined with Mg, due to their synergistic action on the AV node (8, 9).

Whenever Mg salts are given by the i.v. route it is mandatory to frequently check the blood pressure (hypotension), to monitor the ECG (various degrees of heart block) and to closely observe the ventilatory pattern of the patients (respiratory depression) (see below). Sometimes it could be useful to associate *KCl* (20 mEq in 100 ml normal saline in 1-2 h), which may help in suppressing some ventricular arrhythmias, or $CaCl_2$ or Ca-gluconate (10-30 ml of 10% solution in 20 min) when alkalemia or ionized hypocalcemia are associated (tetany, delayed heart repolarization).

Hypermagnesemia

Addison's disease, renal insufficiency and some phases of DKA (contracted diuresis, dehydration, acidemia before starting the therapy) are the main causes of hypermagnesemia in the ICU. Sometimes it could be iatrogenic, due to overenthusiastic therapy of preeclampsia/eclampsia.

Consequences of hypermagnesemia

Any plasmatic Mg concentration in excess of 3 mEq/l could be complicated by hypokinetic arrhythmias (from sinusoid bradycardia to AV blocks), depending on preexisting heart diseases and/or associated antiarrhythmic therapy with Ia, Ic, II, III, IV class drugs.

Moreover, the main clinical manifestations of hypermagnesemia can be quite closely related to the *speed* of the blood level raising (10) and obviously to the *absolute value* of the serum concentration (Table 3).

Table 3. Clinical effects of hypermagnesemia

	Serum Mg (mEq/l)
Normal	1.3-2
Long P-R, bradycardia	3-5
Hypotension	4-6
Respiratory insufficiency	7-9
Heart block	7-9
Respiratory paralysis	> 10

Treatment

The first step in treating symptomatic hypermagnesemia is the i.v. administration of 5-10 mEq of calcium in 5 min to quickly improve the respiratory function and/or the bradycardia and hypotension; the further approach depends on the renal function: if one could hypothesize an effective forced diuresis, furosemide (20 mg/h) and normal saline (300-400 ml/h) can be administered. Otherwise peritoneal dialysis or hemodialysis may be needed.

Potassium

Referring to potassium balance disorders, some principles must be always kept in mind:

1. We usually measure and talk about the small out-of-the-cells K fraction (n.v. = 3.8-5.6 mEq/l), while the intracellular fraction is 40/1 related to the former (11).
2. The extracellular pH strongly influences the [K]p evaluation, almost stoichoiometrically in metabolic disorders, more weakly in the respiratory ones, so that one should evaluate [K]p and plasmatic pH at the same time (12).
3. The electrophysiological effects depend more on the [K]i/[K]e ratio, and the speed of ratio variations, than (on) the plasmatic absolute value (see below).
4. Artificial diets, based on essential amino acids, dextrose and lipids or ketoanalogues can reduce the K input to 40-50 mEq/day: a still serious problem to face, if the diuresis is very reduced.
5. The urinary K elimination is almost the last renal function to be lost (if mineralcorticoid hormones are working normally); in fact one can usually rely on the *kaliuria* to get deeper insights into the potassium balance and – as the major determinant of urinary K excretion is the overall level of body K stores – work out the extent of K depletion (Table 4).

Table 4. Kaliuria and hypokalemia

Kaliuria	
< 20 mEq/day	> 20 mEq/day
• Extrarenal losses	• renal
• Marked K depletion	losses
	renal diseases ↑ ALDO

The main *causes of hypokalemia* can be easily memorized as due to: inadequate input, extra-intracellular redistribution, renal losses, and gastrointestinal losses. As underlined above the simple blood gas analysis associated to the daily kaliuria can strongly suggest the diagnosis and help to correct the disorder.

Consequences

In the ICU setting it is noteworthy to try to focus on the *timing* of the hypokalemia onset (this is also true for hyperkalemia). The reason for that is based on the importance of the Nernst equation, which strictly links the *resting myocardial potential* (E_m) to the potassium intra/extracellular ratio (13):

$$E_M = -61.5 \times \log \frac{[k]i}{[k]e}$$

Normally this value is near -88 mV, modified to -100 mV if the kaliemia is acutely (hours) reduced to 2 mEq/l, but only reduced to -90 mV if the same 2 mEq/l value was reached in some days. This is due to some adaptation mechanism and must be taken in account during the therapeutic approach ("try always to correct with respect to the disorder timing, i.e. slow/slow, fast/fast") (14).

Moreover the hyperpolarizing effect of hypokalemia is associated to a proportional *K-conductance (gk)* reduction: this explains the unhmogeneous and delayed myocardial repolarization (long Q-T or Q-U), with increased probability of *ventricular repetitive arrhythmias* (the most likely cardiac complication due to hypokalemia).

The second main consequence of low [K]p in the critically ill is the influence on transcellular proton shifts, bicarbonate reabsorption, tubular proton secretion, renal ammoniagenesis and aldosterone secretion. The sum of these effects produces a strong tendency toward *metabolic alkalosis*, so that to correct the latter it is almost mandatory to correct the hypokalemia at the same time. Moreover, potassium depletion predisposes susceptible individuals to hepatic encephalopathy and hepatic coma.

Among the other effects (metabolic, muscular, renal, hormonal) perhaps the most remarkable in the ICU setting is the increased risk of *digitalis toxicity*.

Management of hypokalemia

While the chronic K depletion is best treated with oral potassium supplements, sometimes associated with potassium-sparing diuretics or ACE inhibitors, in emergency conditions one has to consider the i.v. route. The theoretical deficit can be calculated as the difference between 4.5 mEq/l (desired value) and the actual one; after that, this difference must be multiplied by the amount of intracellular fluid (ICF) (approximately 1/3 of total body weight) and finally the total amount can safely be given at a rate of 10-20 mEq/h, monitoring the ECG and the diuresis; glucose-containing solutions should not be used as a vehicle, because glucose will stimulate release of insulin, driving potassium into the cells. It is often useful to associate Mg salts, as magnesium is helpful in protecting against ventricular arrhythmias and co-operates in reducing K losses.

Hyperkalemia

Since urinary potassium excretion is basically a secretory function of the distal nephron and is minimally dependent on glomerular filtration, it then follows that, as long as urine output is maintained, renal potassium excretion is essentially adequate to handle dietary load. Obviously in *acute oliguric states* serum potassium levels may increase rapidly in the absence of significant external potassium loads; by contrast, in chronic stable renal failure hyperkalemia may occur when a) the intake is increased, b) mineralocorticoid hormones are decreased (even in normal renal function) or c) following the use of K-sparing drugs. Clinical organic acidosis (more frequently DKA) is commonly associated to hyperkalemia, and *digitalis intoxication* may provoke severe hyperkalemia, by extracellular *shift* of potassium, as digitalis inhibits the Na-K pump (15). When the blood creatine level is normal and the kalemia is high, *aldosterone deficiency* must always be suspected.

Consequences of hyperkalemia

Due to the reduction of the resting potential (less negative) and the increased rate of repolarization, there are two main clinical problems induced by hyperkalemia.

The *neuromuscular manifestations* include paresthesias and weakness in the arms and legs; these may be followed by flaccid paralysis of the extremities, later involving the respiratory muscles up to ventilatory insufficiency. Very often the *cardiac toxicity* is the major source of morbidity and mortality in hyperkalemia patients.

As a consequence of *the reduction of the resting potential* (E_M), the threshold potential (E_T) is reached more easily then normal and the *repolarization is shortened* (increased gk): the end result is a decrease in conduction velocity, with various degrees of AV and intraventricular blocks, producing widening of the QRS complexes and tall T waves. If appropriate therapy is not begun, *ventricular fibrillation* or asystole will follow.

Everyone is well aware of the different approaches available to antagonize the clinical effects of hyperkalemia; but it could be useful to remember the different onset, mechanism and duration of effect of the therapies (16-18) (Fig. 1) (Table 5).

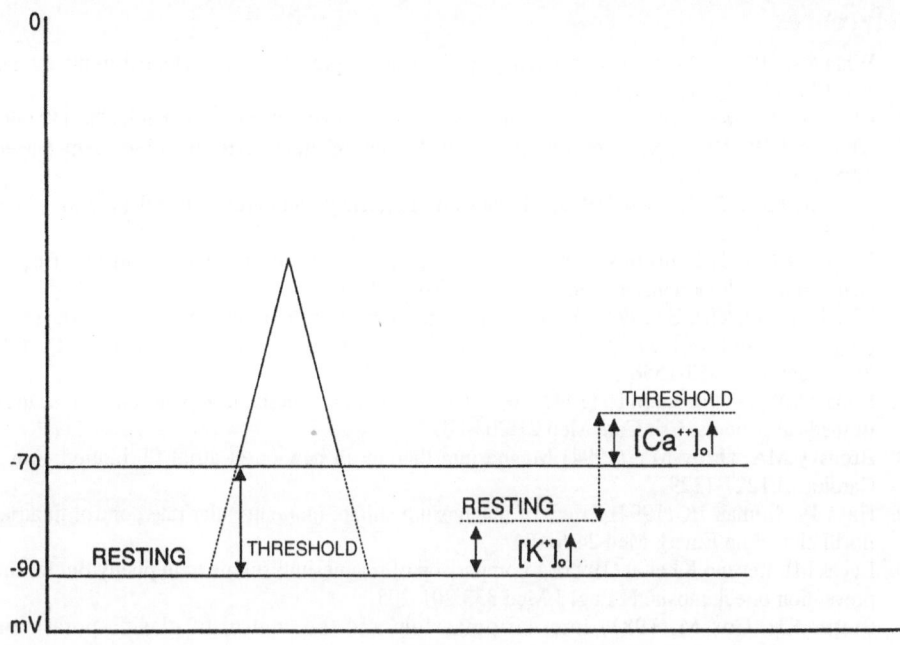

Fig. 1. Ca correction of hyperkalemic depolarization

Table 5. Management of hyperkalemia

Therapy	Mechanism	Onset	Duration
Calcium chloride or Calcium gluconate (6-12 mEq)	Membrane antagonism	1-3 min	30-60 min
Sodium bicarbonate 1 M (50-100 mEq)	Redistribution	3-5 min	120 min
Insulin plus glucose	Redistribution	30 min	4-6 h
Dopexamine (2.5-5 γ/kg/min)	Redistribution	30 min	1-6 h
Kayexalate (25-50 g PO)	Excretion	1-2 h	4-6 h
Dialysis	Excretion	Minutes	Until completed

It is important to notice the specific electrophysiologic antagonizing effect of calcium salts in hyperkalemia. As depicted in Fig. 1, calcium is unique in raising the threshold potential, almost immediately improving AV and intraventricular conduction and myocardial contractility; so it must be used as a first-line drug in such emergencies.

References

1. Whang R (1987) Magnesium deficiency: pathogenesis, prevalence and clinical implications. Am J Med 82 [Suppl 3A]:24-29
2. Chernow B (1989) Hypomagnesemia in patients in post-operative intensive care. Chest 95:391
3. Khnochel JP (1982) Neuromuscular manifestations of electrolyte disorders. Am J Med 72:521-535
4. Iseri LT, Freed J, Bures A (1975) Magnesium deficiency and cardiac disorders. Am J Med 58:837-844
5. Siegel D (1992) Diuretics, serum and intracellular electrolyte levels, and ventricular arrhythmias in hypertensive men. JAMA 267:1083-1089
6. Woods KL, Fletcher S (1992) Intravenous magnesium sulphate in suspected acute myocardial infarction: results of the second Leicester intravenous Magnesium Intervention Trial (LIMIT-2). Lancet 339:1553-1558
7. Rubeiz GY, Baharozian MTh (1993) Association of hypomagnesemia and mortality in acutely ill medical patients. Crit Care Med 21:203-209
8. Brodsky MA, Orlov MY (1994) Magnesium therapy in new-onset atrial fibrillation. Am J Cardiol 73:1227-1229
9. Hays JV, Gilman JK (1994) Effect of magnesium sulfate on ventricular rate control in atrial fibrillation. Ann Emerg Med 24:61-64
10. Lucas MJ, Leveno KJ et al (1995) A comparison of magnesium sulfate with phenytoin for the prevention of eclampsia. N Engl J Med 333:201-205
11. Sterns RH, Cox M (1981) Internal potassium and the control of plasma potassium concentration. Medicine (Baltimore) 60:339-351
12. Adrogué HJ, Madias NE (1981) Changes in plasma potassium concentration during acute acid-base disturbances. Am J Med 71:456-467
13. Schulman M, Narins RG (1990) Hypokalemia and cardiovascular disease. Am J Cardiol 65: 4E-9E
14. Hamill RJ, Robinson LM (1991) Efficacy and safety of potassium infusion therapy in hypokalemic critically ill patients. Crit Care Med 19(5):694-699
15. Bismuth C, Gaultier M (1973) Hyperkalemia in acute digitalis poisoning: prognostic significance and therapeutic implications. Clin Toxicol 6:153-160
16. Blumberg A, Weidmann P (1988) Effect of various therapeutic approaches on plasma potassium and major regulating factors in terminal renal failure. Am J Med 85:507-513
17. Downing HA, Ware RS (1991) Control of hyperkalemia in acute renal failure with dopexamine. Clin Intensive Care 2(6):336-337
18. Fraley DS, Adler S (1977) Correction of hyperkalemia by bicarbonate despite constant blood pH. Kidney Int 12:354-360

Patient Controlled Analgesia (PCA): Clinical Experience

A. Pasetto, A.M. Varutti, V. Bonfreschi, F. Colò

Conventional management of acute postoperative pain with intermittent intramuscular administration of fixed doses of drugs usually fails to produce adequate analgesia for a variety of reasons (1-4):

- Delay between patient's request and need satisfaction by the nurse
- Drug absorption rate from intramuscular depots
- Opioids underprescription for fear of side-effects, mainly respiratory depression
- Wide interpatient variability of analgesic need, related to marked differences of pharmacokinetic and pharmacodynamic factors
- Subjectivity of pain experience that makes difficult the use of any assessment index

. These and other factors make it difficult to accurately predict how much pain a patient will experience after an operation and consequently how much analgesic medication will be required to provide adequate pain relief. Some authors reported an incidence of insufficient postoperative pain relief of 50% (3), even though many of these patients received a larger amount of analgesic medication. Good analgesia can be achieved with a relatively low total drug dose, if the titration of analgesic drug is adequate. The concept of patient controlled analgesia (PCA) was first introduced by Sechzer in 1965 as an objective method of pain measure (5). Soon after PCA became a drug delivery system that allows patients to self-administer small doses of drugs when they feel the need for them. The principle has been accepted as an effective and safe method of postoperative pain relief. It overcomes the inadequacy of traditional analgesic protocols thanks to the individualized treatment (5-12). The patient himself determines his analgesic need within the safety limits fixed by the physician. Repeated self-administrations of small intravenous doses of opioids have the aim to maintain the minimum effective analgesic drug concentration (3). This is a narrow therapeutic window for individual patient, above which side-effects appear and under which the analgesia is inadequate (4).

PCA systems

Most PCA systems are made up of electronically controlled infusion pumps, more or less sophisticated, some of them portable. A thumbswitch (or other mechanism) may be used by the patient to self-administer the bolus dose. All the pumps have a Y connection provided with an antireflux safety-valve; the PCA infusion device must be separated from other i.v. catheters avoiding pharmacologic interferences and flow changes. The brain of sophisticated pumps is a microprocessor interfaced with a digital screen. It allows the physician to program the demand dose and the interval time (or lock-out time) precluding administration of additional doses until such interval has elapsed. This represents a safety feature against accumulation and pharmacological overdose (4, 7, 11, 13). Some pumps are able to fix a maximum dose per time unit (1 or 4 h). The technologically innovating devices are provided with highly sophisticated fail safe features and alarms. The ODAC (on-demand analgesia computer) is connected to a pneumographic sensor, limiting or stopping dosage with a decrease in the patient's respiratory rate (4). Most of the modern PCA devices are able to provide a continuous infusion in combination with the conventional intermittent bolus injection technique. A variety of PCA systems are on the market: the Cardiff Palliator (Graseby Dynamics), the Pharmacia Prominject, the ODAC, the Abbott Life Care PCA infuser, the Bard Harvard PCA (portable pump). The IVAC PCA infuser (Becton Dickinson), the CADD-PCA (Pharmacia), the Provider 5000 (Abbott Pancreatic), all portable, provide PCA by epidural or subcutaneous injection. Single use infusion devices are available (Ex: Infusor Baxter, Infusor Paragon): they are cheap, easy to handle, reliable and suitable in out-patients. Each pump provides for an unchanging bolus dose size and a constant lock-out time; moreover there are no alarm systems. Nevertheless they are accurate enough (10, 14).

The loading dose

The loading dose can be administered over 15-30 min in the recovery-room or in the surgical ward in order to achieve the minimum analgesic plasma concentration in a short time.

Demand dose and lock-out time

They are preset to presumably keep the above-stated concentration. When the patient is sufficiently conscious and cooperating, he is authorized to use the PCA pump. Drug titration must be carefully assessed in the first hours and varied if necessary, according to the onset of inadequate analgesia or excessive sedation. During the sleeping hours some authors suggest increasing the size of the bolus dose, attempting to maximize the intervals (4, 7). The analgesic consumption varies over time: it's high during the first 3-4 postoperative hours; after 12-18 h of stabilization it shows a second peak in the morning of the first postoperative day (1).

Background infusion

Some publications have indicated that the use of continuous opioid infusion would allow a reduction of the bolus size and improve the maintenance of steady plasmatic concentration (3). The concurrent infusion is not considered the best choice, because a real advantage in the pain control is not demonstrated (1, 3, 7, 15, 16). In contrast, other works have pointed out that the presence of a continuous infusion did not decrease the number of patient demands, causing a higher total drug consumption (16-18). Moreover it seems to cause the onset of a tolerance together with a higher increase not only of minor side effects but also of respiratory depression that is extremely rare with demand bolus (1, 3, 7, 15, 16, 19).

Maximum dose

According to some authors, it is not appropriate to fix a maximum limit of consumption, if this isn't adapted for the individual analgesic need (3). There would be the risk of overdose for the patients with low analgesic needs or of inadequate analgesia for the patients with higher consumption (3).

Analgesic choice

In prescribing PCA therapy, the ideal drug would have a rapid onset of analgesic action, an intermediate duration of action, absence of side effects or adverse pharmacologic interactions (3, 4). At the moment a drug with all these characteristics is unavailable.

By intravenous injection, the opioids are still the drugs of largest use (7), mainly morphine, because of the compromise between the duration of the effect and the therapeutic index (3). The loading dose usually prescribed for morphine is 2-10 mg with demand dose size varying from 0.5 to 2 mg and a lock-out time of 5-10 min during the day (3, 4, 7, 9). A study showed that the individual morphine demand after major surgery varied from 0 to 16.5 mg; this demonstrates the high variability of the optimal dose (4). Initially, a 1 mg bolus dose of morphine is prescribed, with the possibility of increasing or reducing 0.5 mg according to the reaction. A 2 mg bolus dose involves the risk of respiratory depression (9). During the sleeping hours some authors suggest a 4 mg bolus with a lock-out time maximized up to 30 min, to prevent the patient from awakening repeatedly (4, 7). The continuous infusion of morphine must be absolutely avoided because of the risk of accumulation and a possible rapid onset of tolerance. Concerning the patients who receive the same dose of opioid, variations of plasmatic rates are documented from two to five times (1). There is the same variability between plasmatic rates and analgesic effect. The interindividual pharmacokinetic differences depending on age, sex, cardiovascular state, simultaneous infusion of other drugs, especially anaesthetics, and surgical stress are not sufficient reasons to explain such a big difference in the analgesic need (1, 3). Experimental studies investigated the question, finding (some other assuming) a linear inverse relation between cerebrospinal fluid endorphin concentrations (or endorphin receptors) during the preoperative period, and the postoperative analgesic demand (3, 4, 20). An important role may be played by the patient's personality, as well as other psychological factors like anxiety and preoperative expectations (3, 4). In contrast, there seems to be no relation between the anthropometric data such as weight, height, and body surface area and analgesic need (20). Fentanyl, sufentanil and alfentanyl are effective in PCA, but their duration of effect is too short and demand bolus too frequent in order to obtain an adequate analgesia (3, 7). An alternative is the association of a background infusion, with additional risks for the patient.

Using meperidine during PCA, the prescribed demand doses are 5-30 mg with a lock-out time of 5-15 min. Some authors have pointed out the possibility of excitatory effects on the central nervous system that cannot be reversed by naloxone. They are caused by normeperidine, an active metabolite of meperidine with an excitatory effect and a long half-life (t 1/2ß 15-20 h) (21). For this reason during PCA with meperidine, the use of high doses for a long period have to be avoided, mainly in patients with impaired renal function.

Methadone is not very manageable either, because it tends to accumulate in the tissues, with slow removal justifying the prolonged half-life (t1/2ß 24-36 h) (4).

A recent alternative to the use of opioids in PCA is represented by ketorolac trometamina, for adequate postoperative pain relief and the absence of relevant side-effects (11, 22).

Administration routes

Analgesic drugs have been used mostly by i.v. injection. The intravenous route of administration eliminates interpatient variability in drug absorption from muscular tissues, allowing a rapid onset of analgesic effect as a rapid reversion of possible side-effects (1, 2, 3, 23). Recently many authors have been interested in epidural (PCEA) and intrathecal PCA. PCEA data are too few to allow a clinically relevant conclusion. It has been demonstrated that opioids in PCEA have a direct spinal effect mechanism together with a systemic action (24, 25). Compared to i.v., epidural morphine allows a reduction of the total dosage up to 80% (23, 26), while using meperidine the reduction is only 30% (23). Likewise, meperidine plasmatic concentrations are relatively high, suggesting an important systemic role (23). The onset of analgesic effect and duration of action are related to differences in opioid lipophilicity. The low lipid solubility of morphine causes a low onset of full analgesic effect (about 1 h) (26, 27) and a higher risk of late respiratory depression, in comparison with fentanyl and sufentanil, more lipophilic substances, that represent a good alternative when administered on demand (24). During PCEA simultaneous use of opioids and anti-inflammatory drugs or local anesthetics enhances the analgesic effects. The latter is appreciated in obstetric analgesia, not only after cesarean section, but most of all during labor, where local anesthetics are basic drugs (23, 28-32). The most used opioids are meperidine and fentanyl. PCA by subcutaneous injection is a simple method, but it needs higher doses than by i.v., with the disadvantage of prolonged kinetics of absorption and elimination (1, 3).

Safety in PCA

Monitoring of sedation level and breathing rate are essential; oversedation regularly anticipates the onset of respiratory depression (3). Instrumental monitoring by pulse-oximetry is to be recommended, in particular with obese patients and during the night (3, 8). Under these conditions respiratory depression is a rare event. An immediate reversal of respiratory depression must be guaranteed by naloxone administration (in case of pure agonist only). Nausea and vomiting would be expected to occur in about 10% of patients (33, 34). Their presence after administration of bolus dose doesn't necessarily have to interrupt PCA. The doctor may change opioid or associate an antiemetic such as metoclopramide (10 mg i.v.) or droperidol in small doses (0.25 mg i.v.) (5, 26, 35). It is demonstrated that opioids administered by PCA cause no more emetic sequelae than the conventional methods. If PCA therapy is to be successful, it is important that the patient understand the concept, as part of the preoperative instructions. In the postoperative period patient collaboration must be checked regularly (4). Many authors propose the introduction of an acute pain service to the general surgical ward. The aim of this structure is to improve the quality of postoperative analgesia, to train skilled physicians and nursing staff, to apply and develop new analgesic techniques and promote research (2, 36, 37).

The low global frequency of incidents (1.6%) demonstrates the relative safety of PCA (3). The documented cases of respiratory depression are attributed to the operator (the most frequent case) and due to misprogramming, to the patient (failure to understand PCA principle or pump device, or intentional abuse), and to mechanical errors (very rare) (8, 34, 38-42).

PCA indications and contraindications

The main indication remains acute postoperative pain. A rational use of PCA must consider cost/effectiveness ratio, owing to the heavy economic impact, being therefore reserved for selected categories of patients, at high risk and pain intensity. More recently PCA has been suggested for other kinds of pain, such as obstetric and medical, but the data are few. Preliminary studies indicate excellent obstetric analgesia without effects on the fetus (3). Data about the treatment of chronic pain (especially oncologic) are also fewer (23, 43). In this case single use and portable PCA devices makes home-treatment possible (14).

It is necessary to exclude from PCA all patients who cannot collaborate for psychic or physical reasons (ex: paralysis), former drug-addicted patients (some authors disagree) (44) and children. However, PCA has been tested on children and teenagers with good results, thanks to the use of devices easy to manage and with a high degree of safety (32). The limiting factor is represented by children age and their psychic development (in the survey the youngest child was 10 years old). Publications indicate that PCA can also guarantee adequate pain relief without increasing risks in the elderly (45).

PCA effectiveness

Many surveys demonstrate better control of postoperative pain with PCA compared to the conventional techniques. Better analgesia would allow early ambulation and physical therapy, reducing hospital stay (4, 12, 46). Many other works confirm the minor total opioid consumption, especially with PCEA, but haven't found real differences in analgesic effectiveness (9, 44, 47). Other authors failed to demonstrate any advantage (48-50). Generally, for the same analgesic effectiveness, patients who have experienced both techniques are more satisfied with PCA for the psychologic advantage of being independent in their own therapy, reducing related pain anxiety (7, 11).

Finally, other comparative studies will be necessary to demonstrate the real cost/effectiveness of PCA in order to justify a widespread acceptance of this therapeutic technique in clinical practice.

References

1. Baubillier E, Bonnet F (1991) Analgésie controlée par le patient. Cah Anesthesiol 39(8): 551-555
2. Riegler FX (1994) Update on perioperative pain management. Section III Regular and special features. Clin Orthop Rel Res 305:283-292
3. Scherpereel PH (1991) Analgésie controlée par le patient (ACP). Ann Fr Anesth Reanim 10:269-283

4. White PF (1988) Use of patient-controlled analgesia for management of acute pain. JAMA 259:243-247
5. Sechzer PH (1990) Patient controlled analgesia (PCA): a retrospective. Anesthesiology 72: 735-736
6. Bennett RL, Batenhorst RL, Bivins BA et al (1982) Patient-controlled analgesia. A new concept of postoperative pain relief. Ann Surg 195(6):700-705
7. Langlade A, Briard C, Bouguet D et al (1994) Analgésie controlée par le patient et douleurs postopératoires. Cah Anesthesiol 42(2):183-189
8. Levin A, Klein SL, Brolin RE et al (1992) Patient-controlled analgesia for morbidly obese patients: an effective modality if used correctly (correspondence). Anesthesiology 76:857-858
9. Owen H, Brose WG, Plummer JL et al (1990) Variables of patient-controlled analgesia. 3. Test of an infusion-demand system using alfentanyl. Anaesthesia 45:452-455
10. Pasetto A, Colò F, Pasqualucci A et al (1993) Control of post-operative pain by a PCA throwaway device. In: Atti APICE, pp 241-245
11. Savoia G (1990) Le basi razionali dell'analgesia controllata dal paziente (PCA). Minerva Anestesiol 56(7-8):349-352
12. Wasylak TJ, Abbott FV, English MJM et al (1990) Reduction of post-operative morbidity following patient-controlled morphine. Can J Anaesth 37(7):726-731
13. Casali R, Di Benedetto M, Masci P et al (1990) Pompa PCA1 Bard nell'immediato dolore post-operatorio. Minerva Anestesiol 56(10):1131-1132
14. Paoletti F, Boanelli A, Falconi S (1995) Ruolo dei presidi infusionali monouso nella terapia antalgica domiciliare. In: Atti Le nuove frontiere dell'impegno anestesiologico: il sistema di emergenza, i trapianti e la terapia antalgica domiciliare. Udine, pp 179-184
15. Owen H, Plummer JL, Armstrong I et al (1989) Variables of patient-controlled analgesia. 1. Bolus size. Anaesthesia 44:7-10
16. Parker PK, Holtmann B, White PF (1991) Patients controlled analgesia. Does a concurrent opioid infusion improve pain management after surgery? JAMA 266:1947-1952
17. Owen H, Szekely SM, Plummer JL et al (1989) Variables of patient-controlled analgesia. 2. Concurrent infusion. Anaesthesia 44:11-13
18. Vercauteren MP, Coppejans HC, Ten Broecke PW et al (1995) Epidural sufentanil for postoperative patient controlled analgesia (PCA) with or without background infusion: a double-blind comparison. Anesth Analg 80:76-80
19. Baubillier E, Leppert C, Delaunay L et al (1992) Analgésie controlée par le patient: effet de l'adjonction d'une perfusion continue de morphine. Ann Fr Anesth Reanim 11:479-483
20. Burns JW, Hodsmann NBA, McLintock TTC et al (1989) The influence of patients characteristics on the requirements for postoperative analgesia. Anaesthesia 44:2-6
21. Stone PA, Macintyre PE, Jarvis DA (1993) Norpethidine toxicity and patient controlled analgesia. Br J Anaesth 71:738-740
22. Rubin P, Yee JP, Murthy VS et al (1987) Ketorolac tromethamine analgesia: no postoperative respiratory depression and less constipations. Clin Pharm Ther 41:182 (abstr)
23. Brasseur L (1992) Analgésie auto-controlée par voie péridurale et méthodes classiques d'analgésie. Cah Anesthesiol 40(7):474-476
24. Chrubasik J, Hans W, Schulte-Monting J (1988) Relative analgesic potency of epidural fentanyl, alfentanyl, and morphine in treatment of postoperative pain. Anesthesiology 68: 929-933
25. Sjostrom S, Hartvig D, Tamsen A (1988) Patient controlled analgesia with extradural morphine or pethidine. Br J Anaesth 60:358-366
26. Marlowe S, Engstrom R, White PF (1989) Epidural patient controlled analgesia (PCA): an alternative to continuous epidural infusions. Pain 37:97-101
27. Chrubasik J, Wiemers K (1985) Continuous plus on demand epidural infusion of morphine for postoperative pain relief by means of a small, externally worn infusion device. Anesthesiology 62:263-267
28. Gambling DR, Christopher JH, Johnathan B et al (1993) Patient controlled epidural analgesia in labour: varying bolus dose and lockout interval. Can J Anaesth 40(3):211-217

29. Gambling DR, Yu P, Cole C et al (1988) A comparative study of patient controlled epidural analgesia (PCEA) and continuous infusion epidural analgesia (CIEA) during labour. Can J Anaesth 35(3):249-254
30. Giangreco R, Rossetto B, Colucci V et al (1990) Inefficacia della PCA endovenosa nel controllo del dolore in travaglio di parto. Minerva Anestesiol 56(10):1127-1128
31. Morisot P, Boureau F (1991) Evaluation de la douleur obstétricale par questionnaire d'adjectifs. Comparison de deux modalités d'analgésie péridurale. Ann Fr Anesth Reanim 10:117-126
32. Murat I, Dubois MC, Esteve C et al (1991) Analgésie auto-contrôlée chez l'enfant. Cah Anesthesiol 39(3):161-164
33. Robinson SL, Fell D (1991) Nausea and vomiting with use of a patient controlled analgesia system. Anesthesia 46:580-582
34. White PF (1987) Mishaps with patient-controlled analgesia. Anesthesiology 66:81-83
35. Sharma SK, Davies MW (1993) Patients-controlled analgesia with a mixture of morphine and droperidol. Br J Anaesthesiol 71:435-436
36. Ball D, Holmes K, Ralph S (1992) Solving the problems with patient controlled analgesia. BMJ 304:1113
37. Gould TH, Crosby DL, Harmer M et al (1992) Policy for controlling pain after surgery: effect of sequential changes in management. BMJ 305:1187-1193
38. Grover ER, Heath ML (1992) Patient-controlled analgesia. A serious incident. Anaesthesia 47:402-404
39. McKanzie R (1988) Patient-controlled analgesia (PCA). Anesthesiology 69:1027
40. Notcutt WG, Knowles P, Kaldas R (1992) Overdose of opioid from patient-controlled analgesia pumps. BMJ 69:95-97
41. Southern DA, Read MS (1994) Overdosage of opiate from patient controlled analgesia device. BMJ 309:1002
42. Thomas DW, Owen H (1988) Patient-controlled analgesia-the need for caution. Anaesthesia 43:770-772
43. Sozio CA, Lorenzelli L (1995) Controllo del dolore oncologico con PCA. In: Atti Le nuove frontiere dell'impegno anesthesiologico: il sistema di emergenza, i trapianti e la terapia antalgica domiciliare (1995). Udine, pp 266-267
44. Howell PR, Gambling DR, Pavy T et al (1995) Patient controlled analgesia following caesarean section under general anaesthesia: a comparison of fentanyl with morphine. Can J Anaesth 42(1):41-45
45. Santangelo E, Savoia G, Scopa C et al (1991) Sicurezza della PCA nel paziente geriatrico. Minerva Anestesiol 57(10):1080-1081
46. De Leon-Casasola OA, Parker BM, Lema MJ et al (1994) Epidural analgesia versus intravenous patient controlled analgesia: differences in the postoperative course of cancer patients. Reg Anesth 19:307-315
47. Testa G, Bozomati V, Rossi A (1994) Impiego del ketorolac in patients controlled analgesia (PCA) nel dolore post-operatorio. Minerva Chir 49:347-362
48. Dahal JB, Daugaard JJ, Larsen HV et al (1987) Patient-controlled analgesia: a controlled trial. Acta Anaesth Scand 31:744-747
49. Eisenach JC, Grice SC, Dewan DM (1988) Patient controlled analgesia following cesarean section: a comparison with epidural and intramuscular narcotics. Anesthesiology 68:444-448
50. Harrison DM, Sinatra R, Morgese L et al (1988) Epidural narcotic and patient-controlled analgesia for post-cesarean section pain relief. Anesthesiology 68:454-457

Management of Acute Myocardial Infarction

G. VOGA

Introduction

Acute myocardial infarction (AMI) could be considered as one of the most important illnesses of our century. In the beginning of the twentieth century, acute coronary occlusion was expected to be immediately fatal, but very soon it became clear that some patients might survive the acute event. After 1960 the medical therapy comprised only analgesia, bed rest and sedation. With the advent of electrocardiographic monitoring, defibrillators and potent antiarrhythmic drugs the hospital mortality secondary to electrical instability was markedly reduced from approximately 30% to 15%. Left ventricular pump failure became the major cause of hospital deaths in late 1960s. As the amount of myocardial necrosis obtained the pivotal role, all attempts were focused toward reducing the myocardial injury by improving the balance between oxygen demand and supply in the jeopardised myocardium. One of the major improvements of the infarction treatment was the development of intracoronary and intravenous thrombolysis. Myocardial salvage became reality and was defined as the act of rescuing and recovering of myocardium following the acute occlusion of the coronary artery. It resulted in reduction of the infarct size, preservation of the ejection fraction and reduction of mortality.

In the last few years a great amount of new information about the pathophysiology and treatment of AMI was published. This paper is a brief review with special emphasis on the clinical importance.

Pathogenesis

AMI had generally been considered a consequence of coronary artery thrombosis until post-mortem studies in the 1970s proved the presence of the coronary thrombi in only 21% to 91% patients with AMI (1, 2). On the basis of these studies the authors claimed that coronary thrombosis is the consequence rather than the cause of the AMI. Controversy was resolved by coronary angiography in the acute phase of myocardial infarction, which demonstrated thrombotic coronary artery occlusion in the majority of patients (3).The general consensus today is that in 80% to 95% of patients coronary thrombotic occlusion can be demonstrated in the early hours after onset of pain.

The initiating event for almost every AMI is a rupture of soft, lipid rich atheromatous plaque in an epicardial coronary artery. This allows free communication between lipid content and blood and the release of macrophages that contain much tissue factor with procoagulant activity. The blood flows into the plaque and causes intraintimal thrombus. Intraluminal thrombus develops over the site of rupture which can later become occlusive or lysed to the healed but larger plaque. The process is dynamic commonly with fluctuation and progression of the occlusion (4, 5). Plaque rupture is usually triggered by increases in catecholamines and platelet aggregation in stress or sudden fright at sites of endothelial abnormality. Exercise itself can thus trigger the onset of AMI, particularly in sedentary persons (6). AMI can occur also in patients with normal coronary arteries (7). Many bioactive mediators such as thromboxane A_2, prostacyclin, serotonin, thrombin, platelet aggregation factor and others have an important role in the pathogenesis of infarction. Recently some substances (PGI_2 stabilising factor - HDL, nitric oxide synthase etc.) that can modulate and prevent the effects of mediators were discovered (1).

Table 1. Mortality (%) related to the time of treatment

Study	Early time	Late time
GISSI I	8.2	11
MITI	1.2	8.7
TIMI II	3.2	5.7
EMIP	9.7	11.1

Prehospital treatment

The most vulnerable and dangerous phase of AMI for the majority of patients occurs before hospital admission. Time is undoubtedly the crucial factor for diagnosis and treatment of AMI due to the benefit of early thrombolytic therapy and to the ever-present threat of sudden death. Treatment in the first hour helps to achieve maximal myocardial salvage and reduction of mortality. More than a half of all deaths from AMI occur in the first hour after onset of pain, mostly because of ventricular fibrillation (5). Despite the widespread knowledge and awareness of the importance of early treatment only few patients (2 to 10%) received treatment in the first hour. This delay, which represents an important barrier to timely treatment, has many factors which can be grouped in three phases: patient/bystander delay (from onset of symptoms to call), prehospital delay (from call to emergency department), hospital delay (from arrival to treatment) (8). The mean decision time for seeking medical care was 111 min and the mean hospital admission time 136 min (9). It was found that the reperfusion and mortality are a function of the length of time between symptom onset and treatment (Table 1) (8, 10).

Therefore a *special, fast track protocol* has been proposed for management of patients with suspected AMI (8). It includes organisational and personnel activities such as: education of personnel and patients, routine ECG registration and proper evaluation in every patient with chest pain, immediate institution of routine therapy and rapid decision for and start of thrombolysis. By using this protocol the mean time from onset of pain to treatment can be reduced and the number of patients treated in the first hour increased (10, 11). Despite focus on thrombolytic therapy, the value of routine, established immediate treatment should not be underestimated and avoided. The following *immediate therapy* should be used in every patient with suspected AMI (8, 12): oxygen, analgesics (opiates given by slow i.v. injections - morphine 5-10 mg), antiemetics (together with opiates), nitrates (immediate sublingual therapy), aspirin (150-300 mg as soon as AMI is suspected), antiarrhythmics (no routine use; atropine, adrenaline and lidocaine must be available). IV line and ECG monitoring should be started as soon as possible.

Hospital treatment

Patients with AMI should be admitted to the coronary care unit (CCU). CCU is a specialised area in hospital with adequate equipment and properly educated and skilled personnel. This enables monitoring of patient's vital functions and immediate interventions to complications.

General measures that should be undertaken in all patients are:

Restricted physical activity: absolute bed rest is mandatory only for first 6-12 h. Later early and individualised mobilisation could be started according to patient's status. Several randomised trials confirmed the safety of early mobilisation and lower complication rate (13).

Supplemental oxygen should be given to all patients by nasal or facial mask in dose 2-4 l/min for the first 24-48 h.

Analgesics (opiates are preferred) should be used in adequate doses to control the pain completely.

Anxiolytics (benzodiazepines) should be liberally provided.

Monitoring of vital signs is one of the most basic CCU activities. *Noninvasive monitoring* usually includes continuous monitoring of patient's ECG for assessment of cardiac rhythm and ST segment deviation, measurement of arterial blood pressure, and arterial oxygen saturation. Such monitoring is sufficient and adequate for most patients with AMI.

For patients with congestive heart failure, right ventricular infarction, cardiogenic shock, and other complications (ventricular septum defect or rupture of papillary muscle), exact determination of systemic and pulmonary pressures, and cardiac output by *invasive monitoring* is mandatory. It can easily be accomplished by bedside insertion of thermodilution flow-directed pulmonary artery catheter and arterial line. Despite much criticism invasive monitoring is becoming routine procedure in the CCU and is used in about 15% patients with AMI and in 26% patients with complicated AMI (14).

In addition to general measures *specific treatment for reduction of infarct size* is routinely used.

Thrombolytic therapy was revolutionised by use of intravenous instead of intracoronary thrombolytic agent. Numerous trials demonstrated a significant decrease in mortality (approximately 25%) by intravenous administration of streptokinase (STK), recombinant human tissue-type plasminogen activator (alteplase; TPA), or anisolated plasminogen streptokinase activator complex (anistreplase; APSAC) (Table 2) (15). Comparative trials have shown only little difference in efficacy between diverse thrombolytic agents (Table 3) (16). The time between onset of symptoms and treatment is far more important factor for successful thrombolysis than the choice of thrombolytic agents (Table 1).

Table 2. Mortality reduction (%) by thrombolysis

Trial	Agent	Reduction %
GISSI	SK	18
ISIS 2	SK	23
ISAM	SK	11
AIMS	APSAC	47
ASSET	TPA	26
LATE	TPA	14

Table 3. Mortality reduction (%) related to different thrombolytic agents

Trial	SK	APSAC	TPA
ISIS 3	10.5	10.6	10.3
GISSI 2	8.6		9
GUSTO	7.2		6.3

The benefit of thrombolytic therapy is well established and definitely outweighs the possible bleeding complications (including cerebral) which occur in about 1% of patients. Thrombolysis is thus indicated in patients within 12 h after onset of typical chest pain and at least 0.1 mm of ST elevation in two contiguous ECG leads (15). Detailed analysis of large randomised trials indicates that fibrinolytic therapy is also beneficial in elderly patients, in patients with cardiogenic shock, history of nontraumatic cardiopulmonary resuscitation and in patients with bundle branch block (15, 17). Contraindications for thrombolysis are: history of severe bleeding, recent internal haemorrhages, major surgery, trauma or delivery within 10 days, cardiopulmonary resuscitation, vascular puncture in a noncompressible site and uncontrolled hypotension (15). The success of thrombolytic therapy can be noninvasively and indirectly assessed by the presence of reperfusion arrhythmias, rapid ST segment resolution (18) and early peak of CKMB and myoglobin (19). Ventricular function and infarct related artery patency have been found to be independent prognostic factors after thrombolytic therapy and therefore must be evaluated (20). The presence and extent of residual stenosis after AMI should be precisely determined by coronary angiography, especially in patients with clinical evidence of myocardial ischemia. Patients with significant residual stenosis should be definitely treated by angioplasty or bypass grafting. Left ventricular function must be assessed as soon as possible with echocardiography or isotopic ventriculography.

Although recent large trials of thrombolysis in AMI reported 30%-40% of patients eligible for thrombolysis it is estimated that only 10% of hospitalised patients in the USA receive this treatment (21). In the majority of patients *other therapeutic options for infarct size limitations* are available. The treatment with intravenous nitroglycerin (22-24), magnesium (25-27), and the use of antiplatelet drugs was found to reduce mortality in AMI (27). In contrast, the use of calcium channel antagonists and beta blockers did not show any important influence on mortality (Table 4) (28-30).

Table 4. Results of meta-analysis of early interventions on mortality after AMI [adapted from (28)]

Drug	Mortality % (treatment)	Mortality % (control)	p-value
Beta blocker	3.4	3.6	NS
Nitrates	13.3	18.9	0.0006
Ca antagonist	8.3	7.6	0.17
Magnesium	3.8	8.2	0.0008
Antiplatelets	9.3	11.7	< 0.0001

In specialised tertiary centres *primary angioplasty* can be performed with better results (lower mortality rate and lower incidence of reinfarction and late interventions) than intravenous thrombolysis (28, 31). Primary angioplasty is currently very expensive and largely unavailable in most countries. Considering the reported results it is obvious that the organisational and financial aspects of the AMI treatment do not meet the possibilities of medical progress. However, even today it offers a chance for survival in high risk patients with contraindications for fibrinolysis. The same is true for immediate bypass grafting as a primary treatment (16). Patients with *serious complications after AMI* (cardiogenic shock, ventricular septum defect, papillary muscle rupture and rupture of free wall) must always be considered as candidates for immediate invasive and surgical procedure. The patients with such complications who could be stabilised and transferred to a specialised cardiac centre for surgical intervention have a much better prognosis than when treated conservatively (32).

Right ventricular infarction (RVI) represents a special subset of AMI, which has an important role in the ICU setting. It is frequently (20%-40%) found as an extension of the inferior left ventricle infarction (33, 34). The most important clinical feature is right ventricular heart failure in the absence of pulmonary congestion with a relatively large incidence of cardiogenic shock and advanced atrioventricular block (35). Patients with cardiogenic shock due to predominant RVI have a much better prognosis than patients with cardiogenic and extensive damage of left ventricle (36). This condition must therefore be recognised early, properly monitored (invasive monitoring!) and adequately treated. The basic treatment of predominant right ventricular failure in RVI setting involves volume expansion, inotropic agents and maintenance or restoration of normal atrioventricular synchronicity (37).

References

1. Kawai C (1994) Pathogenesis of acute myocardial infarction. Circulation 90:1033-1043
2. Roberts WC, Buja LM (1972) The frequency and significance of coronary arterial thrombi and other observations in fatal acute myocardial infarction: a study of 107 necropsy patients. Am J Med 52:425-443
3. DeWood MA, Spores J, Notske R, Mouser LT, Burrugho R, Golden MS, Lang TS (1980) Prevalence of total coronary occlusion during the early hours of transmural myocardial infarction. N Engl J Med 303:897-902
4. Davies MJ, Thomas AC (1985) Plaque fissuring-the cause of acute myocardial infarction, sudden cardiac death and crescendo angina. Br Heart J 53:363-373
5. Vincent R (1994) Pre-hospital management. In: Julian D, Braunwald E (eds) Management of acute myocardial infarction. Saunders, London Philadelphia Toronto Marrickville Tokyo, pp 3-5
6. Mittleman MA, Maclure M, Tofler GH, Sherwood JB, Goldberg RJ, Muller JE (1993) Triggering of acute myocardial infarction by heavy physical exertion. Lancet 329:1677-1683
7. Sharifi M, Frolich TG, Silverman IM (1995) Myocardial infarction with angiographically normal coronary artery arteries. Chest 107:36-40
8. National Heart Attack Alert Program Coordinating Committee (1994) Emergency department: rapid identification and treatment of patients with acute myocardial infarction. Ann Emerg Med 23:311-329
9. Schwartz B, Schoberberger R, Rieder A, Kunze M (1994) Factors delaying treatment of acute myocardial infarction. Eur Heart J 15:1595-1598
10. Cannon CP, Goldhaber SZ (1995) The importance of rapidly treating patients with acute myocardial infarction. Chest 107:598-599
11. Cummings P (1992) Improving the time to thrombolytic therapy for myocardial infarction by using a quality assurance audit. Ann Emerg Med 21:1107-1110

12. Vincent R (1994) Pre-hospital management. In: Julian D, Braunwald E (eds) Management of acute myocardial infarction. Saunders, London Philadelphia Toronto Marrickville Tokyo, pp 17-18
13. Antman EM (1994) General hospital management. In: Julian D, Braunwald E (eds) Management of acute myocardial infarction. Saunders, London Philadelphia Toronto Marrickville Tokyo, p 34
14. Yarzebski J, Goldberg RJ, Gore JM, Alpert JS (1994) Temporal trends and factors associated with pulmonary artery catheterization in patients with acute myocardial infarction. Chest 105:1003-1008
15. International Society and Federation and World Health Organisation Task Force on Myocardial Reperfusion (1994) Reperfusion in acute myocardial infarction. Circulation 90:2091-2101
16. Baker CSR (1994) Myocardial salvage in the ITU. Int J Intensive Care 1:116-119
17. Fibrinolytic Therapy Trialist Collaborative Group (1994) Indications for fibrinolytic therapy in suspected acute myocardial infarction: collaborative overview of early mortality and major morbidity results from all randomised trials of more than 1000 patients. Lancet 343:311-322
18. Dissmann R, Schroeder R, Busse U, Appel M, Brueggemann T, Jereczek M, Linderer T (1994) Early assessment of outcome by ST-segment analysis after thrombolytic therapy in acute myocardial infarction. Am Heart J 128:851-857
19. Ishii J, Nomura M, Ando T, Hasegawa H, Kimura M, Kurokawa H et al (1994) Early detection of successful coronary reperfusion based on serum myoglobin concentration: comparison with serum creatine kinase isoenzyme MB activity. Am Heart J 128:641-648
20. White HD, Cross DB, Elliott JM, Norris RM, Yee TW (1994) Long-term prognostic importance of patency of the infarct related coronary artery after thrombolytic therapy for acute myocardial infarction. Circulation 89:61-67
21. Gossage JR (1994) Acute myocardial infarction. Reperfusion strategies. Chest 106:1851-66
22. Muenzel T, Just H (1991) Nitrate in der Therapie des akuten Myokardinfarktes. Intensivmedizin 28:339-343
23. Werns SW, Rote WE, Davis JH, Guevara T, Lucchesi BR (1994) Nitroglycerin inhibits experimental thrombosis and reocclusion after thrombolysis. Am Heart J 127:727-737
24. Pollak H, Mlczoch J (1994) Effect of nitrates on the frequency of left ventricular wall rupture complicating acute myocardial infarction: a case controled study. Am Heart J 128:466-471
25. Teo KK, Yusuf S, Collins R, Held PH, Peto R (1991) Effects of intravenous magnesium in suspected acute myocardial infarction: overview of randomised trials. Brit Med J 303: 1499-1503
26. Woods KL, Fletcher S, Roffe C, Haider Y (1992) Intravenous magnesium sulphate in suspected acute myocardial infarction: results of the second Leicester intravenous magnesium intervention trial (LIMIT 2). Lancet 339:1553-1558
27. Woods KL, Fletcher S (1994) Long term outcome after intravenous magnesium sulphate in suspected acute myocardial infarction: the second Leicester intravenous magnesium intervention trial (LIMIT 2). Lancet 343:816-819
28. Flather MD, Farkouh ME Yusuf S (1994) Meta-analysis in the evaluation of therapies. In: Julian D, Braunwald E (eds) Management of acute myocardial infarction. Saunders, London Philadelphia Toronto Marrickville Tokyo, pp 393-406
29. Jain P, Lillis O, Cohn PF (1994) Effect of metoprolol on early infarct expansion after acute myocardial infarction. Am Heart J 127:764-773
30. Mathey DG (1986) Betarezeptoren-Blocker und Kalzium-Antagonisten in der Akutphase des Herzinfarktes: Einfluss auf Infarktgroesse und Prognose. Intensivmedizin 23:396-402
31. Boer MJ, Suryapranata H, Hoorntje JCA, Reiffers S, Liem AL, Miedema K et al (1994) Limitations of infarct size and preservation of left ventricular function after primary coronary angioplasty compared with intravenous streptokinase in acute myocardial infarction. Circulation 90:753-761
32. Stomel RJ, Rasak M, Bates ER (1994) Treatment strategies for acute myocardial infarction complicated by cardiogenic shock in a community hospital. Chest 105:997-1002

33. Isner JM, Roberts WC (1978) Right ventricular infarction complicated left ventricular infarction secondary to coronary artery disease. Am J Cardiol 42:885-894
34. Wackers FJT, Lie K, EB, Res J, Van der Schoot I, Durrer D (1978) Prevalence of right ventricular involvement in inferior wall infarction assessed with thallium 201 and technetium-99m pyrophosphate. Am J Cardiol 42:358-362
35. Merx W, Meyer J, Essen R et al (1982) Rechtsherzinsuffizienz beim Infarkt der rechten Kammer. I. Diagnose und Haeufigkeit. Dtsch Med Wochens 107:565-570
36. Gewirtz H, Gold HK, Fallon JT, Pasternak RC, Leinbach RC (1979) Role of right ventricular infarction in cardiogenic shock associated with inferior myocardial infarction. Br Heart J 42:719-725
37. Cohn JN (1979) Right ventricular infarction revisited. Am J Cardiol 43:666-668

Anaesthesia for Abdominal Vascular Surgery

V. PAVER-ERŽEN

Introduction

The goals of anaesthesia for surgery of the abdominal aorta and its major branches are similar to those of any surgical procedure: to minimize patient morbidity and maximize the surgical benefit. To meet these goals, anaesthesia for abdominal vascular surgery demands meticulous attention to every aspect of the procedure, the preoperative assessment of the patients, the anaesthetic management and the postoperative period.

Preanaesthetic assessment

Patients scheduled for surgery of the aorta and/or its major branches are susceptible to atheromatous vascular disease manifested as ischaemic heart disease, cerebrovascular disease or, rarely, renal disease. The heart should be the major focus of the anaesthesiologist's attention as myocardial dysfunction is the single most important cause of morbidity following vascular surgery (1). Particularly coronary artery disease must be identified and addressed preoperatively if one is to achieve optimal results. The prognostic importance of coronary artery disease at the time of elective abdominal aortic aneurysmectomy was evaluated by Roger et al. (2). In this study the presence of uncorrected overt or suspected coronary artery disease was associated with significant increase in perioperative complications and, of factors examined, was the only one that was clinically and statistically significant with respect to both long-term survival and subsequent late events. The results also show that vascular surgery in patients who have undergone coronary revascularization is associated with a lower incidence of perioperative complications. In the study of Hertzer et al. (3) severe correctable coronary artery disease was identified in 31% of patients with abdominal aortic aneurysms who underwent routine coronary arteriography before elective aortic reconstruction. The authors suggested that patients with symptomatic coronary artery disease should undergo coronary arteriography, with the implication that myocardial revascularization should precede aortic surgery. Some authors reserve coronary arteriography for patients with clinically relevant coronary artery disease (4, 5). Those favouring a selective approach argue that patients at risk for ischaemic myocardial events during and after aortic reconstruction can be reliably identified on the basis of clinical criteria (9). In patients without clinical manifestations of coronary artery disease, different centres have different approaches to preoperative evaluation. Noninvasive studies such as stress electrocardiography, continuous Holter monitoring, stress echocardiography, exercise and dipyridamole thalium stress myocardial imaging may be indicated in some subgroups of patients. Decisions to undertake coronary arteriography and myocardial revascularization should be based on the results of these studies (6, 7). The history of a previous myocardial infarction is a consistently reported major risk for perioperative cardiovascular complications (8, 9). A standard electrocardiogram is indicated for all patients scheduled for major vascular surgery. Special attention should be given to the evidence of a previous myocardial infarction, of ventricular strain or hypertrophy, electrolyte or conduction abnormalities, and to that of the presence of myocardial ischaemia and existence of dysrhythmias. The patients undergoing aortic surgery are at greater risk for cardiac complications than those undergoing nonaortic operations (10, 11). Pasternak et al. reported that the incidence of perioperative myocardial infarctions was directly related to the total duration of myocardial ischaemia in patients undergoing peripheral vascular surgery (12). Recent studies have indicated that the rate of reinfarction may be lessened by using invasive monitoring (13, 14). Other coexisting conditions, including pulmonary and renal disease, must also be identified and addressed preoperatively. Marginal pulmonary functions, particularly those below 50% of predicted values for vital capacity and forced expiratory volume in 1 s, may preclude elective aortic reconstruction. Marginal renal function (serum creatinine 229 µmol/l) must be evaluated and corrected if possible.

Patients with mild to moderate diastolic hypertension (95-110 mmHg) or well-controlled hypertension are no more at risk than normotensive patients, provided their antihypertension therapy is maintained, they are adequately monitored during and after surgery, and haemodynamic perturbations are vigorously treated.

Anaesthesia

Virtually all anaesthetic techniques and drugs have been used for aortic reconstructive surgery. For this operative procedure maintaining haemodynamic equilibrium and attending to detail appear to be more crucial to outcome than is the choice of anaesthetic technique. Recent studies by Shah et al., Haku et al., Crosby et al., Baron et al. and Rivers et al., which have compared epidural plus general vs. general, fentanyl vs. sufentanil, regional vs. general, epidural plus general vs. general, and epidural vs. general anaesthesia, respectively, have all failed to demonstrate that anaesthetic technique was associated with a significant effect on outcome (14-18).

Blomberg et al. reported that high thoracic epidural anaesthesia (TEA) (T1-T6) in patients with coronary artery disease was associated with an increase in the diameter of stenotic areas of coronary arteries although coronary perfusion pressure, coronary blood flow distribution, myocardial oxygen consumption and lactate extraction were not altered significantly (19). Kocks et al. investigated the effects of high TEA (T_3-T_5) including the cardiac sympathetic segments on ischaemic ST-segment changes and left ventricular global and regional wall motion abnormalities. They concluded that cardiac sympathetic blockade with TEA in patients with coronary artery disease improves ischaemia - induced left ventricular global and regional wall motion abnormalities at a certain level of physical stress, associated with less pronounced ST-segment depression (20).

A major potential risk of regional anaesthesia is the development of an epidural haematoma. Epidural anaesthesia followed by heparinization for vascular surgery appears to be safe (21) but some authors reported epidural haematoma as a complication of this technique (22).

The study of Benefiel et al. shows that sufentanil anaesthesia alone was associated with less major morbidity than isoflurane anaesthesia in patients undergoing aortic reconstruction (23). For occlusion of the aorta at the supraceliac level, some authors (1) tried to avoid using halothane because the occlusion at this level tends to make the liver hypoxic for a time and in this situation halothane can in theory create a hepatitis-like condition. The results of the study by Colson et al. suggest that anaesthesia with halothane is associated with transient renal vasoconstriction during infrarenal aortic cross-clamping, whereas aortic cross-clamping during isoflurane anaesthesia is not associated with renal haemodynamic impairment (24). Arienta et al. (25) concluded that total intravenous anaesthesia with propofol and fentanyl provided remarkably good haemodynamic stability during major vascular surgery.

Special problems of abdominal aortic surgery

Cross-clamping of the aorta is a major intraoperative cardiovascular stress. The immediate haemodynamic response is an increase of both systolic and diastolic arterial pressures, despite a decrease of stroke volume and of cardiac output. The increased impedance to ejection results in increased left ventricular wall tension, and an increase in myocardial oxygen uptake. Simultaneously, the arteriolar resistance in the upper half of the body decreases as the baroreflex response to the increasing arterial pressure results in arteriolar dilatation. Over a period of 5-10 min after cross-clamping, the normal heart and circulation accommodate to the change. Patients with ischaemic heart disease and susceptibility to acute ischaemic ventricular dysfunction or diminished myocardial contractile reserve frequently develop signs of acute left ventricular decompensation and pump failure after infrarenal aortic cross-clamping (26), characterized by a large decrease in stroke volume and cardiac output and an acute increase in pulmonary artery occlusion pressure, which is often accompanied by cardiac arrhythmias and/or ECG signs of subendocardial ischaemia. Manifestations of acute left ventricular failure are more common following suprarenal or supraceliac cross-clamping of the aorta. Using continuous two-dimensional transoesophageal echocardiography, Roizen et al. (27) demonstrated that supraceliac cross-clamping was associated with large increases in left ventricular end-diastolic pressure and end-diastolic areas and a severe decrease in ejection fraction.

Because of great perturbation which can be imposed on the cardiovascular system with aortic cross-clamping and declamping, the following monitoring is recommended to be used: an intra-radial artery catheter, ECG leads II and V_5 simultaneously, body temperature, pulmonary artery catheter (PA) and/or transoesophageal echocardiography (TEE). When a discrepancy exists between pulmonary capillary filling pressures and end-diastolic dimension (volume) as determined from TEE, the latter has been found to be more reliable and useful (1).

Berlauk et al. (28) reported that when a pulmonary artery catheter was used to optimize patients haemodynamically 3-12 h before peripheral vascular surgery, the perioperative mortality rate was 1.5%, compared to 9.5% in patients who did not receive a pulmonary artery catheter.

Serious blood loss can occur during the period of aortic occlusion from lumbar arteries within the aneurysmal bed, from proximal aortic anastomosis and from coagulopathy. The need for homologous blood transfusion can be reduced by careful surgical technique and autologous transfusion options - preoperative donation, intraoperative phlebotomy and haemodilution, intraoperative blood salvage and return.

Hypotension following release of the aortic clamp may be the result of any combination of events, including: hypovolemia, reactive hyperaemia, washout of acid from the ischaemic areas below the clamp, acid metabolites, release of vasoactive substances and an allergic reaction to the graft material. Raising filling pressure too long before release of the cross-clamp may place an undue and potentially deleterious workload on the heart. To cause a systemic venoconstriction and aid venous return, some anaesthesiologists give 2-4 mg of methoxamine immediately before declamping. Administration of sodium bicarbonate is usually not necessary prior to removal of the cross-clamp.

Intraoperative preservation of renal function

Potential causes of renal dysfunction are: hypovolemia, change in renal perfusion with aortic clamping, embolization of debris or air, and use of nephrotoxic drugs.

When the aorta is cross-clamped at an infrarenal level, serum creatinine has been reported to increase by 0.5 mg/dl or more in 15% of patients. When these patients were compared with those who underwent occlusion at the suprarenal level, there was no difference in postoperative renal function (29).

For preservation of renal function an infusion of mannitol (20 gm, 10% or 20% solution) 30 min before aortic cross-clamping is used. Mannitol possesses vasodilator actions, may increase renal prostaglandin, may decrease renal renin, and it has been reported to shift blood flow to the cortex of the kidney. Loop diuretics inhibit tubular salt reabsorption, have a vasodilator effect and inhibit tubuloglomerular feedback.

Dopamine (1-3 µg/kg/min) inhibits the tubular transport of sodium and increases renal blood flow and urine output.

The use of mannitol, furosemide, ethacrynic acid or low dose dopamine infusion has not been clearly shown to alter the outcome of renal function after aortic surgery.

Fenoldopam – a new dopamine receptor agonist – has been evaluated as an agent for renal preservation. It appears that fenoldopam possesses properties in common with both mannitol and dopamine (30).

The bowel

Manipulation of the bowel can result in the mesenteric traction syndrome, consisting of facial flushing, hypotension and tachycardia. It is mediated by the release of prostacyclin. The syndrome lasts less than 20-30 min but a period of hypertension mediated by increased levels of tromboxan may follow. The treatment for this syndrome is symptomatic and includes the administration of fluids and vasoconstrictor therapy. This syndrome is absent in patients on aspirin or nonsteroidal antiinflammatory drug therapy. Pretreatment with ibuprofen 12 mg/kg by mouth 1-1.5 h preoperatively has been reported to decrease the level of 6-keto PGF1 alpha, which is a metabolite of prostacyclin. Ibuprofen is a cyclooxygenase inhibitor and therefore reduces the formation of prostacyclin (31).

Postoperative management

The patient recovering from aortic surgery requires haemodynamic stabilization, adequate ventilation, oxygenation and tissue perfusion, and effective pain relief. Invasive monitoring, together with pulse oximetry should be continued for as long as it is necessary to ensure stability of the patient's cardiovascular system.

The main recent advance in postoperative management of the patient after aortic surgery has been the introduction of thoracic epidural blockade to provide effective pain therapy during the first postoperative days.

Benefits associated with epidural analgesia in the postoperative period include decreased sedation, better tolerance of chest physiotherapy, earlier ambulation, increased lung volumes and improved arterial oxygenation.

Cardiac complications account for almost all postoperative deaths in the short term. Even long-term morbidity and mortality is related predominantly to coronary artery disease and its sequelae.

Hypercoagulability occurs following abdominal aortic bypass surgery (32). Tumen and coworkers reported that patients who had received a combined general and epidural anaesthesia for major vascular surgery had an attenuated hypercoagulable state postoperatively when compared to patients who had received general anaesthesia. This diminution of their hypercoagulable state resulted in a lower incidence of thrombotic events of peripheral arterial grafts, coronary arteries or deep veins (33). In contrast, the results of Gibbs et al. (34) suggest that epidural blockade with local anaesthetic agents does not prevent the postoperative hypercoagulability response following abdominal aortic bypass surgery.

References

1. Roizen MF, Ellis JE (1992) Anesthesia for vascular surgery. In: Barash PG, Cullen BF, Stoelting RK (ed) Clinical anesthesia. Lippincott, Philadelphia, pp 1059-1094
2. Roger VL, Ballard DJ, Hallett JW, Osmundson PJ, Puetz PA, Gersh BJ (1989) Influence of coronary disease on morbidity and mortality after abdominal aortic aneurysmectomy: a population-based study, 1971-1987. JACC 14:1245-1252
3. Hertzer NR, Beven EG, Young JR et al (1984) Coronary artery disease in peripheral vascular patients: a classification of 1000 coronary angiograms and results of surgical management. Ann Surg 199:223-233
4. Golden MA, Whittemore AD, Donaldson MC, Mannick JA (1990) Selective evaluation and management of coronary artery disease in patients undergoing repair of abdominal aortic aneurysms: a 16-year experience. Ann Surg 212:415-423
5. Reigel MM, Hollier LH, Kazmier FJ et al (1987) Late survival in abdominal aortic aneurysm patients: the role of selective myocardial revascularization on the basis of clinical symptoms. J Vasc Surg 5:222-227
6. McEnroe CS, O'Donnell TF Jr, Yeager A, Konstam M, Mackey WC (1990) Comparison of ejection fraction and Goldman risk factor analysis to dipyridamole-thallium 201 studies in the evaluation of cardiac morbidity after aortic aneurysm surgery. J Vasc Surg 11:497-504
7. Cambria RP, Brewster DC, Abbott WM et al (1992) The impact of selective use of dipyridamole-thallium scans and surgical factors on the current morbidity of aortic surgery. J Vasc Surg 15:43-51
8. Goldman L, Caldera DL, Southwick FS et al (1978) Cardiac risk and complications in noncardiac surgery. Medicine 57:357-370
9. Von Knorring JV (1981) Postoperative myocardial infarction: a prospective study in high-risk group of surgical patients. Surgery 90:55-60
10. Jeffrey CC, Kunsman J, Cullen DJ, Brewster DC (1983) A prospective evaluation of cardiac risk. Anesthesiology 58:462-464
11. Domaingue CM, Davies MJ, Cronin DK (1982) Cardiovascular risk factors in patients for vascular surgery. Anesth Intensive Care 10:324-327
12. Pasternak PF, Grossi EA, Bauman FG, Riles TS, Lamparello PJ, Giangola et al (1989) The value of silent myocardial ischemia monitoring in the reduction of perioperative myocardial infarction in patients undergoing peripheral vascular surgery. J Vasc Surg 10:617-625
13. Rivers SP, Scher LA, Gupta SK, Veith FJ (1990) Safety of peripheral vascular surgery after recent acute myocardial infarction. J Vasc Surg 11:70-76
14. Shah KB, Kleinman BS, Sami H, Patel J, Rao TL (1990) Reevaluation of perioperative myocardial infarction in patients with prior myocardial infarction undergoing noncardiac operations. Anesth Analg 71:231-235

15. Haku E, Hayashi M, Kato H (1989) Anesthetic management of abdominal aortic surgery: a retrospective review of perioperative complications. J Cardiothorac Anesth 3:587-591

16. Crosby ET, Miller DR, Hamilton PP et al (1990) A randomized double blind comparison of fentanyl and sufentanil oxygen anesthesia for abdominal aortic surgery. J Cardiothorac Anesth 4:168-176

17. Baron JF, Bertrand M, Barre E et al (1991) Combined epidural and general anesthesia versus general anesthesia for abdominal aortic surgery. Anesthesiology 75:611-618

18. Rivers SP, Scher LA, Sheehan E, Vieth FJ (1991) Epidural versus general anesthesia for infrainguinal arterial reconstruction. J Vasc Surg 14:764-770

19. Blomberg S, Emanuelsson H, Kvist H, Lamm C et al (1990) Effects of thoracic epidural anesthesia on coronary arteries and arterioles in patients with coronary artery disease. Anesthesiology 73:840-847

20. Kocks M, Blomberg S, Emanuelson H, Lomsky M et al (1990) Thoracic epidural anesthesia improves global and regional left ventricular function during stress-induced myocardial ischemia in patients with coronary artery disease. Anesth Analg 71:625-630

21. Rao TLK, El-Etr AA (1981) Anticoagulation following placement of epidural and subarachnoid catheters: an evaluation of neurological sequelae. Anesthesiology 55:618-620

22. Dickman CA, Shedd SA, Spetzler RF, Shetter AG, Sonntag VK (1990) Spinal epidural hematoma-associated with epidural anesthesia: complications of systemic heparinization in patients receiving peripheral vascular thrombolytic therapy. Anesthesiology 72:942-950

23. Benefiel DJ, Roizen MF, Lampe GH et al (1986) Morbidity after aortic surgery with sufentanil versus isoflurane anesthesia. Anesthesiology 65:A516

24. Colson P, Capdevilla X, Barlet H et al (1992) Effects of halothane and isoflurane on transit renal dysfunction associated with infrarenal aortic cross-clamping. J Cardiothorac Vasc Anesth 6:295-298

25. Arienta G, Patassini V, Angelopulu V, Brunori E (1989) Total intravenous anaesthesia: propofol associated with fentanyl. 43rd SIAARTI Songress 1:115-118

26. Gooding JM, Archic JP, McDowell H (1980) Hemodynamic response to infrarenal aortic cross-clamping in patients with and without coronary artery disease. Crit Care Med 8:382-285

27. Roizen MF, Beaupre PN, Alpert RA, Kremer P, Cahalan MK, Shiller N et al (1984) Monitoring with two-dimensional transesophageal echocardiography. Comparison of myocardial function in patients undergoing suprarenal-infraceliac, or infrarenal aortic occlusion. J Vasc Surg 1:300-305

28. Berlauk JF, Abrams JH, Gilmour IJ et al (1991) Preoperative optimization of cardiovascular hemodynamic improves outcome in peripheral vascular surgery: a prospective randomized clinical trial. Ann Surg 214:289-299

29. Alpert RA, Roizen MF, Hamilton WK, Stoney RJ, Ehrenfeld WK, Poler SM, Wylie EJ (1984) Intraoperative urinary output does not predict postoperative renal function in patients undergoing abdominal aortic revascularization. Surgery 95:707-711

30. Elliott WJ, Weber RR, Nelson KS, Oliner CM, Fumo MT, Gretler DD et al (1990) Renal and hemodynamic effects of intravenous fenoldopam versus nitroprusside in severe hypertension. Circulation 81:970-977

31. Hudson JC, Wurm HW, O'Donnell TF, Kane FR, Mackey WC, Su YF, Watkins WD (1990) Ibuprofen pretreatment inhibits prostacyclin release during abdominal exploration in aortic surgery. Anesthesiology 72:443-449

32. Gibbs NM, Crawford GP, Michalopoulus N (1994) Thrombelastographic patterns following abdominal aortic surgery. Anaesth Intensive Care 22:534-538

33. Tuman KJ, McCarthy RJ, March et al (1991) Effects of epidural anesthesia and analgesia on coagulation and outcome after major vascular surgery. Anesth Analg 73:696-704

34. Gibbs NM, Crawford GP, Michalopoulus N (1992) The effects of epidural blockade on postoperative hypercoagulability following abdominal bypass surgery. Anaesth Intensive Care 20:487-490

Ischemia-Reperfusion in Vascular Surgery

G.P. Novelli, C. Adembri, E. Gandini

Introduction

Many complications occurring in patients submitted to vascular surgery can be attributed to ischemia-reperfusion (I-R) that accompanies vessels clamping and declamping (1). A growing body of evidence indicates that the pathogenesis of I-R can be ascribed to the unbalanced oxygen radical (OR°) generation occurring at reperfusion, when molecular O_2 becomes available (2-4). This process is known as "oxygen paradox".

It has been shown, in fact, that ischemia by itself produces very little damage, which instead appear clearly at reperfusion when OR° are produced. As a consequence, damage is strictly related to the O_2 content of the reperfused blood (5) and is avoided by using free radical scavengers (6-8). Moreover, depletion or inhibition of cells producing OR° protects tissues from I-R (9, 10).

Although a lot of experimental data are available, models of I-R in humans are needed to refine our knowledge and to evaluate the efficacy of pharmacological treatments, in view of their clinical application.

The aim of this paper is to summarize the research performed in the Institute of Anesthesiology and Intensive Care of the University of Florence since 1988 to validate the abdominal aortic surgery as a well controlled model of I-R of skeletal muscle in man and to propose the therapeutic use of antioxidants.

Methods

All the results reported here have been obtained in patients undergoing elective surgery for the repair of abdominal aortic aneurysm. Patients without any clinical or angiographic sign of peripheral vascular insufficiency were selected after informed consent.

Surgical procedures were standardized. Clamping of the abdominal infrarenal aorta was followed by ischemia of both lower limbs which lasted 45-60 min. The right leg was always reperfused first.

Anesthesia was maintained with isoflurane in O_2/air or N_2O avoiding hyperoxia. Mechanical ventilation was set so to prevent hypocapnia. Blood transfusions were not performed.

Venous blood samples from the ischemic-reperfused district and muscle biopsies from the right quadriceps muscle were collected:

1. After the induction of anesthesia (basal samples)
2. At the end of ischemia of the right leg
3. 30 min after reperfusion of the right leg

Investigations

The following aspects of the I-R pathophysiology have been studied:

1. Humoral activation in blood
2. Evidence of cell activation
3. Evidence of muscle peroxidative damage
4. Evidence of systemic damage
5. Protection by antioxidants
6. Sources of RO° in skeletal muscle undergoing I-R

Humoral activation in blood

The aortic clamping creates complete or almost complete ischemia of the lower limbs, as documented by the marked desaturation in the reflowing blood (11).

In blood coming from the I-R district, an enhanced production of $O_2°$ in response to FMLP stimulation was found after reperfusion (Fig. 1). No spontaneous production was observed at any time, so indicating a previous activation or an insufficient sensitivity of the method.

In the same blood samples there was also a significant complement activation ($p < 0.01$) which began in ischemia and was still present at reperfusion (Table 1). Both the classical and the alternative ways were activated, as documented by the decrease in C3 and C4 fractions (1). Complement activated during ischemia plays an important role in attracting granulocytes and activating them. As a consequence, at the end of ischemia, the number of circulating neutrophils in blood reflowing from the ischemic tissue increased significantly over the control values ($p < 0.05$). Thirty minutes after reperfusion, the number of blood neutrophils was furtherly elevated as compared with ischemia and cells occluding capillaries were frequently found, thus contributing to the "no reflow" phenomenon.

Evidence of cell activation

At the end of the ischemic period, light microscopy (L.M.) revealed many granulocytes adhering to the inner and outer capillary wall, in transit across the endothelium or interspersed among the skeletal fibers.

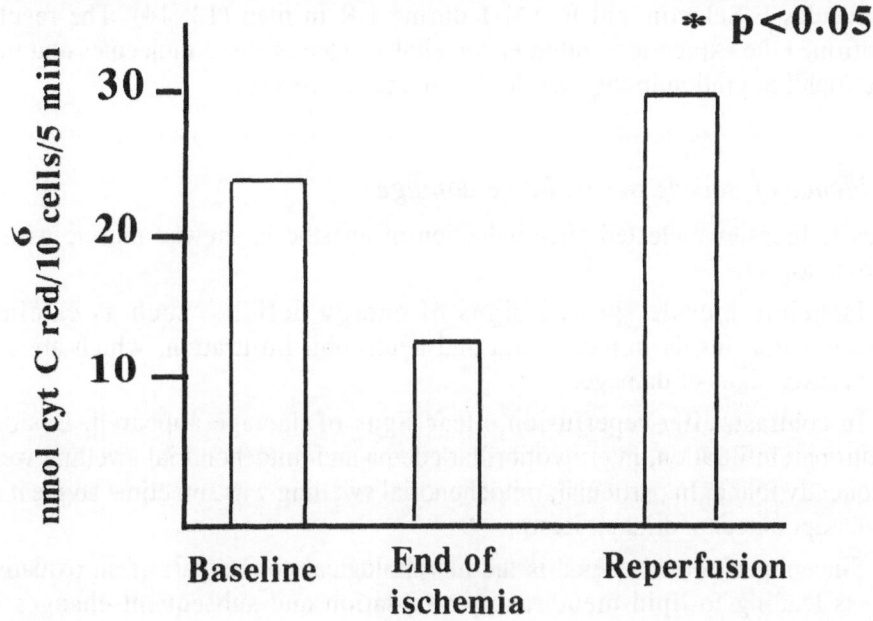

Fig. 1. Superoxide production in venous blood from the ischemic-reperfused lower limbs (12)

Table 1.

	Baseline	Ischemia	
Reperfusion			
Neutrophils	4040	6000 *	8500 *
C3 fraction	115	75 **	70 *
C4 fraction	28	17 **	12 *

* $p < 0.05$.
** $p < 0.01$ (12).

Electron microscopy (E.M.) showed that most of the infiltrating granulocytes were neutrophils which exhibited a normal ultrastructure, forming pseudopodia at their surface.

Neutrophil accumulation in muscle vessels and tissue was furthermore enhanced after 30 min of reperfusion, as observed both at L.M. and E.M. (12).

The absence of endothelial disruption and the strict contact between the endothelium and granulocytes suggested that these cells passed into muscle actively and by reciprocal interaction with endothelial surface in ischemia as well as after reperfusion. Therefore, experiments were performed by immunohistochemical staining to search for the expression of the adhesion molecules E-Selectin and ICAM-1 during I-R in man (13, 14). The results confirmed the expression within endothelial surface of these molecules and that neutrophil migration in the muscle was an active process.

Evidence of muscle peroxidative damage

Muscle biopsies collected after induction of anesthesia showed muscle with a normal aspect.

Ischemic muscle showed signs of energy deficits, such as calcium accumulation inside mitochondria and neutrophil infiltration, which are not themselves signs of damage.

In contrast, after reperfusion, clear signs of damage appeared. Besides neutrophil infiltration, intermyofibrillar edema and mitochondrial swelling were frequently found. In particular, mitochondrial swelling was sometime so great as to disrupt mitochondrial structure.

Since reperfusional edema is the morphological counterpart of an oxidative stress leading to lipid membrane peroxidation and subsequent changes in permeability, we searched for evidence of OR° production directly in skeletal muscle.

As a reliable and clinically useful method for detecting lipoperoxidation in man the malondialdehyde (MDA) content has been previously measured in plasma (15, 3). However, we thought it more exact to monitor MDA content directly in muscle tissue.

A slight but appreciable enhancement of muscle MDA content was also observed during ischemia (Fig. 2), to indicate that, even during clamping of the aorta, the available O_2 is sufficient for a local, limited production of OR°. However, since the OR° production remained low during ischemia, its morphological consequences were scarce, the hallmarks of ischemia being signs of energy deficiency, as mentioned before.

Acute postischemic reperfusion, on the other hand, was responsible for a very strong increase in muscle MDA content, indicating that oxygen reintroduction into the hypoxic tissue is accompanied by a local peroxidative burst, very likely responsible for the damage (16, 17).

To assess the occurrence of lipid peroxidation during aortic surgery, ethane content in exhaled breathing was also measured by quadrupolar mass spectrometry (Fig. 3) (18).

A highly significant increase in ethane concentration in exhaled air was noted after declamping of the first iliac artery, followed by another increase after the declamping of the second artery, i.e. after reperfusion of another area. Ethane in the exhaled air being a good noninvasive marker of lipid peroxidation (19), this datum confirm the OR° generation that accompanies muscle reperfusion during aortic surgery.

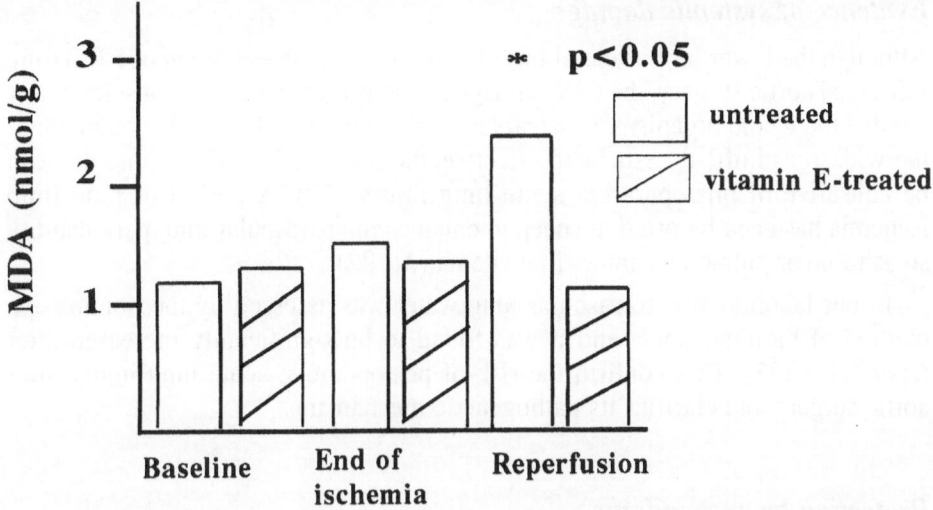

Fig. 2. MDA production in skeletal muscle undergoing I-R: untreated patients and vitamin E-treated patients (18)

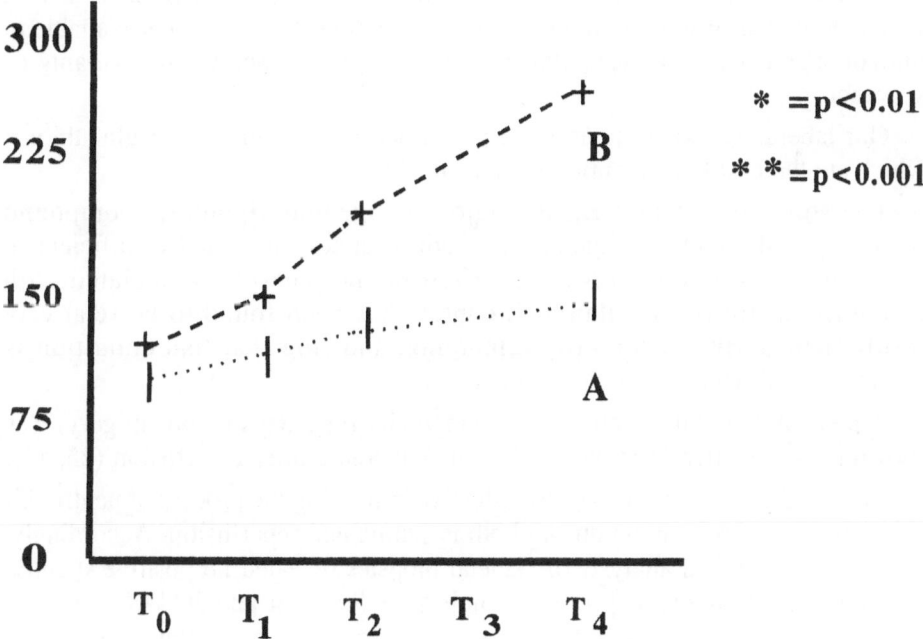

Fig. 3. Ethane in exhaled air of patients submitted to I-R of lower limbs. Group A received GSH; Group B served as control

Evidence of systemic damage

Although the lower limb skeletal muscles are the main target organ of I-R during infrarenal aortic surgery, the OR° damage is not limited to skeletal muscle: it may involve the whole organism, as occurs in declamping shock. Another example of the widespread of I-R associated effects is the involvement of the lung that can be causative of postoperative acute lung injury (20). A period of hind limb ischemia has been reported in sheep to enhance microvascular lung permeability so as to favor pulmonary interstitial edema (21, 22).

In our laboratory, extravascular lung water was assessed by the noninvasive method of bioimpedance, and it was found to be significantly increased after reperfusion (23). This confirm the risk of postoperative acute lung injury after aortic surgery and clarifies its pathogenetic mechanisms.

Protection by antioxidants

The data reported here seem to indicate that OR° and their generation systems are activated during aortic surgery in direct relationship with the evolution of I-R. To make sure of the pathogenetic role of OR°, there was the need to search for the prevention by antioxidants of the above quoted damage.

Several therapeutic approaches have been tried in animal models of I-R. However, it is clear that, up to now, the only pharmacological drugs available in humans against I-R induced damages are drugs that act as antioxidants or scavengers.

Our laboratory experiments were performed with vitamin E or glutathione, which are the best known antioxidant available for clinical use.

The stores of vitamin E, the major endogenous lipophilic compound protecting cell membrane against free radical attack, are usually sufficient in well-nourished patients (24), its deficit being generally associated with malnutrition. However, vitamin E content has been found to be relatively insufficient during aortic cross-clamping, showing that this condition is associated with vitamin E consumption.

A pretreatment with vitamin E (600 mg/daily for 8 days before surgery) was shown to be effective in reducing the MDA increase after reperfusion (25, 17).

Vitamin E pretreatment was also effective in limiting the process of neutrophil infiltration in muscle tissue during both ischemia and reperfusion. Accordingly, immunocytochemical analysis of skeletal biopsies revealed no positive staining for endothelial adhesion proteins, such as E-Selectin and ICAM-1, whose expression is a prerequisite for neutrophils to escape from circulation and enter the muscle.

It is thus conceivable that the absence of biochemical signs of oxidation and of morphological damage is the consequence both of the lack of neutrophil infiltration in skeletal muscle and/or of an antioxidant activity of vitamin E against the OR° produced. Moreover, the release of NO by the endothelium at reperfusion was not affected in patients pretreated with vitamin E, suggesting that this antioxidant molecule blocks the amount of neutrophil adherence to the endothelium and is linked to NO deficit (26).

Vitamin E also protects the lung by preventing the increase in extravascular lung water after reperfusion (23).

Glutathione is another endogenous antioxidant, acting as a redox molecule. A large dose (100 mg/kg) of glutathione before clamping completely prevented the production and exhalation of ethane and the increase in extravascular lung water (27, 18).

The effectiveness of the two antioxidant substances in preventing the I-R associated damages confirm that aortic surgery creates an OR derived disease.

Source of OR° in skeletal muscle undergoing I-R

The question arises of the identification of the mechanisms that provoke the OR° damage during I-R of skeletal muscle in man submitted to aortic surgery. The activated neutrophils, the myofibrils and endothelium itself can be considered.

Neutrophils

Increasing evidence, however, suggests that the activated neutrophils may be the major source of OR° (28, 29, 12).

Muscle cell alterations following I-R appear to be related to neutrophil accumulation in the tissue due to the presence of a membrane-associated enzyme, the NADPH-oxidase, which turns into its active form when cells are triggered; moreover, leukocyte depletion has been reported to protect skeletal muscle from I-R damage in numerous animal models (30, 31).

In the clinical condition of I-R reported here, neutrophils are evidently involved in each phase of the whole process: they are recruited by complement activation, they adhere to the vascular endothelium, and they cross the vascular wall and infiltrate the muscle tissue (12). Moreover, the increase in superoxide anion production (1) in whole blood draining the reperfused muscles was a consequence of activity of granulocytes. Moreover, pretreatment with vitamin E prevented neutrophil infiltration, so also avoiding the production of MDA (25, 17). Evidence suggests that neutrophils – primed when flowing in the ischemic reperfused tissue – spontaneously produce OR° inside the muscle when triggering factors are encountered into the skeletal muscle.

Skeletal muscle (myofibrils)

Another source of OR° might be the ischemic-reperfused muscle itself, due to activity of the xanthine oxidase (XO) system. However, it has been shown that the hypoxanthine content very slowly increases after 15-90 min of reperfusion in human muscle (32), so suggesting a low level of this enzyme in human muscle.

Endothelium

XO content in muscle endothelium is about 100 times the content of myocytes in bovine and in human skeletal muscle (33), thus it might produce OR°. It seems likely that the endothelium contributes to the initial phases of I-R. In fact the OR° locally released induce both the activation of circulating neutrophils and the upregulation of the adhesion molecules (34, 35).

Under normal conditions, neutrophil adhesion to endothelial cells is inhibited by the continuous release of NO which, besides its role in maintaining the basal vascular tone, has also been shown to have an antiinflammatory influence by reducing the activation, the adhesion and the chemotaxis of neutrophils (36, 37). Using NADPH-diaphorase activity as a marker for NO synthase, it has also been evaluated whether changes in NADPH-diaphorase activity of the vascular wall occurred in human skeletal muscle undergoing I-R. We found (26) a slight reduction in NO synthesis even during ischemia that is probably due to the low O_2 levels, as previously reported in another model of I-R (38).

A significant decrease in the activity of NADPH-d was found after reperfusion, which means that an impaired release of NO by the arteriolar and venular walls occurs. This indicates that an impaired NO synthesis, probably due to endothelial dysfunction, accompanies and very likely influences neutrophil adhesion. That is, it is conceivable that even in absence of morphological signs of endothelial damage, a functional alteration may be present and be responsible for the lower amount of NO produced. Otherwise, the impairment of NO production after reperfusion might be due to the inhibitory action of OR° (mainly superoxide) on NO synthase (39, 40).

Conclusions

During aortic vascular surgery, evidence was found of an "oxidative stress" accompanying the I-R associated with this type of surgery.

The main target organ of this oxidative stress is lower limb skeletal muscle, although the damages concern the whole body as demonstrated by the appearance of pulmonary interstitial edema.

I-R associated damage can be prevented or reduced by the administration of drugs which act mainly as antioxidants, thus confirming that aortic reconstruction surgery is an OR° derived disease.

Since it was observed from our preliminary results that the longer the duration of ischemic phase, the more damage results (41), another way to protect patients from I-R is to shorten the duration of ischemia. This is in accordance with the fact that even if damage appears at reperfusion, it is during the ischemic phase that humoral and cellular system involved in OR° production are activated.

Pretreatment with antioxidants – together with shortening the duration of ischemia – is a safe and effective way to reduce skeletal muscle and lung damage in patients undergoing aortic cross-clamping and to improve their recovery in the postoperative period.

References

1. Novelli GP, Adembri C, Brunelleschi S, Livi P, Rossi R, Pratesi C (1990) Oxygen-radicals production during ischemia-reperfusion of the lower limbs in man: inhibitory effects of L-carnitine. Curr Ther Res 48:903-911

2. Odeh M (1991) The role of reperfusion-induced injury in the pathogenesis of the crush syndrome. N Engl J Med 324:1417-1422

3. Rabl H, Khoschsorur G, Colombo T, Tatzber F, Esterbauer H (1992) Human plasma lipid peroxide levels show a strong transient increase after successful revascularization operations. Free Radic Biol Med 13:281-288

4. Grace PA (1994) Ischaemia-reperfusion injury. Br J Surg 81:637-647

5. Korthuis RJ, Smith JK, Carden DL (1989) Hypoxic reperfusion attenuates postischemic microvascular injuries. Am J Physiol 256:H315-319

6. Ferreira RF, Milei J, Llesuy S, Flecha BG, Hourquebie H, Molteni L, De Palma C, Paganini A, Scervino L, Boveris A (1991) Antioxidant action of vitamins A and E in patients submitted to coronary artery bypass surgery. Vasc Surg 25:191-195

7. Abadie C, Baouali AB, Maupoil V, Rochette L (1993) An alpha-tocopherol analogue with antioxidant activity improves myocardial function during ischemia reperfusion in isolated working rat hearts. Free Radic Biol Med 15:209-215

8. Campo GM, Squadrito F, Ioculano M, Altavilla D, Calapai G, Zingarelli B, Scuri R, Caputi AP (1994) Reduction of myocardial infarct size in rat by IRFI-048, a selective analogue of vitamin E. Free Radic Biol Med 16:427-435

9. Kortuis RJ, Grisham MB, Granger DN (1988) Leukocyte depletion attenuates vascular injury in post-ischemic skeletal muscle. Am J Physiol 254:H823-827

10. Weselcouch CD, Grove RI, Demusz CD, Baird AJ (1991) Effect of in vivo inhibition of neutrophil adherence on skeletal muscle function during ischemia in ferrets. Am J Physiol 261:H1178-H1183

11. Novelli GP, Fantozzi R, Livi P, Adembri C, Vanni L, Pieraccioli E, Pratesi C (1988) Generazione di anione superossido nella ischemia chirurgica degli arti inferiori. Acta Anaesth Ital 39:323-331

12. Formigli L, Domenici-Lombardo L, Adembri C, Brunelleschi S, Ferrari E, Novelli G (1992) Ischemia-reperfusion of human skeletal muscle: a role for neutrophils. Hum Pathol 23:627-634

13. Adembri C, Formigli L, Ibba-Manneschi L, Gandini E, Zecchi-Orlandini S, Novelli G (1993) Neutrophil-endothelial cell interactions in I-R of human skeletal muscle. Minerva Anestesiol 59 [Suppl 2]:46

14. Formigli L, Ibba-Manneschi L, Adembri C, Zecchi Orlandini S, Pratesi C, Novelli GP (1995) Expression of E-selectin in ischemic and reperfused human skeletal muscle. Ultrastruct Pathol 19:193-200

15. Draper HH, Hadley M (1990) Malondialdehyde determination as index of lipid peroxidation. Methods Enzymol 186:421-431

16. Adembri C, Gandini E, Papucci L, Pieraccioli E, Rossi R, Vannucci F, Capaccioli S, Novelli GP (1994) Abdominal aortic crossclamping provokes oxidative stress of skeletal muscle as assessed by malondialdehyde. Minerva Anestesiol 60 [Suppl 2]:411
17. Novelli GP, Adembri C, Gandini E, Zecchi Orlandini S, Papucci L, Formigli L, Ibba-Manneschi L, Quattrone A, Pratesi C, Capaccioli S (1995) Vitamin E protects human skeletal muscle from damage during surgical ischemia-reperfusion. Am J Surg (submitted)
18. Scardi S, Rossi R, Pieraccioli E, Tani R, Novelli GP (1993) Reduced glutathione prevents lipid peroxidation as expressed by ethane exhalation during aortic surgery in man. Minerva Anestesiol 59 [Suppl 2]:215
19. Kneepkens CMF, Lepage G, Roy CC (1994) The potential of the hydrocarbon breath test as a measure of lipid peroxidation. Free Radic Biol Med 17:127-160
20. Stallone RJ, Lim RC, Blaisdell FW (1969) Pathogenesis of the pulmonary changes following ischemia of the lower extremities. Ann Thorac Surg 7:539-549
21. Anner H, Kaufman RP, Kobzik L et al (1987) Pulmonary leukosequestration induced by hind limb ischemia. Ann Surg 206:162-167
22. Klausner JM, Paterson IS, Mannick JA et al (1989) Reperfusion pulmonary edema. JAMA 261:1030-1035
23. Rossi R, Fortunati B, Mediati RD, Girardi G, Pieraccioli E, Tani R, Novelli GP (1993) Preoperative high dose alfa-tocopherol prevents the increase of extravascular lung water during ischemia and reperfusion in man. Minerva Anestesiol 59 [Suppl 2]:216
24. Chow CK (1991) Vitamin E and oxidative stress. Free Radic Biol Med 11:215-232
25. Adembri C, Gandini E, Formigli L, Papucci L, Novelli GP (1995) Protection afforded by vitamin E against ischemia-reperfusion damages in human skeletal muscle. Minerva Anestesiol (submitted)
26. Formigli L (1995) Critical events on endothelial surface during ischemia-reperfusion in man. Exp Pathol Practice (submitted)
27. Mediati RD, Girardi G, Rossi R, Pieraccioli E, Tani R, Novelli GP (1993) Glutathione administration prevents the increase of extravascular lung water during ischemia and reperfusion in man. Minerva Anestesiol 59 [Suppl 2]:214
28. Smith JK, Grisham MB, Granger DN, Korthuis RJ (1989) Free radical defense mechanisms and neutrophil infiltration in post-ischemic skeletal muscle. Am J Physiol 256:H789-793
29. Ciuffetti G, Mercuri M, Mannarino E, Lombardini R, Pasqualini L, Ott C, Lupatelli G (1991) Are leukocyte-derived free radicals involved in ischaemia of human legs? Eur J Clin Pharmacol 21:111-117
30. Romson JL, Hook BG, Kunkel SL et al (1983) Reduction of extent of acute myocardial injury by neutrophil depletion in the dog. Circulation 67:1016-1023
31. Korthuis RJ, Grisham MB, Granger DN (1990) Leukocytes depletion attenuates vascular injury in postischemic canine skeletal muscle: role of granulocyte adherence. Circ Res 66:1436-1444
32. Dorion D, Zhong A, Chiu C, Forrest CR, Boyd B, Pang CY (1993) Role of xanthine oxidase in reperfusion injury of ischemic skeletal muscle in the pig and human. J Appl Physiol 75:246-255
33. Jarasch ED, Bruder G, Heid HW (1986) Significance of xanthine oxidase in capillary endothelial cells. Acta Physiol Scand [Suppl]548:39-46
34. Palluy O, Morliere L, Gris JC, Bowne C, Modat G (1992) Hypoxia/reoxygenation stimulates endothelium to promote neutrophil adhesion. Free Radic Biol Med 13:21-30
35. Bulkley GB (1994) Reactive oxygen metabolites and reperfusion injury: aberrant triggering of reticuloendothelial function. Lancet 344:934-936
36. Kubes P, Suzuki M, Granger DN (1991) Nitric oxide: an endogenous modulator of leukocyte adhesion. Proc Natl Acad Sci USA 88:4651-4655
37. Gaboury J, Woodman RC, Granger DN et al (1993) Nitric oxide prevents leukocyte adherence: role of superoxide. Am J Physiol 265:H862-867

38. Tsao PS, Aoki N, Lefer DJ et al (1990) Time course of endothelial dysfunction and myocardial injury during myocardial ischemia and reperfusion in the cat. Circulation 82:1402-1412
39. Mugge A, Elwell JH, Peterson TE et al (1991) Release of intact endothelium-derived relaxing factors depends on endothelial superoxide dismutase activity. Am J Physiol 260:C219-225
40. Rubanyi GM, Ho EH, Cantor EH et al (1991) Cytoprotective function of nitric oxide: activation of superoxide radicals produced by human leukocytes. Biochem Biophys Res Commun 181:1392-1397
41. Gandini E, Adembri C, Formigli L, Papucci L, Novelli GP (1995) Peroxidative damage observed in human skeletal muscle after ischemia-reperfusion are related to duration of ischemia. Minerva Anestesiol (submitted)

Acidosis in the Critically Ill: Interpretation and Significance

J.A. KELLUM

Introduction

To the clinician acidosis is the increased production and/or decreased elimination of acid by the body. To the biochemist or the physiologist acidosis is a process that increases the concentration of hydrogen ion (H^+) in a solution (such as blood). At first glance, this distinction seems minor, but its implications are enormous. The most important implication is that acidosis is not merely the addition (or the decreased elimination) of H^+. One simple example of this is respiratory acidosis. The body "eliminates" most of its H^+ by eliminating CO_2. Yet CO_2 does not contain H^+. Where does the H^+ go? The answer is that it becomes water ($H^+ + HCO_3^- \rightarrow H_2CO_3 \rightarrow CO_2 + H_2O$). This answer seems satisfactory until one asks how an increase in CO_2 produces an increase in H^+ concentration. The answer is that CO_2 is in equilibrium with HCO_3^- and thus an increase in CO_2 produces an increase in H^+ and HCO_3^- (i.e., the reaction is reversible). Here we see that the change in CO_2 *produces* a change in H^+ concentration. The H^+ itself comes from the dissociation of water. This chapter will focus on the other determinates of H^+ concentration in biologic solutions and the clinical effects of changes in these determinants.

Strong ions and the strong ion difference

Stewart (1) reviewed the physical chemical properties of biologic solutions over a decade ago. Although this work has been slow to move into the mainstream of biomedical research (and is virtually unknown in clinical medicine), its implications are far reaching and extremely important to our understanding of acid-base regulation in health and disease. The principles of physical chemistry as outlined by Stewart define the relationship between pH and the three independent variables that control its concentration in biologic solutions. These independent variables are CO_2, the weak acids (protein and phosphate), and the strong ion difference (SID). As the previous example illustrates, we are very familiar with the role of CO_2 in this context. The weak acids (often referred to as buffers) include protein (albumin) and phosphate. These negatively charged molecules also influence the H^+ concentration, although their impact is far less significant (the effect of changes in CO_2 is at least five times greater in most physiologic conditions). The final variable, the SID, has an effect on H^+ concentration that is as great as CO_2.

The SID is defined as the difference between all *strong cations* and all *strong anions*. Here, a strong ion is defined as an ion that is completely or near completely dissociated in water. Na^+, Cl^-, K^+, Mg^{++}, Ca^{++}, and lactate are all *strong ions*. Therefore, for practical purposes SID can be defined as ($Na^+ + K^+ + Mg^{++} + Ca^{++}$) – ($Cl^- +$ lactate). We refer to this as the apparent SID (SIDa) (Table 1). In human blood, the normal SIDa is 40-42 mEq/l. If the concentrations of CO_2 and weak acids are held constant, the pH will be determined by the SID. As the SID increases, H^+ concentration decreases. In this way, differential changes in Na^+ and Cl^-, for instance, will alter the pH predictably if both of the other variables are known. This approach has two major advantages. First, changes in pH can be accurately predicted from changes in these three known variables. For instance, if NaCl is given in sufficient quantity to alter the SID of the blood and CO_2 is held constant, a predictable change in pH will occur. Indeed this is the explanation for the so-called "dilutional" or "rehydration" metabolic acidosis (2) that occurs as a result of resuscitation with large volumes of 0.9% saline. This is because each liter of 0.9% saline contains 154 mEq of Na^+ and Cl^-. Infusing large volumes of this solution will increase both the serum Na^+ and Cl^- concentrations, but the effect on Cl^- will be greater because serum Cl^- concentrations are generally 35-40 mEq/l less than serum Na^+ concentrations. For every mEq/l increase in Cl^- relative to Na^+, the SID will decrease 1 mEq/l. As the SID decreases, the pH will decrease. In this way, changes in electrolytes will have predictable effects on pH. Another example is metabolic alkalosis in the setting of gastric suctioning. As the Cl^- concentration falls (relative to Na^+), the SID increases, as does the pH.

Table 1. The simplified versions of the Stewart and Figge equations

---

- Apparent strong ion difference [SID]a
  [SID]a = $[Na^+] + [K^+] + [Mg^{++}] + [Ca^{++}]$ – ($[Cl^-] +$ [lactate])
- Effective strong ion difference [SID]e
  [SID]e = $\{CO_2, [Albumin], [PO_4]\}$
- Strong ion gas [SIG]
  [SIG] = [SID]a – [SID]e

Urate may also be included in the SIG calculation; however its effect is normally very small

Strong ion gap

A second advantage of this approach is that when the pH, weak acids, CO_2, and SIDa are known, any additional strong ions or weak acids can be quantified (see below). A notable disadvantage of this approach in the past has been the inability to precisely quantify the acid-base impact of serum proteins. However, through the use of NMR techniques, Figge and coworkers were able to determine the charge of albumin (at various pH) and also determined that normal globulins were not significant in terms of acid-base balance (3). Figge and coworkers defined the term effective SID (SIDe) as the sum of charges for CO_2, albumin, and phosphate. An important consequence of the work by Stewart (1) and Figge et al. (3) is that both the SIDa and the SIDe should be exactly equal and opposite. Any "gap" between SIDa and SIDe represents unmeasured anions or, if the "gap" is negative, unmeasured cations. Therefore, the sum of all remaining ions is equal to the size of the remaining gap. We have chosen to refer to this as the *strong ion gap* (SIG) (4), in order to distinguish it from the anion gap. Normally, the SIG should be zero. When it is greater than zero, unmeasured anions outnumber unmeasured cations in the circulation. When it is less than zero, an excess of unmeasured cations exists. When these techniques are applied to various populations (Fig. 1) we appreciate that, although the anion gaps may be very similar, the composition of these gaps vary greatly across patient types. For instance, normal subjects with lactic acidosis induced by exercise have virtually no detectable SIG, whereas patients with similar anion gaps from sepsis have SIGs that account for roughly a third of the total anion gap.

Sources of acidemia in critical illness

It follows then that *acidemia* (arterial pH < 7.36) may occur secondary to an alteration in any of these three independent variables (CO_2, weak acids, SID). The process that alters these variables and produces acidemia is referred to as acidosis. By convention, we refer to those processes that increase CO_2 as respiratory acidosis and all others as metabolic *acidosis*. Of course this is an

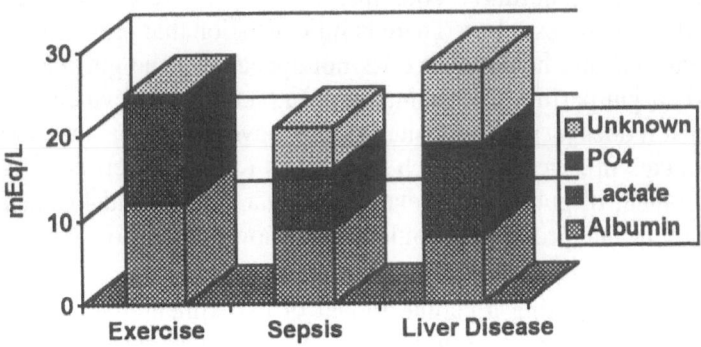

Fig. 1. Anion composition in various populations. This figure shows the contributions various anions make to the total anion gap across different subject types. Adapted from Kellum et al. (4)

oversimplification because metabolic processes that increase CO_2 production may also increase $PaCO_2$, particularly if ventilation is fixed. Still, it is useful clinically to divide disorders into "respiratory", "metabolic" or "mixed". *Metabolic* acidosis is therefore an alteration in the concentration of weak acids or the SID. Although an infusion of phosphoric acid (H_3PO_4) would produce acidemia without a change in the SID, in practice, almost all forms of metabolic acidosis result in a change in the SID. Unfortunately, we cannot measure the SID. We can measure the SIDa, but some strong ions may be missing (causing a change in the SIG). A common example is ketoacidosis. Ketones behave as unmeasured strong anions (they are completely dissociated in solution), and thus, will decrease the SID, but not the measured SIDa. For this reason, reliance on the SIDa alone may be misleading. Decreases in the SID occur in patients with critical illness, particularly from lactate, "unknown" anions and hyperchloremia.

Lactic acidosis

In many forms of critical illness, lactate is the most important cause of metabolic acidosis. Lactate has been shown to correlate with outcome in patients with hemorrhagic (5, 6) and septic shock (7). Conventional wisdom has it that lactic acid is the predominant source of metabolic acidosis occurring in sepsis (8). In this view, lactic acid is released primarily from the muscle and the gut as a consequence of tissue hypoxia. Moreover, the amount of lactate produced is felt to correlate with "the total oxygen debt, the magnitude of the hypoperfusion, and the severity of shock" (9). A series of critical assumptions are implicit in this conventional view (Fig. 2). The assumption that the muscle is involved is based on a long tradition of looking to the muscle as a source of lactic acid during exercise. In this setting, the muscle may be the only significant source of lactate. This observation may be safely generalized to certain patients with trauma or seizures but there the generalization should end. During sepsis, even with profound shock, resting muscle does not produce lactate. In fact, studies by Van Lambalgen and coworkers (10), and more recently by Cain and Curtis (11), show that the muscle may actually consume lactate during endotoxemia. Data concerning the gut are less clear. There is little question that profoundly ischemic gut can release lactate; however, it does not appear that the gut releases lactate during sepsis if gut perfusion is maintained. In fact, there is evidence to support the notion that it does just the opposite. Studies have shown that the gut is neutral to, or even takes up, lactate in such conditions (10, 12). Perfusion is likely a major determinant of gut lactate metabolism. In a canine model of sepsis using endotoxin, gut lactate production could not be shown when flow was maintained with dopexamine hydrochloride (11).

In our laboratory, using a canine model of experimental sepsis induced by endotoxin infusion, we have examined the flux of lactate across various organs. During these experiments, the gut and muscle did not contribute to lactic acidosis (Fig. 3). In fact, both muscle and gut tended to take up lactate in this condition.

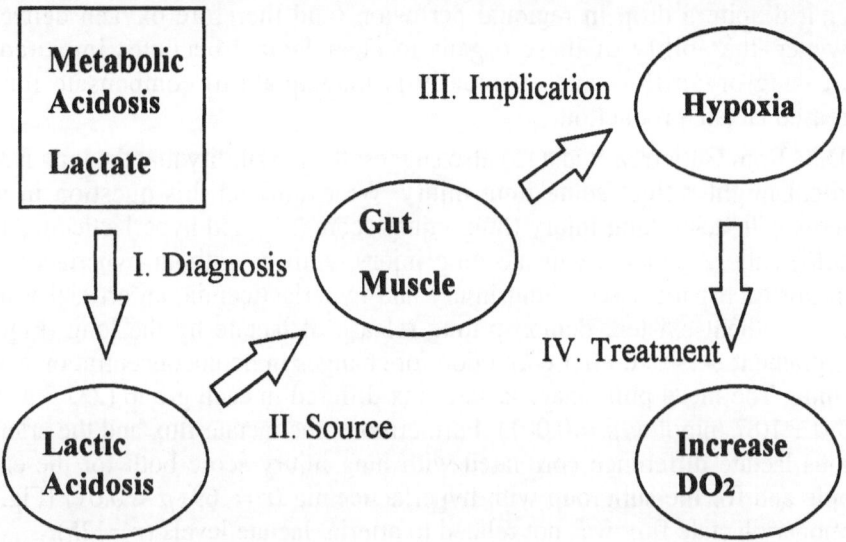

Fig. 2. The four basic assumptions implicit in the conventional view of acidosis in sepsis

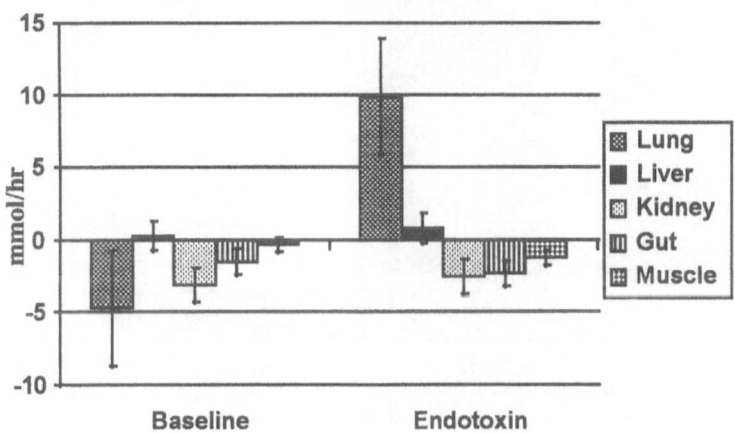

Fig. 3. Transvisceral lactate fluxes. The lactate flux across each organ is shown in mmol/h with standard error bars as shown. The only change from baseline to endotoxemia was for the lung ($p < 0.05$). Adapted from Bellomo et al. (12)

Surprisingly, the lung emerged as the major source of lactate (12). These results are consistent with those of other investigators who have reported lung lactate production in animals during endotoxemia (13) or hemorrhage (14). More recently, Gutierrez and coworkers reported a transpulmonary gradient in patients with sepsis and established ARDS (15). These data suggest a scenario in which the lung is a primary producer of lactate, and the gut and kidneys continue to clear it despite a drop in regional perfusion (and therefore oxygen delivery). However, the ability of these organs to clear lactate becomes impaired by decreasing organ flow and eventually is inadequate to compensate for the increased lactate production.

Data from Gutierrez et al. (15) also suggest the possibility that the lung lactate gradient might reflect acute lung injury. We examined this question in nine patients with acute lung injury (lung injury score ≥ 2) and hyperlacticemia (> 2 mmol/l) and 12 patients with no lung injury, with or without hyperlacticemia (16). For each patient with lung injury and hyperlacticemia, an arterial-venous lactate gradient existed, demonstrating release of lactate by the lung (Fig. 4). This gradient persisted after correction for changes in hemoconcentration across the lung. The mean pulmonary lactate flux differed in each group (231.3 ± 70.4 vs 5.0 ± 10.7 mmol/h; $p = 0.001$). Furthermore, the lactate flux and the arterial-venous lactate difference correlated with lung injury score both for the entire sample and for the subgroup with hyperlacticemia ($r = .69$, $p < 0.01$) (Fig. 5). Pulmonary lactate flux was not related to arterial lactate levels ($r = .25$).

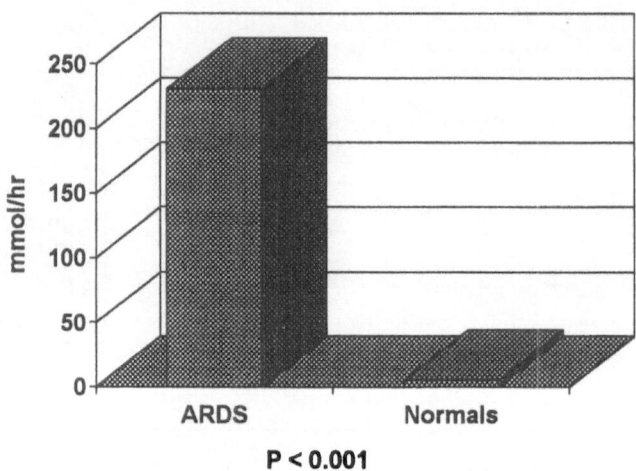

Fig. 4. Mean lactate release by the lung in nine patients with acute lung injury (LIS ≥ 2.5) and hyperlacticemia (arterial lactate > 2 mmol/l) and 12 patients with various lactate levels but without lung injury. Adapted from Kellum et al. (16)

If hyperlacticemia can be equated with anaerobic metabolism, the lung would seem an unlikely source. One possible explanation, however, would be that lung injury is invariably associated with an intense infiltration of activated leukocytes. These cells might easily be operating on anaerobic metabolism for much of the time. Accordingly, we hypothesized that lung inflammation was responsible for this lactate release. However, using a hydrochloric acid installation model of acute lung injury, Lee et al. (17) could not demonstrate lung lactate release.

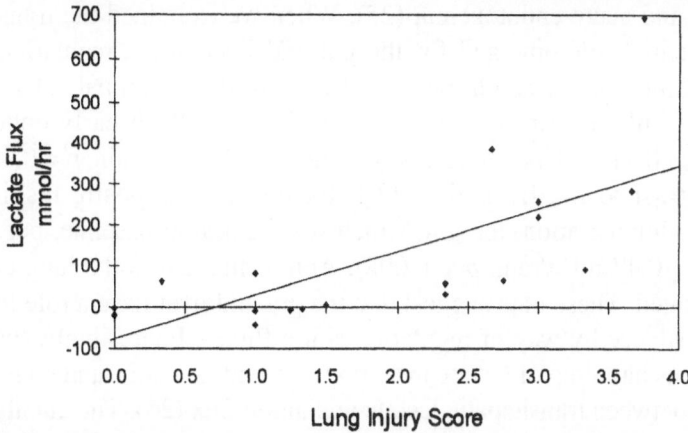

Fig. 5. Relation between lung lactate release and lung injury score ($r = 0.69$, $p < 0.01$). Adapted from Kellum et al. (16)

Therefore, alternative mechanisms for hyperlacticemia would seem to be important. For example, it has previously been shown that endotoxin inhibits pyruvate dehydrogenase activity in vitro (18). Whether this occurs in vivo and is the mechanism responsible for lung lactate release remains to be proven.

Other "unknown" anions

The conventional view of metabolic acidosis in sepsis also relies on the important assumption that lactic acid accounts for all or even most of the acidosis seen. In experimental studies of shock produced by endotoxin injection, lactate accounts for less than half of the acidosis encountered (19, 20). Similarly, in patients with sepsis, an increased anion gap has been observed that is out of proportion to the lactic acid concentration (21, 22). In a prospective study of 30 septic patients, 24 demonstrated a positive anion gap acidosis that was unaccounted for by lactate, ketones, urate, phosphate, or proteins (23). Furthermore, in these patients with sepsis, lactate accounted for less than 50% of the total metabolic acid load seen. Clearly, other forms of acidosis must also be present. Other anions, besides lactate, are well known to cause acidosis in various clinical conditions (ketoacidosis, renal failure, salicylate toxicity, etc.). As shown in Fig. 1, some patients with liver disease (24) and some patients with sepsis (23) have evidence of unexplained anions in their blood (as measured by an increased SIG). These anions would also be expected to decrease the SID and produce acidemia. We became intrigued by the presence of these high SIGs in patients with end-stage liver disease, which led us to explore the liver and gut as potential sources of unexplained anions in septic shock.

Using a canine model of early endotoxemia, we sought to determine the role of the liver in the regulation of anion/cation balance during both stable control conditions and acute endotoxemia (25). When we examined the transorgan ion flux, a potential role emerged for the gut and liver in the regulation of blood anions. During control conditions, the livers of all ten animals cleared anions from the circulation (mean flux -0.34 mEq/min). With early endotoxemia, however, the liver switched to release of anions (0.12 mEq/min, $p = 0.0046$) (Fig. 6). In contrast to the liver, the gut behaved in an opposite fashion. After endotoxin administration, the gut, which was neutral at baseline, began to take up anions (-0.47 mEq/min, $p = 0.008$). Anion flux across the lung and kidney was unchanged. These data suggest that the gut and liver have a role in systemic acid-base balance by way of regulating anion fluxes. Interestingly, the liver did not change its handling of lactate in response to endotoxemia, and no relationship was found between transhepatic lactate and anion flux (25). The gut also appears to play a role in anion balance and its action is opposite to the liver. However, the increase in anion clearance by the gut did not quite offset the increased release by the liver. The total change in anion uptake for these two organs between baseline and endotoxemic conditions was 4.2 mEq/h (25). The results of this study suggest an alternative explanation for the acidosis seen during acute endotoxemia. The switch by the liver from uptake to release of anions during endotoxemia is important because any increase in anions must produce an increase in the H^+ concentration, as any decrease in the SID will result in acidosis (1). This explanation is attractive because it does not require any additional sources of hydrogen (such as ATP hydrolysis), and it is consistent with clinical observations made in both sepsis (23, 26, 27) and liver disease (24).

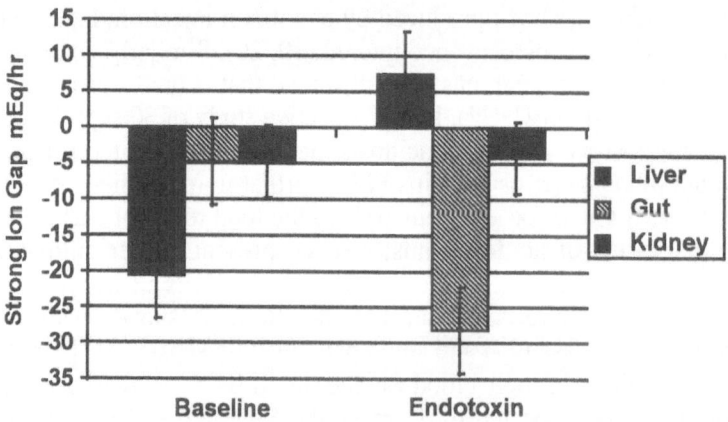

Fig. 6. Change in anion flux with endotoxin. Total fluxes by hour for the various organs studied are shown. Only the liver and gut affect the blood concentrations of unexplained anions ($p < 0.01$). The lung was also studied but did not effect anion concentrations (data not shown). Standard error bars are shown. Both the liver and gut changed their handling of anions significantly from baseline to endotoxemia ($p < 0.01$). Adapted from Kellum et al. (25)

Chloride

It should be clear from the previous sections that the SID may be decreased with resulting acidemia by any addition of anions or removal of cations. Furthermore, we have already eluded to the fact that administration of large amounts of NaCl will lower the SID, and hence produce a decrease in pH. Some authors, citing in vitro studies, have suggested that dilutional acidosis is at best only a minor issue (28). However, our in vivo experiments using endotoxemic animals suggest otherwise (29). Figure 7 shows the total acid loads for six animals given endotoxin and saline resuscitation. These animals were each studied for 3 h following infusion of 1 mg/kg of *E. coli* endotoxin. Interestingly, neither lactate nor other unexplained anions accounted for more than 10% of the total acid load in this resuscitated model. During these experiments, the arterial pH changed from 7.32 to 7.11 ($p < 0.01$), though $PaCO_2$ was unchanged. The mean saline requirement was 1.8 l, and saline infusion increased the serum Cl^- concentration from 127.7 mmol/l to 131.0 mmol/l. There was no significant change in Na^+ concentration; thus, the saline induced a decrease in the SID by 3.3 ± 0.9 mmol/l. This accounted for 37.4% of the total acid load. However, 42% of the total acid load incurred could not be explained by saline, lactate, or other anions. This load was produced by a further increase in Cl^- concentration beyond that caused by saline. The mechanisms responsible for this alteration in Cl^- concentration are unknown. We speculate that the capillary leak produced by endotoxin infusion resulted in an exudation of protein from the vascular space into the interstitial space. This departure of weak anions from the plasma would necessarily be balanced by movement of another anion into the plasma (or of a cation out) in order to conserve charge (i.e., Donnan equilibrium) (30), and could easily explain why the serum Cl^- concentration was higher than predicted.

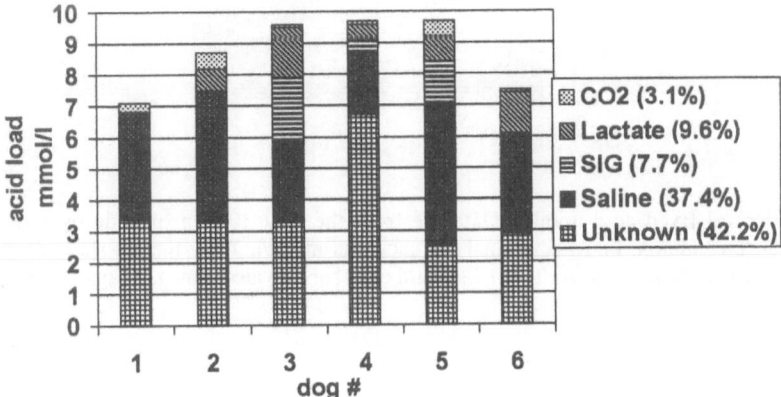

Fig. 7. Acid load by various etiology for six animals treated with endotoxin and resuscitated with 0.9% saline. The mean acid load for the six animals was 8.7 mmol/l. Adapted from Kellum et al. (29)

Visceral fixed acid uptake

Using the SID and SIG techniques, it is also possible to measure the effects of individual tissues on systemic acid-base balance. For instance, by excreting Cl⁻ in excess of Na⁺ the kidney can increase the SID, and thus, increase the pH of the blood. Examination of the electrolytes across the kidney will reveal that, under most conditions, the SID in the renal vein is higher than in the renal artery. Classically, we refer to this as fixed (to distinguish it from volatile, meaning CO_2) acid removal. If another organ were to decrease the SID, this organ could be thought of in the traditional sense as contributing fixed acid to the circulation. For example, working muscle contributes lactate, a strong anion, to the circulation. The result is to decrease the blood SID with a resulting decrease in blood pH. Because metabolic acidosis is so pervasive in sepsis, we sought to determine whether certain organs were contributors of fixed acid (i.e., decreasing the SID) during this condition. Accordingly, we studied the flux of ions across various tissues during endotoxemia (Fig. 8) (31). We found that at baseline, the kidney cleared fixed acid from the circulation (increases the SID) and it continued to do so during endotoxemia. By contrast, the liver was neutral to fixed acid in both conditions (though it did release unexplained anions). Surprisingly, the gut was not the source of fixed acid. In fact, at baseline the gut was neutral, and during endotoxemia the gut actually took up fixed acid (increased the SID).

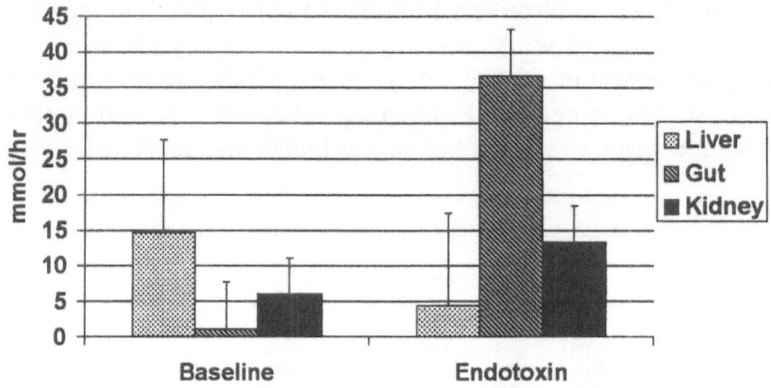

Fig. 8. Visceral fixed acid uptake. Data are from the first 30 min of endotoxemia in the unresuscitated condition. Fixed acid uptake is shown in mmol/h. Only the gut showed a change from baseline to endotoxemia ($p < 0.05$). Standard error bars are also shown. Adapted from Kellum et al. (31)

A body of literature now exists to support the notion that the intracellular pH, as measured by tonometry, increases during critical illness (32-35). Thus, if the gut is taking up acid in conditions that are known to be associated with tissue acidosis, it is interesting to speculate that the two phenomena are in some way linked. This hypothesis is supported by recent work by Salzman and colleagues (36). These investigators have shown that systemic acidosis results in intestinal mucosal acidosis regardless of the cause. In this study, mucosal acidosis increased intestinal permeability even in the absence of tissue ischemia or hypoxia. Thus, during conditions of systemic acidemia, the development of intestinal acidosis may result from fixed acid uptake by the gut. Such findings underscore the importance of systemic acid-base balance to intestinal mucosal integrity.

Summary

The H^+ concentration in the blood is determined by three independent variables: CO_2, weak acids and the SID. Although lactate does decrease the SID, patients with critical illness develop metabolic acidosis as a result of multiple processes, not just hyperlacticemia. An important source of lactate in sepsis appears to be the lung and this may represent acute lung injury. The liver, on the other hand, appears to release unexplained anions during endotoxemia. Finally, increases in Cl^-, either from exogenous sources or from endogenous shifts, appears to be responsible for the majority of acidemia occurring during experimental endotoxemia. One effect of metabolic acidosis may be to produce tissue acidosis in the gut and this may be a direct result of the gut's tendency to take up fixed acid. This gut acidosis may be very important because it has been shown to correlate with increased intestinal permeability even in the absence of tissue ischemia or hypoxia.

References

1. Stewart P (1981) How to understand acid-base: a quantitative acid-base primer for biology and medicine. Elsevier, New York
2. Narins RG, Jones ER, Townsend R, Goodkin DA, Shay RJ (1985) Metabolic acid-base disorders: pathophysiology, classification and treatment. In: Arieff AI, DeFronzo RA (eds) Fluid, electrolyte, and acid-base disorders. Churchill Livingstone, New York, pp 269-384
3. Figge J, Mydosh T, Fencl V (1992) Serum proteins and acid-base equilibria: A follow-up. J Lab Clin Med 120:713-719
4. Kellum JA, Kramer DJ, Pinsky MR (1995) Strong ion gap: a methodology for exploring unexplained Anions. J Crit Care 10:51-55
5. Weil MH, Afifi AA (1970) Experimental and clinical studies on lacate and pyruvate as indicators of the severity of acute circulatory failure (shock). Circulation 41:989-1001
6. Vitek V, Cowley RA (1971) Blood lactate in the prognosis of various forms of shock. Ann Surg 173:308-313
7. Blair E (1971) Acid-base balance in bacteremic shock. Arch Intern Med 127:731-739
8. Madias NE (1986) Lactic acidosis. Kidney Int 29:752-774
9. Mizock BA, Falk JL (1992) Lactic acidosis in critical illness. Crit Care Med 20:80-93
10. van Lambalgen AA, Runge HC, van den Bos GC, Thijs LG (1988) Regional lactate production in early canine endotoxin shock. Am J Physiol 254:E45-51
11. Cain SM, Curtis SE (1991) Systemic and regional oxygen uptake and delivery and lactate flux in endotoxic dogs infused with dopamine. Crit Care Med 19:1552-1560

12. Bellomo R, Ondulick B, Kellum J, Pinsky MR (1994) Visceral lactate fluxes during early endotoxemia in the dog. Am J Respir Crit Care Med 149:A413
13. Sayeed MM (1982) Pulmonary cellular dysfunction in endotoxin shock: metabolic and transport derangements. Circ Shock 9:335-355
14. Bowles SA, Schlichtig R, Kramer DJ, Klions HA (1992) Arteriovenous pH and partial pressure of carbon dioxide detect critical oxygen delivery during progressive hemorrhage in dogs. J Crit Care 7:95-105
15. Gutierrez G, Clark C, Nelson C, Tiu A, Brown S (1993) The lung as a source of lactate in sepsis and ARDS. Chest 104:S12
16. Kellum JA, Kramer DJ, Mankad S, Pinsky MR, Bellomo R, Lee KH (1995) Release of lactate by the lung in acute ARDS. Crit Care Med, 23:A107
17. Lee KH, Rico P, Ondulick BW, Pinsky MR (1995) Hydrochloric acid-induced lung injury is not associated with a positive lung lactate flux. Am J Respir Crit Care Med 151:A761
18. Kilpatrick-Smith L, Dean J, Erecinska M, Silver IA (1983) Cellular effects of endotoxin in vitro. II Reversibility of endotoxic damage. Circ Shock 11:101-111
19. van Lambalgen AA, Bronsveld W, van den Bos GC, Thijs LG (1984) Distribution of cardiac output, oxygen consumption and lactate production in canine endotoxin shock. Cardiovasc Res 18:195-205
20. Rackow EC, Mecher C, Astiz ME, Goldstien C, McKee D, Weil MH (1990) Unmeasured anion during severe sepsis with metabolic acidosis. Circ Shock 30:107-115
21. Gabow P, Kaehny W, Fennessey P, Goodman SI, Gross PA, Schrier RW (1980) Diagnostic importance of an increased serum anion gap. N Engl J Med 303:854-858
22. Mehta K, Kruse JA, Carlson RW (1986) The relationship between anion gap and elevated lactate. Crit Care Med 14:405
23. Mecher C, Rackow EC, Astiz ME, Weil MH (1991) Unaccounted for anion in metabolic acidosis during severe sepsis in humans. Crit Care Med 19:705-711
24. Kellum JA, Kramer DJ, Pinsky MR (1994) Unexplained positive anion gap metabolic acidosis in end stage liver disease. Crit Care Med 22:A209
25. Kellum JA, Bellomo R, Kramer DJ, Pinksy MR (1995) Hepatic anion flux during acute endotoxemia. J Appl Physiol 78:2212-2217
26. Rackow EC, Mecher C, Astiz ME, Goldstien C, McKee D, Weil MH (1990) Unmeasured anion during severe sepsis with metabolic acidosis. Circ Shock 30:107-115
27. Gilfix BM, Bique M, Magder S (1993) A physical chemical approach to the analysis of acid-base balance in the clinical setting. J Crit Care 8(4):187-197
28. Garella S, Chang BS, Kahn SI (1975) Dilution acidosis and contraction alkalosis: Review of a concept. Kidney Int 8:279-283
29. Kellum JA, Bellomo R, Kramer DJ, Pinsky MR (1995) Etiology of metabolic acidosis during saline resuscitation in edotoxemia. Am J Respir Crit Care Med 151:A318
30. Guggenheim EA (1957) Thermodynamics, an advanced treatment for chemists and physicists. North-Holland, Amsterdam, pp 378-382
31. Kellum JA, Bellomo R, Kramer DJ, Pinsky MR (1995) Fixed acid uptake by visceral organs during early endotoxemia. Crit Care Med 23:A173
32. Fiddian-Green R (1989) Splanchnic ischemia and multiple organ failure. Mosby, London, pp 349-363
33. Antonsson JB, Boyle CC III, Kruithoff Kl et al (1990) Validation of tonometric measurement of gut intramural pH during endotoxemia and mesenteric occlusion in pigs. Am J Physiol 259:G519-G523
34. Montgomery A, Almquist P, Arvidsson D et al (1990) Early detection of gastrointestinal mucosal ischemia in porcine E. coli sepsis. Acta Chir Scand 156:613-620
35. Montgomery A, Hartmann M, Jonsson K, Haglund U et al (1989) Intramucosal pH measurement with tonometers for detecting gastrointestinal ischemia in porcine hemorrhagic shock. Circ Shock 29:319-327
36. Salzman AL, Wang H, Wollert PS et al (1994) Endotoxin-induced ileal mucosal hyperpermeability in pigs: role of tissue acidosis. Am J Physiol 266:G633-646

Use of the Gaps in the Critically Ill

F. SCHIRALDI, B. MAGLIONE

The specific diagnosis in acid-base disorders should always start with history, physical examination, electrolyte pattern, full urinary evaluation, and obviously blood gas analysis (BGA) (1-3).

Among all these numbers, the *Na, Cl* and *HCO3 plasmatic* concentrations are very useful to rapidly restrict the diagnostic possibilities in metabolic acidoses; the relative concentrations of these substances in the *urine* are helpful to discover the renal acidifying functionality (*urinary anion gap, UAG*); finally the difference between the measured and the calculated plasmatic osmolarity may help to suspect an intoxicant added to serum (*osmolal gap, OG*) (4, 5).

The anion gap

A starting point to be kept in mind is that the sum of all positively charged ions (cations) must – according to the electroneutrality – equalize the sum of all negatively charged ions (anions). As normally sodium is the only routinely measured cation and both chloride and bicarbonate are the only measured anions, there is a gap to be expected between sodium and such measured anions (anion gap = AG).

$$\text{ANION GAP} = Na - (Cl + HCO_3) = 8 \pm 2 \text{ mEq/l}$$

In simple (= not associated with other acid-base disturbances) metabolic acidoses bicarbonate is always decreased, and – in order to satisfy the principle of electroneutrality – either chloride or any other anion must proportionately increase. So, only if *chloride retention* stoichiometrically matches the HCO_3 consumption will the AG stay within the normal range; otherwise the AG will rise due to over production, underelimination or ingestion of organic or inorganic acids (Fig. 1).

Moreover the AG evaluation will allow a first narrowing of the possible etiologies of metabolic acidoses (Table 1).

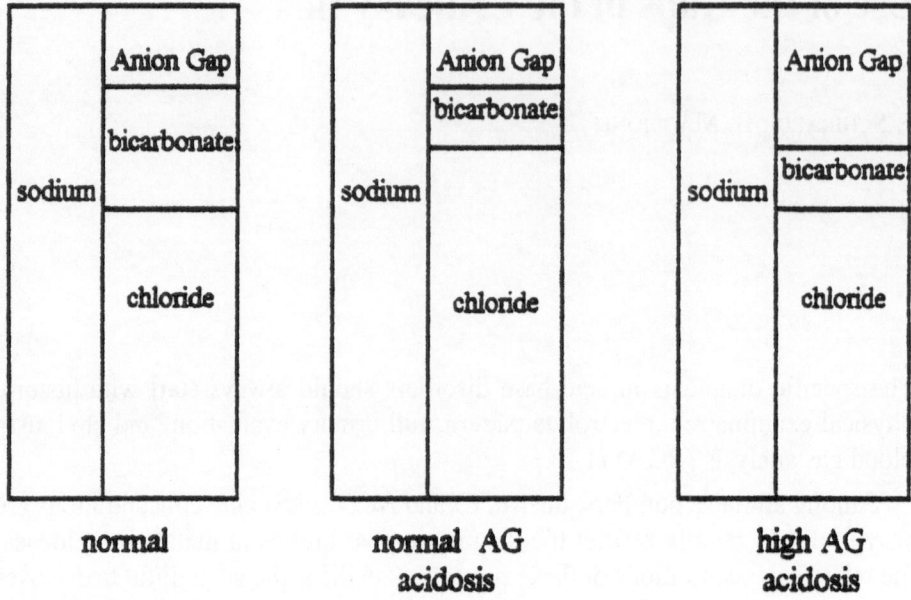

Fig. 1. Anion gap (*AG*) classification of metabolic acidosis

Table 1. Main etiologies of normal AG and high AG acidosis

Normal AG	High AG
1. Gastroenteric HCO_3 loss	1. DKA
2. Ureterosigmoidostomy	2. Alcoholic ketoacidosis
3. Renal tubular acidosis (I, II, IV)	3. Starvation
4. Acetazolamide	4. Lactic acidosis
5. Tubulo-interstitial renal diseases	5. Salicylate intoxication
6. Adrenal insufficiency	6. Methanol intoxication
7. Use of chloride acids	7. Ethylene glycol intoxication
8. Parenteral nutrition	8. Prophylene glycol intoxication
9. Recovery phase of DKA	9. Paraldehyde intoxication
10. Excessive saline administration	10. Inborn errors of metabolism

As the clinical feature usually suggests the correct diagnosis, there are basically three conditions in which the clinician could be helped by the AG evaluation in ICU:

1. To rule out some mixed disorders
2. To suspect any occult intoxications
3. To evaluate any underlying acidosis if alkali have been given (6-8)

The AG in mixed disorders

A patient with *diabetic ketoacidosis (DKA)* complicated by *protracted vomiting* may present with near normal bicarbonate concentration and plasmatic pH, while the clinical picture and the AG, are severely deranged from the normal (Table 2) (9).

Table 2. AG utility in mixed disorders

	Metabolic acidosis (e.g. DKA)	Metabolic alkalosis (e.g. Vomiting)
PCO_2	33	38
pH	7.28	7.40
HCO_3	15	PLUS 25
Cl	100	88
Na	140	138
	AG = 25	AG = 25

It is also possible to find a patient with volume-contracted *metabolic alkalosis*, in such a hypovolemic state to slide toward both marked hypoperfusion and *metabolic (lactic) acidosis*, with blood pH transiently normal and AG usually elevated (10).

The AG in intoxications

Sometimes, in ICU and emergency medicine departments, we have to face non-specific toxic symptoms (dizziness, asthenia, somnolence) associated with metabolic acidosis of unknown origin (11, 12). There are some alcohols and other chemical substances, neither usually detected by routine analyses nor even clinically suspected which interfere with the normal metabolism, producing *high AG metabolic acidosis* or mixed disorders (salicylate, methanol, ethylene, glycol).

In such cases, the diagnosis could be helped and life-saving treatments started, on the basis of the AG evaluations, particularly if there was an associated osmolal gap (see below).

The AG in some "corrected acidoses"

The bicarbonate concentration does not always reflect the underlying metabolic acidosis, as in the case of a patient with DKA (increased AG). If the patient is given sufficient i.v. $NaHCO_3$ to nearly normalize the bicarbonate deficit, the same degree of *ketonemia* could be still present, but not be apparent from the BGA; however, the AG will not be influenced by the *exogenous sodium bicarbonate* and this gap will still serve as a marker of ketone accumulation and ongoing production.

The urinary anion gap

As it is known, there are very large normality ranges concerning *urinary electrolytes*, whose interpretation is strongly linked to the daily balance, pharmacological therapy, endocrine influence and, obviously, renal function.

Nevertheless, as the electroneutrality principle must always be observed, some information can be derived from Na, K and Cl urinary concentrations.

If the clinical picture and patient BGA suggest *normal AG metabolic acidosis*, an evaluation of urine NH_4 excretion could be critical to define the cause of that metabolic acidosis. As the NH_4 is not routinely measured and is usually excreted as NH_4 *chloride*, we can get some useful information from the urinary Cl evaluation if, at the same time, we calculate the urinary Na and K (13, 14).

In metabolic acidosis with normal plasmatic AG, we can broadly suspect two different possibilities (Table 3).

Table 3. Urinary anion gap in metabolic acidosis

A) $[Cl]_u > [Na]_u + [K]_u$ = good NH_4Cl production
(the missing cation, i.e. unmeasured, being H^+)
= good renal acidification
= extrarenal alkali losses
B) $[Cl]_u < [Na]_u + [K]_u$ = poor NH_4Cl production
= very likely renal responsibility in producing metabolic acidosis

The osmolal gap

Normally, sodium, glucose and urea are the major determinants of *plasmatic osmolality* (POSM), which can be variously *calculated*.

One simple formula is:

$$2 \times Na\ (mEq/l) + \frac{GLUC\ (mg/dl)}{18} = POSM\ CALC = 285\ mOsm/l$$

On the other hand, osmolality can be very precisely measured by means of the evaluation of the *freezing point depression* (POSM MEAS).

Normally there is a small *difference* (OSMOLAL GAP) between the measured plasmatic osmolality and the calculated one, due to some usually not measured osmotically active substances, so that

$$\text{OSMOLAL GAP (OG)} = 7 \pm 5 \text{ mOsm/Kg H}_2\text{O}$$

It could be useful to recall some simple physicochemical properties:

1. An *osmol* is the presence of 6.023×10^{23} molecules in 1 kg of water.
2. *Osmolality* is an expression of the number of particles in a given weight of solvent.
3. Osmolality refers not to the size, shape, or weight of a *particle* but only to its *number*.
4. The solutes that are present in the blood or serum are dissolved only in the aqueous phases.

If we suppose that an *intoxicant* of low molecular weight is added to serum, we should find an *increase of the measured osmolality*, leaving the calculated one almost unchanged. In such a case it is very common to find some degree of *metabolic acidosis* (initially of unknown origin) and the finding of a large OG will raise strong suspicion of an *intoxication*. It is interesting to note that the smaller the intoxicant molecular weight is, the wider the OG will be (e.g. if it was more than 50 mOsm/l, think of methanol or ethanol, the largest osmotically contributing alcohols) (Fig. 2).

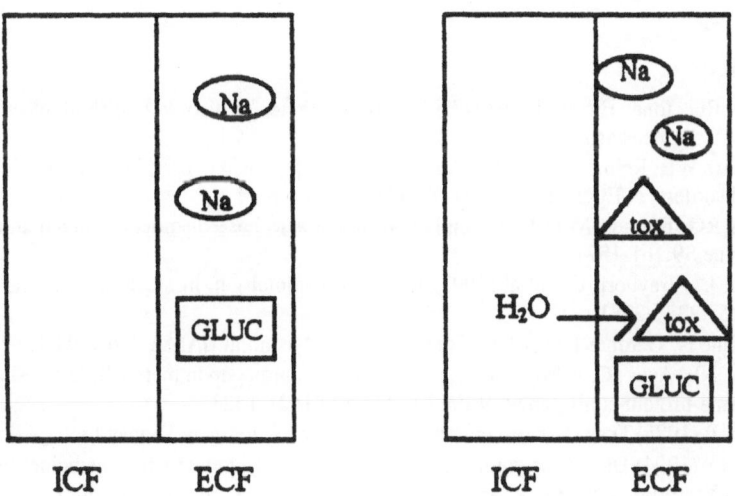

Fig. 2. Effect of intoxicants on osmolality (*ICF*, intracellular fluids; *ECF*, extracellular fluids)

Factors decreasing the anion gap

It is quite obvious that any increase in the serum concentration of an *unmeasured cation* will decrease the AG. Because Ca, Mg and K should be extremely elevated to cause an abnormally low anion gap, i.e., within a life-threatening range, these electrolyte derangements do not in practice interfere with the usual interpretation of the AG. So that the only two clinically relevant conditions resulting in a decrease of the AG are:

1. Some *myelomas* or other *gammopathies* that add strongly positively charged IgG to the serum, reducing to near zero or less the AG.
2. Albumin is usually responsible for 11 mEq/l of the anionic charges. This value would drop to 5-6 if the serum albumin fell to near 2 g/l and that would as a consequence bring about a reduction of the AG to 2-3 mEq/l (15, 16).

Conclusions

The anion gap is not just a bedside diagnostic game; its plasmatic and urinary values may be a useful aid to identify a variety of metabolic disturbances and to suspect some intoxications (if associated to the osmolal gap evaluation). Moreover its use should teach the physician to take more notice of the usually barely known implication of the chloride ion balance, which may sometimes prove to be the very special diagnostic key in ICU.

References

1. Narins RG, Jones ER et al (1982) Diagnostic strategies in disorders of fluid, electrolyte and acid-base homeostasis. Am J Med 72:469-512
2. Schwartz WB, Relman AS (1963) A critique of the parameters used in the evaluation of acid-base disorders. N Engl J Med 268:1382-1388
3. Narins RG, Emmett M (1980) Simple and mixed acid-base disorders: a practical approach. Medicine S9:161-187
4. Braden L, Strayhorn CH et al (1993) Increased osmolal gap in alcoholic acidosis. Arch Int Med 153:2377-2381
5. Smithline N, Gardner KD (1976) Gaps-anionic and osmolal. JAMA 236:1594-1597
6. Madias NE, Ayus JC, Adrogué JH (1979) Increased anion gap in metabolic alkalosis. The role of plasma-protein equivalency. N Engl J Med 300:1421-1423
7. Gabow P (1985) Disorders associated with an altered anion gap. Kidney Int 27:472-483
8. Kruse JA (1994) Use of the anion gap in intensive care and emergency medicine. In: Vincent JL (ed) Yearbook of intensive care and emergency medicine. Springer, Berlin Heidelberg New York, pp 685-696
9. Koch STM, Taylor RW (1992) Chloride ion in intensive care medicine. Crit Care Med 20: 227-240
10. Gamblin GT, Ashburn RW, Kemp DG, Beuttel SC (1986) Diabetic ketocidosis presenting with a normal anion gap. Am J Med 80:758-760
11. Kruse JA (1992) Methanol poisoning. Intensive Care Med 18:391-397

12. Kruse JA (1992) Ethylene glycol intoxication. J Intensive Care Med 7:234-243
13. Kruse JA (1993) Methanol, ethylene glycol, and related intoxications. In: Carlson RW, Geheb MA (eds) Principles and practice of medical intensive care. Saunders, Philadelphia, pp 1714-1723
14. Hruska KA, Ban D (1982) Renal tubular acidosis. Arch Int Med 142:1909-1913
15. Winter SD, Pearson JR, Gabow PA, Schultz AL, Lepoff RB (1990) The fall of the anion gap. Arch Int Med 150:311-313
16. Frohlich J, Adam W, Golbey MJ, Bernstein M (1976) Decreased anion gap associated with monoclonal and pseudomonoclonal gammopathy. Can Med Assoc J 114:231-232

Continuous Noninvasive Aortic Blood Flow Monitoring

M. Singer

Introduction

Haemodynamic monitoring in both operating theatre and intensive care environments remains predominantly pressure-based even though these variables are well recognised as coarse, non-specific and generally late indicators of cardiovascular deterioration. The sensitivity of pressure measurements in detecting changes in flow and ventricular end-diastolic volumes are undermined further by changes in body temperature, ventricular compliance, volaemic status and reflex vasoconstriction. A normal blood pressure frequently masks an inadequate cardiac output while severe hypovolaemia may be present despite normal or even elevated central venous pressures.

The adequacy of organ blood flow is of crucial importance. Appropriate management decisions in the critically ill should ideally be made with knowledge of these flows however we still lack the routine monitoring capability to assess the adequacy or otherwise of organ perfusion. Even the measurement of total body blood flow (cardiac output) often comes a distant and belated second to pressure measurements, although an established and reliable methodology has now been widely available for the last 25 years. In Britain, pulmonary artery catheterisation is rarely performed perioperatively; only 53 of 1616 perioperative deaths had a Swan-Ganz catheter in place during the operation despite 70% being ASA Grade III or above (1). Likewise, in UK intensive care units, on average only 10-20% of patients have a catheter inserted at some time during their stay (2). Shoemaker clearly demonstrated that postoperative complications and mortality can be directly linked to the development of a perioperative tissue oxygen debt and the time taken thereafter for correction (3). An aggressive policy of "supranormalising" the circulation had a dramatic beneficial effect on outcome. His findings in a high-risk surgical group were repeated by Boyd (4) but the same policy was found to be detrimental if the patient had already become critically ill (5).

These studies have highlighted three clear "take home" messages: better monitoring, better use of that monitoring, and more prompt intervention. For all its advantages, pulmonary artery catheterisation does have drawbacks: invasiveness, cost, time and expertise required to place the catheter, and a recognised complication rate. The inclination, therefore, is to wait until the patient shows signs of significant cardiovascular instability (2). Prolonged periods of organ hypoperfusion could elapse before steps are taken to measure and then improve flow, by which time organ dysfunction may have become established.

In the light of the above comments, should we not re-examine our approach to monitoring the ill, or potentially ill, patient? Most would agree that routine pulmonary artery catheter placement in every ICU or operating theatre patient is neither practicable, cost-effective nor justified. To obtain maximal benefit it is not simply a matter of when it is used, but how and in whom. Supranormalisation of haemodynamic variables has been shown to work only in advance of obvious deterioration (3-5). Adverse changes must, therefore, be detected early and acted upon promptly and appropriately. Can relatively non-invasive flow monitoring techniques aid management and indicate at an early stage the need for invasive flow monitoring? Whatever technique is utilised must be safe, reliable and easy to insert and operate. This article will deal with a new haemodynamic monitoring device utilising Doppler ultrasound from an oesophageal approach which offers considerable benefits both in terms of diagnosis and management, in reliability and in ease of use.

The velocity of a moving object is proportional to the shift in reflected frequency of a sound wave of known frequency. An equation was developed (Fig. 1) in which the speed of sound through the medium, and the vector between the directions of the sound wave and the moving object were also taken into account. In the case of arterial blood flow measurement, the moving objects are red blood corpuscles and high frequency ultrasound waves, i.e. frequencies exceeding the upper range of the human ear (> 20 KHz), are used. The density difference between red blood corpuscles and plasma is responsible for the back-scattered Doppler frequency shift signals used to measure blood flow. Processing of these Doppler frequency shift signals can be performed by spectral analysis and depicted as velocity-time waveforms on a real-time monitor (Fig. 2).

Aortic blood flow by Doppler ultrasound measurement was first described in the 1960s, initially via a percutaneous approach below the left second intercostal space (6) and then from a suprasternal position (7). Validations performed against reference techniques such as thermodilution, dye dilution and Fick confirmed its accuracy (8-10). Though non-invasive and painless, quick, and easy to perform, up to 5% of patients cannot be easily measured due to either anatomical (e.g. short neck) or pathological (e.g. emphysema, mediastinal air post-cardiothoracic surgery, aortic valve disease) factors. Sufficient experience is required for accurate measurement and no adequate means has been found to hold the probe in correct position for continuous monitoring.

The oesophageal approach was first described in 1971 (11) and significantly developed since (12-17). The history has been chequered with basic design flaws and inadequate validation studies of some devices often serving to undermine the technique. My major experience has been with the ODM device (Abbott) which

$$V = \frac{c\,f_d}{2\,f_T\,\cos\theta}$$

v = flow velocity

c = speed of sound (in body tissue = 1540 m/sec)

f_d = frequency shift (Hz)

cos θ = cosine of angle between sound beam axis

and velocity vector

f_T = frequency of transmitted ultrasound (Hz)

Fig. 1. Doppler equation

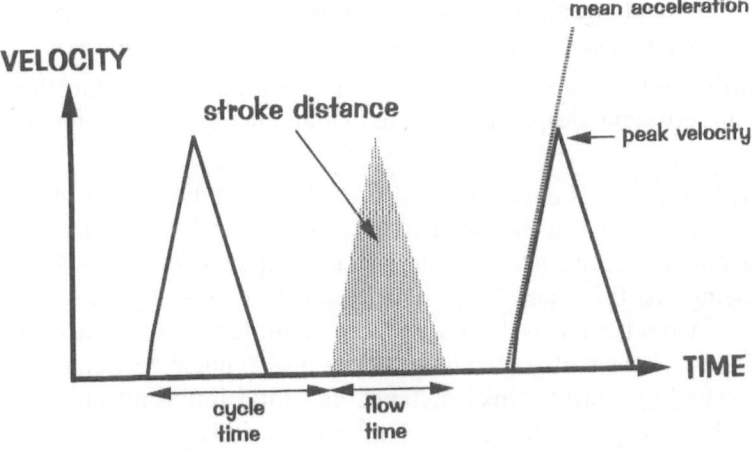

Fig. 2. Doppler flow-velocity waveform

crucially incorporates an on-line monitor to allow visual verification of correct signal measurement and which has undergone the largest number of validation studies against reference techniques (18-21). With the important proviso of adequate training, reliable and reproducible results are obtained. This device consists of a 6-mm diameter 4 MHz continuous wave Doppler transducer which is inserted into the distal oesophagus to a depth of 35-40 cm from the teeth to measure blood flow in the descending thoracic aorta. At this point the oesophagus and aorta are adjacent and run parallel to each other thus the 45° angulation of the probe tip can be taken as the angle of the ultrasound beam to blood flow in the Doppler equation. Blood flow detected in that position will either be aortic, intracardiac or venous (azygos) in origin so the characteristic aortic signal can be readily distinguished on the monitor displaying the flow-velocity waveforms. Insertion and correct positioning is thus simple and quick, usually taking less than two minutes.

The area (integral) of each velocity-time waveform – the *stroke distance* – corresponds to the distance travelled by a column of aortic blood down the descending thoracic aorta with each left ventricular stroke. The stroke volume of blood traversing the descending thoracic aorta is the product of stroke distance and aortic cross-sectional area. Any change in stroke distance represents a proportional change in stroke volume provided the aortic cross-sectional area remains constant during systole. This assumption appears to be valid in adults. Indeed, for purposes of monitoring changes in cardiac output a number of other assumptions have to be made:

– The angle of 45° between ultrasound beam and the direction of blood flow is accurate and remains fixed despite, for example, mediastinal shifts with ventilation.
– The aortic cross-sectional area remains constant during systole despite changes in blood pressure, cardiac output and neurogenic influences.
– The proportion of left ventricular output passing down the descending thoracic aorta remains constant, despite changes in output, pressure, body temperature, etc.

A prototype system was developed and a validation study performed against thermodilution in patients in the intensive care unit or operating theatre (18). Close agreement was found between the two techniques with the mean of the differences being just 0.7% and limits of agreement of ± 14.2%. However, the coefficient of variation was better for the Doppler technique than for thermodilution (4.2% vs 6.4%). A relationship was also noted between absolute values of descending aortic stroke distance and total left ventricular stroke volume provided age (as aortic diameter increases with age) and, to a lesser extent, body surface area were taken into account. A nomogram was developed incorporating these variables and found to produce an estimate of volumetric cardiac output to some 85%-90% accuracy *without* the need for any other measurement to be performed. It should be stressed that this is an estimate and not an absolute; however, it is reliable enough, provided all the rules of insertion and focussing are adhered to, to be now used as a standard monitoring technique on our intensive care unit.

The prototype machine described above was superceded by a dedicated oesophageal Doppler machine (the ODM) which incorporates both the nomogram and software enabling continuous beat-by-beat monitoring of stroke volume. Signals are routinely obtained within minutes and no significant trauma has been recognised despite the probe being left in situ for up to 18 days. Patients with known pharyngo-oesophageal pathology (e.g. varices) are not instrumented yet patients with severe coagulopathy and thrombocytopenia are often monitored without major complication. It cannot be used during aortic balloon counterpulsation which causes turbulent flow, and with severe aortic coarctation. A recent report of its use in critically ill children (22) revealed good trend following compared to thermodilution, however a nomogram to estimate cardiac output has yet to be developed for a paediatric population.

While having a rapid, reliable and relatively non-invasive means of estimating cardiac output is undoubtedly useful, further information is required to direct management. For example, does the patient require fluid, dilators or inotropes for his low output state? The shape of the Doppler flow velocity waveform provides such information to guide therapy. The peak velocity and acceleration are affected by changes in ventricular inotropy and, to a much lesser extent, by alterations in filling. On the other hand, the flow time is more affected by volaemic status while changes in peripheral resistance have an intermediate effect (18, 23, 24) (Fig. 3). The flow time is heart rate-dependent and most haemodynamic interventions will also affect heart rate. In order to study the "pure" effect of a manoeuvre on flow time it is necessary to remove the influence of heart rate. This can be achieved by an adaptation of Bazett's equation (used for correcting the electrocardiographic QT interval for heart rate) (25). This corrected flow time (FTc) is obtained by dividing flow time by the square root of the cycle time.

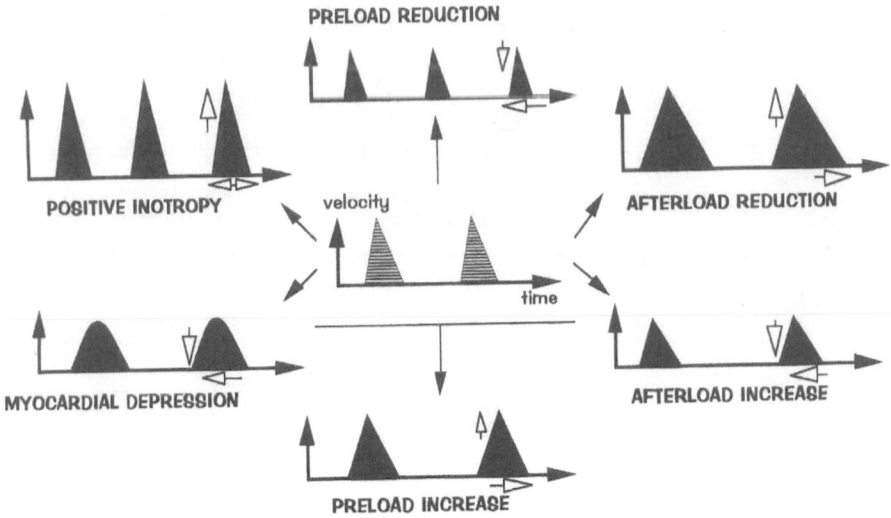

Fig. 3. Change in waveform shape following manoeuvres affecting left ventricular preload, inotropy and afterload

An inverse relationship exists between age and aortic peak velocity as the ventricle becomes less contractile and the aorta dilates with increasing years. The normal range of peak velocity is thus age-related, being approximately 90-120 cm/s at age 20, 70-100 cm/s at age 45 and 50-80 cm/s at age 70. This provides an immediate indication of a hyperdynamic (e.g. sepsis) or hypodynamic (e.g. heart failure) circulation. The corrected flow time gives an idea of left ventricular filling and systemic vascular resistance, the normal range being approximately 330-360 ms. A value below this suggests a hypovolemic or vasoconstricted circulation whereas values in excess are seen with vasodilatation. However, in hypovolaemia, the peak velocity is usually well maintained compared to age-expected values, producing a narrow, peaked waveform. However, with vasoconstriction due to poor ventricular function, the peak velocity is usually reduced producing a narrow but flattened waveform shape (Fig. 4).

These waveform shape changes are consistent (23, 24) and are related to wedge pressure measurements (24). The Doppler technique can thus be used for

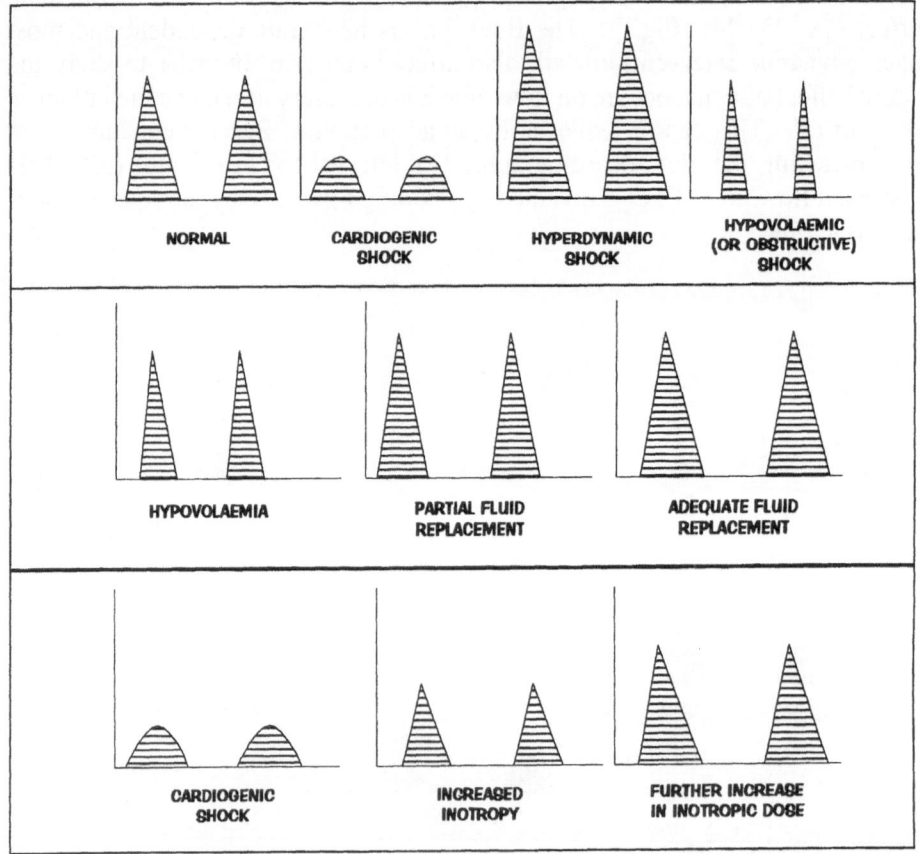

Fig. 4. Effect on waveform shape of hypovolaemia, hypodynamic and hyperdynamic circulations

non-invasive optimisation of left ventricular filling. Challenge by 200 ml colloid or by injection of a small bolus of a short-acting nitrate will produce a haemodynamic effect on stroke volume which can be viewed immediately; this informs the clinician as to whether the patient is adequately filled or not. Occasionally the oesophageal Doppler waveform may even highlight misleading pulmonary artery catheter data (26); for example in mitral stenosis where the PAWP may be grossly elevated or in major pulmonary embolus where the central venous pressure may be very high, the left ventricle is shown to be underfilled by a narrow, peaked waveform.

To date there have been a number of studies published using the ODM. Significant falls in cardiac output can occur at even low levels of positive end-expiratory pressure so that the overall effect on oxygen delivery may be deleterious (27); at least 15 min should elapse before the full short-term cardiorespiratory effect of an increase in PEEP can be assessed (28). Falls in cardiac output are related to the degree of manual lung hyperinflation above pre-set ventilator tidal volumes, rather than to the peak inspiratory pressures generated (29).

The use of cold irrigation fluid during transurethral resection of the prostate (TURP) (30, 31), causing a significant and rapid drop in core temperature, was associated with a marked deterioration in haemodynamic status which was not apparent when observing changes in heart rate or blood pressure. Studies in aortic reconstructive surgery have shown good correlations between Doppler and thermodilution (21) and that the perioperative stroke volume change assessed by Doppler was the best prognostic marker of postoperative outcome (submitted for publication). A randomised study of 60 patients undergoing cardiac surgery (32) revealed that the 30 patients receiving repeated fluid challenges to obtain maximal stroke volume fared significantly better in terms of postoperative outcome than a group of 30 patients managed in conventional fashion. An earlier observational study by the same authors (33) had shown that gastric intramucosal acidosis was much more frequent in those patients whose stroke volume fell during the course of the operation and that this was linked with poor postoperative outcome.

In conclusion, continuous aortic flow monitoring is feasible, quick and reliable. A machine that incorporates an on-line monitor to visualise the flow velocity waveforms is needed to confirm correct probe positioning and satisfactory signal measurement. Proper training is necessary but the technique is rapidly mastered. This allows rapid diagnosis of circulatory status, management of cardiovascular instability, and the possibility of improving outcome.

References

1. Campling EA, Devlin HB, Hoile RW, Lunn JN (1993) National confidential enquiry into perioperative deaths 1991/1992, HMSO, London
2. Singer M, Bennett ED (1989) Invasive hemodynamic monitoring in the United Kingdom. Enough or too little? Chest 95:623-626
3. Shoemaker WC, Appel PL, Kram HB, Waxman K, Lee T-S (1988) Prospective trial of supranormal values of survivors as therapeutic goals in high-risk surgical patients. Chest 94:1176-1186
4. Boyd O, Grounds RM, Bennett ED (1993) A randomised clinical trial of the effect of deliberate perioperative increase of oxygen delivery on mortality in high-risk surgical patients. JAMA 270:2699-2707
5. Hayes MA, Timmins AC, Yau EH, Palazzo M, Hinds CJ, Watson D (1993) Elevation of systemic oxygen delivery in the treatment of critically ill patients. N Engl J Med 330: 1717-1722
6. Light LH (1969) Non-injurious ultrasonic technique for observing flow in the human aorta. Nature 224:1119-1121
7. Light LH (1976) Transcutaneous aortovelography. A new window on the circulation? Br Heart J 38:433-442
8. Huntsman LL, Stewart DK, Barnes SR, Franklin SB, Colocousis JS, Hessel EA (1983) Noninvasive Doppler determination of cardiac output in man. Circulation 67:593-602
9. Chandraratna PA, Nanna M, McKay C et al (1984) Determination of cardiac output by transcutaneous continuous-wave ultrasonic Doppler computer. Am J Cardiol 53:234-237
10. Christie J, Sheldahl LM, Tristani FE, Sagar KB, Ptacin MJ, Wann S (1987) Determination of stroke volume and cardiac output during exercise: comparison of two-dimensional and Doppler echocardiography, Fick oximetry, and thermodilution. Circulation 76:539-547
11. Side CD, Gosling RJ (1971) Non-surgical assessment of cardiac function. Nature 232:335-336
12. Olson M, Cooke JP (1974) A nondestructive ultrasonic technique to measure diameter and blood flow in arteries. IEEE Trans Biomed Eng 168-171
13. Duck FA, Hodson CJ, Tomlin PJ (1974) An esophageal Doppler probe for aortic flow velocity monitoring. Ultrasound Med Biol 1:233-241
14. Daigle RE, Miller CW, Histand MB, McLeod FD, Hokanson D (1975) Nontraumatic aortic blood flow sensing by use of an ultrasonic esophageal probe. J Appl Physiol 38:1153-1160
15. Lavandier B, Cathignol D, Muchada R, Bui Xuan B, Motin J (1985) Noninvasive aortic blood flow measurement using an intraesophageal probe. Ultrasound Med Biol 11:451-460
16. Mark NB, Steinbrook RA, Gugino LD, Madi R, Hartwell B, Shemin R (1986) Continuous noninvasive monitoring of cardiac output with esophageal Doppler ultrasound during cardiac surgery. Anesth Analg 65:1013-1020
17. Stein MS, Barratt SMcG, Purcell GJ (1991) Intraoperative assessment of the Lawrence 3000 Doppler cardiac output monitor. Anaesth Intensive Care 251-255
18. Singer M, Clarke J, Bennett ED (1989) Continuous hemodynamic monitoring by esophageal Doppler. Crit Care Med 17:447-52
19. Lefrant JY, de la Coussaye JE, Bassoul B, Auffray JP, Eledjam JJ (1992) Comparison of cardiac output measured by esophageal Doppler vs thermodilution. Intensive Care Med 18 [Suppl 2]:P238
20. Belot JP, Valtier B, de la Coussaye JE, Mottin D, Payen D (1992) Continuous estimation of cardiac output in critically ill mechanically ventilated patients by a new transoesophageal Doppler probe. Intensive Care Med 18 [Suppl 2]:P241
21. Klotz K-F, Klingsiek S, Singer M et al (1995) Continuous measurement of cardiac output during aortic cross-clamping by the oesophageal Doppler monitor ODM 1. Br J Anaesth 74:655-660
22. Murdoch IA, Marsh MJ, Tibby SM, McLuckie A (1995) Continuous haemodynamic monitoring in children: use of transoesophageal Doppler. Acta Paediatr 84:761-764

23. Singer M, Allen MJ, Webb AR, Bennett ED (1991) Effects of alterations in left ventricular filling, contractility, and systemic vascular resistance on the ascending aortic blood velocity waveform of normal subjects. Crit Care Med 19:1138-1145
24. Singer M, Bennett ED (1991) Non-invasive optimization of left ventricular filling by esophageal Doppler. Crit Care Med 19:1132-1137
25. Bazett MC (1920) An analysis of the time-relations of electrocardiograms. Heart 7:353-364
26. Singer M, Bennett ED (1989) Pitfalls of pulmonary artery catheterisation highlighted by Doppler ultrasound. Crit Care Med 17:1060-1061
27. Singer M, Bennett ED (1989) Optimisation of positive end-expiratory pressure for maximal delivery of oxygen to tissues by using oesophageal Doppler ultrasonography. Br Med J 298:1350-1353
28. Patel M, Singer M (1993) When should the cardiorespiratory effects of PEEP be measured? Chest 104:139-142
29. Singer M, Vermaat J, Hall G, Latter G, Patel M (1994) Hemodynamic effects of hyperinflation in critically ill mechanically ventilated patients. Chest 106:1182-1187
30. Evans JWH, Singer M, Chapple CR, Macartney N, Walker JM, Milroy EJ (1992) Haemodynamic evidence for cardiac stress during transurethral prostatectomy. Br Med J 304:666-671
31. Evans JWH, Singer M, Coppinger SWV, Macartney N, Walker JM, Milroy EJG (1994) Cardiovascular performance and core temperature during transurethral prostatectomy. J Urol 152:2025-2029
32. Mythen MG, Webb AR (1995) Perioperative plasma volume expansion reduces the incidence of gut mucosal hypoperfusion during cardiac surgery. Arch Surg 130:423-429
33. Mythen MG, Webb AR (1994) Intraoperative gut mucosal hypoperfusion is associated with increased post-operative complications and cost. Intensive Care Med 20:99-104

How to Manage Critically Ill Patients After Cardiac Surgery

J.O.C. AULER JR.

Introduction

Acute heart failure after cardiac surgery is a pathophysiologic state in which the heart cannot sufficiently pump blood for tissue requirements. Low cardiac output after cardiac surgery can be related to previous deteriorated ventricular function and perioperative myocardial damage due to ischemia. The principal mechanism responsible for low postoperative cardiac output has been attributed to myocardial damage during cardiopulmonary bypass (CPB). Reduction in oxygen supply relative to demand may cause hypoxia and ischemia, which determines myocardial structural damage manifested by contractility impairment, malignant ventricular arrhythmias and low cardiac output. Acute mechanical contractility dysfunction owing to ischemia may take different amounts of time to recover according to the type of lesion involved (1). Contractility dysfunction that is rapidly reversible with pharmacological agents which are able to reduce oxygen demand indicates viable myocardium defined as "hibernating". On the other hand, contractile dysfunction associated with a short time of ischemia, if slowly reversible, and persisting for days to weeks is termed "stunned myocardium". Therefore, the basic difference between stunned and hibernating myocardium is related to pathophysiological mechanisms and time necessary to recover the contractility. In the stunned myocardium, the period of contractility impairment is slowly reversed and associated to ischemia. In hibernating myocardium the decrease in the contractility is associated to a period of low coronary flow and characterizes to be rapidly reversible (2-4). In addition to increased oxygen demand in the face of reduced supply, another cause of myocardial dysfunction after CPB is the presence of down-regulation of ß-adrenergic receptors. Cardiopulmonary bypass has been known to be a potent stimulus for the release of endogenous catecholamines, and it has been experimentally demonstrated that a reversible ß-adrenergic receptor down-regulation may contribute to difficulty in weaning from CPB after completion of cardiac surgery as well as transitory postoperative cardiac dysfunction (5).

The primary goals in management of severely compromised cardiac function after CPB are combining pharmacological support consisting of inotropes and vasodilators, volume adjustment, control of arrhythmias and possibly mechanical support of the circulation. Furthermore, another important point will be the ventilatory handling. Frequently after cardiac surgery critically ill patients present oxygen disturbances that require elevated levels of PEEP, high peak inspiratory pressure and a long period of ventilation. In this chapter, three aspects that we think to be relevant in the management of critically ill patients after cardiac surgery will be pointed out.

Ventilatory management

The undesirable cardiovascular consequences of mechanical ventilation may be the result of complex changes in venous return, right and left ventricular interactions and modifications in left ventricular afterload, which may decrease cardiac output (6, 7). For the lungs, the distending force to the alveolar opening is the transpulmonary pressure (mouth minus intrapleural pressure); for the chest wall it is the transthoracic pressure (atmospheric minus intrapleural pressure). Airway pressure reflects the average pressure applied by the ventilator; under these same conditions, mean alveolar pressure is the average pressure necessary to recruit the alveoli against the combined recoil of lung and chest wall (8-11).

In this section two aspects are more important to be discussed: first of all, the level of PEEP application and its hemodynamic and respiratory mechanics consequences; secondly, strategies concerning decreasing intrathoracic pressure to improve cardiac output by decreasing inspiratory peak pressure.

Positive end-expiratory pressure (PEEP) has been widely utilized during acute respiratory failure, to provide mechanical stability for distal airspaces and correct hypoxemia (12). Additionally, there is considerable controversy regarding the proper level of PEEP to obtain alveolar stabilization and to improve oxygenation, causing minimal hemodynamic and respiratory compromise (13-15). In postoperative cardiac surgery, lower levels of PEEP (5-6 cm of water) are routinely used to correct intraoperative atelectasis and has also been indicated to control postoperative mediastinal bleeding. Some patients may present an important decrease in blood oxygenation that requires high levels of PEEP; however, the hemodynamic instability present in these patients can be further worsened due to PEEP mechanisms.

To investigate the hemodynamics and respiratory effects of PEEP after cardiac surgery, ten patients, seven male (ages 52.3 ± 8.02 years) were studied. After ICU admittance, before data collection, the patients had their volemia adjusted and myocardial contractility supported by inotropic drugs. Respiratory mechanics and hemodynamics were measured after 15 min of application of three different PEEP levels: 5, 10 and 15 cmH_2O aside from zero end expiratory pressure which was taken as a control. End inflation occlusion method (EIOM) was used to measure the resistive and elastic properties of the respiratory system (16).

Standard hemodynamics consisting of intravascular pressures, cardiac output, arterial and mixed venous blood samples were obtained. Analysis of variance

(ANOVA) for repeated measures was used for comparing the effect of PEEP (p < 0.05) on individual variables. As can be seen in Table 1, there was a significant decrease in total airway resistance as well as in the elastance along with PEEP increase. Significant change occurred in pulmonary elastance or compliance at PEEP levels at 10 and 15 cm of H_2O. The decrease in respiratory elastance can be explained by a supplementary alveolar recruitment. The airway resistance decrease may be caused by a probable increase in airway radius due to the radial forces applied by the alveolar parenchyma on the airway wall. The significant decrease in cardiac index was compensated by an increase in arterial oxygen content owing to a shunt fraction reduction. It is important to point out that PEEP values above 10 cm of H_2O are not commonly recommended after cardiac surgery due to the possible decrease in cardiac output. Although a possible minimal hemodynamic compromise occurred when we changed the PEEP level from 10 to 15 cm of H_2O, the oxygenation improvement owing to the Qs/Qt decrease was able to maintain the DO_2. We observed a significant variation in right and left pressures mainly at 15 cm of H_2O of PEEP that were not corrected for the pleural increased pressure during PEEP application. It is important to note that to obtain accurate values of atrial filling pressure during high levels of PEEP therapy, the value of pleural pressure should be taken in account (Table 1). Lozman et al. (17) observed after cardiac surgery a constant correlation between PCWP and left atrium pressure only at low levels of PEEP. Pinsky et al. (18) found that in the postoperative cardiac patient right atrial pressures do not reflect wedge pressure (PCWP) or change similarly with PEEP induced changes in PCWP; this parameter reflects left atrium pressure only during low levels of PEEP (< 5 cm H_2O). According to our results (19), although PEEP therapy above 10 cm of H_2O substantially increases the oxygenation and compliance, it should be cautiously applied, especially in patients with marginal cardiac function due to contractility disturbances.

Table 1. Respiratory hemodynamic data

	PEEP (cmH$_2$O)			
	0	5	10	15
Ers	23.4 ± 1.2	21.8 ± 0.7	18.8 ± 1.1*	18.4 ± 0.8*
R	13.1 ± 0.7	11.9 ± 0.5*	11.4 ± 0.7*	10.3 ± 0.5*
CI	3.9 ± 0.2	3.4 ± 0.2*	3.3 ± 0.2*	3.1 ± 0.2*
PCWP	8.9 ± 1.2	8.3 ± 0.8	10.3 ± 0.6	11.8 ± 0.8*
RAP	6.3 ± 0.9	5.8 ± 0.78	7.2 ± 0.8	9.1 ± 1.1*
MAP	86.2 ± 4.0	87.8 ± 2.9	86.5 ± 3.2	88 ± 3.8
PVR	61.8 ± 6.0	78.9 ± 6.9*	98.4 ± 13.8*	109.3 ± 11.3*
DO$_2$	481.3 ± 40.1	435.7 ± 35.1	423.0 ± 36.8	432.2 ± 38.6
Qs/Qt	22.2 ± 2.3	19.6 ± 2.1	15.7 ± 1.4*	11.6 ± 1.2*

Elastance (E$_{rs}$; cmH$_2$O/l); Resistance (R; cmH$_2$O/l/sec); Cardiac index (CI; l/min.m^2); Mean pulmonary capillary wedge pressure (PCWP; mmHg); Right atrial pressure (RAP; mmHg); Mean arterial pressure (MAP; mmHg); Pulmonary vascular resistance (PVR; dyne.sec/cm^5); Intrapulmonary shunt (Qs/Qt; %); Oxygen delivery (DO$_2$; ml/min.m^2)
* Significant data

Another important point to be considered is related to the influence of positive airway pressure on cardiovascular function after cardiac surgery. Even being considered in adequate levels, the inspiratory pressure may result in detrimental effects in patients with impaired cardiac function. In this study we compared the influence of two values of peak inspiratory pressure (PIP) by altering the tidal volume (VT), on hemodynamics of patients with impaired contractility after cardiac surgery. Nine patients submitted to coronary artery bypass graft, with low cardiac index and adequate atrial filling pressures, were evaluated under volume controlled ventilation and settled at the following parameters: $FIO_2 = 1.0$, PEEP = 5 cmH_2O, I:E = 1-2, RR = 10/min and VT = 10 ml.kg^{-1}. After 30 min at this condition the VT was changed to 6 ml.kg^{-1}. Hemodynamic and respiratory measurements were obtained in each situation. Statistical analysis was performed by the Student's paired test (* $p < 0.05$) and the data are provided in Table 2.

Ultimately, it is important to consider that this relatively simple maneuver consisting of lowering the VT and PIP can be useful to improve cardiac index in postop patients with impaired cardiac function.

Table 2. Effects of tidal volume on respiratory hemodynamic parameters

	VT = 10 ml.kg^{-1}	VT = 06 ml.kg^{-1}
CI (l.min^{-1}.m^{-2})	2.77 ± 0.5	3.14 ± 0.7*
PCWP (mmHg)	18.0 ± 4.7	18.3 ± 6.5
CVP (mmHg)	15 ± 4.3	14.7 ± 4.2
PaCO$_2$ (mmHg)	35 ± 5.8	42 ± 5.3*
PaO$_2$/FiO$_2$	280 ± 50	290 ± 65
PIP (cmH$_2$O)	24 ± 5.2	19 ± 3.8

CI, cardiac index; PCWP, pulmonary capillary wedge pressure; PIP, peak inspiratory pressure; CVP, central venous pressure

Another point to be emphasized is related to the choice of ventilation mode in hemodynamically unstable patients after cardiac surgery. Recently, it has been demonstrated that pressure controlled ventilation may cause less peak inspiratory pressure elevation (20, 21). This ventilatory mode converts the square wave inspiratory flow to a rapid exponentially decaying curve whereby the tidal volume is delivered in a constant inspiratory time. In this way, the normal lung is ventilated by a fast decelerating flow and the high resistive areas are ventilated by a lower flow rate. Theoretically in this ventilation mode, that results in a suitable decelerating flow pattern, inhomogeneous areas of the lung are ventilated in a more effective way when compared to a normal volume controlled ventilation (22-24). This concept implies that insufflation pressure is responsible for stabilization of lung units, which promotes enhancement of oxygenation while keeping the inspiratory pressure to the lowest acceptable levels as possible

(25, 26). We have demonstrated that pressure controlled ventilation could be quite advantageous over the traditional volume controlled ventilation in patients with low cardiac output after cardiac surgery. Twenty postoperative cardiac patients were alternatively ventilated with the two modes of ventilation. The data were compared with analysis of variance (ANOVA $p < 0.05$) and presented in Table 3. The results showed that pressure controlled and volume controlled modes had comparable effects on patients with preserved (group I cardiac index > 2.5 l/min/m^2) or depressed (group II cardiac index < 2.5 l/min/m^2) cardiac function. The data compared with patients under pressure controlled ventilation showed significantly higher values for cardiac index as well as significantly lower values for inspiratory pressure when compared with those ventilated with volume controlled ventilation. Both ventilation modes had comparable effects on patients with preserved or depressed cardiac output (27).

Table 3. Hemodynamic and respiratory data

	Group I - PCV	Group I - VCV	Group II - PCV	Group II - VCV
CI	3.75 ± 0.7	3.44 ± 0.6	2.4 ± 0.2	2.2 ± 0.2
Paw	13.80 ± 2.4	13.40 ± 2.2	15.0 ± 2.6	14.7 ± 1.7
PIP	31.10 ± 7.8	35.9 ± 8.1	32.7 ± 7.9	40.20 ± 14.1

CI, cardiac index (l.min/m^2); Paw, mean airway pressure (cmH$_2$O); PIP, peak inspiratory pressure (cmH$_2$O)

Pharmacological support

In the last section, we will discuss pharmacological and mechanical support in patients with low cardiac output. In order to investigate the effects of drug association, we evaluated 77 immediate postoperative cardiac patients in whom the cardiac index was lower than 2.5 l/min/m^2. After ICU admission, a standard hemodynamic profile was obtained and according to the infused drugs, the patients were divided in three groups: I ($n = 12$), without any pharmacological therapy; II ($n = 24$), the patients were treated with dopamine; and III ($n = 41$), the patients were under dopamine and sodium nitroprusside infusion. The next step was to add dobutamine 4 to 6 µ/kg/min and the hemodynamic data was again obtained. The data before (B) and after dobutamine infusion (A) were ascribed by analysis of variance (ANOVA) $p < 0.05$. As shown in Table 4, a significant increase in cardiac index as well as a significant reduction in systemic vascular resistance was observed after dobutamine infusion.

Mechanical support

Finally, during the handling of critically ill patients after cardiac surgery it is important to consider some comments about mechanical support of the

Table 4. Dobutamine effects on cardiovascular function

Group	PCWP	CI	SVR
I B	11.1 ± 3.2	2.2 ± 0.5	1410.2 ± 590.4
I A	12.1 ± 4.5	3.0 ± 0.7	1113.1 ± 480.6
II B	16.6 ± 6.4	2.2 ± 0.7	1331.0 ± 586.4
II A	15.1 ± 5.1	3.2 ± 1.0	976.0 ± 288.2
III B	15.0 ± 7.1	2.4 ± 0.8	1322.7 ± 454.0
III A	16.4 ± 5.8	3.1 ± 0.9	1089.5 ± 401.9

PCWP, pulmonary capillary wedge pressure (mmHg); CI, cardiac index (l/min/m²); SVR, systemic vascular resistance (dynes/sec/cm⁵); B, before; A, after

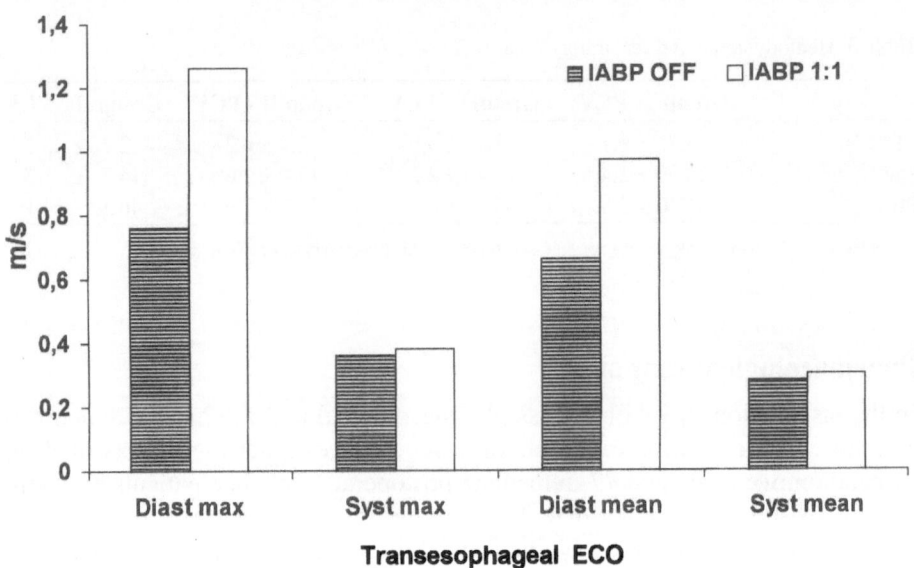

Fig. 1. Coronary flow peak velocity. In this graph, the augmentation in coronary flow peak velocity during the pulse of IABP in the diastolic period can be seen. *Diast max*, maximal peak during diastole; *Diast mean*, mean peak during diastole; *Syst max*, maximal peak during systole; *Syst mean*, mean peak during systole

circulation. Among several kinds of devices, the intra-aortic balloon pump (IABP) is the most extensively used of all cardiac assistance modalities, as it has proven effective, safe and easy to initiate for use in the treatment of patients with low cardiac output, sometimes refractory to pharmacological therapy. The combined effects of IABP support such as increased oxygen supply, afterload reduction and improved systemic perfusion could allow the "hibernating" or "stunned" myocardium after surgery the necessary time to heal and recover function. At the same time, it also provides circulatory support in order to acquire the desirable hemodynamic stability (28, 29). To verify the coronary flow augmentation provided by the IABP, we measured this variable through transesophageal echocardiography. The unpublished data presented in Fig. 1 were obtained in six patients after cardiac surgery. We can see a notable increase in coronary flow during the diastolic time when the pump is on. In conclusion, the management of critically ill patients after cardiac surgery requires direct interventions in the cardiorespiratory system in order to provide enough time for cardiac recovery while maximum cardiac optimization should be sought while trying to avoid negative interference.

References

1. Olthof H, Middelhof C, Meijine NG et al (1983) The definition of myocardial infarction during aortocoronary bypass surgery. Am Heart J 106:631-637
2. Kloner RA, Przyklenk K (1991) Hibernation and stunning of the myocardium. N Engl J Med 325:1877-1879
3. Przyklenk K, Bauer B, Kloner RA (1992) Reperfusion of hibernating myocardium: contractile function, high-energy phosphate content, and myocyte injury after 3 hours of sublethal ischemia and 3 hours of reperfusion in the canine model. Am Heart J 123:575-588
4. Poole-Wilson PA (1991) A possible molecular mechanism for "stunning" of the myocardium. Eur Heart J 12 [Suppl]:25-29
5. Schwinn DA, Leone BJ, Spahn DR et al (1991) Desensitization of myocardial ß-adrenergic receptors during cardiopulmonary bypass. Circulation 84:2559-2567
6. Mathru M, Rao TLK, El-Etr AA, Pifarre R (1982) Hemodynamic response to changes in ventilatory patterns in patients with normal and poor left ventricular reserve. Crit Care Med 10:423-426
7. Sharf SM (1992) Cardiovascular effects of positive pressure ventilation. J Crit Care 7:268-279
8. Marcy TW, Marini JJ (1991) Inverse ratio ventilation in ARDS. Rationale and implementation. Chest 100:494-504
9. Boros S (1979) Variations in inspiratory expiratory ratio and airway pressure wave form during mechanical ventilation: the significance of mean airway pressure. J Pediatr 94:114-117
10. Ciszek T, Modanlou H, Owings D, Nelson P (1981) Mean airway pressure-significance during mechanical ventilation in neonates. J Pediatr 99:121-126
11. Pesenti A, Marcolin R, Prato P, Borelli M, Riboni A, Gattinoni L (1985) Mean airway pressure vs. positive end-expiratory pressure during mechanical ventilation. Crit Care Med 13:34-37
12. Albert RK (1985) Least PEEP Primum non nocere. Chest 87:2-4
13. Gammon RB, Shin MS, Buchalter SE (1992) Pulmonary barotrauma in mechanical ventilation patterns and risk factors. Chest 102:568-572
14. Dreyfuss D, Basset G, Soler P, Saumon G (1985) Intermittent positive-pressure hyperventilation with high inflation pressures produces pulmonary microvascular injury in rats. Am Rev Respir Dis 132:880-884
15. Pinsky MR (1990) The effects of mechanical ventilation on the cardiovascular system. Crit Care Clin 6:663-678
16. Bates JHT, Rossi A, Milic-Emili J (1985) Analysis of the behavior of the respiratory system with constant inspiratory flow. J Appl Physiol 58:1840-1848
17. Lozman J, Powers SR, Older T et al (1974) Correlation of pulmonary wedge and left atrial pressure: a study in the patient receiving positive end-expiratory pressure ventilation. Arch Surg 109:270-277

18. Pinsky M, Vincent JL, Smet De JM (1991) Estimating left ventricular filling pressure during positive end-expiratory pressure in humans. Am Rev Respir Dis 143:25-31
19. Carvalho MJ, Auler Jr JOC, Saldiva PHN, Barbas CSB, Zin WA (1991) The effect of positive end-expiratory pressure (PEEP) on respiratory system mechanics. Annals of 11th International Symposium on Intensive Care and Emergency Medicine, Brussels, Belgium 83
20. Stoller JK, Kacmarek RM (1990) Ventilatory strategies in the management of the adult respiratory distress syndrome. Clin Chest Med 11:755-771
21. Lain DC, Di Benedetto R, Morris SL, Nguyen A, Saulters R, Causey D (1989) Pressure control inverse ratio ventilation as a method to reduce peak inspiratory pressure and provide adequate ventilation and oxygenation. Chest 95:1081-1088
22. Al-Saady N, Bennett ED (1985) Decelerating inspiratory flow waveform improved lung mechanics and gas exchange in patients on intermittent positive-pressure ventilation. Intensive Care Med 11:68-75
23. Tharratt RS, Allen RP, Albertson TE (1988) Positive-pressure ventilation, pressure controlled inverse ratio ventilation in severe adult respiratory failure. Chest 94:755-762
24. Boysen PG, McGough E (1988) Pressure-control and pressure-support ventilation: flow patterns, inspiratory time, and gas distribution. Resp Care 33:126-134
25. Kosecioglu J, Tibboel D, Lachmann B (1994) Advantages and rationale for pressure controlled ventilation. In: Vincent JL (ed) Yearbook of intensive care and emergency medicine. Springer, Berlin Heidelberg New York, pp 524-533
26. Munoz J, Guerrero JE, Escalante JL, Palomino R, De LaCalle B (1993) Pressure-controlled ventilation versus controlled mechanical ventilation with decelerating inspiratory flow. Crit Care Med 21:1143-1148
27. Auler Jr JOC, Carvalho MJ, Silva AMPR, Silva MHC, Dias CA, Jatene AD (1992) Pressure controlled ventilation in patients submitted to cardiac surgery. 12th International Symposium on Intensive Care and Emergency Medicine. Brussels, Belgium. Clin Intensive Care [Suppl]3:64
28. Freedman RJ (1992) Myoconservation in cardiogenic shock - the use of intra-aortic balloon pumping and other treatment modalities. Cardiac Assists 6:1-10
29. Ardehali A, Ports TA (1990) Myocardial oxygen supply and demand. Chest 98:699-705

Transfusion and Thromboembolic Prophylaxis

B. Borghi, M. Montebugnoli, N. de Simone, G. Gargioni, M.A. Feoli

Autotransfusion: predeposit

The number of units and frequency of transfusion is decided by the anesthetist together with the physician performing the transfusion during the first examination, which should take place at least 40 days prior to the operation, according to the clinical condition of the patient (age, weight, basal hemoglobin, any concomitant diseases) and the type of operation and expected perioperative blood loss (1). A subtraction of $350 \pm 10\%$ ml of blood from a patient weighing about 70 kg means a reduction of around 1 g of hemoglobin (Hb) and 3 units of hematocrit (Ht). Before major orthopedic surgery enough units should be predeposited so as to avoid the use of homologous blood in more than 90% of patients. Two units of autologous blood are generally needed for total knee and hip arthroplasty and spine fusion, and 3-4 units for partial or total knee or hip revision.

Intraoperative recovery

In major surgery (i.e. with the likelihood of transfusion) the anesthetist should set the system up for the recovery of blood lost from the wound during the operation. When the drop in intraoperative Hb is more than 1-2 g/dl (2) the kit should be set up so that the blood collected in the reservoir can be reinfused. A peristaltic pump sends the blood from the reservoir to the bowl where it is concentrated by centrifugation at 5000-5600 r.p.m. and the red cells are washed in isotonic saline solution. The blood concentration is then sent automatically to the collection bag where, after microfiltration, it is immediately reinfused into the patient. The Italian made apparatus (BT 795P, Stat, Compact Dideco) gives a better quality wash more quickly thanks to the possibility of mixing the contents in the bowl.

Monitoring postoperative recovery and bleeding

The surgeon places the appropriate number and calibre of drainage tubes along the wound and on each suture plane (1, 2). These tubes are linked by a four way connection to the kit (BT 797 Recovery Dideco). This apparatus consists of a peristaltic pump worked by an adjustable transducer ranging from –100 to +50 mmHg. It has a rechargable battery which enables the patient to be moved while it is in use. It also has an acoustic alarm that switches itself on automatically in case of:

– Blood loss greater than 300 ml/h
– Air in the circuit
– Battery running down

The display with memory shows the time passed from the start of use, the total amount of bleeding, hourly bleeding in the first 8 h and the pressure on the drainage tubes. The first 100-200 ml of blood recovered in the postoperative period and stocked in the bag of the BT 797 Recovery Dideco is treated like the blood recovered during the operation (washing the blood), connecting the collection bag to kit of the apparatus used for intraoperative recovery. When the absence of hemolysis is assured by centrifugation, reinfusion of the red cells after sedimentation and microfiltration proceeds for 6-8 h. It is normally sufficient to connect the drainage tubes to the apparatus for 18-24 h to control early bleeding.

Compression bandage

An external elastic compression bandage can play a decisive part in preventing postoperative hematoma, DVT and controlling bleeding. For hip replacement, this bandage must involve the entire limb up to the iliac crest. To make it more effective, cotton wool pads are placed at the edge of the wound and on the medial surface of the thigh root and also at the back along the sciatic nerve to avoid neurological insufficiency by compressing the nerves. For knee replacement surgery hematoma is prevented by placing two cotton wool pads under the bandage at the sides of *the knee cap*. If the bleeding exceeds 2-3 ml/min it may help to increase the bandage tension. The next step is to progressively decrease the negative pressure on the drainage until it becomes positive, up to + 50 mmHg if necessary and for short spells.

Causes of postoperative bleeding

Postoperative bleeding may be *early* or *late*. The former appears immediately after the operation and is often the result of insufficient surgical hemostasis, mostly due to relative hypotension when it is carried out. Late bleeding is the leakage of blood from the drainage tubes and/or the onset of a hematoma in the surgical site with a significant drop in Hb and protidaemia starting from the day after the operation. It is always the result of an excessive effect by the antithromboembolic drugs used. Therefore, the treatment consists of reducing the dosage or temporary suspension.

Ideal and borderline Hb

Table 1 shows ideal and minimum Hb levels for the various phases of the operation, supplied by the World Health Organisation (WHO) (3) and supported by our experience and that of other Italian institutes (4, 5).

Table 1. Ideal and borderline levels of Hb (g/dl)

Perioperative phases	Ideal	Border
Preadmission	> 11	10
Preoperation	9	8
Intraoperative	8	6
Postoperative immediate	9	7
Postoperative late	9	6
Discharge	10-11	7.5

For patients with heart disease or cerebral vasculopathy it is better to make sure Hb levels always stay above 9-10 g/dl.

Anemia and hypovolemia

Clinical testing of patients with Hb below the ideal level and especially around the borderline level is done in order to exclude the presence of clinical signs of bad tolerance to anemia such as: tachycardia, angina, dyspnea, cephalea, vertigo, insomnia, lipothymia on mobilization, postural hypotension, and state of confusion. The presence of one or more of the above clinical signs combined with borderline Hb and diastolic arterial pressure more than 20 mmHg below the base level should first indicate hypovolemia; therefore, the infusion of crystalloids and possibly plasma expanders should be carried out. If clinical signs of intolerance to anemia persist after volemia has been restored, seen by the normalization of diastolic pressure, red cells are transfused one unit at a time, monitoring the disappearance of symptoms. High frequency tachycardia after lowering Hb with isovolemia points to the possibility of left ventricular hypertrophy. The increase in cardiac output (stroke volume x frequency) required by the lowering of Hb is brought about, above all, by the increase in stroke volume with the increase in left ventricular diastolic volume. In patients with ventricular hypotrophy, the increase in diastolic volume is made difficult by the reduced relaxation of the left ventricle wall; thus the increase in capacity occurs by the increase in frequency (6).

Reinfusion method with autologous blood products

The reinfusion of blood units extracted before the operation must be spread over the first 3 days after the operation to make up for the drop in Hb which normally occurs in major orthopedic surgery. The reinfusion of autologous plasma usually occurs after the operation in case of intraoperative blood loss over 1500 ml, taking care not to cause hypervolemia, hypertension and subsequent increase in postoperative bleeding. Otherwise the plasma is reinfused in the first 24-48 h.

Reinfusion method with homologous blood products

The Hb of the patient influences the type of transfusion according to the availability of autologous blood or only homologous blood:

– Autologous transfusion is carried out whenever the Hb needs taking to the ideal value (see Table 1), always bearing in mind that blood should never be transfused unless it is necessary because of the risks of getting the units and patients mixed up or bad preservation that can occur even with autologous blood.
– Homologous transfusions are used only when Hb is below the borderline level and the anemia is not tolerated. The benefits (immediate) are weighed up against the risks (immediate and long term), such as adverse reaction or transmitted diseases and alloimmunization that can occur with homologous blood.

Antithromboembolic prophylaxis

Due to the decrease in blood donation and the prejudice about transfusion complications spread by the mass media, autotransfusion is becoming a necessary technique in performing surgery when there is a risk of bleeding. Therefore hemodilution is a logical consequence. In planned surgery intentional, moderate hemodilution can be carried out. The degree of hemodilution varies according to the mass withdrawn and the technique of replacing it (crystalloids and/or colloids). In any case it is an effective antithromboembolic prophylaxis (7, 8). Our technique consists of the reintegration of intraoperative blood loss with crystalloids and gelatine (ratio 2:1), while the recovered blood is reinfused after washing during the intraoperative period and after sedimentation in the postoperative period. Normovolemic hemodilution, reducing blood viscosity and vascular resistance stops the formation of platelet and erythrocyte aggregants, compensating the oxygen debt with increased circulation speed (7, 9-11). The blood extracted to induce hemodilution is used as autotransfusion units (concentrated blood and frozen plasma) without compulsory reinfusion. Hemodilution produces a controlled deficit of coagulation factors, i.e., a low level balance similar to that in chronic nephropathy and hepatopathy, useful in the prevention of thrombotic complications, quickly solved with the restoration of protein synthesis, when there is normal hepatic function and protein dispersion (12). The reintegration of only one factor (e.g., ATIII) or a portion of coagulation factors leads to unbalance and a decompensation effect. In the postoperative period there is usually a decrease in prothrombin activity, an increase in activated partial thromboplastin time, a reduction in ATIII, while fibrinogen and platelets increase as a sign of endothelial surgical trauma postoperative hypercoagulability. The reduction of plasmatic coagulation factors subsequent to hemodilution and the loss of plasmatic protein not recoverable during and immediately after the operation influences the dosage of antithromboembolic prophylactic drugs. The need to mediate between the risk of thrombosis and that of hemorrhage, especially in major orthopaedic surgery, calls for the use of:

– Postoperative prophylaxis: a recent study on low molecular weight heparin (LMWH) showed that the incidence of deep vein thrombosis, established by phlebogram, does not vary if the drug is administered before or after the operation.
– Technically manageable drugs: antagonistic (heparin) or with quick wash-out (indobufen).
– Suitable doses reduced according to coagulation control.

Table 2. Regimens of drug prophylaxis, antithromboembolic combined with hemodilution, adopted by our institute

Patient weight	Dose Indo	Patient weight	Dose HeCa	Patient weight	Dose enoxaparin
< 55 kg	100 + 100	< 70 kg	5000 U x 2	< 65 kg	2000 U I
55-65 kg	200 + 200	> 70 kg	5000 U x 3	> 65 kg	4000 U I
> 65 kg	200 + 200				

Calcium heparin (HeCa): used by us in adjusted doses is the most common form of antithromboembolic prophylaxis (13). Combined with hemodilution it does not seem to be the ideal drug due to the low level of antithrombin III, its substrate, obtained in the immediate postoperative period. We advise against its use.

LMWH is now the most used (14), especially in orthopedic surgery. Many authors repute its efficacy in protecting from thromboembolism with a lower risk of hemorrhage compared to classic heparin (15). Our studies also show that it seems to modify thromboplastin time activated in hemodilution, so, its dosage may be adapted. At our institute an enoxaparin is used which is available in doses of 2000 and 4000 I.U. anti XA, and therefore very manageable.

Indobufen: platelet antiaggregant, reversible and selective inhibitor of cyclo-oxygenase (wash-out 24-48 h) (16). Its action is at a peak after 3 h and can still be traced after the 24th hour. With hemodilution it seems to reduce prothrombin activity with anti-vit K-like action and prolong partial activated thromboplastin time more than LMWH.

Case report

From January 1992 to June 1994 in the wards in our anesthesiology department, 980 consecutive patients were treated for total joint replacement: 714 total hips, seven after removal of plates and screws, 145 revisions, and 121 total knee prostheses. Basal Hb was 13.4 ± 1.4 g/dl (range $6.7 - 17.9$ g/dl). In 6.3% of these patients homologous transfusions were carried out. The need to use homologous transfusions was negatively influenced by the female sex, ischemic cardiopathy ($p = 0.005$), the length of surgery and the type of antithromboembolic prophylaxis (indobufen has a significantly low incidence – $p = 0.0001$ – compared to calcium heparin or LMWH). The absence of complications is significantly higher (contingency table $p = 0.0001$) in patients treated with indobufen (94.3% vs 83.5% HeCa vs 85.7% LMWH).

Conclusions

A patient planned for an operation with likelihood of bleeding and thromboembolic complications as in major orthopedic surgery must never enter the operating theater without hemodilution and a suitable number of predeposited blood units (concentrated blood + fresh frozen plasma).

The blood saving and antithromboembolic prophylaxis protocol is the result of 16 years of experience and has been slowly perfected until reaching its present form, consisting of: predeposits possibly combined with medullar stimulation with exogenous erythropoietin, perioperative hemodilution, intraoperative and postoperative recovery, monitoring and limiting bleeding during and, above all, after the operation with the help of special equipment and compression bandages, adapted postoperative drug prophylaxis (PTT and PLT). There has to be a good relationship between the anesthetist, physician performing the transfusion and surgeon aimed at correct assessment and management of the patient and the correct combined application of the various blood saving and antithromboembolic prophylactic techniques.

References

1. Borghi B, Bassi A, de Simone N, Laguardia AM, Formaro G (1993) Autotransfusion: 15 years experience at Rizzoli Orthopaedic Institute. Int J Artif Organs 16(S-5):241-246
2. Borghi B, Bassi A, Grazia M, Gargioni G, Pignotti E (1995) Anaesthesia and autologous transfusion. Int J Artif Organs 18(3):159-166
3. National Resuree Education Program Coordinating Committee National Institute of Health (1989) Summary Report, Bethesda
4. Oriani G, Gaietta T, Meazza D, Ronzio A, Sacchi C (1990) Ematocrito di sicurezza in chirurgia ortopedico-traumatologica. Atti XX Corso Naz. di Aggiornamento in Rianimazione e Terapia intensiva. Ed Piccin, Padova, pp 19-27
5. Borghi B, Oriani G, Bassi A et al (1995) Blood saving program: a multicenter Italian experience. Int J Artif Organs 18(3):150-158
6. Bombardini T, Borghi B, Caroli GC et al (1994) Short term cardiac adaptation to normovolemic hemodilution in normal and hypertensive patients. An echocardiography study. Eur Heart J 15:637-640
7. Vara-Thorbeck R, Rossel Pradas J, Mekinassi KL et al (1990) Prevention of thrombotic disease and post-transfusional complication using normovolemic hemodilution in arthroplasty surgery of the hip. Rev Chir Orthop 76(4):267-271
8. Bombardini T, Borghi B, Montebugnoli M, Picano E, Caroli GC (1995) Normovolemic hemodilution reduces fatal pulmonary embolism: following major orthopaedic surgery. J Vasc Surg (in press)
9. Baron JF et al (1989) Hemodilution, autotransfusion, hemostase. Arnette, Paris, pp 396
10. Messmer K (1988) Haemodilution. Possibilities and safety aspects. Acta Anaesthesiol Scand Suppl 89:49-53
11. Duruble M (1988) Place de l'hemodiluition dans la prevention de la maladie thromboembolique. Phlebografie 41:825-829
12. Caroli GC et al (1994) Profilassi antitromboembolica e rischio emorragico in chirurgia ortopedica. Archivio di Ortopedia e Reumatologia 167(3):125-130
13. Macouillard G et al (1989) Beneficies et risques des differentes methodes des prophylaxis avec ou sans heparinoides. Conferences de Consensus. Ann Fr Anesth Reanim 11:298-299
14. Cosmi B, Hirsh J (1994) Low molecular weight heparin. Curr Opin Cardiol 9(5):612-618
15. Hirsh J (1990) From unfractionated heparins to low molecular weight heparins. Acta Chir Scand Suppl 556:42-50
16. Patrignani P, Volpi D, Ferrario R et al (1990) Effects of racemic, S- and R-indobufen on cyclooxygenase and lipooxygenase activities in human whole blood. Eur J Pharmacol 20; 191(1):83-88

Management of Common Poisoning in the ICU

V. Gašparović, M. Gjurašin, D. Ivanović, R. Radonić, M. Kvarantan, M. Merkler, D. Kakarigi

Poisoning is a clinical condition where one or more organ systems are suddenly or gradually threatened by exposure to a toxic agent. Accidental poisonings are most frequent (herbicides, carbon monoxide, nicotine, alcohol), followed by suicidal poisonings (drugs, less commonly other poisons), while criminal poisonings occur rarely. Acute poisonings are often emergencies demanding an appropriate approach (identification of poison, prevention of further absorption, removal of poison, symptomatic measures as maintenance of vital functions and administration of antidotes).

With the technological advances accompanying the development of civilization man has been confronted with a variety of potentially poisonous substances. Currently, some 12 million chemical compounds are being produced (1). However, in common clinical practice, the number of intoxications is much smaller and may be subdivided in two groups. The first kind is caused by drugs which, in overdose, account for approximately 50% of all serious poisonings (Table 1). The second kind is caused by compounds that man encounters in his surroundings, and which in dependence of the route they enter the organism exert toxic effects (2). Patients admitted to the internal intensive care unit for serious life-threatening poisonings in most cases require additional medical procedures. This review will deal with the treatment of the most common poisonings in the intensive care unit.

Table 1. Incidence of poisonings in ICU in an 8-year period

	F	M	Total	%
Psychotropic drugs	74	53	127	51.0
Antiarrhytmic drugs	4	0	4	1.6
Mushrooms	28	26	54	21.6
Caustics (acids + bases)	16	11	27	10.8
Pesticides	8	12	20	8.0
Ethylene glycol	1	6	7	2.8
Carbon monoxide	2	3	5	2.1
Ethyl alcohol	1	4	5	2.1
Total	134	115	249	100.0

One of the greatest problems in the adequate management of acute poisoning is identification of the toxic substance the patient was exposed to. Severe consciousness disturbances are frequently encountered, and if the case history cannot be obtained, the observance of the clinical syndrome guides further diagnostic procedures and treatment. Among the most frequent toxic syndromes is *cholinergic syndrome*, which is characterized by salivation, bronchorrhoea, lacrimation, urine and stool incontinence, gastrointestinal spasm, confusion and depression of the central nervous system. This syndrome occurs with insecticides, physostigmine and mushrooms poisonings. Prevailing symptoms in *anticholinergic syndrome* are dryness of mucosa, flush, hyperpyrexia, reduced peristalsis, spasms, urine retention, dilated pupils and delirium. These symptoms are mainly the consequence of drug overdose (antihistamines, antiparkinsonian drugs, atropine, scopolamine, antidepressant drugs, antipsychotics, mydiatrics) and of *Amanita muscaria*. *Sympathomimetic syndrome* is characterized by hyperpyrexia, diaphoresis, enhanced reflex activity, hypertension, mydriasis and paranoia. With exception of caffeine and theophylline, most of these substances are stimulant drugs (3). Toxic syndrome characterized by *severe metabolic acidosis* and respiratory acidosis is most frequently caused by methanol, ethylene glycol and formaldehyde. The experience from the intensive care unit points to several specific approaches. Severe poisonings require maintenance of circulation by infusion or vasoactive therapy. Acutely poisoned patients have reduced respiratory function, resulting either from respiratory depression or airway obstruction. Continuous checking of circulation and respiration is essential for the positive outcome in acute poisonings. However, available technological equipment in the intensive care unit has its limitations. Table 2 shows that artificial respiration had favourable effect on survival in drug poisonings. Poisonings caused by caustics and pesticides which required artificial ventilation in most cases had severe prognosis and lethal outcome.

Table 2. Incidence of severe respiratory insufficiency in acutely poisoned patients (8-year follow-up, artificial ventilation)

	Patients	**Death**	**Survived**
Psychotropic	17	1	16
Caustics	4	4	0
Solvents	2	1	1
Other	1		
Pesticides	5	4	1
Total	29 (22.8%)	10	18

Treatment of renal insufficiency by haemodialysis in poisonings with caustics represented a temporary palliative measure, since in six such cases there were four fatalities (Table 3).

Table 3. Incidence of severe renal insufficiency in acutely poisoned patients (8-year follow-up)

	Patients	Death	Survived
Caustics	6	4	2
Solvents	5	1	4
Mushrooms	3	1	2
Pesticides	2	1	1
Total	16	7	9

These data suggest that severe poisonings, particularly those caused by caustics, have poor prognosis regardless of the advanced possibilities of function maintenance.

In the overall survival analysis of acutely poisoned patients, older age is a severe predictor, mostly as a consequence of later complications in the intensive care unit, primarily respiratory nosocomial infections, sepsis due to urinary catheter, etc. (Table 4).

Table 4. Survival of poisoned patients according to age

Age	Survived	Death	Total
< 30	85	1	86
30-59	120	4	124
> 60	27	12	39
Total	232	17	249

Common poisonings

ACIDS. Ingestion of an acid causes irritation, bleeding and severe mucosal lesions with subsequent formation of crusts in mouth and oesophagus. Burns are particularly frequent on the pylorus. Ingestion of a larger quantity is fatal, due to immediate effects. Perforations of hollow organs may occur later, with consequential mediastinitis or peritonitis. In the later stage, survivors develop strictures of the involved organs. Ingested acid is diluted by water or alkali (sodium bicarbonate should not be used). Gastric lavage and induction of vomiting are contraindicated. Diagnostic oesophagoscopy is performed within the first 24 h. Following emergency measures, therapy is administered for pain relief, treatment of shock, infection, and possible perforation.

ALKALIES. Upon ingestion alkalies form proteinates with proteins and soaps with fat, both resulting in penetrating necrosis of tissues. Ingestion of these corrosives has the same early and late effects as with acids. Large amounts of water and milk for the dilution of corrosives must be taken. Gastric lavage and induction of vomiting are contraindicated. Diagnostic oesophagoscopy is performed within the first 24 h. With considerable lesions of oesophagus and stomach, some recommend corticosteroids for the prevention of strictures, but the efficacy of such treatment has yet to be proved. Symptomatic therapy comprises the relief of pain, fluid replacement and clearance of airway obstructions.

CARBON MONOXIDE. This is a colourless, odourless and nonirritating gas produced by incomplete combustion of carbonaceous materials. Its toxicity results from the great affinity of haemoglobin for carbon monoxide with formation of carboxyhaemoglobin which does not carry oxygen and also interferes with the release of oxygen from oxyhaemoglobin to peripheral tissue. Poisoning is characterized by headache, convulsions, coma and respiratory failure. The speed of symptom development depends on the concentration of carbon monoxide in the air. At high concentration, unconsciousness may occur early. Persons poisoned with carbon monoxide have cherry-coloured skin and mucous. Treatment requires breathing of pure oxygen. If necessary, artificial ventilation with pure oxygen should be applied, which improves haemoglobin oxygenation and increases supply of oxygen dissolved in plasma to the peripheral tissues. Red blood cell transfusion is also of value. The patient must be absolutely quiet. If cerebral oedema develops, diuretics and corticosteroids should be administered. Hyperbaric oxygen is helpful in serious cases of carbon monoxide poisoning.

PESTICIDES (insecticides, fungicides, rodenticides, molluscicides, acaricides, herbicides). These are mostly chlorinated diphenyls or chlorinated polycyclic compounds. They are soluble in lipids and organic solvents. Insecticides enter the body through skin, gastrointestinal tract and by inhalation. Signs of poisoning are nausea, vomiting, headache, dizziness, excitement, muscular tremor, central nervous system hyperexcitability, clonic or tonic convulsions, delirium, coma and depression of the central nervous system. Treatment includes induction of vomiting, gastric lavage, charcoal, anticonvulsives and artificial ventilation when necessary. Sympathomimetics should be avoided due to increased myocardial susceptibility.

CHOLINESTERASE INHIBITORS. Most of these compounds are organic phosphates (parathion, malathion, gution), and others are carbamates (carbaril, mactacid). Their toxicity varies. They are prepared for use by dilution with organic solvents and water. Toxic effects occur after absorption from skin, gastrointestinal tract, or inhalation. Toxicity is consequence of acetylcholine accumulation on parasympathetic and motor nerve endings, autonomic ganglions and in the central nervous system, where it is characterized by respiratory depression and coma. Toxic muscarinic effect is manifested by nausea, miosis, sweating, salivation and lacrimation. Nicotinic effects include muscular cramps, fasciculation, fatigue and flaccid paralysis. Nerve poisons mostly inhibit cholinesterase and cause similar clinical features. Patients should be evacuated from the site of poisoning and atropine should be administered in high doses. Treatment consists of induction of vomiting, gastric lavage, charcoal administration and washing of skin with water if poison entered the body by this route. Atropine is applied to block the parasympathetic and central nervous system effects, in the initial dose of 0.5 mg i.v. and simultaneously 1.5 mg i.m. After that a dose of 2 mg is repeated every 10 min until parasympathetic effects are controlled. Atropine is often ineffective against the autonomic ganglion action of acetylcholine and against peripheral muscle paralysis. Oxime releases cholinesterase from its bond with organophosphorus compounds, and this reduces muscular weakness and respiratory paralysis. Pralidoxime is administered intravenously in a dose of 1 g every 8 to 12 h. If cholinesterase inhibition is due to carbamates, pralidoxime is not effective. Symptomatic therapy includes artificial ventilation, anticonvulsives, diazepam orphenobarbital, and if necessary tracheal aspiration (4).

CYANIDES. Toxicity is due to the reaction of cyanide with the trivalent iron of cytochrome oxidase, with consequential blocking of electron transport and inhibition of oxygen utilization in tissues. Signs of poisoning are headache, dizziness, nausea, drowsiness, hypotension, dyspnoea, electrocardiographic changes and convulsion. The breath of the victims has a characteristic bitter almond odour. Amyl nitrate is inhaled every 2 min until blood pressure falls to 80 mmHg. Infusion of 10 ml of 3% sodium nitrite is given over a period of 3 min. Simultaneous infusion of norepinephrine may be useful to maintain blood pressure. Artificial ventilation with 100% oxygen is applied. Therapy should be guided by the methemoglobin value, which should not exceed 40%.

FLUORIDES. These are cellular poisons which inhibit enzymatic reactions, among others degradation of glucose. With calcium they form precipitates and cause hypocalcaemia. In an acid medium fluorides form hydrofluoric acid which is corrosive. Ingestion is followed by nausea, vomiting, diarrhoea, and abdominal pain. Inhalation causes cough, cyanosis and pulmonary oedema. Hypocalcaemia results in hyperirritability, fasciculations, tremors, spasms and convulsions. Death is due to respiratory paralysis or circulatory collapse. Acute poisoning with ingested fluorides is treated with gastric lavage, vomiting, local administration of charcoal. Infusion of 10% calcium gluconate is applied for prevention of hypocalcaemia.

HERBICIDES. Poisons in this group include paraquat and 2.4 dichlorphenoxyacetic acid. Paraquat is a compound used diluted in water as a herbicide. Poisoning causes refractory pulmonary oedema within 24 h. Its metabolism may also provoke pulmonary lesions. Pulmonary fibrosis is a likely sequela in survivors. Treatment includes induction of vomiting, gastric lavage, charcoal or dissolved bentonite 48 h after ingestion (paraquat resorption from gastrointestinal tract is slow and lengthy). Paraquat is effectively removed by forced diuresis, haemodialysis and haemoperfusion. Oxygen administration should be avoided because changes in the lungs may develop (5, 6).

HALOGENATED HYDROCARBONS. Substances in this group are carbon tetrachloride, ethylene dichloride, methyl halide and trichlorethylene. They are lipid soluble and produce cell damage either directly or after conversion to metabolites. Poisonings are most frequently caused by carbon tetrachloride either from inhalation, ingestion or percutaneous absorption. Absorption in the gastrointestinal tract is increased with concomitant use of fats and alcohol. After ingestion, abdominal pain, haematemesis and frequently signs of hepatic lesion develop. Inhalation leads to irritation of upper respiratory tract. Symptoms are nausea, vomiting, headache, dizziness, and in severe poisonings stupor, convulsions, coma, respiratory failure and hypotension. Besides the central nervous system effects, signs of parenchymal damage (centrilobular necrosis with icterus), renal lesion (acute tubular necrosis), pancreatitis and necrosis of adrenal gland occur. Treatment comprises induction of vomiting and gastric lavage. Haemodialysis and haemoperfusion might help in removal of carbon tetrachloride and trichlorethane. Due to increased myocardial susceptibility, sympathomimetics should be avoided.

FORMALDEHYDE. This gas, or solution (formalin), causes cellular lesions due to a chemical reaction with cellular constituents. Poisoning is characterized by nausea and vomiting, diarrhoea and abdominal pain. Metabolic acidosis, collapse and coma develop, and death is due to circulatory failure. Treatment includes ingestion of milk, soup or any organic substance which deactivates formaldehyde. Gastric lavage and induction of vomiting are contraindicated. For correction of metabolic acidosis, infusion of sodium bicarbonate may be administered.

MUSHROOMS. *Amanita muscaria* causes a muscarinic type of poisoning with signs of parasympathetic stimulation: lacrimation, pupillary constriction, salivation, nausea, vomiting, diarrhoea, bronchorrhoea, dyspnoea, bradycardia and hypotension. In severe poisoning, muscular tremors, confusion, excitement and delirium develop. Symptoms of atropine poisoning are rare. With appropriate symptomatic therapy the patient will in most cases recover completely. *Amanita phalloides* contains alpha amanitin, and less toxic phaloidin. Alpha amanitin inhibits RNA polymerase, which hinders synthesis of messenger RNA. Toxins cause parenchymal lesions of liver and kidneys and damage to striped muscles and brain. Poisonings with this kind of mushrooms are characterized by vomiting, diarrhoea and circulatory collapse. Headache, convulsions and coma may develop. Parenchymal lesions lead to hepatocellular icterus or acute renal failure. In poisonings with parasympathomimetic manifestations, atropine is applied every 30 min until symptoms are controlled. When poisoning is caused by cytotoxic mushrooms, fluid and electrolyte balance must be maintained. Hypoglycaemia should be avoided, and symptomatic therapy for convulsions, pain relief and hypotension administered. Thioctic acid and cytochrome-C are supposedly antidotes of alpha amanitin, but this has not been confirmed. In past years administration of penicillin and silibinine has been emphasized, since they are competitive inhibitors of toxin binding to cellular membrane and they prevent parenchymal lesions (7).

PHENOLS. This group comprises, besides phenol, cresols, creosote, hexachlorphene, hydroquinone, lysol, resorcinol and tanninic acid. They are used as antiseptics or caustics. Toxicity is effected through denaturation of cellular proteins. Corrosive action damages skin and mucous. After the initial phase of hyperpnoea, stupor, convulsions and coma occur. Parenchymal lesions are most frequent in liver and kidneys. Treatment consists of administration of olive oil and charcoal. In case of glottal oedema, intubation or tracheotomy is performed.

ALCOHOLS

a) *Glycols*. Ethylene glycol and diethylene glycol are used in antifreeze. They are metabolized in the presence of alcohol dehydrogenase to aldehyde and subsequently to oxalate. These metabolites are responsible for the glycol toxicity. Initial symptoms resemble those of alcoholic intoxication and progress with vomiting to stupor, coma, convulsions and loss of reflexes. Tachypnoea, bradycardia, metabolic acidosis and hypocalcaemia commonly occur. Occasionally, pulmonary oedema or acute renal failure may develop. Treatment is intravenous administration of ethyl alcohol with maintenance of serum concentration of 10 mg/dl, by which alcohol dehydrogenase metabolizes ethyl alcohol. Intravenous pyridoxine, 100 mg i.v., and thiamine, 100 mg i.v., enable conversion to nontoxic metabolites and avoid formation of oxalates. Haemodialysis eliminates glycol well, acidosis is corrected by bicarbonate administration, and hypocalcaemia by calcium infusion.

b) *Isopropyl alcohol*. Its ingestion produces gastric irritation and danger of vomiting with aspiration. Systemic effects are similar to those of ethyl alcohol, but much more potent. Treatment is induction of vomiting, gastric lavage, and symptomatic therapy as appropriate.

c) *Methyl alcohol*. Methyl alcohol is used as a solvent and antifreeze. In the presence of alcohol dehydrogenase, methanol is metabolized to formaldehyde and later to formic acid. These metabolites are responsible for the toxicity of methyl alcohol. There is a particular affinity for optic nerve and retina. Metabolic acidosis is partly the consequence of accumulation of formic acid, and partly of the inhibition of enzymes involved in the oxidation of carbohydrates. Poisonings are characterized by nausea, vomiting, dizziness, headache and vasomotor disturbances. Depression of the central nervous system and respiratory failure develop. Visual disturbances range from blurring vision to blindness. Induction of vomiting and gastric lavage are useful during the first 2 h after ingestion. Large amounts of bicarbonates should be used for correction of metabolic acidosis. Methanol concentration of 50 mg/dl is indication for haemodialysis. Concentration of 20-50 mg/dl demands administration of ethyl alcohol, since alcohol dehydrogenase has a greater affinity for ethyl than methyl alcohol. Ethyl alcohol concentration should be approximately 100 mg/dl, which is achieved by adding 1 g of ethyl alcohol to 5% glucose intravenously over 30 min.

ETHYL ALCOHOL. Ethyl alcohol is metabolized by alcohol dehydrogenase in the liver, and subsequently by catalase in mitochondria and via microsomal oxidation. Clinical features range from drunkenness, characterized by uncoordination of movement and gait, excitement, and in advanced stage stupor and coma. Sometimes a small amount of alcohol may provoke excitation with an outburst of anger, aggressiveness and destructive behaviour, followed by deep sleep, either spontaneous or after sedation. The patient may have no memory of what happened. This state is referred to as "pathologic intoxication". It should be emphasized that the diagnosis of alcoholic coma in the comatose patients with alcohol fetor is made only after exclusion of all other causes of coma.

Mild to moderate degree of intoxication demands no special treatment. Cold shower and forced activity might be helpful, but there is no evidence that they decrease alcohol concentration in the blood. "Pathologic intoxication" may require administration of 10 mg diazepam, repeated once in 20 min. Alcoholic stupor demands no therapy. In the case of coma with respiratory depression, artificial ventilation should be applied. Haemodialysis effectively removes ethyl alcohol from the blood, but it is indicated when alcohol concentration is 500 mg/dl. In metabolic acidosis, bicarbonate is administered.

SEDATIVES. These drugs include two major groups. One comprises barbiturates, bromides, chloral hydrate and paraldehyde, the other meprobamate, other glycerol derivatives and benzodiazepine.

BARBITURATES. According to their action duration they are subdivided into short-acting (hexobarbitone), intermediate-acting (pentobarbitone and cyclobarbitone) and long-acting (phenobarbitone and allobarbitone). Concomitant use of alcohol and barbiturates has an additive effect on symptoms. There are three grades of acute barbiturate intoxication. In the first grade intoxication the patient is drowsy and asleep; he can be roused by calling his name loudly, and reflexes and vital signs are not affected. Moderate or second grade intoxication is characterized by more severe consciousness disturbance, deep reflexes are absent, and respiration is slow. The patient can be roused by vigorous manual stimulation, and when awakened he is dysarthric and confused. In the third grade intoxication, the patient is comatose, he cannot be roused, respiration is slow and shallow, cyanosis, tachycardia, signs of circulatory insufficiency and hypothermia may develop. Treatment consists of induction of vomiting and gastric lavage. In mild or moderate intoxication, no additional procedures are needed. Severe intoxications frequently demand artificial ventilation. Positive pressure in artificial ventilation reduces the incidence of atelectases and subsequent complications. Forced diuresis with more than 5 l glucosaline and urine alkalization to pH 8.2 speeds the barbiturate removal. Haemodialysis removes considerable amounts of barbiturates, and it is applied in deep coma when mentioned procedures have no effect.

Diazepoxide, diazepam and clonazepam are frequently prescribed, thus intoxications occur frequently. Clinical features are confusion, slurred speech, ataxia, drowsiness, respiratory depression, and in older people excitement and coma may develop. Therapy consists of induction of vomiting, gastric lavage, correction of fluid and electrolyte balance, and artificial ventilation as necessary. Flumazenyl is an antidote which rouses the patient (8).

MEPROBAMATE. Meprobamate is a derivative of carbonic acid. Intoxication is manifested by drowsiness, ataxia, stupor, coma and vasomotor collapse. Treatment consists of induction of vomiting or gastric lavage, correction of fluid and electrolyte balance. Artificial ventilation is applied as needed. Haemodialysis and haemoperfusion remove a considerable amount of the substance from the blood.

ANTIPSYCHOTICS. Antipsychotics include phenothiazines, butyrophenones, rauwolfia alkaloids and tioxantines. Commonly used phenothiazines are chlorpromazine, prochlorperazine, promazine, triflupromazine and trifluoperazine. Intoxication is characterized by extrapyramidal symptoms, ataxia, carpopedal spasms, drowsiness, hypothermia, respiratory failure and coma. Treatment includes gastric lavage and induction of vomiting. In extrapyramidal symptoms, intravenous infusion of diphenhydramine 2-3 mg/kg is administered, and in convulsions diazepam 10 mg. Fluid and electrolyte balance should be maintained.

ANTIDEPRESSIVES. These drugs include 3-cyclic antidepressives and monoaminooxidase inhibitors. The 3-cyclic antidepressants comprise imipramine, amitrityline, desipramine, nortryptyline, protryptyline and doxepine. These anticholinergic drugs may cause orthostatic hypotension, urine retention, excitation of the central nervous system, agitation, restlessness and respiratory depression. Treatment is induction of vomiting, gastric lavage, maintenance of fluid and electrolyte balance, and intravenous infusion of 2 mg physostigmine salicylate repeatedly after 20-60 min.

NITROUS GASES. Nitrous gases are combined nitrous oxides. Poisonings occur in cases of fire or explosion. Signs of poisonings appear after 6-12 h and they include respiratory tract irritation, cough, dyspnoea and development of noncardiogenic pulmonary oedema. Treatment includes evacuation of the victim from the poisoning site, resting and oxygen administration.

Role of extracorporeal procedures

A number of studies have described extracorporeal removal of drugs and poisons (9). However, these procedures are questionable, since according to some authors they do not reduce mortality in acutely poisoned patients (10). In our institute, extracorporeal elimination of drugs was performed when supportive therapy could not maintain circulation and respiration. Hypoventilation and hypotension were indications for extracorporeal procedures in emergencies. Specific findings, e.g. previous respiratory disorders (chronic bronchitis, emphysema or lethal drug concentration in the blood) represented an additional indication. The use of extracorporeal removal in drug poisonings is limited by a large distribution volume of some substances. However, this is of a relative importance since there is evidence that clinical features can be significantly affected by extracorporeal procedures in these conditions (11, 12). According to previous descriptions and to our experience, such removal of ethylene glycol and methanol proved to be of vital importance (13). The role of extracorporeal circulation in mushroom poisoning with a long incubation period has been exaggerated, particularly in our country. Removal of toxins by plasmapheresis and haemoperfusion is not disputable, but it has little clinical significance. Conversely, our results confirm significant value of competitive inhibition of either penicillin or silibinine (14). Intoxication with substances like paraquat or poisons with high metabolite toxicity warrant prompt application of an appropriate extracorporeal procedure. Emphasis should be placed on urine alkalization in some drug poisonings (barbiturates) and on additional procedures such as ethyl alcohol administration for competitive inhibition of alcohol dehydrogenase, which results in methanol and ethylene glycol excretion rather than degradation. Acute poisonings remain a field of particular interest in the intensive care unit. Recognition of the poison or drug, clinical features, symptomatic measures, antidotes and removal of toxic substances are essential for the achievement of positive outcome. Once developed irreversible changes in tissues preclude any possibility of successful treatment and may result in lethal outcome, despite all procedures available in an equipped intensive care unit.

References

1. Robertson WO (1994) Coping with poisonings in 1994. Liječ Vjesn (S)1:41-43
2. Gašparović V, Gjurašin M, Ivanović D, Kvarantan M, Radonić R, Merkler M, Puljević D, Pišl Z (1994) Acute poisonings - frequency and prognosis. Liječ Vjesn (S)1:44-46
3. Kulig K (1992) Initial management of ingestion of toxic substances. N Engl J Med 326: 1677-1681
4. Minton NA, Virginia Murrau SG (1988) A review of organophosphate poisoning. Med Toxicol 3:350-375
5. Dearnaley DP, Martin MFR (1978) Plasmapheresis for paraquat poisoning. Lancet 162-162
6. Miller J, Sanders E, Webb (1978) Plasmapheresis for paraquat poisoning. Lancet 875-876
7. Vesconi S, Langer M, Iapichino G, Costantino D, Busi C, Fiume L (1985) Therapy of cytotoxic mushroom intoxication. Crit Care Med 13;5:402-406
8. Kulka PJ, Lauven PM (1992) Benzodiazepine antagonists. An update of their role in the emergency care of overdose patients. Drug Safety 7(5):381-386
9. Gelfand MC, Winchester JF, Knepshield JH (1980) Hemoperfusion is indicated for severe drug overdose? In: Schreiner GE (ed) Controversies in nephrology 1980. Arlington, pp 210-218
10. Garell S, Lorch JA (1981) Hemoperfusion for poisoning: who needs it? In: Schreiner GE (ed) Controversies in nephrology 1980. Arlington, pp 219-230

11. Trafford JAP, Jones RH, Evans, Sharpstone P (1977) Hemoperfusion with R-004 Amberlite resin for treating amitriptyline poisoning. Br Med J 2:1435
12. Duraković Z, Plavšić F, Ivanović D, Gašparović V, Gjurašin M (1982) Resin hemoperfusion in the treatment of trycyclic antidepressant overdose. J Art Org 6:205-207
13. Duraković Z, Gašparović V, Plavšić F (1990) Otrovanje etilen glikolom liječeno hemodijalizom. Arh hig rada toksikol 41:201-207
14. Gašparović V, Puljević D, Radonić R, Gjurašin M, De Wolf F, Pišl Z (1990) Poisoning with mushrooms with long period of incubation. Liječ Vjesn 113:16-20

LARYNGEAL MASK IN CLINICAL ANAESTHESIA

The Role of the Laryngeal Mask in Clinical Practice

A.I.J. Brain, J.R. Brimacombe

Introduction

The laryngeal mask airway (LMA) fills a niche between the face mask (FM) and tracheal tube (TT) in terms of both anatomical position and degree of invasiveness. It has gained widespread acceptance as a general purpose airway and several advanced uses have been described. Recent published data from large studies has confirmed the safety and efficacy of the device for spontaneous or controlled ventilation (1-3). It is also proving cost effective compared with the TT (1, 4). Currently there are in excess of 900 publications, the majority in peer review journals. A number of general (5) and specialized reviews have been published analyzing its use for critical care medicine (6), pre-hospital care (7), neonatal resuscitation (8) and the difficult airway (9).

The current review discusses some of the problems with the LMA literature, focusing on concerns about aspiration. Its potential role in the difficult airway, emergency and intensive care medicine, and neonatal resuscitation will also be briefly discussed.

Concept

Prior to the introduction of the LMA, airway management was primarily restricted to the use of either an FM or TT. From an engineering viewpoint, the way these artificial airways are connected to the respiratory tract is less than ideal (10). Historically, there have been a number of designs in which the lower end of the airway fitted near the larynx, but the LMA is the first to combine ease of insertion with reliability of airway seal. The LMA was designed in 1981 following anatomical studies of the upper airway in human cadavers. It evolved from the search for an airway that was more practical than the face mask (FM), less invasive than the tracheal tube (TT) and could be used as an airway intubator. The LMA became commercially available in the UK in 1988 following an extensive research and development programme which included 60 different prototypes.

Advantages and disadvantages

A meta-analysis of randomized prospective trials conduced by one of the authors revealed that the LMA had 13 significant advantages and four disadvantages compared with the TT and four significant advantages and one disadvantage compared with the FM (11). Advantages over the TT included: increased speed and ease of placement by inexperienced personnel; increased speed of placement by anaesthetists; improved haemodynamic stability at induction and during emergence; minimal rise in intraocular pressure following insertion; reduced anaesthetic requirements for airway tolerance; lower frequency of coughing during emergence; improved oxygen saturation during emergence; and lower incidence of sore throat in adults. Advantages over the FM included: easier placement by inexperienced personnel; improved oxygen saturation during emergence; less hand fatigue; and improved operating conditions during minor paediatric otological surgery. Disadvantages over the TT were lower seal pressures and a higher frequency of gastric insufflation. The only disadvantage compared with the FM was that oesophageal reflux was more likely. It was not possible to assess the significance of these findings in terms of patient outcome.

Safety and efficacy

There have been several large scale studies confirming the safety of efficacy of the LMA. A prospective study of 1500 LMA uses revealed a first time insertion rate of 95.5% with an overall failure rate after three attempts of 0.4% (12). Problems occurred in 6.27%, but oxygen saturation fell below 90% on only ten occasions and below 80% on one occasion. Van Damme studied 5000 day case patients and found the LMA successful in over 99.9% of patients and in only 1.5% was the minimum oxygen saturation less than 90% (1). Braun and Fritz reported its use in 3000 children with a 0.1% incidence of serious complications (3). The anaesthesia department of the first hospital in the world to purchase LMAs estimate uses now totaling over 50000 without mortality or serious morbidity (13). Anaesthesiologists working at this hospital consider they have achieved this remarkable record by simply adhering to the basic contraindications published by the manufacture. Recently in an effort to obtain data in a large patient cohort, an audit of 11910 patients was carried out in the Royal Berkshire Hospital, UK (2). This prospective audit offers the first documented evidence supporting the accumulated experience of district general hospitals in the UK and confirms the safety of the device in both spontaneously breathing ($n = 6674$, 56%) and ventilated patients ($n = 5236$, 44%). There was no statistical difference in complication rate between ventilated or spontaneously breathing patients and no patient required treatment in the intensive therapy unit for complications related to use of the device.

Problems with the LMA literature

It is clear that the scientific appraisal of the LMA is complicated by the existence of a learning curve extending well beyond the experience level of many of those taking part in controlled trials designed to evaluate the device (12, 14). Recent work has shown that there is a 25-fold reduction in the number of problems which occur during the first 75 insertions using the standard technique (Lopez-Gil, p.c., 1995). In a major review, Asai and Morris state that "the true features and role of the LMA will be established only through studies in which the device is used correctly" (5). It has been suggested that adult studies in which first time insertion rates are less than 90%, overall success rates are less than 95%, or median fibreoptic scoring is less than 3.0, may reflect suboptimal use (12).

Data from some large scale studies is limited by the lack of controls and complications were being recorded only when clinically evident. This may in part explain the low complication rate reported in some large series and it is also possible that under-reporting might have occurred. On the other hand, it could equally be argued that there is little merit in recording complications not achieving clinical significance. In addition, more rigorous studies carried out by inexperienced users – which have tended to reveal higher complication rates – may themselves carry less significance if there is a possibility that lack of experience is influencing results. However, carefully a trial is designed and executed, variable user proficiency is likely to invalidate conclusions if the outcome of parameters studied is influenced by user skill.

Future trials

How then can one find a valid method for assessing the intrinsic – as opposed to the learning curve associated – problems related to LMA use? The first step is to recognize the existence of a learning curve, assessing existing publications and designing future studies accordingly. Secondly, it is necessary to agree a standard method of use – particularly of device insertion, fixation and removal – before comparing the results of different patient groups. Although there is evidence that the standard technique is optimal in adults (15), alternatives continue to be described and promoted. Few of the alternative techniques have been tested in randomized controlled trials and, in situations where controlled trials have been attempted, the correct application of the standard technique has not been ensured. It has been suggested that authors should describe the level of experience of personnel placing the LMA and where possible fibreoptic scoring should be conducted (16).

The risk of aspiration

The presence of the mask in the pharynx and the stimulation provoked by insertion inevitably involve the upper gastrointestinal tract reflexes. The degree to which these complex reflexes are aroused depends on the level of anaesthesia and the strength of the applied stimulus, but in addition the nature and quality of the reflex pattern may vary from a more or less coordinated swallow reflex to a more or less coordinated retching or vomiting reflex. For these reasons, the author has always emphasized the need to imitate the physiology of deglutition when inserting the device, in order to arouse a synchronized deglutitive response rather than an uncoordinated or incomplete response, or the even less desirable responses associated with reflux/retching/vomiting. The pharynx contains mechano- and chemo-receptors which play a part in triggering the primary peristaltic wave of deglutition. However, inappropriate stimulation or bypassing of these trigger zones may produce a less coordinated response including secondary peristalsis which lacks both the speed of completion and the coordination of primary peristalsis and can result in relaxation of the lower oesophageal sphincter without subsequent immediate restoration of tone. These effects are complicated by anaesthesia and a further complication is introduced if a local anaesthetic is applied to the mask.

The physiologic interaction between the LMA and the upper gastrointestinal tract has been recently reviewed (17). It has been known for nearly 40 years that sustained distension of the pharynx induced prolonged relaxation of the lower oesophageal sphincter (LOS) (18). There is some evidence from dye studies (19, 20), one study using a pressure probe pull-through technique (21), and two studies using an oesophageal pH probe (20, 22) that LOS tone may be reduced with the LMA when compared to the FM (19-21) or TT (22). However, this theory remains controversial (23-25), and both repeat dye and pH studies in both ventilated and spontaneously breathing patients (26-30) have failed to confirm these findings. The variable figures found in the differing studies may simply reflect the sensitivities of the detection techniques or the skill of the LMA users (25). One factor preventing aspiration may be the persistent function of the upper oesophageal sphincter (UOS). Although the correctly placed LMA tip lies against the UOS, the presence of a mass above the UOS does not necessarily cause it to relax (31). A recent study has suggested that the pharyngo-upper oesophageal sphincter contractile reflex may be enhanced in awake humans (32) and Vanner et al. showed that during spontaneous ventilation anaesthesia UOS pressure does not fall significantly with an LMA in situ (33). This together with the known constrictor reflex of the UOS in response to the presence of acid fluids in the lower oesophagus might explain why acid reflux into the lower oesophagus so rarely results in aspiration during LMA use. In addition, it may be that the presence of the mask blocks passage of alkaline secretions from the upper pharynx from reaching the lower oesophagus. This might explain the greater incidence of acid reflux detected by the use of pH probes when the LMA is compared with the face mask.

A meta-analysis of published literature suggested that the overall incidence of pulmonary aspiration was in the region of 2 per 10000 and similar to that for the tracheal tube and face mask for elective surgery (34). More recently large scale epidemiological studies have confirmed this estimates (1-3). There have been ten confirmed pulmonary aspiration events from published case reports and most cases had one or more predisposing factors. No death or permanent disability occurred.

Difficult airway

Much has been written about the use of the LMA in airway rescue situations and there can be no doubt that it can be life saving in the "failed intubation, failed face-mask ventilation situation" (9). It has been demonstrated in controlled studies that ease of insertion is independent of Mallampati (35) and Cormack and Lehane scoring (35), and is unaffected by manual-in-line traction (36) or the presence of a hard collar (37). Verghese and Brimacombe have estimated the frequency for airway rescue was 1:8300 (2). The nature of such situations precludes evaluation by clinical trial and one is obliged to assess the potential of the device by reference to case reports ($n > 65$). It could be argued that the accumulation of such reports can reach a point beyond which it is no longer appropriate to use the word anecdotal, however the quality of such pooled data is always limited by the possibility that an unknown number of adverse events (i.e. failed LMA use in airway rescue) may have occurred in similar situations but have not been published. One of the authors (AB) can only refer to his own experience during the prolonged development phase (1981-8) when the LMA in various prototype forms was used on 23 occasions where difficulty with intubation was encountered by himself or colleagues. Only one of these cases turned out to be impossible to ventilate with the device because of failed placement and this case was easily ventilated by face mask. This raises the question of whether patients known to be difficult to intubate should be managed with an LMA. Most authors feel this is a contraindication to LMA use (38) and the American Task Force on the Difficult Airway currently recommends awake intubation as the preferred option (39). The authors are unconvinced that this approach is necessarily always correct, fearing that to attempt intubation in someone in whom this is known to be difficult may itself represent an unnecessary risk if the LMA is not otherwise contraindicated. The LMA may be a useful adjunct to awake intubation or may be used to secure the airway prior to induction of anaesthesia.

Emergency medicine

The LMA was first used to resuscitate a patient who suffered a cardiac arrest by a nurse in the Intensive Therapy Unit of St Andrews Hospital in London using a prototype in 1983. As studies showing the relative ease of LMA use by inexperienced personnel began to appear following the launch of the commercial device (40-42) it began to look as if the speed and high success rate it offered might weigh more heavily in the balance than the known lack of protection afforded against aspiration. A pilot study was carried out by Leach et al. which suggested that nurses could easily be taught the technique and that aspiration did not appear to be a major concern (43). Subsequently a multicentre trial was carried out which confirmed these findings, yielding an aspiration rate of 0.4% - the patient concerned being one of the survivors (44). Numbers were too small to reveal any outcome significance, but it was shown that early ventilation could be effectively carried out by non-physicians before the arrival of the resuscitation team. Recently, Grantham et al. trained 30 ambulance officers in the use of the LMA and 233 insertions were attempted in the field over a 12 month period (45). The LMA provided an effective airway in 90% of patients sufficiently comatose to compromise airway care and soiling occurred in ten patients.

As a result of these reports, the concept of training health care workers to use the LMA as part of the Advanced Life Support Training is gradually gaining acceptance in the UK. The utility of the device in CPR is not as a replacement for the TT but as a better alternative than the FM until such time as intubation-competent personnel are available. In Australia and Japan the LMA is already in regular use in some regions by ambulance personnel for pre-hospital care (46). A dedicated LMA is currently being designed which may be more appropriate for emergency use as well as for difficult intubation (47).

Intensive therapy unit

The ideal requirements for any airway device used in this setting are reliability in terms of airway patency and fixation stability, effective protection against aspiration of gastric contents or other secretions, low airflow resistance, lack of trauma when used over a period of days or weeks, ease of insertion and replacement in case of accidental dislodgement, good patient acceptance, preservation of an effective cough reflex and absence of infection transmission risk. Clearly no existing device can claim to fulfil all these desiderata. The LMA does not protect the airway against aspiration of gastric fluids, although it is effective in preventing oral secretions/blood from reaching the larynx and trachea (48). Airway resistance is lower in terms of gas flow since the LMA tube is shorter and wider than the corresponding TT, but because the larynx is not bypassed, overall work of breathing is similar (38). Perhaps the most interesting potential benefit from LMA use in ICU is the lack of interference with the muco-ciliary clearance mechanism, permitting effective coughing in contrast to the endotracheal tube. This subject has not yet been formally studied. However another feature, the relative tolerance of the device compared to the TT is well documented in terms of recovery characteristics and pressor response to insertion and this aspect has led to recent descriptions of use in patients in respiratory failure who would not tolerate an TT (49, 50). Prototypes are currently being assessed which may be more appropriate for ICU use, having both an improved seal and the ability to separate the gastrointestinal and respiratory tracts, potentially reducing the risk of aspiration (51). The LMA has been used for airway rescue (52), bronchoscopy (53) and for endoscopic guided percutaneous tracheostomy in the ICU setting (54).

Neonatal resuscitation

Although the larynx has important differences in the neonate from the adult, study of the neonatal pharynx and hypopharynx during early development work on the LMA indicated that the basic LMA design was likely to be appropriate in neonates. It is well known that neonatal airway management is difficult, even for those with advanced airway control skills. In theory, the LMA offers several advantages over the FM during neonatal resuscitation. It avoids the necessity to form a seal on a slippery surface and manipulation of the head, neck and jaw is not required. It avoids pressure to the eyes and it may free the operator to perform other tasks such as CPR or administer drugs. The advantages over the TT include avoidance of laryngoscopy and its associated adverse effects, less invasion of the respiratory tract and avoidance of the risks of endobronchial or oesophageal intubation. An attenuated haemodynamic stress response to LMA insertion is likely and this may be important in preventing intraventicular haemorrhage. Furthermore, placement is probably independent of factors governing facial and upper airway anatomy making the LMA particularly useful in the "cannot intubate, cannot ventilate" situation in neonates. Tracheal intubation may also cause laryngeal oedema and in the newborn 1 mm of oedema reduces the cross sectional area of the larynx by 65% (55). However, potential limitations of the LMA are that it may not be suitable for removal of meconium aspirate and may be inadequate for neonates who require high airway pressures – in these situations it is not a substitute for an TT.

In a prospective pilot study of neonates born with apnoea or heart rate < 110 min^{-1}, experienced LMA users were able to resuscitate 20/20 neonates with the LMA at the first attempt (56). Mean time for LMA insertion was < 9 seconds and peak circuit pressure was 37 cm H_2O. Oxygenation and restoration of heart rate occurred in most neonates within 30 seconds. Other groups have also reported a rapid increase in oxygen saturation for neonates resuscitated with the LMA (57). Our experience is similar and extends to 39/40 successful resuscitations (58). Three of these neonates weighed 1-1.5 kg (59). Denny et al. used an LMA to successfully resuscitate a 2.75 kg neonate with Pierre-Robin syndrome in whom intubation and face-mask ventilation had failed (60).

Conclusions

The principal factors limiting LMA use in anaesthesiology are the degree of user experience, availability of skilled teaching and/or supervision and known contraindications. Seven years of use of the LMA in the UK has seen steady growth in popularity in an expanding range of applications within the field of anaesthesiology. In spite of a usage rate which may represent approximately 40% of all non-emergency anaesthetics administered in the UK today, no cases of fatality associated with use of the device have yet been reported to the manufacturer or described in the international literature. However, the author wishes to emphasize that this may have as much to do with the high quality and extensive training of UK anaesthesiologists as with the characteristics of the device itself. All new users regardless of seniority should limit their initial experience to the shortest and simplest cases in ASA 1 patients and ensure that very careful and thorough attention is payed to the instruction materials issued with the device. Further research is clearly required to help define the place of the LMA in emergency and intensive care medicine and to decide the safety issues in this context and the level of initial and continued training needed. Training in its use should be considered by anyone involved in airway management and particularly by emergency room and intensive care unit personnel.

References

1. Van Damme E (1994) Die Kehlopfmaske in der ambulanten Anästhesie - Eine Auswertung von 5000 ambulanten Narkosen. Anaesthesiol Intensivmed Notfallmed Schmerzther 29: 284-286
2. Verghese C, Brimacombe J (1995) Survey of laryngeal mask usage in 11,910 patients - safety and efficacy for conventional and nonconventional usage. Anesth Analg (in press)
3. Braun U, Fritz U (1994) Die Kehlopfmaske in der Kinderänasthesie. Anaesthesiol Intensivmed Notfallmed Schmerzther 29:286-288
4. Joshi GP, Smith I, Watcha MF, White PF (1995) A model for studying the cost-effectiveness of airway devices: laryngeal mask airway vs tracheal tube. Anesth Analg 80:S219 (Abstract)

5. Asai T, Morris S (1994) The laryngeal mask airway: its features, effects and role. Can J Anaesth 41:930-960
6. Brimacombe J, Berry A, Verghese C (1995) The laryngeal mask airway in critical care medicine. Intensive Care Med (in press)
7. Sasada MP, Gabbott DA (1994) The role of the laryngeal mask airway in pre-hospital care. Resuscitation 28:97-102
8. Brimacombe J, Berry A (1994) The laryngeal mask airway for obstetric anaesthesia and neonatal resuscitation. Int J Obstet Anesth 3:211-218
9. Brimacombe J, Berry A, Brain A (1995) The laryngeal mask airway. Anesthesiol Clin North Am 13:411-437
10. Brain AIJ (1991) The development of the laryngeal mask - a brief history of the invention, early clinical studies and experimental work from which the laryngeal mask evolved. Eur J Anaesthesiol 4:5-17
11. Brimacombe J (1995) Does the laryngeal mask airway offer any real advantages over the tracheal tube or facemask? A meta-analysis of randomised comparative studies. Can J Anaesth (in press)
12. Brimacombe J (1995) Analysis of 1500 laryngeal mask uses by one anaesthetist in adults undergoing routine anaesthesia. Anaesthesia (in press)
13. Leach AB, Alexander CA (1991) The laryngeal mask - an overview. Eur J Anaesthesiol 4: 19-31
14. Brain AIJ (1991) Studies on the laryngeal mask: first, learn the art. Anaesthesia 46:417-427
15. Brimacombe J, Berry A (1993) Insertion of the laryngeal mask airway - a prospective study of four techniques. Anaesth Intensive Care 21:89-92
16. Brimacombe J, Berry A (1993) Research and the laryngeal mask airway. Anesthesiology 79:411-412
17. Brimacombe J, Berry A (1995) The laryngeal mask airway - anatomical and physiological implications. Acta Anaesthesiol Scand (in press)
18. Ingelfinger FJ (1958) Esophageal motility. Physiol Rev 38:533-584
19. Barker P, Langton JA, Murphy PJ, Rowbotham DJ (1992) Regurgitation of gastric contents during general anaesthesia using the laryngeal mask airway. Br J Anaesth 69:314-315
20. Owens TM, Robertson P, Twomey C, Doyle M, McDonald N, McShane AJ (1995) The incidence of gastroesophageal reflux with the laryngeal mask: a comparison with the facemask using esophageal lumen pH electrodes. Anesth Analg 80:980-984
21. Rabey PG, Murphy PJ, Langton JA, Barker P, Rowbotham DJ (1992) Effect of the laryngeal mask airway on lower oesophageal sphincter pressure in patients during general anaesthesia. Br J Anaesth 69:346-348
22. Valentine J, Stakes AF, Bellamy MC (1994) Reflux during positive pressure ventilation through the laryngeal mask. Br J Anaesth 74:543-545
23. Vanner RG (1993) Regurgitation and the laryngeal mask airway. Br J Anaesth 70:380
24. Brimacombe J, Berry A (1994) Aspiration pneumonitis and the laryngeal mask airway. Anesth Analg 78:816
25. Brimacombe J (1995) Gastroesophageal reflux with the laryngeal mask. Anesth Analg (in press)
26. Akhtar TM, Street MK (1994) Risk of aspiration with the laryngeal mask. Br J Anaesth 72: 447-450
27. El Mikatti N, Luthra AD, Healy TEJ, Mortimer AJ (1992) Gastric regurgitation during general anaesthesia in the supine position with the laryngeal and face mask airways. Br J Anaesth 68:529P-530P (Abstract)
28. Lefort P, Visseaux H, Gabriel R, Palot M, Pire JC (1993) Utilisation du masque larynge pour la coelioscopie. Anales Francaises D'Anesthesie Reanimation 12:R231 (Abstract)
29. Hogu H, Barlas S, Dogu D, Gelis M, Ozay K, Arikan Z (1995) Regurgitation with laryngeal mask airway (LMA) and endotracheal tube (ETT). Br J Anaesth 74:14 (Abstract)

30. Joshi GP, Morrison SG, Okonkwo N, Gajraj NM, Pennant JH, White PF (1994) Continuous hypopharyngeal pH monitoring: use of laryngeal mask airway versus tracheal tube. Anesthesiology 81:A1281 (Abstract)
31. Lund WS (1987) Deglutition. In: Wright DA (ed) Scott-Brown otolaryngology basic sciences. Butterworth, London, pp 284-295
32. Shaker R, Ren J, Zamir Z, Sarna A, Liu J, Sui Z (1994) Effect of aging, position, and temperature on the threshold volume triggering pharyngeal swallows. Gastroenterology 107:396-402
33. Vanner RG, Pryle BJ, O'Dwyer JP, Reynolds F (1992) Upper oesophageal sphincter pressure during inhalational anaesthesia. Anaesthesia 47:950-954
34. Brimacombe J, Berry A (1995) The incidence of aspiration associated with the laryngeal mask airway - a meta-analysis of published literature. J Clin Anesth (in press)
35. Mahiou P, Narchi P, Veyrac P, Germond M, Gory G, Bazin G (1992) Is laryngeal mask easy to use in case of difficult intubation? Anesthesiology 77:A1228 (Abstract)
36. Brimacombe J, Berry A (1993) Laryngeal mask airway insertion. A comparison of the standard versus neutral position in normal patients with a view to its use in cervical spine instability. Anaesthesia 48:670-671
37. Pennant JH, Pace NA, Gajraj NM (1993) Role of the laryngeal mask airway in the immobile cervical spine. J Clin Anesth 5:226-230
38. Boisson-Bertrand D, Hannhart B, Rousselot JM, Duvivier C, Quilici N, Peslin R (1994) Comparative effects of laryngeal mask and tracheal tube on total respiratory resistance in anaesthetised patients. Anaesthesia 49:846-849
39. American Society of Anesthesiologists Task Force on Management of the Difficult Airway (1993). Practice guidelines for management of the difficult airway. Anesthesiology 78: 597-602
40. Wilson RC, Bodenham AR (1993) Percutaneous tracheostomy. Br J Hosp Med 49:123-126
41. Martens P (1994) The use of the laryngeal mask airway by nurses during cardiopulmonary resuscitation. Anaesthesia 49:731-732
42. Baskett PJF (1994) The use of the laryngeal mask airway by nurses during cardiopulmonary resuscitation (a reply). Anaesthesia 49:732
43. Leach A, Alexander CA, Stone B (1993) The laryngeal mask in cardiopulmonary resuscitation in a district general hospital: a preliminary communication. Resuscitation 25:245-248
44. Stone BJ, Leach AB, Alexander CA, Ruffer DR, McBeth C, Warwick JP, Baskett PJF, Nicholls E, Prior-Willeard PFS, Verghese C, Jago RH (1994) The use of the laryngeal mask airway by nurses during cardiopulmonary resuscitation – results of a multicentre trial. Anaesthesia 49:3-7
45. Grantham H, Phillips G, Gilligan JE (1994) The laryngeal mask in pre-hospital emergency care. Emerg Med 6:193-197
46. Brimacombe J (1995) Does the laryngeal mask airway have a role outside the operating theatre? Can J Anaesth 41:258-259
47. Capilla A (1995) A prototype intubating LMA. Br J Anaesth (in press)
48. Cork RC, Depa RM, Standen JR (1994) Prospective comparison of use of the laryngeal mask and endotracheal tube for ambulatory surgery. Anesth Analg 79:719-727
49. Arosio EM, Conci F (1995) Use of the laryngeal mask airway for respiratory distress in the intensive care unit. Anaesthesia 50:635-636
50. Taylor JC, Bell GT (1995) An asthmatic weaned from a ventilator using a laryngeal mask. Anaesthesia 50:454-455
51. Brain AIJ, Verghese C, Strube P, Brimacombe J (1995) A new laryngeal mask prototype - preliminary evaluation of seal pressures and glottic isolation. Anaesthesia 50:42-48
52. Lee JJ, Yau K, Barcroft J (1993) LMA and respiratory arrest after anterior cervical fusion. Can J Anaesth 40:395-396
53. Mabuchi N (1992) Laryngeal mask airway in the ICU. J Clin Experimental Med 162,12,9: 876-878

54. Dexter TJ (1994) The laryngeal mask airway: a method to improve visualisation of the trachea and larynx during fibreoptic assisted percutaneous tracheostomy. Anaesth Intensive Care 22: 35-39
55. Holinger P, Johnston K (1950) Factors responsible for laryngeal obstruction in infants. JAMA 143:1229
56. Paterson SJ, Byrne PJ, Molesky MG, Seal RF, Finucane BT (1994) Neonatal resuscitation using the laryngeal mask airway. Anesthesiology 80:1248-1253
57. Gollo E, Mutani C, Reilia P, Margaria E (1993) Primary resuscitation of the newborn. In: Abstracts of the 2nd World Congress of Perinatal Medicine, Rome, 19-24 September, p 102 (Abstract)
58. Brimacombe J (1995) Resuscitation of neonates with the laryngeal mask - a caution. Pediatrics 95:453-454
59. Brimacombe J (1994) The use of the laryngeal mask airway in very small neonates. Anesthesiology 81:1302
60. Denny NM, Desilva KD, Webber PA (1990) Laryngeal mask airway for emergency tracheostomy in a neonate. Anaesthesia 45:895

CONTROVERSIES IN THE MANAGEMENT
OF CRITICALLY ILL PATIENTS

Pancreas Dysfunction and Related Problems

G. Sganga, M. Castagneto, M. Soiat, A. Gullo

Introduction

The pathophysiological changes following severe acute pancreatitis are well known.

Whatever the etiology, the acute pancreatic inflammation contributes to morbid sequelae leading to a systemic involvement of the whole organism including multiple organ system failure.

The changes in homeostasis are caused both by the acute inflammatory reaction initiated by the enzimatic activation and by the subsequent invasion of bacteria.

Trypsinogen is activated within the pancreas very early in pancreatitis, possibly from localization of intracellular zymogen with lysosomal hydrolases or while accumulating in the interstitium.

The pathologic progression of the pancreatitis has been attributed to these activated enzymes which cause local injury and inflammation leading to edema, haemorrhage and necrosis.

Local activation of inflammatory cells could result in the systemic release of humoral mediators that could not only relate to the severity of the disease but also secondarily influence all organs and tissues.

Products of inflammation have been identified in early pancreatitis in patients including granulocyte elastase and interleukine 6 (IL-6), promptly followed by an elevation of acute phase protein and particularly of C reactive protein.

Both these inflammatory products correlate directly with severity of pancreatitis and with morbidity and mortality of the disease.

The subsequent bacterial colonization could be related to gut macromolecular permeability (1) and bacterial translocation.

The primary pancreatic inflammation represents a huge trigger for systemic reaction leading to multiple organ dysfunction syndrome (MODS) involving the lungs, the kidneys, the heart, the liver, the digestive tract, the central nervous system and the coagulation cascade.

On the other hand, the role of pancreas in the pathophysiology of MODS is more controversial.

However, pancreas is also involved in MODS, despite the fact that failure of this organ is rarely mentioned in MODS studies.

Warshaw et al., in a retrospective study (2) demonstrated an extraordinary incidence of major pancreatic injuries (pancreatitis, focal or widespread pancreatic necrosis and pancreatic abscesses) occurring in patients who have been in shock with a strong positive correlation with the presence of acute tubular necrosis.

Pancreatic lesions in shock and their significance

The extreme vulnerability of the exocrine pancreas to hypovolemic shock and ischemic injury has been found in humans after shock (3) and in experimental studies (4-6).

Extensive studies have been conducted on the rat pancreas (7). In the early phases of shock, mitochondrial swelling and high grade dilatation of granular endoplasmic reticulum (ER), followed by progressive edematous disorganization of the interstitium have been identified. Cells thus damaged will progress step by step to single cell necrosis, releasing larger amounts of lysosomial enzymes during the process.

In electron microscopic studies of pancreatic acinar cells of 22 patients immediately after death in shock (8) Jones et al. evaluated shock duration and intensity and the corresponding submicroscopic alterations. The authors then proposed staging these subcellular changes, ranging from damage of nuclear chromatin via dilatation of ER, mitochondrial swelling, dissolution and calcification, to lysosomal reactions, formation of myelin bodies, karyolysis and fragmentation of the membrane system.

Biochemical manifestations of pancreas injury after shock

The "classic" markers of pancreas damage are: serum amylase, serum lipase (9), amylase/creatinine clearance ratio and serum amylase isoenzymes. They could however be subtle or even absent. The diagnosis of pancreas damage cannot rest with certainty only upon an elevated serum amylase concentration (2). Hyperamylasemia could indeed have many non pancreatic origins and may occur in diseases affecting salivary glands, liver, intestine, genitalia, lungs or kidneys (10, 11) as well as in periods of metabolic derangements such as the postoperative state (12).

As is the case for the other three above mentioned markers whose levels are high in acute pancreatitis, the amylase/creatinine clearance ratio also rises in acute pancreatitis, but not in other diseases causing hyperamylasemia, including mild-to-moderate degrees of renal failure (13).

Pancreatic-type isoamylase is found only in the pancreas (14, 15) and an isolated increase of pancreatic isoamylase is characteristic and specific for pancreatic disease (9, 14).

The role of trypsin

Trypsin represents another specific biochemical marker of pancreatic damage.

Among the circulating forms of trypsin, a study on monitoring intensive care unit patients (16) indicated that high plasmatic levels of immunoreactive trypsin (IRT) were present in about 50% of the monitored patients, together with high values of amylase, persisting for several days and associated with lung injury and sepsis, without clinical signs of pancreatitis.

Further studies (17) on multiple injured patients showed increasing IRT serum levels in the first 24 hours after trauma, followed by a larger release on days 5 to 7, associated with the onset of sepsis. In this case, the study showed a parallel increase of lipase and amylase, indicating a deep involvement of the pancreas.

Trypsin, lipase and ARDS

Another study (18) investigated the relation between serum lipase (SL), IRT and its inhibitors in patients with ARDS of different origin.

The risults of this study showed:
- Marked and prolonged elevation in IRT and SL
- Solely pancreatic origin of IRT (pancreatomized patients showed no IRT) (19)
- High susceptibility of the pancreas to anoxia caused by either arterial PaO_2 and shock, as in ARDS.

Furthermore, other experimental studies (20) showed that in ARDS the complement activation causes aggregation and leukoembolization of granulocytes in the precapillary arteries of the mesenteries. In this case, released pancreatic enzymes are not early markers for cellular injury, but "secondary mediators" for the enhancement of the endothelial increased permeability.

Pancreas disease and coagulation system

In acute pancreatitis, especially in its most severe forms, consumption coagulopathy is commonly found with increased fibrinolysis. This condition may be associated with local deficiency of antiprotease in the peritoneal cavity and high levels of protease-antiprotease complexes in the plasma (21, 22). Because of the involvement of various protease inhibitors and the interaction of various cascade systems, identifying the activation sequence or the possible trigger mechanism is rather difficult, although trypsin is playing a major role. Most affected by changes is the peritoneal fluid, where interaction of protease and antiprotease causes local antiprotease deficiency. In severe cases, the functional capacity of antiprotease practically drops to zero, and may give rise to proteolytic reactions which are no longer limited. Activation of consumption coagulopathy and an increase in fibrinolysis (which may cause haemorrhagic complications) explain disseminated intravascular coagulation (DIC) which is found in severe forms of acute pancreatitis (23). DIC is often involved in the genesis of respiratory failure and MODS, conditions frequently associated with acute pancreatitis. Given the complexity of the various clinical pictures and the differing severity of induced coagulation disorders, the physiopathological alterations rarely lead to DIC or to massive haemorrhage. One of these events may prevail over the other; however, most often thrombotic and haemorrhagic events are more often observed occurring at the same time or in sequence. In view of this, the proper terminology should be intravascular coagulation and fibrinolysis syndrome (ICF). More frequently used in current terminology is the – albeit generic – definition of consumption coagulopathy. The pancreas plays a key role in this context, as is demonstrated by the role of the prekallikrein-kallikrein system which by bypassing the coagulation cascade and directly activating the plasminogen-plasmin system triggers off a series of events which are fundamental in the stimulation of the fibrinolytic system. In critical patient care, the pancreas is therefore to be viewed as having a central role, both as target and as trigger organ.

As to clinical and laboratory data, consumption coagulopathy involves:

- Reduced blood platelet count in medium and severe pancreatitis, especially in presence of complications; after approximately one week plate thrombosis occurs in severe forms.

- Increased prothrombin time (PT) with two-phase progression. During the first 3-5 days this is due to prothrombin consumption (80%-85% in mild forms, 70%-80% in moderate forms, 60%-70% in severe forms). After restoring of the basal value, PT increases yet again between day 9 and 12, due to reduced liver synthesis of vitamin-K-dependent factors.

- Decreased fibrinogen, in severe forms especially during the first 2-3 days. As is shown by experimental studies, fibrinogen depletion from the plasma may be associated with deposits in the lungs, kidneys, liver, pancreas and spleen. Intravascular fibrin thrombi and the early decrease in platelets indicate that intravascular coagulation (IC) contributes to increased fibrinogen catabolism in acute pancreatitis. Fibrinogen – a protein of the acute reaction phase – follows a two-phase trend, subsequently increasing until days 6 and 7 to plasma levels whose height is directly related to the severity of the pancreatitis.

- Minor decrease of factor X during the first 5 days in severe forms, with subsequent increase to levels of the order of 120%-130%.

Increased fibrinolysis involves:
- Plasminogen decrease to levels lower than 75% during the first week since the outbreak of severe forms. Consistently low levels indicate that there is continuing consumption. After infusion with streptokinase i.v., basal levels are restored in less than two days.
- Products resulting from fibrinogen degradation (FDP, D-dimers etc.) are found in the blood during the acute phase only (40% of the cases) and in the peritoneal fluid at all times.

At the plasmatic level, decreased levels of antithrombin III (ATIII) and a_2-macroglobulin (a_2M) are observed, as are increased levels of a_2-antiplasmin (a_2PI) and of the factor-C1-inhibitor of the complement (C_1INH). ATIII irreversibly inhibits trypsin, in addition to thrombin, factor X_a and plasmin. ATIII deficiency – the main endogenous inhibitor of coagulation – reduces the plasma's anticoagulating capacity and increases the risk of microthrombotic phenomena. In pathological conditions, trypsinogen released directly into the blood-stream because of lesion in the pancreas acinar cells can be converted to trypsin, and trypsin – produced in the duodenum by enterokinase – can be reabsorbed (even massively, if there is intestinal ischemia). Trypsin at first is reversibly bound to the inhibitor of a_1-proteinase (a_1PI); then it is released and bound by a_2M in a stable complex that is rapidly (5-10 min) eliminated from the blood-stream by means of the reticulo-endothelial system (RES). The decrease of a_2M in the plasma indicates that proteolytic enzymes have been activated in the blood; persisting presence of these complexes in the blood-stream indicates that there is massive proteolysis (or perhaps altered functions of RES). In severe forms of acute pancreatitis, a_2M levels decrease progressively during the first days, reaching 45% on day 3. Especially in severe cases, a_2PI increases from the initial basal values to approximately 150% at the end of the first week. The high levels of a_2PI have been related to the delay in fibrin elimination from the lungs and to respiratory failure and DIC. Despite a quantitative increase of its levels, a_2PI activity appears to be reduced due to complex formation (found in the peritoneal fluid) or degradation (possibly due to leukocytic elastase). C_1INH – which inactivates factors C_{1s}, 11_a, 12_a, plasmin and kallikrein – behaves like a protein in the acute reaction phase: after a few days it reaches plasmatic levels of the order of 150%-200% in severe forms, although – especially in these – its activity appears to be diminished.

In addition, in acute pancreatitis CI and thromboembolism of lung microcirculation also play an important role with regard to ARDS and renal failure, complications that affect 3% of the cases of acute pancreatitis and involve a mortality rate in excess of 70%.

The pancreas: target or "promoter" of MODS?

The IRT release is part of and simultaneously enhances a complex pathophysiological mechanism, including complement and coagulation cascade activation, inflammatory proenzyme activation, the consequent leukocyte activation and protein destruction, leading to the production of toxic factors and shock specific mediators (such as the miocardial depressant factor - MDF), most likely resulting from the proteolytic breakdown mechanism in intracellular pancreatic proteins. In addition to leukocyte activation, another mechanism is actively studied: the hypoperfusion-ischemia-reperfusion pathway, which leads to cellular damage, release of cellular and soluble mediators and inflammatory reaction. Hypoperfusion – which exocrine pancreas is very sensitive to – and the activation of proteolytic systems trigger off a vicious circle that is self-supporting and in which alterations in microcirculation and coagulation play an active role. These alterations contribute to the development of intravascular coagulation and thromboembolisms which can lead to clear DIC, accompanied by fibrinogen depletion, thrombopenia and reactive hyperfibrinolysis which increases the risk of haemorrhage. As to the treatment of consumption coagulopathy, currently there are no standardized intervention strategies. However, numerous clinical trials – still in the experimental stage – are currently being carried out using drugs such as ATIII, C_1INH, recombinant hirudine and long-acting recombinant hirudine, activated Protein C and gabexate mesylate. Consumption coagulopathy is often the epiphenomenon of complex clinical conditions such as sepsis and MODS; only by setting up ample multi-centre trials based on homogeneous – and therefore comparable – patient data will it in the future be possible to obtain objective data to be used as basis for specific intervention strategies.

Pancreas would not be only a "target" organ in MODS; damage to its structure would also cause the onset or, on the other hand, the enhancement of MODS.

At present, the evaluation of this new role needs further clinical and biological studies.

References

1. Ryan CM, Schmidt J, Lewandrowski K, Compton CC, Rattner DW, Warshaw AL, Tompkins RG (1993) Gut macromolecular permeability in pancreatitis correlates with severity of disease in rats. Gastroenterology 104:890-895
2. Warshaw AL, O'Hara PJ (1978) Susceptibility of the pancreas to ischemic injury in shock. Ann Surg vol 178-II:197-201
3. Hegewald G, Nikulin A, Gmaz-Nikulin E, Plamenac P, Barenwald G (1985) Ultrastructural changes of the human pancreas in acute shock. Path Res Pract 179:610-615
4. Hesch M, Gnidec AA, Bersten AD, Troster M, Rutledge FS, Sibbald WJ (1990) Histologic and ultrastructural changes in nonpulmonary organs during early hyperdinamic sepsis. Surgery 107:397-410
5. Endrich B et al (1990) Gastrointestinal microcirculation. In: Messmer K, Hammersen F (eds) Prog Appl Microcirc. Basel Karger vol 17:141-174
6. Gmaz-Nikulin E, Nikulin A, Plamenac P, Hegewald G, Gaon D (1981) Pancreatic lesions in shock and their significance. J Pathology Vol 135:223-336
7. Donath K, Mitschke H, Seifert H (1970) Ultrastrukturelle Veranderungen am Rattenpankreas beim hämorrhagischen Schock. Beitr Path Anat 141:33-51

8. Jones RT, Garcia JH, Mergner WJ, Pendergrass RE, Valigorsky JM, Trump BF (1975) Effects of shock on the pancreatic acinar cell. Arch Pathol 99:634-644
9. Fernandez-Del Castillo C, Harringer W, Warshaw AL, Vlahakes GJ, Kosky G, Zaslavsky AM, Rattner DW (1991) Risk factors for pancreatic cellular injury after cardiopulmonary bypass. N Engl J Med 325:382-387
10. Warshaw AL, Bellini CA, Lee KH (1976) Electrophoretic identification of isoenzyme of amylase which increases in serum in liver diseases. Gastroenterology 70:572
11. Warshaw AL, Fuller AF Jr (1975) Specificity of increased renal clearance of amylase in diagnosis of acute pancreatitis. N Engl J Med 292:325
12. Morrissey R, Berk JE, Fridhandler L, Pelot D (1974) Nature and significance of hyperamylasemia following operation. Ann Surg 180:67
13. Warshaw AL (1976) The kidney and its changes in amylase clearance. Gastroenterology 71;4:702-704
14. Levette MD, Ellis C, Engel RR (1977) Isoelectric focusing studies of human serum and tissues isoamylase. J Lab Clin Med 90:141
15. Warshaw AL (1977) Serum amylase isoenzyme profiles as a differential index in disease. J Lab Clin Med 90:1
16. Deby-Dupont G, Haas M, Pincemail J, Braun M, Lamy M, Deby C, Franchimont P (1984) Immunoreactive trypsin in adult respiratory distress syndrome. Intensive Care Med 10: 7-12
17. Lamy M, Deby-Dupont G (1994) The role of the pancreas in the multiple organ dysfunction syndrome. In: Hammerle AF (ed) MODS, Maudrich, Wien-Munchen-Bern, 68-69
18. Nicod L, Leuenberger PH, Seydoux C, Van Melle G, Perret CL (1985) Evidence for pancreas injury in adult respiratory distress syndrome. Am Rev Resp Dis 1131:696-699
19. Felber JP, Bambule-Dick J (1980) Radioimmunoessays of plasma trypsin in pancreatic diseases and in juvenile-onset diabetes. In: Podolsky S, Viswanathan M (eds) Secondary diabetes: the spectrum of the diabetic syndromes, Raven, New York, 180:191-196
20. Hammerschmidt DE, Harris PD, Wayland JH, Craddock PR, Jacob HS (1981) Complement-induced granulocyte aggregation in vivo. Am J Pathol 102:146-150
21. Lasson A,Ohlsson K (1986) Comsumptive coagulopathy, fibrinolysis and proteasi-antiproteasi interactions during acute human pancreatitis. Thromb Res 41(2):167-183
22. Ranson JH, Lackner H, Berman IR, Schinella R (1977) The relationship of coagulation factors to clinical complications of acute pancreatitis. Surgery 81(5):502-511
23. Clave P, Guillaumes S, Blanco I, Martines De Hurtado J, Esquius J, Marruecos L, Fontcubert AJ, Perez C, Farré A, Lluis F (1992) Splenic hematoma in acute pancreatitis. Role of coagulation disorders. Z Gastroenterol 30(8):538-542

UPDATING COMPUTER USAGE IN THE ICU

Flow of Information in the ICU - An Overview

W. KOLLER

The challenge of the information age

Information is the major capital nowadays. Also all health care providers have to cope with that fact. At the ICU bedside, the members of the therapeutical team form the link between information about a patient on one side and a correct and goal directed treatment decision on the other side. This patient information is growing rapidly, its mass is too huge to be worked out properly and in time by the human brain. To solve this emerging conflict, three major strategies can be used:

1. A randomized decrease in number and content of information betters the feeling of the overloaded doctor. Still, the now missing information has to be replaced. Dogmatas, rites and other simple yes-no decisions are helpful in finding a way, but lead unevitably to medical fundamentalism.

2. The use of standards is a viable compromise. It is the nature of standards, that they have to be reevaluated continuously, otherwise they result in fixed rules and again lead to dogmatism.

3. Proper and wise use of information, enabled by means of structured presentation, meaningful contexts and "intelligent" abstractions is still the most effective way of making decisions and acting accordingly. This is realized to a great extent in business, stock exchange and in the military field, but medicine is far behind. Doctors tend to accuse industry for this lack of innovation, but mostly the developers interface between the rules of medicine and the tools of information is the weak point.

The birth of information

Pieces of information are created all the time, once a patient has been admitted to an ICU and monitored and treated actively. This process follows the law of action and reaction, both parts being information in itself.

The birth of information

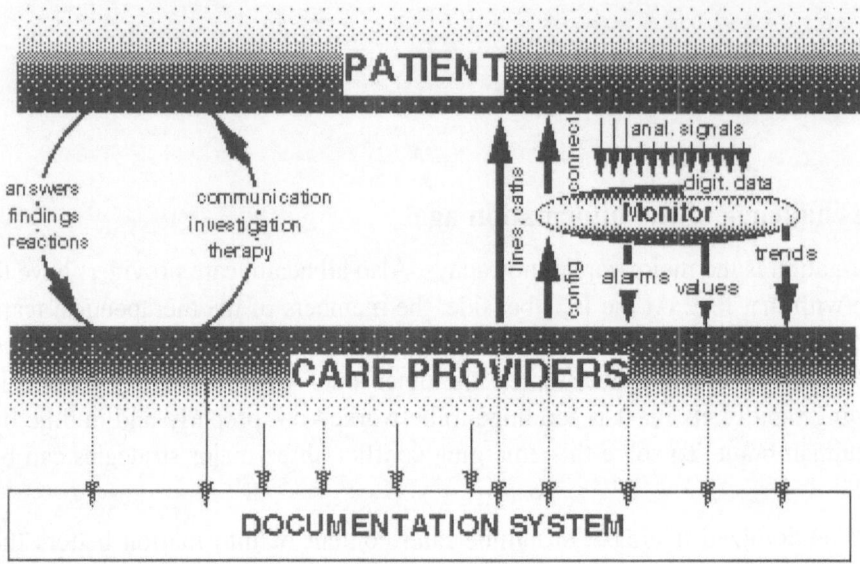

Fig. 1. Information emerges from the patient-care provider interaction. Information is stored as data in the documentation system

Typical situations

Information triggered by the therapeutic team

In the diagnostic situation, the process of investigation and the resulting values or findings are the relevant pieces of information. Once a single blood pressure is recorded in the charts, there is double information in it: the first is the fact that the blood pressure was measured (at a given time), and the second information is the measured value itself. Neglecting the frequency of maneuvers and hanging on to the blank number is called detection bias and has major influence on evaluation and therapy of patients.

Information triggered by the patient

Conscious, unconscious and vegetative expressions from the patient initialize reactions by the staff in this situation. All these signs from the patient become more frequent and important with the use of "soft" techniques in controlling and leading patients toward self-regulating vital functions (early weaning and spontaneous breathing, better understanding of analgosedation...). This very useful information is often drowned in the hectic routine of an ICU, but it may be as important as other findings. Also in many expert systems these patient reactions play no or a minor role in the regulating algorithm.

Information obtained by monitoring

Pieces of information obtained by monitors emerge from a more complex process. The patient needs the information (in the pure sense of the word) that a biological process is being measured. This means adapting the sensors or placing the blood lines and connect the lines and cables. The monitor itself must be informed (configured, setup), and the connection to the patient has to be started (open line). According to these preset devices and rules, the monitor digitizes analog signals into pieces of information (numbers, digital curves, tables, trends). This data can be documented either by read out from the screen and manual writing or routed to a data port and given away to a computer or network (PDM System). This is still a triggered information cycle, yet in a more complex manner.

Information obtained by therapeutic devices

Again, setup and starting connection have do be made. Information received can be either variables of the device (flow of pumps, respirator setups...) or patient reactions (respiratory variables), again read out via screens or data lines.

Structuring information: CIPUs and TRAMs

Another method of structuring information is the structure as given by the acting persons of the therapeutic team. Friesdorf et al. published a model, where a CIPU (Clinical Information Processing Unit) is a piece of information obtained by a person during his/her continuous responsible work for a patient. This CIPU can represent the shift of a nurse, the timed responsibility of an intensivist or even the competence of the surgeon in charge for the treatment of the local operation site. This CIPUs exist in a parallel fashion, representing the different groups of care providers (doctors, nurses, physiotherapists and others) and also in serial fashion, representing the shift changes of one group.

The nature of ICU care is continuous. This means, that between all serial CIPUs a connection must exist. In real life, this is called shift changing. Every ICU employee knows the problems around this field. This changing of shift means information transfer between the shifting people, again a time consuming process. Friesdorf called the bundle of transferred information TRAM (Transfer Module). General visitation rounds are a special form of TRAMs linking parallel running CIPUs (team rounds). The "Grand Rounds" are TRAMs, which include all parallel CIPUs, and therefore the complete therapeutical team. Whenever a patient crosses geographical barriers (admission, discharge, transfers) a special TRAM has to be established (notes, letters, texts, oral transmission...).

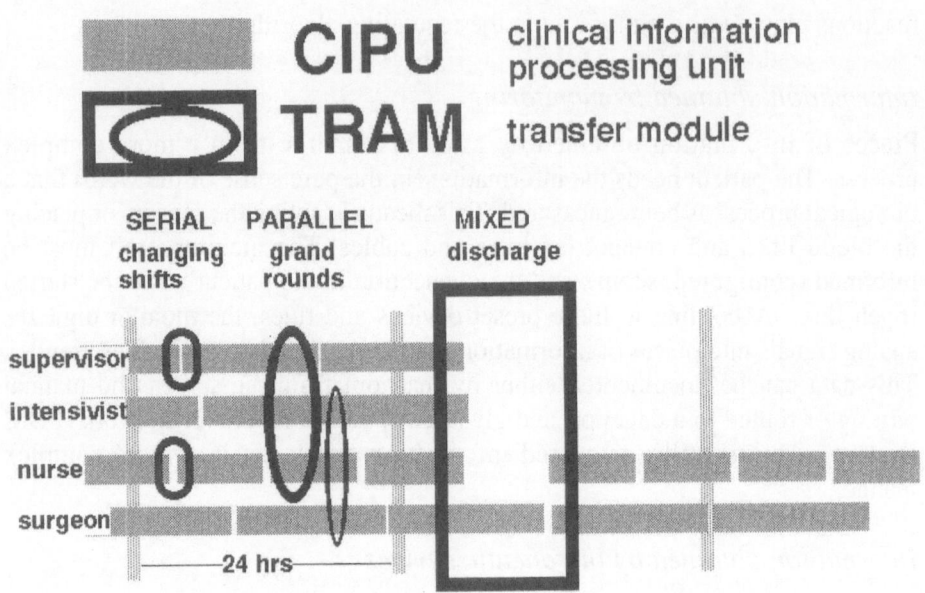

Fig. 2. The interrelationship between CIPUs and TRAMs according to Friesdorf et al

TRAMs have to fulfill the following specifications:

– must include all relevant information of the last CIPUs

– must be shaped according to the need of the recipient

– must be part of the daily routine work (supervised and controlled)

The quality and quantity of TRAMs can be used to describe the general behaviour of an ICU. Emphasize on TRAMs linking serial CIPUs means high performance in information exchange inside a group of care providers. Specialization and high level of profession in the different groups might be the result. Mostly the holistic approach to a patient suffers from a major drawback under these circumstances. This mode of working is often found in highly specialized ICUs (cardiosurgical, neuros).

A ward using more TRAMs linking parallel CIPUs represents a team fashion way of work. This regular information exchange between the layers provides overall information about a patient and tends to form rather mixed teams around the bed. The voice of the specialist in such an environment is often less noisy, but sometimes easily neglected. This way of information exchange is a common finding in general ICUs, treating a wider spectrum of diseases.

Where is all that information finally?
The graveyard of data

Once all pieces of information are collected there must exist a place for storage. If a patient is discharged from the unit, all pieces of paper are collected, filed nicely and additional texts and statistical sheets are added. The convolut is bundled and stored in an archive. Similarly electronic data are stored in mass storage media.

The graveyard of data is an often stated argument against electronic information systems. Regardless whether this archive is used later on or not, it must be considered, that the paper documentation wastes much more human resources than the electronic form. The cardex archive is an even more expensive graveyard than the drives, CD-ROMs, WORMs, MOFs or tapes of any PDM System.

The benefit of information, what is it good for?
Rebuilding information from data

All the documented information is only beneficial if it acts as basis for decision support. The re-synthesis of data into meaningful information takes place mainly at three different levels:

1. At the bedside, decision support for treatment and therapy
2. At the ward level or higher, for management issues, quality control and audit
3. Special requests like legal (lawsuits), clinical studies etc.

The difference between Anesthesia and ICU data management systems

There is a remarkable difference in the goal of information systems between anesthesia and intensive care. Anesthesia systems have been designed to work as quality tools. They should give comprehensive overview about workload, usage of resources, complications and similar staff. Up to now, no anesthesia system is able to give the anesthetist in the OR better support for decisions than the written chart or a monitor. They are made for output at the above levels 2 and 3. ICU systems have been designed from the beginning as treatment tools for use at the bedside. Documentation issues and later retrieval of data is therefore often poor. These systems target primarily to level 1. Now it is easy to understand, why all approaches to generate anesthesia systems from modified ICU systems or vice versa have failed.

Level 1, information prepared for bedside decisions

In paper documentation the way of writing down data is exactly the way of using it. All the flow sheets, order forms, lab entry records have to be reviewed as they are written down. Additional comprehensive sheets (respiratory, nutritional,

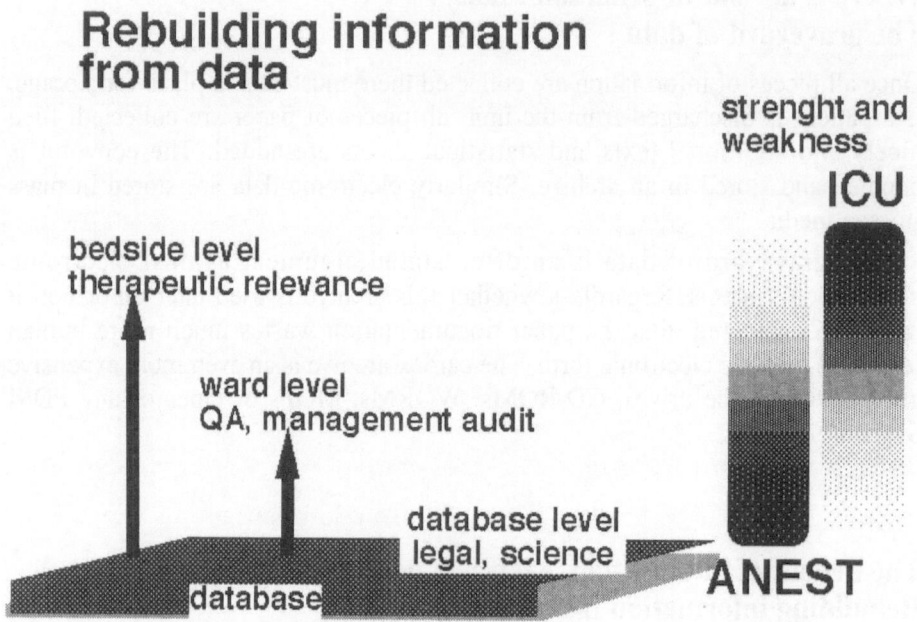

Fig. 3. Useful information is recreated from stored data. Different levels of interest form the main goal of presentation

cardiovascular) are additional papers, taking away manpower and other forms of useful energy. This form of documentation is mostly fixed, only slowly changing in time. Information obtained by use of electronic devices is flexible. By no means has the review to have the same style then the recording act. This is one of the essential advantages of data management systems. Information about a patient used for decision support is decoupled from the mode of data entry. Therefore, the presentation can have lots of different ways:

Texts and events
Simple tables of values vs time (spreadsheets)
Trends of parameters (trend machine) as curves and bars
Organ specific templates
Synoptic presentations (therapy and reaction)
Connecting different organ systems (CV and kidney)

Above this describing methods, all variants of artificial intelligence can be found:

Alerts and alarms (from simple to smart)
Expert systems (deriving diagnosis and treatment suggestion from data) rule based, knowledge based or mixed
Closed loop applications, also simple or smart algorithms

State of the art in the ready for sale systems is the trend machine. Organ specific templates can mostly be configured by the user. Thus the question arises, what makes a PDM System superior to a well equipped monitor, who also gives numerous trends and tables. This question will be asked as long as vendors do not accept the need of further development of their systems toward more intelligence. The knowledge in leading institutions is there.

Level 2, the documentation as tool for management, QA, cost control and audit

As stated before, ICU systems are weak in this field. Just recently quite a few companies offered statistical packages for billing, cost control, shift planning, patient statistics, scoring and similar purposes. The configurability of this tools still must increase, to fit the requirements of more users. Some systems are unable to provide a meaningful stream of data, just producing a real graveyard of electronic informations. Although level 1 information is very important in ICUs, level 2 is increasing in importance, despite the increasing needs for cost controlling and budgeting.

Level 3, data for late requests, legal affairs and science

In the classical scenario generations of students and residents have been sent down to the archives, if there was any request for statistical reviews. They spent days and weeks of precious working time to provide data for lecturers, insurance companies, retrospective studies and hungry hospital administrators.

Meanwhile some researchers have programmed search tools, for retrieval of data from big databases. The key to success is an event triggered search mode, either stating events a priori and searching for them or searching for constellations and naming this later an event. Widespread use of this tools could bring up new information about patients, estimation of goodness of diagnosis, benefit and harm calculations for therapy, prognosis, outcome and more. Also other requests can be fulfilled more easily by means of appropriate database search and browsing tools. As stated for level 2 information, most vendors do not offer that option, or it is billed separately.

Conclusion

In the complete process of information fluxes in ICUs, electronic systems can play a major role in understanding patients, their disease and acute illness. Once used properly and with all the possibilities of modern information processing, they disconnect the cumbersome link from writing down to review of data. They save nursing working time and offer information for understanding complex pathophysiological processes. This systems involve the user, they need active participation and customizing on demand. They are a "hot" medium, changing dramatically the way of working. Therefore all levels of staff have to be prepared to work with, to obtain good results and advance above the paper age.

General references

Systems

Ambroso C, Bowes C, Chambrin MC, Gilhooly K, Green C, Kari A, Logie R, Marraro G, Mereu M, Rembold P, et al (1992) Inform: European survey of computers in intensive care units. Int J Clin Monit Comput 9(1):53-61

Bowes CL, Wilson AJ (1994) Information management systems for intensive care. Comput Methods Programs Biomed 44(1):31-35

Colson AR, Bounds JA, Alt White AC, McDermott S (1995) Preparing for an ICU bedside computer. Nurs Manage 26(5):48A-48B

Friesdorf W et al (1994) Information transfer in high dependency environments: an ergonomic analysis. Int J Clin Monit Comp 11:105-115

Friesdorf W, Gross Alltag F, Konichezky S, Schwilk B, Fattroth A, Fett P (1994) Lessons learned while building an integrated ICU workstation. Int J Clin Monit Comput 11(2):89-97

Friesdorf W, Schwilk B (1992) Patient related data management. J Clin Monit 8(4):308-314

Hohnloser JH, Purner F (1992) PADS (Patient Archiving and Documentation System): a computerized patient record with educational aspects. Int J Clin Monit Comput 9(2):71-84

Kalli S, Ambroso C, Gregory R, Heikela A, Ilomaki A, Leaning M, Marraro G, Mereu M, Tuomisto T, Yates C (1992) Inform: conceptual modelling of intensive care information systems. Int J Clin Monit Comput 9(2):85-94

Lenz K (ed) (1993) Patient data management in intensive care / 11th Vienna Intensive Care Days. Springer, Berlin Heidelberg New York

Morris AH, East TD, Wallace CJ, Orme J Jr, Clemmer T, Weaver L, Thomas F, Dean N, Pearl J, Rasmusson B (1994) Ethical implications of standardization of ICU care with computerized protocols. Proc Annu Symp Comput Appl Med Care 501-505

Data acquisition

Cunningham S, Symon AG, McIntosh N (1994) The practical management of artifact in computerised physiological data. Int J Clin Monit Comput 11(4):211-216

Dawant BM, Manders EJ, Lindstrom DP (1994) Adaptive signal analysis and interpretation for real time intelligent patient monitoring. Methods Inf Med 33(1):60-63

Imhoff M (1992) Acquisition of ICU data: concepts and demands. Int J Clin Monit Comput 9(4): 229-237

Databases and search tools

Laursen P (1994) Event detection on patient monitoring data using Causal Probabilistic Networks Methods. Inf Med 33(1):111-115

Tu JV, Guerriere MR (1992) Use of a neural network as a predictive instrument for length of stay in the intensive care unit following cardiac surgery. Proc Annu Symp Comput Appl Med Care 666-672

Veit C, Tecklenburg A (1992) Computing tools for quality assurance. Qual Assur Health Care 4(1): 3-8

Information, presentation and decision support

Cereijo E (1992) Computer assisted management of information in an intensive care unit. Int J Clin Monit Comput 9(3):159-163

Fackler J, Kohane I (1994) Monitor driven data visualization: Smart Display. Proc Annu Symp Comput Appl Med Care 939-943

Haimowitz IJ (1994) Intelligent diagnostic monitoring using trend templates. Proc Annu Symp Comput Appl Med Care 702-708

Lau F (1994) A clinical decision support system prototype for cardiovascular intensive care. Int J Clin Monit Comput 11(3):157-169

Lau F, Vincent D (1992) Formalized decision support for cardiovascular intensive care. Proc Annu Symp Comput Appl Med Care 442-448

Lesser MF (1994) GIFIC. A graphical interface for intensive care. Proc Annu Symp Comput Appl Med Care 988

Schwaiger J, Haller M, Finsterer U (1992) A framework for the knowledge based interpretation of laboratory data in intensive care units using deductive database technology. Proc Annu Symp Comput Appl Med Care 13-17

Sukuvaara T, Koski EM, Makivirta A, Kari A (1993) A knowledge based alarm system for monitoring cardiac operated patients technical construction and evaluation. Int J Clin Monit Comput 10(2):117-126

Uckun S (1994) Intelligent systems in patient monitoring and therapy management. A survey of research projects. Int J Clin Monit Comput 11(4):241-253

Uckun S, Dawant BM, Lindstrom DP (1993) Model based diagnosis in intensive care monitoring: the YAQ approach. Artif Intell Med 5(1):31-48

From Human Action to Data: Man-Machine Interface in Manual Data Entries

G.H. METNITZ

Introduction

Intensive care units (ICUs) are increasingly confronted with incredibly large amounts of data originating from diagnostic and therapeutic devices as well as from clinical documentation. *Patient Data Management Systems (PDMS)* or *Intensive Care Information Systems (ICIS)* (1) are specialized to collect, visualize and store clinical patient data such as demographics, vital parameters, doctors and nurses plans and notes. Moreover, they are able to facilitate complex calculations for input-output balances, hemodynamic parameters and clinical scores and to support medical decision making through displaying trends and graphs of the patient's course. The man-machine interface builds the base of the interaction between the information system and the user. Its design and implementation plays a large role when defining useability and practicability of an applied system.

System design

Modeling of computer systems has developed especially in the past years. Graphical user interfaces (GUI), which are now included in almost all systems, were invented in the XEROX Palo Alto Research center in the 1970s, based on the work of Jean Piaget and Jerome Bruner (2). Their purpose was to form an operating environment which was able to handle "interface metaphors" – which are graphic representations of "objects" in the computer system in the form of real world objects – to support the illusion that digital data can be manipulated as directly and easy as paper documents. Since interface metaphors use the familiarity with habits and experience of the user, their visual and behavioral characteristics offer a concrete message. Inconsistencies in the mental model of the GUI prevent users from predicting results and are therefore confusing, leading to a lack in confidence. To enable direct manipulation of these metaphors, specialized pointing devices, such as the mouse, trackball, graphical tablets – or last but not least voice input – developed (3). The benefit of these input devices (let's call it a real world simulation) weighs against differences in handling and performance, which are not always easier or faster. Movements of the mouse cursor on the screen, for example, are normally dependent only on user action; neglecting such a convention irritates the user unnecessarily. Computer systems are still not able to process GUI data in real time. Long delays (e.g., after pressing a button) produce anger - no matter how complex ongoing activity might be. To avoid the interpretation of an "ambiguous" behavior of the system, a feedback should be given to the user (like the wellknown "hourglas"). These and other base rules of designing *user interfaces* are often negotiated in available systems.

Measurements done on comparing paper and screen reading show a deficit in performance and accuracy for on-screen reading (4) as well as differences in the "reading process and behavior" on-screen. Seeking information in documents or complex tables seems to be more awkward in electronic media than in conventional paper documents with their flexibility. New features such as hypertext functions, windowing techniques etc. are generally considered for an appropriate system design to overcome these system-inherent properties. But these technical advances also need new and specialized techniques for orientation and navigation. It is therefore assumed that the way in which a problem is presented may have a profound effect on information-acquiring perfomance (5). Visual design of the computer sceen, not only focusing on font types, font size etc. but also on information representation seems to influence man-machine interaction and should be considered. Physiological research data on user attention and processing capabilities have been known (and often revealed) for more than three decades (6). Information systems for intensive care should be designed to support health care personnel with clinical information in situations where attention and processing capabilities of the user are sometimes extremely influenced by activity. Some GUI of available systems appear as if they have never been tested under these conditions. New ways of data presentation and integration have, however, to be developed (and are under development) since the complex dynamic of an ICU patient is being represented by more and more (confusing) data, providing less overview (7).

User performance studies have been initiated to compare graphical screen layouts and to measure user performance in acquiring information and performing tasks (8, 9). Although it seems interesting to provide development tools for screen-design, none of the reviewed approaches takes into account that user performance cannot be defined exactly through measurement of reaction and completion speed of a simulation. This would, for example, completely negotiate the complexity of cognitive models of human behavior and root psychological experiments back to behaviorism theories which have proved not to be adequate. Other facts, like emergency situation and the personal stress response are not included in these models, either. Experimental designs focusing on user performance and application development would therefore be better evaluated in coordination with an appropriate psychosocial modeling rather than simulating clinical patient studies.

Documentation needs and experiences

Critical care is increasingly provided to severely ill patients, producing rapidly increasing costs. This puts pressure on cost control and effective utilization of resources (10) and leads to the necessity of more detailed documentation, which is realistically possible only with the aid of computers (11). The availability of patient data, as in an ICIS, render the extremely time-consuming manual analysis of printed or written data sheets redundant and provides an optimal basis for computerized *audit* programs (11). Whether data input into clinical databases is done automatically or manually, it is never free of artifacts (12, 13). Not all information that suffices as input for simple paper print-outs can easily be processed by a database system. Insufficient or missing validation of manual data input to an ICIS leads to various problems. If the input to text fields is free text, data records are generated which can be printed out, but usually cannot be processed further. In most reviewed ICISs (14) it is possible to enter free text into different fields, consisting of any ASCII character. Artifact management of the input data using default field formats, entry limits and selection lists will improve the quality of the produced database, which is an important condition for a good interpretation. Since it seems almost impossible to remove all artifacts from a clinical database system manually, artifact recognition and handling algorithms have to be developed and integrated further. With a database system like ICDEV (15) it is possible to check the consistency and quality of an existing database. Therefore, recorded data can be examined for their usefulness in answering desired questions. Reviewing the data collected in Vienna since 1993, we found systematic errors in the configuration of the ICISs used at various ICUs. These errors, including missing starting or endpoints of actions, wrong calculations, false counters etc. impaired the analysis of these clinical data for audit purposes. Naturally, the results of the analyses of these data are only as valid as the contents of the database.

Automated data recording is a rapidly expanding and developing technique which supports physicians with almost continuously recorded vital parameters. Moreover, new approaches in the design of the man-machine interface will provide us with fascinating new techniques of data input, display and interpretation. Since manual data entry, however, will at least persist for the next couple of years, attention should also be paid to develop faster and better techniques for manual data handling. An appropriate user interface design, adapted to the special needs of health care personnel, would not only support better data readability and overview, but also help to motivate those persons which are responsible for data entry and handling. Clinical databases, also most are equipped with automated data recording features, need still manual handling. This is valid for information entry as well as for information retrieval. A bad user interface will prevent people from using the system in an appropriate manner.

References

1. Stoutenbeck CP (1994) Dutch specification study of an Intensive Care Information System. In: Vincent JL (1994) Yearbook of intensive care and emergency medicine. Springer, Berlin Heidelberg New York
2. Piaget J (1954) The construction of reality in the child. Basic Books, New York
3. Lynch PJ (1994) Visual design for the user interface, part 1: design fundamentals. J Biocommun 21(1):22-30
4. Dillon A (1992) Reading from paper versus screens: a critical review of the empirical literature. Ergonomics 35(10):1297-1326
5. Kuan Goh S, Coury BG (1994) Incorporating the effect of display formats in cognitive modelling. Ergonomics 37(4):725-745
6. Miller GA (1956) The magical number seven, plus or minus two: some limits on our capacity for processing information. Psychol Rev 63(2):81-97
7. Cole WG, Stewart JG (1993) Metaphor graphics to support integrated decision making with respiratory data. Int J Clin Monit Comput 10:91-100
8. Staggers N, Mills ME (1994) Nurse-computer interaction: staff performance outcomes. Nursing Res 43(3):144-150
9. Chase CR, Ashikaga T, Mazuzan JE (1994) Measurement of user performance and attitude assists the initial design of a computer user display and orientation method. J Clin Monit 10: 251-263
10. Vestrup JA (1992) Critical care audit. Can J Anaesth 39(3):210-213
11. Vassar MJ, Holcroft JW (1994) The case against using the APACHE system to predict intensive care unit outcome in trauma patients. Crit Care Clin 10(1):117-126
12. Friesdorf W, Konichezky S, Gro-Alltag F, Fattroth A, Schwilk B (1994) Data quality of bedside monitoring in an intensive care unit. Int J Monit Comput 11(2):123-128
13. Cunningham S, Symon AG, McIntosh N (1994) The practical management of artifact in computerised physiological data. Int J Clin Monit Comput 11:211-216
14. Metnitz PGH, Lenz K (1995) Patient data management systems in intensive care - the situation in Europe. Intensive Care Med (in press)
15. Metnitz PhGH, Laback P, Popow C, Laback O, Lenz K, Hiesmayr M (1995) Computer assisted data analysis in intensive care: the IC DEV project - development of a scientific database system for Intensive Care. Int J Clin Monit Comput (in press)

From Trends to Multi-Information-Screens in Computing in the ICU

A. Tecklenburg

Computers are becoming a more and more useful tool in the ICU environment. Especially tasks such as computing special algorithms or calculating scores like APACHE II or SAPS II are supported very well by these machines. In these areas computers are effective and easy to use. Whenever one is thinking about computing in the ICU, ideas of patient data management, documentation and information management come to mind. Bedside information systems are the desire of many intensive care medicine physicians and nurses. But to satisfy the staff working at the bedside, an information system must be at least as good as today's paperwork in terms of completeness, evidence, reliability and easiness to use.

This paper discusses computer supported bedside information management and the idea of multi-information-screens. Today only few systems on the market support the staff with more than tables, simple trend lines and graphs on the computer screens. Most of these systems are proprietary and for reasons of age cannot be integrated into modern software technologies, including multimedia.

In the medical environment we are using data of several levels of complexity. A state of the art computer system at the bedside of an intensive care bed has to support all these data:

- Raw data, derived from monitors and other devices at the bedside in form of tables and simple curves and bar graphs
- Calculated data (tables, graphs)
- Complex data such as three-dimensional presentations of organ status
- Compiled information based on figures, graphs, tables
- Custom made graphics (from operations, nursing)
- X-ray images, ultrasound images etc.
- Video
- Sound
  Using some typical routine situations, like
- Daily patient overview
- Patient's vital status

- Routine decision making
- Decision making in an emergency situation
- Shift report
- Final transmission report
- Organ system related detailed report
- Nurse report

an analysis would show, that for any kind of demand a huge amount of different data from various classes, as listed above, are required. The users of an ICU system need a data presentation that comprehends and processes all required information. The philosophy has to be "click and see". If one is forced to go through several screens to obtain what is needed, paper records then are still more handy and much cheaper.

Going through the scenarios one would find out that a lot of different information sources (sheets of paper) have to be used to collect all information together. This is time consuming and involves the risk that important data are not found or simply not seen. On paper records data is ordered in a way that is easy to fill in, but inconvenient to read. Although the raw data for the above scenarios is often the same, the optimal data presentation differs from situation to situation. A solution is a problem oriented data presentation that takes into account the special circumstances and then decides the most comprehensible presentation form. Data can be presented in form of tables, graphs or other more complex compositions. For a computer system it is an easy job to retrieve data from a database and carry out a sophisticated presentation.

Another problem can also be solved by multi-information-screens. Only in few cases are medical problems describable by just one or two figures. Normally data from different sources have to be integrated before a decision can be made. To support this decision making, it is necessary to display several information items in different ways on the same screen: the multi-information-screen.

Multi-information-screens are a composition of different data presentation to inform the user at the right time with the right information in the most understandable form.

Later in this text one scenario will be described in more detail to show how multi-information-screens enhance the possibilities of information management at the bedside of an intensive care unit.

To realize multi-information-screens there are some technical requirements of the hardware and software of computer systems. Very high resolution screens are necessary to display various information, such as alphanumeric or graphics. The huge amounts of data are stored today in relational databases, often in a server-client environment. Using this technology, the bedside computer is only responsible for the data presentation and the user interface, while the server is a bigger machine with a lot of storage capacity. The computers are connected by Ethernet network. But even more important than hardware is software. The development of graphical user interfaces made it possible to realize multi-information-screens. Also well known in the medical field are X-Windows, MacOS, MS-Windows and OS/2. These software packages support modern applications with an intuitive interface and the integration of multimedia in any software. Only with this state of the art graphical user interfaces (GUI) is it possible to provide physicians and nurses with all kinds of data at the bedside.

The ideal solution for a bedside information system that supports multimedia and multi-information-screens consists of the following components:

- Small bedside computer with graphical user interface and net connection to a server and to the bedside medical devices
- Server computer for mass data storage with net connection to the bedside computers and to hospital information system
- Fast and failure tolerable disk operating system on the server
- Relational database system which supports SQL (standard query language) and standard database interfaces like OBDC
- Intensive care information system (PDMS), which is open for interfacing with other applications

With a hard- and software system, which follows the above requirements it is possible to develop an information system that supports most of the needs of intensive care medicine. Because of the open architecture, several software packages, like word processors, spread sheets and database systems, can be integrated into one system. The users are not aware of the different software packages; for the user the system is transparent. The modern GUIs support different kinds of data exchange between applications. The following scenario describes the use and technique of a multi-information-screen system. The task is an overview about the pulmonary status of a ventilated patient:

The user sees a basic screen with some icons to carry out different tasks. In addition there are some actual vital parameters and also an overview about running pumps and infusions. The user presses the icon with a picture of a lung on it. The software now retrieves all data from the database concerning the pulmonary status and the artificial ventilation. After about half a second the software produces different windows on the screen. In the center of the screen the last available chest-X-ray is presented. Above is displayed the written comment of the radiologist to that image. Below are two tables. The left one shows the last available blood gas analysis and the right one the parameters of the ventilator at the time when the blood for the blood gas analysis was taken. Right at the top of the screen one can see a graphic of the bronchus system. This graphic has sensible fields. If the user clicks on the carina a window is opened and a photograph is showed of the last bronchoscope. Also available is a recorded sound of the auscultatory percussion of the lungs from the day before. If the user wants to see more data, he presses at the very bottom the left arrow button, which changes all data to the day before. Also the user can click on the chest-X-ray itself and in a short time the history of all available chest-images shows up on the screen. If the user now wants a printed report, he presses the button labeled printer and all data on the screen are sent to a report writer tool or a text processing system for a printout.

For the user the whole multi-information-system looks as one piece of software. But in this case, a central co-ordination software is responsible for the user interface and data retrieval from the database system. After the data is retrieved, this co-ordination software presents the data by using several data browsers. These browsers receive the data and display them in an appropriate way. The X-ray is presented by an ordinary bitmap viewer. The tables are shown by a spreadsheet software and text is displayed by a simple editor. Sound can be produced by common multimedia software packages in combination with a soundcard and also movies are available for documentation purposes. If all this software were reinvented by one software company with a proprietary operating system, the users would have to pay millions of US $. By using open software standards with intelligent integration of different software tools, the benefit of multi-information-screens for the medical environment can soon become reality at the bedside of an intensive care bed.

Artificial Intelligence for Decision Support: Needs, Possibilities, and Limitations in ICU

S. MIKSCH

The need for decision support

The complexity of medical knowledge has been steadily increasing, the cost of health care services has surged over the years, and growing demands exist for assessing and improving the quality of health care services.

For example, the care of critically ill patients in modern intensive care units (ICUs) is becoming increasingly complex, involving interpretation of many variables, comparative evaluation of many therapy options, and control of many patient-management parameters. Even experienced physicians have difficulties in facing the important and relevant continuous data and in reacting in a time-constrained, critical situation. Not only the amount of information to be processed limits the quality of intensive care, but also human factors, like the problem of vigilance, varying expertise, and human error. These frequently lead to errors in diagnosis and in the selection of appropriate treatments.

Dealing with decision support in medical domains in real-world environments has to be taken into account. Data are usually more faulty than expected and the knowledge available is fuzzy and incomplete. Additionally, data analysis has to deal with different observation frequencies, different regularities, and different data types.

The medical staff has to act and to react in time-constrained and critical situations. Therefore she/he needs the essential and context-relevant information about the health condition of the patient displayed on the screen. The continuous and discontinuous data have to be visualized in a self-explaining form so that the medical staff can cope with the situation as quickly as possible.

Knowledge-based decision support might provide considerable help in solving many of these problems. But it cannot solve management problems or improve the relationship between physician, nurses, patients, and health care administrators. Knowledge-based decision support can promote a deeper level of understanding of the data under investigation and foster new insight into the underlying process.

In my opinion, the need for support is most urgent with regard to the different tasks of monitoring and therapy planning of severely ill patients. I will neglect all administrative and organizational aspects that are covered in patient data management systems (PDMS) and hospital information systems (HIS). Additionally, the decision support presented is mainly concerned with physicians and nurses to improve the patient-oriented medical care. No aspects of health care administrators are involved. In the next sections I will clarify the term AI.

What is AI?

The official birthplace of AI was during a 2-month workshop at Dartmouth in the summer of 1956. AI is one of the extensively and broadly discussed disciplines. Therefore a generally accepted definition is hard to find. According to Russell and Norvig (1) the definitions of AI vary along two main dimensions: first it is concerned with thought processes and reasoning; second it deals with behavior. Additionally, it is concerned with human performance or rationality (an ideal concept of intelligence). Table 1 shows the main four categories.

Table 1. Some definitions of AI organized into four categories

Systems that think like humans	Systems that think rationally
Systems that act like humans	Systems that act rationally

The subareas of AI range from fundamentals, like knowledge representation, knowledge acquisition, problem solving and search, to specific concepts, like knowledge-based systems, intelligent agents, natural language processing, machine learning, computer vision, or impacts. In the following I will not discuss AI in general. My main focus is the use of knowledge-based systems in intensive care medicine.

In 1982 Peter Szolovitz (2) defined the three main aims of knowledge-based systems in medical care in general. Their importance is still relevant and applicable to intensive care medicine:

1. To develop expert computer programs for clinical use, making possible the inexpensive dissemination of the best medical expertise to geographical regions where that expertise is lacking, and making consultation help available to nonspecialists who are not within easy reach of expert human consultants

2. To formalize medical expertise, to enable physicians to understand better what they know and to give them systematic structure for teaching their expertise to medical students

3. To test AI theories in a "real world" domain and to use that domain to suggest novel problems for further AI research

Monitoring and therapy planning

Monitoring and therapy planning involve observing and guiding the behavior of a system with real-time constraints. In contrast to diagnosis, which tries to find the best explanation for the actual situation of a patient, monitoring and therapy planning imply actions: *monitoring* indicates observing the course of a patient's condition under a given therapy, and assessing whether the selected therapeutic action is effective and the predicted improvement of the patient's condition occurs. *Therapy planning* involves selecting which therapeutic actions may improve the patient's condition, predicting the outcome, and adopting a therapeutic plan according to some explicitly defined preferences on the predicted condition of the patient (3).

The building of a knowledge-based monitoring and therapy planning system can be divided into several steps: data selection, data validation, data abstraction (interpretation of the patient's status), determination of proper therapy recommendations and the short- or long-term predictions of the effects of a therapy. All these steps are involved in a single cycle of data interpretation. These knowledge-based techniques are implemented and evaluated in VIE-VENT, a monitoring and therapy planning system of artificially ventilated newborns, which we are currently developing at my institute (4, 5). In the following I will discuss two essential parts, namely, data validation and data abstraction.

Data validation

A critical aspect of effective knowledge-based data analysis is the data validation. The central aim of data validation is to detect faulty or contradictory input data and to arrive at classified data (e.g., reliable, inconsistent, unknown) for further analytic tasks.

Nowadays, data validation does not work well. Several monitors have built-in modules for recognizing faulty data, especially those arising from hardware problems. However, these built-in modules often trigger false alarms and the medical staff, especially the nurses, are suffering under wrong alarms. A context-sensitive examination of the plausibility of input data based on different temporal ontologies improves the data validation process (5). The data validation process uses discontinuously and continuously assessed numerical and qualitative data as well as derived qualitative descriptions. The latter are received from the data abstraction process described in the next section or are given by the users (e.g., user's requests). We distinguish four data validation concepts based on their underlying temporal ontologies: time-point-based, time-interval-based, trend-based, and time-independent validation.

The time-point-based concept uses the value of a variable at a particular time point for the reasoning process. This concept can handle all kinds of data. It benefits from the transparent and fast reasoning process but suffers from neglecting any information about the history of the observed parameters. We apply range checking as well as causal and functional dependencies.

The time-interval-based concept deals with the values of different variables within an interval. We use three methods: temporal validity, allowed changes/values of a single variable during an interval and allowed changes/values of interdependent variables during an interval.

The trend-based concept tries to analyze the development of a variable during an interval. A trend is a significant pattern in a sequence of time-ordered data. Therefore the following methods can only handle continuously observed variables. It benefits from the dynamically derived qualitative trend-categories (descriptions) which overcome the limitations of predefined static thresholds. We apply trend-based functional dependencies of different dependent variables and an assessment procedure of the development of a variable.

The last concept is based on time-independent priority lists of variables and constraints. The data validation process allows identification of less reliable variables or constraints in case of conflicts. The result is a reliability ranking. This method is triggered, for example, if an ambiguous classification of values (e.g., "some are wrong") has been derived.

Data abstraction (interpretation of the patient's status)

Monitoring data are observed by the trained medical staff. However, these single observations may only be recognized for being "normal" or "abnormal". Information about trends, "natural" oscillations, etc. is very difficult to gather. Therefore, inexperienced personnel may have difficulties in interpreting a clinical picture from single monitoring data in a limited time. Some of the variables are influenced by other clinical variables that may not (continuously) be determined (like cardiac output, pulmonary perfusion).

The most common methods to interpret continuous data are time-series analysis techniques (6). Furthermore, probabilistic and fuzzy classifiers are useful approaches to classify values. However, they contain crucial shortcomings. In the absence of an appropriate curve-fitting model time-series analysis techniques are not applicable. Domain specific characteristics, like dynamically changing degrees of parameters' abnormalities depending on the changing states of the environment cannot easily be integrated in probabilistic or fuzzy classifiers. Classifications through value interval assignments (point data abstraction methods) are insufficient in dynamically changing environments where the temporal dimension covering the course of a parameter and the interdependencies of different parameters over time have to be taken into account. These shortcomings require that knowledge-based approaches be applied to solve the troubles.

The data abstraction process should lead to unified qualitative descriptions of point and interval data as well as verbal problem descriptions. The advantage of qualitative values is their unified usability in the data validation, therapy planning, and data visualization, no matter of which origin they are. Adaptation to specific situations can easily be done by specific transformation tables without changing the model of data interpretation. According to our temporal ontologies we define three types of qualitative abstraction: time-point-based, time-interval-based and trend-based abstraction.

The time-point-based abstraction transforms quantitative data points into qualitative values. It is usually performed by dividing the numerical range of a variable into regions of interest. Each region stands for a qualitative category. The time-interval-based abstraction classifies a property of a variable to a time interval. A specific case of the previous abstraction mechanism is the trend-based abstraction, which classifies the development of a variable during a predefined time interval.

Basic requirements for integration in routine clinical practice

Decision support techniques have been available for about three decades. In retrospect, application of knowledge-based techniques are rather limited. Routine clinical use is rather the rare exception (7). To change this situation a set of basic requirements must be put forward:

- Integration into clinical practice is vital
- Integration of diverse information sources to give a coherent picture of the situation of the patient and her/his history
- Assessment of users' needs is necessary (involving the medical staff really using the systems in the future)
- Knowledge-based support systems should deal with defined areas of clinical medicine
- User interface must be easy to use
- Appropriate explanations should be provided
- The user needs to be informed of the quality of the system (intensive evaluation)
- The user needs a secure and legally valid system
- Intensive training of the medical staff (the real end users) and additional support must be guaranteed.

Conclusion

No perfect knowledge-based system will exist in the near future, especially in the field of medicine. The knowledge is changing too quickly. However, we could develop a workbench of useful tools to make the daily routine easier, like tools for data validation, data interpretation, or context-relevant data visualization. We need intelligent assistance to ease the burden of filtering, sorting, filing, and archiving the information that we receive daily.

The presentation is based on the traditional AI method of designing knowledge-based systems. I did not apply methods like neural nets, machine learning, or natural language processing to improve the decision support in medicine. The reason lies in facing the decision making in real-world environments: available data are usually more faulty than expected, data based on different observation frequencies, different regularities, and different data types, and available knowledge is fuzzy and incomplete. Other techniques would not succeed without preprocessing and additional knowledge.

Shortliffe (8) has analyzed the evolving role of computers in medical care and the impact that evolution will have on the delivery of medical care. Starting his paper he tells a typical newspaper story on the clinical use of computers. The story presents a perspective on the future and must quickly attract the public's attention (8).

"The semiconscious patient lies in a futuristic intensive care unit, tubes protruding, wires emerging from under the sheets and connecting to a host of monitor carts or wall-mounted devices, and intravenous fluids with computer-controlled infusion pumps circling the bed. The beeps of the monitors are not interrupted by footfalls of nursing staff, for health workers seldom have to enter the room. Instead, intelligent devices measure every pertinent physiological parameter, deciding how to adjust infusion rates, when to alter the respirator settings, and whether to sound alarms for the intervention of nurses or physicians".

I hope that computer-controlled therapy offering sterile, impersonal, and dehumanizing care will never be reality. The limits of automation will help to avoid such nightmare.

References

1. Russell S, Norvig P (1995) Artificial intelligence: a modern approach. Prentice Hall Series in Artificial Intelligence. Englewood Cliffs, New Jersey
2. Szolovits P (1992) Artificial intelligence and medicine. In: Szolovits P (eds) Artificial intelligence in medicine. Westview, Boulder
3. Stefanelli M (1992) Therapy planning and monitoring. Artificial Intelligence in Medicine 4(2):189-190
4. Miksch S, Horn W, Popow C, Paky F (1993) VIE-VENT: knowledge-based monitoring and therapy planning of the artificial ventilation of newborn infants. In: Andreassen S et al (eds) Artificial intelligence in medicine: proceedings of the 4th Conference on Artificial Intelligence in Medicine Europe (AIME-93). IOS, Amsterdam, pp 218-229
5. Miksch S, Horn W, Popow C, Paky F (1994) Context-sensitive data validation and data abstraction for knowledge-based monitoring. In: Cohn AG (ed) Proceedings of the 11th European Conference on Artificial Intelligence (ECAI 94). Wiley, Chichester, UK, pp 48-52

6. Avent RK, Charlton JD (1990) A critical review of trend-detection methodologies for biomedical monitoring systems. Crit Rev Biomed Eng 17(6):621-659
7. Barahona P, Durinck J, Florin C, Hernandez C, Hucklenbroich P, Rickards A, Stefanelli M (1994) Knowledge processing for decision support: a perspective for the next decade. In: Barahona P, Christensen JP (eds) Knowledge and decisions in health telematics. IOS, Amsterdam, pp 3-58
8. Shortliffe EH (1993) Doctors, patients, and computers: will information technology dehumanize health-care delivery? Proc Am Philosoph Soc 137(3): 390-398

Beyond Trends: Graphics for Decision Support

W.G. COLE

Introduction

It is common to encounter the claim that graphical representation can make data easier to understand, especially large data sets. Large data sets are common in monitoring situations, from nuclear power plants to the operating room. With the rapid proliferation of electronic monitoring devices and the rapid decrease in the cost of computing, we in health care increasingly have the ability to record, store, and manipulate patient data, yet even as we do so we suspect that there may be more useful information within that data than we are discovering. Useful information is gold, because it can be translated into better decisions – decisions that either improve health outcomes or yield outcomes just as good as at present but at lower cost. Thus the claim that graphical representation can reveal useful information in a mountain of patient data is an important claim. It is worthwhile to consider two such claims in some detail, then to go on to analyze exactly why some graphics improve decision making while others do not.

A common graphical representation of medical data: the line graph

Figure 1 shows a line graph representation of some data taken from one patient over a period of twelve epochs of time. At any convention that has booths promoting the products of health care information system vendors, line graphs similar to Figure 1 will be prominently featured, with the claim that "graphic representation of your data will allow you to spot trends quickly and make decisions more easily". The line graph is a good place to start in any consideration of visual data displays because it is so common, has such a long history of use, and is so limited in its usefulness.

Is it easy to spot patterns using the line graph method? Figure 1 is actually a line graph of an invented data set, not a real patient. Figure 1 contains within it a puzzle: two of the lines are in fact the same line, only reversed. That is, one line is the left-right mirror image of another of the lines. It is the same set of numbers, only in reverse order. How easy is it to detect which two lines are identical except for this one aspect, the direction in which they flow? It is surprisingly difficult.

Why is it difficult, even though in Fig. 1 we are only seeing five lines and only 25 epochs? It is because the human perceptual system cannot succeed, in Fig. 1 at least, in finding shapes to compare. The detection of shapes is the first of two steps necessary in interpreting any visual data display. A second graphical representation method, called the polar graph, may be better for detecting shapes.

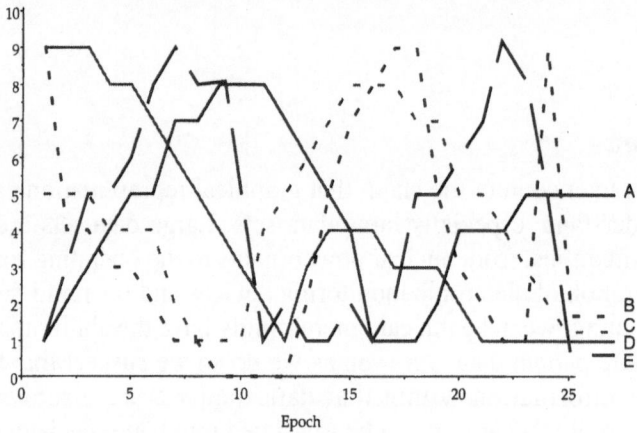

Fig. 1. A line graph. Five patient variables change over 25 epochs. Two of the lines are the same numbers, left-right mirror reversed. Can you tell which two these are? Lines graphs do not always make patterns easily detectable

Innovation in graphical representation of medical data: the polar graph

Within medicine, one graphical method for representing data has been proposed repeatedly. It is perhaps the oldest such method in medicine and is still being put forward today, with minor modifications, as an interesting "new" idea. The method has been proposed in a remarkably broad range of health care disciplines, ranging from epidemiology, through laboratory medicine, to psychiatry. And yet to date there is not one shred of evidence that the method actually improves decision making, nor has the method been reported to be used as a part of the regular decision making procedure in any medical setting. This method, which illustrates both a great strength of health care graphics and a great weakness as well, is called the polar graph.

Figure 2, based on a figure in Williams et al. (1), shows a polar graph for laboratory medicine. A collection of laboratory tests have been carried out on one patient at one moment in time and this graphic summarizes the entire collection at once. Twelve separate tests are represented as twelve spoke-like lines extending radially out from the center of the display. Each line is a scale on which the patient's test value will be plotted as a dot, with low scale values appearing near the center of the display and scale values increasing as you go further out from the center.

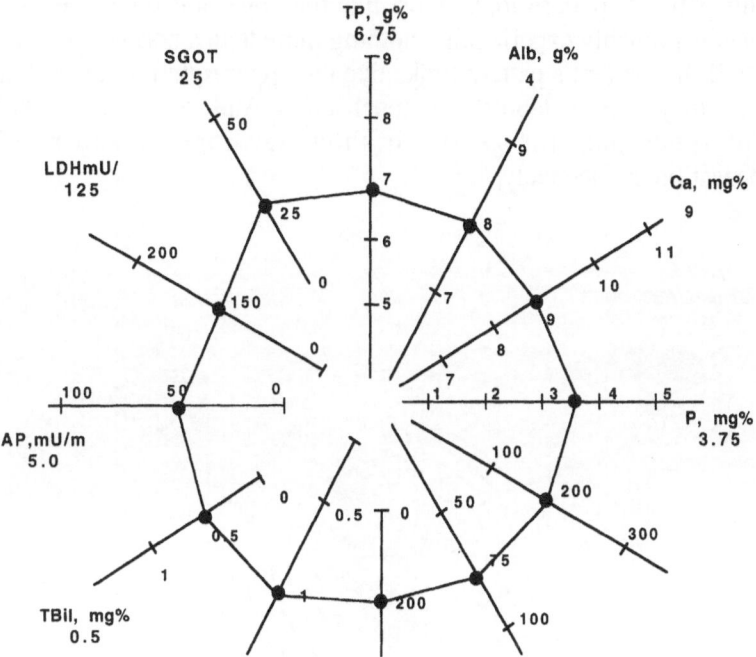

Fig. 2. A polar graph. Twelve laboratory tests have been carried out on a patient, and the results graphed on twelve scales. Normal range for each of the twelve scales is halfway out the line, measured from the center of the display. Since this patient's results are all normal, the data line forms a roughly circular shape

The scales in this particular display are carefully constructed so that the normal range for each test appears about halfway out the line. For the vertical top scale, labelled TP, for example, normal range is around 7 units and this appears about halfway outward from the center of the display. This is important attribute of the display methodology because it means that a patient who is approximately normal on all the tests will have his result dots appearing about halfway out all the lines and when these dots are connected by a data line as shown in this figure, the data line forms a shape that is approximately circular. A caregiver seeing this figure could see the circular shape of the data line about halfway out on the twelve scales and rapidly conclude that this patient was approximately normal on all tests.

Figure 3 shows how the polar graph method has been applied to monitoring of patient parameters in a situation where quick pattern recognition is vitally important. This figure, modeled on a display created by John Siegel (2, 3), shows an emergency room patient's state as a single large polar graph surrounded by four smaller polar graphs that are references for commonly encountered states. That is, this patient's values are all shown on the central, larger graph while all four of the surrounding graphs are there simply to remind the viewer what to look for. If this patient's pattern looks most like the upper left reference shape, then this patient is probably experiencing nothing more than a normal stress response. However, if this patient's pattern looks like the upper right reference shape, then this patient may be in metabolic decompensation. And so on – the lower left and right reference patterns go on to show cardiogenic and respiratory decompensation, respectively.

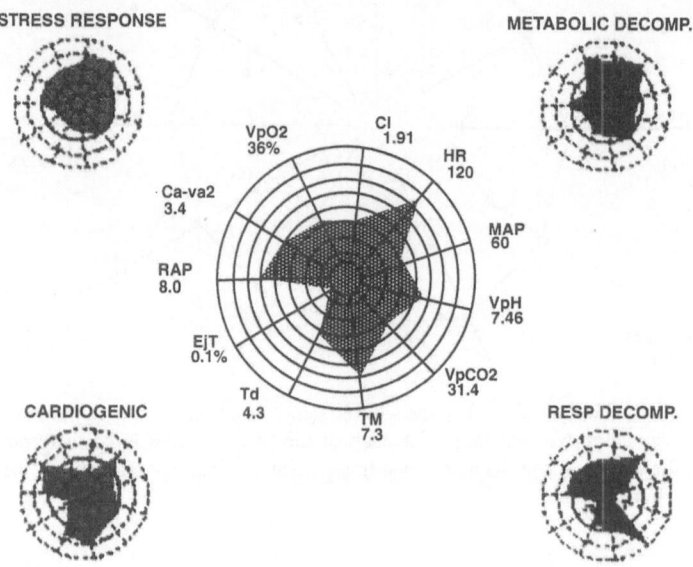

Fig. 3. The large, central polar graph displays several parameters of a patient who has just arrived at the emergency room. The four surrounding polar graphs shows shapes we would expect to see if our patient was in one of these four states. This patient looks most like the lower left reference shape, cardiogenic

The idea of this method is to allow a caregiver who is encountering the patient for the first time to see at a glance a summary of several key patient parameters in such a way that the shape of the graph, rather than careful examination of each parameter value individually, can suggest what might be wrong with the patient and thus where to begin collecting more information or which treatment should be put into motion immediately.

Polar graphs have an advantage over line graphs in that they are more likely to show shapes and thus more likely to reveal patterns. But is this enough?

Siegel's method does something no other polar graph display does – it reminds the viewer of what certain shapes mean. This is a tacit acknowledgement of the second key step in making sense of a visual data display. After the eye has detected that a pattern exists, it next becomes necessary to decide what that pattern means. In Siegel's method, if you are fortunate enough to see a pattern that Siegel anticipated, you can quickly see that this pattern means metabolic decompensation, or stress response, or whatever pattern your patient fits.

Unfortunately, in other settings such as the operating room there may be more patterns of interest than can be conveniently displayed as reference shapes around the actual patient data. How are we to signal the meaning of one of these other patterns? The shape of the patient's pattern is not in itself particularly memorable or recognizable in the absence of a reference shape. The problem with a polar graph is that the axes typically are laid out arbitrarily, so that the axes in the upper right quadrant are no more related to one another than they are to the axes in the lower left. Thus the necessity for Siegel's way of signalling meaning. There is another way of signalling meaning, however, and using this method has some important advantages because it more directly provides support for the human information processing step of decoding the meaning of a detected pattern.

Metaphor graphics: patterns plus meaning

Consider the patient's data pattern in Fig. 3. Does it look like any real world object? Could you give it a name, such as "bird flying northeast" or "ping pong paddle"? Probably not. Suppose, however, we had figured out a way of rearranging the axes on the graph so that whenever the cardiogenic pattern appeared it did not form this unnameable pattern but rather formed a crude heart. Using this new method, whenever the emergency room physician walked in and saw on the display a heart-like pattern, he or she would instantly think that this patient might be a cardiogenic case.

This is the step of creating a *metaphor graphic*, as described by Cole (4-6). Metaphor graphic displays not only form patterns but further form patterns that somehow "look like" the underlying situation. Figure 4, based on a figure by Cole and Stewart (6), shows an example. Each line of Fig. 4 shows 2 h of data taken from a patient on a mechanical ventilator. In each line there are twelve frames within which data appear as rectangular shapes. Each frame shows what went on in a ten-minute epoch of ventilation. Since there are eight lines of data, the entire display shows sixteen hours of data. Each frame has room for two rectangles, one of which shows what the ventilator was doing and the other, if it appears at all, shows the patient's spontaneous contribution. If a frame contains only one rectangle, this means the patient was contributing nothing spontaneously and the ventilator alone was supplying air to the patient. Rectangles are drawn from the top down, so that deeper rectangles represent deeper breathing (greater set volume or spontaneous volume per breath). Wider rectangles represent a larger number of breaths per epoch. Total area of the resulting rectangle represents minute volume. Rectangles also differ in how darkly they are shaded as a function of how much oxygen is being added by the ventilator to the airstream delivered to the patient. Dark rectangles have a great deal of oxyen added, while a blank, unshaded rectangle represents pure room air.

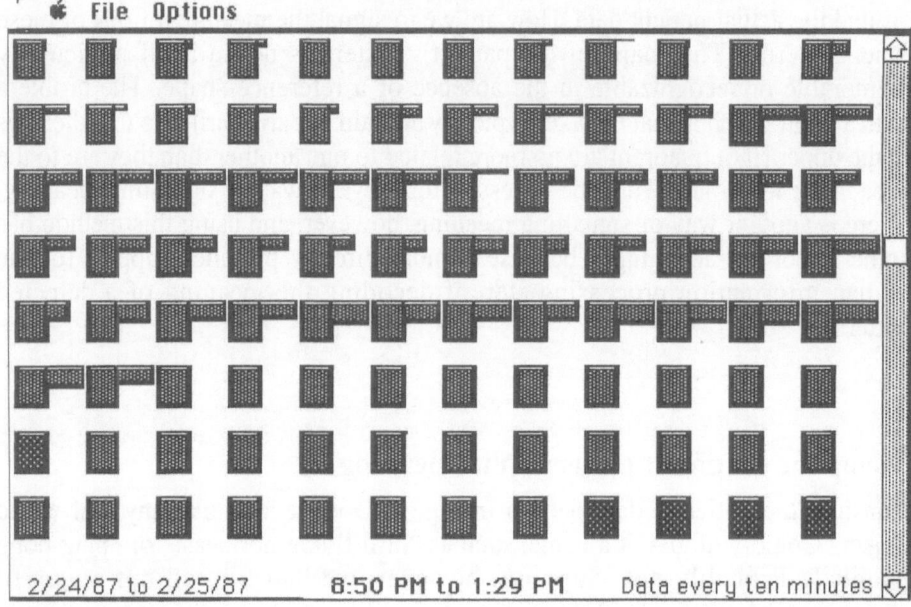

Fig. 4. A metaphor graphic display. Eight lines of twelve frames each are shown. Each frame summarized mechanical ventilation events taking place in a ten minute epoch. A line thus shows a two hour period and this entire display shows sixteen hours of data. In each frame there is room for two rectangles, a left rectangle showing what the ventilator did and a right rectangle summarizing any spontaneous breathing by the patient. Deeper rectangles represent deeper breathing. Wider rectangles represent more breaths per epoch. Darker rectangles have more oxygen added by the ventilator to the room air delivered to the patient. The assignment of these graphical attributes are intended to be metaphoric and thus easily remembered when viewing the display

In Fig. 4, the patient is breathing very little or not at all until about the third line of data (around hour six). For three lines of data (another 6 h), the patient breathes significantly, but then abruptly ceases to spontaneously contribute early in line 6 (around hour 12). Ventilator settings (the left rectangle) do not change greatly during the sixteen hours shown here, although close examination reveals that the ventilator rectangle in the lower right is slightly larger than the initial rectangle in the upper left. Additionally, it is slightly darker, indicating that more oxygen is being added to the airstream.

This particular graphical display method is not the point of the current discussion. The point is to provide an illustration of the second step in human perception of a graphical display, namely grasping the meaning of whatever patterns are detected. Furthermore, Fig. 4 is an illustration of a graphical technique for supporting this second perceptual step. If the graphical representation method creates metaphoric shapes rather than arbitrary shapes, this will speed the second perceptual step of extracting meaning.

Discussion

Line graphs provide relatively crude support for detecting patterns in data. There are two reasons for this and understanding these two reasons both helps us understand how humans perceive graphs and how we should design graphs for most rapid and correct perception. Line graphs often do not allow the eye to detect shapes because lines overlap and it can be difficult to keep track of which line is which. Polar graphs are much more likely to provide a shape that the eye can recognize, but generally polar graph shapes have no immediate meaning. Metaphor graphs are explicitly designed not only to reveal shapes but to suggest the meaning of those shapes as well, thus supporting both of the two key human perceptual steps: shape detection and recognition of the shape meaning.

References

1. Williams BT, Johnson RL, Chen TT (1977) PLATO-based medical information system overview. Proceedings of the First Illinois Conference on Medical Information Systems
2. Siegel JH, Goldwyn RM, Friedman HP (1971) Pattern and process of evolution of human septic shock. Surgery 70:232-245
3. Siegel JH, Coleman B (1986) Computers in the care of the critically ill patient. Urol Clin North Am 13(1):101-117
4. Cole WG (1986) Medical cognitive graphics, Proceedings of CHI '86
5. Cole WG, Stewart JG (1993) Metaphor graphics to support integrated decision making with respiratory data. Int J Clin Monit Comput 10:91-100
6. Cole WG, Stewart JG (1994) Human performance evaluation of a metaphor graphic display for respiratory data. Methods Inf Med 33:390-396

ICU and the Outside World: Multimedia and Networking in the ICU Environment

W. Friesdorf, B. Classen, R. Chr. Reu

Introduction

The main tasks in an intensive care unit are related to information. Information is generated, collected, documented and distributed. An intensive care patient is described by data, curves, pictures (e.g. X-rays), and videos (e.g. ultrasound examination). Information resulting from sounds (e.g. respiratory system) and three-dimensional spaces (e.g. bronchoscopy and surgical intervention) are described in text format. This patient's individual information is analysed in front of general ICU knowledge and experience. Thus by definition the condition of an intensive care patient is described by *multimedia information.*

Where does the patient-related information come from?

The bedside workplace with all its devices for treatment and monitoring is a main source of information. Additional information is provided by other departments, such as the laboratory, X-ray department, and microbiology. Often consultants from other fields are asked for advice: specialists for cardiology, ENT, neurology, pharmacology, etc. These specialists visit the patient in the ward or are just contacted by telephone. A great number of clinicians are involved directly or indirectly in the patient's treatment.

Thus by definition the treatment of a patient is working in an *information network.*

Today's conventional information network uses only few or no electronic facilities with a lot of weak points: collection of information is laboursome, the retrieval is difficult, time-consuming and sometimes impossible. Information may get lost, the transmission may fail, and the transfer of information often lasts too long.

Computing in multimedia quality and electronic networking are promising help. In our contribution we shall focus on the connection of an intensive care unit to the outside world. We do not discuss the workplace network linking the stand-alone devices to a bedside workstation. We also do not address departmental computer systems which are linking the workplaces of an Intensive Care Unit and provide central services such as audit and quality assurance.

In the following we describe some basics of the current state of computer technology, its potential, but also the risks of this new technology.

Technical aspects

Networking of an ICU with the outside world using multimedia requires three things: a local ICU Multimedia TeleCommunication workplace (MTC), connection to an electronic network, and software tools to run the communication.

The MTC requires a powerful computer system such as a workstation (Sun, HP, Deck) or a Pentium-PC with at least a 1-Gbyte hard disk. The processing of video sequences requires at least 64 Mbyte RAM. The video interface should use a compression standard (e.g. MPEG: Motion Pictures Experts Group). Using a compression algorithm, 5 min of a video clip is equivalent to some 45 Mbyte on a hard disk. Many additional input/output devices for capturing and presenting multimedia information are needed: a scanner for loading pictures, a video camera to record video sequences, or to let your dialogue partner see you sitting in front of your MTC. A microphone and a speaker are necessary for sound and speech. Such an MTC costs between 10 and 25 kECU depending on the performance. This MTC can be part of the local area network (LAN) in the ICU (1). The MTC can be a central device in the doctor's room, but it would also be possible to have an MTC in every patient's room.

Via the connection to external networks the MTC and/or the LAN is linked to the wide area network (WAN). This can be done in two steps: first to the hospital network (HIS: hospital information system), which can also be considered a LAN; secondly to the open networks such as Internet. The local MTC needs an interface to the external networks, which – as the simplest one – can be a modem using a conventional analogue telephone line. The transmission rate can be up to 28800 bit/s. For the transmission of texts such as e-mail messages, this performance is sufficient. As far as pictures and videos are concerned, it is not satisfactory. All over Europe the new Euro-ISDN is now available (2). The communication is no longer performed via an analogue but a digitized signal. This technology offers a transfer rate of 64 kbit/s using the old copper cables of the telephone installation. A standard Euro-ISDN connection consists of two data lines (64 kbit/s each) and a control line with 16 kbit/s. Easily the two data lines can be linked together (128 kbit/s), and for extended databases and pictures this performance might be sufficient. These Euro-ISDN connections can be bundled. A standard method is using a multiplexer increasing the capacity 30-fold. The resulting 2 Mbit/s is the absolute minimum for transmitting video sequences at a reduced resolution (3).

Much more powerful are broad-band networks using special lines such as fibreoptic cables with a transmission rate of 155 Mbit/s (B-ISDN: broad-band ISDN) and more. With this performance it is no longer necessary to link communication partners point to point by one line, e.g. a telephone line. The new technology in these high speed networks is using an asynchronous transfer mode (ATM). The transferred message is cut into trunks identified by the sender and the addressee and sent via ATM network (like mailing parcels). The computing system on the other side collects these parcels and puts them together in the right order. With no distance limitations two partners can communicate continuously while the transmission on the high-speed data highway is done asynchronously.

These high-speed networks are growing tremendously, so that all bigger cities in Europe may be expected to be linked soon. Also the connection to other networks, as for instance in the United States, Canada, or Japan will be guaranteed.

Until now the growth of these networks and the communication on these systems are rather chaotic. The requirements of data security (see below) makes it necessary for network participants to defend their computer systems. "Computer security is as important in the information age as were walled cities a millennium ago" (4). This security has to be performed by a firewall, which is an additional computer watching the information transfer to and from your local ICU computer system. In extended hospital networks such as HIS the security requirements are quite different, and maximal, as far as an ICU is concerned. Therefore we consider it necessary to have a special firewall between the ICU and the hospital in addition to a firewall between the hospital and the general networks (WAN) (see Fig. 1) (4).

This technical equipment (workstation, network, and connection) needs software tools for their use. An MTC requires special software for interacting with the different multimedia information. With authoring tools links between bits of information (text, pictures, video, sounds) can be defined. This enables an

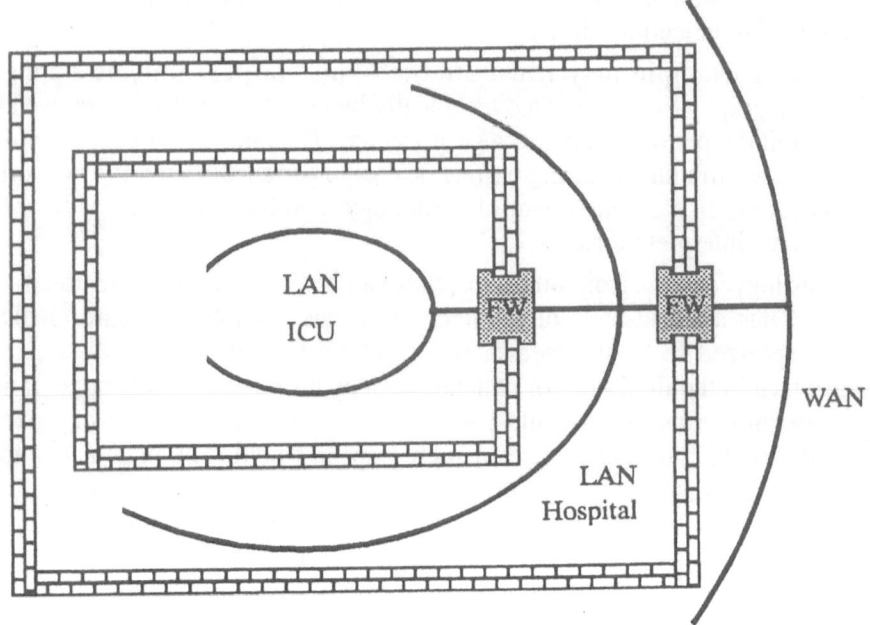

Fig. 1.

easy walk on a structured pathway through a multimedia database well-known from hypertext.

Firewall software is only meant to focus on the safety of data transmission. It has to be installed and maintained very carefully (2).

The communication via the external networks is provided by network services, which establish the connection between communication partners, no matter what physical transmission path is used. They take care of an artefact-free transmission and organize billing (5).

The potential

In a first step we shall have a look at a multimedia network inside the hospital. As described in the introduction, a large number of departments may be involved in the treatment of an ICU patient. Especially in situations when the information to be discussed among specialists consists in curves, pictures or video sequences, multimedia telecommunication would be of great help. Picture archiving and communication systems (PACS) are going to digitize all the pictures and videos supplied by the X-ray department in the near future. The broad-band hospital network can transmit these digitized pictures directly to the ICU in a far more efficient way than the conventional film method. Retrieval is easier, and the picture is available at different places at the same moment.

This development (PACS) is ready for introduction and will provide the basis of a hospital communication net. Our task is to use this opportunity and to extend hospital communication further.

Another example may illustrate the opportunities: transoesophageal echocardiography can be handled technically by an intensive care specialist after a short training period (similar to a gastroscope). The interpretation of the videos may be very difficult, requiring a great deal of experience. Using the network, a specialist (e.g. in the department of cardiology) can be connected via his MTC and give his interpretations.

In analogy, experts from other hospitals can be involved in the treatment of a patient. Thus a world-wide distributed competence of intensive care medicine can be referred to in the treatment of an individual patient. A centre of competence in the field of burn patients, toxicopathology, or multi-organ failure – to give some examples – could control and monitor the treatment of a patient in an ICU with little experience in such a special field. The patient is almost completely presented virtually on a multimedia network and does not need to be transferred to the centre. This takes away the stress of a transport with limited treatment facilities for the patient, treatment can be started earlier, and it also saves money. The possibility of communicating in that manner will support the development of standardized treatment worked out by centres of competence, a precondition for the further improvement of intensive care quality.

The centres of competence may use the network for training purposes as well. On a national or international scale, the training of intensive care specialists may thus be guaranteed at a very high level. This training could be done in real time with interaction facilities between the trainer and trainee. For lack of time, these training sessions may also be stored and recalled whenever they are needed.

The risks

Internet, which is available already today, serves as an example of network communication with some thirty million participants offering and obtaining information. WWW (World Wide Web) is one of the most important tools to support communication. Those having applied these tools for several years are faced with communication problems: lines are disturbed or interrupted, addresses are not available, the partner you are addressing is not answering, and you do not know whether he received your message or not. The "lost-in-hyperspace" syndrome (6) is characteristic of the situation: you may remember a special page in WWW, but you can't find it again even after hours of searching for it. In the clinical environment the time for "surfing" in the world-wide networks is not available. Network services are needed urgently to control and watch the information transfer. A closed and well-organized network is needed for intensive care medicine. In our opinion the quality of intensive care information accessible in the network has to be guaranteed by professional associations such as the European Society of Intensivists.

Data security is the most crucial point. "Security is keeping anyone from doing things you do not want them to do to, with, on, or from your computers or any peripheral devices" (4). As soon as you connect your ICU computer system to an external network, you have to be prepared for a "hacker" to attempt to intrude into your intensive care computer system. An extended HIS of a university hospital, for instance, must be considered insecure. A firewall can protect the local ICU system, but by linking your system to another one using an external network you risk security. Even if the message is decrypted, addresses and contents may be changed, cut, etc. etc. This may be no problem if general medical subjects are discussed, or if the patient is anonymous in the discussion. Anyway these aspects of security are still so complicated that a specialist must take the responsibility.

A lot of additional problems are foreseeable if an extended use of telecommunication among ICUs is established. Take, for example, an expert of a centre of excellence being addressed for consulting. Will he have the time to answer urgent questions? How will this be billed? What is the medicolegal situation if the consultant gives wrong advice? On the other hand, it can be regarded as malpractice if you treat a patient without referring to the most recent knowledge about treatment procedures available due to easy network access.

Considering the potential and the risks of multimedia networking, we are convinced that it is worthwhile introducing this new technology step by step. The first two steps could be: linking an ICU network via a firewall to a hospital network and installing a separated computer system via Euro-ISDN at the same time to obtain experience in using international networks.

References

1. Conrads, Demmelmeier, Halling (eds) (1987) Serielle Busse. Neue Technologien, Standards, Einsatzgebiete. vde-verlag, Berlin Offenbach, Technische Akademie, Wuppertal (TAW)
2. Hooffacker G, Steinmeyer R (1994) Euro-ISDN and ISDN. Der zukünftige Standard. te-wi GmbH, Munich
3. Tempka A (1992) MEDKOM - neue Perspektiven für die Unfallchirurgie? Unfallchirurg 95:488-492
4. Cheswick WR, Bellovin SM (1994) Firewalls and internet security. Repelling the wily hacker. Addison-Wesley, Reading
5. Byerly PF, Denley I et al (1994) A unified method for the design of telecommunication services. Ergonomics 37(10):1729-1747
6. Mesaric G (1995) Hyper-G: Die zweite Generation des Web. Multiuser Multitasking Magazin 3:162-167

Interactive Multimedial Teaching

C. MANNI, R. PROIETTI, C. SANDRONI

Introduction

The aims of interactive multimedial teaching are:

1. To increase the attention of the student by using multiple media (text, graphics, video and sound)
2. To implement self-instruction, allowing the student to participate actively in the learning process
3. To allow the user to evaluate his preparedness
4. To set up computer-simulated environments, in which the user can test his/her capacity to make appropriate decisions and actions (1, 2)

Interactive multimedial teaching derived from the fusion of two distinct experiences: the computer-aided instruction (CAI) and the adoption of new media resources for teaching.

The first experiences of CAI were conducted in early 1960s, but in this early phase their diffusion was limited by the high cost and dimension of computers, and by the lack of a friendly user interface. The systems developed in 1960s and 1970s were sophisticated enough to interact efficaciously with the student, by testing his capability to respond to simple questions and by allowing a dynamic information access based on links (the so-called *hypertext*) (3), but the capability to manage data was still limited mainly to textual information.

In contrast various multimedia self-instruction workstations were developed in the same period. Many of them consisted in a slide projector combined with a cassette player, or a videotape accompanied by written documentation and a set of printed multiple-choice questions (MCQ). The main limitation of these systems was represented by the fact that each of their devices could play only one or two media: for example, slides can include only pictures and a limited amount of text. Coordination among different devices was difficult and based essentially on user control.

After these experiences, it became clear that an efficient and fully interactive multimedia system for self-instruction would require an integrated device capable of controlling either the multiple media and the bidirectional data flow between the "virtual" teacher and the student. This objective was reached with the development of the multimedia personal computer (MPC) supplied with a graphical and intuitive user interface. The use of an MPC allows the user to fully concentrate on the learning process, without distracting his attention for interaction with complex operating systems or uncoordinated media devices.

In the last 15 years, we assisted in an increasing diffusion of multimedia interactive teaching in medicine. This diffusion was only limited by the incomplete knowledge of the many advantages that information technology can produce in the field of teaching and by the unjustified fear that the computer could limit the role of professors or keep them away from the direct interaction with their students. We want to point out, instead, that all computerized self-instruction applications require the active programming and projecting by a teacher familiar with the multiple disciplines involved in the production process (4).

The teaching of anesthesiology and intensive care can greatly benefit from CAI, for many reasons:

1. Large practical component: audiovisual interactive media can be used to teach maneuvers that cannot be clearly described only with words.
2. Standardization of procedures, which can be summarized in a computer-reproducible flow-chart, as for instance in cardiopulmonary resuscitation.
3. Information stored in the computer memory can be rapidly updated, in accordance with the evolution of knowledge and international guidelines.
4. Computer data can be diffused rapidly, either via modem or CD-ROM: this facilitates the exchange of knowledge between teachers and the diffusion on wide geographical area of basic self-instruction courses for rescuers and laypersons.

The multimedia classroom of the "Agostino Gemelli" University Hospital

In 1994 the Department of Anesthesiology and Intensive Care of the Catholic University School of Medicine, in cooperation with the TELEMED Consortium and the National Council for Research, started a research program on CAI in cardiopulmonary resuscitation (CPR). We utilized the multimedia classroom of the Center for Telemedicine Research and Training, located in the "Agostino Gemelli" University Hospital (5).

The classroom's equipment includes 14 MPCs (2 master EISA 486 DX2/66, 1 Gb SCSI HD, 32 Mb RAM and 12 workstations ISA 486 DX2/50, 500 Mb HD, 16 Mb RAM). Every PC is equipped with a 16 bit/44 kHz sound card and a VESA local bus accelerated video card.

The masters are connected with the workstations via LAN on Ethernet adapters. The network operating system is LANtastic for Windows 5.0.

An additional network (IBM Val-Net) is used for sharing of video and keyboard functions among masters and workstations.

The Val-Net allows the teacher, who uses one of the two masters, to take control of the students' system video signals and to show directly on the students' monitor what is on the master's monitor, including video input from an external source (camcorder, VCR, videodisc). The other master is equipped with a video digitizer card and is dedicated to the development of interactive applications using the Multimedia Toolbook authoring program. The educational applications are distributed in runtime form via LAN to the students' workstations for interactive learning purposes.

The 1994 experience of our department

Our first experience with CAI consisted in a 3-day training course on basic and advanced CPR which took place between February and July 1994 and involved 350 MDs (67% males, 33% females, mean age 36 years), graduated at least 2 years previously and trained in emergency facilities.

Lessons were assembled using a multimedia presentation package and delivered to the students' workstations using the Val-Net. Data were organized in a hyerarchical hypertext structure, and links between nodes were activated by buttons and hotwords. CPR maneuvers were displayed directly on the PC screen using digital video sequences and analogic videotapes converted with a video overlay card.

Students' evaluations were made using a computerized multiple choice test including 80 items. Overall performance at the end of course was satisfactory, as shown by pre- and post-test comparison (32.4% versus 58% of correct answers). The greatest improvement in the students' performance was observed for items with the lowest pre-course performances; this result may be explained considering that real-time evaluation allowed teachers to stress subsequently the topics with the worst pre-course scores (6).

Self-instruction: the multimedia courseware

In 1995 we set up an interactive courseware, whose scope is to allow rescuers, medicine students and physicians to teach themselves the procedures of basic CPR (7).

The courseware includes:
1. A preliminary quiz which has the scope to test student knowledge about basic CPR.
2. The Basic CPR Hyperbook, a multimedia manual on basic CPR.

3. A final quiz which verifies the preparedness of the student at the end of the course. The quiz includes all the preliminary questions plus a set of new questions related to topics presented in the Hyperbook.

4. A computer-simulated training that allows the student to learn the correct tempo and number of ventilations and compressions during one-rescuer CPR.

Quizzes

The quizzes are based on different kinds of questions: multiple choice, graphical choice, open-ended, and basket. The program displays hints when an incorrect response is given, acknowledges correct answers, and stores student answers in an ASCII file, which can be imported into spreadsheets or other kinds of applications for research and statistical purposes. Different sounds are also played in response to the student actions.

At the end of the tests, student scores for three different subgroups of questions are automatically calculated and if they are under a preset threshold, the program notifies to the student the subgroups in which performance was insufficient. Final results are displayed in a table and can be printed on paper, along with the student anagraphics.

Hyperbook design

The Basic CPR Hyperbook was designed around a book metaphor. Each screen of the program is a page, and pages are grouped in chapters.

The left hand side of the explanation pages (Fig. 1) contains a written description of the assistance procedure, while the right hand side contains graphic information, as fixed images (pictures or digitized photos) or moving images: in practice brief video clips which demonstrate how to carry out the action correctly.

The student, after having observed an image, can analyze it moving the mouse: each time a significant area is presented, the relative captions come up on the screen one at a time; the advantage of this method is to avoid numerous captions crowding the screen and overlapping each other, so the student's attention can focus on one concept at a time.

Navigation into the book is achieved in two ways:

1. Using buttons located at the bottom of the page: they allow the user to flip to the previous or next page or to browse along the book following links that connect related pages. The function of each button is explained by pop-up legends activated by mouse pointing (somewhat like Microsoft Intellisense function).

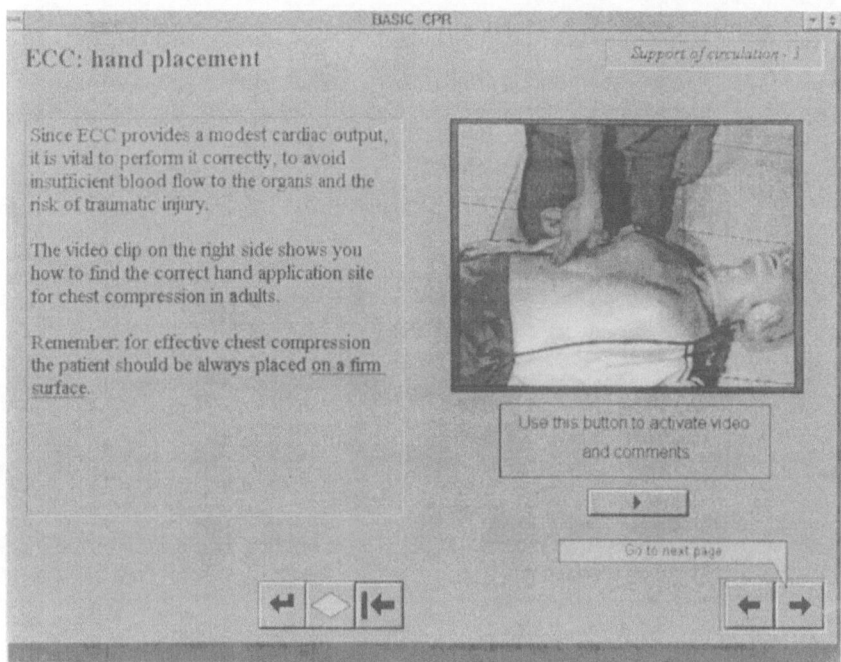

Fig. 1. Explanation page with video and navigation buttons

2. Clicking on or pointing at the key words or phrases of the text (hotwords): related supplementary information is presented as pop-up boxes when small, while larger ones are included in a page where the reader jumps into.

The method of flexible information access described here is called hypertext. Hypertext gives the reader the freedom to absorb topics at his own pace, and it has also the advantage of presenting information in a hierarchical and organized form.

Computer simulation

The computer simulation is a simple exercise book, in which the student can train himself in one-rescuer CPR.

Every time the PC space bar is pressed, the chosen action (ventilation or compression) is performed by a small animated figure on the screen which simulates the student's actions (Fig. 2).

Two counters show the number of actions carried out for each compression or ventilation sequence, and advise the student when that number exceeds the prescribed limit.

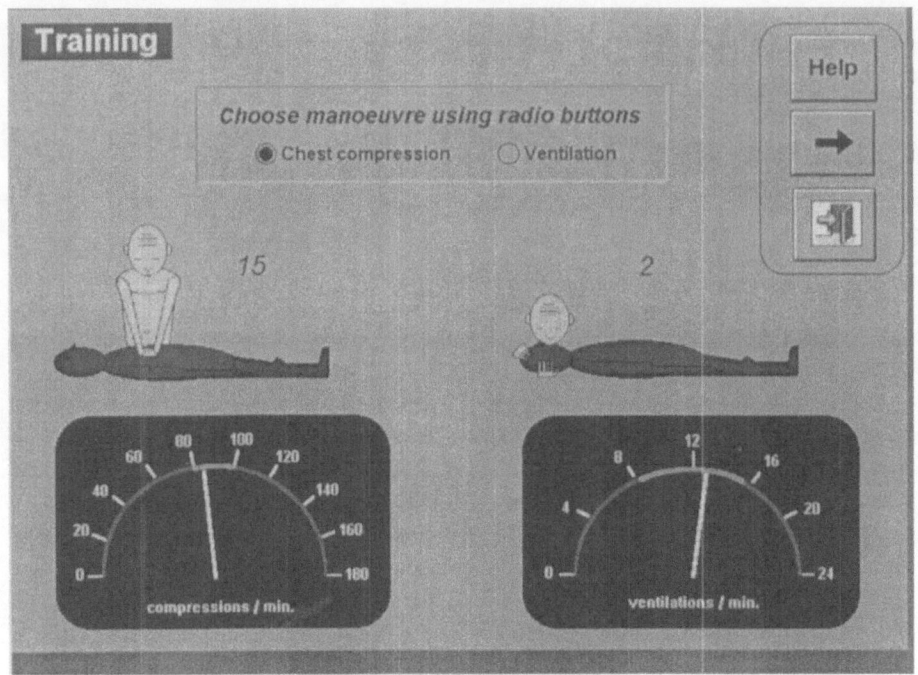

Fig. 2. Computer simulation of one-rescuer CPR

Two dials show in real-time the frequency with which each action is carried out: the correct frequency interval is indicated by a green sector.

The student, making an effort to keep the dials' arrows always in the green sector, can learn the correct tempo and number of compression and ventilation sequences.

The courseware is currently used by the sixth year medicine students of the Catholic University School of Medicine, as a part of the Multidisciplinary Course on Medical and Surgical Emergencies. Courseware sessions are held in multimedia classroom and have a 3-h duration. The analysis of feedback forms filled out by the students showed a 94% rate of global satisfaction rating, while the great majority of students considered this method of teaching more interesting, useful and pleasant (Fig. 3).

Finally, although the self-instruction required the student to use a computer interface for data access, the students considered the courseware easy to use (86%), complete (92%) and clear (94%) (Fig. 4).

Having these positive results in mind, we started to develop a new courseware on advanced CPR, which will be completed by end of 1995. Furthermore, we decided to distribute the courseware on basic CPR, whose target was initially

You think that explanation pages are:

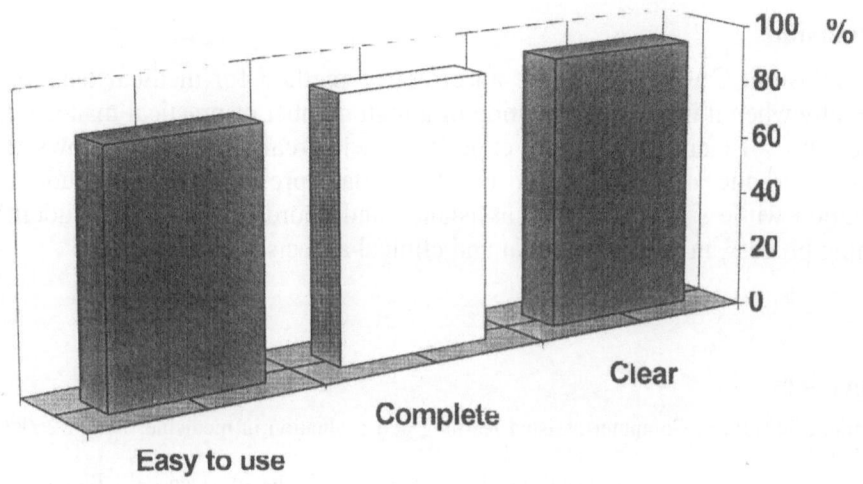

Fig. 3. Feedback forms - 75 students

Comparison between multimedia interactive teaching and traditional teaching

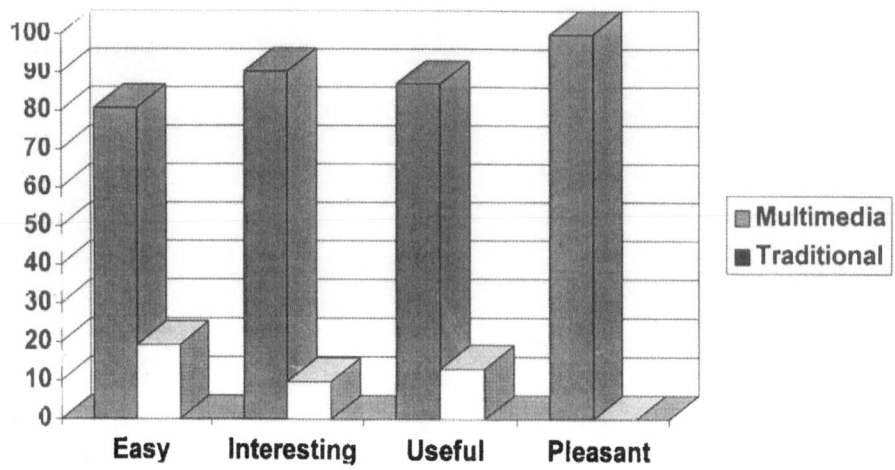

Fig. 4. Feedback forms - 75 students

represented only by the students and residents of the Catholic University School of Medicine. The software is now available on CD-ROM and can be installed on every Windows-based PC.

Conclusions

In conclusion, CAI proved to be an effective method for medical teaching, especially when it implies explanation of a high number of practical maneuvers. Although CAI cannot substitute experience with real patients, it allows the teacher to reduce the time spent merely on data presentation and student's evaluation while saving time for assistance and coordination of the student's learning process, in both theoretical and clinical aspects.

References

1. Piemme TE (1988) Computer assisted learning and evaluation in medicine. JAMA 260(3): 367-372
2. O'Neill P (1992) Instructional multimedia computing in the health sciences. J Biocommun 19:25-29
3. Frisse M (1988) From text to hypertext. BYTE 10:247-253
4. Corvetta A, Pomponio G, Luchetti MM, Salvi A (1991) Hypertext and hypermedia in medical teaching. Artif Intell Med 3:261-263
5. Proietti R (1994) Formazione in Telemedicina. Telemed 5:8-11
6. Sandroni A, Barelli A, Proietti R, Bocci MG (1994) Multimedia interactive teaching of CPR. Resuscitation 28:S45
7. Manni C (1995) Computer-aided instruction (CAI) in medicine. In: Bracale M (ed) Health telematics '95. Ischia, Naples, pp 447-450

ADVANCES IN INHALATORY ANAESTHESIA

How to Detect Cardiovascular Dysfunction in the Perioperative Period

M. MERLI, F. MILAZZO, M.M. VISIGALLI

The evaluation of preoperative risk and the decisions concerning therapeutics, intraoperative monitoring, choice of anaesthetics, postoperative monitoring and care is a major challenge for the anaesthesiologist. Because of the magnitude of the problems of perioperative cardiovascular (CV) morbidity and mortality, many efforts must be made to assess preoperatively CV dysfunction (1-4) and potential intra and postoperative CV adverse events. Unfortunately, with the advent of "come and go-stay" surgery, limited time is available for assessment; patients are older and sicker, the cost containment may limit the number and type of preoperative tests and, last but not the least, the tests are not clearly conclusive. A general six tiered model for determining the efficacy of a medical technology has been suggested by Fryback (5): technical efficacy, diagnostic accuracy, diagnostic thinking efficacy, therapeutic efficacy, patient outcome efficacy and societal efficacy. With regard to this, the need to evaluate and describe clinical events has often placed physicians in the position of using technologies not completely evaluated. Moreover, the importance and applicability of risk indices, because of changes in strategies, in monitoring and therapies are questionable, poorly helpful in everyday practice and there is no statistical evidence strongly suggesting the use of most monitoring technologies; everyday practice and professional skill, clinical judgement and proved guidelines contribute to appropriate decisions.

First of all the matter of perioperative CV dysfunction must be focused, more than obvious perioperative morbidity and mortality.

Adequate perioperative CV functions means no MVO_2/MDO_2 imbalance, no $\dot{V}O_2/DO_2$ imbalance (total body and single organ related), in a regimen of saving energy supply.

From this point of view, perioperative control of energy demands in order not to stress the CV system and CV reserves is mandatory.

This simple but hard to achieve end point must guide perioperative CV evaluation, by means of case history, physical examination and diagnostic technologies, and suggest the best anaesthetic and therapeutic approach.

One more point must be clarified when we discuss about what, when and how to evaluate CV function. Because of the increasing widespread use of expensive

CV testing technologies, often with extremely wide variations in practice between institution, and health-care cost restraints, the main thing to do is to avoid inaccurate and nonessential diagnostic and monitoring practice rather than limit medical care.

Preoperative identification of patients at risk for perioperative cardiovascular adverse events (PCVAE)

The detailed case history is the first step to approach CV dysfunction, then other factors such as predictors of PCVAE must be discussed.

Age

The predictive value of age is still debated (6-10), some authors (11, 12) suggest age not to be as important as the patient's overall physiologic state.

Coronary artery disease (CAD)

Angina. Angina is a controversial predictor of PCVAE (7, 13-15). Other angina related factors (severity, character and therapy) have not been extensively studied but may be more important (7). At the present time, perioperative myocardial ischaemia may be advocated as important for perioperative cardiac morbidity.

Previous myocardial infarction (MI). History of previous MI did not demonstrate a statistically significant independent association with perioperative mortality or morbidity (7, 16), as well as patients with more recent MI (3-6 months old).

Previous CABG surgery does not increase the risk of perioperative cardiovascular morbidity (7, 17, 18).

Congestive heart failure (CHF)

Preoperative CHF is a good predictor (7, 14, 16), while specific signs of CHF are controversial. Only a quantified measure of myocardial contractility is predictive of CV outcome (7, 14, 19, 20).

Valvular heart disease

Aortic and mitral valve dysfunctions (6) are associated with increased perioperative mortality and CHF. More than the type of valvular disease, attention must be addressed to the concomitant ventricular dysfunction and to the degree of valvular dysfunction in order to evaluate the cardiac reserve. Adequate preload and afterload have smaller ranges for optimizing contractility in valvular heart disease patients, namely during and after surgery when increased cardiac work may be called for. The severity of ventricular dysfunction, arrhythmias, pulmonary hypertension and CAD associated with valvular disease are determinant for outcome.

Arrhythmias

Arrhythmias are usually benign in healthy patients with no heart disease, but often they are associated with CAD, CHF, hypertension or valvular heart disease, and sometimes unknown. From this point of view, preoperative premature ventricular contractions (PVC) or rhythm other than normal sinus are predictors of perioperative cardiovascular morbidity (7, 21) while bi-trifascicular blocks, right bundle-branch block or left anterior hemiblock do not increase perioperative risk, unless associated with more serious myocardial conditions (i.e. MI). Moreover, the evidence and the characteristics of dysrhythmias in patients with a known heart disease are often signs of severity of the illness and of the adequacy of CV therapy.

Hypertension and systemic vascular disease

Initially (5-10 years) hypertension is usually asymptomatic; in the following years hypertension, if uncontrolled, causes damage in target organs such as heart, kidneys and brain. Accelerated atherosclerosis and left ventricular hypertrophy increase the risk of myocardial ischaemia and dysfunction; sometimes a disabling peripheral vascular disease may mask a coexisting CAD.

Hypertension and systemic vascular disease are risk factors for perioperative myocardial ischaemia, CHF, and stroke (9, 10, 22-25).

Preoperative withdrawal of antihypertensive medications is associated with blood pressure effects, thus supporting cardiovascular complications.

Pulmonary hypertension (PHT)

Pulmonary hypertension is still a problem for anaesthesiologists because there are many causes of PHT (26), related symptoms are not specific, and physicians, generally attuned to the disease of left heart undervalue this clinical event especially when associated with a more evident lung or cardiac disease. Patients with known or unknown PHT, even if not evidencing "cor pulmonale", are prone to acute right ventricle derangement. Attention therefore must be payed to preoperative recognition and evaluation of PHT.

Cardiovascular therapy

Preoperative investigation concerning cardiovascular therapy may be useful to focus a pre-existent CV disease and to suggest further evaluation and monitoring. Moreover, the beneficial effect of many drugs (ß-blockers, CA channel blockers, clonidine, nitrates, ACE inhibitors) for patients with CAD or CHF, or hypertension are well known, and their withdrawal is associated with an increased incidence of perioperative CV adverse events (27-30).

Diabetes

Diabetes is a predictor of perioperative CV morbidity (7, 14, 31): in diabetics cardiomyopathy and myocardial ischaemia tend to be silent, and the abnormal autonomic tone supports increased perioperative blood pressure effects.

Preoperative CV evaluation

Preoperative evaluation of CAD and coronary reserves

ECG. ST-T changes and Q waves, on a 12-lead preoperative ECG have been identified by some authors as significant predictors of adverse perioperative cardiovascular events (7, 8, 32); others do no support it (33). Q waves and ST-T changes may be useful to detect a previous MI even if radionuclear imaging and echocardiography are more sensitive.

Ambulatory ECG monitoring (AEM). AEM is successful in detecting ST changes during normal daily activity; these events, patterns of ischaemic episodes not always associated with symptomatic angina (34, 35), are correlated with perioperative CV morbidity (36).

Exercise stress testing (EST). The importance of EST as a predictor of PCVAE is under debate (37, 38); nevertheless it has been proved a more sensitive indicator of CAD than history and resting ECG. EST data (ST changes, large, early during stress, sustained during recovery period, associated with low increase of heart pressure and subnormal increase of heart rate during stress) are useful to diagnose chest pain of unknown origin and to evaluate coronary reserves.

In those patients unable to exercise or for a more detailed diagnosis, ECHO dobutamine, ECHO dipyridamole test and dipyridamole thallium imaging has been suggested to be optimal tests (39). Thallium redistribution abnormalities may predict patients most likely to develop wall motion abnormalities when ischaemia favouring haemodynamic events occurs perioperatively (40, 41).

Only in few cases is it advisable to use cardiac catheterization and coronary angiography.

Even if angiographic findings (coronary availability and ventricular function indices) are predictive for PCVAE (17, 42). Expense and morbidity associated with cardiac catheterization and the existence of alternative, less risky and less costly techniques limits its use for preoperative evaluation only in those patients requiring CABG before noncardiac surgery.

Preoperative evaluation of ventricular dysfunction

The ejection fraction (EF) of the left and right ventricles (the ratio of stroke volume to ventricular end diastolic volume) is an efficient tool for quantitative measurement of ventricular performance (43, 44). The cardiovascular system normally maintains the arterial bed in a state of relaxation relative to the state that corresponds with maximal stroke work (45). Experimental and clinical data suggest that maximal efficiency occurs when EF = 0.67 (46).

EF is dependent on contractility and afterload. It is relatively constant, in normal heart, over a wide range of preloads, because of compensation of the entire system with all the endogenous mechanisms; when ventricular function is reduced changes in contractility due to abnormal pre- and/or afterloads are more evident. Thus EF can measure efficiency of the entire cardiovascular system to cope with changes of myocardial contractility, preload and afterload that determine performance of both ventricles.

The enhancement of knowledge concerning cardiac pathophysiology has pointed out the role of lusitropism in influencing the overall cardiac performance. The assessment of diastolic function of both ventricles is difficult because many factors and events can influence it (47, 48).

The indices describing diastolic function, though with inherent potential limitation, provide useful information for evaluating myocardial diastolic function when the patient's history suggests diastolic heart insufficiency. Invasive measurement of end diastolic pressure volume relationship (EDPVR) is the best reference for evaluating diastolic patterns. Nevertheless noninvasive measurements, ECHO derived, are available for clinical use: IVRT (isovolumic relaxation time: the time from the end of systolic ventricular outflow to mitral valve opening), E/A ratio [the ratio of early (E) to late (A) peak blood flow velocity across the mitral valve during diastolic ventricular filling], the enhanced retrograde pulmonary venous blood flow before or during atrial systole and the rate of change of left ventricle diameter and of ventricular thinning during diastole. Nevertheless many pathologic conditions such as pulmonary hypertension, pericardial disease, obesity, hypertension, heart rate and mitral regurgitation may alter transmitral flow patterns that may not yet be adopted for clinical diagnosis of diastolic function unless satisfactory data on sensitivity, specificity and predictivity are available (49). Recognition of ventricular filling patterns, ventricular filling rates and filling time may be also accomplished by radionuclide ventriculography.

Moreover cardiomegaly on chest X-ray (14) (cardiothoracic ratio > 0.5) is predictive of poor ventricular function in approximately 70% of patients.

Preoperative evaluation of arrhythmias

Patient's history, 12-lead ECG, ambulatory ECG monitoring, ECG on stress testing are mandatory to evaluate the type of dysrhythmias, how long lasting, and how severe (LAWN class); moreover the evidence of preoperative dysrhythmias suggests further investigations in order to evaluate any coexisting CV disease.

Preoperative evaluation of hypertension

Hypertension must be confirmed on subsequent visits. If secondary hypertension is suggested, specialized studies such as thyroid function tests, plasma aldosterone and catecholamines, renal vein renin level, intravenous urogram and renal artery angiogram must be planned for a detailed diagnosis.

But for the aim of surgery and preoperative evaluation only simple tests for target organ damage are necessary.

Chest X-ray provides information concerning cardiac enlargement, pulmonary congestion and rib notching.

ECG is useful to evaluate left ventricle hypertrophy, dysrhythmias, conduction defects and previous MI.

TEE or TTE give further data concerning left ventricle volumes, wall thickness, contractility and lusitropism.

EST is mandatory when history and other tests suggest CAD.

Blood and urine tests are useful to evaluate renal damage.

An adequate assessment of the CV state of patients undergoing surgery and the knowledge of surgical procedures should provide sufficient data for planning anaesthesia, intra- and postoperative CV monitoring and postoperative treatment in order to avoid adverse CV events.

Intraoperative CV monitoring

Arterial pressure

Measurement of arterial pressure is an aspecific test to evaluate intraoperative CV state. Measurement of arterial pressure with the use of standard cuff and palpation and auditory or oscillometric techniques varies considerably and becomes inaccurate in the presence of hypotension and of vasoconstriction. Direct catheter transducer pressure measurement may be a more reliable method, even if, because of physiological and extrinsic amplification of arterial pressure, a calibrated transducer may also produce erroneous values in critical haemodynamic conditions. Moreover arterial pressure values and waves vary significantly from a proximal site to a distal site.

Suggested indications for intraarterial pressure monitoring are (50):
– Desirability of a beat to beat display of blood pressure
– Anticipated wide changes in blood pressure
– Anticipated potential significant changes in preload, afterload or contractility
– Overall condition of the patients determined by ASA physical status classification (status III, IV, and V)
– MI within prior 6 months
– Deliberate hypotensive technique
– Open chest procedures
– Frequent blood gas determinations.

The problem is to determine when an increased or decreased arterial pressure become dangerous.

In terms of cardiac work and MVO_2, hypertension and tachycardia are deleterious in the presence of CAD or CHF; however, in terms of organ perfusion, in aged patients with long standing hypertension only a certain degree of hypertension ensures adequate organs perfusion.

Acute hypertension imbalances myocardial oxygen supply and demand. In the normal heart, hypertension elevates diastolic pressure above ventricular end diastolic pressure, thereby raising the coronary perfusion pressure; in the failing heart coronary perfusion pressure is reduced and myocardial ischaemia may be precipitated. In patients with CAD moderate increases of arterial pressure may be well tolerated (16, 34); nevertheless ischaemic episodes and MI often occur during hypertensive episodes (9, 51, 52).

Hypotension reduces myocardial wall tension and MVO_2; nevertheless myocardial ischaemia may occur when coronary autoregolatory mechanism fails to compensate pressure dependent coronary flow reduction, or when critical coronary stenoses are present. Thus a causal relationship between hypotension and ischaemia may exist (16, 53-55); however the severity and duration of hypotension episodes that may precipitate an ischaemic episode may be not predicted. Some authors (56) define sustained hypotension as a 30% decrease in the mean arterial pressure lasting for more than 10 min.

Intraoperative hypo-hypertension may signal acute life threatening events (hypoxaemia, hypercarbia, pneumothorax, heart failure, pulmonary embolism, pulmonary hypertension) or less severe adverse events (insufficient analgesia, stress response, hypothermia, hypo-hypervolaemia) and often confirm a preoperative CV disease.

Finally arterial pressure monitoring is necessary to institute a specific treatment and drug therapy.

Monitoring myocardial ischaemia

Perioperative myocardial ischaemia and its importance in PCVAE are still under debate (57, 58). Intraoperative ischaemic episodes, in CABG and in noncardiac surgery patients, are often uneventful but sometimes develop into MI and may compromise heart performance; therefore they should be regarded by anaesthesiologists as ominous signs in order to prevent such adverse events and worsening of myocardial performance.

Intraoperative ischaemia may be precipitated by impairment of MVO_2/MDO_2 caused by hyper- or hypotension, tachycardia, increased filling pressures, anaemia, hypoxaemia, sympathomimetic drugs, stress, coronary spasm and thrombosis.

Unfortunately there is not an absolute reference standard for ischaemia and different methods are used for this purpose: ECG, TEE, and WP changes. Moreover not all changes interpreted as ischaemia related are really consistent with ischaemia.

Arterial pressure monitoring is an important but too aspecific method. Mean arterial pressure/heart rate quotient (PRQ) (59, 60) and the product of systolic blood pressure and heart rate (RPP) have been suggested as simple, inexpensive methods to alert anaesthesiologists to the presence of myocardial ischaemia; Siraki (60) concluded that in patients with CAD a PRQ value < 1 is a useful indicator of ischaemia. However, it has been shown that methods such as the ratio of the systolic pressure-time index and the diastolic pressure-time index are unreliable predictors of ischaemia during anaesthesia (61-63).

ECG monitoring. ECG, while highly specific, may be relatively insensitive for the diagnosis of ischaemia. Intraoperative ECG used for detection of ischaemia is also subject to physiological factors, electrolytes shifts, temperature, sympathetic stimulation and drugs. This insensitivity may be attributable to the use of 0.1 mV ST displacement criterion; 0.025 mV ST displacement is as sensitive as wall motion abnormalities, once considered diagnostic for intraoperative ischaemia (64). Multiple lead ECG permits identification of most ST changes which are consistent and variable in duration (ST depression and less frequently ST elevation), most commonly in lateral leads (V4-V5) (65).

ST changes may depend on nonischaemic aetiologies (i.e. myocardial hypertrophy) but are chronic and not reversible (66, 67); T waves changes may also occur, but are less specific than ST changes (68, 69).

Intraoperative continuous ECG monitoring is necessary to detect and evaluate arrhythmias. Dysrhythmias, usually benign in healthy patients, are markers of major cardiac events and become dangerous in the presence of heart disease such as ventricular dysfunction with or without CAD (70-72).

Nevertheless the incidence of serious intraoperative dysrhythmias (multifocal premature beats, ventricular tachycardia and fibrillation, supraventricular tachyarrhythmias, AV blocks) is reported up to 10% and its relationship to ischaemia and other postoperative adverse cardiac events has not been clarified. Increased heart rate is itself deleterious for myocardial oxygen supply and may precipitate or worsen ischaemia, especially in the presence of coronary stenosis (34, 52, 73) and hypotension (59).

TEE monitoring. TEE monitoring is suggested to be more sensitive for ischaemia than ECG. TEE wall motion and thickening abnormalities, when acute, are almost consistent with ischaemia (74), and are more sensitive and earlier indices of ischaemic episodes than ECG changes (75-78). Nevertheless, even if in CABG patients TEE wall motion normalities postbypass may predict PCVAE, in noncardiac surgery patients the predictive value of TEE abnormalities is still under debate, because not all wall motion abnormalities result from ischaemia. The incidence of significant new wall motion abnormalities, in high risk patients, is relatively low and the majority of these events are limited to severe and transient hypokinesis infrequently associated with postoperative MI (79).

Moreover, TEE is expensive, requires training and skilled experience for detailed decision making diagnosis, must be placed after laryngoscopy and intubation, and thus is not available during critical periods.

For this reason the discussed sensitivity of ECG can not be simply bypassed by the use of bi- or multiplanar TEE whose role in the "state of the art" for monitoring intraoperative myocardial ischaemia must be critically evaluated.

Wedge pressure (WP) monitoring. Wedge pressure increase in CABG patients has been suggested as an indicator of myocardial ischaemia (80); further studies did not confirm this suggestion (81, 82). For this reason the intraoperative use of pulmonary artery catheters in CAD patients for monitoring myocardial ischaemia is not indicated and is expensive as well.

Intraoperative increase of WP (more than 18 mmHg) is a marker of CHF. Myocardial contractility depression is the main mechanism; in addition preload and afterload increases both affect diastolic and systolic function and may exacerbate CHF.

The presence of impaired ventricular contractility and lusitropism because of CAD, cardiomyopathy, valvular or congenital heart disease suggests a detailed monitoring of myocardial dysfunction in order to prevent further worsening, sometimes developing a low output syndrome.

Continuous monitoring and analysis of ventricular function in terms of pressure volume relationship is the ideal tool for evaluation of heart function. Unfortunately that's possible only in an experimental setting or in selected cases using conductance catheters incorporating a micromanometer providing pressure volume loops (83).

Monitoring ventricular dysfunction

Good performance of left and right ventricle is necessary for optimizing DO_2 to couple O_2 demands.

In this connection arterial pressure (invasive or not invasive) central venous pressure (CVP), SPO_2, plethysmography, $ETCO_2$, ECG, urine output, intermittent blood gases and acid-base status are usually adequate for getting sufficient information. In particular CVP is safe and cost effective; CVP waveform analysis associated with pressure trends and patterns supply useful information concerning right ventricle preload, right ventricle ischaemia and failure, tricuspid valve disease dysrhythmias and conduction disturbances (84).

In several cases because of anaesthesia, surgical procedure and a preexisting CV disease, $\dot{V}O_2/DO_2$ imbalancement may occur; therefore targeted monitoring of intraoperative ventricular contractility, preloads, afterloads, cardiac output, oxygen delivery and consumption by means of further CV monitoring may be extremely important.

Pulmonary artery catheters (PAC). The flow guided PACs and their new adaptations allow clinicians to measure many variables related to cardiac and haemodynamic function: CVP, WP, intermittent or continuous cardiac output, mixed venous oxygen saturation and other calculated variables such as pulmonary and systemic vascular resistances, oxygen delivery and consumption. This helps to choose the appropriate interventions.

More recently a PAC able to measure right ventricular volumes and EF has been introduced into the clinical practice; however, its use is still under debate (85-87); errors in computing volumes especially in presence of high heart rates, arrhythmias and tricuspid insufficiency make this tool less reliable in many cases when heart failure is present.

Continuous cardiac output monitoring by thoracic bioimpedance or suprasternal Doppler ultrasound have been suggested for clinical use. Unfortunately inadequate signals due to electrical noise, mechanical ventilation, surgical manipulation in the operative setting and the underestimating of cardiac output due to the bias of the high standard deviation when compared to thermodilution cardiac output limit the use of these techniques for intraoperative cardiac monitoring; moreover they can't measure filling pressures or permit blood samplings (88, 89).

TEE monitoring. TEE able to detect myocardial wall thickening and motion, ventricular and atrial dimension, valvular function, blood flows and pressure gradient across valves and FAC is a useful tool to evaluate heart dysfunction. It provides an available window through which we can see the anatomy and dynamic cycles of the heart and evaluate the effects of therapeutic interventions.

The usefulness of monitoring left ventricle filling and ejection with TEE is widely accepted. The correlation coefficients between echo and radionuclide estimates is 0.85 for end diastolic volume and 0.96 for EF.

Practically, quantitative analysis requires too much time to be of value during surgery; therefore qualitative estimates of FAC end of end diastolic volume to guide drugs and fluid administration may be used (90). Automated measurement of cardiac output by TEE automated border detection has been suggested as a promising technique; nevertheless the wide limits of agreement and the number of inadequate images increase the need of more technologic refinements to improve the results and to allow an effective extended use (91).

Postoperative CV monitoring

Preoperative identification and evaluation of patients at risk for PCVAE and intraoperative CV course suggest the detailed postoperative CV monitoring approach as described on above.

Postoperative ischaemia, ventricular dysfunction and related events are the items to be focused on again.

Moreover other aspects must be pointed out.

First of all invasive CV monitoring plus continuous ECG (ST analysis) are essential and may not be replaced by other not invasive or semi-invasive techniques. TTE, when indicated, is useful for detailed diagnosis and for intermittent monitoring to support invasive monitoring.

As we have discussed above, the evaluation of left ventricular contractile state, even if very important in selected critical patients, is not feasible because of the technical and invasive demands limitations. Recently Gorcsan and colleagues (92) suggested estimating left ventricular contractility by means of femoral artery pressure coupled with simultaneous echocardiographic automated measure of the left ventricular cross section cavity area. This technique can assess left ventricular performance rapidly when needed, but only in those patients with predominantly normal left ventricular geometry; in fact, the selected TEE mid-ventricular short axis plane and, as a rule, the inadequacy of echocardiography to measure volumes in patients with significant wall motion abnormalities or changing segmental dysfunction limits this technique.

EF and FAC by biplanar TEE in most of cases give a reasonable estimate of the ventricles' function and of therapeutic interventions.

In critical patients with impaired CV function, intravascular volume management must supply an adequate ventricular filling, but not so great as to impair ventricular efficiency.

Whereas echocardiography, invasive arterial pressure and pulmonary catheterization provide data to measure myocardial contractility, cardiac output and afterloads, it is not easy to get adequate information concerning preloads and blood volume status.

Fast circulating blood volume and a slowly perfused compartment have been estimated to be 60% and 40% of total blood volume (93); moreover circulating blood volume is well correlated to total blood volume and to cardiac output (94). Central blood volume (the blood between the pulmonary artery valve and aortic artery valve) is the most reliable guide to left ventricular preload, better than CVP or WP. CVP and WP correlate poorly with intravascular volume because they are affected by the compliance of intra- and extrathoracic low pressure vascular system which may vary during the intra- and postoperative period, mainly in CV critical patients. The use of a new invasive method requiring a central venous line or a PAC and a fibreoptic femoral artery catheter has been suggested by Lewis and Pfeiffer (95) to measure cardiac output, circulating blood volume, central blood volume by means of a double indicator: ice-cold indocyanine green dye.

Conclusion

The assessment of perioperative CV risk is mandatory to improve patient care and prognosis. Anaesthesiologists must focus the problems and request, according to the patient's need, perioperative cardiology consultation with specific and explicit questions in order to get an effective collaboration.

Moreover, not all the patients must be supplied with all the haemodynamic monitoring technologies, because of complications, increasing costs and sometimes not being useful, due to inadequate accuracy and sensitivity for the intended aim. The challenge is to evaluate for the patient the actual risk of developing perioperatively a CV complication, thus tailoring a CV monitoring schedule fit for the patient.

Acknowledgements. The authors wish to thank Miss Angela Stasolla for preparing this manuscript.

References

1. Abraham S, Coles N, Coley C, Strauss H, Boucher C, Eagle K (1991) Coronary risk of non cardiac surgery. Prog Cardiovasc Dis 34:205-234
2. Wong T, Detsky A (1992) Perioperative cardiac risk assessment for patients having peripheral vascular surgery. Ann Intern Med 116:743-753
3. Goldman L (1987) Multifactorial index of cardiac risk in noncardiac surgery. Ten-year status report (review article). J Cardiothorac Anesth 1:237-244
4. Hollenberg M (1992) Predictors of postoperative myocardial ischaemia in patients undergoing noncardiac surgery. JAMA 268:205-209
5. Fryback DG, Thornbyry JR (1991) The efficacy of diagnostic imaging. Med Decis Making 11:88-94

6. Goldman L, Caldera DL, Nussbaum SR, Southwick FS, Krostad D, Murray B, Burke DS, O'malley TA, Goroll AH, Caplan CH, Nolan J, Carabello B, Slater EE (1977) Multifactorial index of cardiac risk in noncardiac surgical procedures. N Engl J Med 297:845-850
7. Foster ED, Davis KB, Carpenter JA, Abele S, Fray D (1986) Risk of noncardiac operation in patients with defined coronary disease. The Coronary Artery Surgery Study (CASS) Registry Experience. Ann Thorac Surg 41:42-50
8. Carliner NH, Fisher ML, Plotnick GD, Garbart H, Rapoport A, Kelemen MH, Moran GW, Gadacz T, Peters RW (1985) Routine preoperative exercise testing in patients undergoing major noncardiac surgery. Am J Cardiol 56:51-57
9. Steen PA, Tinker JH, Tarhan S (1978) Myocardial reinfarction after anaesthesia and surgery. JAMA 239:2566-2570
10. von Knorring J (1981) Postoperative myocardial infarction. A prospective study in a risk group of surgical patients. Surgery 90:55-60
11. Greenberg AG, Saik RP, Pridham D (1985) Influence of age on mortality of colon surgery. Am J Surg 150:65-70
12. Mohr DN (1983) Estimation of surgical risk in the elderly. A correlative review. J Am Geriatr Soc 31:99-102
13. Jamieson WRE, Janusz MT, Miyagishima RT, Gerein AN (1982) Influence of ischaemic heart disease on early and late mortality after surgery for peripheral occlusive vascular disease. Circulation 6 (Suppl I):92-97
14. Larsen SF, Olesen KH, Jacobsen E, Nielsen J, Nielsen AL, Petersen A, Pedersen OJ, Waaben J, Kehket H, Hansen JF, Dalgaard P, Nyobe J (1987) Prediction of cardiac risk in noncardiac surgery. Eur Heart J 8:179-185
15. Wells P, Kaplan JA (1981) Optimal management of patients with ischaemic heart disease for noncardiac surgery by complementary anaesthesiologists and cardiologists interaction. Am Heart J 102:1029-1037
16. Rao TK, Jacobs KH, El-Etr AA (1983) Reinfarction following anaesthesia in patients with myocardial infarction. Anesthesiology 59:499-505
17. Hertzer NR, Beven EG, Young JR, Ohara PJ, Ruschhaupt WF III, Graor RA, Dewolfe VG, Maljovec LC (1984) Coronary-artery disease in peripheral vascular patients. A classification of 1.000 coronary angiograms and results of surgical management. Ann Surg 199:223-233
18. Reul GJ Jr, Cooley DA, Duncan JM, Frazier OH, Ott DA, Livesay JJ, Walker WE (1986) The effect of coronary bypass on the outcome of peripheral vascular operations in 1.093 patients. J Vasc Surg 3:788-798
19. Pasternack PF, Imparato AM, Bear G, Baumann FG, Benjamin D, Sanger J, Kramer E, Wood RP (1984) The value of radionuclide angiography as a predictor of perioperative myocardial infarction in patients undergoing abdominal aortic aneurysm resection. J Vasc Surg 1:320-325
20. Pasternack PF, Imparato AM, Riles TS, Baumann FG, Bear G, Lamparello PJ, Benjamin D, Sanger J, Kramer E (1985) The value of the radionuclide angiogram in the prediction of perioperative myocardial infarction in patients undergoing lower extremity revascularization procedures. Circulation 72 (Suppl II):13-17
21. Cooperman M, Pflug B, Martin EW Jr, Evans WE (1978) Cardiovascular risk factors in patients with peripheral vascular disease. Surgery 35:1-10
22. The 1988 Joint National Committee: The 1988 report of the Joint National Committee on detection, evaluation and treatment of high blood pressure. Arch Intern Med 148:1923-1038
23. Prys-Roberts C, Meloche R, Foex P (1971) Studies of anaesthesia in relation to hypertension. Cardiovascular responses to treated and untreated patients. Br J Anaesth 43:122-137
24. Schneider AJL (1983) Assessment of risk factors and surgical outcome. Surg Clin North Am 63:1113-1125
25. Assidao CB, Donegan JH, Withesell RC, Kalbfleisch JH (1982) Factors associated with perioperative complications during carotid endarterectomy. Anesth Analg 61:631-637
26. Reeves JT, Groves BM (1984) Approach to the patient with pulmonary hypertension. In: Weir KE, Reeved GT (eds) Pulmonary hypertension. Futura, Mounth, Kisco, New York, p 7

27. Magnusson J, Thulin T, Werner O, Jarhult J, Thomson D (1986) Haemodynamic effects of pretreatment with metoprolol in hypertensive patients undergoing surgery. Br J Anaesth 58:251-260
28. Slogoff S, Keats AS (1988) Does chronic treatment with calcium entry blocking drugs reduce perioperative myocardial ischaemia? Anesthesiology 68:676-680
29. Bruce DL, Croley TF, Lee JS (1979) Preoperative clonidine withdrawal syndrome. Anesthesiology 51:90-92
30. Stone JG, Foex P, Sear JW, Johnson LL, Khambatta HJ, Triner L (1988) Myocardial ischaemia in untreated hypertensive patients: effect of a single small oral dose of a ß-adrenergic blocking agent. Anesthesiology 68:495-500
31. Burgos LG, Ebert TJ, Asiddao C, Turner LA, Pattison CZ, Wang-Cheng R, Kampine JP (1989) Increased intraoperative cardiovascular morbidity in diabetics with autonomic neuropathy. Anesthesiology 70:591-597
32. Carliner NH, Fisher ML, Plotnick GD, Moran GW, Kelemen MH, Gadacz TR, Peters RW (1986) The preoperative electrocardiogram as an indicator of risk in major noncardiac surgery. Can J Cardiol 2:134-137
33. Goldman L. Caldera DL, Southwick FS, Nussbaum SR, Murray B, O'Malley TA, Goroll AH, Caplan CH, Nolan J, Burke DS, Krogstad D, Carabello B, Slater EE (1978) Cardiac risk factors and complications in non-cardiac surgery. Medicine 57:357-370
34. Knight AA, Hollenberg M, London MJ, Tubau J, Verrier E, Browner W, Mangano DT (1988) S.P.I. Research Group. Perioperative myocardial ischaemia: importance of the preoperative ischaemic pattern. Anesthesiology 68:681-688
35. Knight AA, Hollenberg M, London MJ, Mangano DT (1989) S.P.I. Research Group. Myocardial ischaemia in patients awaiting coronary artery bypass grafting. Am Heart J 117:1189-1196
36. Raby KE, Goldman L, Creager MA, Cook EF, Weisberg MC, Whittemore AD, Selwyn AP (1989) Correlation between preoperative ischaemia and major cardiac events after peripheral vascular surgery. N Engl J Med 321:1296-1300
37. Cohn PF (1986) Silent myocardial ischaemia. Dimensions of the problem in patients with and without angina. Am J Med 80 (Suppl 4C):1-8
38. Cutler BS, Wheeler HB, Paraskos JA, Cardullo PA (1981) Applicability and interpretation of electrocardiographic stress testing in patients with peripheral vascular disease. Am J Surg 141:501-505
39. Dash H, Massie BM, Botvinick EH, Brundage BH (1979) The noninvasive identification of left main and three vessel coronary artery disease by myocardial stress perfusion scintigraphy and treadmill excercise electrocardiography. Circulation 60:276-284
40. Wackers FJT, Fetterman RC, Mattero JA, Clements JP (1985) Quantitative planar thallium-201 stress scintigraphy: a critical evaluation of the method. Semin Nucl Med 15:46-66
41. Leppo J, Boucher CA, Okada RD, Newell JB, Strauss HW, Pohost GM (1982) Serial thallium-201 myocardial imaging after dipyridamole infusion: diagnostic utility in detecting coronary stenoses and relationship to regional wall motion. Circulation 66:649-657
42. Hertzer NR (1985) Clinical experience with preoperative coronary angiography. J Vasc Surg 2:510-514
43. Mangano DT (1985) Biventricular function after myocardial revascularization in humans: deterioration and recovery pattern during the first 24 hours. Anesthesiology 62:571-577
44. Thys DM, Kaplan JA (1990) Cardiovascular physiology. In: Miller RD (ed) Anesthesia, 3rd edn. Churchill Livingstone, New York, pp 551-553
45. Sagawa K, Maughan L, Suga H, Sunagawa K (eds) (1988) Cardiac contraction and the pressure volume relationship. Oxford University Press, New York
46. Robotham JL, Takada M, Berman M, Harasawa Y (1991) Ejection fraction revisited. Anesthesiology 74:172-183
47. Pagel PS, Grossman W, Haering JM, Waritier DC (1993) Left ventricular diastolic function in the normal and diseased heart. Perspectives for the anaesthesiologists (part 1). Anesthesiology 79:836-854

48. Pagel PS, Grossman W, Haering JM, Waritier DC (1993) Left ventricular diastolic function in the normal and diseased heart. Perspectives for the anaesthesiologists (part 2). Anesthesiology 79:1104-1120
49. Choong CY (eds) (1994) Left ventricular diastolic function. Its principle and evaluation. Principles and practice of echocardiography pp 721-730
50. Blitt CD (1984) Invasive intraoperative haemodynamic monitoring. ASA 12:33-46
51. Roizen MF, Hamilton WK, Sohn YJ (1981) Treatment of stress-induced increases in pulmonary capillary wedge pressure using volatile anasthetics. Anesthesiology 55:446-450
52. Coriat P, Harari A, Daloz M, Viars P (1982) Clinical predictors of intraoperative myocardial ischaemia in patients with coronary artery disease undergoing noncardiac surgery. Acta Anaesthesiol Scand 26:287-290
53. Eerola M, Eerola R, Kaukinen S, Kaukinen L (1980) Risk factors in surgical patients with verified preoperative myocardial infarction. Acta Anaesthesiol Scand 24:219-223
54. Riles TS, Kopelman I, Imparato AM (1979) Myocardial infarction following carotid endarterectomy: a review of 683 operations. Surgery 85:249-252
55. Goldman L, Caldera DL (1979) Risks of general anaesthesia and elective operation in the hypertensive patient. Anesthesiology 50:285-292
56. Ashton CM, Petersen NJ, Wray NP, Kiefe KI, Dunn JK, Wu L, Thomas JAM (1993) The incidence of perioperative myocardial infarction in men undergoing noncardiac surgery. Ann Int Med 118:504-510
57. Nathan H (1994) Perioperative ischaemia is benign. Pro: perioperative ischaemia is benign. J Cardiothorac Vasc Anesth 8:589-592
58. Thomson IR (1994) Perioperative ischaemia is benign. Con: intraoperative myocardial ischaemia is not benign. J Cardiothorac Vasc Anesth 8:593-595
59. Buffington CW (1985) Haemodynamic determinants of ischaemia in myocardial dysfunction in the presence of coronary stenosis in dogs. Anesthesiology 63:651-662
60. Shiraki H, Lee S, Hong Y, Jo Y, Strom J, Goldine P, Oka Y (1989) Diagnostic of myocardial ischaemia by the pressure-rate quotient and diastolic time interval during coronary artery bypass surgery. J Cardiothorac Anesth 3:592-596
61. Moffit EA, Sethna DH, Gray RS, Matloff JM, Bussel JA (1984) Rate-pressure product correlates poorly with myocardial oxygen consumption during anaesthesia in coronary patients. Can Anesth Soc J 31:5-12
62. Gordon MA, Urban MK, O'Connor T, Barash PG (1991) Is the pressure rate quotient predictor or indicator of myocardial ischaemia as measured by ST-segment changes in patients undergoing coronary artery bypass surgery. Anesthesiology 74:848-853
63. Hoffman JIE, Buckberg GD (1978) The myocardial supply: demand ratio. A critical review. Am J Cardiol 41:327-332
64. Slogoff S, Keats AS, David Y, Igo SR (1990) Incidence of perioperative myocardial ischaemia detected by different electrocardiographic systems. Anesthesiology 73:1074-1081
65. London MJ, Hollenberg M, Wong MG, Levenson L, Tubau JF, Browner W, MAngano DT (1988) S.P.I. Research Group: intraoperative myocardial ischaemia. Localization by continuous 12-lead electrocardiography. Anesthesiology 69:232-241
66. Fegert G, Hollenberg M, Browner W, Wellington Y, Levenson L, Franks M, Harris D, Mangano D (1988) Perioperative myocardial ischaemia in the noncardiac surgical patients (abstract). Anesthesiology 69:A49
67. Haggmark S, Hohner P, Ostman M, Friedman A, Diamont G, Lowenstein E, Reiz S (1989) Comparison of haemodynamic, electrocardiographic, mechanical and metabolic indicators of intraoperative myocardial ischaemia in vascular surgical patients with coronary artery disease. Anesthesiology 70:19-25
68. Wong MG, Wellington YC, London MJ, Layug E, Li J, Mangano DT (1988) Prolonged postoperative myocardial ischaemia in high risk patients undergoing noncardiac surgery (abstract). Anesthesiology 69:A56

69. Breslow MJ, Miller CG, Parker SD, Walman AT, Rogers MC (1986) Changes in T-wave morphology following anaesthesia in surgery: a common recovery-room phenomenon. Anesthesiology 64:398-402

70. Bigger JT Jr, Fleiss JL, Kleiger R, Miller JP, Rolnitzky LM (1984) The Multicenter Post-Infarction Research Group. The relationships among ventricular arrhythmias, left ventricular dysfunction and mortality in the 2 years after myocardial infarction. Circulation 69:250-258

71. Olson HG, Lyons KP, Troope P, Butman S, Piters KM (1984) The high risk acute myocardial infarction patient at 1-year follow-up. Identification at hospital discharge by ambulatory electrocardiography and radionuclide ventriculography. Am Heart J 107:358-366

72. McGovern B (1985) Hypokalemia and cardiac arrhythmias. Anesthesiology 63:127-129

73. Kotter G, Kotrly K, Kalbfleish J, Vucins E, Kampine J (1987) Myocardial ischaemia during cardiovascular surgery as detected by an ST segment trend monitoring system. J Cardiothorac Anesth 1:180-199

74. Hertwer NR, Beven EG, Young JR. Ohara PJ, Rushhaupt WF III, Graor PA, Dewolfe VG, Maljovec LC (1984) Coronary-artery disease in peripheral vascular patients. A classification of 1.000 coronary angiograms and results of surgical management. Ann Surg 199:223-233

75. London MJ, Tubau JF, Wong MG, Layug E, Mangano DT (1988) The "natural history" of segmental wall motion abnormalities detected by intraoperative transesophageal echocardiography: a clinically blinded prospective approach (abstract). Anesthesiology 69:A7

76. Wohlgelernter S, Cleman M, Highman HA, Fetterman RC, Duncan JS, Zaret BL, Jaffe CC (1986) Regional myocardial dysfunction during coronary angioplasty: evaluation by two-dimensional echocardiography and 12 lead electrocardiography. J Am Coll Cardiol 7: 1245-1254

77. Smith JS, Cahaln MK, Benefild DJ, Byrd BF, Lurz FW, Shapiro WA, Roizen MF, Bouchard A, Schiller NB (1985) Intraoperative detection of myocardial ischaemia in high-risk patients: electrocardiography versus two-dimensional transesophageal echocardiography. Circulation 72:1015-1021

78. Leung J, O'Kelly B, Browner W, Tubau J, Hollenberg M, Mangano DT (1989) S.P.I. Research Group: prognostic importance of postbypass regional wall-motion abnormalities in patients undergoing coronary artery bypass graft surgery. Anesthesiology 71:16-25

79. London MJ, Tubau JF, Wong MG, Layug E, Hollenberg M, Krupski WC, Rapp JH, Browner WS, Mangano DT (1990) The "natural history" of segmental wall motion abnormalities in patients undergoing non cardiac surgery. Anesthesiology 73:644-655

80. Kaplan J, Wells PH (1981) Early diagnosis of myocardial ischaemia using the pulmonary artery catheter. Anesth Analg 60:789-793

81. Haggmark S, Hohner P, Ostman M, Friedman A, Diamont G, Lowenstein E, Reiz S (1989) Comparison of haemodynamic, electrocardiographic, mechanical and metabolic indicators of intraoperative myocardial ischaemia in vascular surgical patients with coronary artery disease. Anesthesiology 70:19-25

82. Kleinman B, Henkin RE, Glisson SN, El-Etr AA, Balchos M, Sullivan HJ, Mantoya A, Pisarre R (1986) Qualitative evaluation of coronary flow during anaesthesia induction using thallium-201 perfusion scans. Anesthesiology 64:157-164

83. Foex P, Leone BJ (1994) Pressure-volume loops: a dynamic approach to the assessment of ventricular function. Review Article. J. Cardiothorac Vasc Anesth 8:84-96

84. Mark JB (1991) Central venous pressure monitoring: clinical insights beyond the numbers. J Cardiothorac Vasc Anesth 5:163-173

85. Hines R, Rafferty T (1993) Right ventricular ejection fraction catheter: toy or tool? Pro. J Cardiothorac Vasc Anesth 7:236-240

86. Schauble HF (1993) Right ventricular ejection fraction catheter: toy or tool? Con. J Cardiothorac Vasc Anesth 7:241-242

87. Boldt J, Zickmann B, Thiel A, Dapper F, Hempelmann G (1992) Age and right ventricular function during cardiac surgery. J Cardiothorac Vasc Anesth 6:29-32

88. Wong DH, Tremper KK, Stemmer EA, O'Connor D, Wilbur S, Zaccari J, Reeves C, Weidoff P, Trujillo R (1990) Noninvasive cardiac output: simultaneous comparison of two different methods with thermodilution. Anesthesiology 72:784-792

89. Perrino AC, Lippman A, Arivan C, O'Connor TZ, Luther M (1994) Intraoperative cardiac output monitoring: comparison of impedance cardiography and thermodilution. J Cardiothorac Vasc Anesth 8:24-29

90. Leung JM, Levine EH (1994) Left ventricular end-systolic cavity obliteration as an estimate of intraoperative hypovolemia. Anesthesiology 81:1102-1109

91. Pinto FJ, Siegel LC, Chenzbraun A, Shnittger I (1994) On-line estimation of cardiac output with a new automated border detection system using transesophageal echocardiography: a preliminary comparison with thermodilution. J Cardiothorac Vasc Anesth 8:625-630

92. Gorcsan III J, Denault A, Gasior TA, Mandarino WA, Kancel MJ, Deneault LG, Hattler BG, Pinsky MR (1994) Rapid estimation of left ventricular contractility from end-systolic relations by echocardiographic automated border detection and femoral arterial pressure. Anesthesiology 81:553-562

93. Green JF (1979) Determinants of systemic blood flow. In: Guyton AC, Young DB (eds) Cardiovascular physiology III, vol. 18. University Park, Baltimore, pp 33-65

94. Hoeft A, Schorn B, Weyland A, Scholz M, Buhre W, Stepanek E, Allen SJ, Sonntag H (1994) Bedside assessment of intravascular volume status in patients undergoing coronary bypass surgery. Anesthesiology 81:76-86

95. Lewis FR, Pfeiffer UJ (eds) (1990) Practical applications of fiberoptics in critical care monitoring. Springer, Berlin Heidelberg New York

Cardiovascular and Neuroendocrine Reaction During Inhalation Anaesthesia

P. Foëx

The effects of anaesthesia on the circulation have been intensively studied for more than a hundred years. This brief review will address three issues: the effects of anaesthesia on the normal heart, its effect on the ischaemic heart, and the interactions between cardiovascular drugs and anaesthesia.

Effects of anaesthesia on the normal circulation

The effects of volatile and intravenous anaesthetics on the circulation depend upon many factors in addition to the direct effects these drugs exert on the heart, the peripheral vascular beds, and the coronary circulation. This results in haemodynamic responses that are further modified by the effects of artificial ventilation, especially when PEEP is used, and by the sympathetic responses to surgery. Thus, widely different effects of the same anaesthetic agent may be recorded because the prevailing conditions differ.

Effects of anaesthetic agents on the myocardium

With the exception of ketamine, most, if not all, inhalational and intravenous anaesthetics decrease myocardial contractility (1). Indeed, modern inhalational anaesthetics, including desflurane and sevoflurane, cause dose-dependent reductions of myocardial contractility in isolated heart muscle preparations and in the intact heart (2). The resulting myocardial depression is greater when heart muscle preparations are taken from failing hearts (3).

Depression of inotropy relates directly to reductions of calcium fluxes across the sarcolemma of cardiac cells (responsible for the second inward current) and/or across the membrane of the sarcoplasmic reticulum (tail current). These reductions of calcium flux closely correlate with myocardial depression (4, 5). Intravenous agents such as thiopentone, etomidate (6) and propofol (6, 7) cause dose-dependent reductions of contractility also related to decreased calcium fluxes in the myocytes. In addition, a reduction of the amplitude of the delayed rectifier potassium current has been documented for propofol and thiopentone (8).

It must be noted that depression of calcium current through T-type calcium channels is also a feature of the effect of isoflurane on neuronal preparations (9).

Effects of anaesthetics on vascular tone

While a reduction of vascular resistance is a usual feature of the induction of anaesthesia, further reductions in peripheral vascular resistance are observed with isoflurane (10) but hardly with other inhalational anaesthetics. Several studies have shown propofol to cause a dose-dependent reduction of peripheral vascular resistance (11) while others have shown no such effect (12). The initial reduction of vascular resistance with the induction of anaesthesia reflects the decrease in sympathetic activity at the level of the α-adrenergic receptors.

Effects of anaesthesia on sympathetic activity

It has long been recognized that induction of anaesthesia with modern induction agents (with the exception of ketamine), and the administration of inhalational anaesthetics (with the exception of ether and cyclopropane), decreases sympathetic activity (13, 14). In recent years, several studies have documented a marked reduction in sympathetic impulses in humans (15, 16). This reduction is reversed to a significant extent by the surgical stress. At variance with most inhalational anaesthetics, nitrous oxide increases sympathetic activity (17).

Effects of anaesthesia on cardiac output

When both contractility and vascular resistance decrease, cardiac output is well maintained. This is the case with isoflurane (18, 19). However, when vascular resistance is essentially unchanged, the effect of negative inotropy is to cause a dose-dependent reduction of cardiac output (20). At equivalent MAC, enflurane causes more depression of cardiac output than halothane, desflurane (21) or sevoflurane. Intravenous agents, especially thiopentone and propofol cause dose-dependent reductions of cardiac output. However, the effect of etomidate is less pronounced.

Effects of anaesthesia on the coronary circulation

Most anaesthetic agents cause reductions of coronary blood flow that are exactly proportional to the reduction of myocardial oxygen consumption associated with the reduction of arterial pressure and left ventricular inotropy. However, two agents, isoflurane (22) and desflurane (23), appear to cause coronary vasodilatation so that coronary blood flow is maintained in the face of reduced myocardial oxygen demand. This results in a degree of luxury perfusion. This direct effect of isoflurane and desflurane on the regulation of coronary blood flow may have a detrimental effect on regional perfusion when coronary artery lesions are present (see "Coronary Steal").

Effects of anaesthesia on diastolic function

While the effects of anaesthetic agents on contractility have been extensively studied, their effects on diastolic function have been studied only relatively recently. It is now well recognized that diastole is not a passive phenomenon. It requires 15% of the energy of the cardiac cycle. Diastole consists of four phases: isovolumic relaxation, rapid filling, diastasis and atrial contribution to filling. The energy needed for relaxation is used to transport calcium back into the sarcoplasmic reticulum and out of the cardiac cell. Impaired calcium transport is responsible for a delay in the isovolumic relaxation of the ventricle.

The indices of diastolic function which have been studied most frequently are the time constant of isovolumic relaxation (τ), the peak filling rate, and the end-diastolic pressure-dimension relationship (myocardial stiffness).

The time constant of isovolumic relaxation is increased by most inhalational anaesthetics (24, 25) and by both thiopentone and propofol (11). These dose-dependent increases are not surprising as anaesthetic agents alter three major determinants of relaxation, i.e. load (decreased systolic pressure), inactivation (reduced calcium fluxes), and coronary filling (decreased coronary blood flow except with isoflurane and desflurane). An inverse relationship has been found between the halothane-induced increase in the time constant of relaxation and coronary blood flow during isovolumic relaxation (24). It is likely that the reduced load and inactivation brought about by halothane impedes LV relaxation. This in turn prevents the rapid rise in coronary flow during this phase of the cardiac cycle.

The next phase of diastole, i.e. rapid filling, is usually quantified in terms of peak filling rate. Most studies have shown that inhalational anaesthetics decrease the peak filling rate (25, 26). This is not surprising: as inhalational and intravenous anaesthetics such as propofol and thiopentone decrease systolic shortening, they necessarily decrease the scope for lengthening. As a result the peak lengthening rate is reduced.

Stiffness of the left ventricle has also been studied and there is no unanimity as to the effects of anaesthesia on the pressure-dimension relationships at the end of diastole. Some studies have shown stiffness to be increased in a dose-related manner when the concentration of inhalational anaesthetics was increased (25) while other studies have not demonstrated such an effect (26). However, it is quite clear that by comparison with the awake state, cardiac stiffness is increased in the anaesthetized state.

Effects of anaesthesia on the ischaemic myocardium

Early studies of the interactions between anaesthesia and myocardial ischaemia have used models of acute coronary occlusion and examined the extent of infarction or the extent of ST segment elevation (27). In such models the universal conclusion has been that anaesthesia minimises the extent of infarction and reduces the extent of ST segment elevation. As a result, anaesthesia may be regarded as protecting the myocardium against the effect of acute coronary occlusion.

More recently, many studies have used models of coronary stenoses and the effects of anaesthesia have been examined in terms of regional function. Almost universally studies have shown that inhalational anaesthetics cause selectively exaggerated depression of myocardium supplied by a critically or supra-critically constricted coronary artery (28, 29). This detrimental effect of anaesthesia on regional function is unlikely to be a selective effect of the anaesthetic agent on the compromised myocardium. It is much more likely to be a consequence of the reduction of the coronary perfusion pressure because of the negative inotropy of these agents. Indeed, when coronary arteries are critically constricted coronary flow becomes entirely dependent upon the coronary perfusion pressure. Under such circumstances the reduced demand still outstrips the severely compromised supply (30).

Recently, the question of beneficial or adverse effects of anaesthesia on the ischaemic myocardium has changed again as a result of studies of the effects of anaesthesia on the stunned myocardium. After a brief episode of ischaemia, it is well known that systolic function, high energy phosphates, and the ultrastructure of the cardiac cell may be altered for a prolonged period. Studies have shown that recovery of systolic function is faster in the presence of halothane or isoflurane than in the awake state (31) or under fentanyl anaesthesia (32). Thus, the effects of anaesthetic agents on the ischaemic myocardium depend exquisitely upon the model used. Inhalational anaesthetics protect the myocardium against the effect of acute coronary occlusion, facilitate recovery after temporary occlusion, but cause exaggerated depression of myocardium supplied by narrowed coronary arteries.

Coronary steal

An abundance of literature has addressed the issue of an isoflurane induced coronary steal. The controversy surrounding this phenomenon started with the observation by Reiz and colleagues, of ST segment elevation and lactate production in patients with documented coronary artery disease receiving isoflurane (33). Reiz suggested that isoflurane induced a steal phenomenon because of its known coronary vasodilator characteristics. Indeed, in a great many experimental models, isoflurane has been shown to cause redistribution of flow between endo- and epicardium or between compromised and normal myocardium (34, 35). This redistribution is associated with exaggerated reductions of regional function. In clinical practice, however, few studies have shown an adverse effect of isoflurane on outcome (36), while the majority have shown no adverse effect (37, 38). This may be due to the relative rarity of what Buffington and colleagues have termed steal-prone coronary anatomy (39). This term describes the angiographic demonstration of a coronary occlusion of one vessel, a severe stenosis of another and the presence of collateral vessels between them. This configuration of the coronary circulation occurs in about 25% of patients with coronary disease. Another possibility is that clinicians adjust the administration of isoflurane and are unlikely to accept the low perfusion pressures used in experimental models. It is also possible that confounding factors intervene. In particular, in studies of outcome most of the patients enrolled underwent surgery that did not require post-operative ventilation. As patients were allowed to breathe spontaneously post-operatively their PCO_2 must have increased. Carbon dioxide is a potent coronary vasodilator known to override the local control of coronary blood flow (40). Thus, in most if not all studies of outcome, an important confounding factor may have blurred the issue of the possible adverse role of isoflurane in patients with coronary artery disease. Another confounding factor is the afterload reduction that attends the administration of isoflurane. As vascular resistance is decreased, it is likely that some myocardial sparing effect occurs. As desflurane (23) and sevoflurane (41) share with isoflurane a degree of coronary vasodilation, the controversy surrounding the anaesthesia-induced coronary steal is likely to continue.

Interaction between cardiovascular drugs and anaesthesia

For many years it was widely accepted that drugs used in the management of hypertension, especially the beta-blockers, should be stopped before anaesthesia and surgery. This practice was based on anecdotal evidence only. Several studies carried out in the early 1970s have shown that maintenance of the anti-hypertensive medication up until the morning of surgery did not have an adverse effect on the response to anaesthesia (42). Beta-blockers were found to be well tolerated and to protect against the hypertensive response to laryngoscopy and intubation and to reduce the risk of myocardial ischaemia in the immediate peri-operative period (43). Subsequent studies have shown that beta-blockers reduce the risk of silent myocardial ischaemia within 4 h (44), 12 h (45) and up to seven days after surgery (46).

The extensive use of calcium channel antagonists in the management of hypertension and coronary heart disease has raised the possibility of exaggerated hypotension in response to anaesthesia as calcium plays a central role in the control of the extent of the excitation-contraction coupling, both in cardiac cells and in vascular smooth muscle. Experimental evidence of the interactions between verapamil or diltiazem and inhalational anaesthetics shows additive effects as far as negative inotropy is concerned (47-49). Nifedipine is used much more frequently than verapamil or diltiazem, as it causes vasodilatation, exaggerated hypotension may be expected. However, this has not been shown in a recent study of the effects of anaesthesia in patients receiving calcium channel antagonists (50). Similarly, anxiety has been expressed about the possibility of cardiovascular collapse in patients receiving ACE inhibitors. ACE inhibitors decrease the conversion of angiotensin I into angiotensin II, thereby decreasing the concentration of a powerful vasodilator. ACE inhibitors also decrease the conversion of bradykinin into inactive products thereby facilitating vasodilatation. Recent studies give conflicting results. In a study of hypertensive patients receiving ACE inhibitors, the effects of anaesthesia were almost indistinguishable from the effects observed in mildly hypertensive patients on no therapy (50). However, a study comparing the incidence of low blood pressure (systolic less than 90 mmHg) whether enalapril or captopril had been stopped the day before surgery or given in the morning of surgery, showed a higher incidence of hypotension in patients who had received their usual dose of ACE inhibitor in the morning of surgery (51). In a very large study of cardiac surgery, ACE inhibitors were found to be one of the significant predictors for the use of vasopressors after cardio-pulmonary bypass, while no other cardiovascular drug was found to predict the need for vasopressor therapy (52). These discrepancies may reflect differences between groups of patients (cardiac, vascular or general surgical) or differences in the doses of ACE inhibitors.

References

1. Shimosato S, Etsten BE (1969) Effects of anesthetic drugs on the heart: a critical review of myocardial contractility and its relationships with hemodynamics. Clin Anesth 9:17-29
2. Hartman JC, Pagel PS, Proctor LT, Kampine JP, Schmelling WT, Warltier DC (1992) Influence of desflurane, isoflurane and halothane on regional tissue perfusion in dogs. Can J Anaesth 39:877-887
3. Shimosato S, Yasuda I, Kemmotsu O, Shanks C, Gamble C (1973) Effects of halothane on altered contractility of isolated heart muscle obtained from cats with experimentally produced ventricular hypertrophy and failure. Br J Anaesth 45:2-9
4. Terrar DA, Victory JGG (1988) Effects of halothane on membrane currents associated with contraction in single myocytes isolated from guinea-pig ventricle. Br J Pharmacol 94:500-508
5. Terrar DA, Victory JGG (1988) Isoflurane depresses membrane currents associated with contraction in myocytes isolated from guinea-pig ventricle. Anesthesiology 69:742-749
6. Puttick RM, Terrar DA (1992) Effects of propofol and enflurane on action potentials, membrane currents and contraction of guinea-pig isolated ventricular myocytes. Br J Pharmacol 107:559-565
7. Takahashi H, Terrar DA (1994) Effects of etomidate on whole-cell and single L-type calcium channel currents in guinea-pig isolated ventricular myocytes. Br J Anaesth 73:812-819
8. Takahashi H (1994) Effects of general anaesthetics on calcium and potassium channel currents in heart cells. Thesis, Oxford University
9. Study RE (1994) Isoflurane inhibits multiple voltage-gated calcium currents in hippocampal pyramidal neurons. Anesthesiology 81:104-116

10. Horan BF, Prys-Roberts C, Roberts JG, Bennett MJ, Foëx P (1977) Haemodynamic responses to isoflurane anaesthesia and hypovolaemia in the dog, and their modification by propranolol. Br J Anaesth 49:1179-1187

11. Goodchild CS, Serrao JM (1989) Cardiovascular effects of propofol in the anaesthetized dog. Br J Anaesth 63:87-92

12. Puttick RM, Diedericks J, Sear JW, Glen JB, Foëx P, Ryder WA (1992) Effect of graded infusion rates of propofol on regional and global left ventricular function in the dog. Br J Anaesth 69:375-381

13. Roizen MF, Moss J, Henry DP, Kopin IJ (1974) Effect of halothane on plasma catecholamines. Anesthesiology 41:432-439

14. Gothert M, Wendt J (1977) Inhibition of adrenal medullary catecholamine secretion by enflurane. I. Investigation in vivo. Anesthesiology 46:400-403

15. Ebert TJ, Berens RJ, Muzi M, Kampine JP (1991) Direct comparison of etomidate and propofol on sympathetic neural outflow and baroreflex function in man. Anesth Analg 72:S61

16. Sellgren J, Ejnell H, Elam M, Ponten J, Wallin G (1994) Sympathetic muscle nerve activity, peripheral blood flow, and baroreceptor reflexes in humans during propofol anesthesia and surgery. Anesthesiology 80:534-544

17. Millar RA, Warden JC, Cooperman LH, Price HL (1974) Central sympathetic discharge and mean arterial pressure during halothane anaesthesia. Br J Anaesth 41:918-928

18. Stevens WC, Cromwell TH, Halsey MJ, Eger EI, Shakespeare TF, Bahlman SH (1971) The cardiovascular effects of a new inhalation anesthetic, Forane, in human volunteers at constant arterial carbon dioxide tension. Anesthesiology 35:8-16

19. Wolf WJ, Neal MB, Peterson MD (1986) The hemodynamic and cardiovascular effects of isoflurane and halothane anesthesia in children. Anesthesiology 64:328-333

20. Calverley RK, Smith NT, Prys-Roberts C, Eger EI, Jones C (1978) Cardiovascular effects of enflurane anesthesia during controlled ventilation in man. Anesth Analg 57:619-628

21. Pagel, Kampine JP, Schmelling WT, Warltier DC (1991) Comparison of the systemic and coronary hemodynamic actions of desflurane, isoflurane, halothane, and enflurane in the chronically instrumented dog. Anesthesiology 74:539-551

22. Cutfield GR, Francis CM, Foëx P, Jones LA, Ryder WA (1988) Isoflurane and large coronary artery haemodynamics: an experimental study. Br J Anaesth 60:784-790

23. Merin RG, Bernard J-M, Doursout M-FG, Cohen M, Chelly JE (1991) Comparison of the effects of isoflurane and desflurane on cardiovascular dynamics and regional blood flow in the chronically instrumented dog. Anesthesiology 74:568-574

24. Doyle RL, Foëx P, Ryder WA, Jones LA (1989) Effects of halothane on left ventricular relaxation and early diastolic coronary blood flow in the dog. Anesthesiology 70:660-666

25. Pagel, Kampine JP, Schmelling WT, Warltier DC (1991) Alteration of left ventricular diastolic function by desflurane, isoflurane, and halothane in the chronically instrumented dog with autonomic nervous system blockade. Anesthesiology 74:1103-1114

26. Munoz HR, Marsch SCU, Foëx (1995) Regional diastolic left ventricular function under inhalation anaesthesia in dogs. Br J Anaesth 74:479P

27. Bland JHL, Lowenstein E (1976) Halothane-induced decrease in experimental myocardial ischemia in the non-failing canine heart. Anesthesiology 45:287-293

28. Lowenstein E, Foëx P, Francis CM, Davies WL, Yusuf S, Ryder WA (1981) Regional ischemic ventricular dysfunction in myocardium supplied by a narrowed coronary artery with increasing halothane concentrations in the dog. Anesthesiology 55:349-359

29. Philbin DM, Foëx P, Drummond G, Lowenstein E, Ryder WA, Jones LA (1985) Postsystolic shortening of canine left ventricle supplied by a stenotic coronary artery when nitrous oxide is added in the presence of narcotics. Anesthesiology 62:166-174

30. Francis CM, Foëx P, Lowenstein E, Glazebrook C, Davies WL, Ryder WA, Jones LA (1982) Interaction between regional myocardial ischaemia and left ventricular performance under halothane anaesthesia. Br J Anaesth 54:965-980

31. Warltier DC, Al-Wathiqui MH, Kampine JP, Schmelling WT (1988) Recovery of contractile function of stunned myocardium in chronically instrumented dogs is enhanced by halothane or isoflurane. Anesthesiology 69:552-565

32. White JL, Myers AK, Analouei A, Kim YD (1994) Functional recovery of stunned myocardium is greater with halothane than fentanyl anaesthesia in dogs. Br J Anaesth 73: 214-219

33. Reiz S, Balfors E, Sorensen MB, Ariola S, Friedman A, Truedson H (1983) Isoflurane - a powerful coronary vasodilator in patients with coronary artery disease. Anesthesiology 59: 91-97

34. Priebe H-J, Foëx P (1987) Isoflurane causes regional myocardial dysfunction in dogs with critical coronary artery stenoses. Anesthesiology 66:293-300

35. Buffington CW, Romson JL, Levine A, Duttlinger NC, Huang AH (1987) Isoflurane induces coronary steal in a canine model of chronic coronary occlusion. Anesthesiology 66:280-292

36. Inoue K, Reichelt W, El-Banayosy A, Minami K, Dallmann G, Hartmann N, Windeler J (1990) Does isoflurane lead to a higher incidence of myocardial infarction and perioperative death than enflurane in coronary artery surgery? A clinical study of 1178 patients. Anesth Analg 71:469-474

37. Forrest JB, Cahalan MK, Rehder K, Goldsmith CH et al (1990) Multicenter study of general anesthesia. II. Results. Anesthesiology 72:262-268

38. Stuhmeier KD, Mainzer B, Sandmann W, Tarnow J (1992) Isoflurane does not increase the incidence of intraoperative myocardial ischaemia compared with halothane during vascular surgery. Br J Anaesth 69:602-606

39. Buffington CW, Davis KB, Gillispie S, Pettinger M (1988) The prevalence of steal-prone coronary anatomy in patients with coronary artery disease: an analysis of the coronary artery study registry. Anesthesiology 69:721-727

40. Foëx P, Ryder WA(1979) Effect of CO_2 on the systemic and coronary circulations and on coronary sinus blood gas tensions. Bull Europ Physiopath Resp 15:625-638

41. Harkin CP, Pagel PS, Kersten JR, Hettrick DA, Warltier DC (1994) Direct negative inotropic and lusitropic effect of sevoflurane. Anesthesiology 81:156-167

42. Prys-Roberts C, Foëx P, Biro GP, Roberts JG (1973) Studies of anaesthesia in relation to hypertension V. Adrenergic beta-receptor blockade. Br J Anaesth 45:671-681

43. Prys-Roberts C, Meloche R, Foëx P (1971) Studies of anaesthesia in relation to hypertension. I. Cardiovascular responses of treated and untreated patients. Br J Anaesth 43:122-137

44. Stone JG, Foëx P, Sear J, Johnson LL, Khambatta HJ, Triner L (1988) Myocardial ischemia in untreated hypertensive patients: effect of a single small oral dose of a beta-blocker. Anesthesiology 68:495-500

45. Dodds TM, Torkelson AT, Fillinger MP, Tosteson A (1994) Prophylactic beta-blockade reduces perioperative myocardial ischemia in high-risk patients undergoing noncardiac surgery. Anesth Analg 78:S92

46. Wallace A, Layug E, Browner W, Hollenberg M, Jain U, Tateo I, Mangano D (1994) SPI Research Group. Randomized double blinded, placebo controlled trial of atenolol for the prevention of perioperative myocardial ischemia in high risk patients scheduled for noncardiac surgery. Anesthesiology 81:A99

47. Ramsay JG, Cutfield GR, Francis CM, Devlin WH, Foëx P (1986) Halothane-verapamil causes regional myocardial dysfunction in the dog. Br J Anaesth 58:321-326

48. Lehot JJ, Leone B, Foëx P (1987) Calcium reverses global and regional myocardial dysfunction caused by the combination of verapamil and isoflurane. Acta Anaesth Scand 31: 441-447

49. Leone BJ, Philbin DM, Lehot J-J, Wilkins M, Foëx P, Ryder WA (1988) Intravenous diltiazem worsens regional function in compromised myocardium. Anesth Analg 67:205-210

50. Sear JW, Jewkes C, Tellez J-C, Foëx P (1994) Does the choice of antihypertensive therapy influence haemodynamic responses to induction, laryngoscopy and intubation. Br J Anaesth 73:303-308
51. Coriat P, Richer C, Douraki T, Gomez C, Hendricks K, Giudicelli J-F, Viars P (1994) Influence of chronic angiotensin-converting enzyme inhibition on anesthetic induction. Anesthesiology 81:299-307
52. Tuman KJ, McCarthy RJ, O'Connor CJ, Holm WE, Ivankovitch AD (1995) Angiotensin-converting enzyme inhibitors increase vasoconstrictor requirements after cardiopulmonary bypass. Anesth Analg 80:473-479

Common Use and Monitoring of Cardiovasoactive Drugs in General Anesthesia Using Halogenated Agents

R. MUCHADA

Introduction

General anesthesia (GA) has four main objectives: narcosis, analgesia, muscular relaxation, and protection of the visceral reflex system.

It is obviously difficult to meet these objectives with just one drug. The association of curare narcotics and analgesics may provide balanced anesthesia with correct protection of the autonomic nervous system (ANS). Often, however, a sufficient level of anesthesia is obtained at the expense of cardiocirculatory equilibrium (1). The role of halogenated anesthetics in the onset of such changes is not to be ignored: although the new halogenated anesthetics are reputed to exert limited action on myocardial performance and the vascular sector, various authors have described both in vitro and in vivo cardio depressant actions (2, 3).

While not the only mechanisms involved, lowered circulating catecholamine levels and a decrease in B1 receptor sensitivity may be one of the main factors subtending the cardiocirculatory depressant action of halogenated agents (4-6). Certain authors refer to action on the vascular sector conventionally described as vasodilatory; a drop in arterial blood pressure, considered as a vasodilator effect, may in fact be imputable to lowered blood flow with an increase in systemic vascular resistance (7), and in reality correspond to myocardial incompetence.

Cardiocirculatory changes depend on the type of halogenated agent, its concentration, and the adjuvant drugs administered to maintain anesthesia. These changes also depend on an individual response, linked to functional, clinical and pathological events.

When hemodynamic variations under halogenated agents are diagnosed by standard monitoring procedures (arterial blood pressure, heart rate, ECG), the anesthetist tends to implement two measures almost automatically.

1. Lightening of anesthesia by lowering the concentration of the inhaled halogenated agent. This may lead to recovery of hemodynamic equilibrium, but removes ANS protection, requiring onset of the patient's automatic, endogenous reaction to compensate for the resultant imbalance. Hence, this measure eliminates one of the essential aims of general anesthesia, the

protection against stress, and thereby jeopardizes the anesthetic stability required during the surgical procedure.

2. Compensation via vascular filling, which tends to restore blood volume.

Although this maneuver has positive effects on the evolution of cardiovascular parameters, there are three possible explanations for these results:

– First, real hypovolemia exists. In this case, and if treatment is performed on a diagnostic basis, correction should bring about improved hemodynamic status.

– Second, compensation corrects relative hypovolemia due to dilatation of the capacitance system.

– Third, inotropic stimulation occurs via onset of the Frank-Starling mechanism.

In the latter two cases, there is a non-negligible risk of peroperative hydric overload. The corresponding manifestations, particularly dangerous in elderly patients (8, 9) or with a previous cardiovascular pathology, may occur precociously during the surgical procedure, but may be observed above all during the postanesthetic period.

Implementation of these measures, which comply with restricted hemodynamic monitoring, thus apparently does not systematically provide an adequate response to the cardiovascular changes encountered during GA with halogenated agents.

More extensive hemodynamic monitoring seems to be necessary, especially in patients who are elderly, present cardiovascular risk or under particular circumstances (septic and hypovolemic shock, or multiple injury pathology, cardiovascular surgery, enlarged visceral recession, prolonged anesthesia, hemorrhagic risk). Such monitoring should be implemented in order to assist diagnosis, guide therapeutic choices and follow up clinical evolution.

Hemodynamic monitoring

Two kinds of hemodynamic monitoring are currently adopted during GA.

The first calls on invasive techniques, notably emplacement of a Swan Ganz (SW) catheter to monitor cardiac output (CO) by thermodilution (TD), and pressure measurements in the pulmonary region.

This technique, which is well accepted by anesthetists, must be used in patients in whom evaluation of preload by measurement of pulmonary artery pressure (PAP) and pulmonary capillary pressure (PCP) is fundamental.

Yet this technique is reserved for specific cases because it is invasive, expensive, time consuming, and entrains certain risks (injury, hemorrhagic, infection).

Moreover, previously sequential measurement of CO ruled out the acquisition of continuous information. This problem seems to have been solved by the continuous TD method. But inherent errors arise with both sequential and continuous measurement procedures, as has been pointed out recently (10).

The second possibility is use of a noninvasive technique, combining a transesophageal aortic ultrasonography flow-meter (Dynemo 3000 SOMETEC) and satellite apparatus (ECG, noninvasive arterial blood pressure and capnograph monitoring). These devices allow display of a hemodynamic profile with data updating every 8 s, and automatic recording every 2 min or as requested by the operator. Since aortic blood flow (ABF) is influenced by diverse factors, its variations must be interpreted in light of modifications to other parameters, including contractility. In the proposed method, this last one, is monitored by automatic, continuous and objective measurement of the systolic time interval (STI) (11).

On the other hand, preload variations can only be deduced by ongoing analysis of the other parameters, or evaluated at any given moment by a filling test with continuous, evolving control of the hemodynamic profile. Continuous display of evolution of the parameters swiftly alerts the operator as to any hemodynamic changes, thereby allowing assessment of the timeliness of treatment, choice of appropriate therapy, and retrospective evaluation of efficacy of an implemented action.

Integration of the end tidal CO_2 pressure ($PetCO_2$) value into the hemodynamic table may seem questionable. Nevertheless, since the ultimate function of the cardiovascular system is to ensure correct tissular perfusion to maintain normal cell metabolism, any action on the hemodynamic system must be evaluated in terms of the evolution of cardiovascular parameters, but in parallel, in terms of the evolution of cellular perfusion labels. Under certain restrictive observation conditions, $PetCO_2$ may provide highly valuable information with regard to this function (12).

This noninvasive, nonselective method, which is simple to use and very quickly set up, allows easy, continuous monitoring of large adult and pediatric patient series.

This technique is obviously subject to some criticism. Blood flow measurements are performed at the descending aorta, and ABF is on average 18% less than real CO. Consequently, all data calculated on the basis of ABF incorporate a correlative difference with respect to overall CO values. Nevertheless, continuous monitoring and display of evolving tendencies make this a very valuable technique during GA. Moreover, there are contraindications to the use of an esophageal probe (nasal, buccal, oral, or pharyngeal malformations or injury, esophageal lesions or deformations, changes in the aortic-esophageal anatomic ratio, and major thoracic cage malformations).

Halogenated agents and cardiovasoactive compounds

Certain authors have advanced the notion of left myocardial failure during anesthesia with halogenated agents (13), essentially with reference to halothane; this notion has been minimized by other authors, particularly with reference to isoflurane (14, 15). This apparent discrepancy is perhaps attributable to the lack of a specific, easily usable tool designed for hemodynamic monitoring and early detection of myocardial changes. (It should be mentioned that evolution of the STI, analyzed in the hemodynamic context, provides the necessary information for diagnosis of left ventricular failure under GA.)

Once this information becomes readily obtainable, the low output syndrome determined by left ventricular failure is encountered frequently (one of our last studies showed 40% of left venticular failure in 145 patients aged over 60 years, operated on for peripheral arterial pathology under isoflurane).

When this failure is accompanied by a drop in $PetCO_2$, initial compensatory treatment must be envisioned. As mentioned earlier, the drop in circulating catecholamines in this situation may play a major role in the onset of myocardial change. It would thus seem preferable to palliate this deficit by an infusion of exogenous catecholamines, rather than by lightening anesthesia or correcting hypothetical hypovolemia to restore hemodynamic equilibrium. Indeed, the former solution fully upholds the interest of GA, and preserves patient protection against stress-induced phenomena (ANS protection).

On the other hand, if the cardiodepressant action of halogenated agents is frequently recognized during GA, their vasodilator propriety, under certain circumstances, must be remembered because it is an additional fact, determining a cardiovascular alteration and needing a specific compensatory therapeutic (16).

General anesthesia under halogenated agents
Hemodynamic perturbations and cardiovasoactive agents

The summary analysis of use of cardiovasoactive agents during GA with halogenated agents will be limited to the following situations:

– First, low ABF with left ventricular depression and high total systemic vascular resistance (TSVR) (Table 1)
– Second, maintained or high ABF, without left ventricular depression and with collapsed TSVR (Table 2)
– Third, low ABF with left ventricular depression and diminished TSVR (Table 3)

We shall discuss only those cardiovasoactive agents commonly used in our anesthesia department.

Table 1. First situation

ABF	HR	SV	MAP	TSVR	PEPi	PEP/LVET	PetCO$_2$
↓	→	↓	↘	↑	↑	↑	↓

ABF, aortic blood flow; HR, heart rate; SV, stroke volume; MAP, mean arterial pressure; TSVR, total systemic vascular resistances; PEPi, preejection period; LVET, left ventricular ejection time; PEP/LVET, PEP-LVET ratio; PetCO$_2$, end tidal CO$_2$ pressure.

The detection of a hemodynamic profile presenting low ABF, a prolonged preejection period (PEPi) and an increased PEP/LVET ratio (LVET = left ventricular ejection time), a slight drop in mean blood arterial pressure (MAP), increased TSVR, lowered stroke volume (SV), stable or slightly elevated heart rate (HR), and low PetCO$_2$, with alveolar ventilation and stable metabolism, justifies the use of beta-mimetics (17).

Dobutamine

Through its characteristic action (very swift onset of action, average 3 min half-life, dose-dependent modulable action), its pharmacologic properties (beta 1 and beta 2 action, very limited alpha 1 action, lessened chronotropic and bathmotropic effect), and its preservation of the DmO$_2$/VmO$_2$ equilibrium, dobutamine is, in our experience, the treatment of choice for management of the syndrome of lowered left ventricle performance and depressed ABF during GA encountered with halogenated agents.

Hemodynamic parameter recovery is obtained without a major elevation in HR when dosage is modulated from 2.5 to 6 mcg/kg/min, by increasing steps of 0.5 mcg/kg/min every 3 to 5 min, until normalization of the PEPi and the PEP/LVET ratio values.

The correction of hemodynamic parameters, notably ABF and SV, is followed by an almost systematic increase in PetCO$_2$, indicating beneficial therapeutic effects on tissue perfusion (18).

Abnormal response to dobutamine (tachycardia, arterial hypertension, PEPi decrease to below 124 ms) without ABF and SV parameter normalization implies possible hypovolemia, which should be corrected before continuing with treatment. An abnormal response may also be imputable to an individual reaction to dobutamine infusion. The latter situation may lead to adjunctive administration of phosphodiasterase inhibitors or to complete suspension of dobutamine infusion.

The use of dobutamine to manage low ABF during GA necessitates hemodynamic profile monitoring for two reasons:

- First, to diagnose the syndrome. This is essential to ensure that dobutamine is infused on therapeutic grounds, thus avoiding misuse for preventive purposes.
- Second, to follow up hemodynamic response and tissue perfusion benefits, and allow dosage adaptation as a function of objectively measured parameters (PEPi, PEP/LVET, SV, HR, ABF, PetCO$_2$).

Hemodynamic monitoring is thus fundamental. While it is impossible to obtain all the data necessary to build a complete profile, minimum information is nonetheless necessary and indispensable. This minimum can be obtained through monitoring the ECG, HR, systolic blood arterial pressure (SAP), MAP, diastolic blood arterial pressure (DAP), and PetCO$_2$.

Decreased arterial pressure and PetCO$_2$ may indicate a low flow with tissue hypoperfusion. Efficacy of dobutamine can be assessed in terms of recovery of these parameters. Increased dosage must be curbed upon onset of a tachycardia tendency without any improvement in the other parameters.

Dopamine

Dopamine may also be a valuable agent in very specific left myocardial depression with low ABF during GA with halogenated agents. This molecule is endowed with high plasticity, given its dose-dependent dopaminergic, beta-mimetic and alpha-mimetic effects. It is widely established that dopaminergic effects are preponderant with doses under 5 mcg/kg/min. The beta effects occur beyond these doses, and alpha-stimulating, arrhythmogenic and tachycardiac effects occur even at doses not exceeding 10 mcg/kg/min.

Nevertheless, use of low dopamine doses, ranging from 2 to 5 mcg/kg/min, allows obtention of a shortened PEPi and a lower PEP/LVET ratio, accompanied by improved ABF and SV without a substantial increase in HR.

The drawback of this therapy is onset of excess urine secretion compromising the hemodynamic equilibrium by hypovolemia; unless precise, continuous compensation is implemented for urine loss.

It is thus interesting to maintain the dopamine indication for treatment of low ABF during GA, bearing in mind that renal function must be preserved in certain patient categories (over renal aortic clamping, renal failure with maintained diuresis).

Table 2. Second situation

ABF	HR	SV	MAP	TSVR	PEPi	PEP/LVET	PetCO$_2$
↗	→	↓	↓	↓	↘	↘	↓

ABF, aortic blood flow; HR, heart rate; SV, stroke volume; MAP, mean arterial pressure; TSVR, total systemic vascular resistances; PEPi, preejection period; LVET, left ventricular ejection time; PEP/LVET, PEP-LVET ratio; PetCO$_2$, end tidal CO$_2$ pressure.

The presence of elevated ABF with a normal or lowered PEPi and PEP/LVET ratio, collapsed TSVR, and low MAP implies diminished afterload facilitating left ventricular function. Nevertheless, a decline in $PetCO_2$ indicates a change in tissue perfusion, due to either incorrect perfusion pressure or aleatory blood flow distribution. As a collateral element in this situation, it should be pointed out that severe diastolic hypotension (DAP < 30 mmHg) may compromise coronary perfusion with negative consequences in certain patients. An alteration of this kind may be corrected using a vasoconstrictor, the leading agent being norepinephrine. Although this compound presents beta 1 effects, they are masked by the dominant alpha 1 and alpha 2 effects at the administered doses. Usual doses range between 0.5 and 1.5 mcg/kg/min, by continuous infusion.

A second possibility is the use of phenylephrine, specific alpha-mimetic activity of which causes an increase in the pre- and afterload without any coronary ischemia risk in patients with an adequate coronary reserve. Recommended doses vary between 0.3 and 3.5 mcg/kg/min.

Good vasoconstrictor response implies corrected SAP, MAP and DAP values, heightened TSVR with a slight increase in PEPi and in the PEP/LVET ratio, and an occasional decrease in ABF, but increased $PetCO_2$ in all cases.

Table 3. Third situation

ABF	HR	SV	MAP	TSVR	PEPi	PEP/LVET	$PetCO_2$
↓	→	↓	↓	↓	↑	↑	↓

ABF, aortic blood flow; HR, heart rate; SV, stroke volume; MAP, mean arterial pressure; TSVR, total systemic vascular resistances; PEPi, preejection period; LVET, left ventricular ejection time; PEP/LVET, PEP-LVET ratio; $PetCO_2$, end tidal CO_2 pressure.

This situation necessitates simultaneous correction of two concomitant phenomena: myocardial depression and vasoplegia, in order to ensure correct ABF but also to increase TSVR, to maintain the flow/resistance equilibrium which guarantees adequate perfusion pressure and homogeneous blood flow distribution. There are two possible solutions in this case:

– First, combined dobutamine and norepinephrine administration at the doses recommended above.

– Second, use of a two-directional product, cardiac beta 1 action of which is complemented by peripheral alpha 1 action. Etilefrin (Effortil) may prove valuable when used for short periods (risk of tachyphylaxis), by continuous infusion at the average dose of 20 to 40 mcg/kg/min.

Essential points

- One of the main aims of general anesthesia is to protect the patient against autonomous nervous system reactivity (stress).

- The depth of anesthesia needed to meet this aim may compromise cardiovascular system stability. One frequent manifestation is myocardial depression accompanied by a decrease in blood flow and, generally, increased total systemic vascular resistance.

- Use of a noninvasive cardiovascular monitoring method allowing continuous follow-up of the hemodynamic profile, consisting of aortic blood flow, contractility parameters (systolic time intervals), afterload parameters (systolic, diastolic and mean arterial blood pressure, total systemic vascular resistances), heart rate and intramyocardial electric conduction (ECG), constitutes an essential aid for diagnosis, therapeutic choice and follow-up of evolution under treatment. Preload changes can be tested at any time by a filling test with control of evolution of the hemodynamic profile.

- With a stable metabolism and constant alveolar ventilation, the $PetCO_2$ value integrated into this profile provides information on tissue perfusion modifications.

- Modifications in the level or action of endogenous catecholamines undoubtedly occur during the genesis of hemodynamic dysfunction.

- Halogenated anesthetics cause cardiac depression and vasoplegia, partially attributable to this mechanism.

- Although this situation may be correcting by lightening the level of narcosis, this means counting on an automatic, endogenous reaction from the patient, with consequent removal of protection to stress.

- Correction of hypothetical hypovolemia would certainly be useful if such therapy were justified by a positive diagnosis, but it should be superfluous and potentially dangerous if implemented blindly and empirically.

- Infusion of a beta-mimetic agent during general anesthesia using halogenated agents in order to correct diagnosed myocardial depression seems to be justified.

- Dobutamine, through its beta 1 and beta 2 action, limited arrhythmogenic effect, lessened chronotropic effect, lowered of diastolic parietal pressure, and limited increase in myocardial oxygen consumption, in our experience constitutes the treatment of choice in this indication. Doses ranging between 2.5 and 6 mcg/kg/min, adapted as a function of the evolution of hemodynamic parameters, corrects cardiovascular modifications and improves tissue perfusion in the absence of hypovolemia.

- Dopamine can be used for this same purpose, but because of its dopaminergic action and excess urine secretion triggered under these circumstances, use of this agent should be limited to specific indications (over renal aortic clamping, renal failure in patients with maintained diuresis). Compensation for loss is imperative. Dosage should be modulated at 2-5 mcg/kg/min.

- Correct tissue perfusion requires adequate perfusion pressure. Collapsed systemic vascular resistance despite supranormal aortic blood flow may cause general or regional perfusion modifications due to random flow distribution or insufficient pressure. In this situation, vasoconstrictors such as norepinephrine (0.05 to 1 mcg/kg/min) or phenylephrine (0.03 to 4 gamma/kg/min) should be used.

- Treatment of myocardial depression plus vasoplegia calls for either combined administration of two agents (dobutamine-norepinephrine) or punctual, brief use of a two-directional agent (beta- and alpha-mimetic) such as etilefrin (Effortil).

Acknowledgment. The author wishes to thank Mrs. N.J. Norman for her help in the preparation of this manuscript.

References

1. Roizen MF (1981) Anesthetic doses blocking adrenergic (stress) and cardiovascular responses to incision. Anesthesiology 54:390-398
2. Ohqvist N, Sttergren G, Ekeström S, Brodin LA (1985) The influence of isoflurane on blood flow in coronary bypass grafts. Acta Anesthesiol Scand 29:758-763
3. Desmont JM (1986) Halothane, enflurane, isoflurane: que choisir? Cah Anesthesiol 34:79-82
4. Gothert M, Wendet J (1977) Inhibition of medullary cathecholamines secretion by enflurane. Anesthesiology 46:403-403
5. Estanove S (1979) Physiopathology and treatment of hemodynamic disturbance due to cardiac failure during anesthesia. In: Hemodynamic variations. Fifth European Congress of Anesthesia, SFAR, SNP, Paris 3:1279-1330
6. Merin RG (1981) Are the myocardial functional and metabolism effects of isoflurane really different from those of halothane and enflurane? Anesthesiology 55:398-408
7. Muchada R, Piriz H, Cathignol D, Lamazou J, Haro H (1988) Monitorización no invasiva del gasto aórtico y otros parámetros hemodinámicos durante la anestesia con isoflurano y enflurano. Rev Esp Anestesiol Reanim 35:194-198
8. Cooperman LH (1970) Pulmonary edema in the operative and postoperative period: a review of 40 cases. Ann Surg 172:883-889
9. Fleg JL (1986) Alteration in cardiovascular structure and function with advancing age. Am J Cardiol 57:33-44
10. Espersen K, Jense W, Rosenborg D et al (1995) Comparison of cardiac output measurement techniques: thermodilution, Doppler, CO_2-rebreathing and direct Fick method. Acta Anesthesiol Escand 39:245-251
11. Muchada R, Vernier F, Fady JF, Haro D, Lavandier B, Cathignol D (1992) A new automatic measurement method of systolic time intervals (STI). Cardiothorac Vasc Anesthesiol 6[Suppl 1]:22
12. Tournade JP, Moulaire V, Barreiro G et al (1994) Simultaneous monitoring of non invasive hemodynamic profile and capnography for tissue perfusion evaluation. J Anesth 8:400-405

13. Prebe HJ (1987) Differential effects of isoflurane on regional right and left ventricular performances and coronary, systemic and pulmonary hemodynamics in dogs. Anesthesiology 66:262-272
14. Wolf WJ, Neal MB, Peterson MD (1986) The hemodynamic and cardiovascular effects of isoflurane and halothane anesthesia in children. Anesthesiology 64:328-333
15. Lynch C (1986) Differential depression of myocardial contractility by halothane and isoflurane in vitro. Anesthesiology 64:620-631
16. Hess W, Arnold B, Schulte-Sasse U, Tarnow J (1983) Comparison of isoflurane and halothane when used to control intra-operative hypertension in patients undergoing coronary bypass surgery. Anesthesiology 62:15-20
17. Petrucci N, Muchada R (1993) End-tidal CO_2 come indice predittivo della perfusione tissutale. Minerva Anestesiol 59:297-305
18. Muchada R, Litvan H, Galan J, Barreiro G, Vilar Landeira JM, Cathignol D (1993) Evaluación de la perfusión tisular mediante monitorisación simultánea del perfil hemodinámico no invasivo y de la capnografía. Rev Esp Anestesiol Reanim 40:185-192

Circulatory Effects of Desflurane

P. CORIAT

The ideal anesthetic technique for high risk patients should not markedly impair left ventricular function and should not lead to cardiovascular changes which may compromise myocardial oxygen balance. Besides it should provide excellent blood pressure control during surgical manipulations. As regards these aims, both the pharmacokinetic and hemodynamic properties of desflurane which account for the circulatory effects of this new volatile will be presented.

Effects on left ventricular function

In healthy human volunteers maintained normocapnic with controlled ventilation, desflurane decreases systemic vascular resistance and mean arterial pressure in a dose dependant manner similar to isoflurane. Cardiac output and more importantly echocardiographic indices of left ventricular function are well preserved with desflurane up to and at 1.66 MAC (1). When given in young volunteers both desflurane N_2O and isoflurane N_2O can be given at an anesthetic depth up to 1.74 MAC (2) and 2 MAC, respectively. In patients undergoing vascular surgery we found that before surgical stimulation 1 and 1.5 MAC anesthesia with desflurane N_2O anesthesia produced systemic hemodynamic effects (Fig. 1) and changes in the sympathetic tone very similar to those produced by isoflurane. Two MAC concentration of either desflurane-N_2O or isoflurane-N_2O could be obtained in only 30% of the patients in each group. Tachycardia associated with an increased blood pressure was noted in two of the 13 patients receiving desflurane. Thus, associated with tachycardia hypertension which is consistent in young healthy subjects receiving desflurane at 1.5 MAC as the sole anesthetic agent, it is less frequently seen in older patients. The limited coronary and cardiovascular reserves, which characterize patients undergoing vascular surgery (3), account for the fact that anesthetic depth higher than 1 MAC could not be reached before any surgical stimulation in all the patients studied.

In dogs the circulatory response to desflurane is significantly modified by pharmacologic blockade of the sympathetic nervous system. This may explain some differences between volatile anesthetic agents noted in experimental studies in which desflurane appeared to maintain mean arterial pressure and

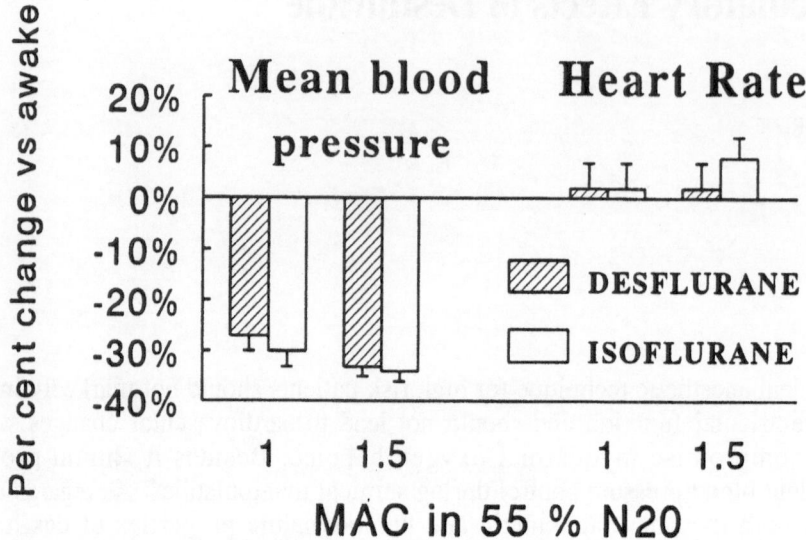

Fig. 1. Percent change (vs awake preoperative value) of mean arterial pressure (MAP) and heart rate (HR) in vascular surgical patients under isoflurane-N_2O ($n = 11$) vs desflurane-N_2O ($n = 13$) anesthesia before surgical stimulation

contractility to a greater degree than equianesthetic concentrations of isoflurane (4, 5).

Control of intraoperative blood pressure changes

The ability of desflurane to blunt the hemodynamic response to perioperative noxious stimulation has been documented. In several studies performed in high risk patients, desflurane effectively controlled blood pressure response to surgical stimulation while maintaining cardiac index and PCWP at pre-induction levels. Consequently, wall tension was stable, which favorably influenced myocardial oxygen balance (2, 6).

Because of its lower blood gas partition coefficient, the effective anesthetic concentration of desflurane is easier to titrate than isoflurane. Vascular hyperreactivity is a common feature in high risk surgical patients, and the marked changes in blood pressure frequently seen intraoperatively can result in serious compromise of the myocardial oxygen balance and left ventricular function (3). An anesthetic agent such as desflurane which can rapidly control blood pressure, but can also rapidly be discontinued, should be well suited for these patients. The effects of desflurane administered intraoperatively to control hypertension under narcotic anesthesia has been confirmed by Thomson et al. (7). In their study, under anesthesia consisting of fentanyl (10 mcg/kg) and vecuronium, desflurane vs isoflurane was administered to control increases in blood pressure associated with sternotomy. Desflurane maintained mean arterial pressure without altering heart rate, stroke index, systemic vascular resistance (SVR) and PCWP. By contrast a significant increase in SVR was noted at sternotomy in patients who received isoflurane. The better control in blood pressure and SVR noted in the desflurane group appears to result from the pharmacokinetic properties of this agent rather than from a different effect on contractility or on the loading condition of the heart. This study emphasizes that desflurane is a safe and effective adjunct to very closely control intraoperative hypertension during anesthesia in high risk patients.

Heart rate response

When considering heart rate response to volatile anesthetic agents it appears that in young volunteers desflurane produces less tachycardia than isoflurane at lower inspired concentration but may lead to tachycardia at higher concentrations.

Unlike isoflurane, heart rate is not altered when anesthesia with desflurane is maintained at light levels (0.83 MAC) (1). However, increasing the concentration of desflurane from 1 to 1.5 MAC may result in hypertension and tachycardia in healthy young volunteers (8). These observations suggest that desflurane has unique effects on the sympathetic nervous system.

This has been confirmed in volunteers by Ebert and Muzi (9). They demonstrated that increasing the inspired concentration of desflurane caused a rise in sympathetic activity and an increase in mean arterial pressure and heart rate. They speculated that this response might be due to a degree of respiratory irritation with desflurane and cautioned that desflurane should be used with caution in patients prone to develop myocardial ischemia. The potential increase in heart rate could be misinterpreted by a clinician who expects deepening of anesthesia but sees instead an increase in blood pressure and heart rate.

Data from clinical studies (1, 9) indicate that this effect is transient, and that it occurs only if desflurane is administered at a concentration greater than 7%. This is the reason why the use of N_2O with desflurane lowers the incidence of this phenomena (2). At a given MAC level, nitrous oxide attenuates the increase in heart rate caused by desflurane. For example, tachycardia does not appear to occur at 1.74 MAC desflurane-N_2O in contrast to 1.66 MAC desflurane-O_2 (2). In addition the increase in heart rate is limited by an adequate premedication (10). A sympathoadrenal activation was also described after rapid increase in isoflurane concentration (11). However, the associated increase in heart rate and blood pressure was seen only when end-tidal isoflurane was increased up to 2.6%.

The sympathoexcitation, which was shown to be consistent in young volunteers if desflurane was given at concentrations greater than 7%, might be less frequent in older people, such as those at risk from suffering from coronary artery disease. Therefore, we designed a study to determine the incidence of this effect in patients scheduled for vascular noncardiac surgery. We compared heart rate and blood pressure response to desflurane-N_2O vs isoflurane-N_2O anesthesia in a randomized clinical trial performed in patients undergoing vascular surgery. In unstimulated patients desflurane vs isoflurane was titrated gradually to the inspired gas over several minutes to 2 MAC anesthesia in N_2O. We employed power spectral analysis (PSA) of heart rate and blood pressure variability and we measured catecholamine plasma levels to better evaluate changes in the autonomic nervous system associated with maintenance of anesthesia with either desflurane or isoflurane in N_2O/O_2 (12).

In the vascular patients studied a stable heart rate was seen under isoflurane-N_2O up to 2 MAC anesthesia (Fig. 1). This is in agreement with previous studies which indicated that in patients older than 50 years isoflurane does not increase heart rate (13).

Heart rate did not change of more than 15% in 11 of the 13 participants who received desflurane-N_2O anesthesia. However, two patients experienced tachycardia which was in both cases associated with hypertension. It occurred suddenly when increasing the anesthetic depth at 1.5 MAC in one case and at 2 MAC in the other. At the preceding lower anesthetic depth sympathetic tone was decreased as indicated by the norepinephrine plasma levels and blood pressure PSA. This suggests that sympathetic hyperactivity was not the result of a progressive increase in the sympathetic tone in response to desflurane but was rather a sudden phenomenon. Combined desflurane-N_2O anesthesia was studied by Cahalan et al. in volunteers (2). Among the 11 patients who received desflurane at 9% together with 60% N_2O, none experienced tachycardia. Our study reveals that in patients who may be placed at risk by an increase in heart rate and blood pressure, sympathetic hyperactivity during desflurane-N_2O anesthesia will not be in clinical practice as frequently seen as in healthy volunteers. Two following reasons account for that conclusion: 1) the sympatho-adrenal activation and its associated hemodynamic response is far from being consistent at 2 MAC anesthesia; 2) the depth of anesthesia at which the phenomena may occur can be reached in only a low percentage of these patients because of the lowering blood pressure effects of this volatile which are similar to those of isoflurane.

The use of desflurane in patients with coronary artery disease

In these patients administration of anesthetic agents for maintenance of anesthesia should be performed in a fashion that minimizes circulatory changes (14). It appears evident that monoanesthetic techniques should be avoided since they inevitably will have negative side effects on the circulation or provide insufficient control of noxious stimuli. The actual trend in anesthesia is therefore to use a basal compound for analgesia, such as fentanyl, and then add one of the volatile agents to avoid awareness and smooth out the effects of noxious stimuli (14). Thereby the side effects of each agents are minimized.

In patients with coronary artery disease (CAD) desflurane has obviously beneficial effects on myocardial oxygen balance when it is used in the treatment of intraoperative hypertension (7). A controversy regarding the use of isoflurane in CAD patients was based on the finding that isoflurane dilated coronary resistance vessels and thus had the potential to produce regional and/or transmural flow maldistribution (15).

This problem is now largely resolved. Under certain experimental and clinical conditions, such flow redistribution might cause myocardial ischemia. However, in the absence of hemodynamic changes (e.g., tachycardia or hypotension), which could exhaust subendocardial vasodilator reserve, ischemia produced by a possible isoflurane or desflurane-induced coronary flow maldistribution would be a rare event in clinical practice. First, isoflurane produces dose dependent coronary vasodilatation in animals and in patients with vascular and coronary disease. In humans, this vasodilatation is significant only if the inhaled dose is above 1.5 MAC, but may occasionally be observed also at lower dose levels. If isoflurane or desflurane is used as an adjunct to opioids rather than as a monoanesthetic, as described above, there is consequently no or negligible coronary vasodilatation in the majority of patients. Besides, desflurane has fewer direct vasodilator properties than isoflurane in vivo. Second, the anatomical condition for regional coronary blood flow redistribution consists of a territory behind a complete coronary occlusion supplied by collaterals from another stenosed artery. This anatomical pattern was observed in 23% of patients in the CASS (Coronary Artery Surgery Study) registry (16), but is considerably less common in an unselected population of vascular or other noncardiac surgical patients. Transmural maldistribution requires a critical stenosis in an epicardial artery, e.g., subendocardial vasodilator reserve should be exhausted. This is why it is essentially patients with a clinical history of previous myocardial infarction and persistent angina pectoris who have the potential for a steal-prone anatomy.

More important and relevant for both transmural and regional flow distribution are those hemodynamic effects produced by anesthetic agents which could exhaust subendocardial vasodilator reserve, e.g., tachycardia and hypotension, and thereby increase the potential for pharmacologically induced flow maldistribution. On the other hand, the negative inotropy produced by isoflurane augments subendocardial vasodilator reserve and thereby counterbalances pharmacologic vasodilatation. Several studies performed in patients undergoing CABG or vascular surgical procedures demonstrate that the risk of myocardial ischemia (as detected using ECG and TEE) is moderate and not significantly increased with desflurane compared with either isoflurane or narcotics when hemodynamics are controlled (7, 8).

In conclusion, desflurane appears to offer some advantages over currently available anesthetics. Its effects on left ventricular function are moderate. The solubility of this agent in blood and tissue is remarkably less than isoflurane, enflurane, or halothane, implying kinetic characteristics that should provide greater hemodynamic control over anesthesia maintenance and recovery. If desflurane is administered at a concentration greater than 7%, transient increase in heart rate and blood pressure may occur. This phenomenon must not be misinterpreted by a clinician who expected deepening anesthesia.

References

1. Weiskopf RB, Cahalan MK, Eger EL et al (1991) Cardiovascular actions of desflurane in normocarbic volunteers. Anesth Analg 73:143-156
2. Cahalan MK, Weiskopf RB, Eger EI, Yasuda N, Pompiliu I, Rampil IJ, Lockhart SH, Freire B, Peterson NA (1991) Hemodynamic effects of desflurane/nitrous oxide anesthesia in volunteers. Anesth Analg 73:157-164
3. Pringle SD, McFarlane PW, McKillop JH, Lorimer AR, Dunn PG (1989) Pathophysiologic assessment of left ventricular hypertrophy and strain in asymptomatic patients with essential hypertension. J Am Coll Cardiol 13:1377-1381
4. Warltier C, Pagel S (1992) Cardiovascular and respiratory actions of desflurane: is desflurane different from isoflurane? Anesth Analg 75:517-531
5. Lowenstein E (1993) Sympathetic nervous system activation and hyperdynamic circulation associated with desflurane: not all isomers are created equal. Anesthesiology 79:419-421
6. Goldman L (1992) Cardiac risk assessment in patients with atheriosclerotic vascular disease. In: J Kaplan (ed) Vascular anesthesia. Churchill Livingstone, New York, pp 1-20
7. Thomson IR, Bowering JB, Hudson RJ et al (1991) A comparison of desflurane and isoflurane in patients undergoing coronary artery surgery. Anesthesiology 75:776-781
8. Helman JD, Leung JM, Bellows WH et al (1992) The risk of myocardial ischemia in patients receiving desflurane versus sufentanil anesthesia for coronary artery bypass graft surgery. Anesthesiology 77:47-62
9. Ebert TJ, Muzi M (1993) Sympathetic hyperactivity during desflurane anesthesia in healthy volunteers: a comparison with isoflurane. Anesthesiology 79:444-453
10. Kelly E, Hartman S, Embree B, Sharp G, Artusio F (1993) Inhaled induction and emergence from desflurane anesthesia in the ambulatory surgical patient: the effect of premedication. Anesth Analg 77:540-543
11. Yli-Hankala A, Randell T, Seppala T, Lindgren L (1993) Increases in hemodynamic variables and catecholamine levels after rapid increase in isoflurane concentration. Anesthesiology 78:266-271
12. Pagani M, Lombardi F, Guzzetti S et al (1976) Power spectral analysis of heart rate and arterial pressure variabilities as a marker of sympatho-vagal interaction in man and conscious dog. Circ Res 59:178-93
13. Tarnow J, Bruckner JB, Eberlin HJ (1976) Haemodynamics and myocardial oxygen consumption during isoflurane anesthesia in geriatric patients. Br J Anaesth 48:669-675
14. Coriat P (1992) Anesthesia for patients with coronary artery disease undergoing non cardiac surgery. In: J Kaplan (ed) Vascular anesthesia. Churchill Livingstone, New York
15. Priebe HJ (1989) Isoflurane and coronary hemodynamics (review article). Anesthesiology 71:860
16. Buffington CW, Davis KB, Gillispie S, Pettinger M (1988) The prevalence of steal-prone coronary anatomy in patients with coronary artery disease: an analysis of the coronary artery surgery study registry. Anesthesiology 69:721

Desflurane: How Does It Work?

R.B. WEISKOPF

Introduction

Desflurane [difluoromethyl-1-fluoro-2,2,2-trifluoroethyl ether (I-653)] was first introduced into clinical practice in the United States in the fall of 1992, and subsequently in several European countries (UK, France, Sweden, Finland, Denmark, Germany, Iceland, Luxembourg, Switzerland, Ireland, and Spain). The pharmacology of this anesthetic, which is chemically similar to isoflurane, was well-summarized by Eger (1) at the time of clinical introduction, as well as more recently (2). This description summarizes the current state of knowledge of the pharmacologic effects of desflurane, with an emphasis on the knowledge accumulated during the past 2 years.

Physical and chemical properties of desflurane and their clinical implications

The seemingly trivial chemical difference between desflurane an isoflurane (the sole difference is that the chlorine atom in isoflurane is replaced by a fluorine atom in desflurane) results in markedly different physical properties. The vapor pressure of desflurane at 20C is 644 mmHg, a value which necessitated the design and production of a new, technologically advanced vaporizer (3), to enable the safe administration of this anesthetic.

The solubility of desflurane in blood (4) (blood/gas partition coefficient = 0.42), brain (5) (brain/gas partition coefficient = 0.5) and other tissues (5) is lower than that of other potent inhaled anesthetics (e.g. for isoflurane these values are 1.41 and 2.1, respectively; for sevoflurane they are 0.6-0.7 and 1.2, respectively). This low solubility confers important clinical pharmacokinetic advantages, including

1. Ability to change alveolar and tissue anesthetic concentrations rapidly and thus take advantage of the anesthetic's dose-dependent pharmacologic effects.
2. Allow for a more rapid emergence from anesthesia than with other anesthetics (6).

3. Suitability for use with low flow administration, thus decreasing cost (7). This more rapid emergence is accentuated with anesthesia of longer duration (6).

Cardiovascular control

Desflurane, in a manner similar to that of other potent inhaled anesthetics, decreases systemic vascular resistance and arterial blood pressure (see below) (8). However, because of the lower solubility of desflurane, one can adjust alveolar, blood, and tissue (including heart) concentrations faster with desflurane than with other potent inhaled anesthetics. This results in a more rapid alteration of systemic vascular resistance and blood pressure. An example of this is depicted in Fig. 1. The same volunteer was anesthetized on two separate occasions, once with desflurane and once with isoflurane. Alveolar anesthetic concentration was rapidly changed from 1.7 MAC to 0.55 MAC. Note the greater rapidity with which blood pressure increased when the volunteer was anesthetized with desflurane than with isoflurane.

Prolonged anesthesia

Many anesthesiologists take advantage of the rapid elimination of desflurane by using desflurane for anesthetics of short duration, typically "same-day" surgery. This allows for rapid emergence and the possibility of early return home.

However, increased duration of anesthesia amplifies the pharmacokinetic advantage of desflurane. With increased duration of anesthesia, increased amounts of anesthetic are taken up by tissues; the increase in uptake is greater with anesthetics of greater solubility. Thus, when the anesthetic is shut off after prolonged anesthesia, more anesthetic must come out of tissues and be eliminated with the more soluble anesthetics than with an anesthetic of lesser solubility (e.g. desflurane). This can be seen in Figs. 2 and 3. The difference in time of emergence from anesthesia for rats anesthetized with desflurane compared to rats anesthetized with other, more soluble, potent anesthetics is greater with increased duration of anesthesia (Fig. 2).

This also occurs in humans. Figure 3 shows data from two patients: one anesthetized with isoflurane for 2 h, the other anesthetized with desflurane for 4 h. When the anesthetic is shut, after 4 h of desflurane anesthesia, the alveolar concentration of desflurane falls to less than 20% of its initial concentration within 2 min. This should be sufficient to allow for awakening. However, after an isoflurane anesthetic half as long (2 h), 10 min after the anesthetic is terminated, the alveolar concentration of isoflurane is still 40%-50% of its initial concentration, which is not likely to allow for awakening.

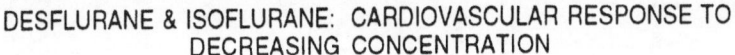

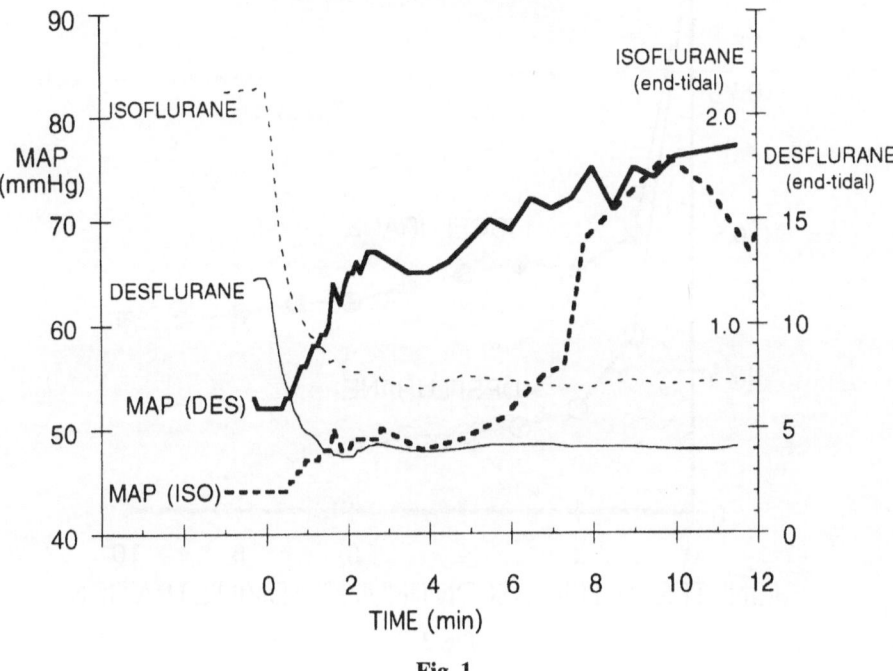

Fig. 1.

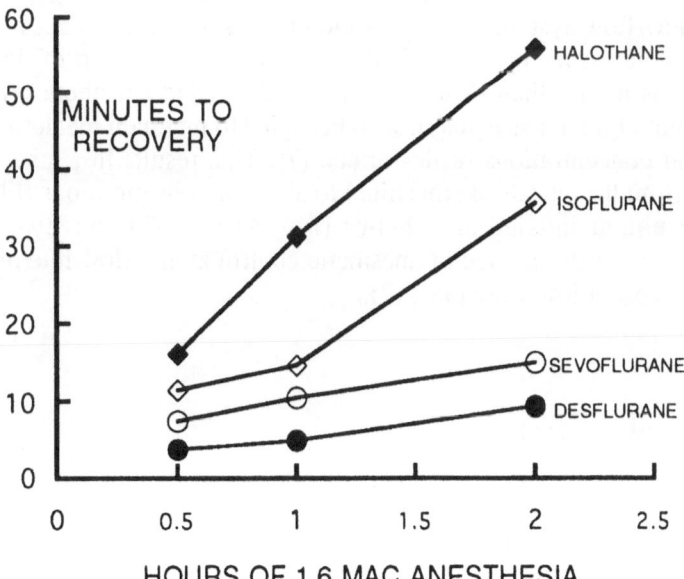

Fig. 2.

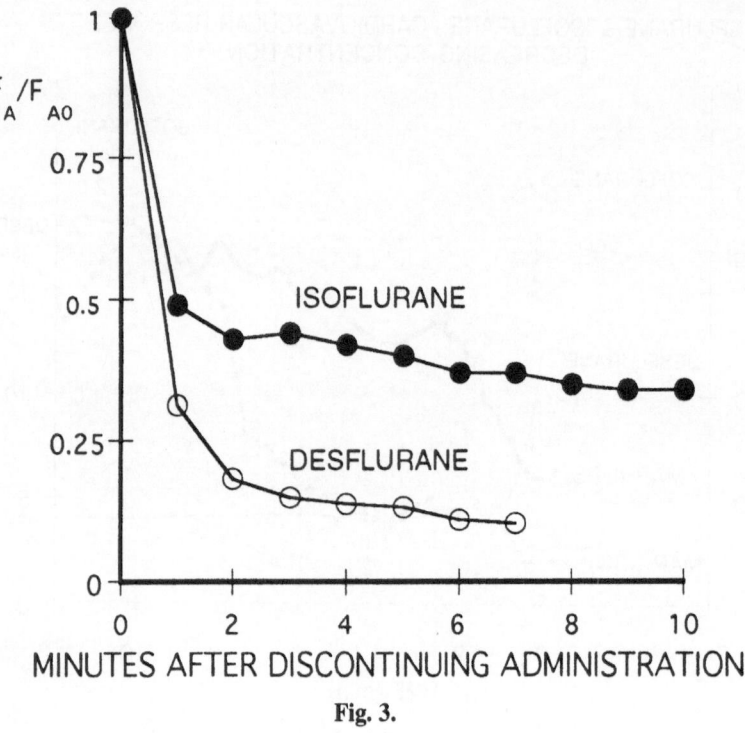

Fig. 3.

Use in low-flow anesthesia and cost

The low blood and tissue solubilities of desflurane make it an agent well-suited for use in low-flow systems. Compared to other potent inhaled anesthetics, little desflurane is taken up by the patient. Thus the concentration of desflurane in expired gas is higher than that of other potent inhaled anesthetics, and thus, a lesser amount of fresh gas is required to be added to maintain the desired inspired and alveolar concentrations of desflurane (7). This results in a smaller ratio of delivered (from the anesthesia machine) to alveolar concentrations (FD/FA) than with other potent inhaled anesthetics (Fig. 4) (7). This has two important implications: a greater degree of anesthetic control at any flow rate of fresh gas, and a lesser cost at low-flow rates (7).

Cardiovascular effects

Largely, the cardiovascular actions of desflurane resemble those of the other potent halogenated inhaled anesthetics. At the time of the introduction to clinical practice of desflurane, its cardiovascular effects of desflurane were well-summarized by Warltier (9). This overview provides an update, including the more recent developments.

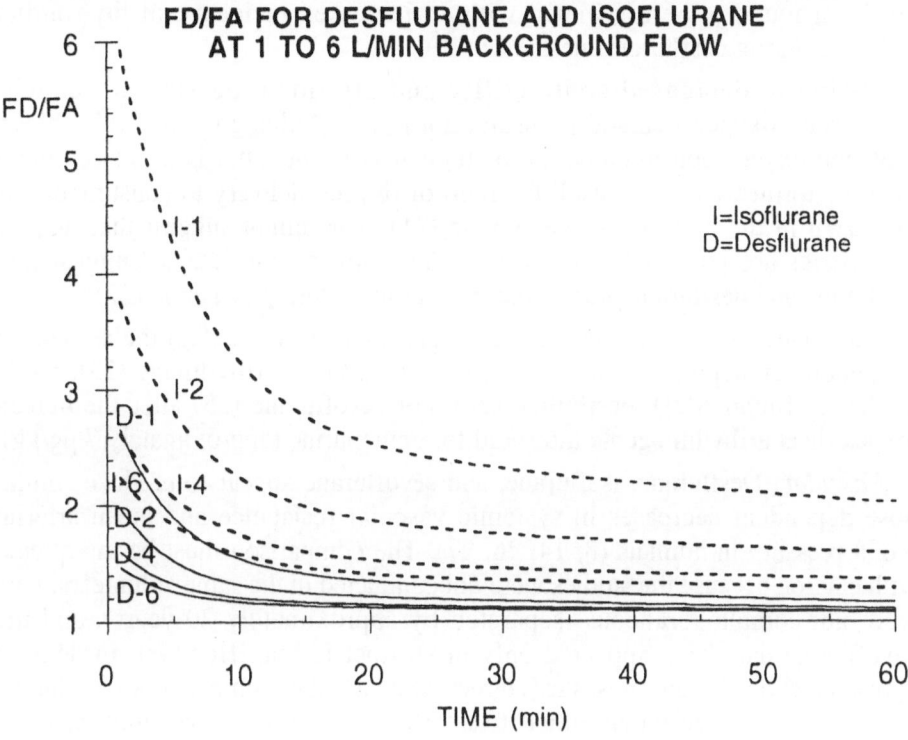

[D = desflurane; I = isoflurane. D-1, D-2, D-4, D-6 indicate desflurane at 1, 2, 4, and 6 L/min fresh gas flow; I-1, I-2, I-4, and I-6 indicate isoflurane at 1, 2, 4, and 6 L/min fresh gas flow].

Fig. 4.

Cardiac: Desflurane directly depresses myocardial contractility in a dose-dependent fashion. Elegant studies from the laboratory of Dr. Warltier have demonstrated that isoflurane, desflurane, and sevoflurane produce approximately equivalent depression of systolic function (10, 11) while other studies have indicated that enflurane and halothane produce somewhat greater depression (12). Similarly, these anesthetics also depress diastolic function, but not compliance, in a dose-dependent fashion (13). Precise analysis of human myocardial contractility is not practical, but studies using less exact measures than those possible in the laboratory have confirmed the myocardial depressant qualities of these anesthetics (8, 14, 15). The halogenated inhaled anesthetics cause coronary arterial dilation (16) and dose-dependent decreases of coronary blood flow (17-19), likely owing to decreased myocardial oxygen demand (see below). Carefully designed and executed laboratory studies clearly demonstrated that when heart rate and blood pressure are maintained at control values, neither isoflurane, desflurane nor sevoflurane produce coronary artery "steal" (17-19). Clinical studies have supported this finding. Steal-prone coronary anatomy has not been found to be associated with an increased incidence of myocardial ischemia during desflurane anesthesia (20).

Owing to decreased contractility and afterload, desflurane reduces myocardial oxygen demand (consumption) (10). Although myocardial blood flow and oxygen consumption are both decreased, the latter is decreased more than the former, and as a result the ratio of oxygen delivery to consumption is *increased* in the presence of desflurane (21). This might suggest that inhaled anesthetics are potentially beneficial. There are recent data to suggest that isoflurane and desflurane *protect* the myocardium during ischemia (22).

Halothane substantially decreases (to approximately 2 µg/kg) the amount of exogenous epinephrine required to cause ventricular arrhythmias (23), while neither isoflurane (23), desflurane (24), nor sevoflurane (25) alter the human myocardical arrhythmogenic threshold for epinephrine (approximately 7 µg/kg).

Vascular: Desflurane, isoflurane, and sevoflurane appear to produce similar dose-dependent decreases in systemic vascular resistance and mean arterial blood pressure in humans (8, 14, 26, 27). The comparison must be interpreted with caution because the studies were not conducted in the same volunteers; they were not comtemporaneous (separated by approximately 20 years), and the sevoflurane data have appeared only in abstract format. However, in dogs, it appears that desflurane causes less direct vascular dilatation than does isoflurane (28). Nitrous oxide when added to desflurane increases systemic vascular resistance and arterial blood pressure (14) likely owing to the sympathomimetic properties of N_2O (29).

Baroreflex: Desflurane and isoflurane produce similar dose-related decreases of the human reflexic increase of heart rate in response to decreased arterial blood pressure (30).

Heart rate and cardiac output: Isoflurane, desflurane and sevoflurane appear to differ in their effects on human heart rate and cardiac output. Again, the published human volunteer data cannot be compared rigorously (see above). Isoflurane increases heart rate at all concentrations from 1.0-2.0 MAC (minimum alveolar anesthetic concentration) in comparison with data obtained when the volunteers were conscious (26). Desflurane (8) and sevoflurane (27) when given in oxygen do not change heart rate at 1 MAC, desflurane increases heart rate at 1.25 MAC, and both desflurane and sevoflurane appear to increase heart rate at 1.7-2.0 MAC. When desflurane 0.8-1.7 MAC is given in a background of 60% nitrous oxide, heart rate is not different from the conscious value (14).

Desflurane in oxygen, 0.8-1.7 MAC, does not alter cardiac output (8). Isoflurane maintains cardiac output unchanged at 1 MAC, but greater anesthetic concentration produces a dose-dependent decrease (26). Sevoflurane appears to decrease cardiac output at 1.0-2.0 MAC (27), as does desflurane when administered with 60% N_2O (14), likely owing to the greater afterload.

Effect of spontaneous ventilation: The results described above were obtained in either laboratory animals or human volunteers with ventilation controlled.

Spontaneous ventilation increases venous return, and thus, cardiac output and arterial blood pressure during isoflurane (31) or desflurane (32) anesthesia, likely owing to a more negative intrathoracic pressure, although increased $PaCO_2$ may also contribute.

Effect of duration of anesthesia: Prolonged inhaled anesthesia with desflurane (8), but not isoflurane (26) appears to result in some reversal of the depressant effects seen earlier during anesthesia. After 7 h of desflurane anesthesia heart rate and cardiac output are greater, but mean arterial blood pressure is unchanged in comparison with the first 2 h of anesthesia.

Effect of inhaled anesthetics on sympathetic activity

The older inhaled anesthetics (nitrous oxide, cyclopropane, diethyl ether, fluoroxene) can produce cardiovascular stimulation during steady-state anesthesia. The modern, potent, halogenated inhaled anesthetics depress sympathetic activity during steady-state conditions. Isoflurane and desflurane decrease sympathetic ganglionic transmission (59) and muscle sympathetic nerve activity (30). At 0.5 MAC desflurane, but not isoflurane depresses the sympathetic response to decreased arterial blood pressure (30). Both anesthetics decrease this response at concentrations equivalent to 1.0 and 1.5 MAC (27). Isoflurane (33, 34) and desflurane (34, 35), but not sevoflurane (65) can produce transient (1-4 min) increases in sympathetic activity, heart rate and blood pressure when the end-tidal concentrations of these anesthetics are increased very rapidly (within 1 min) to concentrations exceeding approximately 1 MAC. It should be noted that these studies were conducted with the intention of producing, and not avoiding stimulation, and thus the method of anesthetic administration was not one usually used clinically. These changes are similar to, but of a greater magnitude, than those produced by isoflurane in volunteers (34), and in patients (33, 36). This response does not occur during rapid change in anesthetic concentration if the anesthetic concentrations remain below 1 MAC (34). In the case of desflurane, this transient response can be blunted substantially by a small dose of fentanyl (1.5 µg/kg iv) (37). Interestingly, repetitive rapid increases of desflurane within 2 h of the initial response produce a markedly decreased response (38). These findings have led to the hypothesis that this response results from activation of receptors in the airways or the lungs (34, 35) and that the receptors are rapidly adapting (38). A more recent finding appears to indicate that although airway/pulmonary receptors may have a role in this response, the more important receptors are located in highly perfused systemic tissue (39).

Three groups of investigators have studied the effect of desflurane in patients undergoing coronary-artery bypass graft surgery. Thomson et al. (40) compared desflurane with isoflurane in groups of 21 and 20 patients. Both groups were given fentanyl 10 µg/kg; during induction of anesthesia the maximum end-tidal anesthetic concentrations were 6% desflurane or 1.2% isoflurane. The groups had similar incidences of ischemia (as detected by Holter monitoring), myocardial infarction, and death. Using echocardiography in addition to Holter monitoring to detect myocardial ischemia, Helman et al. (21) compared desflurane with sufentanil in groups of 100 patients each. The opioid group received a small dose of thiopental, and sufentanil, 5-10 μg/kg and an infusion of 0.07 μg/kg/min, and no halogenated inhaled anesthetic. The desflurane group received no opioid for induction of anesthesia, and after intravenous thiopental had a rapid inhaled induction of anesthesia with desflurane concentrations exceeding 10% end-tidal. The desflurane group had increases of HR and MAP during induction of anesthesia and a 14% incidence of myocardial ischemia during induction of anesthesia which was greater than the zero incidence during induction in the sufentanil group. During maintenance of anesthesia, the sufentanil group had myocardial ischemia of greater duration and intensity than did the desflurane group. There were no differences in incidence of myocardial infarction or death between the two groups. Parsons et al. (41) compared desflurane with fentanyl in groups of 26 and 25 patients. The fentanyl group received 50 μg/kg and no halogenated inhaled anesthetic. The desflurane group received fentanyl 10 μg/kg and a maximum desflurane concentration of 6%. The groups did not differ in the incidence of electrocardiographic changes suggestive of ischemia, myocardial infarction, or death. Although the study by Helman et al. employed more sensitive measures of myocardial ischemia than did the other two studies (which could account for the different results), in retrospect, it now seems reasonable to ascribe their results to the method of anesthetic administration. They increased desflurane concentration rapidly to 10.2% end-tidal, without having administered any opioid, thereby increasing HR and MAP and observing a 14% incidence of myocardial ischemia in their patients with coronary artery disease. We now know that such rapid increases in desflurane concentration without pretreatment with an opioid, increases sympathetic activity, HR and MAP (21, 34, 35, 42) (as does isoflurane) (33, 36, 43). The other two studies by Thomson et al. (40), and Parsons et al. (41) avoided these increases in HR and MAP by applying lower desflurane concentrations (less than 1 MAC), and by administering substantial doses of fentanyl (10 and 50 μg/kg) as part of the induction technique. Standard anesthetic technique for patients with known or suspected coronary artery disease is the administration of an opioid based anesthetic, frequently with addition of relatively low concentrations of an inhaled volatile anesthetic for purposes of blood pressure control. The anesthesia in the studies conducted by Thomson et al. (40) and by Parsons et al. (41) followed this standard clinical practice, while those in the desflurane group of the Helman (43) study did not. Furthermore, the same group reported in an earlier study (44) in patients undergoing CABG surgery, incidences of myocardial ischemia and infarction, and death when isoflurane + fentanyl was used as the anesthetic, which were similar to the incidences described in association with desflurane anesthesia (without fentanyl).

MAC-BAR: "MAC-BAR" is the concentration of inhaled anesthetic which blocks the sympathetic response to a noxious stimulus (skin incision) in 50% of the population (45). Zbinden was unable to find a MAC-BAR value for isoflurane in response to a tetanic stimulus or a skin incision (46) (these stimuli produce equivalent changes in heart rate and blood pressure) (47), suggesting that isoflurane is incapable of blocking the sympathetic response. Desflurane *may* differ from isoflurane in this regard. Yasuda et al. found that 1.66, but not 1.24 MAC desflurane administered to volunteers blocked the heart rate and blood pressure response to a tetanic stimulus (48). In patients undergoing coronary artery bypass surgery anesthetized with either desflurane or isoflurane plus fentanyl, Thomson et al. found similar responses to skin incision, but a lesser increase in blood pressure in response to sternotomy in those patients given desflurane than in those given isoflurane (40), suggesting that desflurane may be better than isoflurane at blocking cardiovascular responses to noxious stimuli.

Respiration

The effects of desflurane on ventilation are similar to those of the other potent, halogenated anesthetics. It is a potent respiratory depressant. In human volunteers, desflurane decreases tidal volume and the ventilatory response to CO_2 and increases resting $PaCO_2$ and the frequency of ventilation (49).

Neuromuscular

As do other potent inhaled halogenated anesthetics, desflurane produces some degree of neuromuscular blockade and potentiates the action of neuromuscular blocking agents (50). Recent data from a well-controlled study in volunteers indicate that desflurane is more potent than isoflurane in potentiating the effects of vecuronium (51). This study also indicated that reduction of the concentration of desflurane produces a more rapid and greater reduction in the neuromuscular blockade afforded by vecuronium than when the concentration of isoflurane is similarly reduced. This has the potential for providing an added safety factor when using desflurane.

Central nervous system

Data thus far accumulated indicate that the effects of desflurane on the central nervous system are similar to those of isoflurane. The effects of desflurane on the electroencephalogram are similar to those of isoflurane in laboratory animals (52) and human volunteers (53). The effects of desflurane on cerebral blood flow resemble those of isoflurane, including a decrease of CBF with a decrease of $PaCO_2$ from 35 mmHg to 27 mmHg (54). In the presence of intracranial masses, 0.5 MAC and 1.0 MAC desflurane do not increase lumbar cerebrospinal fluid pressure in humans. Desflurane at 1.25 MAC can increase lumbar CSF pressure (55). Based on current evidence, it is recommended that for intracranial surgery, desflurane be used in a manner similar to that of isoflurane, in concentrations of 0.5 MAC or less, with the maintenance of hypocapnia.

Pediatrics

The advantageous pharmacokinetic properties described above for adults also pertain to children. However, desflurane should not be used for inhaled induction of anesthesia in children because of a high incidence of significant upper airway difficulties (56). After induction of anesthesia with another anesthetic, desflurane may be used in children to take advantage of its pharmacokinetic properties. Appropriate consideration should be given to postoperative analgesia to obviate the possibility in the child, of a very rapid emergence with pain, which might result in agitation.

Metabolism and toxicity

Desflurane is biodegraded by human hepatic microsomal preparations to a lesser extent than other halogenated anesthetics (57). In vivo metabolism of desflurane is 1/10th to 1/100th that of isoflurane (58). Consequently, even prolonged desflurane anesthesia in humans (> 7 MAC-h), produces no detectable increase in serum F^- (concentration remains less than 1 μM) (58). However, desflurane does undergo very limited metabolism, as demonstrated by small increases in serum (peak concentration = 0.4 μM) and urine concentrations of trifluroacetic acid (60), increases < 10% of those seen after isoflurane anesthesia. Few, if any, substantiated reports of hepatitis have been attributable to isoflurane, after several hundred million isoflurane anesthetics, and thus the potential for desflurane to cause hepatic injury appears to be exceedingly small. Studies in volunteers or patients given desflurane do not reveal alterations in hepatic or renal function (61-63).

However, isoflurane, desflurane, or enflurane placed in contact with soda lime or Baralyme from which the normal moisture has been removed by many hours of high flow of moisture-free gas produce carbon monoxide (64).

Summary

Desflurane has the lowest blood and tissue solubilities of any potent inhaled anesthetic. This produces its clinical advantage: exceedingly rapid recovery from anesthesia, ease of intraoperative titratability, cost control by its use in low flow circuits, and use for prolonged surgery. Its pharmacodynamic properties are quite similar to those of isoflurane, with some differences. Desflurane is the most stable of all potent inhaled anesthetics, implying a low potential for toxicity.

References

1. Eger EI II (1993) Desflurane: a compendium and reference. Healthpress Publishing Group
2. Eger EI II (1994) New inhaled anesthetics. Anesthesiology 80:906-922
3. Weiskopf RB, Sampson D, Moore MA (1994) The desflurane (Tec 6) vaporizer: design, design considerations and performance evaluation. Br J Anaesth 72:474-479
4. Eger EI II (1987) Partition coefficients of I-653 in human blood, saline, and olive oil. Anesth Analg 66:971-973
5. Yasuda N, Targ AG, Eger Ed (1989) Solubility of I-653, sevoflurane, isoflurane, and halothane in human tissues. Anesth Analg 69:370-373
6. Eger EI II, Johnson BH (1987) Rates of awakening from anesthesia with I-653, halothane, isoflurane, and sevoflurane: a test of the effect of anesthetic concentration and duration in rats. Anesth Analg 66:977-982
7. Weiskopf RB, Eger EI II (1993) Comparing the costs of inhaled anesthetics. Anesthesiology 79:1413-1418
8. Weiskopf RB, Cahalan MK, Eger EI II, Yasuda N, Rampil IJ, Ionescu P, Lockhart SH, Johnson BH, Freire B, Kelley S (1991) Cardiovascular actions of desflurane in normocarbic volunteers. Anesth Analg 73:143-146
9. Warltier DC, Pagel PS (1992) Cardiovascular and respiratory actions of desflurane: is desflurane different from isoflurane? Anesth Analg S17-29
10. Pagel PS, Kampine JP, Schmeling WT, Warltier DC (1993) Evaluation of myocardial contractility in the chronically instrumented dog with intact autonomic nervous system function: effects of desflurane and isoflurane. Acta Anaesthesiol Scand 37:203-210
11. Harkin CP, Pagel PS, Kersten JR, Hettrick DA, Warltier DC (1994) Direct negative inotropic and lusitropic effects of sevoflurane. Anesthesiology 81:156-167
12. Pagel PS, Kampine JP, Schmeling WT, Warltier DC (1991) Comparison of the systemic and coronary hemodynamic actions of desflurane, isoflurane, halothane, and enflurane in the chronically instrumented dog. Anesthesiology 74:539-551
13. Pagel PS, Kampine JP, Schmeling WT, Warltier DC (1991) Alteration of left ventricular diastolic function by desflurane, isoflurane, and halothane in the chronically instrumented dog with autonomic nervous system blockade. Anesthesiology 74:1103-1114
14. Cahalan MK, Weiskopf RB, Eger EI II, Yasuda N, Ionescu P, Rampil IJ, Lockhart SH, Freire B, Peterson NA (1991) Hemodynamic effects of desflurane/nitrous oxide anesthesia in volunteers. Anesth Analg 73:157-164
15. Kikura M, Ikeda K (1993) Comparison of effects of sevoflurane/nitrous oxide and enflurane/nitrous oxide on myocardial contractility in humans. Load-independent and noninvasive assessment with transesophageal echocardiography. Anesthesiology 79:235-243
16. Hickey RF, Cason BA, Shubayev I (1994) Regional vasodilating properties of isoflurane in normal swine myocardium. Anesthesiology 80:574-581
17. Hartman JC, Kampine JP, Schmeling WT, Warltier DC (1991) Alterations in collateral blood flow produced by isoflurane in a chronically instrumented canine model of multivessel coronary artery disease. Anesthesiology 74:120-133
18. Hartman JC, Pagel PS, Kampine JP, Schmeling WT, Warltier DC (1991) Influence of desflurane on regional distribution of coronary blood flow in a chronically instrumented canine model of multivessel coronary artery obstruction. Anesth Analg 72:289-299

19. Kersten JR, Brayer AP, Pagel PS, Tessmer JP, Warltier DC (1994) Perfusion of ischemic myocardium during anesthesia with sevoflurane. Anesthesiology 81:995-1004
20. Helman JD, Leung JM, Bellows WH, Pineda N, Roach GW, Reeves Jd, Howse J, McEnany MT, Mangano DT (1992) The risk of myocardial ischemia in patients receiving desflurane versus sufentanil anesthesia for coronary artery bypass graft surgery. The S.P.I. Research Group. Anesthesiology 77:47-62
21. Boban M, Stowe DF, Buljubasic N, Kampine JP, Bosnjak ZJ (1992) Direct comparative effects of isoflurane and desflurane in isolated guinea pig hearts. Anesthesiology 76:775-780
22. Waltier D, personal communication
23. Johnston RR, Eger EI, Wilson C (1976) A comparative interaction of epinephrine with enflurane, isoflurane, and halothane in man. Anesth Analg 55:709-712
24. Moore MA, Weiskopf RB, Eger EId, Wilson C, Lu G (1993) Arrhythmogenic doses of epinephrine are similar during desflurane or isoflurane anesthesia in humans. Anesthesiology 79:943-947
25. Navarro R, Weiskopf RB, Moore MA, Lockhart S, Eger EI II, Koblin D, Lu G, Wilson C (1994) Humans anesthetized with sevoflurane or isoflurane have similar arrhythmic response to epinephrine. Anesthesiology 80:545-549
26. Stevens WC, Cromwell TH, Halsey MJ, Eger Ed, Shakespeare TF, Bahlman SH (1971) The cardiovascular effects of a new inhalation anesthetic, Forane, in human volunteers at constant arterial carbon dioxide tension. Anesthesiology 35:8-16
27. Malan TP, DiNardo JA, Isner RJ, Frink EJ, Goldgerg M, Brown BA, Depa R (1994) Cardiovasular effects of sevoflurane in volunteers. Anesth Analg 78:S262 [abstr]
28. Kersten J, Pagel PS, Tessmer JP, Roerig DL, Schmeling WT, Warltier DC (1993) Dexmedetomidine alters the hemodynamic effects of desflurane and isoflurane in chronically instrumented dogs. Anesthesiology 79:1022-1032
29. Russell GB, Snider MT, Richard RB, Loomis JL (1990) Hyperbaric nitrous oxide as a sole anesthetic agent in humans. Anesth Analg 70:289-295
30. Muzi M, Ebert TJ (1995) A comparison of baroreflex sensitivity during isoflurane and desflurane anesthesia in humans. Anesthesiology 82:919-925
31. Cromwell TH, Stevens WC, Eger Ed, Shakespeare TF, Halsey MJ, Bahlman SH, Fourcade HE (1971) The cardiovascular effects of compound 469 (Forane) during spontaneous ventilation and CO_2 challenge in man. Anesthesiology 35:17-25
32. Weiskopf RB, Cahalan MK, Ionescu P, Eger EI II, Yasuda N, Lockhart SH, Rampil IJ, Laster M, Freire B, Peterson N (1991) Cardiovascular actions of desflurane with and without nitrous oxide during spontaneous ventilation in humans. Anesth Analg 73:165-174
33. Yli HA, Randell T, Seppala T, Lindgren L (1993) Increases in hemodynamic variables and catecholamine levels after rapid increase in isoflurane concentration. Anesthesiology 78: 266-271
34. Weiskopf RBM, Eger EI II MA, Noorani M, McKay L, Chortkoff B, Hart PS, Damask M (1994) Rapid increase in desflurane concentration is associated with greater transient cardiovascular stimulation than with rapid increase in isoflurane concentration in humans. Anesthesiology 80:1035-1045
35. Ebert TJ, Muzi M (1993) Sympathetic hyperactivity during desflurane anesthesia in healthy volunteers. A comparison with isoflurane. Anesthesiology 79:444-453
36. Ishikawa T, Nishino T, Hiraga K (1993) Immediate responses of arterial blood pressure and heart rate to sudden inhalation of high concentrations of isoflurane in normotensive and hypertensive patients. Anesth Analg 77:1022-1025
37. Weiskopf RB, Eger EI II, Noorani M, Daniel M (1994) Fentanyl, esmolol, and clonidine blunt the transient cardiovascular stimulation induced by desflurane in humans. Anesthesiology 81: 1350-1355
38. Weiskopf RB, Eger EI II, Noorani M, Daniel M (1994) Repetitive rapid increases in desflurane concentration blunt transient cardiovascular stimulation in humans. Anesthesiology 81: 843-849
39. Weiskopf RB et al, unpublished data

40. Thomson IR, Bowering JB, Hudson RJ, Frais MA, Rosenbloom M (1991) A comparison of desflurane and isoflurane in patients undergoing coronary artery surgery. Anesthesiology 75: 776-781

41. Parsons RS, Jones RM, Wrigley SR, MacLeod KG, Platt MW (1994) Comparison of desflurane and fentanyl-based anaesthetic techniques for coronary artery bypass surgery. Br J Anaesth 72:430-438

42. Moore MA, Weiskopf RB, Eger EI II, Noorani M, McKay L, Damask M (1994) Rapid 1% increases of end-tidal desflurane concentration to greater than 5% transiently increase heart rate and blood pressure in humans. Anesthesiology 81:94-98

43. Tanaka S, Tsuchida H, Namba H, Namiki A (1994) Clonidine and lidocaine inhibition of isoflurane-induced tachycardia in humans. Anesthesiology 81:1341-1349

44. Leung JM, Goehner P, O'Kelly BF, Hollenberg M, Pineda N, Cason BA, Mangano DT (1991) Isoflurane anesthesia and myocardial ischemia: comparative risk versus sufentanil anesthesia in patients undergoing coronary artery bypass graft surgery. The SPI (Study of Perioperative Ischemia) Research Group. Anesthesiology 74:838-847

45. Roizen MF, Horrigan RW, Frazer BM (1981) Anesthetic doses blocking adrenergic (stress) and cardiovascular responses to incision-MAC BAR. Anesthesiology 54:390-398

46. Zbinden AM, Maggiorini M, Petersen-Felix S, Lauber R, Thomson DA, Minder CE (1994) Anesthetic depth defined using multiple noxious stimuli during isoflurane/oxygen anesthesia. I. Motor reactions [see comments]. Anesthesiology 80:253-260

47. Zbinden AM, Petersen-Felix S, Thomson DA (1994) Anesthetic depth defined using multiple noxious stimuli during isoflurane/oxygen anesthesia. II. Hemodynamic responses [see comments]. Anesthesiology 80:261-267

48. Yasuda N, Weiskopf RB, Cahalan MK, Ionescu P, Caldwell JE, Eger EI II, Rampil IJ, Lockhart SH (1991) Does desflurane modify circulatory responses to stimulation in humans? Anesth Analg 73:175-179

49. Lockhart SH, Rampil IJ, Yasuda N, Eger EI II, Weiskopf RB (1991) Depression of ventilation by desflurane in humans. Anesthesiology 74:484-488

50. Caldwell JE, Laster MJ, Magorian T, Heier T, Yasuda N, Lynam DP, Eger EI 2d, Weiskopf RB (1991) The neuromuscular effects of desflurane, alone and combined with pancuronium or succinylcholine in humans. Anesthesiology 74:412-418

51. Wright PM, Hart P, Lau M, Brown R, Sharma ML, Gruenke L, Fisher DM (1995) The magnitude and time course of vecuronium potentiation by desflurane versus isoflurane. Anesthesiology 82:404-411

52. Rampil IJ, Weiskopf RB, Brown JG, Eger Ed, Johnson BH, Holmes MA, Donegan JH (1988) I653 and isoflurane produce similar dose-related changes in the electroencephalogram of pigs. Anesthesiology 69:298-302

53. Rampil IJ, Lockhart SH, Eger EI II, Yasuda N, Weiskopf RB, Cahalan MK (1991) The electroencephalographic effects of desflurane in humans. Anesthesiology 74:434-439

54. Ornstein E, Young WL, Fleischer LH, Ostapkovich N (1993) Desflurane and isoflurane have similar effects on cerebral blood flow in patients with intracranial mass lesions. Anesthesiology 79:498-502

55. Muzzi DA, Losasso TJ, Dietz NM, Faust RJ, Cucchiara RF, Milde LN (1992) The effect of desflurane and isoflurane on cerebrospinal fluid pressure in humans with supratentorial mass lesions. Anesthesiology 76:720-724

56. Zwass MS, Fisher DM, Welborn LG, Cote CJ, Davis PJ, Dinner M, Hannallah RS, Liu LM, Sarner J, McGill WA et al (1992) Induction and maintenance characteristics of anesthesia with desflurane and nitrous oxide in infants and children. Anesthesiology 76: 373-378

57. Kharasch ED, Thummel KE (1993) Identification of cytochrome P450 2E1 as the predominant enzyme catalyzing human liver microsomal defluorination of sevoflurane, isoflurane, and methoxyflurane. Anesthesiology 79:795-807

58. Sutton TS, Koblin DD, Gruenke LD, Weiskopf RB, Rampil IJ, Waskell L, Eger Ed (1991) Fluoride metabolites after prolonged exposure of volunteers and patients to desflurane. Anesth Analg 73:180-185

59. Boban N, McCallum JB, Schedewie HK, Boban M, Kampine JP, Bosnjak ZJ (1995) Direct comparative effects of isoflurane and desflurane on sympathetic ganglionic transmission. Anesth Analg 80:127-134
60. Koblin DD (1992) Characteristics and implications of desflurane metabolism and toxicity. Anesth Analg S10-6
61. Jones RM, Koblin DD, Cashman JN, Eger Ed, Johnson BH, Damask MC (1990) Biotransformation and hepato-renal function in volunteers after exposure to desflurane (I-653). Br J Anaesth 64:482-487
62. Wrigley SR, Fairfield JE, Jones RM, Black AE (1991) Induction and recovery characteristics of desflurane in day case patients: a comparison with propofol [see comments]. Anaesthesia 46:615-622
63. Weiskopf RB, Eger EI II, Ionescu P, Yasuda N, Cahalan MK, Freire B, Peterson N, Lockhart SH, Rampil IJ, Laster M (1992) Desflurane does not produce hepatic or renal injury in human volunteers. Anesth Analg 74:570-574
64. Fang ZX, Eger EI II, Laster MJ, Chortkoff BS, Kandel L, Ionescu P (1995) Carbon monoxide production from degradation of desflurane, enflurane, isoflurane, halothane, and sevoflurane by soda lime and Baralyme. Anesth Analg 80:1187-1193
65. Ebert TJ, Muzi M, Lopatka CW (1995) Neurocirculatory responses to sevoflurane in humans. A comparison to desflurane. Anesthesiology 83:88-95

TOTAL INTRAVENOUS ANAESTHESIA

Principles and Technique of I.V. Anesthesia

W.F. List

In balanced i.v. anesthesia all necessary components can be managed with i.v. agents – consciousness with hypnotics, pain with opioids, and muscle relaxation with curare type relaxants. An additional stress protection can be achieved with high doses of hypnotics, analgesics or neuroleptics.

The *pharmacodynamics* define the action of an agent in the body over time. The action of a drug has to be related with a specific plasma level instead of a tissue level in the target organ (brain) which cannot be measured. As CP50 (concentration plasma 50%) or ED50 (effective dose 50%) a plasma concentration of a drug is described with which the desired pharmacologic effect is achieved. CP50 means, similar to MAC 50 with volatile anesthetics, that in 50% of the patients 100% of the desired pharmacologic effect, e.g., unconsciousness or analgesia has been attained.

All i.v. hypnotics with the exclusion of ketamine have in common that besides sleep induction a more or less marked direct negative inotropic action on the myocardium and an intracranial pressure lowering action on the cerebrum. Depending on the physiologic variables (e.g., hypovolemia, age) great interindividual differences are possible.

The pharmacodynamic effects of ND muscle relaxants with their action on the neuromuscular endplate and their histamine releasing side action, as well as the opioids, with their specific receptor preference and more or less sedating and vagus stimulating qualities can be assumed as well known.

The *pharmacokinetics* define what the body does with an agent over time. Factors are the plasma volume, biotransformation, different protein binding, ionization, and fat and water solubility. Interindividual kinetic differences are frequent; they explain why in two different patients with the same per kilogram dose different blood levels and brain concentrations are achieved. For a better understanding of i.v. anesthesia a pharmacokinetic simulation with a three-compartment model has been used. With an i.v. bolus in a three-compartment model, an *alpha* phase – fast distribution with a fast concentration fall in blood, a *beta* phase – slow distribution in the tissue and a *gamma* phase – elimination (all phases are expressed as half times) is described. Through an i.v. bolus a plasma level is achieved which is not the target of drug action. After equilibration with the tissue of the target organ brain (biophase) a corresponding action will be found. Tissue levels cannot be measured in reasonable time for clinical practice. Therefore plasma concentrations, e.g. CP50, of a drug are a good reference for a target concentration and potency of a drug.

"Intelligent" computer-driven infusion schemes can, with the knowledge of the kinetics of each drug, attain constant plasma and thereby also constant tissue levels (target control systems). For the infusion pump the following program, similar to the calibrated vaporizer of volatile anesthetics, helps to achieve a desired plasma level CP50 as target concentration: a loading bolus (B) achieves a plasma level after a fast redistribution, a continuous infusion has to replace the drug due to elimination (E) and an exponentially declining infusion is necessary to adapt for the transfer (T) of the drug into other compartments (BET-scheme) (1). Variations of pharmacokinetic parameters are less pronounced than pharmacodynamic variations. Therefore a bolus titration according to clinical necessities and fast changes has to be made.

Similar to the MAC value in inhalation anesthesia, the CP50 value will indicate that in 50% of the population with an i.v. hypnotic or opioid no reaction occurs with a surgical stimulus. It should be clear that different plasma levels do not only indicate interindividual differences but also differences with different surgical simulations, e.g., superficial surgery as compared to large abdominal interventions. So the CP50 with propofol is 3-4 µg/ml, the target concentration for 95% of the population is 6 µg/ml, with 66% N_2O 4.5 µg/ml. Similar to the MAC awake, the CP50 awake for propofol is 1-2 µg/ml.

CP50 are for opioids: fentanyl 1-4 ng/ml, sufentanil 0.15-0.5 ng/ml and alfentanil 40-160 ng/ml. The CP awake for opioids is reached after a 50% reduction of the plasma opioid levels with spontaneous respiration returning; with 80% reduction street readiness can be assumed.

The *elimination half time* is the time in which a drug is eliminated from the body by half. Long elimination half times usually mean a long acting drug as compared to short elimination half times, e.g., diazepam versus midazolam, but a plasma level reduction will be achieved primarily through redistribution and only secondarily through biotransformation and elimination of the drug from the body. If patients awaken after the administration of a hypnotic it is primarily the redistribution of the drug from plasma into tissues, with falling plasma-blood levels and faster awakening. The distribution volume reflects water solubility and especially fat solubility of a drug: the more fat soluble the greater the distribution volume, the faster the drug disappears from plasma.

The *wake up properties* of an i.v. anesthetic depend primarily on the elimination of the drug from plasma. With a given kinetic of a drug it depends on the duration of the continuous administration of the drug. Hughes and Glass et al. (2) defined wake up times as "context sensitive half time", calculated from the duration of infusion and kinetics of different i.v. hypnotics and opioids. The shorter the continuous infusion, the shorter the time until 50% of the plasma level of a drug is achieved and the patient wakes up.

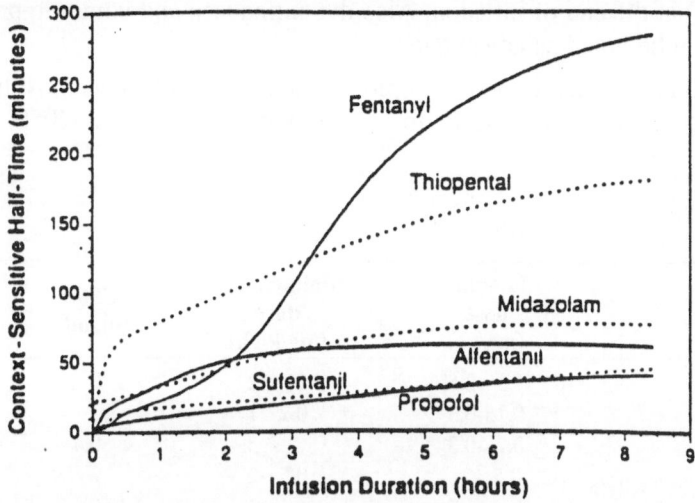

Fig. 1. Wake up properties with different hypnotics and opioids (2)

I.V. anesthesia has absolute indications without other alternatives such as neurosurgery, operations on the larynx and bronchial tree, MH patients, spinal column surgery and ICU sedation. With all other operative interventions the value of i.v. anesthesia has to be determined in comparison to other forms of anesthesia especially volatile anesthetics, as far as indication, performance, wake up properties and cost-effectivity is concerned. I.V. anesthesia is of greatest value in day case surgery, with risk patients and with short surgical interventions because of the low hemodynamic stress, nitrous oxide-free anesthesia and the advantageous wake up properties.

A number of studies on wake up properties and psychomotoric tests have shown that the new inhalation anesthetics sevoflurane and desflurane with their low solution coefficient have improved properties (3). A study with the new inhalation anesthetics and i.v. anesthesia has shown that desflurane had significantly shorter wake up times than propofol. But the time until the patients could be discharged from the recovery room was similar for all patients. A comparison of sevoflurane and propofol in our institution but also other studies showed slightly shorter wake up times with eye opening and orientation for propofol but again the time until patients could be discharged from the recovery room was similar for all patients. In all studies comparing inhalation and i.v. anesthetics a significantly higher incidence of postoperative nausea and vomiting was observed with volatile anesthetics. A comparison of psychomotoric function after hypnotic doses of thiopentone (5 mg/kg), methohexital (1.5 mg/kg) and propofol (2.5 mg/kg) showed for propofol significantly better results (4). An advantage of i.v. anesthesia with propofol for induction and maintenance is the extremely positive wake up properties after the fast fall of blood concentration

(CP awake) at the end of infusion. Also the antinausea and vomiting property of propofol can be noted as advantage.

In the following, i.v. hypnotics, opioids and muscle relaxants most frequently used are listed with their loading doses, maintenance doses and CP50.

Hypnotics

	Loading dose (mg/kg)	Maintenance dose (mg/kg/h)	CP50 (ng/ml)	Protein binding (%)
Propofol	1.5 -2.5	6 -12	3	97
Midazolam	0.15-0.3	0.2- 1	1	94
Etomidate	0.2 -0.3	1 - 3	0.4	77
Ketamine	0.5 -2	0.5- 2	2	12
Methohexital	1 -2.5	1.5- 2	7	73
Thiopental	3 -5	4 - 8	19	83

Modified from Twersky 1992 (5).

Opioids

	CP50 (ng/ml) (ng/ml)	Bolus (µg/kg)	Infusion (µg/kg/h)
Fentanyl	1-4	3-10	2 - 6
Sufentanil	0.15-0.5	1-2	0.5- 2
Alfentanil	40-160	20-80	12 -60

Muscle relaxants

	Intubation bolus (mg/kg)	Onset (mc)	Infusion (mg/kg/h)	95% Recovery (min)
Vecuronium	0.1-0.2	250-90	0.06-0.1	40-60
Atracurium	0.4-0.6	150-90	0.3 -0.5	30-35
Mivacurium	0.15	150-90	0.5	12-15
Rocuronium	0.6-1.0	90-60	0.4 -0.8	45-60

Adapted from Savarese 1992 (6).

Combinations

TIVA, without the use of N_2O, is especially indicated in ileus patients and neurosurgery. IVA with N_2O leads to a dose reduction of i.v. drugs with decreasing hemodynamic stress and is frequently used with success and without increase of nausea and vomiting. With low flow techniques and gas scavenging there should be no significant OP pollution. The most frequent IVA combination could be thiopentone or propofol with fentanyl and a ND muscle relaxant. The cost advantage with the use of thiopentone and fentanyl is reversed through a significant wake up prolongation due to thiopentone and a prolonged respiratory depression with increasing fentanyl doses. Optimal for pharmacokinetic reasons and context sensitive half times is the combination of propofol and sufentanyl.

A combination propofol-ketamine was described by Schüttler et al. (7). For induction ketamine 1 mg/kg and 1 min later propofol 1 mg/kg was given. For maintenance 5-10 mg/kg/h propofol and 1 mg/kg/h ketamine and for increasing depth half the induction bolus of propofol was used. Hemodynamic changes were minimal; psychomimetic phenomena did not occur in the midazolam premedicated patients.

Techniques of i.v. administration

We routinely induce anesthesia with an i.v. bolus of hypnotics in almost all anesthesias except for pediatric patients. For maintenance of i.v. anesthesia, a continuous administration of i.v. hypnotics together with opioids and muscle relaxants should be considered (8). The repeated bolus administration of short acting drugs for maintenance of anesthesia would lead to fluctuation in blood levels which is not desirable. Long acting drugs prolong the wake up phase. Optimal is the continuous administration of i.v. anesthesia with middle or short acting drugs.

The continuous administration can be given with infusions or programmable infusion pumps, for example, according to the BET-scheme whereby the rate of infusion is directed according to the necessary depth of anesthesia with a target blood level and bolus doses as necessary. The controlled continuous apparative infusion can be done with roller-pumps, linear-peristaltic-pumps, and drop-counting devices. Disadvantage of all these forms of controlled infusion is the relatively high inaccuracy with 2% → 10% deviations from the presumed delivery characteristic. Volumetric infusion pumps (1-999 ml/h) are also not exact and not useful for i.v. anesthesia. Optimal are infusion pumps with a delivery rate between 0.1-1600 ml/h with a precision of 1%-2%. These infusion pumps have the disadvantage of small pump volumes (50 ml) and the necessity of repeated refilling during long operative procedures.

Programmable "intelligent" pump systems should have a control setting for bolus administration with a high administration speed (up to 1600 ml/h) and a continuous administration mode for small amounts with falling infusion rates and the possibility of intermittent body weight related bolus doses for increasing depth. There are over 100 systems with a more or less developed software worldwide in use.

Desirable properties of an infusion system

1. Bolus doses with a rate up to 1600 ml/h for automatic or manual administration and continuous delivery rates between 0.1-400 ml/h
2. Inclusion of a pharmacokinetic model for each used drug to achieve a certain CP plus falling delivery rates
3. Internal calculator for dosing of induction, maintenance and bolus doses according to body weight
4. Alarm for end of infusion, occlusion or disconnection
5. Possibility for using three to five syringes with differently programmable channels
6. Each pump with an own screen showing the program dose and total volume
7. Automatic syringe identification and drug library for all i.v. drugs used and their concentrations
8. Battery for patients transport

Computer software programs contain a control algorithm and a pharmacokinetic simulation. They need continuous control by the anesthetist through apparative and clinical supervision and a hand control to rapidly change the depth of anesthesia due to operative necessities and because of kinetic variations between patients.

For the future a closed loop control system especially for the use of muscle relaxants with an apparative feedback control of depth of relaxation is desirable. With the help of a quantitative EEG-analysis (spectral edge frequency 95 or 50) a closed loop feedback control of awareness and depth of anesthesia with propofol as hypnotic has been used (9).

Indications for i.v. anesthesia

Absolute indications are TIVA for neurosurgical patients, operative procedures on larynx, trachea, and spinal column and in patients with MH inclination. Also in burn patients and high risk patients i.v. anesthesia is optimal. In intensive care situations for sedation and relaxation with ventilator patients only i.v. techniques are used. A combination of low dose midazolam or propofol and sufentanil has been extremely useful.

Relative indications are all anesthetics for day case surgery, short procedures and sedation with regional anesthesia. In surgical interventions over 3-4 h i.v. techniques lose their advantage as to wake up properties and costs.

Undesirable side effects and contraindications

All i.v. administered drugs can lead to an unexpected reaction, more frequently induced through stabilizers and solvents than by the drug itself. A premedication with H_1 and H_2 blockers minimizes the occurrence.

Hypnotics: With the exception of ketamine, all i.v. drugs lead to a fall in blood pressure as a consequence of negative inotropic action on the myocardium. Ketamine, on the other hand, leads to blood pressure and intracranial pressure increase and is contraindicated in neurosurgical patients and those with brain trauma.

Muscle relaxants: Succinylcholine can lead to bradycardia and asystole, especially with repeated administration, increased intraocular pressure and frequent postoperative myalgia very rarely to rhabdomyolysis. It is the most important MH trigger. The massive potassium release after tissue trauma and paralysis are important contraindications for its use. With reduced plasma cholinesterases, a prolongation of action has to be considered.

Nondepolarizing muscle relaxants are dose and time dependent histamine liberators. Reddening of the skin, blood pressure fall and tachycardia are registered.

Opioids: Respiratory depression after fentanyl and also after alfentanyl even after hours is possible (silent death). A dose dependent muscle rigidity can be seen after each single opioid, also bradycardia as a consequence of vagus stimulation. Increased pressure in the bile tract and sphincter Oddi have been described. Nausea and vomiting after high doses are frequent. Pruritus and urinary retention may occur.

Awareness during anesthesia: Even with high doses of i.v. anesthetics awareness is possible (1%-2%). No single drug can exclude awareness for certain. Good indications for i.v. anesthesia like operative procedures in polytraumatized patients, cesarean sections, larynx operations and endoscopy are more frequently confronted with the problem. An increase in explicit awareness between 7%-40% was observed (10). Monitoring with EEG and midlatency auditory evoked potentials have been recommended.

Costs of i.v. anesthesia

An analysis of cost effectiveness of intravenous anesthesia has to be seen in comparison to low-flow inhalation anesthesia; not only intraoperative but also postoperative effects of both have to be included. In most studies the low-flow techniques have shown lower costs, especially with a longer duration of anesthesia. I.V. anesthesia has shorter wake up and recovery periods and fewer postoperative problems. PONV, especially in day case surgery, is unpleasant and dangerous and is significantly more frequent with volatile anesthetics. With prolonged operations, intravenous anesthesia loses its advantage and becomes significantly more cost intensive. A short duration in the recovery room, early street fitness and reduced PONV with improved pain management should be the advantages of i.v. anesthesia that make it cost effective.

References

1. Schüttler J, Schwilden H, Stoeckel H (1983) Pharmacokinetics as applied to total intravenous anaesthesia. Anaesthesia [Suppl] 38:53-56
2. Hughes MA, Glass PA, Jacobs JR (1992) Context-sensitive halftime in multicompartment pharmacokinetic models for i.v. anesthetic drugs. Anesthesiology 76:334-341
3. Eger EI II (1994) New inhaled anesthetics. Anesthesiology 80:906-922
4. Mackenzie N, Grant JS (1985) Comparison of the new emulsion formulation of propofol with methohexitone and thipentone for induction of anaesthesia in day cases. Br J Anaesth 57: 725-731
5. Twersky R (1993) The pharmacology of anesthetics used for ambulatory surgery. ASA 1993, annual refresher course lectures: 271
6. Savarese JJ (1992) Review of new and currently available muscle relaxants. ASA 1992, annual refresher course lectures: 253
7. Schüttler J, Schüttler M, Kloos S, Nadstaweck J, Schwilden H (1991) Optimierte Dosierungsstrategien für die totale intravenöse Anästhesie mit Propofol und Ketamin. Anaesthesist 40:199-204
8. Gepts E, Camu F, Cockshott ID, Douglas EJ (1987) Disposition of propofol administered as constant rate intravenous infusions in humans. Anesth Analg 66:125-163
9. Schwilden H, Stoeckl H, Schüttler J (1989) Closed-loop feedback control of propofol anaesthesia by quantitative EEG analysis in humans. Br J Anaesth 62:290-296
10. Ghoneim MM, Block RI (1992) Learning and consciousness during general anesthesia. Anesthesiology 76:279-305

MANAGEMENT IN ANAESTHESIA

Anesthesiologist as Manager in the U.S.A.: The Ambulatory Surgery Experience

B.K. Philip

Introduction

Ambulatory surgical procedures represent a large and increasing fraction of all surgery performed in the U.S.A. Between 1980 and 1990, ambulatory procedures increased from 13% to 51% of all surgery done in U.S.A. hospitals (1). This represents an increase from 3.2 million to 11.7 million operations per year. Also, in 1990 there were 1364 freestanding ambulatory surgery centers which performed an additional 2.3 million procedures. We are seeing the continuing shift of more complex patients and procedures from the inpatient hospital to the outpatient setting.

The Brigham and Women's Hospital, where I work, is a tertiary care teaching hospital of Harvard Medical School, and we too are part of the change. In the year ending May 1995, we performed 9008 ambulatory surgery procedures, which represents 48.3% of the total 18637 operations.

There is a unique philosophy of care which should be used to successfully meet the special needs of ambulatory surgery patients (2). The tenets of this philosophy are:

1. The ambulatory surgery patient is not sick. Patients should be encouraged to feel that they are coming to the facility to have a procedure performed and then continuing with life as usual.

2. The patient is the most important person in his/her health care team. Patients' cooperation is needed in many stages of the ambulatory surgical experience from preparation through recovery from anesthesia.

Patients' expectations about what will happen during their ambulatory surgery and anesthesia must be appropriate so that they are satisfied with their outcome (3). Realistic expectations can be achieved by appropriate perioperative education.

This philosophy helps anesthesiologists make decisions as managers both for the physical organization of the ambulatory surgery facility, and for the function of the facility with its policies and procedures. The majority of ambulatory facilities are located in hospitals, and therefore these discussions will use that example.

Structure - the physical facility

The hospital based surgery unit should be set up to meet the specific needs of the ambulatory patient, and these needs are the patient-driven requirements listed above (4). The patient is "not sick", and it is important to re-enforce this concept so that patients feel safe to go home soon after their surgery. Also, from this arises the need for physical separation from the sick-appearing inpatients. This is important for both ambulatory patients and for their families, who will be the primary caregivers at home. Ambulatory patients also must participate in their health management, and not just be passively cared for. This patient involvement leads to the need for space for preoperative and postprocedural teaching and for family-oriented recovery care. In addition, the ambulatory surgery unit requires a streamlined administration process to expedite patient care and to minimize costs.

Types of physical facilities - a developmental process

Ambulatory surgery units need to provide space for each component of patient care (4). These components are preoperative preparation, operation, postoperative care, including phase 1 (stretcher) and phase 2 (recliner chair) recovery, administration and family waiting room.

Satisfying the specific needs of ambulatory surgery patients requires a balance between the money (in) and the efficiency and satisfaction (out). The simplest ambulatory surgery unit requires no capital outlay. Patients can be seen preoperatively in the emergency ward or the inpatient preoperative or postoperative areas. Operative care is provided in the inpatient surgical and recovery facilities, and the patient can be discharged from there.

The next option is to adapt an available inpatient room ward. This is the system started at the Brigham and Women's Hospital in 1980. Patients were given preoperative preparation in rooms on an inpatient floor. Surgery was done in the inpatient operating suite, in the basement of the hospital. Initial recovery was done in the inpatient area and then the patients returned to the patient lounge area of the inpatient floor for final discharge instructions. In this system, administrative processes were done primarily through the inpatient admitting service. Problems with this system were numerous. Particularly difficult issues were the delays due to patient transport and the timing of patient discharge.

The advantages of adapting available inpatient facilities are:

- Limited capital investment needed
- Quick to setup (no construction)
- Increased flexible use of the facility if program is underutilized or still growing
- The potential to perform more complex procedures in an inpatient facility

Disadvantages of adapting available inpatient facilities are:
- The hospital organization is geared to the sick inpatient, and the administration is too cumbersome
- Limited space and privacy
- Ambulatory patients and their family are mixed with inpatients
- Lack of dedicated staff who know the specific medical, psychological, and nursing needs of ambulatory patients
- Booking priority in the operating suite goes to inpatients because of the perceived increased importance of those procedures
- Ambulatory procedures tend to be "bumped" by inpatient emergencies or partial emergencies
- Delays caused by transportation time from one location in the hospital to another

All of these issues can be improved by use of a dedicated space. Therefore the next consecutive option is to reconstruct areas for separate preoperative and phase 2 postoperative care. A facility of this sort was used at the Brigham and Women's Hospital from 1981-1985 and cared for 20 patients a day. It consisted of an area adjacent to the operating rooms where we built a separate preoperative and postoperative unit. A facility with separated preoperative and phase 2 postoperative care has several advantages: only a moderate expenditure is required, and separate preoperative and phase 2 recovery care can be given which is tailored to the ambulatory patient. Disadvantages of this type of facility are limited space, limited privacy, and lack of dedicated operating room and phase 1 recovery staff.

When the patient census becomes larger, a physically separated unit can be planned and constructed. This unit can be near the main surgical facility, either adjacent to it or nearby within the same hospital complex. Alternatively, the unit may be located as a satellite unit, at sufficient distance to serve an expanded or different market. Planned, dedicated units provide increased satisfaction for patients, anesthesiologists, ambulatory surgery staff and surgeons. Difficulties with this approach are primarily cost. However, there may also be financial pressure for community-wide health cost containment, where adequate numbers of operating rooms may already exist.

In 1987, we built our dedicated adjacent unit at the Brigham and Women's Hospital. The overall space is approximately 60 feet by 40 feet, plus a separate area for preanesthesia interviews located elsewhere in the institution. The capacities of this unit include 12 preoperative stretchers, 10 postoperative stretchers for phase 1 recovery, and 12 phase 2 recovery chairs. This unit provides complete perioperative care for over 7000 patients per year.

As with preoperative and postoperative care, choices need to be made for use of the operating room. The ambulatory surgery program may choose to share the main facility operating rooms. This allows a shared central supply process and may better fill these operating rooms while the ambulatory surgery program is growing. However, dedicated operating rooms are preferable. They are more efficient because specialized care is provided, and turnover (intercase) time can be minimized. Dedicated operating rooms with specialized staff also provide a more friendly, pleasant environment for the patient and the surgeon. In addition, many operating facilities have a separate room for procedures under purely local anesthesia, which needs lower levels of staffing.

Facility administrative issues

There are administrative issues related to the organization of the facility (4). The first issue is scheduling options. Most units have predetermined start and finish times, usually that the first procedures start at 7:30 AM and the last procedures finish at 3:30 PM. Establishing predictable hours allows appropriate scheduling of staff. Many facilities utilize block booking. This means that surgeons who book large numbers of procedures can have a block of time reserved for them, without specifically listing patients' names until shortly before the day of surgery. However, it is also important that these blocks be opened up to other surgeons an adequate amount of time before the day of surgery, so that unused time can be taken by others. Another scheduling issue is the coordination of main operating room and ambulatory surgery unit scheduling. If the operating rooms are shared, they require shared scheduling to avoid surgeons having two simultaneous obligations.

Another administrative issue is the effect on bed occupancy. It is common that when a new ambulatory surgery unit is opened, there is a transient decrease in hospital bed occupancy. This can be a large problem, and needs to evaluated locally. In the U.S.A., there is often no choice whether a procedure is done on an inpatient or outpatient setting. Because ambulatory procedures are mandated, hospitals must close or change the use of inpatient beds. In the U.S.A. we also have developed a large same-day admissions program for patients to be admitted for major surgery on the morning of their operation. This program utilizes the same intake system as the ambulatory program and can increase operating efficiency, but can further decrease bed occupancy.

Staffing for the ambulatory surgery unit consists of its anesthesiologists, surgeons, nurses, and administrative personnel. The anesthesiologists are headed by a Medical Director. Day-to-day responsibilities of the medical director include facilitating the progress of the operating schedule, supervising the recovery areas, and making last minute medical decisions concerning patient appropriateness and safety. All the anesthesiologists who work in this area must be good team members. They must be energetic, enthusiastic, and skilled. Ambulatory anesthesiologists also need personal talents. They have to be able to communicate and gain trust rapidly. They also have to educate patients about all aspects of their preoperative, intraoperative and postoperative anesthetic care, as well as the minor sequelae that are often associated with ambulatory anesthesia.

The surgeons have a pivotal role in the success of an ambulatory program. They too must be able to work smoothly with the other unit personnel. They must be supportive and gentle with patients. Surgeons should inform their patients in detail about what to expect during the operation and for the immediate and short-term postoperative recovery period. They should also work with the unit's nursing staff to develop specific postsurgical and postdischarge instructions.

Ambulatory surgery unit nurses perform a major role in preoperative and postoperative teaching, which supplements preliminary teaching done in the surgeon's office. The nurses explain the expected course of intraoperative and postoperative events, as well as self-care recovery issues. Nursing staff must be chosen for their flexibility, their positive attitude, and the ability to work under pressure. In the operating rooms at my hospital, there are approximately 2.5 nurses per operating room, 1 nurse: three patients in phase 1 recovery and 1 : five to six in phase 2 recovery. Adequate personnel must be available to provide relief and to cover for vacation as well.

Administrative staff must also work cohesively, sharing duties. The required duties include patient registration, patient tracking, and internal and external unit communication, as well as secretarial tasks. Unit administrative staff may also be responsible for operating room scheduling or schedule coordination.

The procedures must also be matched to the ambulatory setting. The length of the planned procedure is important, because the duration of the procedure is directly proportional to the time required for anesthetic recovery, and hence the time to discharge. The need for prolonged postoperative pain management which cannot be provided by oral medication is potentially limiting factor. Significant intrusion into the abdominal cavity may interfere with postoperative oral alimentation. There is also the potential for bleeding or other operative complications which could develop after the patient has been discharged from the brief period of postsurgical supervision. Other limitations result from the need for specialized (and often expensive) surgical equipment. For administrative policy, ambulatory surgery facilities may have inclusion or exclusion lists of acceptable procedures, which must be updated regularly, or may review individual requests as they arise.

Budgeting and fee are determined by local regulations. In the U.S.A., options include patient specific charges for the items and services rendered to an individual, a flat rate per procedure which includes all phases of care, and capitated payments (per person per year).

Facility function - policies and procedures

Clear medical policies must be established for the ambulatory surgery unit (2). There must be an individual Medical Director, who is a physician and who has the authority as well as the responsibility to develop and implement these policies. Some facilities also have a Management Committee. This group includes representatives from all medical, support and administrative staffs involved with the unit, which can provide a smooth, cross-discipline function.

Medical policies must establish the timing of the preoperative anesthesia evaluation. Patients who are not completely healthy should come in for an anesthesia consultation prior to their surgery. These less than healthy patients can receive a thorough preanesthetic evaluation and advance anesthesia planning, which will minimize delays or cancellations on the day of surgery. The evaluation visit should be scheduled sufficiently in advance of surgery, such as one week, in order to complete the additional consultation, testing and treatment which may be needed. Completely healthy patients should have the opportunity to come in for the preanesthetic evaluations on a separate preoperative day, although it may not be required. This separate visit can provide the healthy patient with more information and allay anxiety. At the Brigham and Women's Hospital we obtain separate written informed consent for anesthesia. This discussion is also better done in advance.

Advantages of a separate preoperative visit are the thorough screening and elimination of problems from the day of surgery. A separate preoperative visit also allows nurses to perform their assessment and teaching functions in advance. Disadvantages of a separate preoperative visit are that the patient must take a separate day off from work. This option also requires additional time commitment from the anesthesiology service, apart from providing care in the operating room. In the U.S.A., we see an increasing trend to screening patients by telephone, to identify those individuals who indeed need to make a separate trip to the hospital for medical or psychological evaluations.

Alternatively, completely healthy patients may come in earlier on the morning of surgery, for the first time. It is critical that if patients come in only on the morning of surgery, the information about these patients must be screened in advance. For patients who will be seen only on the day of surgery, we at the Brigham and Women's Hospital require that the history and physical examination and the laboratory results be reviewed several days before by a member of the anesthesia team. A health questionnaire filled out in advance by the patient is also helpful.

Other medical policies are needed to address patient selection criteria. One set of selection criteria is medical. Traditionally, ambulatory surgery units have accepted patients who are basically healthy (American Society of Anesthesiologists [ASA] Physical Status I) and patients who have systemic disease under good control (ASA II). Some hospital based units, such as the Brigham and Women's Hospital, accept patients who have severe systemic disease which limits activity but is not incapacitating (ASA III). Such facilities permit the care of even sicker patients on an ambulatory basis, thereby avoiding a disruptive hospitalization. If the patient's medical diseases are stable and are not likely to be affected by the surgery or anesthetic experience, these patients may be candidates for ambulatory care after consultation with an anesthesiologist. Former premature newborn infants are usually not acceptable candidates. Increased age per se is not a criterion for admission or rejection; it is the patient's health and physical condition that should be considered. The question to be asked when patients are considered for ambulatory surgery is, what specifically will be accomplished during the preoperative admission that could not be done as an outpatient? The answer to this question includes an evaluation of the staff, experience, and facilities available in a particular surgery unit.

It is more difficult to select patients according to the set of psychosocial criteria. Patients have to be willing to participate in their preoperative and postoperative care. They have to be reasonably dependable and cooperative with perioperative instructions. Also, their home situation has to be adequate, and able to provide the help that patients will need while recovering from minor surgery. With advanced planning, social service agencies can provide additional in-home assistance in this country.

Additional policies identify those preoperative evaluations which are required. The surgeon must complete a written history and physical examination for all patients, including those having purely local anesthesia. Written informed consent for the proposed operation must be obtained by the surgeon in advance. A health questionnaire completed by the patient is also recommended. Policies for preoperative laboratory tests must also be established. The trend in the U.S.A. is to limit the number of required tests. Currently, the Brigham and Women's Hospital requires a hematocrit for all [adult] patients and an electrocardiogram for patients 40 years of age and older. These tests may be done at any accredited facility. An additional requirement is for preoperative patient instruction, which includes medical and logistical issues. Many units send patients specific written instructions in a brochure. A general information brochure about anesthesia for ambulatory surgery is available from the American Society of Anesthesiologists. Other policies must address logistics for surgeon's documents, scheduling, and financial screening.

Medical policies must also address intraoperative care. Streamlined efficient care must be provided by all participants to achieve rapid discharge. Specific policies should address surgeon practices, including the duration and complexity of permissible procedures. Policies related to anesthesia care should address N.P.O. requirements and types of anesthesia. At the Brigham and Women's Hospital, we encourage all forms of anesthesia including regional blocks and local with sedation, as well as general anesthesia (5-7). Spinal anesthesia is frequently used, with lidocaine.

There is increasing pressure to provide cost effective anesthesia care, where the choice of anesthetic agent and technique is based on outcomes data. In order to provide efficient care, the anesthesiologists must be truly knowledgeable about pharmacokinetics, to match drug actions with the procedures (8, 9). They must be familiar with specific surgeons' times and requirements. The nursing service must also design efficient care plans for maintaining patient safety and comfort.

In particular, it is important to avoid duplication of patient questions by the several care services. For all services, lengthy notes should be replaced by forms and checklists.

Additional policies address the recovery phase. If there is a shared recovery area with the inpatient units, efficient recovery care is more problematic. Recovery in the inpatient recovery room is usually slow due to benign neglect. This can be combated by increased nursing education and preferably separate ambulatory surgery nurses. If this is not possible, a separate ambulatory recovery area within the main inpatient unit will certainly help. Family members are permitted to rejoin patients in the phase 2 recovery area.

When this hospital unit was first established, we found that surgeons were ordering inappropriate routine postoperative medications based on their inpatient practices. I addressed this issue by writing standardized ambulatory postoperative orders, which were promulgated by the management committee. These preprinted, standard orders address vital signs, intravenous fluid orders, and analgesic and antiemetic medication orders. These orders again highlight the important efficiency concept to reduce paperwork and non-patient care time.

Ambulatory anesthesia requires a redefinition of recovery goals. Patients are not expected to be "street fit"; they should only be "home ready", able to go home and go back to bed. The simplest and most specific definitions of ambulatory recovery can be written in a discharge policy. These criteria do not require complete recovery: pain should be controllable by oral analgesics and nausea or emesis should be mild. Also, patients must be given discharge instructions from their surgeon and anesthesiologist as well as prescriptions. There must be an adult present to accompany the patient home. This point often requires some re-education of both surgeons and patients, but it is critical for patient's safety that they do not go on the streets alone nor drive themselves home. Preferably, the escort should stay with the patient for the postoperative night to provide any needed assistance. The medical policies should include a mechanism for documenting readiness for discharge, again preferably with a simple checklist. Discharge instructions should include appropriate limitations for the first 24 h due to residual anesthetic effects. Discharge instructions after ambulatory anesthesia must be given verbally and in writing to the patient and preferably to the escort as well. In addition to the standard discharge instructions, many facilities have special instructions for specific anesthetic procedures, such as spinal anesthesia or brachial plexus block, and for specific surgical procedures.

The final group of policies relate to patient follow-up. Follow-up is mandatory, both to assess medical outcome and for patient satisfaction. This can be accomplished by a return mail questionnaire, or preferably by a telephone call from by the ambulatory surgery unit nurses. We consider the patients' responses to be an indication of the typical recovery experience, and we have incorporated these responses into an informational handout given at our preanesthesia interview (3). In addition, policies must address the quality of the care being provided in the facility. Quality must be assessed in a regular, ongoing fashion both to identify problems and to improve care.

The anesthesiologist is indeed the individual best suited to be the medical manager of an ambulatory surgery unit. To succeed, this individual must have an energetic attitude, a drive to institute positive change and a determination to complete the details of both structural and procedural management.

References

1. Schneidman DS (ed) (1993) Socio-economic factbook of surgery 1993. American Colleges of Surgeons, Chicago
2. Philip BK (1990) Ambulatory anesthesia. Semin Surg Oncol 6:177-183
3. Philip BK (1992) Patients' assessment of ambulatory anesthesia and surgery. J Clin Anesth 4: 355-358
4. Philip BK (1985) Starting up a hospital-based ambulatory surgery program. In: Successful management of ambulatory surgery programs, Vol II. American Health Consultants, Atlanta, pp 176-184
5. Philip BK, Covino BG (1990) Local and regional anesthesia. In: Wetchler BV (ed) Anesthesia for ambulatory surgery. Lippincott, Philadelphia, pp 309-365
6. Philip BK (1990) Local anesthesia and sedation for adult outpatients. In: White PF (ed) Outpatient anesthesia. Churchill Livingstone, New York, pp 263-291
7. Philip BK (1995) Monitored anesthesia. In: McGoldrick KE (ed) Ambulatory anesthesiology: a problem-oriented approach. Williams and Wilkins, Baltimore, pp 387-398
8. Lichtiger M, Wetchler BV, Philip BK (1985) Management of the adult and geriatric patient. In: Wetchler BV (ed) Anesthesia for ambulatory surgery. Lippincott, Philadelphia, pp 175-224
9. Philip BK (1995) General anesthesia. In: Twersky RS (ed) The ambulatory anesthesia handbook. Mosby, St. Louis, pp 203-207

Day Surgery Experience in the United Kingdom

T.W. Ogg

Over the last decade long surgical waiting lists, shortage of staffing and lack of financial resources have all contributed to the reduction in elective surgery within the British National Health Service (NHS). Several influential reports have been published on day surgery, firstly the Audit Commission (1990) indicated that day surgery provided a quicker, more efficient service with decreased costs (1). Then followed the NHS Management Executive Report on day surgery (1991). Several British day units were studied and the report identified areas of good organisation and management (2). The advantages and disadvantages of day surgery are shown in Table 1.

Table 1. Advantages and disadvantages of day surgery

Advantages	Disadvantages
High volume patient throughput	Pre-operative assessment must be good
Nurse recruitment and retention easier	Still resistance from senior doctors and managers
Patients prefer it especially – Children Elderly – Mothers – Business people	Ideal anaesthetic technique continues to be researched
Minimal major morbidity	Minor sequelae will occur after day case anaesthesia
Reduced cross-infection risk	Community services workload may increase e.g. if geriatric and more major surgery
Reduced surgical waiting lists	Medicolegal problems . patient recovery and driving
Psychological benefits	Good equipment and facilities required for day surgery
Economic benefits (dependent on a reduction of inpatient beds)	Education, audit and research into the subject should be supported
Smaller hospitals required	
Acceptable to doctors, nurses, GPs and managers	
Day surgery lends itself to audit	

The Royal College of Surgeons of England (1992) has also supported the expansion of day surgery and this initiative has stimulated the development of many day units (3). Recently a British NHS Task Force Report on Day Surgery (1993) concluded that day surgery represented the best care for 50% of all those undergoing elective surgery and that this target figure should be reached by all British hospitals by the year 2000 (4). And finally the Royal College of Anaesthetists (1994) has just published its training objectives for anaesthetic trainees and they have been advised to spend an 8 week module learning all aspects of day surgery and anaesthesia (5).

British day surgery

The number of day operations has increased annually to approximately 2 million (1994-1995) and several British units now perform 50%-60% of their elective, non-emergency cases on a day basis. The formation of the British Association of Day Surgery (1990) has assisted this rapid expansion as the Association advises on all matters of day surgery and it organises regular seminars and conferences to instruct others (Table 2). At present throughout Europe there is a great deal of variation in the amount of day surgery performed but the recent formation of an International Association of Ambulatory Surgery (1995) in Brussels may stimulate the future European expansion of short stay surgery.

Table 2. Role of British Association of Day Surgery

• Multidisciplinary
• Advisory: promotes day surgery
• Education/training
• Monitors standards
• Holds national conferences
• Produces a journal

Establishing a purpose built day surgery unit

The author has designed two day surgery units at Addenbrooke's Hospital in Cambridge. The first unit cost £ 300,000 and the facilities of one operating theatre and 12 recovery trolleys successfully treated 30000 patients between 1983-1992 with a hospital admission rate of 0.5%. Again in 1992 Dr. Ogg secured a sum of money with the remit to build a two-theatre, 18 bed demonstration day surgery unit separate from the main operating theatre suite but within the hospital environment. It is acknowledged that initially such units require high capital expenditure but over the years it has been shown that a separate day unit can provide efficient, high quality and cost-effective patient care (6).

The new demonstration day surgery unit incorporated extensive design input from patients and staff. The waiting and treatment areas were separated with special facilities for children. Great effort was taken to make the unit as "un-hospital" as possible and a seminar room for teaching was established. The new unit is outlined diagramatically (Fig. 1).

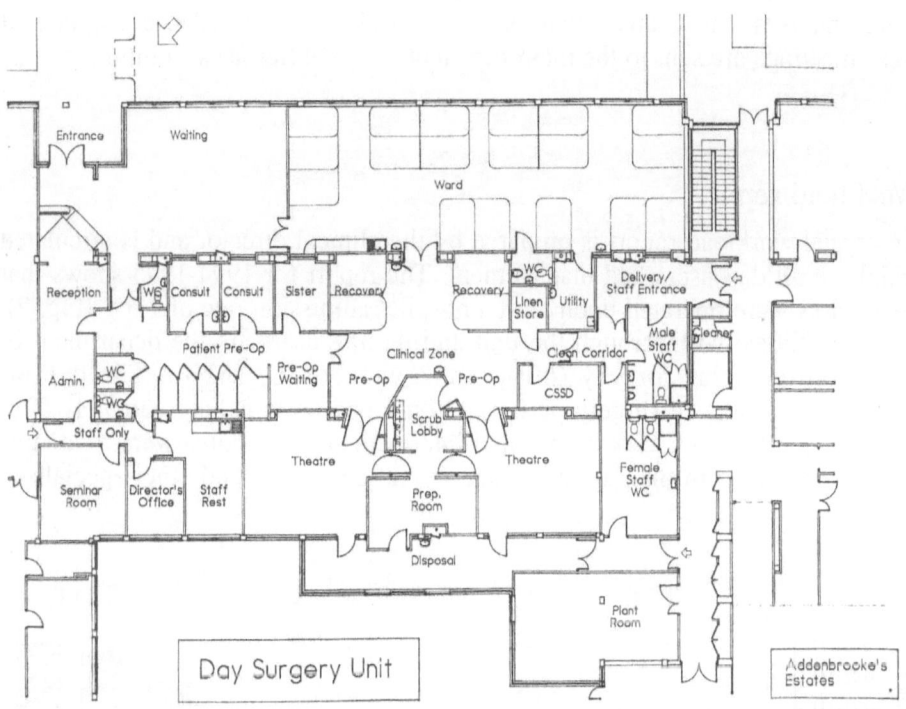

Fig. 1. The new purpose built National Demonstration Day Surgery Unit: Addenbrooke's Hospital, Cambridge 1992

Organisation

The Addenbrooke's unit functions with a multi-disciplinary team including doctors, nurses, managers and office staff. An operational policy was written and is regarded as a most important document. All future day unit users were sent a copy of this document and it includes details of appropriate procedures, booking arrangements, allocation of operating elective sessions, discharge criteria, pre-operative patient selection criteria, patient information, staffing requirements, paediatric arrangements and programmes of research, audit and education. There is more to day surgery than first meets the eye!

The medical director is a consultant anaesthetist and he spends the majority of his contract in the day surgery unit. He is supported by an experienced manager and a specialised team of day surgery nurses. The latter perform most of the routine pre-operative patient assessment and they rotate through the operating theatres, recovery and ward areas. These nurses also discharge patients from the day unit but the medical staff still retain final responsibility.

The day to day running of the unit is supervised by the manager and senior staff meetings are held once per fortnight. Monthly audit and educational meetings are open to all staff and there is a Day Surgery Users' Committee chaired by the unit director. This committee meets quarterly and includes representatives from management, surgery, nursing and anaesthesia. Minutes of these meetings are sent to the main Inpatient Surgical Services Committee.

Workload report

An annual workload report is prepared by the clinical director and is circulated widely to all day users and management. The report for 1994-1995 shows that 4940 cases were operated upon with a hospital admission rate of 1.5% (Fig. 2). Ten specialities work through the unit and the big users are the department of oro-maxillo-facial surgery (60%) and gynaecology (52%). The overall proportion of elective surgery performed on a day basis is approximately 57% and during 1994-95 13,500 minor and intermediate procedures were treated as day surgery cases in the day unit, main operating theatre and other specialised clinics.

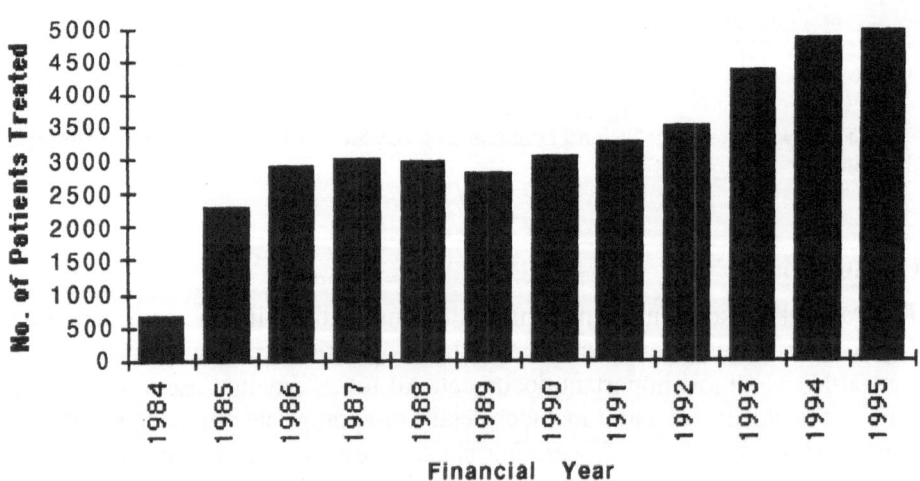

Fig. 2. Day surgery unit patient throughput 1983-1995 Addenbrooke's NHS Trust, Cambridge, England

Safety

In 1987 Natof reported a series of 1.1 million day case anaesthetics with a mortality of 0.15 per 10000 cases (7). This figure is decidedly below the mortality following inpatient anaesthesia (8). Minor post operative morbidity following day surgery has been reported by Ogg (1972) (9) and these sequelae still arise e.g. drowsiness, dizziness, headache, nausea and vomiting and pain (10). All complications following day surgery should be audited but there is a high level of patient satisfaction with day surgery (11). Furthermore in this series less than 6% of general practitioners questioned were against further day surgery expansion.

Good practices to run an efficient day unit

Pre-operative patient selection and assessment

This is of vital importance and Table 3 outlines those selection criteria. At Addenbrooke's there is no upper age limit for day surgery and the patients initially complete a pre-operative questionnaire with 26 yes/no answers prior to meeting a senior nurse. Patients should be selected on surgical, medical and social grounds. Cambridge day patients are not over-investigated and clear fluids may safely be given orally 2-3 h prior to general anaesthesia (12).

Table 3. Day surgery unit preoperative selection guidelines April 1995

1. Patients must be accompanied home
2. Age > 6 months - all patients are judged on physiological and not chronological age
3. Patients should be fit and healthy: American Association of Anaesthesiologists (ASA) class 1, 2, and stable class 3
4. Avoid operations where severe post-operative pain or haemorrhage may arise
5. Exclude all patients who are grossly obese (Body Mass Index "BMI" > 36), have imperfectly controlled diabetes, chronic respiratory or cardiovascular disease
6. Laparoscopy patients should have a body mass index < 30
7. No solid food orally for 6 h prior to general anaesthesia
   Clear fluids can be ingested up to 3 h preoperatively
8. Operations should not normally exceed 60 min duration
9. Patients should have access at home to a telephone, indoor toilet and bathroom
10. Patients undergoing major day surgery should have a friend or relative to:
    a) Drive them home
    b) Look after them for 24-48 h

Ask your anaesthetist if in doubt. Patients who are ASA 3 and stable e.g. diabetics, asthmatics or epileptics will be considered for day surgical procedures.

Post-operative nausea and vomiting

The causes of post-operative nausea and vomiting are many and sickness has economic implications both from the prophylactic use of antiemetic drugs and the increased hospital admission rate. At Addenbrooke's total intravenous anaesthesia (TIVA) with propofol and alfentanil reduces the incidence of PONV (13). Should day patients require prophylaxis the following three antiemetics are in routine use, droperidol 10 mcg/kg, metaclopramide 0.15 mg/kg and ephedrine 0.15 mg/kg. Recently the 5 HT_3 antagonist, ondansetron has been used effectively with orally or i.v. doses of 4-8 mg. All surgeons and anaesthetists working in a day unit environment should establish PONV protocols.

Post-operative analgesia

Certain day operations are painful and these include hernia repair, laparoscopy, varicose vein stripping, circumcision and bilateral bat ear correction. Few anaesthetists have examined the value of pre-emptive analgesia (14). Again pain protocols are required and the extensive use of infiltrated local anaesthetic solutions is recommended. Day units should also ensure that patients receive enough oral analgesia once they have been discharged into the community. Simple analgesics e.g. paracetamol and non-steroidal anti-inflammatory drugs e.g. ibuprofen are satisfactory take home analgesics.

Quality assurance

Day surgery should deliver high quality patient care and audit is about measuring how far you are from where you would like to be. All aspects of day unit activity have been reported recently (15) and after implementing specific recommendations the audit loop was then closed (16). Audit should be an ongoing process and all day unit staff should be involved in the collection of data.

What does the future hold for day surgery?

With the development of robotics and telecommunications the range of day case activity will increase. Already minimal access surgery is flourishing throughout Europe and perhaps the future will see development of minimally-nursed patient hotels or hostels. With the present economic health climate all doctors are being encouraged to increase their efficiency and an expansion of short stay surgery is high on the agenda.

Conclusions

The modern day anaesthesiologist has an important role to play in any future health-care scheme. Essentially day surgery is an organisational exercise and the anaesthesiologist of the future will have to re-consider their duties. In British hospitals anaesthesiologists frequently become the directors of day surgery units. At Cambridge the author supervises a twin operating theatre suite with 18 beds and is in administrative charge of 33 surgeons, 10 anaesthetists and a nursing staff of 25. In addition to his clinical role he pursues an active programme of audit, research and education. Finally the future management role within day units for European anaesthetists will involve economic analysis, personnel selection, negotiating patient contracts, maintaining discipline, dealing with complaints, purchasing equipment and formulating business plans. Already North American anaesthesiologists are firmly in control of ambulatory surgicentres but the European scene is rapidly changing with fresh challenges for anaesthesiologists.

References

1. Audit Commission (1990) A short cut to better services. Day Surgery in England and Wales. HMSO, London
2. NHS Management Executive Value For Money Unit (1991) Day Surgery: Making it happen. HMSO, London
3. Commission on the provision of surgical services (1992) Guidelines for day case surgery. Revised ed; Royal College of Surgeons of England, London
4. NHS Management Executive Day Surgery Task Force (1993) HMSO, London
5. Report on specialist training in anaesthesia (1994) Royal College of Anaesthetists, London
6. Ogg TW, Heath PJ, Brownlie GS (1988) A case for the expansion of day surgery. Health Trends 21:114-117
7. Natof HE (1987) FASA survey results revised, as reported by Wetchler BV, Outpatient anaesthesia, no double standard. Anaesth Patient Safety Foundation Newsletter 2:8
8. Keenan RL (1988) Anaesthetic disasters: causes, incidence and preventability. Refresher course of lectures, American Society of Anaesthesiologists. Lippincott, Philadelphia, pp 242
9. Ogg TW (1972) An assessment of post-operative outpatient cases. Br Med J 4:573
10. Ching F, Baylon GJ (1993) Persistent symptoms delaying discharge after day surgery. Can J Anaesth 40:A21
11. Hitchcock M, Ogg TW (1994) A quality assurance initiative in day case surgery: general considerations. Ambulatory Surgery 2:181-192
12. Goodwin APL, Rowe WL, Ogg TW, Samaan A (1991) Oral fluids prior to day surgery. Anaesthesia 46:1066-68
13. Ogg TW, Hitchcock M (1994) Post-operative nausea and vomiting. J One Day Surg Spring 18-19
14. McQuay HJ (1992) Pre-emptive analgesia. Br J Anaes 69:1-3
15. Hitchcock M, Ogg TW (1994) Quality assurance in day case anaesthesia. Ambulatory Surg 2:193-204
16. Watson B, Hitchcock M, Ogg TW, Dutton K (1994) Closing the audit loop. Ambulatory Surg 2:205-211

Sanitary Organization and Safety

I. Salvo, I. Colombo

Since the law no. 724 was passed on December 23, 1994, on cost containment which changed medical reimbursement and introduced in our country the "diagnosis-related groups" system (DRGs), hospitals and physicians have seen dramatic changes in health care delivery.

What is happening now here nearly resembles what happened for the same reasons (the need of health care cost containment) in the USA in the 1980s where the DRG reimbursement system was first introduced by the Federal Government (Medicare). Hospitals had then to face financial pressures and a lot was achieved by opening and expanding outpatient facilities. Performing surgery on an outpatient basis was demonstrated in those years to reduce the cost of medical care, increase the availability of hospital beds for those who need them and offer a level of care for many procedures that is comparable with that received on a inpatient basis with less stress (especially for children) and a lower risk of hospital-acquired infections (1-3).

Surgical day hospital (also referred to as same-day or day surgery) is defined as the provision of surgical services that require anesthesia (general anesthesia, local-regional anesthesia and deep sedation) with a period of postoperative observation to patients who are not expected to need overnight hospitalization.

Slowly through the 1980s day surgery came into acceptance and physicians and patients realized that hospitalization was not the only method of providing quality care. This shift towards the day hospital setting was made possible and successful thanks to the improvement and changes in surgical techniques and to the development and the use of short-acting anesthetic and analgesic agents (e.g., propofol and midazolam as intravenous agents, sevoflurane and desflurane as inhalation agents and alfentanil as a short-acting analgesic).

As a matter of fact, anesthesia has played a major role in the growth of day surgery in the USA and the success of any day surgery program depends on continuous involvement and leadership of the anesthesiologist.

Now in the USA the number of day surgery procedures has exceeded the number of inpatient procedures: in 1981 only 16% of all surgical procedures were performed on a day hospital basis; today almost 60% are delivered this way (4, 5) and according to the SMG Marketing Group Project, 65% will be reached by the end of 1995. In 1984 only 50% of US hospitals had day hospital units, while in 1991 86% and today almost all hospitals have day hospital facilities.

In Table 1 19 of the most common procedures (now exceeding 800 different operations) performed in an outpatient setting in the US in 1986 are listed (6). The first nine procedures comprised about 30% of total surgery performed in this country. The Federal Government and the insurance companies are still pushing towards the use of day surgery for more and more procedures. Many insurance companies are now using financial pressure (higher percent of reimbursement for day surgery) to encourage physicians and patients to this setting except in high-risk situations.

Table 1. The most common surgical procedures performed on an outpatient basis in the USA (6)

Breast biopsy	Appendectomy
Dilatation and curettage	Cesarean section
Knee arthroscopy	Hysterectomy
Cystoscopy	Transurethral resection of prostate
Myringotomy	Bronchoscopy
Inguinal hernia repair	Cholecystectomy
Tonsillectomy	Laminectomy
Cataract procedures	Major joint procedures
Fallopian tube ligation	Major artery/vein procedures
	Coronary revascularization

Over the decade from 1981 to 1991 the number of hospitals and inpatient beds declined considerably (–8.1% and –7.9%, respectively), as did the total number of annual admissions to the hospital (admissions to hospitals fell from 36.4 to 31.1 million - 14.7%) (Table 2). The average occupancy rate dropped over this period from 76% to 66% (7). Between 1980 and 1992, 642 hospitals had to close.

Table 2. Hospital changes in the USA from 1981 to 1991

Characteristics	1981	1991	Change (%)
Hospitals	5.813	5.342	– 8.1
Beds*	1.003	924	– 7.9
Admissions*	36.438	31.064	–14.7
Occupancy (%)	76	66	–13.1
Surgical operations*	19.236	22.405	+16.5
Outpatient visits*	202.768	322.048	+58.8

* Thousands
[Modified from Hospital Statistics (7)]

The financial consequences of this decline were softened considerably by the explosive growth of outpatient visits and total number of surgical procedures (7, 8).

Table 3 shows data published by the Organization for Economic Cooperation and Development (OECD) on the availability and use of inpatient medical services in Italy (1989) and the USA (1990) (9). In Italy we have 7.2 hospital beds/1000 people as compared with 4.7 in the US; the average length of stay in the hospital is 11.7 days in our country and 9.1 in the US. There is a similar occupancy rate in the two countries while the number of employees per bed is 1.4 in Italy as compared with 3.4 in the US. This is due to a higher number of administrative personnel in the US hospitals.

Table 3. Data from the OECD on inpatient medical services in Italy (1989) and the USA (1990) (9)

Country	Hospital beds/1000 population	Average length of stay (Days)	Occupancy rate (%)	Employees/ bed
Italy	7.2	11.7	68.4	1.4
USA	4.7	9.1	69.5	3.4

Now in the 1990s a considerable part of the surgical pie is moving out of the hospital to "Freestanding Surgical Centers". These surgical centers are private, profit-making, open only daytime, highly efficient and competitive with traditional hospitals.

While in 1984 hospitals controlled nearly 90% of all day hospital activities, in 1990 they control little over 70% (10, 11). Prior to 1985 reimbursement to hospitals for day surgery was considerably greater than to freestanding units. Since 1985, there has been an equalizing of the rate. The volume of cases performed by freestanding centers is expected to increase very quickly in the future.

At last, to meet the capability of performing more significant surgical procedures on a day hospital basis, an increasing number of postoperative health care facilities (hospital hotels, home care nursing services and freestanding recovery centers) have been introduced in the past years.

Coming back to what is happening now in Italy, what we know is that from January 1, 1995, medical reimbursement to hospitals will be set on a DRG basis and that the Italian government will contribute to the expenses for the activation of day hospital facilities within hospital wards. The rate for day surgery procedures, including preoperative evaluation and tests, should be equal to 70%-75% of the corresponding DRG rates for inpatient care (12-17).

Though the ultimate success of a day surgery program depends on its ability to provide cost-effective care without jeopardizing quality and patient safety. This is accomplished when the unit mixes appropriate patients with appropriate procedures, performed by cooperative surgeons and anesthesiologists who fully understand the foregoing prerequisites for the patient and the procedure. And, although the surgeon sees potential day surgical patients first, the true gatekeeper, who assumes a managerial role in the day surgery setting, is the anesthesiologist. This because the anesthesiologist is constantly present, from the selection of the patient down to his safe discharge from the unit. Besides, anesthesia for day surgery offers an unusual opportunity for the anesthesiologist to relate to conscious patients and their families, become more active in their perioperative assessment, and once again function more fully as physicians.

References

1. Steward DJ (1973) Experience with an outpatient anesthesia service for children. Anesth Analg 52:877-882
2. Otherson AB, Clatworthy HW (1968) Outpatient herniorraphy for infants. Am J Dis Child 78:116-122
3. Wetchler BV (ed) (1990) Anesthesia for ambulatory surgery, Lippincott, 2nd edn Philadelphia
4. Berk AA, Chalmers TC (1981) Cost and efficacy of substitution of ambulatory for inpatient care. N Engl J Med 304:396-397
5. AHA Annual Surveys of Hospital (1992)
6. National Centre for Health Statistics (1989) Detailed diagnosis and procedure for patient discharge from short-stay hospital, US, 1986. Vital and health statistics, series 13, no 95. US Government Printing Office, Washington
7. American Health Association Hospital Statistics (ed) (1993) A comprehensive study of US hospitals, 1992-93. Chicago
8. Iglekart JK (1993) Health policy report: the American care system. N Engl J Med 329: 372-376
9. Organization for Economic Cooperation and Development (1993) OECD health systems: facts and trends. Organization for Economic Cooperation and Development, Paris
10. Joint Commission on Accreditation of Health Care Organization (1990)
11. Henderson J (1986) Freestanding outpatient surgery centers: a market in transition. Health Industry Today
12. Gruppo di studio SIAARTI per la Sicurezza in Anestesia (1995) Raccomandazioni per l'anestesia nel Day Hospital. Ed SIAARTI
13. Gruppo di studio SIAARTI per la Sicurezza in Anestesia (1990) Raccomandazioni per gli standard di monitoraggio in anestesia e rianimazione. Ed La Mandragola, Siena
14. Gruppo di studio SIAARTI per la Sicurezza in Anestesia (1992) Controllo dell'apparecchio di anestesia. Ed La Mandragola, Siena
15. Gruppo di studio SIAARTI per la Sicurezza in Anestesia (1992) Il Consenso informato per l'anestesia. Ed La Mandragola, Siena
16. Gruppo di studio SIAARTI per la Sicurezza in Anestesia (1994) Raccomandazioni per la valutazione preoperatoria. Ed La Mandragola, Siena
17. Gruppo di studio SIAARTI per la Sicurezza in Anestesia (1994) Raccomandazioni per la sorveglianza postoperatoria. Ed SIAARTI

Recommendations for Anesthesia in Day Hospital

I. SALVO AND THE STUDY GROUP FOR SAFETY IN ANESTHESIA*

The following "Recommendations for Anesthesia in Day Hospital", elaborated by the Study Group for Safety in Anesthesia and published by SIAARTI in June 1995 (1), were written to provide anesthesiologists with the information needed to understand and meet the challenges of day hospital anesthesia, actually a sub-speciality of anesthesia.

Anesthesia in day hospital, which includes general anesthesia, local-regional anesthesia and deep sedations, must allow a safe return of the patient to his home the same day of the surgical procedure. Together with guidelines for a careful selection of the right patient and the right procedure, and the introduction of specific discharge criteria, anesthesiologists are recommended to follow all the general standards for safety in anesthesia previously published by SIAARTI (2-6). It is important that all safety measures are implemented and well documented in the patient's medical record.

This document was made possible thanks to the contribution of other American and European Societies of Anesthesia that experienced day hospital anesthesia before us and thanks to many other colleagues who worked in this Study Group and that I now have the opportunity to acknowledge.

Surgical procedures

The anesthesiologist and the surgeon decide together the list of surgical procedures to be performed in a day hospital setting.

Procedures should be:

- Elective, short (not exceed 2 h)
- With minimal physiological disorders and with low incidence of complications (particularly blood loss and respiratory distress)
- With simple postoperative course (minimal or at least readily controlled postoperative pain, nausea and vomiting)

The list of acceptable procedures may include, according to the operators' experience and after careful risk evaluation:

– Some simple emergencies
– Longer procedures (but only if suitable with postanesthetic care)

These procedures require previous agreement between surgeon and anesthesiologist.

Selection of patients

Patient selection must follow social and clinical standards.

Social standards

Patients who are candidates for day hospital anesthesia must:
– Understand and truly accept the procedure performed on this basis
– Be able to follow medical instructions
– Assure home hygienic conditions compatible with postoperative instructions
– Be accompanied by responsible adult who will transport and supervise the patient the first 24 h after surgery
– Be brought in a place not too far from the hospital or from other medical facilities assuring emergency care (less than 1 h distance)
– Have a telephone

Clinical standards

Age

Chronologic age should not be part of the selection criteria.

Selection must be based on patient's general condition.

The only absolute contraindication about age is represented by infants with a history of respiratory distress syndrome, particularly those born prematurely and less than 60 postconceptual weeks old. These patients are at greater risk of developing life-threatening perioperative apnea.

Physical status

Anesthesia in day hospital must preferably be performed in patients classified as ASA I and II.

ASA III patients are appropriate candidates for day surgery only when:
– Health problems are well under control
– The surgical procedure does not interfere with these problems or with their treatment

– Preliminary agreement between anesthesiologist and surgeon is reached
– Specific plans have been made for postoperative monitoring and treatment

Other conditions

In women possible pregnancy must be considered.

Preoperative evaluation

Anesthesia in day hospital must follow the safety guidelines published by SIAARTI (1994) in "Recommendations for pre-operative evaluation" (16).

The preoperative evaluation should be performed in order to allow a specific evaluation and, when necessary, the accomplishment of integrative visits and tests.

The patient should be informed that, if the preoperative evaluation takes place the same day of the operation, the procedure could be deferred for the need of further analyses or because hospitalization is required.

The choice of the tests to be performed must be related to the kind of surgery and to the physical status of the patient.

Much attention must be placed on possible postoperative complications.

The patient must be informed about his clinical conditions, the anesthetic technique chosen (with its risks and complications) and that this technique could be modified during surgery, if required.

The patient should be informed about possible transfusions (with connected risks), though it is recommended not to perform procedures with significant blood losses in a day hospital setting.

The patient must give his written consent once all questions have been answered.

During the preoperative evaluation the patient should be given all information about preoperative preparation (fasting hours, drug treatments, etc.) and postoperative care (a responsible adult with him 24 h after surgery; absolute rest; no driving, signing documents, doing dangerous work, etc.).

It is recommended to give these written instructions to the patient and have them signed when entering the hospital.

Anesthesia

Recommendations about patient monitoring in anesthesia and about the control of the anesthesia machine are indicated in the SIAARTI guidelines published in 1990 and 1992 (13, 14).

The clinician should try to avoid long-acting drugs with prolonged residual effects. The choice of the anesthesia technique should consider the length of the postoperative care time available.

Recovery

Recommendations about postoperative care are indicated in the SIAARTI guidelines published in 1994 (17).

After general anesthesia patients must be monitored until airway protection reflexes, space and time orientation and vital parameter stability are achieved.

After local-regional anesthesia patients must be monitored until normal muscolar tone has been re-established (i.e., deambulation) and there is no orthostatic hypotension.

It is necessary to foresee a possible hospitalization, for the patients who at the end of the procedure require it, in the unit itself or in a nearby hospital.

Discharge criteria

Patient must be discharged by both the anesthesiologist and the surgeon when the following conditions are satisfied:
- Complete psycho-motor recovery (or same preoperative conditions)
- Complete cardio-vascular stability (or same preoperative conditions)
- No orthostatic hypotension
- Complete airway protection reflexes recovery
- No respiratory distress (or the same preoperative conditions)
- Able to void
- No bleeding
- No excessive pain, nausea or vomiting
- Able to tolerate oral fluids
- Able to stand unaided and walk

Before being discharged the patient with his escort must be informed, verbally and by written postoperative instructions, about problems and complications that could appear during the following days.

Complications that can represent a danger for the patient must be clearly distinguished by discomforts considered as normal consequences of surgery. Clear indications must be given in these cases.

Data concerning preanesthetic evaluation, anesthesia, recovery and patient discharge conditions must be recorded on the patient's clinical record.

The day hospital unit must be able to guarantee for emergencies a 24-h contact place (in the unit or in a near hospital) and a 24-h anesthesiological and surgical telephone availability.

References

1. Gruppo di studio SIAARTI per la Sicurezza in Anestesia (1995) Raccomandazioni per l'anestesia nel Day Hospital. Ed SIAARTI
2. Gruppo di studio SIAARTI per la Sicurezza in Anestesia (1990) Raccomandazioni per gli standard di monitoraggio in anestesia e rianimazione. Ed La Mandragola, Siena
3. Gruppo di studio SIAARTI per la Sicurezza in Anestesia (1992) Controllo dell'apparecchio di anestesia. Ed La Mandragola, Siena
4. Gruppo di studio SIAARTI per la Sicurezza in Anestesia (1992) Il Consenso informato per l'anestesia. Ed La Mandragola, Siena
5. Gruppo di studio SIAARTI per la Sicurezza in Anestesia (1994) Raccomandazioni per la valutazione preoperatoria. Ed La Mandragola, Siena
6. Gruppo di studio SIAARTI per la Sicurezza in Anestesia (1994) Raccomandazioni per la sorveglianza postoperatoria. Ed SIAARTI

* **The Study Group for Safety in Anesthesia**: Accorsi A (Bentivoglio, Bologna), Bellucci G (Siena), Bianchetti L (Torino), Calderini E (Milano), Fiori R (Milano), Frova G (Brescia), Giuliani R (Bari), Gregorini P (Bologna), Messori P (Piacenza), Peduto AV (Cagliari), Paolillo GM (Milano), Pietropaoli P (Ancona), Salvo I (Milano), Stella L (Milano), Tavola M (Lecco), Torri G (Milano), Tufano R (Napoli), Verderio C (Milano), Zuccoli P (Parma)

Pharmacoeconomics in Anaesthesia

A. GASPARETTO, P. ORSI

"Pecuniae omnia parent" [Or.]

The new science *pharmacoeconomics* has been defined as the "description and analysis of the costs of drug therapy to health care system and society" (1). It examines the total impact of the price of drugs on resources.

Anaesthesia practice is not immune to demands for cost containment in health care. Thus the anaesthetist, like other specialists, will be under increasing pressure to achieve the same successful outcome at less expense.

Cost can be defined as the irreversible use of a resource. There are a variety of costs included in cost analyses (2):

– *Direct costs* (the actual payments for goods or services). Direct costs can be divided into *fixed* (e.g. the rent on a building or personnel wages) and *variable* (e.g. to acquire the anaesthesia drugs).
– *Indirect costs* (e.g. temporary loss of work days).
– Intangible costs (which include items difficult to measure, e.g. pain and suffering).

Moreover, several types of cost analysis should be considered:

– *Cost identification* (which merely identifies costs in money).
– *Cost-benefit analysis* (net costs and benefits of the individual strategy, usually presented in currency. It is used to decide which project will deliver the greatest value, e.g. whether to buy a new anaesthetic machine or a transoesophageal echocardiographic equipment).
– *Cost-effectiveness analysis* (it calculates how much a nonmonetary effectiveness, e.g. absence of a particular postoperative side effect, would cost).

The easiest and most popular examples of cost-benefit and cost-effectiveness analysis in anaesthesia address comparison a) of local and regional with general anaesthesia and b) of new anaesthesia agents with older drugs.

Typical arguments are that local or regional anaesthesia is usually more economical than general anaesthesia, mostly due to shorter hospital stay and less postanaesthesia care. This is well documented for many procedures, e.g. inguinal hernia repair, tonsillectomy, carotid endoarterectomy, as well as for several categories of high-risk surgical patients (3).

In the case of outpatient surgical procedures, the use of local and regional techniques or the employment of very short-acting drugs and proper antiemetics both allow patients to recover more quickly from the immediate effects of the anaesthetic.

In terms of cost analysis, the avoidance of a cost is entered as a negative cost. Therefore, it should result in a greater *net benefit*.

However, shorter hospital stay or shorter recovery time is not automatically translated into savings for the hospital. In many analysis lists there is a tendency to mix costs and charges. From the hospital's point of view, *costs* are the revenues spent on providing care, while *charges* are costs from payers' (patients') point of view. Thus, *where the reimbursement mechanism is represented by billing*, a shorter hospitalization may decrease charges but not reduce staffing and personnel time, which normally represent a fixed cost. Therefore, *unless overtime is avoided*, the loss in potential revenues may not be offset by a reduction in variable costs, leading to an unfavourable cost-benefit ratio.

Yet, one might assume that, in a busy outpatient centre, delay in discharge, e.g. caused by postoperative nausea and vomiting (PONV), other than increasing costs due to the use of resources such as beds and nursing time in the postanaesthesia care unit, limits the number of cases performed in a given time period, preventing the treatment of additional patient (4). However, the assumption does not seem to be adequately supported by data in a prospective study, as well as the cost to the patient from lost wages.

Another North American study on the same subject found that prophylactic administration of the recent and expensive antiemetic ondansetron, substantially free of side effects, was *cost-effective* if the expected incidence of PONV exceeded 33%, whereas the considerably cheaper droperidol, which does present some uncomfortable side effects, was cost-effective when the incidence of PONV was 10% (5).

Nevertheless, the foremost question is represented by the value of patient comfort. In cost-effectiveness analysis the benefit is abstract. *Is the highest probability of avoiding PONV worth 10? 100? 1.000? 10.000?*

Identifying factors involved in the cost of anaesthetic practice, e.g. *to apportion OR costs among anaesthesia and surgery*, undoubtedly challenge any OR management system.

By far the largest part of *total operating theatre costs* are associated with the utilization of OR personnel, e.g. *salaries* (6).

Varying case load, inefficient scheduling of cases due to unrealistic estimates of operating time, unpredictable length of many procedures, and urgent or emergency cases all render futile any other cost containment strategies in anaesthesia and surgery.

Another highly significant cost in OR is related to *wastage of the surgical supplies*, mainly due to the opening of unnecessary items, e.g. sutures. In addition, *preoperative laboratory tests* enormously increase operating costs. Indeed, most of the leading institutions in the USA are going to definitely eliminate indiscriminate laboratory testing, as well as routine preoperative ECG and chest X-ray (7). *Therefore, drug costs may represent a quite small part of the entire OR budget.*

In fact, while OR accounts for 40%-60% of hospital revenues, *anaesthesia - related drug costs* only account for 1.4% of the total operating expenses of the hospital (8).

Other authors calculate that anaesthesia drugs represent less than 1% of the hospital costs even in cases where the ten times more expensive anaesthetic technique is used (9).

Two very different approaches have been used to calculate the cost of an anaesthetic:

a) To calculate all drugs, gases and consumable items used for *a particular anaesthetic*; these variable costs are also called *"running costs"*

b) To *total the costs* of staff salaries, preoperative assessment and recovery, postoperative analgesia, anaesthetic capital and equipment maintenance, insurance and administration and all anaesthetic drugs and consumable items, (i.e. both variable *and* fixed costs) *for a year divided by the total number of patients*, which takes no account of the anaesthetic technique used in any particular patient (*"overhead costs"*)

However, direct costs such as cost of land, lighting, heating, porters, which are common to both surgery and anaesthesia, are usually not included. Overheads are generally apportioned to patients by the *duration* that each patient uses the service. Pricing structure, however, might also be related to the patient's preoperative ASA status score (10).

The aim of this task is to evaluate the running costs alone of different anaesthetics.

Acquisition costs of drugs should be considered together with the element of *waste*. The practice of discarding multidose vials after each case to prevent cross-infections is common, although not supported by evidence.

However, drug cost should be calculated as cost per *unit* effectiveness. Of course, all prices are dependent on the amount purchased by each hospital (bulk discount).

Table 1 reports the purchase prices in Lit. per unit in June 1995 of the most common anaesthesia agents, together with fluids, blood products and consumable adult items. Comparisons *of examples* of different anaesthetics are indicated in Tables 2 and 3.

Table 1. Cost of anaesthesia drugs, blood products and consumables, in Lit.

Sedatives, neuroleptics	Diazepam 10 mg	1.166	*Reversal*	Naloxone 0.4 mg	2.749
	Droperidol 2.5 mg (*)	315		Doxapram 50 mg	700
Anticholinergics	Atropine 0.5 mg	126		Flumazenil 1 mg	38.800
Opioids	Fentanyl 0.05 mg (*)	200	*Antishiverings*	Nefopam 4 mg	416
	Morphine 10 mg	463	*Antiemetics*	Metoclopramide 10 mg	240
Hypnotics	Thiopentone 500 mg	2100		Ondansetron 4 mg	13.350
	Propofol 200 mg	6220	*Postop. analgesics*	Ketorolac 30 mg	2.016
	Propofol 1000 mg (*)	32	*Osmotic diuresis*	20% Mannitol 250 ml	945
	Ketamine 50 mg (*)	535	*Local anaesthetics*	Bupivacaine 0,5% 10 ml	14.850
Neuromuscular blocking	Suxamethonium 500 mg	185		Mepivacaine 2% 10 ml	11.340
	Pancuronium 4 mg	1275		Lidocaine 2% 10 ml	8.550
	Atracurium 25 mg	1840		Hyperbaric al bupivacaine	12.150
	Vecuronium 4 mg	2650	*Vasopressors*	Metaraminol 10 mg	2.600
Anticholinesterasic	Neostigmine 2.5 mg	700	*& needles*	Sprotte spinal needle	23.000
Gases	Oxygen 1 l	1.69		Tuohy epidural needle	12.500
	Nitrous oxide 1 l	7.65	*Fluids*	0.9% Saline 500 ml	700
Halogenated	Halothane 250 ml/1ml	119		Dextrose 5% 500 ml	635
	Isoflurane 100 ml/1ml	888		Hemmaccel 500 ml	5700
Soda lime	/g	13.5			
Blood products	Human albumin 20% 50 ml: Lit. 65.800; packed cells (&filter): Lit. 165.000; fresh frozen plasma: Lit. 28.000; platelets 5 U: Lit. 300.000 (procurement costs plus associated costs, e.g., waste, extra cross matches, blood administration sets)				
Disposable	Syringes: from 2.5 to 20 ml: from Lit. 60 to Lit. 152; intravenous infusion tubing: Lit. 300; simple cannula 16 g: Lit. 570; profile tracheal tube (disposable): Lit. 3.400; 5 ECG electrodes: Lit. 1025; airway filter (Dar): Lit. 19.740; suction catheter: Lit. 315; urinary catheter: Lit. 920; surgical gloves: Lit. 420				
Special	Transducer set per channel (disposable): Lit. 15.000; CV catheter: Lit. 99.000; pulmon. artery catheter & introducer: Lit. 287.000				

(*) Multidose vials, weight and cost/ml

Table 2. Cost of anaesthesia drugs and consumables, in Lit. Example of a typical operation: hernia repair in a 70 kg, healthy adult patient; duration 45 min

	Intravenous	Inhalat., High-flow	Inhalat. Low-flow	Epidural	Spinal	Local
Diazepam (mg)	(10) 1.166	(10) 1.166	(10) 1.166	(10) 1.166	(10) 1.166	(10) 1.166
Atropine (mg)	(0.5) 126	(0.5) 126	(0.5) 126	(0.5) 126	(0.5) 126	(0.5) 126
Propofol (mg) *	(140) 6.220	(140) 6.220	(140) 6.220	(100) 6.620	(100) 6620	(100) 6620
Droperidol (mg)	(5) 630	(5) 630	(5) 630			
Fentanyl (mg)	(0.5) 2.000	(0.1) 400	(0.1) 400			
Norcuron (mg)	(12) 7.950	(12) 7.950	(12) 7.950			
Muscle relax. reversal	3.626	3.626	3.626			
Naloxone (mg)	(0.4) 2.749					
Nefopam (mg)	(20) 416	(20) 416	(20) 416			
Oxygen (l/min)	(3) 228	(3) 228				
Nitrous oxide (l/min)	(5) 1.721	(5) 1.721				
Isoflurane (%)		(1,2) 19.180	9.590 (§)			
Tuohy needle				12.500		
Sprotte needle					23.000	
Bupivacainc 0.5%(ml)				(20) 29.700		
Hyperb. bupivac. (mg)					(20) 12.150	
Metaraminol (mg)					(10) 2.600	
Mepivacaine 1% (ml)						(30) 22.680
0.9% Saline (ml)	(1000) 1.400	(1000) 1.400	(1000) 1.400	(2000) 2.800	(2000) 2.800	(1000) 1.400
Consum. (average) #	25.652	25.652	25.652	2.207	2.207	2
Ketorolac (mg)	(30) 2.016	(30) 2.016	(30) 2.016	(30) 2.016	(30) 2.016	(30) 2.016
Total Lit.	55.900	70.731	59.192	57.135	52.685	34.010

(*) 200 mg vials, wastage is included; (§) most cautious estimates: high-flow/2 (see text); (#) 3 siringes, 1 intravenous infusion tube and 1 cannula, 3 ECG electrodes (or 5 in case of periph. nerve stim.) common to general and locoregional anaesthesia. The former needs also 1 endotracheal tube, 1 airway·filter and 1 suction catheter, the latter just surgical gloves

Table 3. Cost of anaesthesia drugs and consumables, in Lit. Examples of cheap (fentanyl/N$_2$O/pancuronium) vs expensive (high-flow isoflurane/N$_2$O/vecuronium) anaesthetics for a long case: craniotomy in a 70 kg, healthy adult patient; duration 12 h

Diazepam (mg)	(10) 1.166	(10) 1.166
Atropine (mg)	(0.5) 126	(0.5) 126
Propofol (mg) *		(140) 6.220
Thiopentone (mg)	(280) 2.100	
Droperidol (mg) (§)	(6) 1.890	(2) 630
Fentanyl (mg) (§)	(6,23) 24.920	(0.5) 2.000
Norcuron (mg)		(47,6) 31.800
Pancuronium (mg)	(23,8) 7.650	
Oxygen (l/min)	(3) 3.650	(3) 3.650
Nitrous oxide (l/min)	(5) 27.540	(5) 27.540
Isoflurane (%)		(1,2) 306.893
0.9% Saline (ml)	(4.000) 5.600	(4.000) 5.600
Mannitol 20% (ml)	(250) 945	250 945
Consum. (#)	31.154	31.154
Muscle relax. reversal	3.625	3.625
Naloxone (mg)	(0.8) 5.498	
Nefopam (mg)	(20) 416	(20) 416
Total Lit.	116.280	421.765

(*) 200 mg vials, wastage is included; (#) 6 siringes, 2 intravenous infusion tubes and cannulas, 1 endotracheal tube, 3 ECG electrodes, 1 airway filter and 1 suction catheter

With respect to current costs, local anaesthesia is undoubtedly economical, otherwise regional techniques appear as much expensive as intravenous or inhalational, low-flow anaesthesia. Indeed, one of the simplest ways to save on anaesthesia costs should be to use *low-flow anaesthesia.*

With modern equipment and agent analyser, fresh gas flow (FGF) can safely be reduced to 1 l/min (apart from higher flows both at induction and at emergence). In comparison to high-flow techniques, cost saving should be up to 75% for N$_2$O and O$_2$ and 50 to 75% for inhalational agents (3). The saving in N$_2$O alone balances the cost of soda lime.

For practical purposes, the amount of vapors used (in ml/h) is approximately FGF in l/min times 3 times percent of drug. *Cost-benefit analysis* would help to decide whether to buy an open circuit anaesthetic machine or a more expensive low-flow, closed circuit system together with gas monitor. In fact, depending on surgical case-load, equipment capital and maintenance costs are amenable to be calculated on an hourly basis.

We might calculate cost-benefit ratio in the following manner: for example, an open circuit system costs about Lit. 40.000.000 (Ohmeda 7800), while the price of closed circuit anaesthetic machine and gas and volatile agents monitor is about Lit. 90.000.000 (Ohmeda Modulus CD).

Assuming write-off time is 7 years, estimating maintenance at 8% of capital cost per year and expecting a *full* 8-h day, 5 days per week and 52 weeks per year utilization using vapours (10), one might not unrealistically calculate: [(90.000.000 – 40.000.000) * 7 * 0.08 * 50.000.000]/14.560 h = Lit. 5.358. This represents the total hourly cost difference between the two types of anaesthetic equipment capital and maintenance.

Considering the *minimal saving of* inhalation agent to be 50% using a low-flow, closed circuit system, one could *roughly* calculate, for example in the case of isoflurane, whose purchase cost is Lit. 888/ml: 0.5 * 8 * 3 *1 = 12 ml = Lit. 10.656/h drug cost saving. Assuming that inflation affects all costs similarly, *net benefit* is Lit. 10.656 – 5.358 = Lit. 5.298/h, that is to say, Lit. 11.019.840/year.

However, while the calculation is realistic, the assumption that exclusively inhalational anaesthesia is carried out on a full-time basis and that all the patients are suitable for low-flow technique *is not*. Probably, its expected utilization should be halved. This, unfortunately, abolishes the benefit.

Nevertheless, even in event of worthless benefit, the closed circuit technique probably is *cost-effective*. In fact, a closed circuit offers the advantage of decreased environmental pollution and possible risks to the health of staff working in the operating theatre. Moreover, it provides ideal inspired humidity and allows measurement of oxygen consumption and anaesthetic uptake.

Muscle relaxant may account for up to 30% of the total anaesthesia drug budget. In the USA, vecuronium, which is still protected by patent, is almost eleven times more expensive than pancuronium on a weight basis, and even more on an ED95 basis (0.05 and 0.07, respectively). Thus, substitution of pancuronium for vecuronium is recommended when anaesthesia time is greater than 90' (11). Moreover, 25% of vecuronium may be wasted due to improper labelling or techniques. In Italy, vecuronium is only twice as expensive as pancuronium on a weight basis. Therefore the impact of cost-effectiveness analysis on the anaesthesia drug budget seems really poor.

Therefore, even in particularly long procedures, the selection of the neuromuscular blocking drug would appear to be better based upon autonomic and cardiovascular impact, as well as patient's health status. In fact, in the example reported in Table 3, the money saved by substituting pancuronium for vecuronium, even with a weight ratio 1 : 2, is Lit. 24.150.

This represents a meaningless saving within the entire cost of anaesthesia and surgery. However, during lengthy cases, *one might use both drugs*. Pancuronium would be preferred at regimen *and* noncumulative, shorter-acting vecuronium near emergence, to avoid bradycardia and unintentional prolonged curarization, respectively. Since muscle relaxants are combined, careful assessment of neuromuscular blockade throughout the procedure is even more mandatory. The customary peripheral nerve stimulator costs about Lit. 400.000 (the cost of two ECG-type electrodes Lit. 410, should also be considered for each procedure).

This strategy is also expected to be more cost-effective, as well as result in more net, although minute, benefit.

Finally, some other aspects must doubtlessly be considered. Appropriate perioperative antibiotic prophylaxis is probably cost-effective. However, the price of any new antibiotic used may be significantly higher for what may be only minimal, if any, enhancements in outcome (3). The choice is with the surgeon and the infectivologist, although on this matter the opinion of anaesthetist could be requested.

Other than selection of drugs, the use of medical equipment in OR and recovery also can affect anaesthesia cost containment. As an example, routine use of pulmonary artery catheterization (PAC) or oximetric PAC versus CVP monitoring increases costs and *does not* ameliorate outcome and hospital stay even in cardiac patients (12).

Finally, the use of blood salvage instruments seem to be cost-effective when limited to procedures in which it is certain that more than 2 units of packed red blood cells will be reinfused (3).

Conclusions

As expected, anaesthetic choices do not significantly affect direct, indirect and intangible costs, really representing a small item in a hospital's financial picture. Therefore, anaesthesia drug costs do not seem to warrant extensive analysis.

Some authors calculate that, with respect to overheads and salaries and preoperative assessment and recovery, drugs and consumables may represent between 30% and 50% of the cost of an anaesthetic lasting from 45 to 120 min (10). However, even using sixfold more expensive anaesthesia drugs for a 12-h neurosurgical procedure (Table 3), Lit. 420.000 is undoubtedly far less than 1% of the global hospital cost for such a case. Indeed, global hospital costs for each individual case are hard to determine in most instances.

Nevertheless, several aspects should be considered:

a) Although the item "drugs" is a minute part of the anaesthesia department's or OR budget, it is undoubtedly one of the easiest to calculate and therefore most amenable to immediate reduction in anaesthesia costs.

   In fact, most of the anaesthetic expenses (salaries, capital and maintenance) are often charged to other departmental budgets.

   On the other hand, it may be difficult to apportion the anaesthetic salaries between giving anaesthetic and ICU, research, audit, teaching, pain therapy.

b) Even though the percentage is a minute part of the revenue, the reduction in anaesthesia drug expenditure could represent a significant part of the hospital's profit.

c) As hospital profit margins narrow, the amount of savings in the anaesthesia department becomes much more important.

d) Saved money might be used for a project delivering value.

e) As *reimbursement* is bundled and *based on capitation* plans (instead of billing), attention is shifted to controlling cost rather than increasing revenue. Clinical departments and service are now viewed as *cost centres* rather than profit centres.

f) Immediate drug cost reduction in an anaesthesia department budget is easier and probably better accepted than loss of subsidies, support personnel, equipment, or work space.

g) Ability to perform cost studies is essential for planning any negotiation under new reimbursement schemes. The anaesthetist should take his share of the responsibility for finding solutions to the financial crisis in health care.

h) Questionnaires issued to anaesthetists to test their present knowledge of the prices of the commonest anaesthesia items have shown the costs of some more expensive drugs and consumables to be consistently underestimated, whereas the cheaper ones are overestimated (13). Educational programmes on cost containment should be set up.

i) Finally, lowering the cost of medical care will not automatically lower the quality of care, but will simply allow the best outcome at a *reasonable* cost to be achieved, that is to say, optimize knowledge and resources.

References

1. Bootman JL, Larson LN, McGhan WF, Townsend RJ (1989) Pharmacoeconomic research and clinical trials: concepts and issues. Ann Pharmacother 23: 693-7
2. Vitez TS (1994) Principle of cost analysis. J Clin Anaesth 6:357-363
3. Becker KE Jr, Carrithers J (1994) Practical methods of cost containment in anaesthesia and surgery. J Clin Anaesth 6:388-399
4. Carroll NV, Miederhoff PA, Cox FM (1994) Cost incurred by outpatient surgical centers in managing postoperative nausea and vomiting. J Clin Anaesth 6:364-369
5. Mehernoor FW, Smith I (1995) Cost-effectiveness analysis of antiemetic therapy for ambulatory surgery. J Clin Anaesth 6:370-377
6. White PF, Withe LD (1994) Cost containment in the operating room: who is responsible? J Clin Anaesth 6:351-356
7. Narr BJ, Hansen TR, Warner MA (1991) Preoperative laboratory screening in healthy Mayo patients: cost-effective elimination of tests and unchanged outcomes. Mayo Clin Proc 66: 155-159
8. Johnstone RE, Jozefczyk KG (1994) Costs of anaesthetic drugs: experiences with a cost education trial. Anaesth Analg 78:766-771
9. Todd MM, Warner DS, Sokoll MD, Maktabi MA, Hindman BJ, Scamman FL, Kirschner J (1993) A prospective, comparative trial of three anaesthetics for elective supratentorial craniotomy. Propofol/fentanyl, isoflurane/nitrous oxide, and fentanyl/nitrous oxide. Anaesthesiology 78:1005-1020

10. Broadway PJ, Jones JG (1995) A method of costing anaesthetic practice. Anaesthesia 50: 56-63
11. Szocik JF, Learned DW (1994) Impact of a cost containment program on the use of volatile anaesthetics and neuromuscular blocking drugs. J Clin Anaesth 6:378-382
12. Naylor CD, Sibbald WJ, Sprung CL, Pinfold SP, Calvin JE, Cerra FB (1993) Pulmonary artery catheterization. Can there be an integrated strategy for guideline development and research promotion? JAMA 269:2407-2411
13. Bailey CR, Ruggier R, Cashman JN (1993) Forum. Anaesthesia: cheap at twice the price? Anaesthesia 48:906-909

INDEX